About This Treatment Guide

The Oncology Group of UBM Medica, publisher of *ONCOLOGY, ONCOLOGY Nurse Edition,* and *Oncology NEWS International,* and the website, **cancernetwork.com**, is pleased to present *Cancer Management: A Multidisciplinary Approach,* 13th edition.

Cancer Management: A Multidisciplinary Approach is designed to present important clinical information concisely, uniformly, and logically, emphasizing the natural history of the malignancy, screening and diagnosis, staging and prognosis, and treatment.

The fundamental principle behind this comprehensive treatment guide is the importance of a truly integrated, multidisciplinary approach to the management of the patient with cancer. Accordingly, the discussion of each disease site combines the perspectives of medical oncology, surgical oncology, and radiation oncology, as appropriate. Further, each of the book's medical editors represents a particular discipline.

The Oncology Group would like to thank the contributors and all involved in the development and production of this important handbook. In particular, we thank the book's principal editors:

Richard Pazdur, MD (Medical Oncology)
US Food and Drug Administration

Lawrence D. Wagman, MD (Surgical Oncology)
Center for Cancer Prevention and Treatment, St. Joseph Hospital

Kevin A. Camphausen, MD (Radiation Oncology)
National Cancer Institute

William J. Hoskins, MD (Gynecologic Oncology)
Memorial Sloan-Kettering Cancer Center

We also thank the staff of The Oncology Group and in particular wish to recognize the efforts of Angela Cibuls, Susan Reckling, and Marie Best.

This 13th edition has been produced in an effort to keep pace with the rapidly changing field of oncology. Be sure to visit **www.cancernetwork.com**, where the full text of this edition will be made available online, with important updates as appropriate.

Please let us know how you use this book, and how we can make it even more valuable. We look forward to hearing from you.

Sincerely,

Rachel Warren
Editorial Director
rachel.warren@ubm.com

Amy Birnbach
Publisher
amy.birnbach@ubm.com

13TH EDITION

Cancer Management: A Multidisciplinary Approach

Medical, Surgical, & Radiation Oncology

Edited by

Richard Pazdur, MD
Director, Office of Oncology Drug Products
Center for Drug Evaluation and Research
US Food and Drug Administration

Lawrence D. Wagman, MD
Executive Medical Director
The Center for Cancer Prevention and Treatment
St. Joseph Hospital

Kevin A. Camphausen, MD
Chief, Radiation Oncology Branch
National Cancer Institute

William J. Hoskins, MD
Executive Director of Surgical Activities
Memorial Sloan-Kettering Cancer Center

And the publishers of the journal *ONCOLOGY*

UBM Medica

www.cancernetwork.com

Note to the reader

The information in this volume has been carefully reviewed for accuracy of dosage and indications. Before prescribing any drug, however, the clinician should consult the manufacturer's current package labeling for accepted indications, absolute dosage recommendations, and other information pertinent to the safe and effective use of the product described. This is especially important when drugs are given in combination or as an adjunct to other forms of therapy. Furthermore, some of the medications described herein, as well as some of the indications mentioned, had not been approved by the US Food and Drug Administration at the time of publication. This possibility should be borne in mind before prescribing or recommending any drug or regimen.

The views expressed are the result of independent work and do not necessarily represent the views or findings of the US Food and Drug Administration or the United States Government.

Library of Congress Catalog Card Number 2010941140
ISBN Number 9780615418247

For information on purchasing additional copies of this publication, visit www.cancernetwork.com/cancer-management.

UBM Medica

Publishers of

ONCOLOGY

ONCOLOGY Nurse Edition

Oncology NEWS International

cancernetwork.com

Contents

GYNECOLOGIC MALIGNANCIES

SKIN CANCERS

SARCOMAS

BRAIN TUMORS

OTHER SOLID TUMORS

HEMATOLOGIC MALIGNANCIES

PALLIATIVE AND SUPPORTIVE CARE

Contributors

Nathan B. Adams, MD
Division of Medical Oncology
The University of Vermont

Peter Ahn, MD
Department of Radiation Oncology
Thomas Jefferson University

Steven R. Alberts, MD
Division of Medical Oncology
Mayo Clinic

Erika Masuda Alford, MD
Department of Endocrine Neoplasia and Hormonal Disorders
M. D. Anderson Cancer Center

Andrew J. Armstrong, MD
Divisions of Medical Oncology and Urology
Duke University Medical Center

Al B. Benson III, MD
Division of Hematology/Oncology
Robert H. Lurie Comprehensive Cancer Center, Feinberg School of Medicine/Northwestern University

J. Sybil Biermann, MD
Department of Orthopaedic Surgery
University of Michigan Comprehensive Cancer Center

Charles D. Blanke, MD
Division of Medical Oncology
The University of British Columbia

Mary S. Brady, MD
Division of Surgery
Memorial Sloan-Kettering Cancer Center

Julie R. Brahmer, MD
Department of Oncology
The Sidney Kimmel Comprehensive Cancer Center at Johns Hopkins

Eduardo Bruera, MD
Department of Palliative Care and Rehabilitation Medicine
M. D. Anderson Cancer Center

Mark Buyyounouski, MD, MS
Department of Radiation Oncology
Fox Chase Cancer Center

Antonio Calles, MD
Division of Medical Oncology
Centro Integral Oncológico Clara Campal

Emiliano Calvo, MD, PhD
Division of Medical Oncology
Centro Integral Oncológico Clara Campal

Kevin A. Camphausen, MD
Radiation Oncology Branch
National Cancer Institute

Brian C.-H. Chiu, PhD
Department of Health Studies
The University of Chicago

Warren A. Chow, MD
Department of Medical Oncology and Therapeutics Research/ Department of Molecular Pharmacology
City of Hope National Medical Center

Deborah E. Citrin, MD
Radiation Oncology Branch
National Cancer Institute

Jay S. Cooper, MD
Department of Radiation Oncology
Maimonides Medical Center

Jorge E. Cortes, MD
Department of Leukemia
M. D. Anderson Cancer Center

Sanjeet Dadwal, MD
Division of Infectious Diseases
City of Hope National Medical Center

Atreya Dash, MD
Department of Urology
University of California, Irvine Medical Center

Lisa M. DeAngelis, MD
Department of Neurology
Memorial Sloan-Kettering Cancer Center

John F. de Groot, MD
Department of Neuro-Oncology
M. D. Anderson Cancer Center

Kieron Dunleavy, MD
Center for Cancer Research
National Cancer Institute

Carmen P. Escalante, MD
Department of General Internal Medicine
M. D. Anderson Cancer Center

Andrew M. Evens, DO, MSc
Division of Hematology/Oncology
Robert H. Lurie Comprehensive Cancer Center, Feinberg School of Medicine/Northwestern University

Steven Feigenberg, MD
Department of Radiation Oncology
University of Maryland Medical Center

Paul Fisher, MD
Department of Radiology and Surgery
Stony Brook University Medical Center

Keith Flaherty, MD
Division of Hematology/Oncology
Massachusetts General Hospital

Stephen J. Forman, MD
Department of Hematology and Hematopoietic Cell Transplantation
City of Hope National Medical Center

Jorge A. Garcia, MD
Departments of Solid Tumor Oncology and Urology
Cleveland Clinic Taussig Cancer Institute

Guillermo Garcia-Manero, MD
Department of Leukemia
M. D. Anderson Cancer Center

Leda Gattoc, MD
Gynecology and Obstetrics
Emory University School of Medicine

Bonnie S. Glisson, MD
Department of Thoracic/ Head and Neck Medical Oncology
M. D. Anderson Cancer Center

Shari B. Goldfarb, MD
Breast Cancer Medicine Service
Memorial Sloan-Kettering Cancer Center

Leo I. Gordon, MD
Division of Hematology/Oncology
Robert H. Lurie Comprehensive Cancer Center, Feinberg School of Medicine/Northwestern University

Sharad Goyal, MD
Department of Radiation Oncology
Robert Wood Johnson Medical School
The Cancer Institute of New Jersey

Richard J. Gralla, MD
Division of Hematology/Oncology
North Shore University Hospital and LIJ Medical Center

Frederic W. Grannis, Jr., MD
Section of Thoracic Surgery
City of Hope National Medical Center

Kathryn M. Greven, MD
Department of Radiation Oncology
Wake Forest University School of Medicine

Steven M. Grunberg, MD
Division of Medical Oncology
The University of Vermont

Karl Haglund, MD, PhD
Radiation Oncology Branch
National Cancer Institute

John D. Hainsworth, MD
Oncology Research Program
Sarah Cannon Research Institute

William J. Hoskins, MD
Department of Surgery
Memorial Sloan-Kettering Cancer Center

Mimi I. Hu, MD
Department of Endocrine Neoplasia and Hormonal Disorders
M. D. Anderson Cancer Center

Mark Hurwitz, MD
Department of Radiation Oncology
Dana-Farber/Brigham and Women's Cancer Center

Jimmy J. Hwang, MD
Division of Hematology/Oncology
Lombardi Comprehensive Cancer Center
Georgetown University Medical Center

James I. Ito, MD
Division of Infectious Diseases
City of Hope National Medical Center

Rajesh V. Iyer, MD
Department of Radiation Oncology
Community Medical Center
Saint Barnabas Health Care System

Sundar Jagannath, MD
Multiple Myeloma Program
The Mount Sinai Medical Center

Ishmael Jaiyesimi, DO
Division of Hematology/Oncology
William Beaumont Hospital

Lori Jardines, MD
Division of Surgery
Albert Einstein Medical Center

Aminah Jatoi, MD
Department of Medical Oncology
Mayo Clinic

Hagop Kantarjian, MD
Department of Leukemia
M. D. Anderson Cancer Center

Aradhana Kaushal, MD
Radiation Oncology Branch
National Cancer Institute

Kemp H. Kernstine, MD, PhD
Department of Thoracic Surgery
City of Hope National Medical Center

Christine Ko, MD
Radiation Oncology Branch
National Cancer Institute

Jane Kriengkauykiat, PharmD
Division of Infectious Diseases
City of Hope National Medical Center

Mario E. Lacouture, MD
Department of Dermatology
Memorial Sloan-Kettering Cancer Center

Lily Lai, MD
Division of General and Oncologic Surgery
City of Hope National Medical Center

Nicole Lamanna, MD
Department of Medicine/ Leukemia Service
Memorial Sloan-Kettering Cancer Center

Jeffrey P. Lamont, MD
Division of Surgery
Baylor University Medical Center

Miriam N. Lango, MD
Department of Surgical Oncology
Fox Chase Cancer Center

Joseph Lattanzi, MD
Department of Radiation Oncology
Southern Ocean County Hospital
Meridian Health System

Alan List, MD
Department of Hematologic Malignancies
H. Lee Moffitt Cancer Center and Research Institute

Jay S. Loeffler, MD
Department of Radiation Oncology
Massachusetts General Hospital

Patrick J. Loehrer, MD
Division of Hematology/Oncology
Indiana University Melvin and Bren Simon Cancer Center

Sharmila Makhija, MD
Department of Gynecology and Obstetrics
Emory University School of Medicine

Robert Maki, MD, PhD
Department of Medicine
Memorial Sloan-Kettering Cancer Center

Ellen Manzullo, MD
Department of General Internal Medicine
M. D. Anderson Cancer Center

Maurie Markman, MD
Cancer Treatment Centers of America
Eastern Regional Medical Center

David Scott Miller, MD
Division of Gynecologic Oncology
University of Texas Southwestern Medical Center

Ronald T. Mitsuyasu, MD
UCLA CARE Center
University of California, Los Angeles

Judd W. Moul, MD
Division of Urologic Surgery
Duke University Medical Center

Benjamin Movsas, MD
Department of Radiation Oncology
Henry Ford Health System

Michael S. Mulligan, MD
Division of Surgery
University of Washington

Nikhil C. Munshi, MD
Department of Medical Oncology
Dana-Farber Cancer Institute

Robert J. Myerson, MD, PhD
Department of Radiation Oncology
Washington University

Margaret R. O'Donnell, MD
Department of Hematology and Hematopoietic Cell Transplantation
City of Hope National Medical Center

Bert O'Neil, MD
Department of Medicine
University of North Carolina at Chapel Hill

Channing J. Paller, MD
Department of Oncology
The Sidney Kimmel Comprehensive Cancer Center at Johns Hopkins

Richard Pazdur, MD
Office of Oncology Drug Products
Center for Drug Evaluation and Research
US Food and Drug Administration

Carlos A. Perez, MD
Department of Radiation Oncology
Washington University School of Medicine

Louis L. Pisters, MD
Department of Urology
M. D. Anderson Cancer Center

Peter W. T. Pisters, MD
Department of Surgical Oncology
M. D. Anderson Cancer Center

Laura Raftery, MD
Division of Hematology/Oncology
University of North Carolina at Chapel Hill

Deepa Reddy, MD
Division of Hematology/Oncology
University of California, Los Angeles

Paul Richardson, MD
Department of Medical Oncology/Hematologic Malignancies
Dana-Farber Cancer Institute

John Andrew Ridge, MD, PhD
Department of Surgical Oncology
Fox Chase Cancer Center

John M. Robertson, MD
Department of Radiation Oncology
William Beaumont Hospital

Miguel A. Rodriguez-Bigas, MD
Department of Surgical Oncology
M. D. Anderson Cancer Center

Steven T. Rosen, MD
Division of Hematology/Oncology
Robert H. Lurie Comprehensive Cancer Center, Feinberg School of Medicine/Northwestern University

Melanie Royce, MD, PhD
Division of Hematology/Oncology
University of New Mexico Cancer Center

Stephen C. Rubin, MD
Division of Gynecologic Oncology
Hospital of the University of Pennsylvania

Paul Sabbatini, MD
Gynecologic Medical Oncology Service
Memorial Sloan-Kettering Cancer Center

Aaron R. Sasson, MD
Division of Surgery
University of Nebraska Medical Center

Roderich E. Schwarz, MD, PhD
Division of Surgical Oncology
University of Texas Southwestern Medical Center

Walter Scott, MD
Division of Thoracic Surgical Oncology
Fox Chase Cancer Center

Nicole A. Shonka, MD
Division of Oncology and Hematology
University of Nebraska Medical Center

Richard T. Silver, MD
Department of Medicine
Weill Cornell Medical College

Douglas Skarecky, BS
Department of Urology
University of California, Irvine Medical Center

Philippe E. Spiess, MD
Department of Genitourinary Oncology
H. Lee Moffitt Cancer Center and Research Institute

David Straus, MD
Department of Medicine
Memorial Sloan-Kettering Cancer Center

William Tew, MD
Division of Gynecologic Oncology
Memorial Sloan-Kettering Cancer Center

Richard Tsang, MD
Department of Radiation Oncology
Princess Margaret Hospital

Akila Viswanathan, MD
Department of Radiation Oncology
Dana-Farber Cancer Institute

Lawrence D. Wagman, MD
Division of Surgery
The Center for Cancer Prevention and Treatment, St. Joseph Hospital

Sharon M. Weinstein, MD
Departments of Anesthesiology, Neurology, and Internal Medicine (Oncology)
Huntsman Cancer Institute

Lawrence M. Weiss, MD
Division of Pathology
City of Hope National Medical Center

Mark A. Weiss, MD
Department of Medical Oncology
Kimmel Cancer Center

Mitchell Weiss, MD
Department of Radiation Oncology
Monmouth Medical Center

Jeffrey Weitzel, MD
Division of Clinical Cancer Genetics
City of Hope National Medical Center

Jane N. Winter, MD
Division of Hematology/Oncology
Robert H. Lurie Comprehensive Cancer Center, Feinberg School of Medicine/Northwestern University

Joachim Yahalom, MD
Department of Radiation Oncology
Memorial Sloan-Kettering Cancer Center

Alan W. Yasko, MD
Department of Orthopaedic Oncology
Robert H. Lurie Comprehensive Cancer Center, Feinberg School of Medicine/Northwestern University

Sriram Yennurajalingam, MD
Department of Palliative Care and Rehabilitation Medicine
M. D. Anderson Cancer Center

Editorial and publishing staff: *Angela Cibuls, Project Manager; Susan Reckling and Marie-Louise Best, Sr. Editors; Anne Landry, Editor; Ian Ingram, Editorial Assistant; Nancy Bitteker, Creative Director; Andrew Barkus, Group Production Manager; Rachel Warren, Editorial Director; Amy Birnbach, Publisher*

CONTRIBUTOR DISCLOSURE INFORMATION

The following contributors have no significant financial interest or other relationship with the manufacturers of any products or providers of any service mentioned in their respective chapters: Nathan B. Adams; Peter Ahn; Steven R. Alberts; Erika Masuda Alford; J. Sybil Biermann; Charles D. Blanke; Mary S. Brady; Eduardo Bruera; Mark Buyyounouski; Antonio Calles; Kevin A. Camphausen; Brian C.-H. Chiu; Deborah E. Citrin; Jay S. Cooper; Sanjeet Dadwal; Atreya Dash; Kieron Dunleavy; Carmen P. Escalante; Steven J. Feigenberg; Stephen J. Forman; Guillermo Garcia-Manero; Leda Gattoc; Shari B. Goldfarb; Sharad Goyal; Frederic W. Grannis, Jr; Kathryn M. Greven; Karl Haglund; William J. Hoskins; Mimi I. Hu; Mark Hurwitz; Rajesh V. Iyer; Ishmael Jaiyesimi; Lori Jardines; Aminah Jatoi; Aradhana Kaushal; Kemp H. Kernstine; Christine Ko; Jane Kriengkauykiat; Lily Lai; Jeffrey P. Lamont; Miriam N. Lango; Joseph Lattanzi; Jay S. Loeffler; Patrick J. Loehrer; Sharmila Makhija; Ellen Manzullo; Maurie Markman; Michael Mulligan; Robert J. Myerson; Margaret R. O'Donnell; Channing J. Paller; Richard Pazdur; Carlos A. Perez; Peter W. T. Pisters; Laura Raftery; Deepa Reddy; John Andrew Ridge; John M. Robertson; Miguel A. Rodriguez-Bigas; Stephen C. Rubin; Aaron R. Sasson; Roderich E. Schwarz; Walter Scott; Nicole A. Shonka; Richard T. Silver; Douglas Skarecky; David Straus; William Tew; Richard Tsang; Akila Viswanathan; Sharon M. Weinstein; Mitchell Weiss; Joachim Yahalom; Alan W. Yasko; Sriram Yennurajalingam

The following contributors disclosed a financial interest or other relationship with manufacturers of products or providers of a service(s) mentioned in their respective chapters:

Andrew J. Armstrong: Consultant or paid advisory board: Active Biotech AB, Amgen, Cougar Biotechnology/Johnson & Johnson, Novartis; Research support: Active Biotech AB, Bristol-Myers Squibb, Dendreon, ImClone Systems, Inc, Medivation, Novartis, Pfizer, sanofi-aventis; Lecture fees: Dendreon, Pfizer, sanofi-aventis

Al B. Benson III: Consultant or paid advisory board: Amgen, Bristol-Myers Squibb, Genentech, ImClone, Pfizer, Roche, sanofi-aventis; Lecture fees: Amgen; Grant support: Amgen, Bayer/Onyx, Genentech, NCCN, sanofi-aventis, Schering-Plough, Taiho

Julie R. Brahmer: Consultant or paid advisory board: Astra Zeneca, Cephalon, Lilly, Genentech, GlaxoSmithKline, ImClone; Research support: Bristol-Myers Squibb, Merck, Regeneron, Synta, TGD Pharma

Emiliano Calvo: Consultant or paid advisory board: Cephalon, Novartis, Pfizer; Lecture fees: GlaxoSmithKline, Novartis

Warren Chow: Research support: Ariad

Jorge E. Cortes: Consultant or paid advisory board: Ariad, Bristol-Myers Squibb, Chemgenex; Research support: Ariad, Bristol-Myers Squibb, Chemgenex, Deciphera, Novartis, Pfizer

Lisa M. DeAngelis: Consultant or paid advisory board: Genentech

Andrew M. Evens: Consultant or paid advisory board: Celgene, Millennium, Seattle Genetics, Spectrum, Ziopharm; Research support: Lilly, Millennium, Ortho-Biotec, Ziopharm

Paul Fisher: Grant support: Siemens

Keith Flaherty: Consultant or paid advisory board: GlaxoSmithKline, Novartis, Plexxikon, Schering-Plough

Jorge A. Garcia: Consultant or paid advisory board: Novartis, Onyx, Pfizer, Roche; Research support: Amgen, Genentech, ImClone, Novartis, Pfizer

Bonnie S. Glisson: Research support: Amgen, ImClone, Pfizer

Leo I. Gordon: Consultant or paid advisory board: Cure Tech, Ltd; Lecture fees: Genentech; Research support: Millennium

Richard J. Gralla: Consultant or paid advisory board: Eisai, GlaxoSmithKline, Helsinn, Merck; Lecture fees: Helsinn, Merck; Grant support: Helsinn

Steven M. Grunberg: Consultant or paid advisory board: Helsinn, Merck, SNBL; Equity ownership/stock options: Merck; Lecture fees: Merck, Ono Pharmaceuticals; Grant support: Merck

John D. Hainsworth: Grant support: bioTheranostics, Genentech

Jimmy Hwang: Consultant or paid advisory board: Genentech; Lecture fees: Genentech, sanofi-aventis

James I. Ito: Lecture fees: Astellas, Cubist, Pfizer

Sundar Jagannath: Consultant or paid advisory board: Celgene, Millennium

Hagop Kantarjian: Grant support: Bristol-Myers Squibb, Genzyme, Novartis

Mario E. Lacouture: Consultant or paid advisory board: Amgen, Bayer, Boehringer-Ingelheim, Bristol-Myers Squibb, Genentech, Genzyme, GlaxoSmithKline, Hana, ImClone, Lilly, Onyx, OSI, Pfizer, Roche, Wyeth

Nicole Lamanna: Consultant or paid advisory board: Celgene; Research support: Bayer, Biogen Idec, Celgene, Genentech, Hospira

Alan List: Lecture fees: Celgene; Grant support: Celgene

Robert Maki: Consultant or paid advisory board: Eisai, Lilly, Novartis; Honoraria: Novartis, Ziopharm; Research support: Hoffmann LaRoche, Pfizer

Maurie Markman: Consultant or paid advisory board: Amgen, Boehringer-Ingelheim, Celgene, Genentech, Hana Pharmaceuticals, Lilly, Ortho Biotech

David Scott Miller: Equity ownership/stock options: Agilent Technologies, Baxter Healthcare Corp, Cardinal Health Inc, Covidien Ltd, CVS Caremark Corp, Elan Pharmaceuticals, Procter & Gamble; Lecture fees: Lilly, Merck, MGI Pharma, sanofi-aventis; Other support: Marshall Edwards Pty Limited, Genentech, Fujirebio Diagnostics, GlaxoSmithKline

Ronald T. Mitsuyasu: Consultant or paid advisory board: Merck; Grant support: Bionor Immuno, Sangamo

Judd W. Moul: Consultant or paid advisory board: Astra-Zeneca, Bayer, Theralogix; Lecture fees: Dendreon, Ferring, sanofi-aventis

Benjamin Movsas: Research support: Resonant Inc, Varian Inc, Philips Inc

Nikhil C. Munshi: Consultant or paid advisory board: Celgene, Millennium, Novartis

Bert O'Neil: Consultant or paid advisory board: Bayer; Grant support: Bayer

Paul Richardson: Consultant or paid advisory board: Bristol-Myers Squibb, Johnson & Johnson

Steven T. Rosen: Consultant or paid advisory board: Abbott Laboratories, Allos, Celgene, CTI, Genentech; Grant support: Celgene; Honorarium: Genentech, Therakos

Melanie Royce: Contracted research: Amgen, Novartis, Pfizer, Roche; Lecture fees: Novartis, Genentech, Pfizer

Paul Sabbatini: Research support: Genentech, Menarini

Philippe E. Spiess: Consultant or paid advisory board: Endo Pharmaceuticals; Lecture fees: Endo Pharmaceuticals; Research support: Endo Pharmaceuticals

Lawrence D. Wagman: Consultant or paid advisory board: MedWaves Inc; Lecture fees: AngioDynamics Inc, sanofi-aventis

Lawrence M. Weiss: Consultant or paid advisory board: Clarient Inc, Pathwork Diagnostics; Equity ownership/stock options: Clarient Inc; Lecture fees: Clarient Inc

Mark A. Weiss: Consultant or paid advisory board: Celgene

Jeffrey Weitzel: Lecture fees: Myriad Genetics

Jane N. Winter: Consultant or paid advisory board: Antisoma, Bristol-Myers Squibb, CVS Caremark, Eisai, Hana Bioscience, Novartis; Equity ownership: GlaxoSmithKline, Merck, Medco Health Solutions

Preface

In writing and editing the first edition of *Cancer Management: A Multidisciplinary Approach*, published in 1996, three consistent goals guided our editorial policies. These goals continue to direct this 13th edition:

- To provide practical information for physicians who manage cancer patients;
- To present this information concisely, uniformly, and logically; and
- To emphasize a collaborative multidisciplinary approach to patient management that involves surgical, radiation, and medical-hematologic oncologists, as well as other health care professionals, working as a cohesive team.

Chapters in the current volume have been authored jointly by practicing medical-hematologic, surgical, and radiation oncologists. In some cases, other specialists have been asked to contribute their expertise to a particular chapter. The 40 chapters and four appendices in the Handbook represent the efforts of more than 100 contributors from approximately 50 cancer treatment centers. All of our contributors personally manage patients using a multidisciplinary approach in their respective institutions. These chapters reflect the recommendations of practitioners cognizant that decisions and recommendations regarding therapies must be founded on evidence-based research directed at practical patient care in a cost-effective manner.

Over the 15-year period since the first edition was published, important advances have occurred in our understanding of cancer and the treatment of patients with malignant diseases. Quality cancer care is dependent on this integrated approach involving the medical and hematologic, surgical, and radiation oncologists, along with numerous other health professionals. The 13th edition of *Cancer Management: A Multidisciplinary Approach* reflects the ongoing commitment of the authors, editors, and publisher to disseminate to oncologists and the cancer care community the most current information on the multidisciplinary management of patients with cancer.

In this latest edition the editors and contributors make every effort to bring you the newest clinical data relevant to the day-to-day care of patients with cancer. To present this information in the most concise and practical manner possible, we focus solely on the clinical management of disease. The more than 10,000 clinicians and cancer specialists who receive this publication annually have helped us craft the current edition. Many of these clinicians told us that they use this publication daily as a practical resource for clinical information where and when they need it most: in the clinic and with the patient. Therefore, we have updated the staging systems tables in all tumor types, with major changes in a few.

Recent scientific advances in the field of molecular oncology have led to the identification of large numbers of potential targets for novel anticancer therapies. "Personalized medicine" is frequently included in the discussion of breast, sarcoma, lung, and colorectal cancers. This has resulted in an expansion of the drug development pipeline, and the number and diversity of clinically useful novel anticancer therapeutic agents is growing at an unprecedented rate. The 13th edition of *Cancer Management:*

A Multidisciplinary Approach focuses on the agents currently available and includes information that is emerging at peer-reviewed meetings. Other advances include the advent of high-quality invasive diagnostic approaches guided by radiologic imaging modalities; combination therapy with both chemotherapy and molecularly targeted drugs, and the use of charged particles, most commonly, protons; and better tumor targeting using intensity modulated radiotherapy (IMRT) and image-guided radiotherapy (IGRT). Finally, the use of combinations of chemotherapy/radiation and surgery to limit functional losses has become a guiding principle. All of these advances have contributed to improvements in the multidisciplinary approach to cancer management detailed further within the 13th edition of the Handbook.

The substantial changes that were made in previous editions to the chapters on breast cancer, non–small-cell lung cancer, colon, rectal, and anal cancers, cervical cancer, and melanoma were well received by our readers. The 13th edition of *Cancer Management: A Multidisciplinary Approach* has major additions to the chapters dealing with non-Hodgkin lymphoma; soft-tissue sarcomas; and cancers of the prostate, ovary, uterine cervix, rectum, colon, and brain. All chapters have been updated to reflect the latest information about cancer treatment, and the most current data on novel therapies and clinical trials. Changes to TNM staging systems have been noted in this Handbook. Readers are referred to the *AJCC Cancer Staging Manual*, 7th edition (Edge SB et al, eds, Springer, New York, 2010) for a comprehensive review of updates or changes to TNM staging systems. Watch also for updates to individual chapters online at www.cancernetwork.com/cancer-management.

Important new drugs and new indications have emerged and changed our treatment paradigms. New therapies for prostate cancer, including cabazitaxel (Jevtana) and the first-approved autologous cellular immunotherapy (sipuleucel-T [Provenge]) have been introduced into clinical practice. New therapies for hematological malignancies, including romidepsin (Istodax) for the treatment of cutaneous T-cell lymphoma and ofatumumab (Arzerra) for the treatment of patients with refractory chronic lymphocytic leukemia (CLL), have been approved.

Drugs that have been previously used in the treatment of hematological malignancies have been investigated for new indications and have received acceptance in our treatment plans. This includes an expanded indication for nilotinib (Tasigna) for the treatment of adult patients with newly diagnosed chronic myeloid leukemia in chronic phase and the expanded use of rituximab ([Rituxan] in combination with fludarabine and cyclophosphamide) for the treatment of CLL. Women with breast cancer whose tumors are hormone receptor–positive with HER2 overexpression now have the option of being treated with lapatinib (Tykerb) in combination with letrozole (Femara). Selected patients with non–small-cell lung cancer now have treatment options for "maintenance therapy" with erlotinib (Tarceva) or pemetrexed (Alimta).

In addition to discussions of many of these new anticancer agents, new indications for existing drugs, and new standards of care for a variety of malignancies, appendix 3 of the 13th edition of the Handbook provides a snapshot of selected cancer drugs newly approved or newly labeled by the US Food and Drug Administration, from October 2009 through September 2010. We hope you find this year's edition of *Cancer Management: A Multidisciplinary Approach* valuable in your daily practice.

To write, edit, and publish this 1,000+-page 13th edition of *Cancer Management: A Multidisciplinary Approach* requires the dedication of all of the authors, as well as a professional publication staff to coordinate the technical aspects of editing and publishing. We acknowledge the following individuals at UBM Medica: Angela Cibuls, project manager; Susan Reckling, Marie-Louise Best, and Anne Landry, editors; Ian Ingram, Editorial Assistant; Nancy Bitteker, Creative Director; and Rachel Warren, Editorial Director.

Richard Pazdur, MD
Director, Office of Oncology Drug Products
Center for Drug Evaluation and Research
US Food and Drug Administration

Lawrence D. Wagman, MD
Executive Medical Director
The Center for Cancer Prevention and Treatment
St. Joseph Hospital
Orange, California

Kevin A. Camphausen, MD
Chief, Radiation Oncology Branch
National Cancer Institute

William J. Hoskins, MD
Executive Director of Surgical Activities
Memorial Sloan-Kettering Cancer Center
New York, New York

See the following page for a timeline outlining
"15 Years of Advances in Cancer Management, 1996–2010"

15 Years of Advances in Cancer Management, 1996–2010[a]

1996 **FDA approves:**

- Topotecan (Hycamtin), for the treatment of metastatic ovarian cancer, becoming the first of a class of drugs that interferes with the enzyme topoisomerase I. Topotecan is derived from the bark of a Chinese tree known as *Camptotheca acuminata*.
- Irinotecan (Camptosar), another topoisomerase inhibitor, for the treatment of metastatic colorectal cancer.

1997 It is recommended by the National Cancer Advisory Board that NCI advise all women age 40 years and older to receive screening mammograms every 1 to 2 years.

Cancer stem cells are first identified in acute myelogenous leukemia.

FDA approves:

- Rituximab (Rituxan) to treat non-Hodgkin lymphoma (NHL), becoming the first biotechnology product approved by the FDA to treat patients with cancer.

1998 Tamoxifen can reduce the incidence of breast cancer by 50% in women who are at increased risk of the disease, according to data from the Breast Cancer Prevention Trial. Tamoxifen is subsequently approved by the FDA for the prevention of breast cancer.

FDA approves:

- Trastuzumab (Herceptin), for the treatment of metastatic breast cancer.

1999 **FDA approves:**

- Hybrid Capture II human papillomavirus (HPV), a DNA test that can be used in conjunction with the Pap smear in screening for cervical cancer.

2000 The most common form of NHL, diffuse large B-cell lymphoma (DLBCL), is identified as two distinct diseases, germinal center B-like DLBCL and activated B-like DLBCL. In the pre-rituximab (Rituxan) era patients with germinal center B-like DLBCL had significantly improved overall survival; this prognostic difference between these two groups is less apparent now.

2001 Imatinib mesylate (Gleevec) is shown to be effective against chronic myelogenous leukemia (CML), becoming the first anticancer drug developed specifically to target the molecular defect that causes a particular type of cancer.

FDA approves:

- Letrozole (Femara), for first-line treatment of advanced breast cancer in postmenopausal women with estrogen-dependent tumors.

2002 The National Lung Screening Trial (NLST) is launched by the NCI to determine whether spiral computed tomography is better than single-view chest x-ray in reducing deaths among current and former heavy smokers. Second-hand smoke is classified as carcinogenic to humans by the International Agency for Research on Cancer.

FDA approves:

- Zoledronic acid (Zometa) for multiple myeloma and bone metastases from solid tumors.

2003 Daily use of aspirin for as little as 3 years reduces the development of colorectal polyps by 19% to 35% in individuals at high risk for colorectal cancer.

Men taking finasteride (Proscar) had 25% fewer diagnoses of prostate cancer than men taking a placebo, indicating that prostate cancer can be prevented, according to results from the Prostate Cancer Prevention Trial (PCPT).

Postmenopausal women diagnosed with early-stage breast cancer who took the aromatase inhibitor letrozole after completing an initial 5 years of adjuvant tamoxifen had a significantly reduced risk of cancer recurrence compared with women taking a placebo, according to results from an NCI-supported international clinical trial.

FDA approves:

- Bortezomib (Velcade), for the treatment of multiple myeloma.

2004 Women who take estrogen in combination with the hormone progestin have a greater risk of developing breast cancer than women who take estrogen alone, according to data from the Women's Health Initiative (WHI) study.

FDA approves:

- Letrozole for the adjuvant treatment of early-stage breast cancer after 5 years of tamoxifen therapy.
- Palifermin (Kepivance), to decrease the incidence and duration of severe oral mucositis in patients with hematologic malignancies who receive high doses of chemotherapy and radiation therapy followed by stem cell rescue.
- Three drugs for metastatic colorectal cancer: bevacizumab (Avastin), cetuximab (Erbitux), and oxaliplatin (Eloxatin).

2005 The addition of trastuzumab (Herceptin) to chemotherapy in women with early-stage HER2-positive invasive breast cancer significantly decreases the risk of cancer recurrence compared with chemotherapy alone, according to data reported in two large NCI-sponsored randomized clinical trials.

FDA approves:

- A nanoparticle formulation of paclitaxel (Abraxane) for use in women with metastatic or recurrent breast cancer.

2006 Raloxifene (Evista) is reported to reduce the incidence of invasive breast cancer by approximately 50% and is less likely to cause some potentially dangerous side effects found with tamoxifen, according to initital results from the STAR Trial.

FDA approves:

- Gardasil vaccine, for protection against persistent infection by two types of HPV that cause approximately 70% of cervical cancers worldwide.
- Trastuzumab (Herceptin), for use with other drugs in the adjuvant treatment of women with early-stage, node-positive, HER2-overexpressing breast cancer.

2007 The addition of arsenic trioxide following standard chemotherapy resulted in longer disease remissions and better overall survival than standard chemotherapy alone in patients with previously untreated acute promyelocytic leukemia, according to data from a large phase III trial.

FDA approves:

- Three drugs for metastatic renal cell carcinoma, including sunitinib (Sutent), sorafenib (Nexavar), and temsirolimus (Torisel).

2008 Virtual colonoscopy is reported to be similar to conventional, optical colonoscopy in detecting intermediate-size and large colorectal polyps, suggesting that the procedure could serve as an initial screening exam for colorectal cancer.

2009 Results of a preliminary phase II study show a PARP inhibitor (poly ADP ribose polymerase), BSI-201, to have unprecedented effects on inducing tumor responses, delaying time to progression, and improving survival in women with advanced triple-negative breast cancer.

An antibody-based immunotherapy (chimeric anti-GD2 antibody ch.14.18) is reported to reduce the risk of relapse and improved overall survival among children with high-risk neuroblastoma.

Early use of ginger supplements, in combination with traditional antinausea drugs, significantly reduces chemotherapy-related nausea in patients with cancer.

A new gene signature assay predicts risk of recurrence among patients with stage II colon cancer.

EGFR status predicts response to first-line gefitinib (Iressa) for lung cancer.

FDA approves:

- Bevacizumab (Avastin), for renal cell carcinoma and glioblastoma.
- HPV vaccine (Cervarix), a new vaccine to prevent cervical cancer and precancerous lesions caused by HPV types 16 and 18.

- Pemetrexed (Alimta) for maintenance treatment of locally advanced or metastatic nonsquamous non–small-cell lung cancer (NSCLC) patients.
- Pazopanib (Votrient), for the treatment of patients with advanced renal cell carcinoma.

2009 / 2010

FDA approves[b]:

- Ofatumumab (Arzerra, also known as HuMax-CD20) for the treatment of patients with chronic lymphocytic leukemia (CLL) whose disease does not respond to treatment with fludarabine (Fludara) and alemtuzumab (Campath).
- Lapatinib (Tykerb) in combination with letrozole (Femara) for women with HER2-postive, ER-positive metastatic breast cancer.
- Erlotinib (Tarceva) for first-line maintenance treatment of locally advanced or metastatic NSCLC in patients whose disease has not progressed after 4 cycles of platinum-based therapy.
- Sipuleucel-T (Provenge), a dendritic cell–based vaccine for the treatment of asymptomatic or minimally symptomatic metastatic castrate-resistant (hormone-refractory) prostate cancer.
- Cabazitaxel (Jevtana), in combination with prednisone, for treatment of men with advanced, hormone-refractory prostate cancer that has worsened during or after treatment with docetaxel (Taxotere).

[a] Adapted from the National Cancer Institute, 100 Years of Advances Against Cancer. For the full report, visit http://www.cancer.gov/aboutnci/100-years-advances

[b] See Appendix 3 for a comprehensive list of new drugs approved by the FDA from October 2009 through September 2010.

CHAPTER 1

Head and neck tumors

John Andrew Ridge, MD, PhD, Bonnie S. Glisson, MD,
Miriam N. Lango, MD, and Steven Feigenberg, MD

In 2010, approximately 36,540 men and women (25,420 men and 11,120 women) in the United States were diagnosed with cancer of the oral cavity and pharynx, and 7,880 will succumb to these diseases. Further, an estimated 12,720 men and women (10,110 men and 2,610 women) in the United States were diagnosed with laryngeal cancer, and approximately 3,600 died from this malignancy. Most patients with head and neck cancer have metastatic disease at the time of diagnosis (regional nodal involvement in 43% and distant metastasis in 10%).

Head and neck cancers encompass a diverse group of uncommon tumors that frequently are aggressive in their biologic behavior. Moreover, patients with a head and neck cancer often develop a second primary tumor. These tumors occur at an annual rate of 3% to 7%, and 50% to 75% of such new cancers occur in the upper aerodigestive tract or lungs.

The anatomy of the head and neck is complex and is divided into sites and subsites (Figure 1). Tumors of each site have a unique epidemiology, anatomy, natural history, and therapeutic approach. This chapter will review these lesions as a group and then individually by anatomic site.

MALIGNANCIES OF THE HEAD AND NECK

EPIDEMIOLOGY

Gender

Head and neck cancer is more common in men; 66% to 95% of cases occur in men. The incidence by gender varies with anatomic location and has been changing as the number of female smokers has increased. The male-female ratio is currently 3:1 for oral cavity and pharyngeal cancers. In patients with Plummer-Vinson syndrome, the ratio is reversed, with 80% of head and neck cancers occurring in women.

Age

The incidence of head and neck cancer increases with age, especially after 50 years of age. Although most patients are between 50 and 70 years old, younger patients can develop head and neck cancer. There are more women and fewer smokers in the younger patient group.

It is controversial whether head and neck cancer is more aggressive in younger patients or in older individuals. This "aggressiveness" probably reflects the common delay in diagnosis in the younger population, since, in most studies, younger patients do not have a worse prognosis than do their older counterparts.

Race

The incidence of laryngeal cancer is higher in African-Americans relative to the white, Asian, and Hispanic populations.

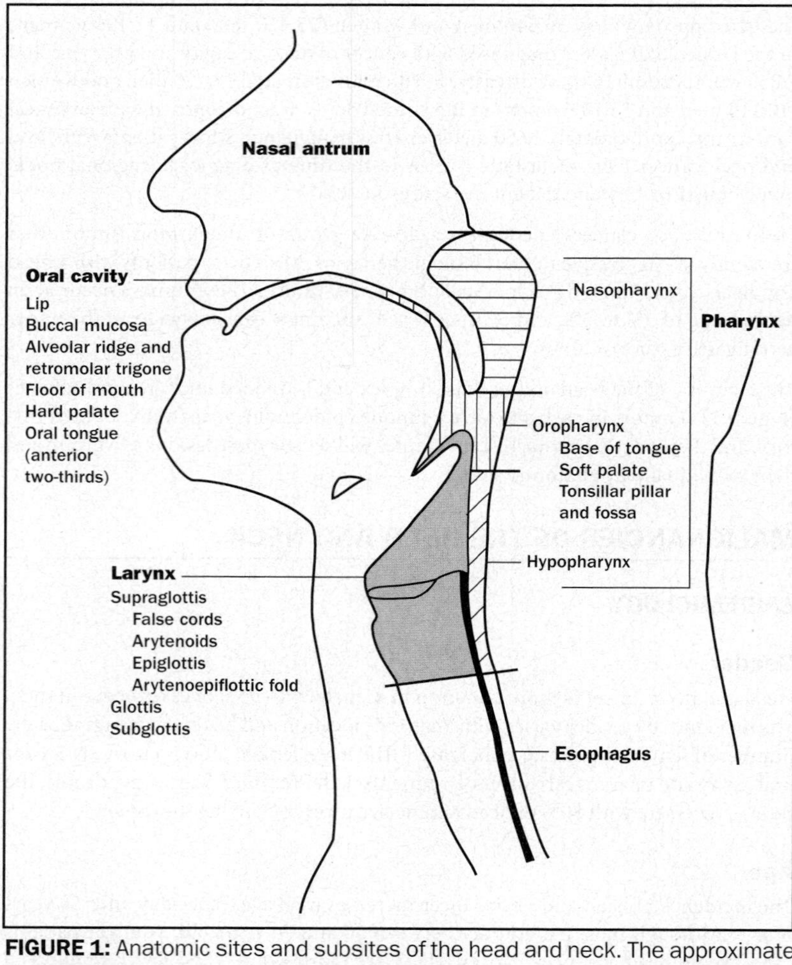

FIGURE 1: Anatomic sites and subsites of the head and neck. The approximate distribution of head and neck cancer is oral cavity, 44%; larynx, 31%; and pharynx, 25%.

Additionally, in African-Americans, head and neck cancer is associated with lower survival for similar tumor stages. The overall 5-year survival rate is 56% in whites and 34% in African-Americans.

Geography

There are wide variations in the incidence of head and neck cancer among different geographic regions. The risk of laryngeal cancer, for example, is two to six times higher in Bombay, India, than in Scandinavia. The higher incidence of the disease in Asia is thought to reflect the prevalence of risk factors, such as betel nut chewing and use of smokeless tobacco. In the United States, the high incidence among urban males is thought to reflect exposure to tobacco and alcohol. Among rural women, there is an increased risk of oral cancer related to the use of smokeless tobacco (snuff).

Nasopharyngeal carcinoma is another head and neck tumor with a distinct ethnic predilection. Endemic areas include southern China, northern Africa, and regions of the far Northern Hemisphere—areas in which the diet of inhabitants includes large quantities of salted meat and fish. When people from these regions migrate to areas with a lower disease incidence, their risk falls but remains elevated. Cancer of the nasopharynx in these geographic areas also has been associated with Epstein-Barr virus (EBV) infection (see section on "Etiology and risk factors").

ETIOLOGY AND RISK FACTORS

Risk factors for head and neck cancer include tobacco and alcohol use, ultraviolet (UV) light exposure, viral infection, and environmental exposures.

Tobacco

The incidence of head and neck tumors correlates most closely with the use of tobacco.

Cigarettes

Head and neck tumors occur six times more often among cigarette smokers than nonsmokers. The age-standardized risk of mortality from laryngeal cancer appears to rise linearly with increasing cigarette smoking. For the heaviest smokers, death from laryngeal cancer is 20 times more likely than for nonsmokers. Furthermore, active smoking by head and neck cancer patients is associated with significant increases in the annual rate of second primary tumor development (compared with former smokers or those who have never smoked). Use of unfiltered cigarettes or dark, air-cured tobacco is associated with further increases in risk.

Cigars

Often misperceived as posing a lower health risk than cigarette smoking, cigar smoking results in a change in the site distribution for aerodigestive tract cancer, according to epidemiologic data. Although the incidence of cancer at some sites traditionally associated with cigarette smoking (eg, larynx, lungs) is decreased in cigar smokers, the incidence of cancer is actually higher at other sites where pooling of saliva and associated carcinogens tends to occur (oropharynx, esophagus).

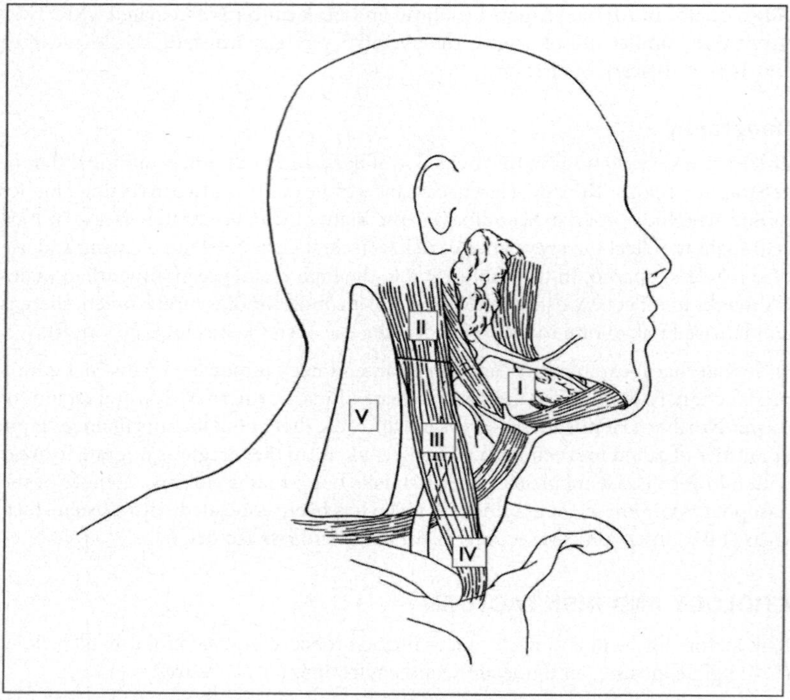

FIGURE 2: Levels of the neck as determined by lymphatic drainage patterns.

Smokeless tobacco

Use of smokeless tobacco also is associated with an increased incidence of head and neck cancer, especially in the oral cavity. Smokeless tobacco users frequently develop premalignant lesions, such as oral leukoplakia, at the site where the tobacco quid rests against the mucosa. Over time, these lesions may progress to invasive carcinomas. The use of snuff has been associated with an increase in cancers of the gum and oral mucosa.

Alcohol

Alcohol consumption, by itself, is a risk factor for the development of pharyngeal and laryngeal tumors, although it is a less potent carcinogen than is tobacco. For individuals who use both tobacco and alcohol, these risk factors appear to be synergistic and result in a multiplicative increase in risk.

UV light exposure

Exposure to UV light is a risk factor for the development of cancer of the lips. At least 33% of patients with lip cancer have outdoor occupations.

Occupational exposures

A small group of head and neck cancers may be attributable to occupational exposures. Nasal cancer has been associated with wood dust exposure, and squamous cell cancer of the maxillary sinus, has been linked to nickel exposure. Petroleum exposure may be associated with pharyngeal cancer, but the relationship has not been proven.

Radiation exposure

Exposure to radiation is clearly an important risk factor for thyroid cancer and has been associated with cancer of the salivary glands.

Viruses

There is a strong link between EBV exposure and the development of nasopharyngeal cancer. The potential etiologic role of human papillomavirus (HPV) in oropharyngeal cancer is supported by a growing body of evidence. A case-control study of 100 patients with squamous cancer of the oropharynx documented that HPV DNA, type 16, was found in 72% of tumor specimens. Further, 64% of the patients had antibodies to HPV-16 oncoproteins. Oral infection with HPV increased the risk of oropharyngeal cancer with an odds ratio of 14.6 (95% confidence interval [CI], 6.3–36.6). This risk was independent of tobacco and alcohol use. These patients appear to have a better outcome following surgery, radiotherapy, and chemotherapy. In addition, these patients have a lower incidence of second cancers and a lower risk of death from other tobacco-related illnesses (eg, heart and lung disease).

Diet

Epidemiologic studies suggest that dietary intake of vitamin A, β-carotene, and α-tocopherol may reduce the risk of developing head and neck cancer.

Marijuana

Smoking marijuana is associated with the development of head and neck cancer, but the degree of risk is unknown.

ANATOMY

The anatomy of the head and neck region is complex. The anatomic sites are illustrated in Figure 1. More detailed descriptions are included below in the discussions of specific sites and subsites.

Levels of the neck

The anatomy of the neck is relevant to the treatment of all head and neck cancers. The neck may be divided into levels (Figure 2). The lymphatic drainage of the unmanipulated neck is systematic and predictable; knowledge of these drainage patterns assists the clinician in locating the primary tumor that has given rise to a neck metastasis (Table 1).

TABLE 1: Lymphatic drainage of the head and neck and associated sites of primary tumors

Lymphatic drainage	Likely primary sites
Level I: Includes the submental and submandibular triangles	
Submental	Lower lip, chin, anterior oral cavity (including anterior one-third of the tongue and floor of the mouth)
Submandibular	Upper and lower lips, oral tongue, floor of the mouth, facial skin
Level II: Includes the superior jugular chain nodes extending from the mandible down to the carotid bifurcation and posterior border of the sternocleidomastoid muscle	Oral cavity and pharynx (including soft palate, base of the tongue, and piriform sinus)
Level III: Consists of the jugular nodes from the carotid bulb inferiorly to the omohyoid muscle	Larynx, hypopharynx, and thyroid
Level IV: Continues from the omohyoid muscle inferiorly to the clavicle	Larynx, hypopharynx, thyroid, cervical esophagus, and trachea
Level V: Represents the posterior border of the sternocleidomastoid anteriorly, the anterior border of the trapezius posteriorly, and the clavicle inferiorly	Nasopharynx, thyroid, paranasal sinuses, and posterior scalp
Supraclavicular	Infraclavicular sites (including lungs, esophagus, breasts, pancreas, gastrointestinal tract, gastrointestinal and genitourinary sources)

SIGNS AND SYMPTOMS

Head and neck cancer typically produces symptoms referable to the upper aerodigestive tract, including alterations in deglutition, phonation, hearing, and respiration. In particular, patients should be questioned about dysphagia, odynophagia, globus sensation, hoarseness, a change in the ability to form words, epistaxis, epiphora, otalgia, hemoptysis, stuffiness of the ears, and trismus. (Signs and symptoms of cancer at specific anatomic sites and subsites can be found in the respective discussions of these tumors.)

It is important to ascertain the duration and course (progression or improvement) of symptoms. Progression of disease is often noted during the evaluation and worsens the prognosis.

SCREENING AND DIAGNOSIS

Screening

Since many patients with head and neck cancer are unlikely to be engaged in the health-care system, the means by which patient screening would be achieved remains a fundamental problem.

Diagnosis

The need for expeditious diagnosis of head and neck cancer and referral to a skilled head and neck specialist cannot be overemphasized, as early diagnosis can lead to a reduction in mortality. One study suggested that in the 24 months prior to the diagnosis of head and neck cancer, patients had a median of 10.5 health-care visits. These visits provide an opportunity to evaluate patients' symptoms and underscore the important role of dentists and primary care physicians in the early diagnosis of head and neck cancer.

History

Risk factors as outlined previously, including a history of tobacco and alcohol use and environmental exposures, should be reviewed. Any adult patient with symptoms referable to the upper aerodigestive tract that have lasted longer than 2 weeks or with an asymptomatic neck mass should undergo a thorough examination with a high index of suspicion for carcinoma.

Physical examination

The physical examination is the best means for detecting lesions of the upper aerodigestive tract. Frequently, the initial assessment also will indicate the severity and chronicity of the disease. Due to the frequent occurrence of multiple primary tumors in patients with a head and neck tumor, careful evaluation of the entire upper aerodigestive tract is necessary at the time of diagnosis. The examination should always follow a systematic approach.

Skin/scalp A search should be made for ulcers, nodules, and pigmented or other suspicious lesions. This part of the evaluation is frequently overlooked.

Cranial nerves A cranial nerve evaluation is essential for any patient with a head and neck tumor or neck mass (which may be a manifestation of occult cancer). This evaluation should include assessing eye motion (cranial nerves [CN] III, IV, and VI); testing sensation of the face (CN V); examining the muscles of facial expression by having the patient grin, grimace, raise eyebrows, close eyes tightly, show teeth, and puff out the cheeks (CN VII); testing of hearing (CN VIII); assessing gag reflex (CN IX); evaluating vocal cord mobility (CN X); and having the patient fully abduct the shoulder (CN XI) and protrude the tongue (CN XII). Even the slightest abnormality may be helpful in identifying a primary tumor.

Eyes/ears/nose The eyes, ears, and nose should be evaluated for any sign of mass effect, abnormal drainage/discharge, bleeding, or effusion.

Oral cavity Halitosis may be the first indication of a lesion in the upper aerodigestive tract. The teeth, gingivae, and entire mucosal surface should be inspected. (Dentures should be removed.) The lymphoid tissue of the tonsillar pillars should be inspected and any asymmetry noted. Tongue mobility also should be evaluated.

The floor of the mouth, tongue, and cheeks should be palpated using a bimanual technique (one gloved finger inside the mouth and the second hand under the mandible). Palpation should be the last step of the examination due to stimulation of the gag reflex. Worrisome lesions should be biopsied.

Neck A systematic examination of the neck consistently documents the location of any mass. Palpation is the cornerstone of the examination. It is performed by grasping the tissue and feeling the nodes between the thumb and index and long fingers. The relationship of a mass to major structures, such as the salivary gland, thyroid, and carotid sheath, should be considered.

Important qualities of a mass include location, character, tenderness, size, mobility, and associated thrill or bruit. The thyroid should be palpated.

Laryngoscopy The nasopharynx, hypopharynx, and larynx should all be examined with care. The vocal cords should be visualized and their mobility evaluated. Mirror examination provides an overall impression of mobility and asymmetry, which may point to a hidden tumor. Nasopharyngoscopes permit a thorough inspection of the upper aerodigestive tract in the office setting. Attention should be focused individually on the piriform sinuses, tongue base, pharyngeal walls, epiglottis, arytenoids, and true and false vocal cords. Also, any pooling of secretions should be noted.

Examination under anesthesia with endoscopy Approximately 5% of patients with head and neck cancer have a synchronous primary squamous cell cancer of the head and neck, esophagus, or lungs. Examination with the patient under anesthesia with endoscopy (which may include direct laryngoscopy, esophagoscopy, and bronchoscopy) and directed biopsy should be performed in all patients with an occult primary squamous cell cancer and in many patients with a *known* head and neck primary. Examination with the patient under anesthesia also can provide information regarding the extent of the tumor.

The most common sites of silent primary tumors are the tonsils, base of the tongue, and piriform sinuses. Tumors of the nasopharynx have become easier to identify with the increased use of flexible nasopharyngoscopy. Biopsies should be performed in common areas of silent primaries in addition to the primary anatomic sites associated with lymphatic drainage of any neck mass.

Laboratory evaluation

There are no specific screening laboratory tests other than preoperative studies performed in the diagnostic evaluation of most head and neck carcinomas. EBV, anticapsid antibodies, and serum immunoglobulin G are tumor markers for nasopharyngeal carcinomas.

Diagnostic imaging

Plain x-rays Posteroanterior and lateral chest x-rays should be obtained in all adult patients to eliminate the possibility of occult lung metastasis or a second primary. A Panorex film may be helpful in delineating bony involvement in some cases of oral cavity lesions.

CT The CT scan is probably the single most informative test in the assessment of a head and neck tumor. It may delineate the extent of disease and the presence and extent of lymphatic involvement. CT scans of the chest, abdomen, and pelvis sometimes may identify the site of an occult primary tumor presenting with a node low in the neck. CT offers high spatial resolution and discriminates among fat, muscle, bone, and other soft tissues and surpasses MRI in the detection of bony erosion.

In a multicenter, prospective study of patients with newly diagnosed and untreated head and neck cancers, PET scanning results were discordant with standard imaging (eg, CT scan, MRI) in 43% of cases, and they altered the therapeutic plan in 14% of patients. Nuanced judgment in adding PET scanning to conventional imaging seems to be warranted *(Lonneux M et al: J Clin Oncol 28:1190–1195, 2010)*.

MRI may provide accurate information regarding the size, location, and soft-tissue extent of tumor. It provides limited information regarding bony involvement, unless there is gross involvement of the marrow space. Relatively greater sensitivity of MRI in relation to CT is offset by its decreased specificity. The main disadvantage of MRI is movement artifact, which is a particular problem in the larynx and hypopharynx. Gadolinium-enhanced MRI is probably superior to CT for imaging tumors of the nasopharynx and oropharynx.

PET has been evaluated in both primary and recurrent squamous cell carcinomas of the head and neck. ^{18}F-fluorodeoxyglucose (FDG) is the most commonly used PET radiotracer. It enters the cell and undergoes the first step in glycolysis to produce FDG-6-phosphate, which reflects the metabolic rate of the tissue. The metabolic rate of malignancies is higher than that of most benign tumors or normal tissues. FDG imaging therefore has the potential to distinguish between benign and malignant processes, grade tumors, identify metastases, and diagnose tumor recurrence. In head and neck cancer, FDG imaging has been useful in detecting clinically occult recurrences, although it has proved less useful in identifying an occult primary site for metastatic cervical disease.

Biopsy

Biopsies of the primary tumor often can be performed in an outpatient setting.

Punch or cup forceps biopsy is important in the diagnosis of mucosal lesions. The biopsy should be obtained at the border of the lesion away from areas of obvious necrosis.

Fine-needle aspiration (FNA) is a useful diagnostic modality. Multiple passes are made through the lesion with a fine-gauge (22-gauge) needle while suction is applied. Suction should be released before withdrawing the needle through surrounding soft tissue of the neck. FNA has an associated false-negative rate as low as 7%. The diagnostic accuracy depends on the physician's skill and the cytopathologist's experience.

Cytology is particularly useful in distinguishing a metastatic squamous cell carcinoma from other malignant histologies. However, a negative result should not be interpreted as "absence of malignancy."

Core biopsy should not be performed on a neck mass, with the rare exception of a proven lymphoma.

Open biopsy should be performed only when a diagnosis has not been made after extensive clinical evaluation and FNA is nondiagnostic. The operation should be performed only by a surgeon prepared to conduct immediate definitive surgical treatment at that time (which may entail radical neck dissection).

PATHOLOGY

Squamous cell carcinoma

More than 90% of all head and neck cancers are squamous cell carcinomas.

Histologic grade

There are three histologic grades based on the amount of keratinization: A well-differentiated tumor is characterized by > 75% keratinization; a moderately differentiated tumor, by 25% to 50%; and a poorly differentiated tumor, by < 25%.

Histologic grade has not been a consistent predictor of clinical behavior. Features that predict aggressive behavior include perineural spread, lymphatic invasion, and tumor spread beyond the lymph node capsule.

Morphologic growth patterns

Four morphologically distinct growth patterns have been recognized. The ulcerative type, the most common form, begins as a round or oval ulcer that is friable. Ulcerative lesions progress toward infiltration. Infiltrative lesions extend deeply into underlying tissues. The exophytic type tends to grow more superficially and metastasize later than the other types. It begins as an area of thickened epithelium.

Verrucous cancer is an uncommon variant that, in the United States, typically occurs in elderly patients with poor oral hygiene or ill-fitting dentures. It is characterized by a warty, bulky, elevated, fungating appearance. Verrucous cancers seldom metastasize.

Molecular markers

The inactivation of *TP53*, a central event in head and neck carcinogenesis, occurs by means of several prognostically significant mechanisms. Over 50% of head and neck squamous cell carcinomas have been found to harbor a mutation of the *TP53* gene and linked to diminished survival. HPV, which causes inactivation of *TP53* via elaboration of *E6* and *E7* oncogenes, has been identified in 35% to 75% of oropharyngeal squamous cell carcinomas and has been associated with an improved clinical outcome.

In 2007, a case-control study providing epidemiologic evidence of a causal role for HPV in oropharyngeal cancer was published. Oral infection with HPV-16 or any other 37 subtypes was independently associated with oropharyngeal cancer. HPV-16 was identified in 72% of oropharyngeal tumors. Patients without a history of smoking and/or ethanol abuse were more likely to harbor oral HPV-16. The development of oropharyngeal cancer was associated with high-risk sexual behaviors, including a high lifetime number of sexual partners, casual sexual relations, young age at first intercourse, and infrequent condom use. An HPV vaccine may reduce the incidence of oropharyngeal cancer.

Other tumor types

Other less common head and neck cancers include mucoepidermoid carcinoma, adenoid cystic carcinoma, and adenocarcinoma, all of which may arise in the salivary glands. Head and neck cancers with neuroendocrine features include small-cell undifferentiated cancer and esthesioneuroblastoma (olfactory neuroblastoma). Both Hodgkin lymphoma and non-Hodgkin lymphoma may also be diagnosed as head and neck tumors, often involving the lymph nodes of the neck or Waldeyer's ring.

Precancerous lesions

There is a sequence of disease progression from atypia/dysplasia through carcinoma in situ to frankly invasive cancer. Leukoplakia and erythroplakia are terms applied to clinically identifiable lesions that may harbor invasive cancer or undergo malignant transformation.

Pathology

Leukoplakia results from chronic irritation of mucous membranes by carcinogens; this irritation stimulates the proliferation of white epithelial and connective tissue. Histopathologic examination reveals hyperkeratosis variably associated with underlying epithelial hyperplasia. In the absence of underlying dysplasia, leukoplakia rarely (< 5%) is associated with progression of disease to malignancy.

Erythroplakia

This is characterized by superficial, friable, red patches adjacent to normal mucosa. It is commonly associated with underlying epithelial dysplasia and has a much greater potential for malignancy than leukoplakia. Carcinoma is found in nearly 40% of erythroplakia cases.

Dysplasia

Dysplasia is characterized by cellular atypia, loss of normal maturation, and loss of normal epithelial stratification. It is graded as mild, moderate, or severe, based on the degree of nuclear abnormality present. In the transition from mild to severe dysplasia, nuclear abnormalities become more marked, mitoses become more apparent, and these changes involve increasing depth of epithelium. The likelihood of developing a carcinoma relates to the degree of dysplasia. In the case of severe dysplasia, as many as 24% of patients may develop invasive squamous cell cancer.

Carcinoma in situ

This is characterized by the presence of atypical changes throughout the epithelium with complete loss of stratification. It is estimated that approximately 75% of invasive squamous cell carcinomas have an associated in situ component. Specific DNA mutations have also been identified in the sequence of disease progression from mild dysplasia to atypia to carcinoma in situ to invasive carcinoma.

Field cancerization

Field cancerization is an important concept related to the natural history of head and neck cancer. This term describes the diffuse epithelial injury throughout the head and neck, lungs, and esophagus that results from chronic exposure to carcinogens.

Clinically, field cancerization is manifested by the frequent occurrence of (1) mucosal abnormalities, such as leukoplakia and dysplasia, beyond the margins of a head and neck cancer, and (2) second primary tumors within this exposed field. The lifetime risk of a patient with head and neck cancer developing a new cancer is 20% to 40%. Over time, as the risk of relapse of the initial cancer declines, the development of a new cancer represents the greatest risk for these patients.

Regional and distant metastases

The incidence of lymph node metastases is related to the size and thickness of the primary tumor. If the primary site is near the midline, contralateral or bilateral metastases should be anticipated. In the presence of lymph node metastases, extracapsular spread of tumor is an important prognostic factor.

STAGING AND PROGNOSIS

Staging system

The TNM staging system of the AJCC maintains uniformity in the staging of head and neck tumors. The staging of primary mucosal tumors of the head and neck varies with the anatomic location and will be covered later by site. However, the staging system for metastases and stage groupings are nearly uniform for all mucosal sites.

Prognosis correlates strongly with stage at diagnosis. For many head and neck cancer sites, survival for patients with stage I disease exceeds 80%. For patients with locally advanced disease at the time of diagnosis, (ie, stages III and IV disease), survival drops below 40%. Development of nodal metastases reduces survival of a patient with a small primary tumor by ~50%. Involvement of even a single lymph node is associated with a marked decline in survival. Most patients with head and neck cancer have stage III or IV disease at diagnosis.

Pattern of relapse

Despite aggressive primary treatment, the majority of relapses that occur following a head and neck cancer are within the head and neck. Locoregional relapse accounts for ~80% of primary treatment failures. Distant metastases increase as the disease progresses and most often involve the lungs, and, to a lesser extent, the bones and liver, which is why the addition of PET scans is of minimal utility in evaluating for distant cancer spread. By the time of death, 10% to 30% of patients will have clinically detected distant metastases.

TREATMENT APPROACHES

In general, head and neck tumors may be treated using a single modality for early-stage disease (stage I or II) but may require multimodality therapy for advanced disease (stage III or IV).

The best therapeutic approach for the primary tumor depends on the anatomic site. The approach to treatment of the neck also varies with the site and treatment of the primary tumor. When the primary tumor is treated with irradiation, the "at-risk" regional lymphatics are incorporated into the treatment fields. Neck dissections should remain standardized (ie, complete anatomic dissections, as opposed to "berry picking" or random biopsy) in these settings so as to avoid incomplete surgery.

Preoperative assessment

Before surgical resection, preoperative assessment of the extent of disease is essential. Complete physical examination and appropriate radiologic evaluation are necessary. Direct laryngoscopy and esophagoscopy are frequently performed to determine tumor extent and to rule out the presence of a second primary tumor. A chest x-ray or CT scan may be obtained to screen for distant metastases or a primary lung cancer.

Surgical principles

Classic principles of surgical oncology apply to head and neck cancer. Complete resection is necessary. Securing sufficient margins may be challenging due to the many structures in this area. Reconstruction is complex after resection of head and neck tumors, as the surgery may have an impact on appearance, speech, and swallowing. Decisions regarding the extent of resection should be made by experienced surgeons.

Surgery plus radiation therapy

The combination of radical surgery and radiation therapy has been used for several decades to treat patients with advanced head and neck cancers.

Postoperative versus preoperative radiation therapy

Postoperative radiation therapy (60 to 70 Gy in 6 to 7 weeks) reduces the rate of locoregional recurrence from ~50% to 15% for tumors with pathologic features predictive of locoregional recurrence. The indications for postoperative radiation therapy are well established and include a large primary tumor (T4); close or positive margins; an involved lymph node > 3 cm or multiple involved lymph nodes; extracapsular extension; an open lymph node biopsy not followed by an immediate neck dissection; perineural invasion; invasion of the lymphovascular space, cartilage, bone, or deep soft tissue; and surgeon unease (an experienced surgeon's recommendation to deliver post-operative radiation should be credited by the radiation oncologist because the surgeon will often appreciate worrisome features not documented in a pathology report). The addition of postoperative radiation therapy reduces the risk of locoregional failure but does not decrease the risk of developing distant metastases.

Preoperative radiotherapy (45–50 Gy in 4–5 weeks) has been used for patients with advanced primary tumors, but rates of locoregional recurrence appear to be lower and complications fewer as compared with postoperative radiation therapy; however, this observation was based upon a study performed in the 1970s. Preoperative radiotherapy with or without chemotherapy is indicated for marginally resectable tumors, such as those with fixed cervical lymph nodes. In this setting, preoperative irradiation often permits resection of an otherwise unresectable tumor. However, this approach is used rarely due to the improvements in outcome with chemoradiation and the poor functional outcomes of patients requiring trimodality therapy.

Postoperative chemotherapy/radiation therapy

Two randomized clinical trials were launched to determine whether the addition of chemotherapy to radiation therapy enhanced locoregional tumor control and survival in high-risk patients with head and neck cancer following definitive surgical resection. The results of these trials were published in 2004. In the RTOG 95-01/Intergroup trial, patients with high-risk features including two or more involved lymph nodes, extracapsular extension, or positive margins following definitive surgical resection were randomized to receive 6,000 to 6,600 cGy of postoperative irradiation with or without cisplatin (100 mg/m^2 given on days 1, 22, and 43). With a median follow-up of 45.9 months, the estimated 2-year rate of local and regional tumor control was 82% in the combined-therapy group versus 72% in the radiotherapy group ($P = .01$). The disease-free ($P = .04$), but not overall ($P = .19$), survival was significantly longer in the combined-treatment group, although the primary endpoint was locoregional control and was not powered to demonstrate a survival advantage. The incidence of acute adverse effects (grade 3 or greater) was higher in the combined-treatment group (77% vs 34%; $P < .001$).

In the EORTC 22931 trial, similar conclusions were reported. This study included patients with T3 or T4 disease, perineural invasion, and involvement of the lymphovascular space in addition to positive margins and extracapsular extension. The overall survival rate was significantly improved in the combined-therapy group compared with the radiotherapy group. After a mean of 60 months, the overall survival of 334 randomized patients was 53% in the combined-treatment group versus 40% in the radiation-alone group ($P = .02$). The discrepancy in effect on overall survial was thought to be related to different entry criteria used in the RTOG and EORTC trials.

In a comparative analysis of the two trials, the presence of extracapsular extension and/or microscopically involved surgical margins were the only risk factors for which the impact of chemoradiation therapy significantly improved survival in both trials.

Curative radiation therapy

Radiation therapy with curative intent usually involves daily treatment for 6–7 weeks (total dose: 60 to 70 Gy). Although there is no tissue loss with radiation therapy, as there is with surgery, potential complications include dry mouth, tissue fibrosis, trismus, bone necrosis, hypothyroidism, and dysphasia. Some problems are common and sufficiently debilitating that they require significant care during treatment planning. Surgery often produces less morbidity in the oral cavity; whereas radiotherapy produces less morbidity in the oropharyngeal, laryngeal, and nasopharyngeal regions.

Radiation fractionation

The RTOG 90-03 trial was conducted to determine the efficacy of various fractionation schemes in the treament of locally advanced head and neck cancer. Four schedules were tested: (1) standard fractionation at 2 Gy/fraction/d, 5 d/wk, to 70 Gy/35 fractions/7 wk; (2) hyperfractionation at 1.2 Gy/fraction, twice daily, 5 d/wk to 81.6 Gy/68 fractions/7 wk; (3) accelerated fractionation with split at 1.6 Gy/fraction, twice daily, 5 d/wk to 67.2 Gy/42 fractions/6 wk, including a 2-week rest after 38.4 Gy; or (4) accelerated fractionation with a concomitant boost at 1.8 Gy/fraction/d, 5 d/wk, and 1.5 Gy/fraction/d to a boost field as a second daily treatment for the last 12 treatment days to 72 Gy/42 fractions/6 wk. A total of 1,113 patients were entered in the study, with a median follow-up of 23 months.

Patients treated with both hyperfractionation and accelerated fractionation with a concomitant boost had significantly increased locoregional tumor control rates (the primary endpoint) on RTOG 90-03 compared with patients on the other two arms. All three groups treated with the altered fractionation schemes had more acute, but not late, side effects. The study concluded that hyperfractionation and accelerated fractionation with a concomitant boost were both superior to conventionally fractionated radiotherapy.

An update of this trial further demonstrated that the hyperfractionated arm showed a trend towards an overall survival benefit; the accelerated fractionation arm using the concomitant boost, showed a trend toward increased late side effects ($P = .06$).

A recent, large meta-analysis that analyzed different fractionation schedules demonstrated an 8% improvement in overall survival with hyperfractionation similar to benefit of added concurrent chemotherapy seen in the 1995 meta-analysis.

Intensity-modulated radiation therapy (IMRT)

IMRT is a more sophisticated approach for obtaining highly conformal radiation dose distributions needed to irradiate complex targets positioned near sensitive normal structures. Treatment planning for IMRT (also known as inverse planning) is extremely complex and different from that of conventional or three-dimensional radiation therapy planning. The starting point with IMRT is a description of the desired dose distribution rather than the application of traditional fields and beam modifiers to generate an acceptable plan. Conventional radiation treatment utilizes relatively uniform beams of radiation (typically between 2 and 4 beams), whereas IMRT, instead of using 4 beams of 50 cGy each, could use 50 beams of 4 cGy each. Each beam direction is divided into multiple segments to modulate the radiation dose.

The role of IMRT continues to evolve, although its use should not be considered standard for all head and neck tumors. One randomized trial in patients with early nasopharyngeal cancer showed a small improvement in salivary function. IMRT in head and neck cancer is ideal in the setting of a tumor adjacent to a critical structure (eyes, optic nerve, spinal cord, brainstem, optic chiasm, or spinal cord), which would not otherwise be treated adequately with conventional planning.

Various groups have examined dosimetric and quality-of-life differences between IMRT and conventional radiation techniques. The group at MSKCC compared its IMRT planned treatment for nasopharyngeal cancer with conventional treatment with a conformal boost. Locoregional tumor control was 97%, versus 78%, respectively, at 2 years. The University of Michigan and Washington University have reported reductions in late xerostomia with IMRT.

Proper patient selection is imperative when using IMRT. Marginal failures have been reported in the postoperative setting where there is no consensus guidelines on optimal target volume and in the setting of bulky adenopathy. The postoperative setting is difficult, because disruption of normal draining lymphatics makes the appropriate target volume much more difficult to define. Bulky adenopathy may change the typical drainage pattern and lead to the base of the skull or parotid metastases.

In addition, the RTOG-0234 group reported that IMRT in the postoperative setting increased acute side effects in high-risk patients when compared with three-dimensional conformal radiotherapy. This increase in side effects may be related to such dosimetric parameters such as "hot spots" or a greater volume of normal structures receiving low doses.

In the definition setting, all series have demonstrated improved outcomes. RTOG H-0022 was a multi-institutional study using IMRT for T1 or T2, N0 or N1 squamous cell carcinoma of the oropharynx to 66 Gy in 30 fractions. Investigators found that moderately accelerated hypofractionated IMRT without chemotherapy for early oropharyngeal cancer is feasible, achieving high tumor control rates and reduced salivary toxicity when compared with treatment of similar patients in previous RTOG studies.

Chemotherapy

Induction (neoadjuvant) chemotherapy versus concomitant chemotherapy and radiation therapy

A rationale for using induction chemotherapy for treating advanced-stage laryngeal cancer involves using chemotherapy as a marker of radiation sensitivity to select potentially radiocurable patients. In the VA Laryngeal Cancer Cooperative Study, the major benefit for two-thirds of patients in the experimental arm was laryngeal preservation. In this study, the lack of a substantial tumor response to induction chemotherapy was not associated with reduced survival. Patients who failed to respond to induction chemotherapy underwent surgery, which had the advantage of not being performed in an irradiated field. One problem with this approach is that radiation sensitivity may not be related to chemotherapy. For example, in the RTOG 91-11, 11 of 12 patients who refused laryngectomy due to lack of a response to chemotherapy were nevertheless salvaged with radiotherapy, suggesting response to induction chemotherapy may not predict radioresponsiveness.

The use of concurrent treatment (opposed to induction) using chemotherapy and irradiation is associated with an increased locoregional tumor control and survival. When used concurrently with radiotherapy, the function of chemotherapy is thought to "radiosensitize" the tissue in the radiation field. The RTOG 91-11 trial demonstrated improved locoregional tumor control as well as an increased rate of laryngeal preservation in patients with stage III and IV resectable laryngeal cancer who underwent concurrent chemoradiation therapy (for details, see discussion later in chapter). However, the rate of mucosal toxicity in those receiving concomitant chemotherapy was double that of either of the other two arms. Patients with extensive T4 primaries, such as those with cartilage invasion or those with involvement of the tongue base, were not included in the study due to poor outcomes in the VA larynx study.

Biologic agents

The toxicity of chemotherapeutic agents has prompted the development of molecular agents with potentially greater tumor specificity and diminished toxicity. In one study, 424 patients with locoregionally advanced head and neck cancer were randomly assigned to receive treatment with high-dose radiotherapy alone or with weekly cetuximab. The primary endpoint was locoregional control; secondary endpoints included overall and progression-free survival. The median duration of locoregional tumor control was 24.4 months among patients treated with cetuximab plus radiotherapy and 14.9 months among those given radiation therapy alone (HR for locoregional progression or death, 0.68; $P = .005$). With a median follow-up of 54.0 months, the median duration of overall survival was 49.0 months among patients treated with combined therapy and 29.3 months among those treated with radiation therapy alone (HR for death = 0.74; $P = .03$). Radiotherapy plus cetuximab significantly prolonged progression-free survival (HR for disease progression or death = 0.70; $P = .006$) In March 2006, cetuximab received FDA approval for use in combination with radiotherapy for patients with squamous cell cancer of the head and neck as well as for monotherapy for metastatic disease. Combined-modality treatment was not associated with any increased mucosal toxicity or long-term differences in measured quality of life. Other agents are currently being investigated.

The cooperative groups are evaluating the benefit of cetuximab and conventional chemotherapy with radiation in the locally advanced and high-risk postoperative setting, since the added effects from cetuximab are low and not overlapping.

Chemotherapy and survival

Numerous clinical trials have shown an improvement in locoregional tumor control using concurrent chemoradiation therapy, but a survival benefit has been observed less consistently. Recently published information from an updated meta-analysis of chemotherapy in head and neck cancer reports individual patient outcomes for 50 trials of concomitant chemoradiation therapy compared with irradiation alone. The pooled hazard ratio (HR) was 0.81, with a $P < .0001$ and an absolute survival benefit of 8% at 5 years for concomitant treatment. In contrast, neoadjuvant chemotherapy with cisplatin and fluorouracil (5-FU) prior to radiation did not improve survival, demonstrating the importance of timing with respect to the integration of chemotherapy in primary management.

> **At ASCO 2007, investigators presented data on excision repair cross-complementation group 1 (ERCC-1) enzyme, which appears to be related to resistance to platinum-based chemotherapy in other cancer sites in patients treated with head and neck cancer. In this study, patients who had low levels of ERCC-1 expression had four times greater odds of benefiting from an objective response to chemotherapy (*P* = .01), which corresponded to a lower risk of cancer-related death *(Mountzios G et al: J Clin Oncol 25[18S]:6011, 2007)*. A second study demonstrated a 54% ERCC-1 expression rate, which similarly translated into poor outcomes in terms of progression-free survival and overall survival *(Jun H et al: J Clin Oncol 25[18S]:6061, 2007)*.**

In the RTOG 91-11 randomized trial, chemotherapy given concurrently with irradiation, or sequentially prior to irradiation, suppressed the incidence of distant metastases and improved disease-specific survival relative to irradiation alone. However, overall survival was not different between all three arms.

Concurrent chemoradiation therapy has the greatest impact on survival in the setting of unresectable squamous cell cancer, based on a head and neck Intergroup study. In this study, 295 patients with stages III and IV head and neck cancer were randomized to participate in one of three arms: (A) radiotherapy alone to 70 Gy in 35 fractions; (B) 70 Gy in 35 fractions plus concurrent cisplatin on days 1, 22, and 43; and (C) split-course radiotherapy and 3 cycles or concurrent cisplatin/5-FU chemotherapy, with 30 Gy given with cycle 1 and 30–40 Gy given with cycle 3. Grade 3 or worse toxicity occurred in 53% of arm A patients, 86% of arm B patients, and 77% of arm C patients. The 2- and 3-year Kaplan-Meier projected survivals for arm A are 30% and 20%, compared with 43% and 37% for arm B (*P* = .016) and 40% and 27% for arm C (*P* = .13). Median survival is 12.6 months for arm A, 19.1 months for arm B, and 14.0 months for arm C. The addition of concurrent, high-dose, single-agent cisplatin to conventional radiotherapy significantly improved survival with acceptable toxicity. Additionally, concurrent multiagent chemotherapy did not offset the loss of efficacy resulting from split-course irradiation.

The impact of adjuvant concomitant chemotherapy and radiotherapy on survival was assessed in two similarly designed trials in high-risk, postoperative head and neck cancer patients that tested adjuvant chemoradiation therapy against standard postoperative radiotherapy. In the RTOG 95-01 trial, disease-free survival was significantly increased in patients treated with adjuvant chemoradiation therapy relative to those treated with radiotherapy alone, but overall survival was not affected. In the EORTC trial published at the same time as the RTOG trial, the 5-year overall survival was also significantly improved in the group receiving concomitant chemotherapy and radiotherapy.

Induction chemotherapy in combination with concomitant chemoradiation therapy

Concurrent chemoradiation therapy is the current standard of care for patients with locally advanced squamous cell carcinoma of the head and neck. Many think this paradigmatic shift has influenced patterns of failure, and distant metastasis has become more important. Several phase I/II studies have tested this approach and shown its feasibility and efficacy. In fact, now several phase III studies have demonstrated superiority (response rate and survival) of a taxane-based triplet (docetaxel [Taxotere], cisplatin, and 5-FU) as induction therapy as opposed to the historic standard induction therapy (cisplatin and 5-FU) when combined with concurrent therapy. To date, however, there have been no data suggesting that this combination is better than concurrent chemoradiation alone. Physicians who oppose this approach are concerned about the risk of tumor progression on chemotherapy (10%) and, ultimately, the 30% of patients who are not able to initiate and/or complete the definitive chemoradiation component of this treatment. If induction therapy impairs the ability to control local disease, then induction therapy will not have a positive impact on outcomes. Two studies are currently enrolling patients evaluating this question; the initial findings of one were presented at the 2010 ASCO meeting.

Adjuvant chemotherapy following surgery or irradiation

Adjuvant chemotherapy has been given following initial surgery or radiation therapy to eliminate microscopic residual disease and distant metastases. Although this approach has resulted in a reduced rate of distant metastasis, it has not been associated with improved locoregional tumor control or survival, except in a large meta-analysis. As concomitant approaches evolve and locoregional tumor control for advanced disease becomes the rule rather than the exception, the value of additional chemotherapy (as induction or adjuvant therapy) will need to be reexplored to address the problem of distant metastasis.

In September 2007, docetaxel (Taxotere) in combination with cisplatin and fluorouracil (TPF) was approved by the FDA for use as induction therapy for patients with locally advanced squamous cell cancer of the head and neck. The trial that led to this indication was a multicenter, open-label, randomized, phase III evaluation of TPF compared with cisplatin and fluorouracil for 3 cycles prior to chemoradiation with weekly carboplatin. A total of 501 patients with stages III or IV disease, deemed either unresectable or candidates for organ preservation, were randomized. Locoregional control was improved in the TPF arm (70% vs 62%). This translated into an improvement in overall survival with median survival rates of 71 vs 30 months and a HR for survival in the TPF arm of .70 (*P* = .006). Distant failure was similar in both arms and uncommon, observed in less than 10% of patients. Neutropenia and neutropenic fever were more common in the TPF group. With the addition of prophylactic antibiotics, the regimen was, however, safe and feasible *(Posner MR et al: N Engl J Med 357:1705–1715, 2007)*.

Locally advanced head and neck cancer

Data from prospective trials continue to support the use of altered fractionation and concurrent chemotherapy and irradiation as an alternative to surgery or conventionally fractionated irradiation alone for locally advanced cancers of the head and neck. The long-term results of RTOG 90-03, which randomized 1,113 patients with stages III and IV squamous cell carcinoma of the oral cavity, oropharynx, or supraglottic larynx and stages II to IV squamous cell carcinoma of the base of the tongue or hypopharynx to receive one of four different schedules of irradiation alone, revealed locoregional tumor control and disease-free survival were superior for the hyperfractionated arms and accelerated fractionation with the concomitant boost compared with the conventional fractionated radiotherapy arm.

A prospective study of 98 patients who underwent radiation for head and neck cancer did not support the use of FDG-PET/CT rather than CT imaging alone in evaluating treatment response early after the completion of radiotherapy. Overall, CT imaging is more sensitive when used during the early postradiation period However, for high-risk patients (eg, current or former smokers, those with HPV-negative and nonoropharyngeal cancers), PET/CT scans enhanced the positive predictive value when compared with CT scan alone (100% in the primary site and 75% in the cervical lymph nodes compared with 71% and 37%, respectively, for CT imaging). This suggested that early PET/CT scanning may accurately identify patients at high risk of failure who may benefit from salvage surgery *(Moeller BG et al: J Clin Oncol 27:2509–2515, 2009).*

The hyperfractionated arm demonstrated a trend toward improved overall survival.

Updated results for RTOG 99-14, a phase II prospective study designed to integrate the altered fractionated radiation regimen using concomitant boosts from RTOG 90-03 with chemotherapy, were also reported in 2005. Cisplatin was given during weeks 1, 3, and 5. Longer-term results for 76 of 84 patients were reported, and the 3-year disease-free, overall, and cause-specific survival rates were 45.8%, 57.7%, and 61.2%, respectively. The 3-year local recurrence and distant metastasis rates were 38.7% and 23.3%, respectively. Of the 35 patients who were alive, 22 had a temporary feeding tube, and 17% (6 patients) still required a feeding tube at the time of their last follow-up.

RTOG 97-03, a three-arm randomized phase II trial, evaluated the feasibility of concurrent, multi-agent chemotherapy with radiation therapy. In this study, three different regimens of chemotherapy were used with irradiation (70 Gy/35 fractions) for oral cavity, oropharyngeal, and hypopharyngeal cancers. Arm 1 received cisplatin (10 mg/m^2) and 5-FU (400 mg/m^2) via continuous infusion daily for the final 10 days of radiotherapy. Treatment on arm 2 consisted of hydroxyurea (1 g/d) and 5-FU (800 mg/m^2) via continuous infusion delivered concurrently with radiation therapy. Arm 3 received paclitaxel (30 mg/m^2) and cisplatin (20 mg/m^2) weekly. The incidence of acute toxicity was high, with the lowest incidence of persistent feeding tube dependence in arm 3. Arm 2 was associated with a slightly higher rate of grade 4 toxicity and treatment interruption. All arms demonstrated improved survival relative to historic controls treated with radiation therapy alone.

To diminish toxicity in locally advanced oropharyngeal and laryngeal cancers, a phase II trial using taxane-based induction followed by concurrent chemoradiation therapy was conducted through the ECOG E2399 group. A total of 111 patients (T2, N+ or T3–4N0–3) underwent induction therapy with 2 cycles of paclitaxel (175 mg/m^2) and carboplatin followed by concurrent weekly paclitaxel (30 mg/m^2) and 70 Gy of radiotherapy. Patients with progressive or stable disease at the primary site after induction therapy underwent surgery. Patients with primary laryngeal cancers fared significantly worse using this regimen. Patients with laryngeal cancer had a lower rate of major response to induction chemotherapy, a lower 2-year progression-free survival, and a trend toward higher distant failure than did those with primary oropharyngeal cancer. The 2-year progression-free survival was 50% for patients with laryngeal cancer, as compared with 75% for those with oropharyngeal cancer (P = .05). The indications for induction chemotherapy remain poorly defined.

Determination of tumor response after chemoradiation

For patients with persistent disease after radiation, prompt diagnosis and treatment may improve survival. However, the sensitivity of the physical examination is poor as a result of the presence of submucosal disease and inflammatory changes in the upper aerodigestive tract from radiation. The best method for assessing tumor response to radiation remains under investigation. The sensitivity of CT imaging in the early postradiotherapy period (ie, within 10 weeks of the completion of radiation) is 80% for the primary site and 87% for the regional lymphatics. This modality, however, lacks specificity. FDG-PET/CT imaging has been shown to improve the positive predictive value of CT scans in determining response to radiation.

Chemotherapy for recurrent or metastatic disease

The combination of cisplatin/5-FU produces overall response rates of approximately 30% and survival rates of 6 months. In randomized trials comparing this combination with single-agent cisplatin, 5-FU, or methotrexate, response rates with the single agents are lower, but survival is equivalent. However, because many practitioners believe response is a surrogate for palliation, cisplatin/5-FU has been used widely in this setting.

The taxanes are the most active cytotoxins yet identified in head and neck cancer, with overall response rates of approximately 35% in patients with recurrent or incurable disease. In one randomized trial, the combination of paclitaxel/cisplatin was compared with cisplatin/5-FU in patients with recurrent disease. A total of 194 patients who were therapy-naive for recurrent disease with an ECOG performance status of 0–1 were randomized. Efficacy outcomes were similar in the two arms, with median survival rates of 8 and 9 months for arms 1 and 2, respectively. Paclitaxel/cisplatin was less toxic and more convenient, representing an effective and safe alternative to the traditional 5-FU–containing regimen.

Based on nearly universal expression of EGFR in squamous cell cancer of the head and neck, EGFR-targeted agents have been evaluated in patients with recurrent disease. Although the single agent response rates of the monoclonal antibody cetuximab and the tyrosine kinase inhibitors erlotinib (Tarceva) and gefitinib (Iressa) in this setting are only in the range of 5% to 15%, their use in combination with chemotherapy, particularly cetuximab, holds more promise. Results of the EXTREME trial, which accrued 442 patients with recurrent or metastatic squamous cell cancer of the head and neck, showed that when compared with platinum-based chemotherapy alone, the combination with cetuximab improved median (7.4 months vs 10.1 months) and 1-year (31% vs 39%) survival rates, with a HR of 0.8 ($P = .036$). Similar promising, albeit preliminary, results have been reported from phase II, single-arm studies of cetuximab/paclitaxel and erlotinib/docetaxel/cisplatin. Overall, these observations lend impetus to further investigation of EGFR-targeted therapy in combination with neoadjuvant chemotherapy and with chemoradiation therapy in patients with curable disease. Many such trials are ongoing.

Photodynamic therapy

Photodynamic therapy may have some promise in the treatment of mucosal dysplasia and small head and neck tumors.

Small studies of photodynamic therapy, performed at several institutions, suggest that widespread areas of carcinoma in situ or severe dysplasia, as well as cancer, are often extirpated after photodynamic therapy. Some patients have experienced durable remissions, but the long-term efficacy of this modality remains uncertain.

Pulsed dye laser therapy for early laryngeal lesions

The pulsed dye laser initially used to treat vascular lesions has recently been investigated in the treatment of respiratory papillomatosis, dysplastic cancers, and early invasive glottic carcinomas. The efficacy of the laser is mediated through its antiangiogenic properties. The nontoxic treatment preserves the laryngeal microarchitecture, and preserves or restores near-normal vocal quality. Additionally, this modality can be utilized in an outpatient clinic setting. Preliminary findings are favorable. At this time, however, pulsed dye laser therapy should be considered investigational.

Chemoprevention

The area of chemoprevention has received a great deal of attention in recent years, and the concept of field cancerization is important in this context. As mentioned previously, this concept refers to the diffuse epithelial injury incurred by upper aerodigestive tract mucosa due to chronic exposure to carcinogens (most commonly, alcohol and tobacco). These mucosal changes increase the risk of developing premalignant lesions (leukoplakia and erythroplakia), as well as multiple primary lesions.

Retinoids (vitamin A analogues) have been investigated as chemopreventive agents in the aerodigestive tract based on their efficacy in tumor models, such as the hamster buccal pouch. Retinoids mediate changes in gene expression through interaction with nuclear retinoic acid receptors, which function as transcription factors. Nutritional epidemiology studies also have indicated that low serum levels of both carotenoids and retinoids contribute to the risk of cancer development in the epithelium of the upper aerodigestive tract.

The role of retinoids in the prevention of second primary tumors in patients treated with curative intent for an early-stage index squamous cell cancer of the head and neck has been investigated in three randomized trials. The initial study was a small, single-center, phase III trial of *cis*-retinoic acid (1–2 mg/kg/d) by Hong et al. Although this study demonstrated decreased second primary tumors in the experimental arm, compliance and morbidity with this high dose were problematic. A second study using a low dose of *cis*-retinoic acid (10 mg/d) was performed by ECOG and was negative. Results from a third large, multicenter trial with an intermediate dose of 30 mg/d have been reported in abstract form and are also negative in regard to second primary prevention.

Rehabilitation

Rehabilitation also is very important in the care of patients with head and neck cancer. It includes physical and occupational therapy, speech and swallowing rehabilitation, and nutritional support. For example, resection of the spinal accessory nerve, which innervates the trapezius muscle, leads to scapular winging, an inability to abduct the arm fully, and, eventually, severe pain around the shoulder. These symptoms may be ameliorated with appropriate physical therapy.

Adapting to the loss of the larynx also requires intensive rehabilitation and patient motivation. Voice rehabilitation options include esophageal speech, artificial larynges (portable, battery-operated devices), and tracheoesophageal shunts.

Patients who undergo nonsurgical treatment also benefit from early swallowing rehabilitation. Intensive chemoradiation protocols are associated with prolonged feeding tube dependence in 20% of patients. Early swallowing therapy improves treatment-related dysphagia.

Nutritional support is facilitated by temporary nasoduodenal tubes or gastrostomy tubes (which impose added morbidity but are more socially acceptable and ease the patient's transition to normal activities).

Management of symptoms and treatment side effects

Photodynamic therapy

At the time of diagnosis, many patients with head and neck cancer will have lost a significant amount of weight. Maintaining adequate nutrition is a major problem for these patients, as both the tumor and treatment side effects, such as mucositis from chemotherapy and radiation therapy, may be contributory. For patients who are unable to eat or who are being treated with aggressive concomitant chemotherapy and radiation therapy protocols, placement of a gastrostomy tube is often necessary to maintain caloric intake and adequate hydration.

Pain

Clinicians must also be aware of the significant pain associated with these lesions and use narcotic analgesics appropriately to relieve discomfort.

Mucositis

The use of chemotherapy concomitantly with radiation therapy increases the occurrence of mucositis.

Nephrotoxicity and ototoxicity

For patients treated with cisplatin-containing regimens, renal insufficiency and ototoxicity are potential serious side effects.

Xerostomia

Following radiation therapy of a head and neck cancer, xerostomia may be a significant long-term side effect. In some patients, pilocarpine has been useful in stimulating the production of saliva.

The use of organic thiophosphates, such as amifostine (Ethyol), in patients undergoing radiotherapy for head and neck cancer reduces the severity of late xerostomia without compromising the antitumor activity of the irradiation.

TABLE 2: Types of neck dissection and structures removed in the treatment of head and neck cancer

Type of neck dissection	Structures removed
Comprehensive neck dissection	
"Classic" radical neck dissection	All lymph-bearing tissue (levels I-V), spinal accessory nerve (cranial nerve [CN] XI), sternocleidomastoid muscle, and internal jugular vein
Modified radical neck dissection	Neck dissection with sparing of one or more of the above structures
Type I	CN XI spared
Type II	CN XI and internal jugular vein spared
Type III (functional neck dissection)	All three structures spared (CN XI, internal jugular vein, and sternocleidomastoid muscle)
Selective neck dissection	Removal of lymph-bearing tissue from:
Lateral	Levels II-IV
Posterolateral	Levels II-V
Supraomohyoid	Levels I-III

From Medina JE, Rebual NM: Neck dissection, in Cummings CW, Fredrickson J, Harker LE, et al (eds): Otolaryngology: Head and Neck Surgery, pp 1649–1672. St. Louis, Mosby Yearbook, 1993.

Gastroesophageal reflux disease (GERD)

Often asymptomatic or "silent," GERD is a common finding in patients treated for pharyngolaryngeal squamous cell carcinoma. In addition, cisplatin-containing chemotherapy may aggravate GERD.

Treatment of the neck

Either irradiation alone or radical neck dissection will control metastatic squamous cell cancer to a single small neck node more than 90% of the time if there is no extracapsular tumor spread. Hence, radiation treatment may easily provide prophylactic treatment of the neck if control of the primary tumor is undertaken with irradiation. Traditionally, if the tumor in the neck was N2 or greater, or if there was tumor beyond the confines of a node, neck dissection and irradiation were combined for optimal control of the neck tumor. The need for neck dissection in patients clinically staged N2–N3 with a complete clinical and radiographic response following radiation therapy remains under investigation.

Types of dissection

There are several approaches to the surgical treatment of the neck nodes in patients with head and neck cancer (Table 2). This discussion will be limited to two types of neck dissection: comprehensive and selective.

Comprehensive neck dissection entails complete removal of all lymphatic tissue from the neck (levels I–V). A radical neck dissection includes comprehensive node dissection with removal of the sternocleidomastoid muscle, jugular vein, and spinal accessory nerve. Modified radical neck dissection was developed to diminish the morbidity of the classic operation. The most important structure to preserve is the spinal accessory nerve.

Selective neck dissection consists of the removal of lymph node groups at highest risk of containing metastases from a primary cancer. In such procedures, the lymph nodes removed correspond to the most significant drainage basins of specific head and neck tumor sites. These are staging operations usually performed in patients with clinically N0 neck cancer. If metastases are identified, further treatment to the neck will be required. A selective neck dissection should not be employed as the sole treatment of clinically palpable disease.

Sentinel lymph node biopsy for oral cavity lesions has been evaluated. Forty patients with clinically N0 neck cancer underwent sentinel lymph node biopsy followed by complete neck dissection. A sentinel node was identified in 90% of necks, with a 97% accuracy rate in predicting the nodal status of the remainder of the neck. This finding corresponded to a sensitivity of 94% and a specificity of 100%. Although these results are encouraging, they need to be validated in a larger trial. The completed ACOSOG study (Z0360) examined this technique in patients with T1 or T2, N0 oral cavity cancer. The final conclusions are pending, but sentinel lymph node biopsy may prove useful in small lesions without deep penetration, but it remains investigational.

FOLLOW-UP OF LONG-TERM SURVIVORS

As mentioned, head and neck cancers are aggressive tumors. The majority (80%) of recurrences will develop within 2 years. Since many recurrences are treatable with curative intent, patients should be followed closely during the months following their treatment. This period coincides with the time of greatest need from the standpoint of rehabilitation.

After 2 years, second primary tumors of the head and neck and lungs become important causes of death and morbidity. Late complications of treatment, such as radionecrosis, radiation-induced fibrosis, hypothyroidism, and sequelae of spinal accessory nerve sacrifice or injury, may develop even after years. Complications and second primary cancers are more common in patients who continue to smoke.

Timing of follow-up evaluations

Follow-up evaluations at regular intervals should be complete and should include a focused history and examination, as outlined previously. Physicians who are able to perform a head and neck examination (including laryngoscopy) should direct follow-up. After surgical treatment, this evaluation will usually require visits with the head and neck surgeon. Patients treated with irradiation should be followed by both their radiation oncologist and a head and neck surgeon or otolaryngologist.

Evaluations should be scheduled every 1 to 2 months during the first year after treatment, every 2 to 4 months during the second year, every 3 to 6 months during the third year, and every 6 months thereafter for several more years.

TABLE 3: TNM staging system for cancers of the lips and oral cavity

Primary tumor (T)	
TX	Primary tumor cannot be assessed
T0	No evidence of primary tumor
Tis	Carcinoma in situ
T1	Tumor ≤ 2 cm in greatest dimension
T2	Tumor > 2 cm but ≤ 4 cm in greatest dimension
T3	Tumor > 4 cm in greatest dimension
T4	(lip) Tumor invades through cortical bone, inferior alveolar nerve, floor of mouth, or skin of face, ie, chin or nose[a]
T4a	Moderately advanced local disease[a] (lip) Tumor invades through the cortical bone, mouth, or skin of the face (ie, chin or nose) (oral cavity) Tumor invades adjacent structures (eg, through cortical bone [mandible or maxilla] into the deep [extrinsic] muscle of the tongue [genioglossus, hyoglossus, palatoglossus, and styloglossus], maxillary sinus, or skin of the face)
T4b	Very advanced local disease Tumor involves masticator space, pterygoid plates, or skull base and/or encases internal carotid artery
Regional lymph nodes (N)	
NX	Regional nodes cannot be assessed
N0	No regional lymph node metastasis
N1	Metastasis in a single ipsilateral lymph node, ≤ 3 cm in greatest dimension
N2	Metastasis in a single ipsilateral lymph node, > 3 cm ≤ 6 cm in greatest dimension; or in multiple ipsilateral lymph nodes, none > 6 cm in greatest dimension; or in bilateral or contralateral lymph nodes, none > 6 cm in greatest dimension
N2a	Metastasis in a single ipsilateral lymph node, > 3 cm but ≤ 6 cm in greatest dimension
N2b	Metastasis in multiple ipsilateral lymph nodes, none > 6 cm in greatest dimension
N2c	Metastasis in bilateral or contralateral lymph nodes, none > 6 cm in greatest dimension
N3	Metastasis in a lymph node, > 6 cm in greatest dimension

[a] Superficial erosion alone of bone/tooth socket by gingival primary is not sufficient to classify a tumor as T4.

continued

Imaging and laboratory studies

Any mucosal abnormality should be biopsied. There are no tumor markers or other useful laboratory studies to follow. Chest x-rays should be obtained yearly. There is little justification for performing CT scans or MRI in the follow-up of asymptomatic patients. Thyroid-stimulating hormone (TSH) should be measured yearly in patients who have received irradiation to the larynx or nasopharynx.

HEAD AND NECK TUMOR REGIONS

As mentioned previously, tumors occurring at different anatomic sites and subsites of the head and neck vary considerably with regard to epidemiology, risk factors, anatomy, natural history, staging of the primary tumor, and therapy. The following sections highlight these differences.

ORAL CAVITY

Sites of the oral cavity include the lips, hard palate, floor of the mouth, buccal mucosa, and tongue. Cancers at these sites comprise < 5% of all malignancies in the United States.

TABLE 3: TNM staging system for cancers of the lips and oral cavity *(continued)*

Distant metastases (M)

M0	No distant metastasis
M1	Distant metastasis

Stage grouping

Stage 0	Tis	N0	M0
Stage I	T1	N0	M0
Stage II	T2	N0	M0
Stage III	T3	N0	M0
	T1	N1	M0
	T2	N1	M0
	T3	N1	M0
Stage IVA	T4a	N0	M0
	T4a	N1	M0
	T1	N2	M0
	T2	N2	M0
	T3	N2	M0
	T4a	N2	M0
Stage IVB	Any T	N3	M0
	T4b	Any N	M0
Stage IVC	Any T	Any N	M1

From Edge SP, Byrd DR, Compton CC, et al (eds): AJCC Cancer Staging Manual, 7th ed. New York, Springer, 2010.

Anatomy

The oral cavity extends from the cutaneous vermilion junction of the lips to the junction of the hard and soft palates above and to the line of the circumvallate papillae below. It includes the lips, buccal mucosa, upper and lower alveolar ridges, retromolar trigone, floor of the mouth, hard palate, and anterior two-thirds of the tongue (the "oral" tongue). The primary lymphatic drainage is to the submental triangle, submandibular nodes, and upper deep jugular nodes.

Natural history

The most common presenting complaint is a sore in the mouth or on the lips. One-third of patients present with a neck mass.

The differential diagnosis includes other malignancies and benign diseases or lesions. Other malignancies to be considered include salivary gland tumors, sarcoma, lymphoma, and melanoma. Benign diseases include pyogenic granuloma, tuberculous disease, aphthous ulcers, and chancres.

Benign mucosal lesions include papillomas and keratoacanthomas, which may be exophytic or infiltrative. The exophytic lesions are less aggressive. The infiltrative papillomas and keratoacanthomas are more often associated with destruction of surrounding tissues and structures. These lesions may progress to malignancy. The TNM staging system for cancers of the lips and oral cavity is outlined in Table 3. T4 lesions have been divided into T4a (resectable) and T4b (unresectable) in the seventh edition of the *AJCC Cancer Staging Manual.*

Treatment

Management of cancers of the oral cavity involves surgery or radiotherapy for T1 or T2 lesions or combined-modality treatment that includes surgical resection and postoperative radiation therapy (60–70 Gy in 6–7 weeks) for advanced disease. For early-stage disease, surgery and radiotherapy are considered to have equivalent efficacy, although surgery is associated with less morbidity. Supraomohyoid neck dissection is performed in surgically treated patients with N0 necks. Bilateral neck dissection is performed if the tumor approaches the midline. Neck dissection is recommended for tumor thickness that is at least 4 mm, although some investigators believe that 2 to 3 mm should be the cutoff.

The lips

The lips are the most common site of oral cavity cancer. There are approximately 4,000 new cases per year in the United States. The lower lip is affected most often. The vast majority of patients (90%) with lip cancer are men, and 33% have outdoor occupations.

Natural history

The most frequent presentation is a slow-growing tumor of the lower lip that may bleed and hurt. Physical examination must include assessment of hypoesthesia in the distribution of the mental nerve (cutaneous sensation of the chin area). Currently, fewer than 10% of American patients with squamous cell carcinoma of the lower lip have cervical metastases.

Treatment

The primary tumor Patients with early-stage lip cancers are usually treated with surgery. Radiation therapy may be utilized in patients who are medically unsuited for surgery or who refuse surgical resection.

Resection involves excision with at least 0.5 cm of normal tissue circumferentially beyond the recognized border of the tumor. After the resection of larger lesions, reconstruction may pose a major challenge. Small tumors are excised with a V incision.

Patients with advanced disease (stage III or IV) are usually managed with a combination of surgery and postoperative radiation therapy.

The neck Elective treatment of the neck is seldom recommended for patients with squamous cell carcinoma of the lower lip and a clinically negative neck because few of these patients have cervical metastases. Neck dissection is recommended only in patients with palpable cervical metastases. Neck dissection is followed by postoperative radiation therapy.

Results The cure rate for T1–T3 tumors is 90% with surgical excision alone. Smaller lesions (T1–T2) may be treated equally well with radiation therapy. Survival rates for patients with T1 and T2 lesions are 90% and 80%, respectively. Overall, younger patients have a poorer prognosis, as do those with involvement of the mandible and extension of the tumor within the oral cavity.

The tongue

The oral tongue (anterior two-thirds) is the site of 75% of all tongue cancers. In 2009, approximately 10,530 men and women (7,470 men and 3,060 women) will be diagnosed with cancer of the tongue, and 1,910 will succumb to the disease.

Natural history

The most common presenting symptom in patients with cancer of the tongue is a persistent, nonhealing ulcer with or without associated pain. Other symptoms include difficulty with deglutition and speech. There may be a history of leukoplakia, especially in younger women.

Rate of growth Cancer of the tongue seems to grow more rapidly than other oral cavity cancers. Tongue cancers may grow in an infiltrative or exophytic fashion. The infiltrative tumors may be quite large at presentation.

Lesion thickness Thicker lesions have a worse prognosis than thin cancers, and lesion thickness is a more important prognostic factor than is simple tumor stage. The incidence of clinically occult cervical metastases to the neck is significantly higher when the tumor thickness exceeds 4 mm.

Cervical metastases occur more frequently from tongue cancer than from any other tumor of the oral cavity. At initial evaluation, 40% of patients have node metastases.

Treatment

Early-stage disease Treatment usually entails partial glossectomy. Margins should be assessed at the time of resection, as the disease spreads along muscle bundles, leading to more extensive tumor than is appreciated grossly.

Radiation therapy using external-beam radiation or an interstitial implant is a suitable option for small or minimally infiltrating tumors. In general, morbidity appears to be less with surgery. Small cancers are resected without reconstruction. Following larger resections, reconstruction with a skin graft or with free tissue transfer produces good function.

Large, infiltrative lesions should be treated with combined-modality therapy (radiation therapy and surgical resection).

Advanced disease More advanced tumors with mandibular involvement require composite resection, including a partial glossectomy, mouth floor resection, and mandibulectomy.

The neck A selective neck dissection is often recommended for clinically N0 neck cancer. Comprehensive neck dissection is required in the presence of palpable cervical metastases.

Results Control of disease closely correlates with the extent of the primary tumor and the presence of metastases. Rates of local tumor control using radiation therapy or surgery are similar for T1 (~85%) and T2 (~80%) tumors. T3 tumors should be treated using surgery and radiation therapy. Only 10% to 15% of local recurrences are amenable to repeated resection.

Overall survival is approximately 50%. Rates of survival at 5 years by stage follow: stage I, 80%; stage II, 60%; and stages III and IV, 15% to 35%. For equivalent primary cancers, the presence of lymph node metastases decreases the survival rate by 50%.

The floor of the mouth

There are approximately 4,000 cases of floor of the mouth cancer in the United States annually. Mouth floor cancer accounts for 10% of head and neck cancer.

Pathology

Most lesions are moderately differentiated to well-differentiated squamous cell cancers and are exophytic.

Natural history

Patients usually present with a painful mass located near the oral tongue. Because these lesions do not cause pain until they are deep, they are frequently advanced at presentation.

Extension of disease into the soft tissues of the submandibular triangle is not uncommon. Fixation of the tumor to bone suggests possible mandibular involvement, which may be evaluated further with CT imaging. Changes in the mental foramen can be distinct or demonstrate slight asymmetry when compared with the contralateral anatomy. Restricted tongue mobility reflects invasion into the root of the tongue. Palpation demonstrates the depth of infiltration much better than does inspection alone.

Tumors near the midline may obstruct the duct of the submandibular gland, leading to swelling and induration in the neck, which may be difficult to distinguish from lymph node metastases. Level I nodes are the first-echelon metastatic sites.

Multifocality Multifocal cancers are more common in the floor of the mouth than in other oral cavity sites. Approximately 20% of patients with mouth floor tumors have a second primary tumor, half of which are in the head and neck.

Treatment

Early invasive lesions (T1–T2) involving the mucosa alone may be treated with either surgery or irradiation alone with comparable results. Primary tumors with mandibular involvement should be surgically resected.

Cancer invades the mandible through tooth sockets. Hence, if the tumor merely abuts the mandible, a marginal mandibulectomy (which removes the bone margin but preserves continuity) may be performed. Otherwise, a segmental resection is needed. Selective neck dissection for treatment planning is advisable for thick stage I or II cancers.

Advanced disease The treatment of choice for advanced disease is combined-modality therapy with surgery and radiation therapy. Complete surgical resection may require a composite resection of the mandible, including a partial glossectomy and neck dissection for advanced primary cancers. Lesions near the midline with a clinically positive lymph node require ipsilateral comprehensive neck dissection with a contralateral selective (supraomohyoid) neck dissection.

Results Overall, ~40% of patients are cured of their disease; 80% of recurrences appear within the first 2 years. Survival rates at 5 years by stage follow: stage I, 85%; stage II, 75%; stage III, 66%; and stage IV, 30%. Signs of poor prognosis include involvement of both the tongue and mandible and extension of the tumor beyond the oral cavity.

OROPHARYNX

Carcinoma of the oropharynx affects 4,000 patients in the United States annually. The incidence of oropharyngeal cancer is increasing.

Anatomy and pathology

The opening to the oropharynx is a ring bounded by the anterior tonsillar pillars (faucial arch), extending upward to blend with the uvula and inferiorly across the base of the tongue (behind the circumvallate papillae). The walls of the oropharynx are formed by the pharyngeal constrictor muscles, which overlie the cervical spine posteriorly. The superior boundary is the soft palate, which separates the oropharynx from the nasopharynx.

Subsites of the oropharynx include the base of the tongue, soft palate, tonsillar area, and posterior pharyngeal wall. The extent of a primary tumor may be difficult to assess due to its location.

The jugulodigastric nodes (levels II and III) constitute the first echelon of lymphatic drainage. Metastases may also appear in the parapharyngeal and retropharyngeal nodes and may be detected only through imaging studies.

Premalignant lesions occur in the oropharynx but are less common than in the oral cavity.

Improved prognosis for HPV-associated squamous cancer of the head and neck has been suggested by multiple, single-institution, retrospective analyses. In ECOG 2399, a phase II trial, patients with locally advanced oropharyngeal and laryngeal cancers were treated with neoadjuvant paclitaxel and carboplatin followed by radiation with weekly paclitaxel. These data indicated that 40% of evaluable cases were positive for HPV. Patients who were HPV-positive had a higher response rate to both neoadjuvant chemotherapy and chemoradiation and had improved survival. For patients with HPV-positive tumors, HRs for progression and death were 0.27 and 0.36, respectively. These preliminary prospective data strongly confirmed previous retrospective analyses identifying HPV association as a favorable prognostic indicator, especially for oropharyngeal primary tumors *(Fakhry C et al: J Natl Cancer Inst 100:261–269, 2008).*

Treatment

Radiation therapy

External-beam radiation therapy (65–70 Gy over 7 weeks) and interstitial irradiation have been used in the curative treatment of oropharyngeal carcinomas for over 70 years. Radiation therapy represents a reasonable alternative to surgery and may also be required following radical resection of tumors with poor pathologic features to reduce the likelihood of local recurrence.

Altered fractionation schedules (accelerated and/or hyperfractionated) have gained interest in the past several decades based on both theoretical grounds and the results of mainly retrospective data. One prospective, randomized trial in patients with oropharyngeal cancer (excluding base of the tongue cancer) documented a 20% increase in locoregional tumor control and a 14% survival benefit at 5 years in patients who received 8,160 cGy at 120 bid in a hyperfractionated schedule, as opposed to 7,000 cGy in a conventionally fractionated schedule, specifically for intermediate-risk patients with T2 or T3 N0 or N1 squamous cell carcinomas. This improvement in outcome was not offset by any significant increase in acute or late tissue toxicity.

Local tumor control rates with radiation therapy alone for all primary sites (including the tonsils, soft palate, base of the tongue, and posterior oropharyngeal wall) follow: T1, 90%; T2, 80%; T3, 65%; and T4, 55%. Cancers of the tonsillar fossa are better controlled with irradiation than are cancers arising in other subsites of the oropharynx; this phenomenon may be related to tumors linked to HPV.

Chemoradiation therapy

A number of studies supporting the use of multimodality therapy with radiation therapy and chemotherapy as an alternative to surgery with postoperative irradiation or irradiation alone have been published. In an Intergroup trial by Adelstein et al, cisplatin (100 mg/m^2) given every 3 weeks with standard irradiation was found to be safe and effective. Induction therapy followed by concurrent chemoradiation regimens has the potential for diminishing distant failure while maintaining the local tumor control achieved via concurrent regimens. Such regimens are currently under active investigation.

Surgery

Surgical extirpation of relatively inaccessible tumors in the oropharynx traditionally required radical surgery, including mandibulotomy or mandibulectomy, and, occasionally laryngectomy. These surgical procedures were associated with worse functional outcomes relative to nonsurgical approaches. Radical surgery, however, has been supplanted by minimally invasive approaches. Using bivalved laryngoscopes for tumor exposure, surgical resection using the carbon dioxide laser coupled to a microscope has led to complete pathologic resections and high local control rates for oropharyngeal cancer. The reported functional results have been good, with few patients requiring placement of a feeding tube or tracheotomies.

The use of the line-of-sight carbon dioxide (CO_2) laser beam has been limited by inadequate exposure of the pathologic lesion in patients with short or stiff necks, retrognathia, full dentition, trismus, or obesity. Limited access to pathology has precluded use of transoral CO_2 laser surgery in many patients. A flexible, photonic, band-gap fiber for the delivery of CO_2 laser energy that was developed by OmniGuide Inc, allows video-assisted visualization and extirpation of previously poorly accessible pathology. Limited access has also been surmounted by the adaptation of the surgical robot for transoral applications. The daVinci Surgical System (Intuitive Surgical; Sunnyvale, CA), originally designed as a three-armed robotic device controlling "wristed" surgical microinstruments and angled telescopes, has now been FDA–approved for a variety of general, cardiac, gynecologic, and urologic procedures.

Improved surgical exposure to tumors in the upper aerodigestive tract have been reported relative to those obtained with more traditional transoral approaches. In 2009, transoral robotic surgery received FDA approval for T1 and T2 lesions. Minimally invasive surgery is safe and effective for early-stage disease (stages I and II), but its role in treating advanced-stage disease has yet to be defined.

The base of the tongue

Cancer of the base of the tongue is far less common than that of the oral tongue, but its incidence is increasing.

Anatomy

The base of the tongue is bordered anteriorly by the circumvallate papillae and posteriorly by the epiglottis. There is a rich lymphatic network, with metastases frequently seen in levels II to V.

Natural history

The base of the tongue is notorious for lesions that infiltrate deeply into muscle and are advanced at diagnosis. This finding is probably due to the relatively asymptomatic anatomic location. Thus, bimanual oral examination with digital palpation is a critical part of the physical examination.

Most patients present with pain and dysphagia. Other symptoms include a neck mass, weight loss, otalgia, and trismus.

All oropharyngeal cancers have a strong propensity to spread to the lymph nodes, and tumors arising at the base of the tongue are no exception. Approximately 70% of patients with T1 primary base of the tongue tumors have clinically palpable disease in the neck, and 20% to 30% have palpable, bilateral lymph node metastases. The risk of nodal metastases increases with increasing T stage and approaches 85% for T4 lesions.

Treatment

Early-stage disease Stage I or II cancers may be treated equally effectively with either surgical resection or radiation therapy alone. If irradiation of the primary tumor is employed, both sides of the neck should be treated, even if the nodes do not seem to be involved. Surgical management of an oropharyngeal malignancy includes lymphadenectomy. For patients clinically staged N0, selective neck dissection encompassing levels II–IV is sufficient. For patients with cancers at the base of the tongue, bilateral neck dissection is required.

Advanced disease More advanced disease may require total resection of the tongue base with or without laryngectomy to ensure complete removal of disease. Total resection of the tongue base is associated with severe oropharyngeal dysphagia with aspiration, but even subtotal resection of the base of the tongue may result in significant aspiration, which is exacerbated by postoperative radiotherapy. Total laryngectomy may be the only way to isolate the airway from oral secretions and eliminate the risk of aspiration. Chemoradiation therapy via external-beam irradiation or irradiation alone combined with an implant can be curative for patients with advanced tumors of the tongue base.

Results In general, the prognosis of cancers of the tongue base is poor due to their advanced stage at presentation. The extent of nodal disease predicts survival. For T1 and T2 cancers, local tumor control rates approach 85%. The major determinant of treatment failure is the tumor's growth pattern, with a high local tumor control rate for exophytic lesions and a far worse rate for infiltrative tumors.

Tonsils and tonsillar pillar

The tonsils and tonsillar pillar are the most common locations for tumors of the oropharynx.

Natural history

Tonsillar fossa tumors tend to be more advanced and more frequently metastasize to the neck than do tonsillar pillar cancers. At presentation, 55% of patients with fossa tumors have N2 or N3 disease, and contralateral metastases are common. Symptoms include pain, dysphagia, weight loss, a mass in the neck, and trismus.

Treatment

Single-modality therapy (irradiation or surgery alone) is acceptable for T1 and T2 tumors. Irradiation alone may be curative for more advanced tumors, although chemotherapy is often added in a concurrent fashion for T3 or T4 disease or in the setting of N2 or N3 disease. The neck should always be included in treatment planning. More advanced disease usually requires surgery combined with irradiation. Well lateralized cancers of the tonsillar fossa (minimal to no involvement of the soft palate or base of the tongue) may be treated with unilateral irradiation, since contralateral neck failure is rare (< 10%).

HYPOPHARYNX

Hypopharyngeal cancers are approximately one-third as common as laryngeal cancers.

Anatomy

The hypopharynx (or laryngopharynx) is the entrance to the esophagus. The superior aspect (above the plane of the hyoid bone) communicates with the oropharynx, and the inferior border is situated in the plane of the lowest part of the cricoid cartilage (the esophageal inlet). The anterior surface (postcricoid area) is contiguous with the posterior surface of the larynx, adjacent to the lamina of the cricoid cartilage. The pharyngeal musculature forms the lateral and posterior walls. The piriform sinuses are within the hypopharynx on each side of the larynx.

The hypopharynx contains three subsites: the paired piriform sinuses (lateral, pear-shaped funnels); the posterior pharyngeal wall, from the level of the vallecula to the level of the cricoarytenoid joints; and the postcricoid area (pharyngoesophageal junction), which begins just below the arytenoids and extends to the inferior border of the cricoid cartilage. The piriform sinuses are composed of a medial wall, which abuts the aryepiglottic fold, and a lateral wall. Seventy percent of hypopharyngeal cancers occur in the piriform sinuses.

Natural history

Hypopharyngeal tumors produce few symptoms until they are advanced (> 70% are stage III or IV at presentation). They may cause a sore throat, otalgia, a change in voice, odynophagia, or an isolated neck mass. Subtle changes on physical examination, including pooling of secretions, should be regarded with concern.

Nodal metastases

Diffuse local spread is common and is due to tumor extension within the submucosa. Abundant lymphatic drainage results in a higher incidence of lymph node metastases than with other head and neck tumors. At presentation, 70% to 80% of patients with hypopharyngeal tumors have palpable cervical lymph node metastases; in half of these patients, palpable cervical nodes are the presenting complaint. Levels II and III are most commonly involved. Bilateral metastases are seen in only 10% of patients with piriform sinus cancers but in 60% of those with postcricoid tumors.

Synchronous lesions

These are common. Overall, 20% to 25% of patients with hypopharyngeal cancer develop a second primary tumor within 5 years, usually in the head and neck.

Chemotherapy and external-beam radiotherapy

Similar in design to the VA Cooperative Laryngeal Cancer Study, a randomized EORTC trial has shown that initial therapy with cisplatin and 5-FU, followed by definitive irradiation in patients with complete remissions (or, alternatively, surgical salvage), results in at least equivalent survival relative to immediate pharyngolaryngectomy. Of patients treated with initial chemotherapy, 28% retained a functional larynx at 3 years (approximately two-thirds of survivors).

Though directed to laryngeal cancers (rather than hypopharyngeal cancers), the RTOG 91-11 trial results have been widely interpreted as applying to hypopharyngeal cancer, increasing enthusiasm for concomitant chemoradiation therapy for patients with advanced cancers of the hypopharynx.

Transoral laser surgery for piriform sinus carcinoma

Organ-sparing approaches such as transoral laser microsurgery for piriform sinus carcinomas have been used in several institutions for the past 25 years. Long-term follow-up in a retrospective review of 129 previously untreated patients has been published (Steiner et al). In this series, which included mostly advanced-stage disease, the reported 5-year local control rate was 82% for patients with stages I and II cancers and 69% for those with stages III and IV cancers. Radiation therapy was administered after surgery. Laryngeal preservation rates were comparable to the local tumor control rates. The 2-year overall survival rates were 91% for patients with stages I and II cancer and 75% for patients with stages III and IV cancer. These oncologic and functional results compare favorably with those obtained with either nonsurgical or surgical approaches requiring opening the neck and pharynx.

TABLE 4: TNM staging system for cancers of the larynx

Primary tumor (T)

TX	Primary tumor cannot be assessed
T0	No evidence of primary tumor
Tis	Carcinoma in situ
Supraglottis	
T1	Tumor limited to one subsite of the supraglottis with normal vocal cord mobility
T2	Tumor invades mucosa of more than one adjacent subsite of the supraglottis or glottis or region outside the supraglottis (eg, mucosa of base of the tongue, vallecula, medial wall of piriform sinus) without fixation of the larynx
T3	Tumor limited to the larynx with vocal cord fixation and/or invades any of the following: the postcricoid area, pre-epiglottic space, paraglottic space, and/or inner cortex of thyroid cartilage
T4a	Moderately advanced local disease
	Tumor invades through the thyroid cartilage and/or invades tissues beyond the larynx (eg, trachea, soft tissues of neck, including deep extrinsic muscle of the tongue, strap muscles, thyroid, or esophagus)
T4b	Very advanced local disease
	Tumor invades prevertebral space, encases carotid artery, or invades mediastinal structures
Glottis	
T1	Tumor limited to the vocal cord(s) (may involve anterior or posterior commissure) with normal mobility
T1a	Tumor limited to one vocal cord
T1b	Tumor involves both vocal cords
T2	Tumor extends to the supraglottis, and/or subglottis or with impaired vocal cord mobility
T3	Tumor limited to the larynx with vocal cord fixation and/or invasion of paraglottic space, and/or inner cortex of the thyroid cartilage
T4a	Moderately advanced local disease
	Tumor invades through the outer cortex of the thyroid cartilage and/or invades tissues beyond the larynx (eg, trachea, soft tissues of the neck, including deep extrinsic muscle of the tongue, strap muscles, thyroid, or esophagus)
T4b	Very advanced local disease
	Tumor invades prevertebral space, encases carotid artery, or invades mediastinal structures
Subglottis	
T1	Tumor limited to the subglottis
T2	Tumor extends to vocal cord(s) with normal or impaired mobility
T3	Tumor limited to the larynx with vocal cord fixation
T4a	Moderately advanced local disease
	Tumor invades cricoid or thyroid cartilage and/or invades tissues beyond the larynx (eg, trachea, soft tissues of the neck, including deep extrinsic muscles of the tongue, strap muscles, thyroid, or esophagus)
T4b	Very advanced local disease
	Tumor invades prevertebral space, encases carotid artery, or invades mediastinal structures

continued

TABLE 4: TNM staging system for cancers of the larynx (*continued*)

Regional lymph nodes (N)	
NX	Regional lymph nodes cannot be assessed
N0	No regional lymph node metastasis
N1	Metastasis in a single ipsilateral lymph node, ≤ 3 cm in greatest dimension
N2	Metastasis in a single ipsilateral lymph node, > 3 cm but ≤ 6 cm in greatest dimension; or in multiple ipsilateral lymph nodes, none > 6 cm in greatest dimension; or in bilateral or contralateral lymph nodes, none > 6 cm in greatest dimension
N2a	Metastasis in a single ipsilateral lymph node, > 3 cm but ≤ 6 cm in greatest dimension
N2b	Metastasis in multiple ipsilateral lymph nodes, none > 6 cm in greatest dimension
N2c	Metastasis in bilateral or contralateral lymph nodes, none > 6 cm in greatest dimension
N3	Metastasis in a lymph node(s), > 6 cm in greatest dimension
Distant metastases (M)	
MX	Distant metastasis cannot be assessed
M0	No distant metastasis
M1	Distant metastasis

Stage grouping			
Stage 0	Tis	N0	M0
Stage I	T1	N0	M0
Stage II	T2	N0	M0
Stage III	T3	N0	M0
	T1	N1	M0
	T2	N1	M0
	T3	N1	M0
Stage IVA	T4a	N0	M0
	T4a	N1	M0
	T1	N2	M0
	T2	N2	M0
	T3	N2	M0
	T4a	N2	M0
Stage IVB	T4b	Any N	M0
	Any T	N3	M0
Stage IVC	Any T	Any N	M1

From Edge SP, Byrd DR, Compton CC, et al (eds): AJCC Cancer Staging Manual, 7th ed. New York, Springer, 2010.

LARYNX

Laryngeal cancers constitute approximately 1.2% of all new cancer diagnoses in the United States. Approximately 12,720 new cases were expected in 2010, and some 3,600 died from the disease.

Anatomy and pathology

The laryngeal anatomy is complex and includes cartilages, membranes, and muscles. The three subsites of the larynx are the glottis, or true vocal cords; the supraglottis, which includes the false cords, epiglottis, and aryepiglottic folds; and the subglottis, which is the region below the glottis and within the cricoid cartilage. The TNM staging system for cancers of the larynx is outlined in Table 4.

Treatment

Surgery

Surgical treatment for laryngeal cancer includes transoral or open approaches. Treatment is dictated by the site and extent of the lesion. All or part of the larynx may need to be removed to achieve surgical control of laryngeal cancer. Decision-making for partial laryngectomy is complex and depends on the patient's overall health, the extent of local disease, the skill of the surgeon, and patient preference.

External-beam radiation therapy and chemoradiation therapy

With improvements in techniques and fractionation schedules, external-beam radiation therapy, which allows for laryngeal preservation, is an option for all but the most advanced tumors.

Results

As in other head and neck sites, patients with early laryngeal cancer may be treated with surgery or radiation therapy, and those with advanced-stage disease require multimodal therapy, including surgery and postoperative radiation therapy or chemotherapy and radiation therapy. For T1 and T2 tumors of the glottic or supraglottic larynx, radiation therapy is associated with local tumor control rates of 75% to 95%. Open partial laryngectomy for early laryngeal cancer is associated with local tumor control rates of 84% to 98% but requires a temporary tracheotomy and may be associated with postoperative vocal and swallowing dysfunction. Transoral laser surgery for early laryngeal cancer has yielded local tumor control rates of 82% to 100%, without significant dysphagia or a need for a temporary tracheotomy. However, transoral laser surgery requires technical expertise limited to a small number of institutions.

Select patients with T3 or T4 laryngeal cancers may be candidates for larynx preservation surgery, but most require total laryngectomy as the surgical option. The VA Cooperative Laryngeal Cancer Study was the first trial to test the efficacy of chemotherapy and radiation therapy in the management of stages III and IV laryngeal cancer, assess the possibility for laryngeal preservation using such a regimen, and compare its efficacy against the historic standard of surgery and postoperative radiation therapy. The VA Cooperative Laryngeal Cancer Study randomized patients with resectable squamous cell carcinoma of the larynx to receive either total laryngectomy followed by radiation therapy or neoadjuvant therapy with cisplatin and 5-FU followed by radiation therapy for those achieving a good response to chemotherapy.

Approximately two-thirds of patients survived 2 years following the combination of either chemotherapy plus irradiation or resection plus irradiation. Of those patients initially treated with chemotherapy and irradiation, one-third required total laryngectomy because of a lack of response to treatment; the larynx was successfully preserved in two-thirds of these patients. In this study, the increased local recurrence rate in the chemoradiation therapy group was offset by the decreased incidence of distant metastases and second primary tumors, and the 2-year survival rate was comparable between the groups. Advanced T stage was a risk factor for local failure in this study. Salvage total laryngectomy was required for 56% of T4 laryngeal cancers, suggesting that patients with bulky primary tumors may not be optimal candidates for organ-preservation therapy.

Data from the RTOG 91-11 trial demonstrated an improvement in locoregional tumor control using concurrent chemoradiation therapy relative to induction chemotherapy followed by radiotherapy or radiotherapy alone. There was no primarily surgical or altered fractionated arm in this study. This three-armed study randomized 517 patients with stages III and IV laryngeal cancer to receive one of the following regimens: induction chemotherapy (with cisplatin/5-FU) followed by radiation therapy or concurrent chemoradiotherapy (with cisplatin given on days 1, 22, and 43) or radiation therapy alone. Locoregional tumor control for the three arms was 61%, 78%, and 56%, respectively. The larynx preservation rate was 75%, 88%, and 70%, respectively. At 2 years, the proportion of patients in whom the larynx was preserved after irradiation and concurrent cisplatin (88%) differed significantly from the proportion in groups given induction chemotherapy followed by irradiation (75%; $P = .005$) or irradiation alone (70%; $P < .001$). The authors concluded that the combination of irradiation and concurrent cisplatin was superior to induction chemotherapy followed by irradiation or irradiation alone for laryngeal preservation and locoregional tumor control. Notably, patients with T4 laryngeal cancers comprised only 10% of patients in this study, compared with 25% in the original VA Cooperative Laryngeal Cancer Study, accounting for the improved local tumor control with surgery. Follow-up studies revealed that local failure nevertheless remained the predominant initial site of failure, and the survival of patients who underwent salvage laryngectomy was somewhat diminished.

The cure rate for early cancers of the larynx approaches 80% or more. Half of patients with T3 cancer are cured, whereas more than two-thirds of patients with T4 cancer will die of the disease.

SUPRAGLOTTIS

Supraglottic tumors occur less frequently than tumors of the true vocal cords. The epiglottis is the most common location for supraglottic cancers.

Natural history

Tumors close to the glottis produce symptoms earlier than do tumors at other subsites. In contrast, nearly 60% of patients with supraglottic tumors have T3 or T4 primary tumors at presentation.

The supraglottis has a rich lymphatic network. There is an associated high incidence of lymph node metastases in early-stage tumors (40% for T1 tumors). The incidence of metastases in patients with clinically N0 neck cancer is about 15%. The incidence of bilateral cervical lymph node involvement is about 10%, and this rate increases to 60% for anterior tumors. The neck is a frequent site of recurrence in patients with supraglottic malignancies.

Treatment

Appropriate cancers may be treated with partial laryngectomy. Supraglottic laryngectomy removes the upper portion of the thyroid cartilage and its contents, including the false vocal cords, as well as the epiglottis and aryepiglottic folds. This approach preserves speech and swallowing, but more extensive resections are not well tolerated by patients with impaired lung function who are not able to tolerate the inevitable postoperative aspiration. Supracricoid partial laryngectomy is suitable for supraglottic tumors that cross the ventricle to involve the glottis. Select T3 tumors with limited pre-epiglottic space involvement may be approached with this procedure. Patients must have sufficient pulmonary reserve to be able to tolerate the chronic aspiration associated with this procedure. The local tumor control rates of transoral laser supraglottic laryngectomy are between 75% and 100% for T1 and T2 lesions in recent series and are associated with less postoperative dysphagia than open approaches. Significant technical expertise is needed, and patients must have the proper habitus to assure adequate exposure.

The high incidence of cervical metastases makes treatment of the neck a necessity. About one-third of cases of clinically negative neck cancer contain involved nodes, and the incidence of recurrence in untreated patients is high. For patients undergoing surgical treatment of T1 or T2 primary tumors, bilateral selective neck dissection is advisable.

Supraglottic laryngectomy is seldom appropriate as salvage therapy following irradiation due to complications, including swelling, difficulty swallowing, and poor wound healing. The usual salvage operation for persistent supraglottic cancer following radiation therapy is total laryngectomy. However, some patients remain candidates for larynx-preservation surgery.

Advanced-stage laryngeal cancer usually requires multinodal treatment, as noted previously. Laryngeal preservation frequently is not possible using primary surgical approaches. The use of primary radiation enables preservation of the larynx. The use of combined radiation concurrently with chemotherapy is the treatment of choice for many patients.

GLOTTIS

The glottis is the most common location of laryngeal cancer in the United States, comprising more than half of all cases. The incidence of laryngeal cancers and other malignancies related to smoking has been declining.

Natural history

The cure rate for tumors of the true vocal cords is high. These cancers produce symptoms early, and, thus, most are small when detected. Approximately 60% are T1 and 20% are T2. Normal cord mobility implies invasion of disease limited to the submucosa. Deeper tumor invasion results in impaired vocal cord motion; this finding is most common in the anterior two-thirds of the vocal cord.

The true vocal cords have very little lymphatic drainage. Cervical metastases are infrequent with T1 (1%) and T2 tumors (3% to 7%).

Treatment

Carcinoma in situ is highly curable and may be treated equally well with microexcision, laser vaporization, or radiation therapy. Treatment decisions should be based upon the extent of local disease. Serial recurrences should heighten suspicion of an invasive component, and a more aggressive approach, such as partial or total laryngectomy or irradiation, should be employed. Hypofractionated (> 2 Gy/d) radiotherapy is preferred to conventional fractionation (1.8–2 Gy). Local tumor control for T1 using surgery or irradiation is comparable, usually greater than 90%. Local tumor control for T2 glottic lesions is reported between 70% and 85% with radiotherapy and 85% and 95% with open partial laryngectomy. Partial laryngectomy can be performed in selected patients after irradiation failure of some T1 or T2 glottic cancers.

Advanced T4 disease is best treated with total laryngectomy. Most T3 lesions are now being treated with concomitant chemoradiotherapy, with salvage laryngectomy required in ~20% of patients for residual/recurrent disease or laryngeal dysfunction.

Results Cure rates by tumor size alone follow: T1, 90%; T2, 80%; T3, 50%; and T4, 40%. Neck involvement worsens the prognosis dramatically.

SUBGLOTTIS

Subglottic cancer is unusual, accounting for fewer than 10% of all laryngeal cancers.

Natural history

These cancers tend to be poorly differentiated, and, as the region is clinically "silent," most present as advanced lesions (~70% are T3–T4). The subglottis also has rich lymphatic drainage, and the incidence of cervical metastases is 20% to 30%.

Treatment

Partial laryngectomy is not practical for the treatment of tumors in the subglottis, and, thus, therapy usually includes total laryngectomy plus neck dissection. Combination therapy (surgery plus radiation therapy [60–65 Gy in 6–7 weeks]) is recommended for more advanced disease.

Results The cure rate for the uncommon T1 and T2 tumors is ~70%. Most failures occur in the neck. The cure rate for more advanced lesions is ~40%.

UNKNOWN HEAD AND NECK PRIMARY SITE

The cervical lymph nodes are the most common metastatic site at which squamous cell carcinoma is found.

Natural history

Most patients who present with squamous cell carcinoma involving cervical lymph nodes, especially in the upper or middle portion of the cervical chain, will have a primary site within the head and neck. When the lower cervical or supraclavicular lymph nodes are involved, a primary lung cancer should be suspected.

In the overwhelming majority of these cases, the primary lesion will be discovered based on history, physical examination, proper radiographic evaluation (CT and/or

MRI), and examination with the patient under anesthesia with endoscopy (direct laryngoscopy and nasopharyngoscopy), targeted biopsies, and tonsillectomy. Esophagoscopy and bronchoscopy seldom yield a diagnosis in patients with upper cervical lymph node involvement. "Silent" primary tumors are most often discovered in the base of the tongue or within tonsillar crypts.

Treatment

A substantial percentage of patients achieve long-term disease-free survival after treatment of the involved side of the neck. Locoregional control and survival are diminished by multiple lymph nodes and the presence of extracapsular extension of disease in the involved neck.

Irradiation alone Patients with early-stage neck disease (N1 disease) can be treated with surgery alone if an open biopsy has not been performed. Recurrences in mucosal sites occur in 20% to 30% of cases, and radiotherapy is used for to lower the risk of recurrence in the neck, not the primary. Radiation therapy dosages and techniques should be similar to those used in patients with early-stage (ie T1), primary head and neck cancer. Dosages ranging from 5,760 to 6,480 cGy are acceptable. The nasopharynx, and oropharynx, with or without the hypopharynx, should be included in the irradiated field.

Surgery alone When neck dissection is used at the initial treatment, a primary tumor in the head and neck subsequently becomes obvious in about 20% of patients when radiation therapy is not employed.

Irradiation alone or combined with surgery Combination therapy (surgery plus radiation therapy [60–65 Gy in 6–7 weeks]) is recommended for patients found at surgery to have multiple involved nodes or extracapsular extension or for those who have suspected residual microscopic disease in the neck without a clinically detectable tumor. Open nodal biopsy does not appear to compromise outcome as long as adequate radiotherapy is delivered subsequently.

In most modern series utilizing predominantly combination therapy, 5-year survival rates exceed 50%. The volume of tumor in the involved neck influences outcome, with N1 and N2 disease having a significantly higher cure rate than N3 disease or massive neck involvement. Regional relapse is usually predicted by extranodal disease.

Chemotherapy The role of chemotherapy in treating patients with an unknown primary metastatic squamous carcinoma in cervical lymph nodes remains undefined. The benefit of concurrent chemoradiation therapy of these patients is uncertain (because their primary sites are small or absent), and neck control after resection followed by irradiation, or after irradiation alone, is excellent in patients with cancers of an unknown primary site.

NASOPHARYNX

Nasopharyngeal carcinoma is uncommon in most of the world. Endemic areas include southern China, northern Africa, and regions of the far Northern Hemisphere. The incidence (per 1,000 population) ranges from 25.6 in men and 10.2

in women in Hong Kong to 0.6 in men and 0.1 in women in Connecticut.

Epidemiology and risk factors

Gender and age

The incidence of nasopharyngeal cancer peaks in the fourth to fifth decades of life, and the male-female ratio is 2.2:1. Both patient age at disease onset and male-female ratio are lower for nasopharyngeal cancer than for other head and neck malignancies.

Risk factors

Nasopharyngeal carcinoma WHO types 2 and 3 (see section on "Anatomy and pathology") appears to have different determinants than do other head and neck cancers. They include diet, viral agents, and genetic susceptibility. Populations of endemic areas have a diet characterized by high consumption of salt-cured fish and meat. Studies reveal an association between EBV and nasopharyngeal carcinoma. Anti-EBV antibodies have been found in the sera and saliva of patients with this type of carcinoma. Major histocompatibility (MHC) profiles associated with an increased relative risk include H2, BW46, and B17 locus antigens.

Anatomy and pathology

The nasopharynx communicates anteriorly with the nasal cavity and inferiorly with the oropharynx. The superior border is the base of the skull. The lateral and posterior pharyngeal walls are composed of muscular constrictors. Posteriorly, the nasopharynx overlies the first and second cervical vertebrae. The eustachian tubes open into the lateral walls. The soft palate divides the nasopharynx from the oropharynx.

Cancers arising in the nasopharynx are classified using WHO criteria: type 1 denotes differentiated squamous cell carcinoma; type 2, nonkeratinizing carcinoma; and type 3, undifferentiated carcinoma. The TNM staging system for cancers of the pharynx is outlined in Table 5.

Natural history

A mass in the neck is the presenting complaint in 90% of patients. Other presenting symptoms include a change in hearing, sensation of ear stuffiness, tinnitus, nasal obstruction, and pain.

Cranial nerve involvement

Invasion of disease into the base of the skull is seen in ~25% of cases and may lead to cranial nerve involvement. CN VI is the first cranial nerve to be affected, followed by CN III and CN IV. Deficits are manifested by changes in ocular motion. Involvement of CN V may also occur; this is manifested by pain or paresthesia high in the neck or face.

Level V metastases

Unlike malignancies of the oral cavity and oropharynx, nasopharyngeal cancers often metastasize to level V lymph nodes. Bilateral metastases are common.

TABLE 5: TNM staging system for cancers of the nasopharynx, oropharynx, and hypopharynx

Primary tumor (T)

TX	Primary tumor cannot be assessed
T0	No evidence of primary tumor
Tis	Carcinoma in situ
Nasopharynx	
T1	Tumor confined to the nasopharynx, or tumor extends to the oropharynx and/or nasal cavity without parapharyngeal extension[a]
T2	Tumor with parapharyngeal extension[a]
T3	Tumor involves bony structures of skull base and/or paranasal sinuses
T4	Tumor with intracranial extension and/or involvement of cranial nerves, hypopharynx, or orbit or with extension to the infratemporal fossa/masticator space
Oropharynx	
T1	Tumor $\leq$ 2 cm in greatest dimension
T2	Tumor > 2 cm but $\leq$ 4 cm in greatest dimension
T3	Tumor > 4 cm in greatest dimension or extension to lingual surface of the epiglottis
T4a	Moderately advanced local disease
	Tumor invades the larynx, deep/extrinsic muscle of the tongue, medial pterygoid, hard palate, or mandible[b]
T4b	Very advanced local disease
	Tumor invades the lateral pterygoid muscle, pterygoid plates, lateral nasopharynx, or skull base or encases the carotid artery
	Mucosal extension to the lingual surface of the epiglottis from primary tumors of the base of the tongue and vallecula does not constitute invasion of the larynx.
Hypopharynx	
T1	Tumor limited to one subsite of the hypopharynx and/or $\leq$ 2 cm in greatest dimension
T2	Tumor invades more than one subsite of the hypopharynx or an adjacent site or measures > 2 cm but $\leq$ 4 cm in greatest dimension without fixation of the hemilarynx
T3	Tumor measures > 4 cm in greatest dimension or with fixation of the hemilarynx or extension into the esophagus
T4a	Moderately advanced local disease
	Tumor invades thyroid/cricoid cartilage, hyoid bone, thyroid gland, or central compartment soft tissue[c]
T4b	Very advanced local disease Tumor invades prevertebral fascia, encases carotid artery, or involves mediastinal structures

[a] Parapharyngeal extension denotes posterolateral infiltration of tumor beyond the pharyngobasilar fascia.
[b] Mucosal extension to the lingual surface of the epiglottis from primary tumors of the base of the tongue and vallecula does not constitute invasion of the larynx.
[c] Central compartment soft tissue includes prelaryngeal strap muscles and subcutaneous fat.

continued

TABLE 5: TNM staging system for cancers of the nasopharynx, oropharynx, and hypopharynx *(continued)*

Regional lymph nodes (N):	
Nasopharynx	
NX	Regional lymph nodes cannot be assessed
N0	No regional lymph node metastasis
N1	Unilateral metastasis in cervical lymph node(s), ≤ 6 cm in greatest dimension, above the supraclavicular fossa and/or unilateral or bilateral, retropharyngeal lymph nodes, ≤ 6 cm in greatest dimension[d]
N2	Bilateral metastasis in cervical lymph node(s), ≤ 6 cm in greatest dimension, above the supraclavicular fossa[d]
N3	Metastasis in a lymph node(s) > 6 cm and/or to the supraclavicular fossa
N3a	> 6 cm in dimension
N3b	Extension to the supraclavicular fossa[e]
Oropharynx and hypopharynx[f]	
NX	Regional lymph nodes cannot be assessed
N0	No regional lymph node metastasis
N1	Metastasis in a single ipsilateral lymph node, ≤ 3 cm in greatest dimension
N2	Metastasis in a single ipsilateral lymph node, > 3 cm but ≤ 6 cm in greatest dimension; or in multiple ipsilateral lymph nodes, none > 6 cm in greatest dimension; or in bilateral or contralateral lymph nodes, none > 6 cm in greatest dimension
N2a	Metastasis in a single ipsilateral lymph node, > 3 cm but ≤ 6 cm in greatest dimension
N2b	Metastasis in multiple ipsilateral lymph nodes, none > 6 cm in greatest dimension
N2c	Metastasis in bilateral or contralateral lymph nodes, none > 6 cm in greatest dimension
N3	Metastasis in a lymph node, > 6 cm in greatest dimension
Distant metastases (M)	
MX	Distant metastasis cannot be assessed
M0	No distant metastasis
M1	Distant metastasis

[d] Midline nodes are considered ipsilateral nodes.

[e] The supraclavicular zone or fossa is relevant to the staging of nasopharyngeal carcinoma and is the triangular region originally described by Ho. It is defined by three points: the superior margin of the sternal end of the clavicle, the superior margin of the lateral end of the clavicle, and the point where the neck meets the shoulder. Note that this would include the caudal portions of levels IV and VB. All cases with lymph nodes (whole or part) in the fossa are considered N3b.

[f] Metastases at level VII are considered regional lymph node metastases.

continued

Treatment

Treatment of nasopharyngeal cancer usually involves radiation therapy for the primary tumor and draining lymph nodes. Overall survival is 50% at 5 years. Surgical resection has high morbidity and is seldom entertained.

Nasopharyngeal cancer is distinguished from other sites of head and neck cancer by its radiosensitivity and chemosensitivity. Advanced nodal disease can be controlled by irradiation alone in ~50% of patients, but eventual distant metastasis remains a problem.

TABLE 5: TNM staging system for cancers of the nasopharynx, oropharynx, and hypopharynx *(continued)*

Stage grouping:

Nasopharynx			
Stage 0	Tis	N0	M0
Stage I	T1	N0	M0
Stage II	T1	N1	M0
	T2	N0	M0
	T2	N1	M0
Stage III	T1	N2	M0
	T2	N2	M0
	T3	N0	M0
	T3	N1	M0
	T3	N2	M0
Stage IVA	T4	N0	M0
	T4	N1	M0
	T4	N2	M0
Stage IVB	Any T	N3	M0
Stage IVC	Any T	Any N	M1
Oropharynx and hypopharynx			
Stage 0	Tis	N0	M0
Stage I	T1	N0	M0
Stage II	T2	N0	M0
Stage II!	T3	N0	M0
	T1	N1	M0
	T2	N1	M0
	T3	N1	M0
Stage IVA	T4a	N0	M0
	T4a	N1	M0
	T1	N2	M0
	T2	N2	M0
	T3	N2	M0
	T4a	N2	M0
Stage IVB	T4b	Any N	M0
	Any T	N3	M0
Stage IVC	Any T	Any N	M1

From Edge SP, Byrd DR, Compton CC, et al (eds): AJCC Cancer Staging Manual, 7th ed. New York, Springer, 2010.

The final report of the Intergroup trial 0099 confirmed that for patients with locally advanced nasopharyngeal cancer, concurrent cisplatin chemotherapy with radiation therapy (followed by systemic chemotherapy) provided a clear survival benefit when compared with treatment with irradiation alone. At 5 years, patients who received combined-modality therapy had an overall survival rate of 67%, compared with 37% with radiation therapy alone ($P = .001$). Disease-free survival at 5 years was 74% for the chemoradiation therapy arm versus 46% for the radiation therapy-alone arm.

RECURRENT HEAD AND NECK CANCER

As mentioned previously, surveillance after treatment of head and neck cancer is mandatory, as early detection of second primary cancers or locoregional recurrence affords the best chance for disease control. Nearly two-thirds of patients whose head and neck cancer recurs develop a tumor at (or near) the primary site or in the neck nodes. Eighty percent of head and neck cancer recurrences eventuate within 2 years.

After surgery for head and neck cancer, patients remain at high risk of locoregional recurrence. Having undergone surgery for recurrent disease, 130 patients were randomized to receive postoperative reirradiation combined with concomitant hydroxyurea and fluorouracil or undergo observation. A higher incidence of treatment-related mortality and severe acute and chronic toxicity was found in the treatment group. The disease-free, but not overall, survival was improved in the treatment arm ($P = .006$ and .5, respectively) ***(Janot F et al: J Clin Oncol 26:5518–5523, 2008).***

DIFFERENTIATING RECURRENCE FROM LATE COMPLICATIONS OF IRRADIATION

Differentiating between recurrent carcinoma and significant sequelae of radiotherapy is a difficult clinical problem at all sites within the head and neck. Any suspicious mucosal changes, enlarged nodes in the neck, or discrete subcutaneous nodules warrant prompt biopsy.

CANDIDATES FOR SURGERY

Different choices of first treatment (ie, surgery or radiation therapy) and the intensity of follow-up influence success in treating recurrence. Aggressive surgical intervention should be offered to two groups of patients with recurrent local or regional disease: those whose therapy is chosen with curative intent and those who have the prospect for significant palliation.

The types of recurrence that may be approached surgically with the greatest likelihood of success include (1) metastases in the neck after initial treatment limited to the primary tumor alone and (2) reappearance or persistence of cancer at a site previously treated with radiotherapy alone. Salvage resection may also be considered in other situations, however. They include the appearance of cancer in the neck after prior irradiation or neck dissection, at the margins after previous resection, and even at the base of the skull.

Surgery is the standard of care for the treatment of recurrent disease, but there is a growing body of evidence suggesting that reirradiation with concurrent chemotherapy can cure selected patients when resection is not possible. Several institutions have reported experiences retreating patients, and these results led to the development of the first multi-institution reirradiation study.

A single-arm, phase II study (RTOG 96-10) evaluated toxicity and therapeutic results for patients with recurrent squamous cell carcinoma of the head and neck. Eighty-six patients received four weekly courses of 1.5-Gy fractions twice daily with concurrent 5-FU and hydroxyurea. Each cycle was separated by 1 week of rest. The median survival was 8.1 months, and the 1- and 2-year survival rates were 41.7% and 16.2%, respectively. Compared with patients who experienced early recurrences, patients whose disease recurred 3 years after the original irradiation fared better, with 1- and 2-year survival rates of 48.1% and 32.1%, respectively.

The first results for the entire cohort of patients for RTOG 99-11, the successor trial to RTOG 96-10, were presented in 2005. In this study, patients with locally recurrent or second primary head and neck tumors, who previously received radiation therapy were treated with split-course hyperfractionated radiotherapy (60 Gy total; 1.5 Gy/fraction twice daily for 5 days every 2 weeks for 4 cycles) in combination with cisplatin (15 mg/m^2 IV daily) for 5 courses and paclitaxel (20 mg/m^2 IV daily) for 5 courses every 2 weeks for 4 cycles. Granulocyte colony-stimulating factor (G-CSF) support was administered on days 6 through 13 of each 2-week cycle. Of the 105 patients enrolled, 99 were eligible for analysis, and 23% of the patients had second primary head and neck tumors. The median prior dose of radiotherapy was 65.4 Gy (range: 45–75 Gy), and the median time from prior radiotherapy was 40 months.

Of eight patients with grade 5 (fatal) toxicities, five occurred during the acute period (dehydration, pneumonitis, neutropenia [2 cases], and cerebrovascular accident) and three during the late period (two of three attributable to carotid hemorrhage). Other acute toxicities included leukopenia (30% grade 3/4), anemia (21% grade 3/4), and GI toxicity (48% grade 3/4). The median follow-up for patients was 23.6 months, and the median survival was 12.1 months.

The estimated 1- and 2-year overall survival rates were 50.2% and 25.9%, respectively. The median and 1-year progression-free survival rates were 7.8 months and 35%, respectively. Overall survival was significantly better ($P = .044$) than for the historic control in RTOG 96-10 (estimated 1- and 2-year overall survival rates 41.7% and 16.7%, respectively).

Despite significant toxicity and high mortality, hyperfractionated split-course reirradiation with concurrent cisplatin and paclitaxel chemotherapy proved feasible in this select patient population. This approach was to be tested in an RTOG 04-21, a phase III trial, which was to randomize patients between this arm and chemotherapy alone; however, this trial was closed due to a lack of accrual in early 2007.

Unless a patient cannot tolerate an operation, resection of discrete local or regional recurrent tumors should be entertained as the first course of treatment. Management of recurrences involves complex decision-making and requires familiarity with multidisciplinary care.

SUGGESTED READING

Ang K, Pajak T, Wheeler R, et al: A phase III trial to test accelerated versus standard fractionation in combination with concurrent cisplatin for head and neck carcinomas (RTOG 1209): Report of efficacy and toxicity. 51st Annual ASTRO Meeting; November 1–5, 2009; Chicago, Illinois. Abstract LB2.

Ang KK, Harris J, Garden AS, et al: Concomitant boost radiation and concurrent cisplatin for advanced head and neck carcinomas: Radiation Therapy Oncology Group Phase II Trial 99-14. J Clin Oncol 23:3008–3015, 2005.

Bernier J, Cooper JS Pajak TF, et al: Defining risk levels in locally advanced head and neck cancers: A comparative analysis of concurrent postoperative radiation plus chemotherapy trials of the EORTC (#22931) and RTOG (#9501). Head Neck 27:843–850, 2005.

Bonner JA, Harari PM, Giralt J, et al: Radiotherapy plus cetuximab for squamous-cell carcinoma of the head and neck. N Engl J Med 354:567–578, 2006.

Bourhis J, Lapeyre M, Tortochaux J, et al: Phase III randomized trial of very accelerated radiation therapy compared with conventional radiation therapy in squamous cell head and neck cancer: A GORTEC trial. J Clin Oncol 24:2873–2878, 2006.

Cooper JS, Pajak TF, Forastiere AA, et al: Postoperative concurrent radiotherapy and chemotherapy for high-risk squamous-cell carcinoma of the head and neck. N Engl J Med 350:1937–1944, 2004.

Curran D, Giralt J, Harari PM, et al: Quality of life in head and neck cancer patients after treatment with high-dose radiotherapy alone or in combination with cetuximab. J Clin Oncol 25:2191–2197, 2007.

D'Souza G, Kreimer A, Viscidi R, et al: Case-control study of human papilloma virus and oropharyngeal cancer. N Engl J Med 356:1944–1956, 2007.

Eisbruch A, Harris J, Garden AS, et al: Multi-institutional trial of accelerated hypofractionated intensity-modulated radiation therapy for early-stage oropharyngeal cancer (RTOG 00-22). Int J Radiat Oncol Biol Phys 76:1333–1338, 2010.

Fakhry C, Westra WH, Li S, et al: Improved survival of patients with human papillomavirus-positive head and neck squamous cell carcinoma in a prospective clinical trial. J Natl Cancer Inst 100:261–269, 2008.

Forastiere AA, Goepfert H, Maor M, et al: Concurrent chemotherapy and radiotherapy for organ preservation in advanced laryngeal cancer. N Engl J Med 349:2091–2098, 2003.

Garden AS, Morrison WH, Rosenthal DI, et al: Patterns of disease recurrence following radiation for oropharyngeal cancer. Int J Radiat Oncol Biol Phys 75:S32, 2009.

Hockstein NG, Nolan NP, O'Malley BW Jr, et al: Robot-assisted pharyngeal and laryngeal microsurgery: Results of robotic cadaver dissections. Laryngoscope 115:1003–1008, 2005.

Horwitz EM, Harris J, Langer CJ, et al: Combination with split course concomitant hyperfractionated re-irradiation in patients with recurrent squamous cell cancer of the head and neck: Results of RTOG 99-11. Int J Radiat Oncol Biol Phys 63(suppl 1):S72–S73, 2005.

Jemal A, Siegel R, Xu J, et al: Cancer statistics, 2010. CA Cancer J Clin 60:277–300, 2010.

Jun H, Ahn M, Kim H, et al: Clinical significance of ERCC1 expression in advanced squamous cell carcinoma of the head and neck treated with cisplatin-based concurrent chemoradiation. J Clin Oncol 25(18S):6061, 2007.

Kies MS, Harris J, Rotman MZ, et al: Phase II randomized trial ofpostoperative chemoradiation plus cetuximab for high-risk squamous cell carcinoma of the head and neck (RTOG 0234). Int J Radiat Oncol Biol Phys 75:S14–S15, 2009.

Lonneux M, Hamoir M, Maingon P, et al: Positron emission tomography with [18F] fluorodeoxyglucose improves staging and patient management in patients with head and neck squamous cell carcinoma: A multicenter prospective study. J Clin Oncol 28:1190–1195, 2010.

Mountzios G, Handra-Luca A, Hernandez J, et al: ERCC1 immunohistochemical expression and cancer-specific survival in patients with locally advanced squamous-cell carcinoma of the head and neck treated by cisplatin-based induction chemotherapy. J Clin Oncol 25(18S):6011, 2007.

O'Malley BW Jr, Weinstein GS, Snyder W, et al: Transoral robotic surgery (TORS) for base of tongue neoplasms. Laryngoscope 116:1465–1472, 2006.

Pignon JP, le Maitre A, Bourhis J: Meta-analyses of chemotherapy in head and neck cancer (MACH-NC): An update. Int J Radiat Oncol Biol Phys 69:S112–S114, 2007.

Posner MR, Hershock DM, Blajman CR, et al: Cisplatin and fluorouracil alone or with docetaxel in head and neck cancer. N Engl J Med 357:1705–1715, 2007.

Trotti A, Fu KK, Pajak TF, et al: Long-term outcomes of RTOG 90-03: A comparison of hyperfractionation and two variants of acclerated fractionation to standard fractionation radiotherapy for head and neck squamous carcinoma. Int J Radiat Oncol Biol Phys 63:S70–S71, 2005.

Urba S, Wolf G, Eisbruch A, et al: Single-cycle induction chemotherapy selects patients with advanced laryngeal cancer for combined chemoradiation: A new treatment paradigm. J Clin Oncol 24:593–598, 2006.

Vermorken J, Mesia R, Vega V, et al: Cetuximab extends survival of patients with recurrent or metastatic SCCHN when added to first line platinum based therapy: Results of a randomized phase III (EXTREME) study. J Clin Oncol 25(18S):6091, 2007.

Yom SA, Machtay M, Biel MA, et al: Survival impact of planned restaging and early surgical salvage following definitive chemoradiation for locally advanced squamous cell carcinomas of the oropharynx and hypopharynx. Am J Clin Oncol 28:385–392, 2005.

Abbreviations in this chapter

ACOSOG = American College of Surgeons Oncology Group; AJCC = American Joint Committee on Cancer; ASCO = American Society of Clinical Oncology; ASTRO = American Society for Therapeutic Radiology and Oncology; ECOG = Eastern Cooperative Oncology Group; EORTC = European Organisation for Research on the Treatment of Cancer; EXTREME = Erbitux in First-Line Treatment of Recurrent or Metastatic Head and Neck Cancer; FDA = US Food and Drug Administration; MSKCC = Memorial Sloan-Kettering Cancer Center; RTOG = Radiation Therapy Oncology Group; VA = Veterans Administration; WHO = World Health Organization

CHAPTER 2

Thyroid and parathyroid cancers

Erika Masuda Alford, MD, Mimi I. Hu, MD, Peter Ahn, MD, and Jeffrey P. Lamont, MD

Endocrine malignancies, although relatively uncommon, are often difficult to diagnose and treat effectively. According to American Cancer Society (ACS) estimates, more than 46,930 new cases of endocrine neoplasms will be diagnosed in the United States in 2010, and approximately 2,570 deaths will result from these cancers. This chapter will focus on thyroid and parathyroid cancers. (A discussion of carcinoid tumors, insulinomas, gastrinomas, and other gastrointestinal neuroendocrine tumors, as well as adrenocortical cancer, can be found in chapter 11.)

THYROID CANCER

Thyroid cancer is the most common endocrine cancer. The number of deaths from thyroid cancer estimated for 2010 is 1,690, or 3.8% of all new thyroid cancer cases.

The prevalence rate for occult thyroid cancers found at autopsy is 5% to 10%, except in Japan and Hawaii, where the rate can be as high as 28%. Autopsy rates do not correlate with clinical incidence.

The prevalence of thyroid nodules in the general population is 4% to 7%, with nodules being more common in females than males. The prevalence of thyroid cancer in a solitary nodule or in multinodular thyroid glands is 10% to 20%; this increases with irradiation of the neck in children and older men (see section on "Etiology and risk factors").

TUMOR TYPES

Thyroid cancer is classified into four main types according to its morphology and biologic behavior: papillary, follicular, medullary, and anaplastic. Differentiated (papillary and follicular) thyroid cancers account for > 90% of thyroid malignancies and constitute approximately 0.8% of all human malignancies. Medullary thyroid cancers represent 3% to 5% of all thyroid neoplasms. About 75% of patients with medullary cancer have a sporadic form of the disease, whereas the remaining 25% have inherited disease. Anaplastic carcinoma represents < 3% of all thyroid carcinomas.

Papillary thyroid carcinoma is the most common subtype and has an excellent prognosis. Most papillary carcinomas contain varying amounts of follicular tissue.

THYROID

When the predominant histology is papillary, the tumor is considered to be a papillary carcinoma. Because the mixed papillary-follicular variant tends to behave like a pure papillary cancer, it is treated in the same manner and has a similar prognosis.

Papillary tumors arise from thyroid follicular cells, are unilateral in most cases, and are often multifocal within a single thyroid lobe. They vary in size from microscopic to large cancers that may invade the thyroid capsule and infiltrate into contiguous structures. Papillary tumors tend to invade the lymphatics, but vascular invasion (and hematogeneous spread) is uncommon.

Up to 40% of adults with papillary thyroid cancer may present with regional lymph node metastases, usually ipsilateral. Distant metastases occur, in decreasing order of frequency, in the lungs, bones, and other soft tissues. Older patients have a higher risk for locally invasive tumors and for distant metastases. Children may present with a solitary thyroid nodule, but cervical node involvement is more common in this age group; up to 10% of children and adolescents may have lung involvement at the time of diagnosis.

Follicular thyroid carcinoma is less common than papillary thyroid cancer, occurs in older age groups, and has a slightly worse prognosis. Follicular thyroid cancer can metastasize to the lungs and bones, often retaining the ability to accumulate radioactive iodine (which can be used for therapy). Metastases may be appreciated many years after the initial diagnosis.

Follicular tumors, although frequently encapsulated, commonly exhibit microscopic vascular and capsular invasion. Microscopically, the nuclei tend to be large and have atypical mitotic figures. There is usually no lymph node involvement.

Follicular carcinoma can be difficult to distinguish from its benign counterpart, follicular adenoma. This distinction is based on the presence or absence of capsular or vascular invasion, which can be evaluated after surgical excision but not by fine-needle aspiration (FNA).

Thyroglobulin, normally synthesized in the follicular epithelium of the thyroid, is present in well-differentiated papillary and follicular carcinomas and infrequently in anaplastic carcinomas but not in medullary carcinomas. Therefore, thyroglobulin immunoreactivity is considered to be indicative of a follicular epithelial origin.

Hürthle cell, or oxyphil cell, carcinoma is a variant of follicular carcinoma. Hürthle cell carcinoma is composed of sheets of Hürthle cells and has the same criteria for malignancy as does follicular carcinoma. Hürthle cell carcinoma is thought to have a worse outcome than follicular carcinoma and is less apt to concentrate radioactive iodine.

Medullary thyroid carcinoma originates from the C cells (parafollicular cells) of the thyroid and secretes calcitonin. Secretory diarrhea and flushing, related to calcitonin secretion, can be clinical features of advanced medullary thyroid carcinoma. On gross examination, most tumors are firm, grayish, and gritty.

Sporadic medullary thyroid carcinoma usually presents as a solitary thyroid mass; metastases to cervical and mediastinal lymph nodes are found in half of patients and may be present at the time of initial presentation. Distant metastases to the lungs, liver, bones, and adrenal glands most commonly occur late in the course of the disease.

Hereditary medullary thyroid carcinoma typically presents as a bilateral, multifocal process. Histologically, hereditary medullary carcinoma of the thyroid does not differ from the sporadic form. However, the hereditary form is frequently multifocal, and it is common to find areas of C-cell hyperplasia in areas distant from the primary carcinoma. Another characteristic feature of hereditary medullary carcinoma is the presence of amyloid deposits.

There are three hereditary forms: familial medullary thyroid carcinoma; multiple endocrine neoplasia type 2A (MEN-2A), characterized by medullary thyroid cancer, pheochromocytomas, and hyperparathyroidism; and multiple endocrine neoplasia type 2B (MEN-2B), characterized by medullary thyroid cancer, marfanoid habitus, pheochromocytomas, and neuromas. These syndromes are associated with germ-line mutations of the *RET* proto-oncogene, which codes for a receptor tyrosine kinase (RTK). Hereditary medullary thyroid carcinoma is inherited as an autosomal-dominant trait with high penetrance and variable expression. In addition, approximately 40% of sporadic medullary thyroid carcinomas contain somatic *RET* mutations, which may represent potential therapeutic targets. (For a discussion of genetic testing to screen for *RET* mutations in MEN kindreds, see section on "Diagnostic workup.")

Anaplastic carcinoma Anaplastic tumors are high-grade neoplasms characterized histologically by a high mitotic rate and lymphovascular invasion. Aggressive invasion of local structures is common, as are lymph node metastases. Distant metastases tend to occur in patients who do not succumb early to regional disease. Occasional cases of anaplastic carcinoma have been shown to arise from preexisting differentiated thyroid carcinoma or in a preexisting goiter.

Other tumor types Lymphomas of the thyroid account for < 5% of primary thyroid carcinomas. Other tumor types, such as teratomas, squamous cell carcinomas, and sarcomas, may also rarely cause primary thyroid cancers.

EPIDEMIOLOGY

Age and gender Most patients are between the ages of 25 and 65 years at the time of diagnosis of thyroid carcinoma. Women are affected more often than men (2:1 ratio for the development of both naturally occurring and radiation-induced thyroid cancer).

ETIOLOGY AND RISK FACTORS

Differentiated thyroid cancer

Therapeutic irradiation External low-dose radiation therapy to the head and neck during infancy and childhood, frequently used between the 1940s and 1960s for the treatment of a variety of benign diseases, has been shown to predispose an individual to thyroid cancer. The younger a patient is at the time of radiation exposure, the higher is the subsequent risk of developing thyroid carcinoma. Also, as mentioned previously, women are at increased risk of radiation-induced thyroid cancer. There is a latency period ranging from 10 to 30 years from the time of low-dose irradiation to the development of thyroid cancer.

As little as 11 cGy and as much as 2,000 cGy of external radiation to the head and neck have been associated with a number of benign and malignant diseases. It was once thought that high-dose irradiation (> 2,000 cGy) to the head and neck did not increase the risk of neoplasia. However, it has been shown that patients treated with mantle-field irradiation for Hodgkin lymphoma are at increased risk of developing thyroid carcinoma compared with the general population, although they are more likely to develop hypothyroidism than thyroid cancer.

Radiation-associated thyroid cancer has a natural history and prognosis identical to sporadic thyroid cancer.

Other factors Besides radiation-induced thyroid cancer, there are only sparse data on the etiology of differentiated thyroid cancer. There has been intensive research on distinguishing molecular factors important for cell differentiation, growth, and motility. Considerable attention has focused on BRAF, a member of the RAF family of serine/threonine kinases that mediates cellular responses to growth-promoting signals via the RAS-RAF-MEK-MAPK signaling pathway. *BRAF* mutations so far have only been documented in papillary thyroid carcinoma (45%) and papillary thyroid carcinoma-derived anaplastic thyroid carcinoma (25%). The presence of *BRAF* mutations in FNA biopsy specimens of papillary thyroid caricinoma is highly predictive of extrathyroidal extension, thyroid capsular invasion, and lymph node metastases and an increased risk for persistent or recurrent disease over 3 years of follow-up. Because of this, *BRAF* mutations have been implicated as potential prognostic factors and therapeutic targets. Over the past few years, *BRAF* mutations have been implicated as potential prognostic factors and therapeutic targets.

SIGNS AND SYMPTOMS

Most thyroid cancers present as asymptomatic thyroid nodules. Patients may feel pressure symptoms from nodules as they begin to increase in size. A change in the voice can be caused by a thyroid cancer or benign goiter. The voice change usually occurs when there is compression of the larynx or invasion of the recurrent laryngeal nerve.

On physical examination, a thyroid nodule that is hard or firm and fixed may represent a cancer. The presence of palpable enlarged nodes in the lateral neck, even in the absence of a palpable nodule in the thyroid gland, could represent metastases to the lymph nodes.

DIAGNOSTIC WORKUP

As mentioned previously, thyroid nodules are present in 4% to 7% of the general population and in a higher percentage of individuals who have had irradiation to the head and neck region. Most thyroid nodules are benign (colloid nodules or adenomas); therefore, it is important for the workup to lead to surgical resection for malignant nodules and to avoid unnecessary surgery for benign lesions. Although most solid nodules are benign, thyroid carcinomas usually present as solid nodules. A cystic nodule or a "mixed" (cystic-solid) lesion is less likely to represent a carcinoma and more likely to be a degenerated colloid nodule.

History The history is important in the evaluation of thyroid nodules. If there is a history of irradiation to the head and neck, the risk of there being cancer in the nodule is higher (as great as 50%) than in nonirradiated patients (10% to 20% risk).

Age also is important in the evaluation of thyroid nodules. Nodules that occur in either the very young or the very old are more likely to be cancerous, particularly in men.

A new nodule or a nodule that suddenly begins to grow is worrisome as well.

> A recent study demonstrated that 97% of indeterminate thyroid nodule biopsies with mutations of *BRAF, RAS, RET/PTC*, and *PAC8/PPAR-gamma* had a malignant diagnosis after surgical resection. Molecular testing of a nodule for specific mutations can be useful in the analysis of an indeterminate FNA cytology *(Nikiforov YE et al: J Clin Endocrinol Metab 94:2092–2098, 2009).*

FNA has become the initial diagnostic test for the evaluation of thyroid nodules. FNA can determine whether the lesion is cystic or solid. For solid lesions, cytology can yield one of three results: benign, malignant, or indeterminate. The accuracy of cytologic diagnosis from FNA is 70% to 80%, depending on the experience of the person performing the aspiration and the pathologist interpreting the cytologic specimen.

In a series of 98 "suspicious" FNAs, findings of cellular atypia (pleomorphism, enlarged nuclei, nuclear grooves, coarse or irregular chromatin, prominent or multiple nucleoli, or atypical or numerous mitotic figures) or follicular lesions with atypia were associated with malignancy 20% and 44% of the time, respectively. Follicular lesions without atypia have a 6.7% risk of malignancy. Core needle biopsy has been used as an alternative method for diagnosis. Some studies have shown the adequacy of sample may be greater with core biopsy than FNA. However, there are conflicting reports as to whether a core biopsy offers greater accuracy in the diagnosis of a thyroid nodule. Thus, the 2009 guidelines by the American Thyroid Association recommend ultrasound-guided FNA for evaluating thyroid nodules. Ultrasound guidance is preferred over FNA by palpation for nodules with a higher likelihood of nondiagnostic cytology (> 25% to 50% cystic component) or sampling error (difficult to palpate or posteriorly located nodules) whereas predominantly solid nodules that are palpable and confirmed with diagnostic ultrasound may have FNA by ultrasound or palpation. However, a prospective study showed that ultrasound-guided FNA was more cost-effective than FNA by palpation.

Imaging modalities Ultrasonographic and radionuclide (radioiodine and technetium) scans are also used in the evaluation of thyroid nodules.

Ultrasonography is now widely considered an essential tool in the assessment of thyroid nodules. The presence of certain features is associated with malignancy and can guide physicians in deciding which nodules should be biopsied. Although there is a decrease in cancer rate per nodule in patients with multiple nodules, the overall rate of thyroid cancer per patient is similar to that seen in patients with a solitary nodule.

Thyroid cancer is most often found in the dominant, or largest, nodule in multinodular glands; however, approximately one-third of the cases of cancer are found in nondominant nodules. Nodule size is a poor predictor of malignancy, as the likelihood of cancer has been shown to be the same regardless of nodule size.

A consensus statement from the Society of Radiologists in Ultrasound outlined various features of solitary nodules associated with thyroid cancer: microcalcifications, hypoechogenicity, irregular margins or no halo, solid composition, intranodule vascularity, and more tall than wide dimensions. No single feature has both high sensitivity and specificity; however, the combination of more than one factor can increase the likelihood of cancer. Other than characterization of thyroid nodules, ultrasonography can guide the FNA biopsy, which increases the diagnostic efficacy of the procedure. Additionally, ultrasonography can identify abnormal cervical lymph nodes, which should prompt a biopsy of the lymph node and possibly an ipsilateral thyroid nodule.

Thyroid isotope scans cannot differentiate absolutely a benign from a malignant nodule but can, based on the functional status of the nodule, assign a probability of malignancy. "Hot" thyroid nodules (ie, those that concentrate radioiodine) represent functioning nodules, whereas "cold" nodules are nonfunctioning lesions that do not concentrate the isotope. Most thyroid carcinomas occur in cold nodules, but only 10% of cold nodules are carcinomas. It is not necessary to operate on all cold thyroid nodules. CT or MRI scan of the neck may be appropriate in some cases.

Calcitonin level Medullary thyroid carcinomas usually secrete calcitonin, which is a specific product of the thyroid C cells (parafollicular cells). In patients who have clinically palpable medullary carcinoma, the basal calcitonin level is almost always elevated. In patients with smaller tumors or C-cell hyperplasia, the basal calcitonin level may be normal, but administration of synthetic gastrin (pentagastrin) or calcium results in marked elevation of calcitonin levels. The use of calcitonin levels as a tumor marker and stimulation screening in hereditary forms of medullary cancers has been largely replaced by genetic testing (see below).

Carcinoembryonic antigen (CEA) Serum CEA levels are elevated in patients with medullary thyroid cancer.

Ruling out pheochromocytoma Medullary thyroid carcinoma can be associated with MEN-2A, MEN-2B, or familial non-MEN. Both the MEN-2A and MEN-2B syndromes are characterized by medullary thyroid cancer and pheochromocytoma. Thus, in any patient with hereditary medullary thyroid carcinoma, it is imperative that the preoperative workup include a determination of 24-hour urinary catecholamine and metanephrine levels to rule out the presence of a pheochromocytoma. Fractionated plasma metanephrine levels have been demonstrated to have a high sensitivity and may be included in the initial assessment.

Genetic testing Germ-line mutations in the *RET* proto-oncogene are responsible for familial non-MEN medullary thyroid carcinoma in addition to MEN-2A and MEN-2B. DNA analysis performed on a peripheral blood sample is a highly reliable method for identifying the presence of a *RET* mutation. The 2009 Management Guidelines for the American Thyroid Association regarding MTC recommend all patients with FNA or calcitonin diagnostic or suspicious for MTC undergo *RET* mutation analysis, ideally performed with genetics counseling and completed preoperatively. Approximately 95% of patients with a *RET* mutation will eventually develop medullary carcinoma of the thyroid; thus, prophylactic surgical treatment is recommended. The specific mutated codon of *RET* may correlate with the aggressiveness of medullary carcinoma of the thyroid. This should be considered when counseling affected individuals and their families regarding prophylactic thyroidectomy and the age at which to perform such surgery. Long-term data regarding the effectiveness of prophylactic thyroidectomy based on *RET* testing are scarce at this time. In a recent report of 50 patients (ages 19 years and younger) treated surgically after positive *RET* mutational analysis, 33 patients had carcinoma identified in the surgical specimen. At the time of the publication, 44 patients were found to be free of disease more than 5 years after surgery.

Recommended ages for prophylactic surgery range from within the first 6 months of life to 10 years of age, depending on the mutation. The prophylactic surgical procedure of choice is total thyroidectomy with or without central lymph node dissection.

Periodic determinations of stimulated calcitonin levels may help make the early diagnosis of medullary thyroid carcinoma in those who do not undergo surgery but will not always prevent the development of metastatic medullary thyroid carcinoma.

SCREENING

At this time, no organization recommends periodic screening for thyroid cancer using neck palpation or ultrasonography in average-risk, asymptomatic adults. However, the ACS recommends examination of the thyroid during a routine checkup, since this surveillance can result in case findings.

STAGING AND PROGNOSIS

Unlike most other cancers, in which staging is based on the anatomic extent of disease, the American Joint Committee on Cancer (AJCC) and International Union Against Cancer (UICC) staging of thyroid cancer also takes into consideration patient age at the time of diagnosis and tumor histology (Table 1).

Differentiated thyroid cancers Recurrence and death following initial treatment of differentiated thyroid cancer can be predicted using a number of risk classification schemes. The most commonly used systems are the AMES (age, metastases, extent, and size) and AGES (age, grade, extent, and size) classifications.

Low-risk patients are generally those < 45 years of age with low-grade nonmetastatic tumors that are confined to the thyroid gland and are < 1 to 5 cm. Low-risk patients enjoy a 20-year survival rate of 97% to 100% after surgery alone.

High-risk patients are those ≥ 45 years old with a high-grade, metastatic, locally invasive tumor in the neck or with a large tumor. Large size is

The 2009 American Thyroid Association management guidelines for MTC recommends monitoring of doubling time of CEA and calcitonin. Frequency of surveillance has been recommended based on the DT calculation for CT and CEA. Patients with calcitonin or CEA doubling times of greater than 2 years typically do not require systemic therapy and initiation of such treatment should only be done after thorough discussion. Patients with rapidly progressing disease with doubling time of < 2 years should be considered for treatment *(Kloos RT et al: Thyroid 19:565–612, 2009).*

TABLE 1: AJCC/UICC staging of thyroid cancer

Primary tumor (T)

TX	Primary tumor cannot be assessed
T0	No evidence of primary tumor
T1	Tumor ≤ 2 cm in greatest dimension limited to the thyroid
T1a	Tumor ≤ 1 cm, limited to the thyroid
T1b	Tumor > 1 cm but ≤ 2 cm in greatest dimension, limited to the thyroid
T2	Tumor 2 cm to 4 cm in greatest dimension, limited to the thyroid
T3	Tumor > 4 cm in greatest dimension limited to the thyroid, or any tumor with minimal extrathyroid extension (eg, extension to sternothyroid muscle or perithyroid soft tissues)
T4	All anaplastic carcinomas are considered T4 tumors
T4a	Moderately advanced. Intrathyroidal anaplastic carcinoma. Tumor of any size extending beyond the thyroid capsule to invade subcutaneous soft tissues, larynx, trachea, esophagus, or recurrent laryngeal nerve
T4b	Very advanced. Anaplastic carcinoma with gross extrathyroid extension. Tumor invades prevertebral fascia or encases carotid artery or mediastinal vessels

Note: All categories may be subdivided: (s) solitary tumor, (m) multifocal tumor (the largest determines the classification).

Regional lymph nodes (N)

NX	Regional lymph nodes cannot be assessed
N0	No regional lymph node metastasis
N1	Regional lymph node metastasis
N1a	Metastasis to level VI (pretracheal, paratracheal, and prelaryngeal/Delphian lymph nodes)
N1b	Metastasis to unilateral, bilateral, or contralateral cervical (Levels I, II, III, IV, or V) or retropharyngeal or superior mediastinal lymph nodes (Level VII)

Distant metastasis (M)

MX	Distant metastasis cannot be assessed
M0	No distant metastasis
M1	Distant metastasis

Stage grouping:

	Papillary or follicular < 45 years old				Papillary or follicular (≥ 45 years old) or medullary (any age patient)		
Stage I	Any T	Any N	M0	Stage I	T1	N0	M0
Stage II	Any T	Any N	M1	Stage II	T2	N0	M0
Stage III				Stage III	T3	N0	M0
					T1	N1a	M0
					T2	N1a	M0
					T3	N1a	M0
Stage IVA				Stage IVA	T4a	N0	M0
					T4a	N1a	M0
					T1	N1b	M0
					T2	N1b	M0
					T3	N1b	M0
					T4a	N1b	M0
					T4a	Any N	M0
Stage IVB				Stage IVB	T4b	Any N	M0
Stage IVC				Stage IVC	Any T	Any N	M1

Stage grouping: Undifferentiated (anaplastic)[a]

Stage IV	Any T	Any N	Any M

AJCC = American Joint Committee on Cancer; UICC = International Union Against Cancer

[a] For undifferentiated cancers, all cases are classified as stage IV.

From Edge SB, Byrd DR, Compton CC, et al (eds): AJCC Cancer Staging Manual, 7th ed. New York, Springer, 2010.

defined by some authors as > 1 cm and by other authors as > 2 or > 5 cm. The 20-year survival rate in the high-risk group drops to between 54% and 57%.

Intermediate-risk patients include young patients with a high-risk tumor (metastatic, large, locally invasive, or high grade) or older patients with a low-risk tumor. The 20-year survival rate in this group of patients is ~85%.

Medullary thyroid carcinoma is associated with an overall 10-year survival rate of 40% to 60%. When medullary carcinoma is discovered prior to becoming palpable, the prognosis is much better: patients with stage I medullary tumors (ie, tumors ≤ 2 cm or nonpalpable lesions detected by screening and provocative testing) have a 10-year survival rate of 95%.

Stage II medullary cancers (tumors > 2 but < 4 cm) are associated with a survival rate of 50% to 90% at 10 years. Patients who have lymph node involvement (stages III and IVA disease) have a 10-year survival rate of 15% to 50%. Unfortunately, approximately 50% of patients have lymph node involvement at the time of diagnosis.

When there are distant metastases (stages IVB and IVC), the long-term survival rate is compromised. In patients with metastatic medullary thyroid cancer, the disease often progresses at a very slow rate, and patients may remain alive with disease for many years. Doubling time of calcitonin and CEA are predictive of prognosis. Doubling time of < 6 months has a survival of 25% at 5 years and 8% at 10 years versus doubling time of > 2 years.

The ATA has a calculator for CEA and calcitonin doubling time (see http://www.thyroid.org/professionals/calculators/CDTC.php).

Anaplastic thyroid cancer does not have a generally accepted staging system, and all patients are classified as having stage IV disease. Anaplastic carcinoma is highly malignant and has a poor 5-year survival rate (0% to 25%). Most patients die of uncontrolled local disease within several months of diagnosis.

TREATMENT

As most thyroid nodules are not malignant, it is important to differentiate malignant from benign lesions to determine which patients should undergo surgery. If the cytologic result from FNA indicates that the nodule is benign, which is the case most of the time, the nodule can be safely followed.

SURGERY

Malignant or indeterminate cytologic features are the main indications for surgery.

Malignant nodule

Differentiated thyroid cancer If the cytologic result shows a malignant lesion, thyroidectomy should be performed. There is significant debate in the literature regarding the extent of thyroid surgery for primary tumors confined to one lobe. The surgical options include total lobectomy, total lobectomy with contralateral subtotal lobectomy (subtotal thyroidectomy), or total thyroidectomy. The decision about which procedure to perform should be based on the risk of local recurrence and the anticipated use of radioactive iodine (see section on "Radioactive I-131").

Most authorities agree that a good-risk patient (age < 45 years) with a 1-cm or smaller papillary thyroid cancer should undergo ipsilateral total lobectomy alone. Most experts also agree that total thyroidectomy (or at least subtotal thyroidectomy) is appropriate for high-risk patients with high-risk tumors. Intermediate-risk patients are treated with total lobectomy alone or total (or subtotal) thyroidectomy plus postoperative radioactive iodine. Preoperative neck imaging may help plan the surgery. Patients with radiation-induced thyroid malignancies can be treated similarly, as their cancers have a similar prognosis; however, a total thyroidectomy may be preferable in these patients because of the increased risk of multicentric tumors.

The neck should be palpated intraoperatively. If positive nodes are found, a regional lymph node dissection should be performed.

Medullary carcinoma Patients with medullary thyroid cancer should be treated with total thyroidectomy and a sampling of the regional nodes. If there is involvement of the nodes, a modified neck dissection should be performed (see section on "Lymph node dissection"). If the cancer is confined to the thyroid gland, the patient is usually cured. Postoperative adjuvant external irradiation may be used in certain circumstances (see section on "External radiation therapy").

Anaplastic carcinoma A tracheostomy often is required in patients with anaplastic thyroid cancer because of compression of the trachea. If the tumor is confined to the local area, total thyroidectomy may be indicated to reduce local symptoms produced by the tumor mass. Radiation therapy is used to improve locoregional tumor control, often together with radiosensitizing chemotherapy.

Indeterminate or suspicious nodule

Indeterminate and suspicious FNA should be treated as possible cancers and removed for histologic evalution. The initial operation performed in most patients should be total lobectomy, which entails removal of the suspicious nodule, hemithyroid, and isthmus. There is no role for nodulectomy or enucleation of thyroid nodules. The specimen can be sent for frozen-section analysis during surgery. If frozen section is clearly benign no further resection is required.

Follicular lesion If frozen-section biopsy results indicate a follicular lesion in a patient who is a candidate for total thyroidectomy, and a decision cannot be made as to whether the lesion is benign or malignant, two options are available: (1) stop and wait for final confirmation of the diagnosis, which may require a future operation; or (2) proceed with subtotal or total thyroidectomy, which obviates the need for a later operation. The diagnosis of follicular carcinoma requires identification of vascular or capsular invasion, which may not be evident on frozen-section biopsy.

Hürthle cell carcinoma If the nodule is diagnosed as a Hürthle cell carcinoma, total thyroidectomy is generally recommended for all large (> 4 cm) invasive lesions. Small lesions can be managed with total lobectomy. However, controversy remains over the optimal treatment approach for this cancer.

Lymph node dissection

Therapeutic dissection Therapeutic central neck node dissection should be performed for medullary carcinomas and other thyroid neoplasms with nodal involvement. The dissection should include all the lymphatic tissue in the pretracheal area and along the recurrent laryngeal nerve and anterior mediastinum. If there are clinically palpable nodes in the lateral neck, a modified neck dissection is performed.

Prophylactic dissection There is no evidence that performing prophylactic neck dissection improves survival. Therefore, aside from patients with medullary thyroid cancer, who have a high incidence of involved nodes, only therapeutic neck dissection is indicated.

Removal of individual abnormal nodes ("berry picking") is not advised when lateral neck nodes are palpable because of the likelihood of missing involved nodes and disrupting involved lymphatic channels.

Metastatic or recurrent disease

Survival rates from the time of the discovery of metastases (lung and bone) from differentiated thyroid cancer are less favorable than those associated with local recurrence (5-year survival rates of 38% and 50%, respectively). Survival also depends on whether the metastatic lesions take up I-131.

Surgery, with or without I-131 ablation (discussed below), can be useful for controlling localized sites of recurrence. Approximately half of patients who undergo surgery for recurrent disease can be rendered free of disease with a second operation.

RADIOACTIVE I-131

Uses in papillary or follicular thyroid carcinoma

There are two basic uses for I-131 in patients diagnosed with papillary or follicular thyroid carcinoma: ablation of normal residual thyroid tissue after thyroid surgery and treatment of thyroid cancer, either residual disease in the neck or metastasis to other sites in the body. It should be emphasized that patients with medullary (in the absence of a concomitant epithelial cell-derived differentiated thyroid cancer), anaplastic, and most Hürthle cell cancers do not benefit from I-131 therapy.

Postoperative ablation of residual thyroid tissue should be considered in high-risk patients and patients with high-risk tumors. Ablation of residual normal thyroid tissue allows for the use of I-131 scans to monitor for future recurrence, possibly destroys microscopic foci of metastatic cancer within the remnant, and improves the accuracy of thyroglobulin monitoring.

Ablation must also be accomplished in patients with regional or metastatic disease prior to the use of I-131 for treatment, as the normal thyroid tissue will preferentially take up iodine compared with the cancer. Some states permit the use of I-131 for ablation and treatment on an outpatient basis, but administration is strictly governed by national guidelines, which minimize the risk of radiation exposure to the public.

Following surgery, the patient can be treated with liothyronine for a duration of 2 weeks. The TSH level should be determined approximately 4 to 6 weeks after surgery; in patients who undergo total or subtotal thyroidectomy, TSH levels will generally be > 50 μU/mL. A postoperative iodine scan can then be performed. If this scan documents residual thyroid tissue, an ablative dose of I-131 should be given. The patient should be advised not to undergo any radiographic studies with iodine during ablation therapy and to avoid seafood and vitamins or cough syrups containing iodine. Patients are prepared with a specific diet prior to the I-131 therapy. Iodine-123 may also be used in the postoperative setting. It may produce a better quality image than I-131 scans.

For patients who have contraindications for thyroid hormone withdrawal, administration of recombinant human thyroid-stimulating hormone (rTSH) is an alternative for preparation for radioiodine ablation of a post-surgical thyroid remnant. Currently, there are no long-term data ascertaining the maintenance of a low tumor recurrence rate using rTSH, which may have a quality-of-life advantage compared with thyroid hormone withdrawal and is the subject of a clinical trial.

In general, doses of I-131 up to 75 to 100 mCi will ablate residual thyroid tissue within 6 months following ingestion. In some patients, it may take up to 1 year for complete ablation to occur. Patients should be monitored following ablation, and when they become hypothyroid, hormone replacement therapy should be given until they are clinically euthyroid and TSH is suppressed. Recently, lower doses have been found to be effective, and some authors have recommended doses between 25 and 50 mCi, assuming they achieve euthyroid levels with TSH suppression to < 0.1 μU/mL.

Approximately 6 to 12 months after ablation of the thyroid remnant, a follow-up I-131 scan should be performed. Recombinant human thyrotropin alpha (Thyrogen) is now available. Patients may continue on thyroid replacement and receive two doses of thyrotropin prior to I-131 scanning; this approach can prevent the symptoms of hypothyroidism.

Treatment of residual cancer For disease in the tumor bed or lymph nodes that was not surgically resectable, an I-131 dose of 100 to 150 mCi is given. For disease in the lungs or bone, the I-131 dose is 200 to 250 mCi. Following this therapy, the patient is again put on thyroid hormone replacement, and adequate suppression is maintained by monitoring TSH levels.

Some clinicians advocate obtaining a repeat scan in 1 year, along with a chest x-ray, and repeating this procedure yearly until a normal scan is obtained. However, the frequency of repeat scans and the dose of I-131 are rather controversial and should be guided by the individual's risk profile.

Various preclinical studies evaluating the effects of other novel therapies have shown promising results. PTC cell lines carrying a *RET/PTC* rearrangement or a *BRAF* mutation treated with CI-1040 (a MEK1/2 inhibitor) in vitro and in vivo demonstrated inhibition of PTC cell growth *(Henderson YC et al: Arch Otolaryngol Head Neck Surg 135:347–354, 2009)*. Treatment with AZD0530 (a Src inhibitor) inhibited the growth and invasion of human PTC and ATC cell lines *(Schweppe RE et al: J Clin Endocrinol Metab 94:2199–2203, 2009)*. Anaplastic and follicular thyroid cancer cell lines incubated with gefitinib (Iressa, an EGFR inhibitor) resulted in a dose-dependent decrease in colony formation. Additionally, ionizing radiation combined with gefitinib reduced cell proliferation; thus, this combination may be promising for anaplastic and follicular thyroid carcinomas *(Lopez JP et al: Laryngoscope 118:1372–1376, 2008)*.

Following thyroid remnant ablation, serum thyroglobulin measurements are useful in monitoring for recurrence. Since thyroglobulin in a patient receiving thyroid hormone replacement may be suppressed, a normal test may be incorrect ~10% of the time. In general, the presence of disease is accurately predicted by a thyroglobulin value > 5 ng/mL while the patient is in the suppressed state and by a value > 10 ng/mL in the hypothyroid state. However, measurable disease may not be identified in many patients. Whether or not they should be treated on the basis of the thyroglobulin value if the I-131 scan is normal is a subject of current debate. Any rise in the thyroglobulin level from the previous value should increase the suspicion of recurrent disease.

Neck ultrasonography is useful to evaluate locoregional tumor recurrence and should be performed at yearly intervals for 5 to 10 years after initial therapy depending upon the stage of disease. Continued monitoring is necessary, as late recurrence can occur. It should be pointed out that certain aggressive tumors may neither be radioactive iodine–avid nor synthesize thyroglobulin. PET scanning may contribute to localization of disease in some cases and may even carry prognostic value. PET/CT may be more useful than other imaging techniques; in a recent study, additional information was obtained with PET/CT in up to 67% of cases.

Side effects and complications

Acute effects The acute side effects of I-131 therapy include painful swelling of the salivary glands and nausea. Ibuprofen or other pain relievers are usually used to decrease salivary gland discomfort. Nausea may be treated with standard antiemetics.

Rarely, in patients with significant residual thyroid tissue, radioactive iodine may cause acute thyroiditis, with a rapid release of thyroid hormone. This problem can be treated with steroids and β-blockers.

Patients must also be cautioned not to wear contact lenses for at least 3 weeks following ingestion of I-131, as the tears are radioactive and will contaminate the lenses and possibly lead to corneal ulceration.

Long-Term Complications Long-term risks of radioactive iodine are not well understood. They can include effects on the salivary glands consisting of sialadenitis and xerostomia, and possible increased risk of bladder tumors and colon cancers with repeat administrations.

Bone marrow suppression and leukemia are potential long-term complications of I-131 therapy but are poorly documented and appear to be extremely rare. Patients should have a CBC count performed prior to ingestion of an I-131 dose to ensure adequate bone marrow reserve. They should also have yearly blood counts. Leukemia occurs rarely with doses of I-131 < 1,000 mCi.

Pulmonary fibrosis may be seen in patients with pulmonary metastases from papillary or follicular thyroid cancer who are treated with I-131. Those with a miliary or micronodular pattern are at greater risk, as a portion of normal lung around each lesion may receive radiation, leading to diffuse fibrosis.

Effects on fertility Data have documented an increase in follicle-stimulating hormone (FSH) levels in one-third of male patients treated with I-131. Changes in FSH after one or two doses of I-131 are generally transitory, but repeated doses may lead

> **T**wice-daily radiation therapy may be of benefit over once-a-day treatment for local tumor control and possibly survival. Multimodality therapy with R0/R1 resection followed by doxorubicin with twice-daily radiation therapy had the highest rates of local tumor control and median survival in this retrospective comparison of 75 patients *(Swaak-Kragten AT et al: Radiother Oncol 92:100–104, 2009).*

to lasting damage to the germinal epithelium. Sperm banking should be considered in male patients likely to receive cumulative doses of I-131 higher than 500 mCi.

The effects of I-131 on female fertility have been investigated. A published article showed no significant difference in the fertility rate in women receiving radioactive iodine. Exposure to > 100mCi of I-131 was also not associated with increased miscarriages, congenital malformations, or thyroid disease or cancer in offspring. However, it is generally recommended to avoid pregnancy for 1 year after therapeutic I-131 administration.

No ill effects have been noted in the offspring of treated patients.

EXTERNAL RADIATION THERAPY

Papillary or follicular thyroid cancer

There are a number of indications for external irradiation of papillary or follicular thyroid carcinoma. Surgery followed by radioactive iodine may be used for disease that extends beyond the capsule. However, if all gross disease cannot be resected, or if residual disease is not radioactive iodine–avid, external irradiation is used as part of the initial approach for locally advanced disease in older patients. The benefit of adjuvant external irradiation for cause-specific survival is inferred from institutional series. Intensity-modulated radiation therapy is associated with decreased severe late toxicities in an institutional series and provides the best target coverage in dosimetric studies.

Unresectable disease External irradiation is useful for unresectable disease extending into the connective tissue, trachea, esophagus, great vessels, and anterior mediastinum. For unresected disease, doses of 6,000 to 6,500 cGy are recommended. The patient should then undergo I-131 scanning, and, if uptake is detected, a dose of I-131 should be administered.

> **S**tereotactic radiosurgery for unresectable nodal recurrences was used in a small study to a dose of 30 to 39 Gy in one to three fractions in nine patients and found to be safe. However, four of these nine patients developed other nodal recurrences *(Kim JH et al: Oto-Head and Neck Surg 142:338-343, 2010).*

Recurrence after resection External irradiation may also be used after resection of recurrent papillary or follicular thyroid carcinoma that no longer shows uptake of I-131 , or for gross unresectable disease. In this situation, doses of 5,000 to 6,600 cGy are delivered to the tumor bed to prevent local recurrence. Multiple-field techniques and extensive treatment planning are necessary to deliver high doses to the target volume to minimize the risk of significant complications.

Recurrences to regional lymph nodes that are not resectable can be salvaged with regional external radiation therapy. In either situation, the radiation fields extend from cervical lymph node stations to the superior mediastinum, with esophageal stricture reported as a common long-term morbidity of treatment.

Palliation of bone metastases External radiation therapy is useful in relieving pain from bone metastasis. If the metastasis shows evidence of I-131 uptake, the patient should be given a therapeutic dose of I-131 followed by local external radiation therapy to the lesion of up to 4,000 to 5,000 cGy. The use of intravenous bisphosphonate therapy has been shown to decrease the pain of bone metastasis and improve reported quality of life.

Anaplastic thyroid carcinoma

Anaplastic carcinoma of the thyroid is an exceptionally aggressive disease, with few long-term survivors. It often presents as a rapidly expanding mass in the neck and may not be completely resected. External irradiation to full dose (6,000 to 6,500 cGy) may slow the progress of this disease but rarely controls it.

Chemoradiation therapy There are reports of the use of accelerated fractionation regimens of external irradiation (160 cGy twice daily to 5,700 cGy) with weekly doxorubicin in patients with anaplastic thyroid cancer, as well as reports of the combination of doxorubicin and cisplatin with external irradiation. These regimens have improved local tumor control but at the expense of increased toxicity. Unfortunately, the majority of patients die of local and/or distant recurrence.

Medullary thyroid carcinoma

External irradiation has been used for medullary thyroid cancer in the postoperative setting, but only retrospective series are available therefore this technique is controversial. However, much of the available literature has indicated that indications would include positive surgical margins, gross residual disease, or extensive lymph node metastasis. Further controversy exists in the setting of elevated postoperative calcitonin levels in patients

A phase I study of XL184 (a c-Met, VEGFR2, and RET kinase inhibitor) has been shown to achieve PR or SD in metastatic MTC *(Sherman SI et al: 2008 Symposium on Molecular Targets and Cancer Therapeutics; Geneva, Switzerland)*. A phase II XL184 placebo controlled trial is currently ongoing. Vandetanib used in an open-label phase II trial of patients with locally advanced or metastatic hereditary MTC showed PR in 20%, SD ≥ 24 weeks in 53%, decreased calcitonin by 50% in 80%, and decreased CEA by 50% in 53% *(Wells SA et al: J Clin Oncol 28:767–772, 2010)*. Results of a randomized, double-blind phase III trial of vandetanib in advanced hereditary or sporadic MTC were presented at the 2010 ASCO annual meeting. Statistically significant prolongation of the primary endpoint of progression-free survival was observed for vandetanib vs placebo (HR = 0.45). Additionally, vandentanib exhibited a significant objective response rate compared with placebo *(Wells SA et al: ASCO 2010, abstract 5503)*. Sunitinib, in a phase II trial with continuous dosing in patients with differentiated thyroid cancer and MTC with FDG-PET avid disease, showed a disease control rate of 83% (CR 7% + PR 25% + SD 48%) *(Carr L et al: J Clin Oncol 27[15s]:6056, 2009)*. Sorafenib, in a phase II clinical trial of metastatic MTC, showed 6.3% PR, and 87.5% with SD in sporadic MTC with median PFS survival of 17.9 months with common AEs of diarrhea, hand-foot-skin reaction, rash, and hypertension *(Lam ET et al: J Clin Oncol 2010 Apr 5 EPub)*.

> **I**matinib (Bcr-Abl and PDGF inhibitor) studied in a phase II trial in patients with anaplastic thyroid carcinoma showed partial response in 25%, stable disease in 50%, and progressive disease in 25% at 8 weeks, with a 6-month progression free survival of 27% and 6-month overall survival of 46% *(Ha HT et al: ASCO 2009, abstract 6057)*. Sorafenib, in a phase II trial in patients with progressive anaplastic thyroid carcinoma, showed 13% partial response and 27% stable disease, with median survival of 3.5 months; this trial is ongoing *(Nagaiah G et al: ASCO 2009, abstract 6058)*.

who have undergone macroscopically complete resection, without radiographic evidence of distant disease. The recommended dose is 5,000 to 7,000 cGy in 5 to 7 weeks. Radiation is also used for palliation of different sites of metastatic disease.

ROLE OF MEDICAL THERAPY

Differentiated thyroid cancer

As mentioned previously, thyroid hormone is used to suppress TSH in most patients with differentiated thyroid cancer after surgery and I-131 (as appropriate) treatment. Greater TSH suppression has been associated with improved progression-free survival in patients with high-risk papillary thyroid carcinoma. Modest TSH suppression in patients with stage II disease yields similar results. Patients with stage I disease do not appear to have any change in outcomes based on the degree of TSH suppression.

Systemic chemotherapy is used for widespread disease, although reproducibly effective regimens have not been identified to date.

Over the past few years, molecularly targeted treatments have been studied in patients with advanced thyroid carcinoma no longer responsive to radioactive iodine. They include multitargeted tyrosine kinase inhibitors, a DNA methylation inhibitor, histone deacetylase inhibitors, a proteasome inhibitor, and a heat-shock protein-90 inhibitor. These agents are still being investigated in clinical trials.

According to 2008 National Comprehensive Cancer Network Guidelines, patients with metastatic differentiated or medullary thyroid carcinoma not amenable to surgery or radioiodine should be referred to a clinical trial investigating targeted therapies or recommended to off-label use of sorafenib (Nexavar), if a trial is not available to the patient, or maintained with best supportive care (www.nccn.org, Thyroid Carcinoma, v.1.2008).

Medullary thyroid carcinoma

In patients with medullary thyroid carcinoma, the usual treatment is surgery. Various oral, small molecule tyrosine kinase inhibitors have been investigated in patients with locally advanced, metastatic, or progressive hereditary and sporadic medullary thyroid carcinomas. The responses have been variable among agents and have consisted of partial response as the best outcome. However, the development of these novel agents and others offers much promise in the targeted treatment of metastatic medullary thyroid carcinoma, which currently has no effective cure. In patients with hereditary medullary carcinoma who have a coexisting pheochromocytoma, appropriate control of catecholamine hypersecretion should precede thyroid surgery.

Anaplastic thyroid carcinoma

As mentioned previously, the usual treatment for patients with resectable or localized anaplastic thyroid cancer is surgery. Like radiotherapy, chemotherapy is an important alternative approach, but further evaluation is needed to optimize its effectiveness. Patients with unresectable local tumors should be referred to clinical trials, treated with radiotherapy and chemotherapy, or maintained with best supportive care.

Several molecular targeted tyrosine kinase inhibitors are showing promising results for thyroid cancer. Sorafenib was used to clinically treat patients with progressive radioactive iodine–resistant differentiated thyroid cancer, with partial response in 20%, stable disease in 60%, and most noticeable response in the lungs, suggesting a tissue-specific response (*Cabanillas ME et al: J Clin Endocrinol Metab 95:2588–2595, 2010*). Motesanib (inhibitor of VEGFR, PDGFR, and KIT) given in a phase II study showed stable disease of ≥ 24 weeks in 48%, and decreased target lesion measurement in 76%, with median progression free survival of 48 weeks (*Schlumberger MJ et al: J Clin Oncol 27:3794–3801, 2009*). In a phase II study of Sunitinib (a RET, VEGFR, and PDGFR inihibitor), 2 cycles of therapy showed partial response in 13%, stable disease in 68%, and progressive disease in 10% with most common adverse events of fatigue, diarrhea, palmar-plantar erythrodysesthesia, and GI events (*Cohen EE et al: J Clin Oncol 26[15S]:6025, 2008*).

PARATHYROID CARCINOMA

Parathyroid carcinoma is a rare cause of hypercalcemia, accounting for < 2% of cases with primary hyperparathyroidism.

EPIDEMIOLOGY AND ETIOLOGY

The disease presents in midlife and occurs with similar frequency in both genders. The etiology of parathyroid carcinoma is obscure; an association with prior neck irradiation is not apparent. Parathyroid carcinoma can be associated with the hereditary hyperparathyroidism–jaw tumor syndrome, which is due to an inactivating mutation of the *HRPT2* gene that encodes the parafibromin protein. In addition, somatic mutations of the *HRPT2* gene have been demonstrated in sporadic parathyroid carcinomas (66% to 100%) but have not been seen with sporadic adenomas.

SIGNS AND SYMPTOMS

Most patients with parathyroid cancer have symptomatic moderate to severe hypercalcemia (mean serum calcium level, 15 mg/dL) and high parathyroid hormone levels. They often present with a palpable neck mass. Unlike benign hyperparathyroidism, renal and bone abnormalities are more common in patients with parathyroid cancer.

Rarely, nonfunctioning tumors may present as neck masses; their clinical course is similar to that of functioning tumors. Clinical concern about parathyroid cancer should be raised in the presence of a palpable neck mass and severe hypercalcemia, recurrent hyperparathyroidism, or associated vocal cord paralysis.

PATHOLOGY

The principal features of parathyroid cancer include a trabecular pattern, mitotic figures, thick fibrous bands, and capsular or vascular invasion of disease. Other important features include lymphatic or hematogenous metastases and histologic evidence of tumor infiltration into the surrounding tissues (including macroscopic adherence or vocal cord paralysis).

Although cytologic evidence of mitoses is necessary to establish the diagnosis of carcinoma, mitotic activity alone is an unreliable indicator of malignancy. The only reliable microscopic finding of malignancy is invasion of surrounding structures or metastasis to lymph nodes or other organs.

TREATMENT

Surgical treatment of primary hyperparathyroidism

The diagnosis of parathyroid carcinoma is sometimes made during surgical exploration for primary hyperparathyroidism. Most surgeons advocate identification of all four parathyroid glands. In most cases, the upper glands can be found on the posterior aspect of the upper third of the thyroid lobe, just cephalad to the inferior thyroid artery and adjacent to the recurrent laryngeal nerve as it enters the larynx.

The inferior parathyroid glands are more variable in location. Most are found on the posterior or lateral aspect of the lower pole of the thyroid gland, but the inferior parathyroid glands may be ectopically placed in the superior or true mediastinum, often within the thymus.

The inferior and, less commonly, superior glands can be found in an ectopic location in the upper or lateral neck, adjacent to the esophagus, or within the carotid sheath.

Surgical exploration for primary hyperparathyroidism Most cases of primary hyperparathyroidism are caused by a single hyperfunctioning parathyroid adenoma. If the surgeon finds one (or occasionally two) enlarged abnormal gland(s) and the remaining glands are normal, the enlarged gland should be removed.

If four enlarged glands are found, indicating the rare case of primary parathyroid hyperplasia, subtotal parathyroidectomy including 3.5 glands should be performed. Consideration should be given to transplanting the remaining gland remnant to an ectopic location that would be easily accessible to the surgeon if hyperparathyroidism recurs.

If only normal glands are found at exploration, a missed adenoma in an ectopic location should be suspected. Thorough intraoperative neck and superior mediastinal exploration should be performed, and if the missing gland cannot be found, thymectomy and hemithyroidectomy should be performed to exclude an intrathymic or intrathyroidal adenoma. Localization studies, including CT/MRI or radionuclide imaging, should precede reexploration for a missed adenoma.

Intraoperative parathyroid hormone (ioPTH) levels are increasingly used to guide surgery for primary hyperparathyroidism. A 50% or greater decrease in the ioPTH level from the preexcision value to the 10-minute postexcision value is used as a predictor of successful surgery. The advent of ioPTH monitoring, coupled with preoperative localization studies (sestamibi scanning), has facilitated less invasive surgical techniques, such as minimally invasive parathyroidectomy. This has resulted in shorter average hospitalization stays and reduced postoperative recovery times.

> **Loss of parafibromin and *Rb* expression and overexpression of *galectin-3* can be distinguishing features of parathyroid carcinoma vs other parathyroid tumors** *(Fernandez-Ranvier GG et al: Cancer 115:334–344, 2009).*

The use of ioPTH with parathyroid hyperplasia requires more strict evaluation of ioPTH levels. Siperstein et al performed a prospective evaluation of ioPTH and bilateral neck exploration and found that up to 15% of cases will have additional "abnormal" glands that were not predicted by ioPTH or preoperative imaging. This study demonstrates the need for long-term follow-up of patients undergoing focused parathyroid surgery.

If parathyroid carcinoma is suspected, based on the severity of hyperparathyroidism or invasion of surrounding tissues by a firm parathyroid tumor, aggressive wide excision is indicated. This procedure should include ipsilateral thyroidectomy and en bloc excision of surrounding tissues as necessary.

Patterns of recurrence of cancer The average time from initial surgery to the first recurrence of cancer is approximately 3 years but may be as long as 10 years. The thyroid gland is the usual site of involvement, with disease "seeding" in the neck a common pattern. Other sites of involvement include the recurrent nerve, strap muscles, esophagus, and trachea.

Distant metastases can be present at the time of initial surgery, or local spread to contiguous structures in the neck may be followed subsequently by distant metastases to the lungs, bone, and liver.

In a recent analysis, 85% of patients with parathyroid carcinoma were alive 5 years after diagnosis; death usually results from complications of the hypercalcemia rather than from the tumor burden.

Treatment of isolated metastases Isolated metastases should be aggressively resected to enhance survival and control hypercalcemia.

Medical therapy

Morbidity and mortality are generally caused by the effects of unremitting hypercalcemia rather than tumor growth. Medical treatment provides temporary palliation of hypercalcemia. Drugs used include bisphosphonates, such as pamidronate (60 to 80 mg every 4 to 6 days) or zoledronic acid (Zometa); calcitonin, 4 to 8 IU/kg every 6 to 12 hours; mithramycin (plicamycin [Mithracin]), 25 μg/kg every 4 to 6 days; and gallium nitrate (Ganite), 100 to 200 mg/m^2/day IV for 5 days. Cinacalcet (Sensipar), a calcimimetic that targets the calcium-sensing receptor on parathyroid cells and reduces parathyroid hormone secretion, is an FDA-approved oral treatment of hypercalcemia associated with parathyroid carcinoma (up to 90 mg bid) in patients who do not respond to surgery or other medical treatments.

Radiation therapy

There is little evidence for an effect of adjuvant radiation therapy in achieving locoregional control. Some institutions have used surgical margin status to determine whether patients receive adjuvant radiation therapy including elective nodal irradiation.

SUGGESTED READING

ON THYROID CARCINOMA

Bal CS, Kumar A, Pant GS: Radioiodine dose for remnant ablation in differentiated thyroid carcinoma: A randomized clinical trial in 509 patients. J Clin Endocrinol Metab 89:1666–1673, 2004.

Can AS, Peker K: Comparison of palpation-versus ultrasound-guided fine-needle aspiration biopsies in the evaluation of thyroid nodules. BMC Res Notes 1:12, 2008 [Epub May 15, 2008].

Cooper DS, Doherty GM, Haugen BR, et al: Revised American Thyroid Association management guidelines for patients with thyroid dodules and differentiated thyroid cancer. Thyroid 19:1167–1214, 2009.

David A, Blotta A, Rossi R, et al: Clinical value of different responses of serum thyroglobulin to recombinant human thyrotropin in the follow-up of patients with differentiated thyroid carcinoma. Thyroid 15:267–273, 2005.

Frates MC, Benson CB, Charboneau JW, et al: Management of thyroid nodules detected at US: Society of Radiologists in Ultrasound consensus conference statement. Radiology 237:794–800, 2005.

Garsi JP, Schlumberger M, Rubino C, et al: Therapeutic administration of 131-I for differentiated thyroid cancer: Radiation dose to ovaries and outcome of pregnancies. J Nucl Med 49:845–852, 2008.

Hall NC, Kloos RT: PET imaging in differentiated thyroid cancer: Where does it fit and how do we use it? Arq Bras Endocrinol Metab 51:793–805, 2007.

Jimenez C, Hu MI, Gagel RF: Management of medullary thyroid carcinoma. Endocrinol Metab Clin North Am 37:481–496, 2008.

Kloos RT, Eng C, Evans DB, et al: Medullary thyroid cancer: Management guidelines of the American Thyroid Association. Thyroid 19:565–612, 2009.

Meadows KM, Amdur RJ, Morris CG, et al: External beam radiotherapy for differentiated thyroid cancer. Am J Otolaryngol 27:24–28, 2006.

Sampson E, Brierley JD, Le LW, et al: Clinical management and outcome of papillary and follicular (differentiated) thyroid cancer presenting with distant metastasis at diagnosis. Cancer 110:1451–1456, 2007.

Sawka AM, Lea J, Alshehri B, et al: A systematic review of the gonadal effects of therapeutic radioactive iodine in male thyroid cancer survivors. Clin Endocrinol (Oxf) 68:610–617, 2008.

Sherman SI: Advances in chemotherapy of differentiated epithelial and medullary thyroid cancers. J Clin Endocrinol Metab 94:1493–1499, 2009.

Sherman SI: Molecularly targeted therapies for thyroid cancers. Endocr Pract 15: 605-611, 2009.

Sherman SI: Tyrosine kinase inhibitors and the thyroid. Best Pract Res Clin Endocrinol Metab 23:713-722, 2009.

Sherman SI, Angelos P, Ball DW, et al: Thyroid carcinoma. J Natl Compr Canc Netw 5:568–621, 2007.

Silverberg SJ, Rubin MR, Faiman C, et al: Cincalet hydrochloride reduces the serum calcium concentration in inoperable parathyroid carcinoma. J Clin Endocrinol Metab 92:3803–3808, 2007.

Torlontano M, Attard M, Crocetti U, et al: Follow-up of low risk patients with papillary thyroid cancer: Role of neck ultrasonography in detecting lymph node metastases. J Clin Endocrinol Metab 89:3402–3407, 2004.

United States Nuclear Regulatory Commission: Medical, industrial, and academic uses of nuclear materials: Regulations, guidance, and communications. Available at: www.nrc.gov.

Urhan M, Dadparvar S, Mavi A, et al: Iodine-123 as a diagnostic imaging agent in differentiated thyroid carcinoma: A comparison with iodine-131 post-treatment scanning and serum thyroglobulin measurement. Eur J Nucl Med Mol Imaging 34:1012–1017, 2007.

Verburg FA, de Keizer B, Lips CJ, et al: Prognostic significance of successful ablation with radioiodine of differentiated thyroid cancer patients. Eur J Endocrinol 152:33–37, 2005.

Ying AK, Huh W, Bottomley S, et al: Thyroid cancer in young adults. Semin Oncol 36:258–274, 2009.

ON PARATHYROID CARCINOMA

Marcocci C, Cetani F, Rubin MR, et al: Parathyroid carcinoma. J Bone Miner Res 23:1869–1880, 2008.

Munson ND, Foote RL, Northcutt RC, et al: Parathyroid carcinoma: Is there a role for adjuvant radiation therapy? Cancer 98:2378-2384, 2003.

Silverberg SJ, Rubin MR, Faiman C, et al: Cinacalcet hydrochloride reduces the serum calcium concentration in inoperable parathyroid carcinoma. J Clin Endocrinol Metab 92:3803–3808, 2007.

Siperstein A, Berber E, Mackey R, et al: Prospective evaluation of sestamibi scan, ultrasonography, and rapid PTH to predict the success of limited exploration of sporadic primary hyperparathyroidism. Surgery 136:872–880, 2004.

CHAPTER 3

Non–small-cell lung cancer

Benjamin Movsas, MD, Julie Brahmer, MD, Channing Paller, MD, and Kemp H. Kernstine, MD, PhD

Lung cancer has been the leading cause of cancer death among men in the United States for years, and since 1988, it has become the number-one cause of cancer death among women. An estimated 222,520 new cases of lung cancer are expected in 2010, and 157,300 deaths due to this disease are expected to occur, roughly 28% of all cancer deaths. This exceeds the combined number of deaths from the next leading causes of cancer (breast, prostate, and colon cancers). It accounts for 6% of all deaths in the United States.

Lung cancer develops from pulmonary parenchymal or bronchial supportive tissues. Although multiple cell types are often found within a single lung tumor, one type usually predominates. Based on the therapeutic approach, there are two major subdivisions of lung cancer: small-cell lung cancer (SCLC), for which chemotherapy is the primary treatment, and non–small-cell lung cancer (NSCLC), which in its early stages (I and II) is treated primarily with surgery.

This chapter provides basic information on the epidemiology, etiology, screening, prevention, and signs and symptoms of lung cancer in general and then focuses specifically on the diagnosis, staging, pathology, and treatment of NSCLC and carcinoid tumors of the lungs, as well as the pulmonary evaluation of lung cancer patients and follow-up of long-term survivors.

Chapter 4 provides information on the staging, pathology and pathophysiology, and treatment of the far less common SCLC and concludes with brief discussions of mesothelioma and thymoma.

EPIDEMIOLOGY

Gender

In the United States, the estimated number of new lung cancer cases for 2010 is 116,750 for men and 105,770 for women. Although the incidence of lung cancer had been rising in women, the rate of increase has begun to slow recently. The incidence is decreasing in men.

Age

The age at which lung cancer patients are diagnosed varies widely, but the median age at diagnosis is approximately 70 years.

Race

In the United States, the highest incidence of lung cancer in men and women is found in African Americans (107.6/100,000 for men and 54.9/100,000 for women), followed by Caucasians (79.3/100,000 for men and 54.9/100,000 for women).

Geography

There are geographic variations in the incidence of lung cancer, with the highest rates worldwide observed in North America and Eastern Europe; in the United States, the highest rates are found in northern urban areas and along the southern coast from Texas to Florida. The state with the highest incidence of lung cancer is Kentucky, with an incidence of 136.2/100,000 in men and 76.2/100,000 in women.

NSC LUNG

Survival

The overall 5-year survival rate for lung cancer is 15%, of which there has been a 1% improvement each decade for the past 30 years.

ETIOLOGY AND RISK FACTORS

Cigarette smoking

Approximately 87% of all cases of lung cancer are related to cigarette smoking. There is a relatively strong dose-response relationship between cigarette smoking and the development of this cancer. The greater the number of cigarettes smoked on a daily basis and the greater the number of years of smoking, the greater is the risk of lung cancer. An individual who smokes one pack of cigarettes daily has a 20-fold increased risk of lung cancer compared with a nonsmoker.

The overall incidence of cigarette smoking decreased from 1974 through 1992. Smoking cessation decreases the risk of lung cancer, but a significant decrease in risk does not occur until approximately 5 years of discontinuation, and the risk remains higher in former smokers than in nonsmokers for at least 25 years. The benefit of smoking cessation is greater if it occurs at a younger age.

Smoking cessation is difficult. Recent data have suggested that a variety of hereditary factors increase the risk of addiction to nicotine among some individuals. Nevertheless, millions of former smokers have quit successfully. Smoking cessation programs that address both physical withdrawal from nicotine and psychological dependence appear to be more effective than either of these approaches alone. In addition, continued efforts are needed to prevent adolescents and preadolescents from beginning to smoke or to encourage them to quit after a brief period of experimentation.

Several cancer centers have recently reported that more than half of their patients with newly diagnosed lung cancer are former smokers, having quit more than 1 year before diagnosis. Healthy ex-smokers represent a large group of individuals who may benefit from effective tools for early detection and/or chemoprevention of lung cancer.

Secondhand smoke

Not only is smoking risky for those who smoke, but it also poses a hazard to nonsmokers who either live or work with smokers. It is estimated that approximately 3,000 lung cancer deaths per year in the United States are due to secondhand smoke. Individuals who live in a household with a smoker have a 30% increase in the incidence of lung cancer compared with nonsmokers who do not live in such an environment.

Asbestos exposure

Exposure to asbestos is another risk factor for lung cancer. Cigarette smokers who are exposed to asbestos develop lung cancer at an extremely high rate. There is a 90-fold increase compared with unexposed individuals. Exposure to asbestos is also a major risk factor for the development of mesothelioma (see discussion of this cancer in the following chapter).

Radioactive dust and radon exposure

Uranium miners who have been exposed to radioactive dust and radon gas also have an increased incidence of lung cancer. Although there has been some controversy about the risk posed by exposure to residential radon gas, a study conducted in Sweden showed an increased incidence of lung cancer in individuals who were exposed to a high level of radon in their homes.

SCREENING AND PREVENTION

Screening

Currently, screening for lung cancer among asymptomatic individuals at elevated risk due to smoking history or occupational exposures is not recommended. An unfortunate result of this policy is that most patients present in advanced stage, and cure rates have improved little over the past 30 years. Only 7% of NSCLC patients are diagnosed in stage IA.

Three randomized screening trials conducted in the United States in the 1970s failed to show a reduction in lung cancer mortality among the smokers who were screened by sputum cytology and chest x-ray for lung cancer. Despite the fact that these American trials were not designed to evaluate chest x-ray as a screening tool, the results led most experts to conclude that screening for lung cancer was not worthwhile. In addition, most investigators recommended that research efforts and resources be allocated to the *prevention* of lung cancer. A recent, randomized, prospective trial from Czechoslovakia showed that screening with a chest x-ray increased the diagnosis of early-stage lung cancer but failed to reduce the mortality from lung cancer.

The potential to screen for lung cancer has received renewed interest due to the superior performance of low-dose helical CT compared with chest radiography in detecting small lesions. Although there is insufficient evidence to establish policy related to routine screening for lung cancer with spiral CT, there is a growing trend toward promoting screening with this new technology to individuals at increased risk for lung cancer.

Numerous studies are currently under way to evaluate chest CT scan for lung cancer screening. Several recent reports from Japan, Germany, and the United States have documented the ability of low-dose spiral CT scans to detect lung cancer at an early stage. In some recent trials, more than 80% of lung cancers detected by screening were diagnosed in stage I.

Kaneko screened male smokers > 50 years of age. Of the 15 cancers detected by CT scan, only 4 were seen on chest x-ray; 14 of the 15 cancers were stage I, with an average diameter of 1.6 cm. Ohmatsu found 35 lung cancers (0.37% detection rate) with 9,452 CT scans. Of these cancers, 27 were stage IA. These patients had a 3-year survival rate of 83%.

The I-ELCAP (http://www.ielcap.org/professionals.htm) is a single-arm prospective study that has accrued more than 35,000 study subjects from 30 sites and documented that a high percentage of lung cancers are detected in stage I, a stage in which long-term survival can reasonably be anticipated in more than 60% of patients. These studies provide early evidence to suggest that CT lung cancer population screening has the potential to reduce lung cancer mortality in the near future.

In a controversial article from I-ELCAP, Henschke et al presented the results of their low-dose CT screening trial in 31,567 high-risk participants. CT was performed every 7 to 18 months. Lung cancer was found in 484 (1.5%), of whom 412 (85%) were stage I, with an 88% 10-year survival rate estimated in that cohort. Noncalcified pulmonary nodules were detected in 233 participants (23% [95% confidence interval (CI): 21–26]) by low-dose CT at baseline, compared with 68 (7% [95% CI: 5–9]) by chest radiography. Lung cancer was detected by CT in 27 patients (2.7% [95% CI: 1.8–3.8]) and by chest radiography in 7 patients (0.7% [95% CI: 0.3–1.3]).

Of the 27 CT-detected cancers, 26 were resectable. Stage I cancers were diagnosed in 23 of 27 patients (85%) by CT and 4 of 7 patients (57%) by chest radiography. In addition, low-dose CT detected four more nonparenchymal cases of lung cancer: two with endobronchial lesions and two in the mediastinum. These cases show an added benefit of low-dose CT over chest radiography, although the data were not included in the analysis. (The study primarily focused on malignant disease in noncalcified pulmonary nodules detected by low-dose CT or radiography.) It remains to be seen, however, whether lung cancer screening with low-dose spiral CT will reduce the lung cancer mortality of the study population or only improve the 5-year survival rate of the patients diagnosed with lung cancer.

Based on growing evidence that spiral CT may truly provide for a successful early detection strategy, NCI launched the NLST (http://www.nci.nih.gov/NLST) in September 2002. NLST has accrued 50,000 current and former smokers (aged 55–74) into a prospective trial, randomizing participants to receive annual spiral CT or annual chest x-rays. Survival data will not be available for a number of years.

The efficacy of lung cancer screening is also being evaluated as part of the PLCO. Men and women were randomized to receive annual chest x-ray vs usual care. Eligibility was not based on risk of lung cancer, because given the large size of the study (> 100,000 participants), it was expected that there would be appreciable numbers of current and former smokers among the participants.

In response to the I-ELCAP results, Bach et al reviewed the collective results of three prospective concurrently run randomized screening trials in 3,246 high-risk patients. They found no reduction in lung cancer deaths or advanced cancer in the screened groups.

The increased use of CT scanning in the United States, currently more than 62 million scans per year, has significantly increased the exposure to radiation in the population and may be a future health issue. The exposure to radiation from two to three CT scans in an adult is similar to that experienced by survivors of atomic bombs dropped on Japan in 1945. The risks associated with exposure to radiation are highest in children.

Biomarkers, proteomic evaluations, and circulating endothelial cells are currently under intensive investigation within and outside the Early Detection Research Network (http://edrn.nci.nih.gov/). The lack of demonstrated benefit for the earlier radiographic screening approaches should not be misinterpreted as nihilism about the early detection of lung cancer. Individuals at risk (current and former smokers) who present with symptoms consistent with lung cancer deserve appropriate evaluation. A lack of resolution of radiographic abnormalities on a chest x-ray obtained after the completion of empiric antibiotic therapy for pneumonia should prompt further evaluation for possible lung cancer.

Chemoprevention

The concept of field carcinogenesis was originally developed for the aerodigestive tract in the early 1950s. Reducing the exposure of the epithelial mucosa to carcinogens, predominately cigarette smoke, has the greatest impact on reducing the incidence of cancer in high-risk individuals.

The Finnish Alpha-Tocopherol Beta-Carotene Study evaluated 29,133 male smokers over 5 to 8 years, and there was an 18% increased incidence of lung cancer in the group taking beta-carotene. Other chemopreventative agents studied in a phase III fashion include retinol, aspirin, retinyl palmitate, etretinate, isotretinoin, α-tocopherol, 4-hydroxyphenyl retinamide, anethole dithiolethione, and N-acetylcysteine. None of them showed any preventive benefit.

Second primary lung tumors develop at a rate of 1% to 3% annually for the first 5 years following resection of stage I NSCLC.

The intergroup randomized trial that assessed the ability of 13-*cis*-retinoic acid to prevent the occurrence of a second primary cancer in patients with completely resected stage I NSCLC showed no impact of treatment on the incidence of second primary tumors. Furthermore, patients who continued to smoke and who received isotretinoin had a higher risk of recurrence of the index cancer. Also, there was no reduction in second primary tumors in the 13-*cis*-retinoic acid-treated group. Trials using cyclooxygenase-2 inhibition are yet to be reported in former and current smokers. Tyrosine kinase inhibition is currently being studied to reverse bronchial premalignant lesions and Ki-67 levels in the Lung Cancer Biomarkers Chemoprevention Consortium trial.

Selenium as L-selenomethionine has been shown to inhibit cell growth, induce apoptosis in vitro, and retard carcinogenesis at higher dose levels in animal models.

Epidemiologic data suggest an inverse relationship between selenium intake and lung cancer.

In a study by Clark et al designed to determine the effects of selenium on the incidence of basal or squamous cell carcinomas, nutritional supplementation with this agent showed no consequences on the incidence of skin cancer; however, secondary analyses revealed that it was associated with significantly fewer cases of lung cancer.

A phase III intergroup selenium prevention trial has been designed to follow the lung cancer isotretinoin prevention trial. To reduce the incidence of second primary tumors, this double-blind design is randomizing patients by a 2:1 ratio to receive either selenomethionine (200 μg/d) vs placebo daily for 48 months. Patients are monitored for safety, development of second primary tumors, and recurrence. A total of 1,552 patients have been entered into the run-in phase, and of them, 1,375 have been enrolled in the trial. Based on enrollment to date, the projected goal of 1,960 patients should be reached by February 2011.

Educational programs

Although the information from the intergroup randomized chemoprevention study is being collected, it is important to continue educational efforts to prevent adolescents from smoking cigarettes and to advocate smoking cessation in active smokers. Some experts believe that educational programs must begin during childhood, probably between the ages of 6 and 10 years. Targeting children and young adults is a significant priority of any lung cancer reduction program.

SIGNS AND SYMPTOMS

The clinical manifestations of lung cancer depend on the location and extent of the tumor. In patients who have localized disease, the most common symptoms are related to obstruction of major airways; infiltration of lung parenchyma; and invasion of surrounding structures, including the chest wall, major blood vessels, and viscera.

Cough

Cough is a major manifestation of lung cancer and is present in nearly 80% of patients with symptomatic lung cancer. It is important to remember, however, that most lung cancer patients are current or former smokers and may have a cough related to chronic irritation of the upper and/or lower airways from cigarette smoke. Therefore, smokers should be asked whether there has been a change in their cough, such as an increase in frequency or severity.

Dyspnea and hemoptysis

Increasing dyspnea and hemoptysis may be signs of lung cancer, although in the case of hemoptysis, 70% of patients bleed from nonmalignant causes, mostly infection, and more frequently, bronchitis. In patients who present with hemoptysis, are older than age 40, and have a history of smoking and chronic obstructive pulmonary disease without an abnormality on chest radiograph, lung cancer should be considered in the differential diagnosis.

Pneumonia

Postobstructive pneumonia secondary to partial or complete bronchial obstruction occurs relatively frequently in association with lung cancer. It is important to obtain repeat chest x-rays in adults who have been treated for pneumonia to be certain that the radiographic abnormalities have cleared completely.

Pleural effusion

Lung cancer may spread to the pleural surface or may obstruct segmental or lobar lymphatics, resulting in pleural effusion and increased dyspnea.

Chest pain

Approximately 5% of lung tumors invade the chest wall. The resultant pain is a better predictor of chest wall invasion than are chest CT findings. An individual who complains of persistent chest pain should have a chest x-ray to exclude the presence of peripheral lung cancer that has invaded the chest wall.

Shoulder and arm pain

Apical tumors that infiltrate surrounding structures (also called Pancoast tumors) produce shoulder and/or arm pain as a result of brachial plexus compression. Tumors in the apical lung segments may be difficult to detect on a routine chest x-ray; therefore, a person who complains of persistent shoulder pain, particularly with signs of neurologic involvement, should have a CT scan of the chest to look for an apical tumor. An MRI scan of the chest apex may be beneficial. It is also important to examine the lung apex in bone films obtained to evaluate shoulder pain.

Horner's syndrome

Invasion of the sympathetic ganglion by an apical lung tumor causes Horner's syndrome (ptosis, myosis, and ipsilateral anhidrosis).

Hoarseness

Hoarseness secondary to vocal cord paresis or paralysis occurs when tumors and lymph node metastases compress, cause dysfunction in, or invade the recurrent laryngeal nerve. This situation is more common on the left side, where the recurrent laryngeal nerve passes under the aortic arch, but it may also occur with high lesions on the right side of the mediastinum.

Other symptoms of tumor compression

Lung tumors may also cause dysphagia by compression or invasion of the esophagus or superior vena cava syndrome by compression or invasion of this vascular structure.

Some tumors may result in wheezing or stridor secondary to compression or invasion of the trachea and may also cause signs of cardiac tamponade secondary to involvement of the pericardial surface and subsequent accumulation of pericardial fluid.

Signs and symptoms of metastatic disease

Lung cancer can metastasize to multiple sites, most commonly to bone, liver, brain, lungs (contralateral or ipsilateral), and adrenal glands.

A lung cancer patient who has brain metastases may complain of headaches or specific neurologic symptoms, or family members may notice a decrease in the patient's mental acuity. Also, metastatic lung cancer may cause spinal cord compression, resulting in a characteristic sequence of symptoms: pain, followed by motor dysfunction, and then sensory symptoms. The patient may have any or all of these symptoms.

Patients who complain of band-like pain encircling one or both sides of the trunk may have spinal cord compression. In addition, coughing and sneezing may cause significant exacerbation of pain from spinal cord compression.

Bone x-rays and/or a bone scan are warranted in lung cancer patients who complain of persistent pain in the trunk or extremities. If performed in the evaluation of lung cancer, ^{18}F-fluorodeoxyglucose (FDG)-PET supplants the need for a bone scan in most patients. PET appears to be more sensitive but less specific for bone metastases. If plain films are normal or equivocal for metastases, CT and/or MRI may be helpful to evaluate suspicious areas. MRI of the spine is the most effective way to evaluate suspected spinal cord compression.

Systemic paraneoplastic symptoms

Lung cancer is commonly associated with systemic manifestations, including weight loss (with or without anorexia). In addition, patients frequently complain of fatigue and generalized weakness. SCLC is associated with hormone production, which causes endocrine syndromes in a subset of patients, such as SIADH (syndrome of inappropriate antidiuretic hormone secretion) and via secretion of ACTH (adrenocorticotropic hormone) hypercortisolism.

Specific neurologic syndromes

Such syndromes, such as Lambert-Eaton syndrome (see chapter 39), cortical cerebellar degeneration, and peripheral neuropathy, may occur in lung cancer patients but are relatively rare.

Clubbing

Although clubbing may occur in a variety of conditions, it is important for the clinician to evaluate a patient's hands. If clubbing is noted, obtaining a chest x-ray may result in the early diagnosis of lung cancer.

Hypertrophic pulmonary osteoarthropathy

A relatively small percentage of patients with lung cancer may present with symptomatic hypertrophic osteoarthropathy. In this syndrome, periosteal inflammation results in pain in affected areas, most commonly the ankles and knees. It is frequently associated with clubbing.

Carcinoid syndrome

This syndrome is extremely uncommon in patients who have a bronchial carcinoid tumor. Most of these patients are asymptomatic (tumors are found by x-ray), and a few have cough from an endobronchial lesion.

TABLE 1: TNM7 staging of lung cancer

Description	Definitions
T	**Primary tumor**
T0	No primary tumor
T1	Tumor ≤ 3 cm[a], surrounded by lung or visceral pleura, no bronchoscopic evidence of invasion, more proximal than the lobar bronchus
T1a	Tumor ≤ 2 cm[a]
T1b	Tumor > 2 but ≤ 3 cm[a]
T2	Tumor > 3 but ≤ 7 cm[a] or tumor with any of the following[b]: Invades visceral pleura, involves main bronchus ≥ 2 cm distal to the carina, atelectasis/obstructive pneumonia extending to hilum but not involving the entire lung
T2a	Tumor > 3 but ≤ 5 cm[a]
T2b	Tumor > 5 but ≤ 7 cm[a]
T3	Tumor > 7 cm or directly invading chest wall, diaphragm, phrenic nerve, mediastinal pleura, or parietal pericardium; or tumor in the main bronchus < 2 cm distal to the carina[c]; or atelectasis/obstructive pneumonitis of entire lung; or separate tumor nodules in the same lobe
T4	Tumor of any size with invasion of heart, great vessels, trachea, recurrent laryngeal nerve, esophagus, vertebral body, or carina; or separate tumor nodules in a different ipsilateral lobe
N	**Regional lymph nodes**
N0	No regional node metastasis
N1	Metastasis in ipsilateral peribronchial and/or perihilar lymph nodes and intrapulmonary nodes, including involvement by direct extension
N2	Metastasis in ipsilateral mediastinal and/or subcarinal lymph nodes
N3	Metastasis in contralateral mediastinal, contralateral hilar, ipsilateral or contralateral scalene, or supraclavicular lymph nodes
M	**Distant metastasis**
M0	No distant metastasis
M1a	Separate tumor nodules in a contralateral lobe; or tumor with pleural nodules or malignant pleural dissemination[d]
M1b	Distant metastasis
Special situations	
T, N, M	T, N, or M status not able to be assessed
Tis	Focus of in situ cancer
T1	Superficial spreading tumor of any size but confined to the wall of the trachea or mainstream bronchus

From Detterbeck FC, Boffa DJ, Tanoue LT: Chest 136:260–271, 2009; Goldstraw P, Crowley J, Chansky K, et al: J Thorac Oncol 2:706–714, 2007; Rami-Porta R, Ball D, Crowley J, et al: J Thorac Oncol 2:593–602, 2007.

These subgroup labels are not defined in the IASLC publications but are added here to facilitate a clear discussion.

[a] In the greatest dimension.

[b] T2 tumors with these features are classified as T2a if ≤ 5 cm.

[c] The uncommon superficial spreading tumor in central airways is classified as T1.

[d] Pleural effusions that are cytologically negative, nonbloody, transudative, and clinically judged not to be due to cancer are excluded.

TABLE 1: TNM7 staging of lung cancer ***(continued)***

TNM Elements in Staged Groups			
Stage groups	**T**	**N**	**M**
Ia	T1a, b	N0	M0
Ib	T2a	N0	M0
IIa	T1a, b	N1	M0
	T2a	N1	M0
	T2b	N0	M0
IIb	T2b	N1	M0
	T3	N0	M0
IIIa	T1–3	N2	M0
	T3	N1	M0
	T4	N0, 1	M0
IIIb	T4	N2	M0
	T1–4	N3	M0
IV	Any T	Any N	M1a, b

T and M		N0	N1	N2	N3
6th edition TNM	**7th edition TNM**	**Stage**	**Stage**	**Stage**	**Stage**
T1 (≤ 3 cm)	T1a (≤ 2 cm)	IA	IIA	IIIA	IIIB
	T1b (> 2–3 cm)	IA	IIA	IIIA	IIIB
T2 (> 3 cm)	T2a (> 3–5 cm)	IB	IIA (IIB)[a]	IIIA	IIIB
	T2b (> 5–7 cm)	IIA (IB)[a]	IIB	IIIA	IIIB
	T2c (> 7 cm)	IIB (IB)[a]	IIIA (IIB)[a]	IIIA	IIIB
T3 (invasion)	T3	IIB	IIIA	IIIA	IIIB
T4 (same lobe nodules)	T4	IIB (IIIB)[a]	IIIA (IIIB)[a]	IIIA (IIIB)[a]	IIIB
T4 (extension)	T4	IIIA (IIIB)[a]	IIIA (IIIB)[a]	IIIB	IIIB
M1 (ipsilateral lung)	T4	IIIA (IV)[a]	IIIA (IV)[a]	IIIA (IV)[a]	IIIA (IV)[a]
T4 (pleural effusion)	M1a	IV (IIIB)[a]	IV (IIIB)[a]	IV (IIIB)[a]	IV (IIIB)[a]
M1 (contralateral lung)	M1a	IV	IV	IV	IV
M1 (distant)	M1b	IV	IV	IV	IV

[a] Change in classification with the 7th edition.

TUMOR BIOLOGY

Non–small-cell tumors account for approximately 85% of all lung cancers. The three major tumor types included under this category are adenocarcinoma, squamous cell carcinoma, and large-cell carcinoma.

STAGING AND PROGNOSIS

Staging

2009 changes to TNM The staging of lung cancer must be conducted in a methodical and detailed manner. The TNM staging system (Table 1) applies equally well to all histologies of NSCLC, but TNM for SCLC is less helpful. Most patients have advanced disease at the time of presentation.

Stage is commonly reported as either clinical or pathologic, designated as c or p, respectively. Clinical stage is based on noninvasive (or minimally invasive) tests, whereas pathologic stage is based on tissue obtained during surgery (see section on "Diagnosis and staging evaluation").

The IASLC has developed changes in the TNM system (TNM 7) based on an international collection and review of 100,809 patients.

1. Moving tumors > 7 cm from T2 to T3
2. Reassigning the category given to additional pulmonary nodules in some locations
3. Reclassifying pleural effusion as an M descriptor.

In addition:

1. T2b, N0, M0 cases can be moved from stage IB to stage IIA
2. T2a, N1, M0 cases can be moved from stage IIB to stage IIA
3. T4, N0–1, M0 cases can be moved from stage IIIB to stage IIIA.

Prognostic factors

Stage

The most important prognostic factor in lung cancer is the stage of disease.

Performance status and weight loss

Within a given disease stage, the next most important prognostic factors are performance status and recent, unexplained weight loss. The two scales used to define performance status are the ECOG performance status system and the Karnofsky system (see Appendix 1) or the Zubrod system. Simply, patients who are ambulatory have a significantly longer survival than those who are nonambulatory. Similarly, patients who have lost > 5% of body weight during the preceding 3–6 months have a worse prognosis than patients who have not lost a significant amount of weight.

The ongoing CALGB 14020 and SWOG 0720 are two examples of prospective trials using molecular information to guide therapy. Patients less likely to benefit from adjuvant therapy are monitored for recurrence, and those exhibiting certain molecular features receive treatment. "Personalized medicine" is expected to have a greater role in preventing recurrence in early-stage lung cancer.

Molecular prognostic factors

Several studies published over the past decade have indicated that mutations of *ras* proto-oncogenes, particularly *KRAS*, portend a poor prognosis in NSCLC, and in the case of adenocarcinomas, are more frequently found in smokers. Accordingly, selective research has focused on developing molecularly targeted therapeutic approaches to the *ras* proto-oncogenes, in particular, the farnesyl transferase inhibitors as well as epidermal growth factor receptor (EGFR) inhibitors and antiangiogenic approaches (see section on "Novel and promising agents").

Of equal relevance was the completion of large studies by Pastorino et al and Kwiatowski et al evaluating the prognostic importance of immunocytochemical and molecular pathologic markers in stage I NSCLC.

In the study by Pastorino et al, gene-expression profiles were performed in 198 tumor samples to develop a predictive model for recurrence, the lung metagene model. The model was then tested in three cohorts of stage IA patients and was found to be highly accurate in predicting the likelihood of recurrence. By identifying patients who are likely to experience recurrence, adjuvant therapy is more likely to be effective. In the study by Kwiatowski et al, gene-expression profiles were performed in 185 frozen samples, and a 5-gene signature that correlated with relapse-free and overall survival was identified.

The findings of these two studies suggest that pathologic stage and completeness of surgical resection may yield the most critical prognostic information, but mutation of the *KRAS* oncogene and absence of expression of the *HRAS* p21 proto-oncogene may augment the pathologic information. Further data indicate that a molecular prognostic model differentiating patients with lung cancer may be possible using proteomics or other molecular biology techniques.

Molecular profiling has been described as a means to molecularly characterize tumors and to identify the metastatic potential and regional growth character. Other molecular markers that portend a poor prognosis include reduced expression of RASSF1A and FHIT (fragile histidine triad); reduced expression of catenins and E-cadherin; reduced ERCC1 and RRM1; reduction in tumor suppressor genes *p53*, retinoblastoma gene, *p16INK4A*, and *p15INK4B*; increased telomerase activity; overexpression of EGFR (c-ErbB-1), matrix metalloproteinase, HER2/*neu* (c-Erb-2), and vascular endothelial growth factor (VEGF); c-Met overexpression; overexpression of mutated *p53*; urokinase plasminogen activator overexpression; promoters of angiogenesis; reduced expression of *nm23* gene; and low KAI1/CD82.

Potti et al used microarray techniques to study prognosis in stage I NSCLC. Their results indicated that the lung metagene model offers a potential mechanism to estimate a patient's risk of disease recurrence and, in principle, to affect decisions regarding the use of adjuvant chemotherapy in early-stage NSCLC.

Quality of life (QOL)

RTOG reanalyzed the results of RTOG 9801 to assess the added value of QOL as a prognostic factor for overall survival. On multivariate analysis, they found that the global QOL score superseded the classic predictors of survival (eg, Karnofsky performance status, stage, etc) in patients with locally advanced NSCLC. Patients with a global QOL score less than the median (66.7 of 100) had a 70% higher rate of death than patients with a QOL ≥ 66.7 ($P = .002$). Of note, patients who were married or had a partner had higher QOL scores than those who were not ($P = .004$). A clinically meaningful increase in the QOL score (of 10 points) corresponded to a decrease in the hazard of death by 10% ($P = .002$). This study highlights the "added value" of patient-reported outcomes and the need to incorporate QOL measures into clinical oncology trials.

DIAGNOSIS AND STAGING EVALUATION

History and physical examination

The diagnosis and preoperative staging of lung cancer begin with a good history and physical examination. When obtaining the history, the clinician should keep in mind the tendency for lung cancer to involve major airways and other central structures. Similarly, the patterns of metastatic dissemination and systemic manifestations must be considered when conducting the physical examination.

Patients should be questioned specifically about the presence of palpable masses, dysphagia, bone pain, headache, or changes in vision. Careful auscultation and percussion may suggest the presence of atelectasis or pleural effusion. Auscultation of the chest also may provide evidence of large airway obstruction and pulmonary consolidation. Rhonchi and wheezing may provide some helpful treatment planning information. An enlarged liver may indicate hepatic metastases.

Palpation of the neck and supraclavicular fossa

Discovery of adenopathy of the neck and supraclavicular fossa may allow both diagnosis and staging, by needle or open biopsy.

Imaging studies

Chest x-rays

These provide initial helpful information in patients with new respiratory symptoms. Posteroanterior and lateral chest x-rays are fundamental in assessing the local extent of the primary tumor and also may provide valuable information regarding metastatic disease.

The chest x-ray should be inspected for the presence of a pleural effusion or synchronous pulmonary nodules, and the bones should be examined for evidence of osseous metastases. A widened mediastinum usually indicates metastatic disease within the mediastinal lymph nodes. Comparison with previous x-rays is helpful and well worth the effort expended in their retrieval.

Chest CT from the lower neck to the mid level of the kidneys

Testing of this area, including the entire liver and adrenal glands with 5- to 10-mm slices, is performed routinely to further define the primary tumor and to identify lymphatic or parenchymal metastases. In a review of 20 studies that assessed the value of CT scan to determine mediastinal lymph node involvement, with an average prevalence of 28%, CT had a pooled sensitivity of 57%, a specificity of 82%, and a negative predictive value (NPV) of 83%. Benign enlargement of mediastinal nodes is more common in patients with postobstructive infection. Histologic confirmation of the presence or absence of tumor within the mediastinal lymph nodes is necessary whenever this information will change treatment recommendations. In patients who are considered surgical candidates, metastatic tumor is found in approximately 15% to 20% of mediastinal lymph nodes < 1 cm in greatest diameter.

In mediastinal nodes > 1 cm by CT that are negative by FDG-PET, the false-negative rate is 13% to 25%, and the false-positive rate is approximately 56%.

It is important to remember that patients with persistent symptoms, such as cough and dyspnea, who have a normal chest x-ray may be harboring a central lesion that is not obvious on chest x-ray but can be easily detected by chest CT. Also, as previously mentioned, apical tumors (Pancoast tumors) may be difficult to detect on a chest radiograph but are usually readily apparent on a CT scan.

PET

For lung masses, FDG accumulation on PET implies a significant likelihood of malignancy.

The maximum standardized uptake value (SUV) threshold of 2.5 within the region of interest optimizes the sensitivity and specificity of PET in assessing suspicious lung lesions larger than 1 cm. An FDG-avid lesion on PET should never be assumed to be malignant, and a PET-negative lesion is not absolutely benign. Bronchioloalveolar and carcinoid are two cell types that do not readily accumulate FDG. Furthermore, higher SUV lesions do not imply a greater likelihood of cancer; the highest SUVs have been found in inflammatory lesions, such as granulomas and infections.

A review of 18 studies of the utility of PET to assess the mediastinal lymph nodes demonstrated a pooled sensitivity of 84% and a specificity of 89%, with a positive predictive value (PPV) of 79% and an NPV of 93%. Combining the results of CT and PET, the PPV and NPV were 83% to 93% and 88% to 95%, respectively. Thus, FDG-PET is superior to CT scanning in staging the mediastinal lymph nodes. An estimated 15% to 20% of patients with a known or suspected diagnosis benefit from a preoperative FDG-PET, because previously unrecognized metastatic disease will be discovered.

The false-negative rate can be as high as 25% to 30% for CT, PET, and PET-CT when the prevalence of mediastinal involvement is higher, such as in cases of lesions being large and/or more centrally located and/or when there is hilar lymph node involvement.

Several trials have evaluated the prognostic significance of FDG uptake on PET scan in NSCLC. Utilizing multivariate Cox analysis, these studies noted that SUV_{max} (maximum SUV within the region-of-interest) of the primary lesion, particularly when > 7 to 10, was an independent prognostic factor.

PET scanning may also prove a valuable tool for staging and evaluating patients undergoing radiation therapy and patients with NSCLC treated with chemoradiotherapy or irradiation. In a study by MacManus et al, the PET response after treatment was found to be a powerful predictor of survival.

Adrenal gland

The adrenal gland may be the sole site of metastatic disease in as many as 10% of patients with NSCLC, though patients with adrenal masses should not be assumed to have metastatic disease and should not be denied a potentially curative surgery on the basis of a scan alone. Less than 1% of adrenal masses at least 1 cm that are negative on FDG-PET are malignant. Contrast-enhanced MRI-weighted images may assist in achieving a diagnosis. Suspicious adrenal masses should be either biopsied or resected in potentially operable patients to confirm the stage of disease.

Obtaining a tissue diagnosis

The next step is to obtain a histologic or cytologic diagnosis of the radiologically revealed lesion, although preoperative histologic diagnosis need not be obtained in a highly suspicious lung mass without evidence of distant or locoregional metastases (see below).

Central lesions

Collecting daily sputum cytologies for 3 consecutive days provides a cytologic diagnosis for central lesions 71% of the time and for peripheral lesions 49% of the time. In clinically suspicious lung nodules/masses, a negative sputum cytology result warrants further clinical investigation. Flexible bronchoscopy is commonly required to achieve a diagnosis. For central lesions that are exophytic, at least three direct forceps biopsies should be performed to achieve a 74% sensitivity. Washings and brushings add to the sensitivity but by themselves have a sensitivity of 48% and 59%, respectively. Further improved sensitivity is obtained with bronchoscopic fluoroscopically directed transbronchial needle aspiration biopsies. For central lesions, the overall sensitivity for flexible bronchoscopy is, in experienced hands, 88%.

In addition, bronchoscopy may provide important staging information, such as whether the tumor involves the distal trachea or carina, and may help surgeons to plan the appropriate operation (lobectomy or sleeve resection vs pneumonectomy). Determining the degree of bronchial involvement assists surgical planning. Bronchoscopy-directed biopsies should be performed to assist in determining the intended line of resection, especially when evaluating for submucosal involvement. One to two percent of patients with lung cancer will have an endobronchial synchronous primary or metastatic lesion.

Peripheral lesions

Bronchoscopy is less likely to yield a diagnosis in patients with peripherally located lesions. Bronchoscopic ability to make a diagnosis of malignancy in peripheral lesions is dependent upon size; for those less than 2 cm, the sensitivity is 33%, and for lesions greater than 2 cm, it is 62%. If a bronchiole is seen traversing or extending to the mass on CT, the sensitivity is reported to be twice as high, nearly 60%.

TABLE 2: Selective indications for mediastinoscopy

Enlarged N1, N2, or N3 lymph nodes on chest CT scan
FDG-PET–positive mediastinal disease
Centrally located tumors
T2–T4 tumors

Newer image-guided bronchoscopic technologies are being investigated to improve diagnostic capabilities.

Electromagnetic-directed navigational bronchoscopy uses CT-derived information and corresponding anatomic features to accurately direct bronchoscopic biopsies. For patients with solitary pulmonary nodules that are ≤ 3 cm in maximum diameter, there is an intermediary risk of malignancy, and diagnosis can be a challenge. Electromagnetic navigation bronchoscopy may offer an additional diagnostic means of achieving brushings, washings, and directed biopsies.

A CT-guided needle biopsy may diagnose up to 90% of peripheral lung cancers but is dependent on the quality of the CT scan and the experience of the radiologist performing the procedure. The false-negative rate is 20% to 30%. Needle biopsy is usually reserved for patients who are not candidates for an operation due to distant metastatic disease or poor health or performance status. If the patient is a candidate for surgery, resection is generally recommended for any suspicious mass, whether the result of needle biopsy is positive or nondiagnostic. Therefore, for patients with a suspicious peripheral lesion that is not associated with pleural effusion, mediastinal adenopathy, or other evidence of metastatic disease, it is reasonable to proceed directly to surgery.

Mediastinoscopy

Mediastinoscopy is a time-tested technique whereby the middle (cervical mediastinoscopy) and the anterior mediastinum may be assessed for direct or metastatic lymph node involvement. In the hands of a specialist, the risk of biopsy trauma to local structures (great vessels, trachea, or esophagus), bleeding, recurrent nerve paresis, infection, or death is minimal. Whole-node biopsies may be taken, achieving a great deal of information about the location, number of nodal stations involved, number of metastatic lymph nodes within each station, degree of nodal involvement, and lymph node capsular invasion. There is no evidence that mediastinoscopic biopsy spreads tumor within the mediastinum, worsens the prognosis, or renders eventual surgical mediastinal dissection difficult. The sensitivity of mediastinoscopy is estimated to be between 85% and 92%, with a specificity of 100% and a false-negative rate of 3% to 10%.

With the advent of videoscopic technology, the video-assisted mediastinal lymphadenectomy (VAMLA) and the transcervical extended mediastinal lymphadenectomy (TEMLA) have been described, whereby extensive mediastinal evaluation and lymph node resection are performed. The additional 1 to 2 hours required to perform these procedures and slightly increased patient discomfort are offset by the significant improvement in the access to the nodal stations, acquisition of lymph nodes, and improved staging and therapeutic potential. The sensitivity of TEMLA (94%) is superior to that of mediastinoscopy, with a negligible false-negative rate.

> In a group of 151 NSCLC patients at high risk for mediastinal nodal involvement, EBUS and EUS were falsely negative in 28% and 22%, respectively *(Cerfolio RJ et al: 46th Annual Meeting of the Society of Thoracic Surgeons; January 24–26, 2010; Fort Lauderdale, Florida; abstract 34).*

Selective indications for mediastinoscopy are listed in Table 2. To assess response to therapy, repeat mediastinoscopy has been performed, with few complications. Patients with N2 disease may potentially benefit from neoadjuvant treatment. Patients with N3 disease are considered to be stage IIIB and less likely to benefit from surgical resection. A few retrospective reports have demonstrated survival from induction therapy in patients with microscopic N3 involvement.

Endobronchial ultrasonography (EBUS) and endoesophageal ultrasonography (EUS) staging

EBUS is a real-time means of directly evaluating mediastinal masses and lymph nodes to direct transtracheal and transbronchial fine-needle and core aspiration/biopsy. Often performed under general anesthesia and combined with EUS, it provides access to all of the paratracheal, subcarinal, and proximal hilar lymph node stations. It may reduce the need for mediastinoscopy.

Real-time transesophageal biopsies by EUS can be performed on mediastinal tumors and the lymph nodes with sensitivity and accuracy comparable to EBUS. EUS provides access to lymph node stations in the posterior mediastinum in the mid to distal periesophageal lymph nodes, involved in 10% to 15% of patients. Both are minimal-access procedures that can be performed with little risk.

Thoracentesis and thoracoscopy

Individuals who have pleural effusions should undergo thoracentesis. Video-assisted thoracoscopic surgery (VATS) should be used to assess patients who have cytology-negative effusions. Sixty percent of patients with known pleural disease and effusions will have cytology-negative effusions. However, lung cancer patients with exudative cytology-negative effusions and their cytology-positive counterparts appear to have equally poor survival. VATS permits direct visualization of the pleural surface, enables direct biopsy of the pleural nodules, and also may facilitate biopsy of ipsilateral mediastinal lymph nodes. The role of VATS to assess effusions remains to be elucidated.

Measurement of serum tumor-associated antigens

This has no current role in the staging of NSCLC.

Diagnosis and evaluation of suspected carcinoid tumor

A carcinoid tumor of the lungs may be suspected in a patient with a slowly enlarging pulmonary mass and a prolonged history of respiratory symptoms. Patients usually have no symptoms. Most tumors are located centrally and exist endobronchially. When they occur, symptoms may include wheezing, recurrent pneumonia, dyspnea, and potentially paraneoplastic syndromes. Bronchoscopy frequently assists in diagnosing the lesion. The finding of a polypoid, pale, firm mass should not lull the bronchoscopist into taking a large-forceps biopsy. First, these masses are frequently vascular, and massive bleeding has been reported; second, the entire mass can be accidentally removed, making it difficult to identify the site of the original location of the polyp.

Given the bleeding potential, rigid bronchoscopy may be a better way to assess these lesions. Especially with cytology, carcinoid tumors may be difficult to differentiate from small-cell and atypical carcinoid tumors. Carcinoid tumor should be suspected when a small-cell tumor diagnosis by fine-needle aspiration does not respond to therapy. True carcinoids will have metastatic nodal disease in 5% to 10% of patients and have an excellent prognosis with surgical resection. Atypical carcinoid tumors are differentiated from typical tumors in that they have more than two mitotic figures per high-powered field and areas of necrosis.

Unlike its infradiaphragmatic counterpart, pulmonary carcinoid tumors rarely present with paraneoplastic syndromes, including carcinoid syndrome, acromegaly, and Cushing syndrome. Therefore, it is only necessary to measure urinary 5-hydroxyindoleacetic acid (5-HIAA) excretion prior to surgery in symptomatic patients. Less than 3% of all patients with pulmonary carcinoid tumors have detectable urinary 5-HIAA.

Intraoperative staging

Intraoperative staging is an integral part of any operation for lung cancer. In addition to the thorough visual and tactile inspection of the lungs, diaphragm, and pleura, the ipsilateral mediastinal lymph nodes must be either completely removed or at least sampled.

The American Thoracic Society has assigned numbered levels to locations in which lymph nodes are regularly found, defined by their relation to constant anatomic structures. A complete mediastinal lymph node dissection is associated with little morbidity and lengthens the operation only slightly.

Pulmonary evaluation

To determine the volume of lung that can be removed without rendering the patient a pulmonary cripple and to identify those individuals at risk for postoperative complications, each patient may undergo pulmonary function testing, spirometry, and potentially a diffusing capacity. The results of pulmonary testing should be referenced to the normal values for ethnicity, height, age, and gender rather than the absolute value.

Forced expiratory volume in 1 second

Postoperative respiratory failure rarely occurs if the postresection forced expiratory volume in 1 second (FEV_1) is > 30% of predicted. Regardless of the extent of the scheduled resection (lobectomy or pneumonectomy), if the preoperative FEV_1 is < 60% of predicted, a split-function perfusion scan may be obtained to determine the contribution of each lung region to overall pulmonary function. This information may be critical when an unplanned pneumonectomy is required to achieve complete tumor resection.

TABLE 3: WHO and IASLC guidelines for the histologic classification of lung cancer

I Adenocarcinoma
- i. Adenocarcinoma with mixed subtypes
  1. Well-differentiated fetal adenocarcinoma
  2. Mucinous adenocarcinoma
  3. Mucinous cystadenocarcinoma
  4. Clear cell adenocarcinoma
  5. Signet ring adenocarcinoma
- ii. Acinar
- iii. Papillary
- iv. Bronchioloalveolar carcinoma
  1. Mucinous
  2. Nonmucinous
  3. Mixed mucinous and nonmucinous
- v. Solid adenocarcinoma with mucin

II Squamous cell carcinoma
- i. Papillary
- ii. Small-cell
- iii. Clear cell
- iv. Basaloid

III Large-cell carcinoma
- i. Large-cell neuroendocrine carcinoma
- ii. Basaloid carcinoma
- iii. Lymphoepithelioma-like carcinoma
- iv. Mixed large-cell neuroendocrine carcinoma
- v. Clear cell carcinoma with rhabdoid phenotype

IV Adenosquamous carcinoma

V Carcinomas with pleomorphic, sarcomatous characteristics
- i. Carcinosarcoma
- ii. Pulmonary blastoma
- iii. Carcinomas with spindle and/or giant cells
  1. Giant cell carcinoma
  2. Spindle cell carcinoma
  3. Pleomorphic carcinoma
- iv. Other

VI Carcinoid
- i. Typical carcinoid
- ii. Atypical carcinoid

VII Carcinomas of salivary gland origin
- i. Adenoid cystic carcinoma
- ii. Mucoepidermoid carcinoma
- iii. Others

VIII Unclassified

Adapted from the World Health Organization (WHO): Histologic typing of lung tumors. In: International Classification of Tumors. Geneva, Switzerland: WHO, 1991; Travis WD, Colby TV, Corrin B, et al: World Health Organization: Histological Typing of Lung and Pleural Tumours, 3rd ed. Berlin: Springer-Verlag, 1999; Detterbeck FC, Boffa DJ, Tanoue LT: Chest 136:262–271, 2009.
IASLC = International Association for the Study of Lung Cancer

> An analysis of 18,800 patients from the Society of Thoracic Surgeons National Database showed the odds ratios for morbidity and mortality for surgical resection of NSCLC patients to be unavailable and 3.9, respectively, for pneumonectomy, 2.5 and 3.1 for poor performance status (Zubrod ≥ 3), 2.0 and 3.6 for poor physical status (ASA ≥ 4), 2.0 and 2.1 for induction therapy; 1.9 and unavailable for lobectomy vs wedge resection, 1.7 and 2.5 for renal insufficiency, 1.6 and 1.9 for treatment with steroids, 1.6 and unavailable for thoracotomy vs VATS, 1.5 and unavailable for heart failure; 1.5 and unavailable for smoking within 30 days, 1.2 and 1.8 for every 10 years of age, unavailable and 1.7 for urgent surgery, 1.1 and 1.1 for every 10% reduced in FEV_1, unavailable and 1.4 for male gender, and 0.8 and 0.7 for every increase of 10 kg/m^2 in body mass index *(Kozower BD: 46th Annual Meeting of the Society of Thoracic Surgeons; January 24–26, 2010; Fort Lauderdale, Florida; abstract 2)*.

Other pulmonary function tests

A diffusing capacity of the lung for carbon monoxide (D_LCOa; a = adjusted for the patient's hemoglobin level) < 60% of the predicted value or a maximum voluntary ventilation < 35% is associated with increased postoperative morbidity. All presurgical patients should have DLCO measured, because a surprising number have a normal FEV1 and an abnormally low DLCO that might have an impact on the surgical management. Patients with a baseline oximetry saturation of less than 90% and those who desaturate more than 4% with exercise have a greater likelihood of postoperative complications. Arterial blood gas Pco_2 > 45 mm Hg is an independent risk factor for increased operative morbidity and mortality.

In patients with borderline lung function, further physiologic testing may be required to better estimate pulmonary reserve prior to and after surgery. Quantitative pulmonary ventilation-perfusion scanning may assist in this endeavor. The perfusion portion is used to calculate the percentage of lung to be removed and the estimated postoperative percentage of normal. An additional test is exercise pulmonary function testing. Patients are monitored for heart rate, rhythm, blood pressure, and oxygen consumption. Patients who reach their target heart rate and exercise capacity and who have a maximal oxygen consumption > 15 mL/kg/min are less likely to have a postoperative complication and mortality.

Pathology

The WHO and the IASLC have devised guidelines for the histologic classification of lung cancer, which are revised as necessary (Table 3). The different cell-type classifications are performed using light microscopy and do not require electron microscopy or immunohistochemistry. There are variations in the natural history of the different cell types and potential differences in response to treatment and survival. Overall, 90% to 95% of NSCLCs are adenocarcinomas, squamous, or large cell, with 3% to 4% being mixed tumors, such as adenosquamous carcinomas. Three major types of tumors are included under the NSCLC category: adenocarcinomas, squamous cell carcinomas, and large-cell carcinomas.

Adenocarcinomas

These are the most common type of NSCLC, accounting for approximately 30% to 40% of cases. Of all the types of lung cancer, adenocarcinomas are most likely to occur in nonsmokers or former smokers. They are also the most common tumors in women.

Typically, adenocarcinomas present as small peripheral lesions that have a high propensity to metastasize to both regional lymph nodes and distant sites. Because of the tendency of the primary tumor to occur in peripheral locations, it frequently produces no symptoms. In contrast with their metastatic lesions, the primary adenocarcinoma tumor is histologically heterogeneous in 80% of patients, consisting of numerous histologic subtypes, and is classified as "mixed-" or "indeterminate-adenocarcinoma."

During the past decade, it has become apparent that the incidence of bronchioloalveolar adenocarcinoma (BAC) is increasing. This tumor originates from type II pneumocytes, and it may present as a pneumonic infiltrate, as multiple nodules scattered throughout the lungs, and, occasionally, as a single nodule.

Squamous cell carcinomas

These comprise approximately 30% of all cases of lung cancer. These tumors tend to occur in a central location and tend to spread to regional lymph nodes; they are the most likely of all lung cancers to remain localized and to cavitate. In fact, autopsy studies have shown that about 15% to 30% of patients with squamous cell carcinoma may die of local disease without evidence of distant metastases.

Large-cell carcinomas

These account for approximately 10% to 15% of all lung cancers. They tend to present as relatively large peripheral lesions and, like adenocarcinomas, have a high propensity to metastasize to regional lymph nodes and distant sites.

TREATMENT

In operable candidates, clinically staged IA, IB, IIA, and IIB NSCLC should undergo anatomic complete surgical resection. Primarily, patients with stages IIIB and IV disease are treated nonoperatively. Although multimodality therapy is routinely recommended for stage IIIA disease, it is recommended that it be performed within a clinical trial.

Surgical approach

Over the last two decades, the new subspecialty of general thoracic surgery has evolved in the United States. Surgeons in this specialty have completed their cardiothoracic surgery training and have obtained further subspecialty training in malignant and benign diseases of the chest.

The appropriate surgical treatment of NSCLC is resection of the lobe containing the tumor to achieve a negative surgical margin (R0), 16–20 lymph nodes pathologically assessed from at least three lymph node stations (two from the ipsilateral and contralateral mediastinum), and a pleural wash of the affected side. Tumor spillage is avoided. Occasionally, a bilobectomy or pneumonectomy is required. Mortality approximates 3% following lobectomy and 7% following pneumonectomy. A wedge or segmental resection is associated with a three to five times higher incidence of local recurrence and a lower 5-year survival rate than a lobectomy. Therefore, if the patient can tolerate the procedure, the standard operation should be a lobectomy, rather than a wedge resection or segmentectomy. As a curative resection, segmentectomy, though, has not been sufficiently evaluated, and more recent investigation demonstrates that in selected tumors, when the bronchus and vascular supply are individually ligated with a regional node resection, survival appears to be comparable and it salvages lung parenchyma.

A retrospective evaluation based on the SEER database found that in stage I lung cancer, the difference in long-term survival between a wedge resection and lobectomy was negligible after 71 years of age.

A radiologic and PET evaluation has demonstrated that lesions smaller than 2 cm, peripheral ground-glass opacity with a PET maximum SUV of less than 2.5, and no evidence of metastatic disease may be considered for a more limited resection if the surgical margin is approximately the size of the lesion. A prospective randomized clinical trial (CALGB 140503) is currently accruing patients to assess whether anatomic lobectomy provides superior survival compared with sublobar resection in peripheral stage I NSCLC < 2 cm.

VATS

Traditionally, lung cancers have been resected through a posterolateral thoracotomy incision. Muscle-sparing incisions may reduce pain. The current trend is toward an even less invasive approach: lobectomy and lymph node dissection with VATS. This approach appears to offer the same cancer operation and survival with perhaps lower morbidity.

Two VATS methods have been described: the mass hilar ligation technique and individual ligation of the vasculature and airway. Patients with peripheral tumors up to 4 to 6 cm without clinical hilar or mediastinal adenopathy appear to be good candidates for a VATS procedure. Conversion rates to open thoracotomy are 10%, and hospital stays are usually 3 to 5 days.

The results of several VATS series show lower complication rates than for reported series for thoracotomy; granted, a selection bias may have occurred. One small randomized trial showed a significant benefit favoring VATS. Patients have better shoulder function, better performance on the 6-minute walk, and less impairment of vital capacity after VATS than after thoracotomy. A VATS approach may be better tolerated than other approaches for older patients.

Patients with pathologic stage IA disease have a 70% to 80% 5-year survival rate after resection, whereas 5-year survival rates are 60% in those with stage IB disease and 40% to 50% in those with stage IIA/IIB disease. Patients found to have N2 (stage IIIA) disease located at a single nodal level have a 25% to 30% 5-year survival rate.

Mediastinal lymph node involvement

The standard lung cancer operation should include sampling or dissection of mediastinal lymph nodes. The presence of metastases in any of the mediastinal lymph nodes (N2 and/or N3 disease) is indicative of advanced disease and is thought by some to represent a contraindication to surgery. Resection of mediastinal disease may have prognostic significance, implications for postoperative care, and potential therapeutic value. Some series of patients with N2 disease have shown a 5-year survival rate of 20% to 30%, but patients in these series are highly selected.

Patients with N2 disease may potentially benefit from neoadjuvant treatment. Patients with N3 disease are considered to be stage IIIB and less likely to benefit from surgical resection. A few retrospective reports have demonstrated survival from induction therapy in patients with microscopic N3 involvement. The American College of Surgeons has completed accrual to a randomized, prospective study comparing survival following mediastinal lymph node sampling vs dissection. Complications and operative mortality appear equivalent between the sampling and dissection groups. Long-term survival is under investigation. Also, clinical trials are currently testing preoperative chemotherapy and chemoradiation therapy in patients with mediastinal node involvement.

Preoperative histologic assessment of the mediastinal lymph nodes is essential if multilevel metastases are suspected, as there have been few long-term survivors among patients with metastatic disease at more than one level. Nonsurgical treatment appears preferable, or patients should be offered participation in a trial designed to assess the benefits of neoadjuvant therapy. Although patients with stage IIIB tumors are usually treated with irradiation and chemotherapy (see later discussions), the occasional patient with isolated involvement of the vena cava or atrium can undergo resection.

Carcinoid tumors

Although the majority of carcinoid tumors remain localized, regional lymph node metastases are identified in 5% to 10% of patients. The surgical approach, therefore, should be similar to that used in NSCLC. If a small tumor in a proximal airway is identified and there is no histologic evidence of lymph node disease, a bronchoplastic procedure with preservation of lung tissue can sometimes be performed. Rates of survival at 10 years are > 90% for patients with stage I disease and 60% for patients with stage II disease.

Adjuvant therapy

Chemotherapy

Classic postoperative adjuvant chemotherapy has been tested in three randomized trials conducted by the LCSG. For almost 20 years, the relative value of adjuvant chemotherapy for resectable NSCLC has been disputed and debated. In a randomized, prospective study involving 488 patients, Keller et al showed no benefit to adjuvant chemotherapy. The ALPI study of 1,209 patients also showed no survival benefit. In contrast, the IALT randomized 1,867 patients to receive cisplatin-based adjuvant chemotherapy or no treatment. At 5 years, the treatment arm showed a survival advantage of 4.1% ($P = .003$), compared with the observation arm. However, that benefit appeared to diminish with longer follow-up. With 3 additional years of follow-up, there was a significant difference between the results of overall survival before and after 5 years (hazard ratio = 0.86; $P = .01$ vs hazard ratio = 1.45; $P = .04$). Similar results were observed with disease-free survival and confirmed the efficacy of chemotherapy for the first 5 years after surgery; however, they suggested possible late adjuvant chemotherapy-related mortality and underscored the need for long-term follow-up of adjuvant lung cancer trials.

> **A** meta-analysis by the LACE group found that in completely resected NSCLC patients, the 5-year overall survival benefit of cisplatin-containing adjuvant regimens was 5.4% (hazard ratio = 0.89; *P* = .004). There appeared to be a survival advantage of 8.9% for cisplatin-vinorelbine, which was superior to other regimens containing cisplatin. The greatest benefit of adjuvant therapy was seen in patients having disease of a higher stage (14.7% for stage III, 11.6% for stage II, 1.8% for stage I; *Douillard JY et al: J Clin Oncol 5:220–228, 2010*).

Two trials, the Canadian BR-10 and CALGB 9633, both demonstrated initial clinically significant improvement in survival, with minimal chemotherapy side effects; cisplatin and vinorelbine were used in the BR-10 trial and carboplatin and paclitaxel were used in CALGB 9633. These results, in combination with the recent positive findings of the adjuvant trial of UFT (a drug composed of tegafur and uracil mixed at the ratio of 1:4) in patients with stage IB NSCLC, increase the likelihood of adjuvant platinum-based therapy becoming the standard of treatment for patients with stages IB–IIIB NSCLC. Recent results of a prospective phase III trial from the SLCG NATCH trial compared the use of adjuvant and neoadjuvant and surgery alone in 616 patients with stages I (> 2 cm), II, and T3 N1. For those who received chemotherapy, three 3-week cycles of paclitaxel (200 mg/m^2), and carboplatin (at an area under the concentration-time curve [AUC] of 6) were given. Despite an excellent safety profile, a major radiologic response at 59%, and a complete response of 9% of induction patients, there was no difference found in survival. Again, it appears that the survival advantage in the treatment arm was lost, except in those patients with larger primary tumors (> 4 cm) or more advanced disease (stage IIIA).

Based on these results from adjuvant chemotherapy trials, the initial enthusiasm has been somewhat tempered. The potential benefits are higher efficacy of chemotherapy early in the natural history of disease, facilitation of subsequent local therapy, and early eradication of distant micrometastases. Further investigation in the use of adjuvant therapy is under way to determine which patients will benefit and what is the optimal treatment.

Stage I disease Currently approved chemotherapeutic regimens do not appear to provide any survival benefit in this patient population and are not advised outside of the clinical trial setting. From the subset analysis of CALGB 9335, patients with tumors > 4 cm may have some benefit, given the likelihood for recurrence. Currently under investigation is the use of tumor histology and marker evaluation to select the appropriate patient and the ideal chemotherapeutic plan with the greatest efficacy and least toxicity.

The current trend is to provide involvement in a chemopreventive clinical trial for stage IA patients. For patients with stage IB disease, platinum-based adjuvant chemotherapy (cisplatin or carboplatin combined with a taxane or vinorelbine) should be strongly considered.

JBR.10, which included 532 stage Ib or II completely resected patients who were randomized to cisplatin/vinorelbine or observation, demonstrated that the survival benefit appears to be confined to N1 patients over 9 years of prolonged follow-up.

Stage II/III disease In two earlier trials, postoperative adjuvant chemotherapy with six courses of CAP (cyclophosphamide, Adriamycin [doxorubicin], and Platinol [cisplatin]), given alone in one study and following postoperative radiation therapy in the other, resulted in a modest improvement in median survival but had no impact on long-term survival. In contrast, the IALT, ANITA, CALGB 9623, and Canadian BR-10 trials demonstrated an initial clinically significant survival advantage, justifying consideration for adjuvant chemotherapy. In contrast to IALT, which included all resectable disease and showed a decrease in survival after 5 years, JBR.10, which included stage IB/II patients, continues to show a survival benefit with over 9 years of follow-up. While there does not appear to be a clear survival advantage to adding adjuvant mediastinal radiotherapy to chemotherapy, this is reasonable to consider when there are particularly high risk factors for local recurrence. Potential indications for postoperative radiotherapy include:

- mediastinal involvement
- multiple positive lymph nodes or lymph node stations
- extracapsular nodal extension
- bulky nodal disease
- grossly positive surgical margins
- close or microscopically positive margins

Radiation therapy

A trial conducted by the LCSG showed that in patients with squamous cell carcinoma of the lungs and resected N1/N2 disease, administration of postoperative radiation therapy reduced the risk of recurrence in the chest from 20% to 1%. Although there was no improvement in overall survival, postoperative irradiation was associated with a significant improvement in disease-free survival for patients with N2 disease. A trial by the BMRC reached similar conclusions.

A meta-analysis of nine randomized trials assessing postoperative radiation therapy in lung cancer reported a 21% increase in mortality in patients receiving this therapy. However, many of the patients in these trials had N0 disease, for which few would advocate radiation therapy. Also, most of the patients were treated with cobalt-60 beams and technically limited treatment planning, not with modern radiation therapy techniques.

Recently, the impact of radiation therapy on survival was reanalyzed in the ANITA trial, in which postoperative radiation therapy was optional, based on each center's practice. Interestingly, in patients with N2 (mediastinal) disease, adjuvant radiation therapy improved overall survival in both arms: 21% vs 17% in the observation arms and 47% vs 34% in the adjuvant chemotherapy arms (with or without radiation therapy, respectively). Based on this descriptive analysis, radiation therapy appeared to provide a benefit in addition to adjuvant chemotherapy in patients with N2 disease (whereas the converse was true in patients with N1 disease). A randomized trial with and without postoperative radiation therapy in patients with resected N2 disease is under way in Europe.

RTOG 0214 studied the role of prophylactic cranial irradiation (PCI) in patients with stage III NSCLC. The study opened in September 2002 and closed due to slow accrual in August 2007. The total accrual was 356 patients (of the targeted 1,058), of whom 340 were eligible. One-year overall survival (75.6% vs 76.9%; *P* = .86) and 1-year disease-free survival (56.4% vs 51.2%; *P* = .11) for PCI vs observation, respectively, were not significantly different. However, the incidence of CNS metastases at 1 year was 7.7% for PCI vs 18% for observation (*P* = .004). Thus, PCI in stage III NSCLC significantly decreases the risk of CNS metastases, with no significant difference in overall survival or disease-free survival *(Gore EM et al: J Clin Oncol 27: abstract 7506, 2009).*

These results created a lack of consensus about treatment recommendations, with some experts advocating the use of postoperative radiation therapy to reduce local recurrence, and others avoiding it because of the absence of an effect on survival.

At present, therefore, the appropriate role of postoperative radiation therapy remains controversial. Such therapy should be seriously considered, however, in patients at high risk for locoregional relapse. In patients who are receiving adjuvant chemotherapy, it is reasonable to administer the chemotherapy first (as it has been associated with a survival benefit) followed by radiation therapy (for enhanced local tumor control).

Moreover, in a randomized trial by Keller et al, no benefit was shown for concurrent chemoradiation therapy over radiation therapy when in the adjuvant setting for completely resected patients with stage II/IIIA NSCLC. An exception may be in patients with microscopic residual disease (ie, positive margins or extracapsular extension), for whom a delay in radiation therapy may be detrimental.

Neoadjuvant chemotherapy or chemoradiation therapy

During the past decade, numerous phase II trials showed that, in general, it is feasible to perform pulmonary resection following chemotherapy or chemoradiation therapy. Although surgery can be more difficult after preoperative treatment, morbidity and mortality are acceptable.

Stage IIIA/IIIB disease

The greater effectiveness of current chemotherapeutic regimens to reduce disease bulk suggested that their use prior to surgery, either alone or in combination with radiation therapy, might increase both resectability and survival in patients with stage IIIA NSCLC. Multiple phase II trials have shown such an approach to be feasible; however, it is not clear whether such a strategy improves median or long-term survival over best nonsurgical chemoradiotherapy among patients who initially have more than minimal N2 disease.

In 2009, Albain et al reported on Intergroup 0139, a phase III study of 202 stage IIIA patients that showed improved progression-free survival in the trimodality group with neoadjuvant chemoradiation followed by surgery (12.8 months vs 10.5 months; *P* = .017) but no difference in overall survival. The lack of survival benefit was thought to be possibly related to the high mortality rate following pneumonectomies, particularly on the right side.

Current recommendations

In selected patients, preoperative treatment may have a favorable effect on outcome in surgically resectable stage IIIA NSCLC. Although aggressive neoadjuvant approaches may have increased treatment-associated mortality, in experienced institutions, potential benefits seem to outweigh the risks. The results of the intergroup randomized trial comparing preoperative chemoradiation therapy with definitive chemoradiation therapy (in pathologic N2 disease) showed a significant improvement in progression-free survival (but not overall survival) in the surgical arm (P = .02). This approach, however, may not be optimal if a pneumonectomy is required, as this procedure was associated with a high rate of treatment-related deaths (> 20%). However, in a subset analysis, survival was improved for patients who underwent lobectomy, but not pneumonectomy, vs chemotherapy plus radiation alone. In this trial, it is not clear whether patients with persistently positive N2 disease after neoadjuvant therapy will benefit from surgical resection.

Stage I–IIIA disease

Neoadjuvant chemotherapy may have a role in early-stage disease. A multicenter trial from France randomized 373 patients with stage I to IIIA NSCLC to undergo either surgery alone or chemotherapy (mitomycin [6 mg/m^2 on day 1], ifosfamide [1.5 g/m^2 on days 1 to 3], and cisplatin [30 mg/m^2 on days 1 to 3]) at 3-week intervals for three cycles followed by surgery. Disease-free survival was significantly longer in the patients randomized to receive neoadjuvant chemotherapy than in those treated with surgery alone (P = .02). The most striking benefit of chemotherapy was seen in patients who had minimal lymphadenopathy (either N0 or N1; P = .008). No excessive complications were seen in the chemotherapy-treated patients.

> **In the Intergroup 0139 trial, 202 operable NSCLC patients (T1–3, pN2, M0) were randomly assigned to either two cycles of induction cisplatin and etoposide and concurrent 45 Gy of radiotherapy followed by surgery or to four cycles of the same therapy with concurrent 61 Gy of radiation. The median overall survival was 34.4 months for surgical patients who had complete regression of nodal disease. The 5-year overall survival was 27% for surgically treated patients and 20% for those not given surgery. There did not appear to be a significant advantage among patients treated with pneumonectomy (*Albain KS et al: Lancet 374:378–386, 2009*).**

Cumulative data support a difference in treatment, but no one study is statistically significant. Pooled analyses suggest positive benefit to neoadjuvant therapy, with all individual studies showing a trend toward improved overall survival, and significant differences in disease-free survival.

Following on previous trials was a study presented by Scagliotti in which 270 patients with stage IB–IIIA NSCLC were randomized to undergo surgery and follow-up vs induction chemotherapy with cisplatin and gemcitabine (Gemzar) followed by surgery. This trial closed early due to accrual problems, after only 270 of a projected 700 patients enrolled. Overall survival at 3 years favored the chemotherapy plus surgery arm with (P = .053). Overall survival at 3 years for the neoadjuvant arm was 67% vs 60% for surgery alone (P = .053).

A subset analysis suggested that for stage IIB–IIIA, 3-year overall survival was 70% vs 40% in favor of chemotherapy ($P = .001$), whereas there was no difference for patients with stage IB–IIA who were treated. This continues to support data suggesting that for stage IIB–IIIA disease, chemotherapy, either in the adjuvant or neoadjuvant setting, provides a significant survival advantage.

Treatment of patients with medically inoperable stage I/II disease

Some patients with resectable stage I or II NSCLC are high-risk operative candidates because of poor cardiopulmonary function or other medical problems. Other patients refuse to undergo surgery despite the recommendation of their treating physicians. In such patients, an attempt should be made to optimize pulmonary function by encouraging smoking cessation and initiating vigorous treatment, such as with bronchodilators. Evaluation by an experienced general thoracic surgeon is warranted before discounting a surgical approach. For many of these patients, stereotactic body radiation therapy (SBRT) has emerged as a safe and effective noninvasive treatment option (see box).

Radiation therapy

Several institutions have reported their experience with definitive radiation therapy for such patients. Although the results are not as good as those reported in patients selected for surgery (possibly due to differences in patient selection and between clinical vs pathologic staging), patients with medically inoperable early-stage NSCLC clearly should be offered radiation therapy, with a reasonable expectation of cure. For patients with early-stage (I/II) NSCLC, surgical resection is the standard of care. However, many patients with lung cancer are not eligible for surgery because of various comorbidities. In the past, the main treatment alternative for these medically inoperable patients has been conventional radiation therapy, typically requiring once-daily treatments every weekday for approximately 7 weeks. Results with conventional radiation therapy have not been encouraging, with local tumor control rates of only 50%.

As mentioned, SBRT has evolved as another treatment option for patients with medically inoperable, peripheral stage I NSCLC. SBRT involves the delivery of high doses of highly precise radiation therapy in a hypofractionated scheme over three to five fractions, administering biologically equivalent doses (BEDs) > 100 Gy over 1 to 2 weeks, with promising local tumor control rates of 85% to 90%.

Onishi et al reported the clinical outcomes of approximately 250 patients treated in Japan with SBRT for stage I NSCLC. They reported a cumulative 5-year local tumor control rate of 84% for those treated with a BED > 100 Gy vs 37% for those receiving a BED < 100 Gy ($P < .001$). Interestingly, among operable patients, the 5-year overall survival rate was 72% for those treated with a BED > 100 Gy vs 50% for those receiving a BED < 100 Gy ($P < .05$). These promising results have led to the European ROSEL study, which is enrolling patients with early-stage NSCLC (eligible for surgery) and randomizing them to undergo surgery or SBRT to evaluate tumor control, quality of life, survival, and cost of treatment.

Timmerman et al reported the results of a phase I study of SBRT in patients with medically inoperable stage I NSCLC. SBRT was delivered in three fractions over

2 weeks, with a starting dose of 800 cGy per fraction. The dose was escalated to 2,000 cGy per fraction for three fractions. Recently, excellent results have been reported in a phase II cooperative group study with this approach (see box). The investigators found that although this treatment was safe and effective for patients for peripheral lung lesions, there was a significantly higher rate of grade 3 toxicity in patients with central lung lesions. Other institutional studies, such as those conducted at Henry Ford Hospital, suggest that early central NSCLC lesions can be treated safely and effectively with SBRT by using smaller fraction sizes of 10 to 12 Gy per session for three to four sessions. A prospective trial, RTOG 0813, will further study this issue in a dose escalation trial.

In 2010, Timmerman et al reported on a phase II North American multicenter study (RTOG 0236) of 59 patients with biopsy-proven, peripheral T1–2, N0, M0 NSCLC tumors (measuring < 5 cm in diameter) and medical conditions precluding surgical treatment. Patients were treated with a total of 54 Gy in three fractions over a 1- to 2- week period with a median follow-up of 34.4 months. The rates for disease-free survival and overall survival at 3 years were 48.3% (95% CI, 34.4%–60.8%) and 55.8% (95% CI, 41.6%–67.9%), respectively. The estimated 3-year primary tumor control was 97.6%, and the median overall survival was 48.1 months. The 2-year local control rate was excellent at 94% *(Timmerman R et al: JAMA 303:1070–1076, 2010).*

RFA

RFA in patients who are not operative candidates is actively being studied. Although there is considerable experience with RFA for cancer in other organs, further evaluation of RFA and cryotherapeutic techniques for lung cancer is under way to assess complications related to the therapy, local recurrence, and survival.

Treatment of patients with stage IIIA/IIIB disease

Radiation therapy

In the past, radiation therapy was considered the standard therapy for patients with stage IIIA or IIIB disease. Long-term survival was poor, in the range of 5%, with poor local tumor control and early development of distant metastatic disease.

A randomized trial compared standard daily radiation therapy (66 Gy) with a continuous hyperfractionated accelerated radiation therapy regimen (CHART) that delivered 54 Gy over 2.5 weeks. The altered fractionation schedule resulted in improved 2-year survival.

Various efforts have assessed combining altered fractionation schema with chemotherapy. Although the results of RTOG 94-10 did not favor altered fractionation (see section on "Concurrent vs sequential chemoradiation therapy"), the long-term results of another study support this strategy.

Jeremic et al compared hyperfractionated radiation therapy (bid to 69.6 Gy) and concurrent low-dose daily carboplatin/etoposide with or without weekend carboplatin/etoposide in a randomized trial of approximately 200 patients. Although investigators found no benefit with the addition of weekend carboplatin/etoposide, both arms demonstrated promising median survival times of 20 and 22 months and excellent 5-year survival rates of 20% and 23%.

Conformal radiation therapy

Hayman et al reported updated results of the Michigan phase I dose-escalation trial of three-dimensional (3D) conformal radiation therapy for NSCLC. In this study, the radiation dose was escalated based on the effective volume of irradiated lung (up to 102.9 Gy). Such doses produced acceptable toxicity and no cases of isolated failures in purposely nonirradiated, clinically uninvolved nodal regions. This strategy is now being integrated with chemotherapy.

Socinski et al reported a dose-escalation radiotherapy (from 60 Gy up to 74 Gy) trial, using 3D computer-assisted planning techniques, in patients receiving induction carboplatin and paclitaxel and concurrent weekly carboplatin/paclitaxel. Ninety-seven percent (31 of 32) of the patients completed therapy to 74 Gy, as planned. The grade 3/4 esophagitis rate overall was relatively low at 11%. Moreover, the results showed a promising median survival of 26 months and a 3-year survival of 47%.

Indeed, several analyses support the importance of radiation therapy dose escalation in stage III NSCLC. Movsas et al analyzed data from more than 1,400 patients treated in nine prospective RTOG nonoperative NSCLC studies activated during the 1990s. The analysis was stratified by the presence of chemotherapy and the accrual year. On multivariate analysis, they found that a higher BED significantly predicted for higher overall survival and higher locoregional tumor control. For an increase in BED of 10 Gy, there was a dramatic 14% reduction in the hazard of death. Similarly, researchers at the University of Michigan found a significantly improved survival in patients treated with a higher BED. To test this important hypothesis prospectively, an RTOG/intergroup phase III trial has recently opened to compare concurrent chemoradiation therapy with either 60 Gy or 74 Gy with or without cetuximab (Erbitux).

Chemoradiation therapy

Chemoradiation therapy vs radiation therapy alone At least 11 randomized trials have compared thoracic irradiation alone with chemoradiation therapy in patients with stage III NSCLC. Several meta-analyses have demonstrated a small, but statistically significant, improvement in survival with the combined-modality regimens.

Concurrent vs sequential chemoradiation therapy Furuse et al evaluated mitomycin, vindesine, and Platinol (cisplatin; MVP), administered either concurrently or prior to thoracic irradiation (56 Gy), in patients with unresectable stage III NSCLC. With more than 300 patients randomized, survival favored concurrent over sequential therapy (median survival, 16.5 months vs 13.3 months, and 5-year survival rates, 15.8% vs 8.9%; *P* = .04). Furuse et al also reported the patterns of failure, which demonstrated a benefit of concurrent chemoradiotherapy in improving the local relapse-free survival (*P* = .04) but not the distant relapse-free survival (*P* = .6).

> Govindan et al reported on CALGB 30407, a phase II study of pemetrexed, carboplatin, and thoracic radiation with or without cetuximab in patients with locally advanced, unresectable NSCLC. Preliminary efficacy data showed no difference in complete or partial response, median failure-free survival, or 18-month survival *(Govindan R et al: J Clin Oncol 27[15S]: abstract 7505, 2009)*.

Curran et al presented the long-term results of a larger randomized trial (> 600 patients) comparing sequential and concurrent chemoradiotherapy (RTOG 9410). The 4-year survival with concurrent cisplatin/vinblastine and once-daily irradiation was 21% vs 12% with sequential treatment ($P = .04$). The third treatment arm (concurrent cisplatin/oral etoposide and hyperfractionated irradiation) was intermediate, with a 4-year survival of 17%.

The role of altered radiation therapy fractionation may deserve further study. ECOG 2597 randomized patients after induction chemotherapy (with carboplatin and paclitaxel) to receive either standard radiation therapy (64 Gy/2 Gy fraction) vs hyperfractionated accelerated radiation therapy (HART), 57.6 Gy delivered 1.5 Gy three times daily over 2.5 weeks. Although the study closed prematurely due to poor accrual (only 111 patients were eligible), the median survival in the investigational arm appeared promising (22 months).

Several randomized phase II trials also appear to support the use of concurrent chemoradiation therapy for locally advanced NSCLC. For example, Belani et al performed a randomized phase II study in 276 patients of three chemoradiation therapy regimens with paclitaxel, carboplatin, and thoracic irradiation in their locally advanced multimodality protocol (LAMP). They found that concurrent chemoradiation therapy followed by adjuvant chemotherapy appeared to have the best therapeutic outcome, with a median survival of 16.3 months, compared with either induction chemotherapy followed by concurrent chemoradiation therapy (median survival, 12.7 months) or sequential chemotherapy followed by irradiation (median survival, 13 months).

Similarly, in another randomized phase II study, Zatloukal et al studied 102 patients treated with concurrent chemoradiation therapy and sequential chemotherapy followed by irradiation. The chemotherapy consisted of four cycles of cisplatin and vinorelbine. The investigators reported a median survival in the concurrent arm of ~20 months, vs ~13 months in the other arm ($P = .02$).

Movsas et al reported the results of the first Patterns of Care Study (PCS) for lung cancer, which was conducted to determine the national patterns of radiation therapy practice in patients treated for nonmetastatic lung cancer. As supported by clinical trials, the PCS for lung cancer demonstrated that patients with clinical stage III NSCLC received chemotherapy plus radiation therapy more than radiation therapy alone ($P < .0001$). In clinical stage I NSCLC, though, radiation therapy alone was the primary treatment ($P < .0001$). Factors correlating with increased use of chemotherapy included lower age ($P < .0001$), histology (SCLC > NSCLC; $P < .0001$), increasing clinical stage ($P < .0001$), increasing Karnofsky performance status ($P < .0001$), and lack of comorbidities ($P = .0002$) but not academic vs nonacademic facilities ($P = .81$). Of all patients receiving chemotherapy, approximately three-quarters received it concurrently with radiation therapy. Only 3% of all patients were treated on Institutional Review Board–approved trials, demonstrating the need for improved accrual to clinical trials. Future PCSs will be done as part of the Quality Research in Radiation Oncology (QRRO) project.

The HOG reported the results of the phase III trial of cisplatin plus etoposide plus concurrent chest radiation therapy with or without consolidation docetaxel (Taxotere) in patients with inoperable stage III NSCLC. In a study of 203 patients (of whom 147 were randomized to receive or not receive docetaxel) with a median

TABLE 4: Active newer agents for NSCLC chemotherapy

Agent	Number of studies	Number of patients	Response rate (%) (range)
Irinotecan	3	150	34 (32–37)
Docetaxel	7	257	33 (21–54)
Paclitaxel	4	151	22 (10–24)
Gemcitabine	7	566	21 (20–26)
Vinorelbine	4	501	21 (12–32)

follow-up of 25.6 months, they reported a median survival time in the docetaxel arm of 21.6 months vs 24.2 months in the observation arm ($P = .94$). They concluded that consolidation docetaxel does not further improve survival and is associated with significant toxicity (including an increased rate of hospitalization and premature deaths) and should not be used in this setting.

Current treatment recommendations

At present, it is reasonable to consider concurrent chemoradiation therapy (with once-daily radiation therapy) as a new treatment paradigm in stage III (inoperable) lung cancer patients with an ECOG performance status of 0/1 who have not lost more than 5% of their usual body weight. The results of a meta-analysis using individual patient data from randomized clinical trials showed that concomitant chemoradiation therapy, as compared with sequential chemotherapy and radiation therapy, improved survival of patients with locally advanced NSCLC, primarily due to a decrease in locoregional tumor progression. Overall, there was an absolute benefit in survival of 6% at 3 years.

Novel biologic agents The results of SWOG 0023 were updated. This was a randomized phase III trial of gefitinib (Iressa) vs placebo maintenance after chemoradiation therapy followed by docetaxel in patients with stage III NSCLC. With a median follow-up of 27 months in 243 randomized patients, the median survival for the gefitinib arm (n = 118) was 23 months vs 35 months for the placebo arm (n = 125; $P = .013$). The authors concluded that in this unselected population, gefitinib did not improve survival. The decrease in survival was likely due to cancer, not to gefitinib toxicity. A recent secondary analysis of SWOG 0023 found that V20 (which represents the percentage of total normal lung volume that received > 20 Gy of radiation) was the greatest predictor for radiation pneumonitis. This finding is consistent with other studies showing V20 to be a reliable predictor of pneumonitis in patients who are treated with radiation therapy for lung cancer. They found that patients with a V20 >35% had a higher rate of grade > 3 pneumonitis than patients with a V20 < 35% (14% vs 6%, respectively; $P = .02$) and a shorter median survival (11 vs 23 months, respectively; $P = .0001$). Of note, there was no imbalance of the V20 parameter between the two arms of this SWOG 0023. It is now considered standard for radiation oncologists to formally evaluate dose vs volume parameters in the treatment of lung cancer.

Blumenschein et al combined cetuximab with paclitaxel and carboplatin with radiation therapy. This phase II RTOG trial accrued 87, with a promising median survival of 23 months. This represents an approximately 30% increase in survival from the 17 to 18 months usually observed with chemoradiation therapy alone. This novel strategy of adding cetuximab to chemoradiation therapy in locally advanced NSCLC is being tested in a 2 × 2 randomized phase III study (also investigating the role of radiation dose escalation).

Treatment of patients with stage IV disease

Until recently, there was considerable controversy over the value of treating stage IV NSCLC patients with chemotherapy. Treatment with older cisplatin-containing regimens, such as cisplatin/etoposide, showed only a modest effect on survival, improving median survival by approximately 6 weeks, according to a meta-analysis, and yielding a 1-year survival rate of approximately 20% (as compared with a rate of approximately 10% for supportive care).

However, several chemotherapeutic agents have produced response rates in excess of 20% in NSCLC (Table 4). The potentially useful newer agents include the taxanes (paclitaxel and docetaxel), vinorelbine, gemcitabine, and irinotecan. Several of these drugs have unique mechanisms of action. Paclitaxel and docetaxel increase the polymerization of tubulin; gemcitabine is an antimetabolite; and irinotecan is a topoisomerase I inhibitor.

Furthermore, randomized trials demonstrated that a combination of a newer agent plus cisplatin significantly improves the response rate over cisplatin monotherapy (historically considered the most active agent for NSCLC). This increase in response rate translates into significant, although modest, improvement in survival.

> Over the last 5 years, histology subtyping has helped to improve survival in NSCLC. Pemetrexed is a relatively new antifolate agent and is a potent inhibitor of thymidylate synthase. Scagliotti et al published a noninferiority, phase III, randomized study of 1,725 chemotherapy-naive patients with stage IIIB or IV NSCLC who received cisplatin/gemcitabine on days 1–8 or cisplatin/pemetrexed on day 1 every 3 weeks for up to six cycles. Overall survival for cisplatin/pemetrexed was noninferior to cisplatin/gemcitabine (median survival, 10.3 vs 10.3 months, respectively; hazard ratio = 0.94; 95% CI, 0.84–1.05). Overall survival was statistically superior for cisplatin/pemetrexed vs cisplatin/gemcitabine in patients with adenocarcinoma (n = 847; 12.6 vs 10.9 months) and large-cell carcinoma histology (n = 153; 10.4 vs 6.7 months). Patients with squamous cell histology (n = 473) had significantly improved survival with cisplatin/gemcitabine vs cisplatin/pemetrexed (10.8 vs 9.4 months; *Scagliotti GV et al: J Clin Oncol 26:3543–3551, 2008*).

Optimal chemotherapy for advanced NSCLC

Until the early 1990s, regimens of cisplatin plus a vinca alkaloid or etoposide were most common. More recently, regimens that employ newer agents are more widely used. However, choosing one regimen from many options is a difficult task because there is no survival advantage documented for one regimen over another or standard regimen vs regimens containing newer agents.

Table 5 summarizes the results of selected randomized trials in which combination regimens

TABLE 5: Results of selected randomized trials evaluating chemotherapy regimens of newer agents in advanced NSCLC

Initial investigator	Chemotherapy regimen	No. of patients	Response rate (%)	Median survival	1-yr survival rate (%)
LeChevalier (1994)	Vinorelbine + cisplatin	206	30	40 wk	35
	Vindesine + cisplatin	200	19	32 wk	27
	Vinorelbine	206	14	31 wk	30
Bonomi (1996)	Etoposide + cisplatin	600 (total)	12	7.7 mo	32
	Paclitaxel + cisplatin		27	9.6 mo	37
	Paclitaxel + cisplatin + G-CSF		32	10.0 mo	39
Giaccone (1997)	Teniposide + cisplatin	157	28	9.9 mo	41
	Paclitaxel + cisplatin	152	41	9.7 mo	43
Belani (1998)	Etoposide + cisplatin	179	14	9.9 mo	37
	Paclitaxel + carboplatin	190	22	9.5 mo	32
Crino (1998)	Mitomycin + ifosfamide + cisplatin	152	28	38 wk	NA
	Gemcitabine + cisplatin	154	40	35 wk	NA
Georgoulias (1999)	Docetaxel + cisplatin	152	32	10 mo	42
	Docetaxel + gemcitabine	144	34	9 mo	34
Masuda (1999)	Irinotecan + cisplatin	378 (total)	43	50 wk	48
	Vindesine + cisplatin		31	47 wk	38
	Irinotecan		21	46 wk	41
Kelly (1999)	Paclitaxel + carboplatin	184	27	8 mo	36
	Vinorelbine + cisplatin	181	27	8 mo	33
Schiller (2000)	Paclitaxel + cisplatin	1,163 (total)	21	7.8 mo	31
	Gemcitabine + cisplatin		21	8.1 mo	36
	Docetaxel + cisplatin		17	7.4 mo	31
	Paclitaxel + carboplatin		15	8.2 mo	35
Frasci (2000)	Gemcitabine + vinorelbine	60	22	29 wk	30
	Vinorelbine	60	15	18 wk	13
Lilenbaum (2002)	Paclitaxel + carboplatin	292	29	10 mo	NA
	Paclitaxel	290	17	8.6 mo	NA
Gronberg (2009)	Pemetrexed + carboplatin	225	NA	NA	34
	Gemcitabine + carboplatin	221	NA	NA	31

G-CSF = granulocyte colony-stimulating factor; NA = data not available

containing a newer agent are compared with old "standard" regimens or regimens containing another newer agent. Subtle differences in the eligibility criteria (eg, inclusion of patients with stage III tumors or those with poor performance status) make it difficult to directly compare the trial results. Nevertheless, there is a trend indicating that regimens containing newer agents show higher response rates and also better survival outcomes in some series than do older regimens.

Vinorelbine plus cisplatin combination Vinorelbine was the first agent that demonstrated improved activity against NSCLC in combination with cisplatin. The European multicenter trial reported by LeChevalier showed the results favoring a cisplatin plus vinorelbine combination (vinorelbine, 30 mg/m^2 weekly; cisplatin, 120 mg/m^2 on days 1 and 29, then every 6 weeks) over a vindesine plus cisplatin combination (vindesine, 3 mg/m^2 weekly; cisplatin, 120 mg/m^2 on days 1 and 29, then every 6 weeks) and vinorelbine alone (30 mg/m^2 weekly). The median survival duration of 40 weeks in the vinorelbine/cisplatin treatment arm was significantly longer than the 32 weeks in the vindesine/cisplatin arm ($P = .04$) and 31 weeks in the vinorelbine monotherapy arm ($P < .001$). This trial, however, did not confirm the role of vinorelbine in NSCLC therapy, even though it confirmed the role of cisplatin.

To address this issue, SWOG conducted a study comparing cisplatin alone (100 mg/m^2 every 4 weeks) with the vinorelbine/cisplatin combination (cisplatin, 100 mg/m^2 every 4 weeks; vinorelbine, 25 mg/m^2 weekly × 3 every 4 weeks). Survival outcome was analyzed for 415 patients, 92% with stage IV tumors. The vinorelbine/cisplatin treatment significantly improved the disease progression-free (median, 2 months vs 4 months; $P = .0001$) and overall survival (median, 6 months vs 8 months; 1-year survival 20% vs 36%; $P = .0018$).

Comella et al reported interim analysis results of a phase III trial of the SICOG. A three-drug regimen (cisplatin, gemcitabine, and vinorelbine) was associated with a substantial survival gain over the cisplatin and vinorelbine regimen (median survival time, 51 weeks and 35 weeks, respectively).

Paclitaxel plus platinum compound A number of studies demonstrate promising results with paclitaxel in combination with cisplatin or carboplatin and other agents. Two large randomized trials compared paclitaxel plus cisplatin with standard regimens. In a three-arm, randomized trial (ECOG 5592) reported by Bonomi et al, 600 eligible patients with chemotherapy-naive stages IIIB–IV NSCLC were randomly assigned to receive a combination of cisplatin (75 mg/m^2) plus etoposide (100 mg/m^2 daily on days 1 to 3) vs either low-dose (135 mg/m^2 over 24 hours) or high-dose (250 mg/m^2 over 24 hours with growth factor) paclitaxel plus cisplatin (75 mg/m^2). The response rates for the low-dose and high-dose paclitaxel arms were 26.5% and 32.1%, respectively, significantly better than the cisplatin/etoposide arm (12.0%). Superior survival was observed with the combined paclitaxel regimens (median survival time, 9.99 months; 1-year survival, 39%) compared with etoposide plus cisplatin (median survival, 8 months; 1-year survival rate, 32%; $P = .048$). Comparing survival rates for the two dose levels of paclitaxel revealed no significant differences.

In a European trial of similar design reported by Giaccone et al, cisplatin/paclitaxel improved the response rate and QOL parameters. There was no improvement in overall survival, however, compared with a standard regimen of cisplatin/teniposide (Vumon).

Paclitaxel/carboplatin has been the most widely favored regimen for first-line chemotherapy in all NSCLC stages among US medical oncologists, mainly due to promising phase II trial results and the ease of administration for outpatients, with manageable toxicity profiles compared with those of cisplatin-containing regimens. One of the early phase II trials, for example, reported a response rate of 62%, a median survival duration of 53 weeks, and a 1-year survival rate of 54%. However, a randomized trial sponsored by the manufacturer of paclitaxel failed to demonstrate a survival advantage over the standard cisplatin plus etoposide regimen. Nevertheless, paclitaxel plus carboplatin may remain a community standard because a SWOG trial reported results equivalent to the time-tested vinorelbine/cisplatin regimen (see Table 5).

Combination vs single-agent chemotherapy A randomized phase III study conducted by CALGB further supported the superiority of combination chemotherapy over single-agent therapy. Previous trials had indicated that a platinum plus a novel agent was superior to a platinum alone. Lilenbaum et al demonstrated that for patients with stage IIIB or IV NSCLC, carboplatin and paclitaxel are superior to paclitaxel alone, even for patients with an ECOG performance status of 2. This randomized trial showed a median survival advantage for the combination therapy.

Gemcitabine plus cisplatin Gemcitabine has also been approved by the FDA for use against NSCLC based on a series of successful phase II trials of cisplatin/gemcitabine and three major phase III trials. The Hoosier Oncology Group study, reported by Sandler et al, compared gemcitabine/cisplatin with cisplatin alone and showed a modest improvement in median and 1-year survival comparable to those seen in the vinorelbine trials. The Spanish and Italian trials, reported by Cardenal et al and Crino et al, compared gemcitabine plus cisplatin with standard-regimen cisplatin plus etoposide and mitomycin plus ifosfamide plus cisplatin, respectively. Although there was a significant improvement in overall response, these two studies failed to demonstrate a survival benefit.

Because gemcitabine is relatively well tolerated without dose-limiting myelosuppression, it is being evaluated for use as a single agent or in combination with other agents in older or medically compromised patients. Italian investigators report that gemcitabine combined with the vinorelbine regimen is associated with significantly better survival than single-agent vinorelbine in elderly patients with NSCLC.

Other combination regimens that contain cisplatin plus newer agents, such as docetaxel or irinotecan, also showed similar results when compared with other two-drug regimens of either two newer or two older agents.

Major randomized trials comparing cytotoxic regimens

To identify a better chemotherapy regimen for advanced-stage NSCLC, the US cooperative study groups conducted large phase III trials. The SWOG investigators compared paclitaxel/carboplatin with vinorelbine/cisplatin (the time-tested regimen in previous European and SWOG trials). A total of 404 evaluable patients were randomized to receive either paclitaxel (225 mg/m^2 over 3 hours) plus carboplatin (at an area under the curve [AUC] of 6 mg/mL/min on day 1) every 21 days or vinorelbine (25 mg/m^2 weekly) plus cisplatin (100 mg/m^2 on day 1) every 28 days. Overall response rates were 27% for both groups. The median survival times were also identical (8 months), with virtually identical 1-year survival rates (35% and 33%, respectively). Although both regimens provided effective palliation for advanced NSCLC, the investigators identified paclitaxel/carboplatin for future studies because of a favorable toxicity profile and better tolerability and compliance.

The ECOG 1594 trial compared three platinum-based regimens containing new agents in the treatment of NSCLC with a control arm of cisplatin and paclitaxel. The regimens were gemcitabine (1,000 mg/m^2 on days 1, 8, and 15) plus cisplatin (100 mg/m^2 on day 1) every 4 weeks, docetaxel (75 mg/m^2) plus cisplatin (75 mg/m^2 on day 1) every 3 weeks, and paclitaxel (225 mg/m^2 over 3 hours) plus carboplatin (at an AUC of 6 mg/mL/min on day 1) every 21 days; the reference regimen was paclitaxel (175 mg/m^2 over 24 hours) plus cisplatin (75 mg/m^2 on day 1) every 21 days.

Analysis of 1,163 eligible patients showed no statistically significant differences in overall response, median survival, and 1-year survival rates when compared with the control arm, paclitaxel and cisplatin. Gemcitabine plus cisplatin was associated with a statistically significant prolongation of time to disease progression when compared with the control arm (4.5 months vs 3.5 months; $P = .002$) but was also associated with a higher percentage of grade 4 thrombocytopenia, anemia, and renal toxicity.

Recent randomized trials have begun to suggest that differentiating treatment regimens by histology may be important. A phase III trial by Scagliotti et al randomized 1,725 patients to receive a combination of cisplatin and gemcitabine vs cisplatin and pemetrexed (Alimta). In patients who did not have a squamous cell histology, the combination of cisplatin and pemetrexed had a superior overall survival. On the other hand, in patients with a squamous cell histology, the combination of cisplatin and gemcitabine had a superior survival. These and other data suggest that pemetrexed and platinum appear to be superior in non-squamous cell populations. The investigators reported that this is the first prospective phase III study in NSCLC to show survival differences based on histologic type. Overall survival was statistically superior for cisplatin/pemetrexed than for cisplatin/gemcitabine in patients with adenocarcinoma vs squamous histology (12.6 vs 10.9 months; $P = .03$). In addition, cisplatin/pemetrexed provided similar efficacy to cisplatin/gemcitabine with better tolerability, a reduced need for supportive therapies, and more convenient administration than cisplatin. This was the first phase III study in NSCLC to prospectively demonstrate a survival difference between platinum doublets based on histology. Based on the results of this study, the FDA approved pemetrexed, in combination with cisplatin, in the first-line treatment of locally advanced and metastatic NSCLC, for patients with a nonsquamous histology.

Because all the regimens showed similar efficacy, QOL becomes a critical issue in choosing a particular regimen. The decision to use one regimen over another will depend not only on ease of administration and side effects, but also on the personal preference and experience of the treating oncologist.

Second-line chemotherapy for NSCLC

Before the new generation of more effective agents became available, few, if any, significant benefits were expected from second-line chemotherapy. As a result, reports in the literature seldom address this issue specifically or systematically. The most experience with second-line chemotherapy in NSCLC is with docetaxel, which has received FDA approval for this indication based on two randomized phase III trials confirming the promising phase II results of docetaxel monotherapy in patients with advanced NSCLC previously treated with platinum-based chemotherapy.

The PASSPORT trial is designed to evaluate the safety of bevacizumab (Avastin) in the first- and second-line settings. The primary endpoint is safety, based on the rate of grade 2 or greater CNS hemorrhage. A combined report presented at ASCO 2008 included patients entered onto the PASSPORT trial (n = 65) and patients on the ATLAS trial (n = 26), which was amended to include patients with treated and controlled brain metastases. PASSPORT also allowed patients treated in either the first- or second-line setting; ATLAS included only patients treated in the first-line setting. During active treatment, no grade 2 or greater CNS hemorrhagic events were reported; one grade 2 CNS hemorrhage was reported in a patient whose disease progressed following cessation of bevacizumab treatment. The PASSPORT trial has completed accrual with approximately 110 patients. This early analysis suggests bevacizumab is safe in the setting of brain metastases provided patients are treated effectively and definitively and that they retain a good performance status *(Akerley WL, et al: J Clin Oncol 26: abstract 8043, 2008).*

In a multicenter US trial reported by Fossella et al, 373 patients were randomized to receive either docetaxel (100 mg/m^2 [D100] or 75 mg/m^2 [D75]) or a control regimen of vinorelbine (30 mg/m^2/wk) or ifosfamide (2 g/m^2 × 3 days) every 3 weeks. Overall response rates were 10.8% with D100 and 6.7% with D75, each significantly higher than the 0.8% response of the control arm (P = .001 and P = .036, respectively). Although overall survival was not significantly different among the three groups, the 1-year survival was significantly higher with D75 than with the control treatment (32% vs 19%; P = .025).

In a phase III trial led by Hanna et al, 572 previously treated patients were randomized to receive pemetrexed with vitamin B_{12}, folic acid, and dexamethasone or docetaxel with dexamethasone. The overall response rate in the pemetrexed arm was higher, 9.1% vs 8.8%. The median disease progression–free survival was 2.9 months for each arm, and the median survival favored pemetrexed (8.3 months vs 7.9 months). The 1-year survival for each arm was 29.7%. Adverse reactions (grade 3/4) were more severe with docetaxel.

The second trial reported by Shepherd et al compared single-agent docetaxel with best supportive care. The initial docetaxel dose was 100 mg/m^2, which was changed to 75 mg/m^2 midway through the trial because of toxicity. A total of 204 patients were enrolled; 49 received D100, 55 received D75, and 100 received best supportive care. Treatment with docetaxel was associated with significant prolongation of survival (7.0 months vs 4.6 months; log-rank test, P = .047) and time to disease progression (10.6 weeks vs 6.7 weeks; P < .001).

Hanna et al conducted a noninferiority trial to test whether pemetrexed was equivalent to docetaxel in the second-line setting. They randomized 571 patients to receive 500 mg/m^2 of pemetrexed or 75 mg/m^2 of docetaxel preceded by a vitamin B_{12} injection every two cycles. The median survival on the two arms was equivalent, but the pemetrexed arm had significantly less grade 3/4 neutropenia and fewer hospitalizations overall. On the basis of this study, the FDA approved pemetrexed for second-line therapy for NSCLC.

Duration of chemotherapy

ASCO has recommended that no more than eight cycles of chemotherapy be administered to patients with stage IV NSCLC. However, therapy should be individualized depending on the quality of tumor response and the patient's tolerance.

Two trials during the past 2 years have suggested that there may be some benefit to maintenance chemotherapy in patients who have response or stable disease after front-line therapy. Fidias et al suggested that adding docetaxel as maintenance therapy after platinum-based front-line chemotherapy can delay tumor progression and lead to improvements in disease-free survival. Data by Ciuleanu et al presented at the 2008 ASCO meeting utilized maintenance pemetrexed after front-line response to chemotherapy and also showed a significant improvement in progression-free survival from 2 months for placebo to 4 months for pemetrexed. In both these trials, subpopulation analysis showed that certain groups of patients tend to benefit especially from maintenance chemotherapy. This phenomenon is currently being explored by investigators.

Evidence for maintenance therapy

Recently, there has been interest in maintenance therapy using both classical cytotoxic chemotherapy and biologics. Belani et al presented data for pemetrexed maintenance therapy. The trial compared best supportive care plus pemetrexed or placebo in 663 patients with stage IIIB/IV NSCLC whose disease had not progressed after four cycles of platinum-based induction chemotherapy. The pemetrexed group had significantly better progression-free and overall survival (13.4 vs 10.6 months, respectively), with a median survival of 15.5 months vs 10.3 months with placebo. A subgroup analysis noted that the primary effect was seen with nonsquamous histology. The FDA approved pemetrexed for nonsquamous NSCLC in patients whose disease has not progressed after four cycles of platinum-based first-line therapy. Since pemetrexed was not given as a first-line treatment in this study, it is unclear if the same benefit will be seen with pemetrexed given for induction and maintenance therapy.

> The IPASS study was a phase III, multicenter, randomized, open-label, parallel-group study of 1,217 selected never- or light-smoking patients in East Asia who had advanced NSCLC and received either gefitinib or carboplatin plus paclitaxel as first-line treatment. The primary endpoint was progression-free survival; the secondary endpoints included overall survival, for which the analysis is ongoing. The 12-month rates of progression-free survival were 24.9% with gefitinib and 6.7% with carboplatin-paclitaxel ($P < .0001$). Based on these data and those of SATURN, the FDA approved erlotinib as maintenance therapy for patients with the *EGFR* mutation and for first-line maintenance treatment of locally advanced or metastatic NSCLC in patients whose disease has not progressed after four cycles of platinum-based chemotherapy *(Mok TS et al: N Eng J Med 2009;361:947–957, 2009)*.

SATURN was an international, phase III study of 889 patients that compared maintenance erlotinib (Tarceva) with placebo in patients who had received four cycles of front-line therapy. Cappuzzo et al demonstrated that maintenance erlotinib given immediately after first-line chemotherapy significantly increased progression-free survival in both wild-type and *EGFR* mutation–positive patients with hazard ratios of 0.78 and 0.10, respectively. Maintenance erlotinib is a reasonable option for patients without an *EGFR* mutation, but the benefit is not quite as dramatic as for patients with the mutation.

The BETA trial had previously compared bevacizumab in combination with erlotinib vs erlotinib alone for the treatment of advanced NSCLC after failure of first-line chemotherapy. This phase III trial demonstrated improved progression-free survival in the combination arm. Thus, ATLAS was designed to compare maintenance therapy using bevacizumab and erlotinib with bevacizumab alone following first-line therapy using bevacizumab and a platinum-containing doublet in patients with stage IIIB/IV NSCLC. The data safety monitoring committee stopped the trial early, because it met the primary endpoint, showing that the median progression-free survival was 4.8 months for the combination arm and 3.7 months for the bevacizumab-only arm. Bevacizumab has known side effects, including impaired wound healing, proteinuria, and hypertension. Survival data will be available in the next few years.

Novel and promising agents

Several novel agents are being developed for the treatment of solid tumors, including lung cancer. These novel agents include signal transduction inhibitors, such as tyrosine kinase inhibitors (eg, erlotinib, gefitinib; antiangiogenic agents, including both monoclonal antibodies, such as bevacizumab, and small molecule tyrosine kinase inhibitors of vascular endothelial growth factor (VEGF), such as sunitinib (Sutent) and sorafenib (Nexavar); and monoclonal antibodies (C225 [antiepidermal growth factor receptor antibody] and trastuzumab [Herceptin]). Many of these novel agents are being tested in combination with chemotherapeutic agents, as their mechanisms of action suggest that they may be far more effective as chronic inhibitors of cancer progression than as classic cytotoxics.

Combinations of cetuximab with chemotherapy also appear promising. Pirker et al showed that adding cetuximab to cytotoxic chemotherapy with cisplatin and vinorelbine improved median survival from 10.1 to 11.3 months in a randomized trial of 1,125 patients with advanced and metastatic NSCLC. This statistically significant (P = .044) 1.2-month improvement in median survival was not duplicated when cetuximab was added to taxane/platinum-based chemotherapy. However, in both of these studies, adding cetuximab to chemotherapy improved response rate, and these data are currently being evaluated in their totality as physicians integrate this epidermal growth factor receptor into the therapeutic arm of NSCLC.

Gefitinib and erlotinib To date, most phase I studies of these various compounds have suffered from a difficulty in developing pharmacologically or molecularly driven endpoints that will serve as reasonable intermediate biomarkers of efficacy or even surrogates for toxicity. Further research has focused on the novel small molecule tyrosine kinase inhibitors erlotinib and gefitinib. Two phase II trials of gefitinib in the second- and third-line settings were conducted in Europe and Japan. Patients were randomized to receive either 250 or 500 mg daily. The drug was found to be active, with an 11% to 18% response rate, and there was no superiority for the higher dose. Similar data were seen for erlotinib.

Unfortunately, randomized combination trials of gefitinib at 250 and 500 mg daily with cytotoxic chemotherapy, either paclitaxel and carboplatin in one trial or gemcitabine and cisplatin in the other study vs placebo in front-line therapy, failed to demonstrate any survival advantage. These results have cast a pall over the development of tyrosine kinase inhibitors in combination with chemotherapy. Regardless, the question of whether or not to approve these new agents for third-line therapy of lung cancer in cisplatin/docetaxel-refractory patients remains open for debate.

The activity demonstrated by gefitinib and erlotinib as single agents in advanced NSCLC generated much optimism, including a recent trial indicating that erlotinib improved survival (by a median of 2 months) in the second- and third-line treatments of NSCLC, with a substantial increase in 1-year survival ($P < .001$). After the initial successes with chemotherapy and promising results from targeted tyrosine kinase inhibitors in stages IIIB and IV NSCLC, several large phase III trials of either gefitinib or erlotinib in combination with conventional platinum-based chemotherapy were conducted as the INTACT 1 and INTACT 2 trials or the TALENT and TRIBUTE trials.

The phase III trials of single-agent erlotinib and gefitinib, when compared with best supportive care in the second- and third-line settings, had dramatically different results. Shepherd et al conducted a randomized trial of erlotinib (150 mg daily) vs placebo in 723 patients previously treated with front- or second-line chemotherapy for NSCLC. A total of 488 patients received erlotinib and 243 received placebo.

The median overall survival significantly favored the erlotinib arm (6.7 months vs 4.7 months), with a reduction in the hazard ratio of 0.73 ($P > .001$), as did the 1-year survival rate (31% vs 21%; $P > .01$). QOL and median time to deterioration also significantly favored erlotinib. On the other hand, the phase III trial of gefitinib vs best supportive care in more than 1,600 patients was reported and showed no significant advantage to gefitinib at 250 mg daily in a patient population with a significant number of active smokers.

For patients who have the classic exon 19 or 21 mutation, erlotinib and gefitinib provide a significant advantage over standard chemotherapy. However, some patients are resistant or develop a *T790M* mutation; this adds a bulky methionine group in the ATP binding pocket, which sterically hinders the attachment of tyrosine kinase inhibitors. Newer, irreversible EGFR tyrosine kinase inhibitors are believed to be able to bind in spite of this mutation. In a phase II study of 67 stage IIIB/IV NSCLC patients with *EGFR* mutation–positive disease, BIBW 2992 is showing promise, with a disease control rate of 95%.

Bevacizumab When combined with chemotherapy, bevacizumab appears to result in a significant survival advantage for patients with advanced NSCLC. Based on promising phase II data of bevacizumab in combination with carboplatin and paclitaxel, Sandler et al randomized 878 patients to receive either bevacizumab with carboplatin and paclitaxel or carboplatin and paclitaxel alone.

There was a significant increase in the response rate for the combination (27.2%) with bevacizumab vs paclitaxel and carboplatin alone (10%; $P < .0001$), and both median and progression-free survival significantly favored the bevacizumab combination arm (overall survival: 12.5 months vs 10.2 months; $P = .007$; hazard ratio = 0.77; 95% CI = 0.65–0.93; progression-free survival: 6.4 months vs 4.5 months; $P < .0001$; hazard ratio = 0.62; 95% CI = 0.53–0.72). As in the phase

TABLE 6: Single-agent chemotherapy regimens for NSCLC

Drug	Dose and schedule
Vinorelbine	30 mg/m² IV weekly
LeChevalier T, Brisgand D, Douillard J-Y, et al: J Clin Oncol 12:360–367, 1994.	
Vinorelbine	For patients 70 years old or older: 30 mg/m² IV on days 1 and 8, every 21 days
Gridelli C, Perrone F, Cigolari S, et al: Proc Am Soc Clin Oncol [abstract] 20:308a, 2001.	
Docetaxel	75 mg/m² IV on day 1 every 3 weeks
Shepherd FA, Dancey J, Ramlau R, et al: J Clin Oncol 18:2095–2103, 2000.	
Pemetrexed	500 mg/m² IVPB every 3 weeks
Dexamethasone (4 mg by mouth twice daily) should be started a day before and a day after pemetrexed. All patients should also receive folic acid (350–1,000 mg/d) started about a week before and thereafter while taking pemetrexed. Vitamin B_{12} (1,000 mg IM) should be started about 1 to 2 weeks before pemetrexed and every 9 weeks while taking pemetrexed.	
Hanna N, Shepherd F, Fossella FV, et al: J Clin Oncol [abstract] 22:1589–1597, 2004.	
Erlotinib	150 mg orally once a day
Perez-Soler R, Chachoua A, Hammond LA, et al: N Engl J Med 22:3238–3247, 2004.	
Gefitinib	250 mg orally once a day
Kris MG, Natale RB, Herbst RS, et al: JAMA 290:2149–2158, 2003.	
Gemcitabine	1,000 mg/m² IV on days 1, 8, and 15 every 4 weeks
Vansteenkiste J,Vandebroek J, Nackaerts K, et al: Proc Am Soc Clin Oncol [abstract] 19:1910a, 2000.	

IVPB = intravenous piggyback
Table prepared by Ishmael Jaiyesimi, DO.

II trial, this study reported a total of eight treatment-related deaths on the bevacizumab arm vs two on the paclitaxel and carboplatin arm. A second phase III randomized trial testing the value of adding bevacizumab to gemcitabine and cisplatin therapy showed an improvement in disease-free survival, but not overall survival.

Other promising novel agents currently being investigated in lung cancer include inhibitors of the insulin-like growth factor receptor. Karp et al showed that these agents appear to be particularly promising in patients with squamous cell lung tumors, with response rates in a small study as high as 70%. As more pathways involved in NSCLC are found, more clinical trials involving inhibitors of phosphoinositide 3-kinase, c-MET (where sensitivity is predicted by a mutation in *BRAF* [B-*Raf* proto-oncogene serine/threonine-protein kinase]), and insulin-like growth factor (IGF) are being initiated. In addition, PF-02341066 is a promising agent being tested in early-phase clinical trials that inhibits both MET and anaplastic lymphoma kinase (ALK).

Personalized therapies

Evaluation of NSCLC involves distinction between a squamous lesion or adenocarcinoma and of actual genetic differences. Pemetrexed and bevacizumab are used in nonsquamous histology, and erlotinib is given for *EGFR* mutations, but other oncogene addictions are becoming apparent. *ALK* gene rearrangement occurs in 4% of NSCLC patients with *EML4* (echinoderm microtubule associate protein like 4) as its most common fusion partner. *EML4-ALK* is seen in up to 20% of nonsmokers and about 30% of patients who are never-smokers and *EGFR* wild-type. It is strongly associated with signet ring cell histology. PF-02341066 is now being studied in a phase I trial in patients with a mutation in *EML4-ALK*; the overall response rate was 59% with ongoing analysis.

Current treatment recommendations

It is important to note that patients who have lost significant amounts of weight or who have a poor performance status are at greater risk for toxicity, including a higher likelihood of lethal toxicity, when they are treated with modest doses of chemotherapy. Based on currently available data, a reasonable approach for patients with stage IV NSCLC who have a good performance status (ECOG performance status 0/1) and have not lost a significant amount of weight (< 5% of usual weight) would be to encourage them to participate in a clinical trial. However, it would also be appropriate to treat this group of patients with etoposide plus cisplatin or with one of the newer combination regimens, such as gemcitabine/cisplatin, vinorelbine/cisplatin, paclitaxel/cisplatin, paclitaxel/carboplatin, or docetaxel/cisplatin (Tables 6 and 7).

Role of photodynamic therapy (PDT)

PDT, which combines Photofrin (a hematoporphyrin derivative in which the less active porphyrin monomers have been removed) with an argon-pumped dye laser, has been explored in a variety of different tumors, with varying results. Several investigators have reported excellent results with PDT in early-stage head and neck cancers as well as intrathoracic tumors. However, initial studies have involved a limited number of patients.

Although this novel technique seems to be extremely promising, it appears to be applicable to a minority of patients with NSCLC. Nevertheless, PDT appears to be particularly useful for the treatment of early-stage lung cancer for a variety of reasons. First, it appears to preserve lung function and can be repeated as additional tumors appear—an important consideration as such patients appear to be at high risk for developing other new tumors. Second, this technique does not preclude ultimate surgical intervention when deemed necessary.

Results in early-stage NSCLC

Perhaps most striking are the results reported by Furuse et al, who treated 54 patients with 64 early-stage lung cancers using Photofrin (2.0 mg/kg) and 630-nm illumination of 100 to 200 J/cm^2. Of 59 accessible tumors, 50 responded completely and 6 showed partial responses. Five of the complete responders developed recurrences 6 to 8 months after treatment.

TABLE 7: Combination chemotherapy regimens recommended for NSCLC

Regimen	Agents	Dose and schedule	Treatment interval
PT	Platinol	75 mg/m² IV on day 2	3 weeks
	Taxol	135 mg/m² IV on day 1 (24-h infusion)	
CP	Carboplatin	AUC of 6 mg/mL/min IV on day 1	
	Paclitaxel	225 mg/m² IV on day 1 (3-h infusion)	3 weeks
PG	Platinol	100 mg/m² IV on day 1	4 weeks
	Gemcitabine	1,000 mg/m² IV on days 1, 8, and 15	
PD	Platinol	75 mg/m² IV on day 1	3 weeks
	Docetaxel	75 mg/m² IV on day 1	
PV	Platinol	100 mg/m² IV on day 1	4 weeks
	Vinorelbine	25 mg/m² IV on days 1, 8, 15, and 22	
PCB	Paclitaxel	200 mg/m² IV on day 1 (3-hr infusion)	3 weeks
	Carboplatin	AUC of 6 mg/mL/min IV on day 1	
	Bevacizumab	15 mg/kg IV	
PC[a]	Pemetrexed	500 mg/m² IV on day 1	3 weeks
	Cisplatin	75 mg/m² IV on day 1	

AUC = area under the concentration-time curve

[a]Carboplatin may be substituted in patients with poor performance status. Dexamethasone (4 mg by mouth twice daily) should be started a day before and a day after pemetrexed. All patients should also receive folic acid (350–1,000 mg/d) started about a week before and thereafter while taking pemetrexed. Vitamin B_{12} (1,000 mg IM) should be started about 1 to 2 weeks before pemetrexed and every 9 weeks during therapy.

The major predictor of response in this study was tumor length. The likelihood of achieving a complete response was 97.8% if the tumor was < 1 cm, as opposed to only 42.9% if the lesion was > 1 cm. The overall survival rate in these patients was 50% at 3 years.

A similar study by Kato et al also indicated a 96.8% complete response rate for tumors < 0.5 cm but only a 37.5% rate for tumors > 2 cm. The overall 5-year survival rate for the 75 patients treated in this study was 68.4%, which is acceptable by current standards.

Results in advanced-stage NSCLC Two prospective, randomized trials (European and US/Canadian) compared PDT with the neodymium:yttrium-aluminum-garnet (Nd:YAG) laser for partially obstructive, advanced NSCLC. Investigators analyzed results from the two trials both individually and collectively. Collective analysis included data from 15 centers in Europe and 20 centers in the United States and Canada and involved a total of 211 patients. In the European trial, 40% of the patients had received prior therapy, whereas in the US/Canadian trial, all of the patients had received previous treatment.

TABLE 8: Percentage of patients with symptoms of NSCLC palliated by external-beam irradiation

Symptom	Standard RT (24–30 Gy in 6–10 fractions)	17 Gy in 2 fractions (first trial/second trial)	1 fraction of 10 Gy
Cough	56	65/48	56
Hemoptysis	86	81/75	72
Chest pain	80	75/59	72
Anorexia	64	68/45	55
Depression	57	72/NA	NA
Anxiety	66	71/NA	NA
Breathlessness	57	66/41	43

NA = data not available; RT = radiation therapy
Data from Bleehen NM, Girling DJ, Fayers PM, et al: Br J Cancer 63:265–270, 1991; Bleehen NM, Bolger JJ, Hasleton PS, et al: Br J Cancer 65:934–941, 1992.

Tumor response was similar for both therapies at 1 week. However, at 1 month, 61% and 42% of the patients treated with PDT in the European and US/Canadian trials, respectively, were still responding, compared with 36% and 19% of patients who underwent laser therapy in the two trials.

PDT also produced more dramatic improvements in dyspnea and cough than did Nd:YAG therapy in the European trial, but the two treatments had similar effects on these symptoms in the US/Canadian trial. Both sets of investigators concluded that PDT appears to be superior to laser therapy for the relief of dyspnea, cough, and hemoptysis. Also, the overall incidence of adverse reactions was similar with the two therapies (73% for PDT vs 64% for Nd:YAG therapy). Early-stage lung cancer, most specifically endobronchial squamous cell carcinoma smaller than 1 cm, is effectively treated with PDT, with a complete response rate of 75% and a recurrence rate of 30% over 5 years.

Palliation of local and distant symptoms

Radiation therapy

Many patients with lung cancer experience distressing local symptoms at some time. They may arise from airway obstruction by the primary tumor, compression of mediastinal structures by nodal metastases, or metastatic involvement of distant organs. Radiation therapy is effective in palliating most local symptoms, as well as symptoms at common metastatic sites, such as bone and brain. For selected patients with a solitary brain metastasis and controlled disease in other sites, resection followed by irradiation appears to be superior to radiation therapy alone in improving both survival and QOL. (For more information regarding management of brain metastases, see chapter 23.)

Doses In the United States, radiation oncologists often use doses of ~30 Gy in 10 fractions for palliative thoracic treatment in lung cancer. Data from the United

Kingdom suggest that similar efficacy without greater toxicity may be achieved with more abbreviated schedules, such as 17 Gy in two fractions 1 week apart or single fractions of 10 Gy (see Table 8). Such schedules may facilitate the coordination of irradiation and chemotherapy and also reduce patient travel and hospitalization.

Just over 400 patients with inoperable NSCLC (stage III/IV) were randomized to receive three different fractionation regimens (8.5 Gy × 2, 2.8 Gy × 15, or 2.0 Gy × 25). Using the EORTC Quality-of-Life Questionnaire (QLQ) C-30 with the lung cancer–specific module (LC-13), Sundstrom et al found the effect of hypofractionated irradiation (17 Gy in two fractions) was comparable to that achieved with longer fractionation schemes with regard to symptom relief and survival.

Endobronchial irradiation with cobalt-60 or iridium-192 has been used to palliate symptoms arising from partial airway obstruction, including cough, dyspnea, and hemoptysis. The dosimetric advantage of being able to deliver a high radiation dose to the obstructing endobronchial tumor while sparing adjacent normal structures, such as the lungs, spinal cord, and esophagus, has clear appeal, particularly in the patient whose disease has recurred following prior external-beam irradiation. Although good rates of palliation have been reported with endobronchial irradiation, significant complications, including fatal hemoptysis, are seen in 5% to 10% of patients. It remains unclear, however, how often this complication is actually due to the irradiation or the underlying disease itself.

Endobronchial irradiation should be considered as one of several approaches (including laser excision, cryotherapy, and stent placement) used in the management of patients with symptomatic airway obstruction, and management should be individualized. All of these approaches are more suitable for partial than for complete airway obstruction.

Chemotherapy

Several trials have explored the use of chemotherapy to palliate specific symptoms in patients with lung cancer. In general, these trials have found that rates of symptomatic improvement were considerably higher than objective response rates and were not dissimilar to symptomatic response rates with local radiation therapy.

Thus, although radiation therapy remains the most appropriate modality for the treatment of such problems as superior vena cava obstruction, spinal cord compression, brain metastases, or localized bone pain, patients who have more extensive disease without these local emergencies may be considered for palliative chemotherapy, which may relieve local symptoms and prolong survival.

Bisphosphonates

Approximately 30% to 65% of patients with advanced lung cancer develop bone metastases. The median survival following development of bone metastases is 6 months. Bone disease is associated with significant morbidity, including severe pain, hypercalcemia of malignancy, pathologic fracture, and spinal cord or nerve root compression. Treatment of bone metastases may include surgical intervention, radiation therapy, and chemotherapy. Bisphosphonate treatment can decrease skeleton-related complications, delay progressive disease, and relieve bone pain.

Bisphosphonates such as clodronate, pamidronate, and zoledronic acid (Zometa) exhibit strong affinity for the hydroxyapatite crystal of bone and preferentially accumulate at sites of active bone remodeling, where they prevent bone resorption. They provide effective treatment for hypercalcemia of malignancy and have been shown to delay the onset of progressive bone disease and relieve bone pain in studies largely performed in patients with metastases secondary to breast cancer, multiple myeloma, and prostate cancer. Nitrogen-containing bisphosphonates, such as pamidronate and zoledronic acid, appear to exert antitumor effects. Zoledronic acid has also been found to have pronounced antinociceptive effects, which have been absent with other bisphosphonates in preclinical studies. Zoledronic acid is the only bisphosphonate shown to be effective in reducing skeletal complications in patients with bone metastases from lung cancer and solid tumors other than breast and prostate cancers.

FOLLOW-UP OF LONG-TERM SURVIVORS

At present, no standard follow-up protocol exists for patients with cured NSCLC or SCLC. However, long-term follow-up should at least include serial physical examinations once the patient has reached the 5-year mark. Controversy currently exists about the value of utilizing CT scanning or even chest x-rays for the long-term follow-up of these patients.

In this vein, retrospective reviews of the literature have revealed that patients with SCLC appear to have the highest rate of second primary tumor development—as high as 30%—over the course of their lifetime, with some studies reporting annual second primary tumor rates of 5% to 10%. Therefore, the concept of chemoprevention appears to have particular merit in these patients.

A randomized chemoprevention study of patients with stage I NSCLC showed a surprisingly high annual recurrence rate of 6.5% in patients with T1 tumors, as opposed to 11.2% in patients with T2 tumors. Whether retinoids are effective chemopreventive agents remains to be seen. Nevertheless, there is clearly a need for effective chemoprevention for both of these tumor subsets, as well as the establishment of consistent guidelines for routine long-term follow-up. Given the current controversy over lung cancer screening, however, it is unlikely that this issue will be resolved without the performance of another prospective screening trial.

SUGGESTED READING

Albain KS, Swann RS, Rusch VW, et al: Radiotherapy plus chemotherapy with or without surgical resection for stage III non-small-cell lung cancer: A phase III randomised controlled trial. Lancet 374:379–386, 2009.

Arriagada R, Bergman B, Dunant A, et al: Cisplatin-based adjuvant chemotherapy in patients with completely resected non-small-cell lung cancer. N Engl J Med 350:351–360, 2004.

Arriagada R, Dunant A, Pignon JP, et al: Long-term results of the international adjuvant lung cancer trial evaluating adjuvant cisplatin-based chemotherapy in resected lung cancer. J Clin Oncol 28:35–42, 2010.

Bach PB, Jett JR, Pastorino U, et al: Computed tomography screening and lung cancer outcomes. JAMA 297:953–961, 2007.

Belani CP, Brodowicz T, Ciuleanu T, et al: Maintenance pemetrexed plus best supportive care (BSC) versus placebo plus BSC: A randomized phase III study in advanced non-small cell lung cancer. J Clin Oncol 27(18S): abstract CRA8000, 2009.

Blumenschein GR Jr, Khuri FR, von Pawel J, et al: Phase III trial comparing carboplatin, paclitaxel, and bexarotene with carboplatin and paclitaxel in chemotherapy-naive patients with advanced or metastatic non–small-cell lung cancer: SPIRIT II. J Clin Oncol 26:1879–1885, 2008.

Brenner DJ, Hall EJ: Computed tomography—An increasing source of radiation exposure. N Engl J Med 357:2277–2284, 2007.

Capuzzo F, Ciuleanu T, Stelmakh L, et al: SATURN: A double-blind, randomized, phase III study of maintenance erlotinib versus placebo following non-progression with first-line platinum-based chemotherapy in patients with advanced NSCLC. J Clin Oncol 27(15S): abstract 8001.

Ciuleanu T, Brodowicz T, Zielinski C, et al: Maintenance pemetrexed plus best supportive care versus placebo plus best supportive care for non-small cell lung cancer: A randomized, double-blind, phase 3 study. Lancet 374:1432–1440, 2009.

Douillard JY, Tribodet H, Aubert D, et al: Adjuvant cisplatin and vinorelbine for completely resected non-small cell lung cancer: subgroup analysis of the Lung Adjuvant Cisplatin Evaluation. J Clin Oncol 5:220–228, 2010.

Giaccone G, Herbst RS, Manegold C, et al: Gefitinib in combinaton with gemcitabine and cisplatin in advanced non-small-cell lung cancer: A phase III–INTACT 1. J Clin Oncol 22:777–784, 2004.

Govindan R, Bogart J, Wang X, et al: Phase II study of pemetrexed, carboplatin, and thoracic radiation with or without cetuximab in patients with locally advanced unresectable non-small cell lung cancer: CALGB 30407. J Clin Oncol 27(15S): abstract 7505, 2009.

Gronberg BH, Bremnes RM, Flotten O, et al: Phase III study by the Norwegian lung cancer study group: pemetrexed plus carboplatin compared with gemcitabine plus carboplatin as first-line chemotherapy in advanced non-small-cell lung cancer. J Clin Oncol 27:3217–3224, 2009.

Hanna NH: Phase III trial of cisplatin plus etoposide plus concurrent chest radiation with or without consolidation docetaxel in patients with inoperable stage III non-small cell lung cancer: HOG LUN 01-24/USO-023. J Clin Oncol 26:5755–5760, 2008.

Herbst RS, Giaccone G, Schiller JH, et al: Gefitinib in combination with paclitaxel and carboplatin in advanced non-small -cell lung cancer: A phase III trial–INTACT 2. J Clin Oncol 22:785–794, 2004.

I-ELCAP; Henschke CI, Yankelevitz DF, et al: Survival of patients with stage I lung cancer detected on CT screening. N Engl J Med 355:1763–1771, 2006.

Jemal A, Siegel R, Xu J, et al: Cancer statistics, 2010. CA Cancer J Clin 60:277–300, 2010.

Karp DD, Paz-Ares LG, Novello S, et al: High activity of the anti-IGF-IR antibody CP-751,871 in combination with paclitaxel and carboplatin in squamous NSCLC. J Clin Oncol 26:8015, 2008.

Kato H, Ichinose Y, Ohta M, et al: A randomized trial of adjuvant chemotherapy with uracil-tegafur for adenocarcinoma of the lung. N Engl J Med 350:1713–1721, 2004.

Kawahara M: Irinotecan in the treatment of small cell lung cancer: A review of patient safety considerations. Expert Opin Drug Saf 5:303–312, 2006.

Komaki R, Sejpal SV, Wei X, et al: Significant reduction of bone marrow toxicity for patients with locally advanced NSCLC treated with concurrent chemotherapy and proton beam therapy compared to intensity modulated radiation therapy. Radiother Oncol 90:S61, 2009.

Kuzdzat J, Zielinski M, Papla B, et al: The transcervical extended mediastinal lymphadenectomy versus cervical mediastinoscopy in non-small cell lung cancer staging. Eur J Cardiothorac Surg 31:88–94, 2007.

Lilenbaum RC, Herndon J, List M, et al: Single-agent versus combination chemotherapy in advanced NSCLC: The Cancer and Leukemia Group B (study 9730). J Clin Oncol 23:190–196, 2005.

Miller VA, O'Connor P, Soh C, et al: A randomized, double-blinded, placebo-controlled, phase IIIb trial (ATLAS) comparing bevacizumab therapy with or without erlotinib after completion of chemotherapy with B for first-line treatment of locally advanced, recurrent, or metastatic non-small cell lung cancer. J Clin Oncol 27(18S): abstract LBA8002, 2009.

Mok TS, Wu YL, Thongprasert S, et al: Gefitinib or carboplatin-paclitaxel in pulmonary adenocarcinoma. N Eng J Med 361:947–957, 2009.

Movsas B, Bae K, Meyers C, et al: Phase III study of prophylactic cranial irradiation versus observation in patients with stage III non-small cell lung cancer: Neurocognitive and quality of life analysis of RTOG 0214. 2009 Annual ASTRO Meeting; September 11–12, 2009; St. Louis, Missouri.

Movsas B, Moughan J, Sarna L, et al: Quality of life supersedes the classic prognosticators for long-term survival in locally advanced non-small-cell lung cancer: an analysis of RTOG 9801. J Clin Oncol 27:5816–5822, 2009.

Peng G, Tinner RG, Wang Y, et al: Comparison of patient outcomes stratified by histology among pemetrexed-treated patients with stage IIIB/IV non-small cell lung cancer in two phase II trials. J Clin Oncol 26(15S): abstract 8096, 2008.

Pirker R, Szczesna A, von Pawel J, et al: FLEX: A randomized, multicenter, phase III study of cetuximab in combination with cisplatin/vinorelbine (CV) versus CV alone in the first-line treatment of patients with advanced non–small-cell lung cancer (NSCLC). J Clin Oncol 26:[abstract 3], 2008.

Pisters K, Vallieres E, Bunn PA, et al: S9900: Surgery alone or surgery plus induction paclitaxel/carboplatin chemotherapy in early stage non-small cell lung cancer: Follow-up on a phase III trial. J Clin Oncol 25:[18S]:7520, 2007.

Ramlau R, Zatloukal P, Jassem J, et al: Randomized phase III trial comparing bexarotene (L1069-49)/cisplatin/vinorelbine with cisplatin/vinorelbine in chemotherapy-naive patients with advanced or metastatic non–small-cell lung cancer: SPIRIT I. J Clin Oncol 26:1886–1892, 2008.

Sandler AB, Gray R, Brahmer J, et al: Randomized phase II/III trial of paclitaxel plus carboplatin with or without bevacizumab in patients with advanced non-squamous non-small-cell lung cancer: An Eastern Cooperative Oncology Group trial. N Engl J Med 355:2542–2550, 2006.

Scagliotti GV, Parikh P, von Pawel J, et al: Phase III study comparing cisplatin plus gemcitabine with cisplatin plus pemetrexed in chemotherapy-naive patients with advanced-stage non-small-cell lung cancer. J Clin Oncol 26:3543–3551, 2008.

Shaw AT, Yeap BY, Mino-Kenudson M, et al: Clinical features and outcome of patients with non-small-cell lung cancer who harbor EML4-ALK. J Clin Oncol 27:4247–4253, 2009.

Shepherd FA, Rodrigues Pereira J, Ciuleanu T, et al: Erlotinib in previously treated non-small-cell lung cancer. N Engl J Med 353:123–132, 2005.

Shih J, Yang C, Su W, et al: A phase II study of BIBW 2992, a novel irreversible dual EGFR and HER2 tyrosine kinase inhibitor, in patients with adenocarcinoma of the lung and activating EGFR mutations after failure of one line of chemotherapy (LUX-Lung 2). J Clin Oncol 27(15s): abstract 8013.

Simon G: Personalized chemotherapy may favorably alter intrinsic disease biology to produce a higher proportion of long term survivors in patients with advanced NSCLC. 2009 Annual Meeting of the International Association for the Study of Lung Cancer; July 31–August 4, 2009; San Francisco, California. Abstract D7.6.

Strauss GM: Adjuvant chemotherapy of lung cancer: Methodologic issues and therapeutic advances. Hematol Oncol Clin North Am 19:263–281, 2005.

Strauss GM, Herndon JE, Maddaus MA, et al: Adjuvant chemotherapy in stage IB non-small cell lung cancer: Update of Cancer and Leukemia Group B protocol 9633. J Clin Oncol 24[18S]:7007, 2006.

Sundstrom S, Bremnes RM, Aasebo U, et al: Hypofractionated palliative radiotherapy (17 Gy/2 fractions) in advanced NSCLC is comparable to standard fractionation for symptom control and survival: A national phase III trial. J Clin Oncol 22:801–810, 2004.

Timmerman R, McGarry R, Yiannoutsos C, et al: Excessive toxicity when treating central tumors in a phase II study of stereotactic body radiation therapy for medically inoperable early-stage lung cancer. J Clin Oncol 24:4833–4839, 2006.

Timmerman R, Paulus R, Galvin J, et al: Stereotactic body radiation therapy for inoperable early stage lung cancer. JAMA 303:1070–1076, 2010.

Vincent MD, Butts C, Seymour L, et al: Updated survival analysis of JBR.10: A randomized phase III trial of vinorelbine/cisplatin versus observation in completely resected stage IB and II non-small cell lung cancer. J Clin Oncol 27(15S): abstract 7501, 2009.

Winton T, Livingston R, Johnson D, et al: Vinorelbine plus cisplatin vs. observation in resected non-small cell lung cancer. N Engl J Med 352:2589–2597, 2005.

Abbreviations in this chapter

ALPI = Adjuvant Lung Project Italy; ANITA = Adjuvant Navelbine International Trialist Association; ASA= American Socity of Anesthesiologists; ASCO = American Society of Clinical Oncology; ATLAS = A Study Comparing Bevacizumab Therapy With or Without Erlotinib for First-Line Treatment of Non-Small Cell Lung Cancer; BETA = Bevacizumab/ Tarceva; BMRC = British Medical Research Council; CALGB = Cancer and Leukemia Group; B ECOG = Eastern Cooperative Oncology Group; EORTC = European Organisation for Research on the Treatment of Cancer; FDA = US Food and Drug Administration; HOG = Hoosier Oncology Group; IALT = International Adjuvant Cancer Trial; IASLC = International Association for the Study of Lung Cancer; I-ELCAP = International Early Lung Cancer Action Project; INTACT = Iressa NSCLC Trial Assessing Combination Treatment; IPASS= Iressa Pan-Asia Study; LACE = Lung Adjuvant Cisplatin Evaluation; LCSG = Lung Cancer Study Group; MADeIT = Molecular Analyses Directed Individualized Therapy for Advanced Non-Small Cell Lung Cancer; NCI = National Cancer Institute; NLST = National Lung Screening Trial; PASSPORT = A Study of Bevacizumab in Combination With First- or Second-Line Therapy in Subjects With Treated Brain Metastases Due to Non-Squamous NSCLC; PLCO = Prostate, Lung, Colorectal, and Ovarian Cancer Screening Trial; ROSEL = Radiosurgery or Surgery for Operable Stage I NSCLC; RTOG = Radiation Therapy Oncology Group; SATURN = Sequential Tarceva in Unresectable NSCLC; SEER = Surveillance, Epidemiology, and End Results; SICOG = Southern Italy Cooperative Oncology Group; SLCG = Spanish Lung Cancer Group; SWOG = Southwest Oncology Group; TALENT = Tarceva Lung Cancer Investigation; TRIBUTE = Tarceva Responses in Conjunction with Paclitaxel and Carboplatin; WHO = World Health Organization

CHAPTER 4

Small-cell lung cancer, mesothelioma, and thymoma

Bonnie S. Glisson, MD, Benjamin Movsas, MD, and Walter Scott, MD

As discussed in chapter 3, there are two major subdivisions of lung cancer: small-cell lung cancer (SCLC), for which chemotherapy is the primary treatment, and non–small-cell lung cancer (NSCLC). SCLC is decreasing in frequency in the United States, with recent data showing it represents only 14% of lung cancers. This chapter provides information on the staging and prognosis, pathology and pathophysiology, treatment, and follow-up of long-term survivors of SCLC and concludes with brief discussions on mesothelioma and thymoma.

Chapter 3 provides information on the epidemiology, etiology, screening and prevention, and diagnosis of lung cancer in general and covers NSCLC and carcinoid tumors of the lungs.

SMALL-CELL LUNG CANCER

STAGING AND PROGNOSIS

An international database consisting of 8,088 patients with SCLC was developed by the International Society for the Study of Lung Cancer (IASLC). Their analysis showed that the 7th edition of the TNM staging system is applicable to SCLC. IASLC recommends that the 7th edition of the AJCC lung cancer should be applied to both NSCLC and SCLC (see chapter 3, Table 1). SCLC has previously been described as either limited (M0) or extensive (M1), although these general terms are inadequate when evaluating the role of surgery. Patients with SCLC who have stages I–III disease, excluding those with a malignant pleural effusion, are classified as having limited disease. These patients constitute approximately one-third of all SCLC patients. The remaining SCLC patients fall into the extensive-disease category, which includes any patient with a malignant pleural effusion or any site of distant disease, such as the brain, liver, adrenal gland, bone, and bone marrow.

The staging of lung cancer must be conducted in a methodical and detailed manner to permit appropriate therapeutic recommendations and to allow comparison of treatment results from different institutions.

Stage is commonly reported as either clinical or pathologic. The former is based on noninvasive (or minimally invasive) tests, whereas the latter is based on tissue obtained during surgery (see chapter 3).

The most important prognostic factor in lung cancer is the stage of disease. Within a given disease stage, the next most important prognostic factors are performance status and recent weight loss. The two scales used to define performance status are the ECOG performance status system and the Karnofsky performance index (see Appendix 1). In short, patients who are ambulatory have a significantly longer survival. Those who have lost ≥ 5% of body weight during the preceding 3 to 6 months have a worse prognosis.

PATHOLOGY AND PATHOPHYSIOLOGY

SCLC tends to present with a large central lung mass and associated extensive hilar and mediastinal lymphadenopathy. Clinically evident distant metastases are present in approximately two-thirds of patients at diagnosis. Additionally, data from autopsy examination indicate micrometastatic disease in 63% of patients who died within 30 days of attempted curative resection of SCLC. Thus, it is a systemic disease at presentation in the majority of patients.

SCLC is a small, blue, round cell tumor that is primitive and undifferentiated at the light microscopic level. Electron microscopy demonstrates its neuroendocrine derivation by the presence of dense core granules. The immunohistochemical evidence of neuroendocrine derivation includes positive staining for chromogranin, synaptophysin, and other proteins. The amine precursor uptake and decarboxylation machinery present in the dense core granule leads to the production of biologically active amines and promotes the synthesis of polypeptide hormones such as ADH and ACTH. Paraneoplastic syndromes due to hormone excess result. The most common of these syndromes, syndrome of inappropriate antidiuretic hormone secretion, occurs in approximately 10% of patients with SCLC. Hypercortisolism and a Cushing-like syndrome are more rare, seen in only 1% to 2% of patients.

TREATMENT

TREATMENT OF DISEASE LIMITED TO LUNG PARENCHYMA

Surgery

The majority of patients with SCLC present with advanced-stage disease. In the 5% to 10% of patients whose tumor is limited to the lung parenchyma, very often the diagnosis is established only after the lung mass has been removed. If, however, the histology has been determined by bronchoscopic biopsy or fine-needle aspiration and there is no evidence of metastatic disease following extensive scanning, examination of the bone marrow, and biopsy of the mediastinal lymph nodes, resection should be performed. Adjuvant chemotherapy is recommended because of the high likelihood of the development of distant metastases following surgery.

The surgical approach in SCLC is similar to that used in NSCLC: A lobectomy or pneumonectomy should be followed by a thorough mediastinal lymph node dissection. Tumor resection in SCLC should be limited to patients who have no evidence of mediastinal or supraclavicular lymph node metastases. Data suggest that patients with SCLC presenting as a solitary pulmonary nodule and proven pathologically to be stage I have a 5-year survival rate of ~70% when treated with resection and adjuvant chemotherapy.

TREATMENT OF DISEASE LIMITED TO THE THORAX

Approximately one-third of SCLC patients present with disease that is limited to the thorax and can be encompassed within a tolerable radiation portal. In early studies in which either radiation therapy or surgery alone was used to treat such patients, median survival was only 3 to 4 months, and the 5-year survival rate was in the range of 1% to 2%. The reason for the failure of these therapies was both rapid recurrence of intrathoracic tumor and development of distant metastasis.

Chemotherapy

During the 1970s, it became apparent that SCLC was relatively sensitive to chemotherapy. Various combination chemotherapy regimens were used to treat limited SCLC. Although none of the regimens was clearly superior, median survival was approximately 12 months, and the 2-year survival rate was approximately 10% to 15%. It appears that maintenance chemotherapy adds little to survival in patients with limited SCLC.

Chemotherapy plus thoracic irradiation

One of the major advances in treating SCLC in the past 15 years is the recognition of the value of early and concurrent thoracic chemoradiation therapy. This advance was clearly facilitated by the increase in therapeutic index when PE (cisplatin [Platinol]/etoposide) chemotherapy is given with thoracic irradiation, as opposed to older anthracycline- or alkylator-based regimens. Although the major impact from this approach is improved locoregional tumor control, there are hints from randomized trials that early control of disease in the chest can also reduce the risk of distant metastasis.

An Intergroup trial directly compared once-daily with twice-daily fractionation (45 Gy/25 fractions/5 weeks vs 45 Gy/30 fractions/3 weeks) given at the beginning of concurrent chemoradiation therapy with PE. Initial analysis showed excellent overall results, with median survival for all patients of 20 months and a 40% survival rate at 2 years. With a minimum follow-up of 5 years, survival was significantly better in the twice-daily than in the once-daily irradiation group (26% vs 16%). The only difference in toxicity was a temporary increase in grade 3 esophagitis in patients receiving twice-daily radiation therapy.

Outcomes for patients with limited-stage SCLC have improved significantly over the past 20 years. In an analysis of phase III trials during this period, median survival was 12 months in the control arm in 26 phase III studies initiated between 1972 and 1981, compared with 17 months in studies between 1982 and 1992 ($P < .001$). Five studies demonstrated a statistically significant improvement in survival in the experimental arm compared with the control arm. Interestingly, all five studies involved some aspect of thoracic radiation therapy (three trials compared chemotherapy alone vs chemoradiation therapy; one compared early with late radiation therapy; and one compared daily vs twice-daily thoracic radiation therapy). Similarly, data from the SEER database demonstrate that the 5-year survival rate has more than doubled from 1973 to 1996 (5.2% vs 12.2%; $P = .0001$).

Current recommendations

Although important questions remain as to the optimal radiation doses, volumes, and timing with regard to chemotherapy, a reasonable standard is to deliver thoracic irradiation concurrently with PE chemotherapy (cisplatin [60 mg/m^2 IV on day 1] and etoposide [120 mg/ m^2 IV on days 1 to 3]). An attempt is made to integrate thoracic irradiation as early as possible, during cycle 1 (or 2).

Fried et al performed a meta-analysis evaluating early vs late timing of radiation therapy in limited-stage SCLC. Earlier radiation therapy was defined as prior to 9 weeks after initiation of chemotherapy vs late radiation therapy (≥ 9 weeks). Seven trials (n = 1,542 patients) were included in the analysis. They reported a small but significant improvement in 2-year overall survival for early vs late radiation therapy (5.2%; $P = .03$). This finding is similar to the benefit of adding radiation therapy or prophylactic cranial irradiation (PCI) to chemotherapy. A greater difference was evident for the subset of patients receiving early rather than late hyperfractionated radiation therapy and platinum-based chemotherapy. Hyperfractionated accelerated fractionation should be considered, given the results of the Intergroup 0096 trial. An Intergroup phase III study is under way to compare twice-daily radiation therapy to 45 Gy vs once-daily with radiation therapy to a higher dose (70 Gy) vs a modified regimen combining these strategies.

Irradiation can be incorporated sequentially with chemotherapy; however, this approach appears to be inferior to early concurrent therapy and should be reserved for use in those for whom concurrent approaches are predicted to be excessively toxic.

Takada et al reported on a randomized trial of concurrent vs sequential thoracic radiotherapy in combination with PE in over 200 patients with limited-stage SCLC; they demonstrated a benefit to concurrent therapy, with a median survival of 27.0 months (30%, concurrent arm) vs 19.7 months (20%, sequential arm; $P = .097$). Thoracic radiation therapy consisted of 45 Gy over 3 weeks, starting either with the first cycle of PE in the concurrent arm or after the fourth cycle in the sequential arm.

Results of an intergroup trial indicate that radiation therapy strategies that increase biologic dose can improve tumor local control and survival. Further exploration of accelerated fractionation or conventional doses > 45 Gy is warranted and is currently being investigated in prospective trials.

Komaki et al have reported both phases I and II data with a "concomitant boost" chemoradiation approach (RTOG 0239). This therapy involves treating the initial large field in daily fractions and boosting the small field to a higher dose (61.2 Gy in 5 weeks), with a second daily fraction on the last 9 days of treatment. The chemotherapy regimen included etoposide and cisplatin. The locoregional tumor control rate at 2 years was 80%, though the 2-year survival rate of 37% is not as promising.

Severe grade esophagitis occurred in 18% of patients, which is lower than the rate of 27% observed in the accelerated arm of Intergroup 0096.

Movsas et al reported the results of the first Patterns of Care Study (PCS) for lung cancer in the United States. This study was conducted to determine the national patterns of radiotherapy practice in patients treated for nonmetastatic lung cancer in 1998 and 1999. As supported by clinical trials, patients with limited-stage SCLC received chemotherapy plus radiotherapy more often than radiotherapy alone (92% vs 5%; $P < .0001$). However, the median radiotherapy dose was 50 Gy, 80% at 1.8 to 2.0 Gy per fraction. Only 6% of patients received hyperfractionated (twice-daily) radiotherapy. A total of 22% received PCI, with a median dose of 30 Gy in 15 fractions.

Interestingly, Choi et al reported long-term survival data from their phase I trial assessing chemotherapy with either standard daily radiotherapy or accelerated twice-daily radiotherapy as from the CALGB 8837 trial. They previously reported that the maximum tolerated dose was 45 Gy in 30 fractions for twice-daily radiotherapy and > 70 Gy in 35 fractions for once-daily radiotherapy. The 5-year survival estimated (from this phase I trial) for the twice-daily arm was 20%, vs 36% for the once-daily radiotherapy arm. The CALGB and RTOG are accruing patients to a large trial testing three chemoradiation regimens for limited-disease SCLC (CALGB 30610/RTOG 0538). This study includes the accelerated regimen from Intergroup 0096, the concomitant boost from RTOG 0239, and the daily conventional fractionation as studied by Choi et al, with etoposide and cisplatin in all three arms.

Surgery

Although surgical resection is not usually part of the standard therapy for SCLC, the JCOLCSG reported the results of a phase II trial of postoperative adjuvant PE in patients with completely resected stages I–IIIA SCLC. The 5-year survival rates (in a cohort of 62 patients) for pathologic stages I, II, and IIIA SCLC were 69%, 38%, and 40%, respectively.

The role of surgery for stage II or IIIA SCLC has evolved from a number of phase II trials and retrospective case series to include specific indications; they include resection of tumors with mixed histology (containing both SCLC and NSCLC components), salvage surgery for chemoresistant localized SCLC or local relapse after initial response to chemoradiotherapy, or second primary tumors after cure of initial SCLC. Johnson has shown that the rate of second primary NSCLC in patients treated for SCLC can be as high as 2% to greater than 10% per year.

Prospective, randomized trials are ongoing in Europe and Japan to examine the role of surgery as part of multimodality therapy for patients with stages II and IIIA SCLC.

Prophylactic cranial irradiation

Recognition that patients with SCLC were at high risk for the development of brain metastases led to the suggestion that they be given PCI to prevent the clinical manifestation of previously present but occult CNS disease. The role of PCI has been controversial. Most trials have shown a reduction in CNS relapse rates but little effect on survival with PCI. There also has been concern about the contribution of PCI to the late neurologic deterioration seen in some patients with SCLC, although studies show neurologic impairment in many patients with SCLC prior to any treatment.

A meta-analysis of all randomized trials of PCI in patients with SCLC who achieved a complete or near-complete response to induction chemotherapy (alone or combined with thoracic irradiation) showed a statistically significant improvement in survival in patients treated with PCI (20.7% at 3 years vs 15.3% in those not given PCI). The survival improvement with PCI was seen in all patient subgroups, regardless of age, stage of disease, type of induction treatment, or performance status. Approximately 85% of the patients included in the meta-analysis had limited disease, and recommendations for use of PCI have been applied generally to this subgroup. One randomized trial, however, suggests benefit for PCI in patients with responding extensive disease as well.

Given the high incidence of symptomatic brain metastases and the relatively short survival following this event in patients with extensive SCLC, the EORTC randomized 286 patients after response to chemotherapy to receive PCI or not. Irradiation reduced the risk of symptomatic brain metastases, with a hazard ratio of 0.27 (95% CI = 0.16–0.44; $P < .001$). The cumulative incidence of brain metastases was reduced from 40% in the control group to 15% within 1 year of follow-up. From the time of randomization, patients who were radiated had an approximate 2-month increase in median survival (6.7 vs 5.4 months) and double the 1-year survival rate (27% vs 13%); progression-free survival was less affected (14.7 vs 12.0 weeks). PCI was reasonably well tolerated, with expected acute effects of headache, nausea and vomiting, and fatigue. Radiated patients were more frequently given chemotherapy at the time of extracranial disease progression (68% vs 45%). Further, only 59% of patients in the control group who developed brain metastases were treated with whole-brain irradiation. These latter factors may have contributed to the observed survival differences.

Current recommendations

Patients should be offered PCI after completion of chemotherapy/chemoradiation therapy if they have clear regression of disease and a retained ECOG performance status of 0 to 2. It should optimally be integrated within 3 to 5 weeks of the last cycle of chemotherapy.

Radiation doses for PCI should probably be in the range of 25 to 30 Gy, with a daily fraction size of 2.0 to 2.5 Gy (see sidebar on page 130).

TREATMENT OF EXTENSIVE DISEASE

As mentioned previously, two-thirds of SCLC patients have extensive disease at diagnosis. Without treatment, median survival in this group of patients is 6 to 8 weeks. Treatment with combination chemotherapy increases the median survival duration to approximately 8 to 10 months.

Induction chemotherapy

The combination of cisplatin or carboplatin/etoposide (see Table 1 for common dose ranges) is considered the standard of care in the United States at this time. This standard is primarily based on therapeutic index, as randomized trials have not demonstrated a survival benefit for this combination relative to the older regimen of cyclophosphamide, doxorubicin, and vincristine. The regimen is repeated at 3-week intervals for 4 to 6 courses. In North America, multiple randomized trials of newer cytotoxins replacing etoposide in a doublet with cisplatin, or added to the etoposide/platin base, have not provided a survival benefit. Japanese data that showed a 3.4-month survival advantage for irinotecan, as opposed to etoposide, with cisplatin were not confirmed in a trial in the United States.

> The role of consolidative extracranial irradiation for patients with one to three sites of extensive SCLC is being studied in a randomized, phase II study (RTOG 0937). This research is based on an earlier randomized study *(Jeremic B et al: J Clin Oncol 17:2092–2099, 1999)* indicating that adding consolidative radiation therapy to the treatment of the most favorable subset of patients with extensive SCLC led to improved survival when compared with use of chemotherapy alone.

Another large North American study, SWOG S0124, and a trial from Germany comparing irinotecan with etoposide, when both are combined with platinating agents, were recently reported. Both showed equivalence in major efficacy outcomes. A Scandinavian trial with a similar design demonstrated a 1.4-month increase in the median survival rate for irinotecan-based treatment. However, these results are suspect due to an imbalance of elderly patients between the arms and a mandated dose reduction for etoposide in the elderly group. Overall, the data suggest efficacy is equivalent with either approach. Due to problematic severe diarrhea with irinotecan, the therapeutic index may be improved with etoposide-based therapy.

TREATMENT OF PROGRESSIVE DISEASE

Progressive SCLC is classified based on response and duration of response to initial induction therapy. Patients whose tumors do not regress or progress up to 60 to 90 days following the last cycle of chemotherapy are considered to have refractory disease.

TABLE 1: Common chemotherapy regimens for SCLC

Drug/combination	Dose and schedule
Etoposide + cisplatin or carboplatin	
Etoposide	100–120 mg/m^2 IV on days 1–3
Cisplatin	60–75 mg/m^2 IV on day 1
	or
Etoposide	100 mg/m^2 IV on days 1–3
Carboplatin	Area under the concentration-time curve of 5 mg/mL/min IV on day 1
Repeat cycle every 3 weeks.	
Irinotecan + cisplatin	
Irinotecan	60 mg/m^2 on days 1, 8, and 15
Cisplatin	60 mg/m^2 IV on day 1
Repeat cycle every 4 weeks for 4 cycles.	

Noda K, Nishiwaki Y, Kawahara M, et al: N Engl J Med 346:85–91, 2002.
Table prepared by Ishmael Jaiyesimi, DO.

Recently, a randomized trial studied the issue of standard-dose vs higher-dose PCI in patients with limited-stage SCLC. One-half of 720 patients with limited-stage SCLC in complete remission were randomly assigned to receive a standard-dose PCI regimen (25 Gy in 10 fractions). The other half received a higher PCI total dose (36 Gy) delivered using either conventional (18 daily fractions of 2 Gy) or accelerated hyperfractionated (24 fractions in 16 days of 1.5 Gy) radiation. With a median follow-up of 39 months, there was no significant difference in the 2-year incidence of brain metastases between the arms. The 2-year survival was 42% in the standard-dose group and 37% in the higher-dose group (P = .05).The lower overall survival in the higher-dose group was thought to be due to an increase in cancer-related mortality. Overall, this randomized study showed no significant reduction in brain metastases after higher-dose PCI, but there was a significant increase in mortality. Therefore, standard doses of PCI should remain the standard of care in limited-stage SCLC *(Le Pechoux C et al: Lancet Oncol 10:467–474, 2009)*. In reporting on RTOG 0212, Wolfson et al noted that 36 Gy delivered once or twice daily resulted in a greater risk of neurocognitive toxicity than did 25 Gy of PCI. Age > 60 years was significantly predictive for the possibility of this complication *(Wolfson AH, Bae K, Komaki R, et al: Int J Radiat Oncol Biol Phys Aug 26, 2010 [Epub ahead of print])*.

Conversely, patients whose tumors respond and who have an unmaintained progression-free interval longer than 60 to 90 days, are deemed to have sensitive relapse. This categorization is based on the probability of objective response to additional cytotoxic therapy, which is uncommon, typically less than 15%, in the case of platin-refractory SCLC.

Topotecan (Hycamtin) is the only drug approved by the FDA for the treatment of recurrent disease. Its initial indication in 1998 was for patients with sensitive relapse and was based on similar efficacy compared with an older three-drug regimen. A subsequent trial compared IV administration with oral topotecan capsules, documenting similar efficacy and tolerance.

Most recently, a randomized trial of 141 patients, with an ECOG performance status of 0 to 2, compared oral topotecan with best supportive care. Patients with both refractory and sensitive disease were accrued. Median survival was nearly doubled on the topotecan arm, 26 vs 14 weeks (P = .0104), as was 6-month survival, 49% vs 26%. Benefit was seen in all subgroups analyzed, including patients with refractory cancer and an ECOG performance status of 2. Despite a low rate of response to topotecan of 7% and typical side effects, treated patients had slower deterioration of quality of life and improved symptom control. Based on these data, the FDA granted topotecan in capsule form a broad indication for treatment of recurrent SCLC in October 2007.

More limited data with irinotecan suggest its activity is probably similar to that of topotecan; however, it has never been evaluated in a randomized trial in the recurrent setting. Amrubicin, a synthetic anthracycline, has been studied extensively in recurrent SCLC in Japan and has been approved there. Initial data published in abstract form in North American patients suggest promising response rates with amrubicin in patients with refractory disease and a similar survival benefit as observed with topotecan in sensitive relapse. Amrubicin remains investigational in the United States.

Other cytotoxins, known more for their efficacy in NSCLC, such as docetaxel (Taxotere) and paclitaxel, gemcitabine (Gemzar), and vinorelbine, do not have high single-agent response rates in therapy-naive SCLC and are not recognized as standard in management.

Integration of biologics in therapy

Ongoing clinical research is focused on integration of molecularly targeted therapy in an effort to make progress in treating this stubborn malignancy. At this time, data from completed trials do not indicate an active strategy with a biologic, whether in combination with induction chemotherapy, as maintenance following induction, or as single agents for recurrent disease.

High-dose chemotherapy plus bone marrow transplantation (BMT)

Most phase II trials using high doses of chemotherapy plus BMT appear to show no advantage to the high-dose approach over standard doses of chemotherapy.

Alternating chemotherapy regimens

These have been used to overcome drug resistance. In randomized trials, alternating chemotherapy regimens have shown a slight improvement in terms of median survival (4 to 6 weeks) when compared with a single chemotherapeutic regimen but no improvement in long-term survival.

PALLIATION OF LOCAL AND DISTANT SYMPTOMS

Radiation therapy

Many patients with lung cancer have distressing local symptoms at some point in their disease course. These symptoms may arise from airway obstruction by the primary tumor, compression of mediastinal structures by nodal metastases, or metastatic involvement of distant organs. Radiation therapy is effective in palliating most local symptoms as well as symptoms at common metastatic sites, such as in bone and the brain.

In the United States, most radiation oncologists use doses in the vicinity of 30 Gy in 10 fractions for palliative treatment. Data from the United Kingdom suggest that similar efficacy without greater toxicity may be achieved with more abbreviated schedules, such as 17 Gy in 2 fractions 1 week apart or single fractions of 11 Gy (see chapter 3, Table 8). Such schedules may facilitate the coordination of irradiation and chemotherapy and also may reduce patient travel and hospitalization.

Endobronchial irradiation with cobalt-60 or iridium-192 has been used to palliate symptoms arising from partial airway obstruction, including cough, dyspnea, and hemoptysis. The dosimetric advantage of being able to deliver a high radiation dose to the obstructing endobronchial tumor while sparing adjacent normal structures, such as the lungs, spinal cord, and esophagus, has clear appeal, particularly in the patient whose disease has recurred following prior external-beam irradiation. Although good rates of palliation have been reported with endobronchial irradiation, significant complications, including fatal hemoptysis, are seen in 5% to 10% of patients. Whether this represents a true treatment complication vs the underlying disease remains unclear.

Other local approaches

Endobronchial irradiation should be considered as only one of several approaches (including laser excision, cryotherapy, and stent placement) in the treatment of patients with symptomatic airway obstruction, and management should be individualized. All of these approaches are more suitable for partial than for complete airway obstruction.

Chemotherapy

Several trials have explored the use of chemotherapy to palliate specific symptoms in patients with lung cancer. In general, these trials have found that rates of symptomatic improvement were considerably higher than objective response rates and were not dissimilar to symptomatic response rates with local radiation therapy. Chemotherapy in the newly diagnosed patient is highly palliative for relief of symptoms related to superior vena cava syndrome, obstructive lung disease, and painful bony metastases. In the patient with recurrent disease, irradiation is more commonly associated with symptomatic relief from these localized problems. Radiation therapy remains the standard of care for even chemotherapy-naive patients with spinal cord compression or symptomatic brain metastasis.

FOLLOW-UP OF LONG-TERM SURVIVORS

At present, no standard follow-up protocol exists for patients with cured SCLC or NSCLC. However, at least long-term follow-up should include serial physical examinations once the patient has reached the 5-year mark. Controversy currently exists about the value of utilizing CT scanning or even chest x-rays for the long-term follow-up of these patients.

In this vein, retrospective reviews of the literature have revealed that patients with SCLC appear to have the highest rate of second primary tumor development, as high as 30% over the course of their lifetimes, with some studies reporting annual second primary tumor rates of 5% to 10%. Therefore, the concept of chemoprevention appears to have particular merit in these patients.

MESOTHELIOMA

Mesotheliomas are uncommon neoplasms derived from the cells lining the pleura and peritoneum. Currently, 2,000 to 3,000 new cases are diagnosed in the United States each year.

EPIDEMIOLOGY

Gender

Men are affected five times more commonly than women.

Age

The median age at diagnosis is 60 years.

ETIOLOGY AND RISK FACTORS

Asbestos exposure

The relationship between asbestos exposure and diffuse pleural mesothelioma was first reported by Wagner, who documented 33 pathologically confirmed cases from an asbestos mining region in South Africa. Selikoff and colleagues documented a 300-fold increase in mortality from mesothelioma among asbestos insulation workers in the New York metropolitan region when compared with the general population. The interval between asbestos exposure and tumor formation is commonly 3 to 4 decades.

Asbestos fibers are generally divided into two broad groups: serpentine and amphibole. The latter includes crocidolite, the most carcinogenic form of asbestos. The inability of phagocytic cells to digest the fiber appears to initiate a cascade of cellular events that results in free-radical generation and carcinogenesis.

DIAGNOSIS

Patients with mesothelioma usually seek medical attention while the disease is limited to a single hemithorax and commonly complain of dyspnea and pain. Dyspnea results from diffuse growth of the tumor on both the parietal and visceral pleurae, which encase the lung in a thick rind. Pain is caused by direct tumor infiltration of intercostal nerves.

Chest x-ray demonstrates pleural thickening, pleura-based masses, or a pleural effusion. Chest CT scanning more accurately portrays the extent of disease and frequently reveals chest wall invasion, as well as pericardial and diaphragmatic extension.

Thoracentesis and pleural biopsy establish the diagnosis in 26% of cases, however thoracoscopic biopsy yields a diagnosis in 98% of cases and is the gold standard.

Light microscopy is often insufficient for differentiating among mesothelioma, metastatic adenocarcinoma, and sarcoma. Immunohistochemistry and electron microscopy are frequently necessary to establish the diagnosis.

Small retrospective series have studied three biomarkers: soluble mesothelin-related peptide (SMRP), megakaryocyte potentiation factor (MPF), and osteopontin (Table 2). SMRP may predict the development of mesothelioma in asbestos-exposed individuals. Prospective studies are required to validate the utility of these biomarkers for early detection, predicting the extent of disease and determining prognosis.

PATHOLOGY

Mesotheliomas may contain both epithelial and sarcomatoid elements and are classified by the relative abundance of each component. Epithelial mesotheliomas are most common (50%), followed by mixed (34%) and sarcomatoid (16%) tumors. Survival for the epithelial type is 22 months, compared with only 6 months for patients with other types.

STAGING AND PROGNOSIS

The IMIG has developed a staging system based on TNM descriptors. This was adopted by the American Joint Committee on Cancer (Table 3). Another commonly utilized staging system for mesothelioma, that of Butchart, is based on inexact descriptions of the extent of local tumor growth or distant metastases (Table 4).

TABLE 2: Potential uses for mesothelioma serum biomarkers

Variables	SMRP	MPF	Osteopontin
Screening in asbestos-exposed population (retrospective study)	Yes	Not done	Yes
Screening in asbestos-exposed population (prospective study)	High false-positive rate	Not done	Not done
Monitoring treatment effect	Yes	Yes	Yes
Predicting prognosis	Yes	Yes	Yes
Differentiating MM from benign pleural disease	Yes	Yes	Yes
Differentiating MM from other cancers	Yes	Not done	No
Determining duration of asbestos exposure	Not done	Not done	Yes
Sensitivity for detecting MM (at a specificity of 95%)	73%	34%	47%

MM = mesothelioma; SMRP = soluble mesothelin-related peptide; MPF = megakaryocyte potentiation factor

Ray M, Kindler HL: Chest 136:888-896, 2009.

Other, more detailed staging systems based on TNM criteria have been proposed.

The median survival following diagnosis ranges from 9 to 21 months. Although autopsy series have demonstrated distant metastases in as many as 50% of patients with mesothelioma, death usually results from local tumor growth.

TREATMENT

Treatment rarely results in cure and should be considered palliative.

Combined-modality treatment options

Surgical procedures (pleural fluid drainage and talc pleurodesis, or pleurectomy and decortication) to control symptomatic pleural effusions are well accepted. Otherwise, the role of surgery in the potentially curative treatment of mesothelioma remains controversial. In this setting, the goal of surgery is to remove all gross disease; however microscopic disease is likely to remain. Therefore surgery is most commonly performed in combination with other treatments (multimodality therapy). The type of operation is also controversial. Pleurectomy and decortication (PD) is designed to remove both the visceral and parietal pleura while preserving underlying lung tissue. Extrapleural pneumonectomy (EPP) removes the pleural envelope and the lung en bloc. The advantages of PD are that the lung is preserved and morbidity and mortality are less, however adjuvant radiation may be difficult because the lung remains. EPP has a higher mortality rate but adjuvant radiation to the pleural cavity is possible without the risk of radiation pneumonitis because the lung is removed. Recent retrospective studies have reported no difference in overall survival between PD and EPP; however patients undergoing PD may have had a lower volume of disease at the time of surgery than the patients who underwent EPP.

TABLE 3: New international staging system for diffuse MPM

Primary tumor (T)

TX	Primary tumor cannot be assessed
T0	No evidence of primary tumor
T1	Tumor limited to the ipsilateral parietal pleura with or without mediastinal pleura and with or without diaphragmatic pleural involvement T1a No involvement of the visceral pleura T1b Tumor also involving the visceral pleura
T2	Tumor involving each of the ipsilateral pleural surfaces (parietal, mediastinal, and diaphragmatic, and visceral) Involvement of diaphragmatic muscle Extension of tumor from visceral pleura into the underlying pulmonary parenchyma
T3	Locally advanced but potentially resectable tumor; tumor involving all of the ipsilateral pleural surfaces (parietal, mediastinal, diaphragmatic, and visceral) with at least one of the following features: Involvement of the endothoracic fascia Extension of tumor into mediastinal fat Solitary, completely resectable focus of tumor extending into the soft tissues of the chest wall Nontransmural involvement of the pericardium
T4	Locally advanced technically unresectable tumor; tumor involving all of the ipsilateral pleural surfaces (parietal, mediastinal, diaphragmatic, and visceral) with at least one of the following features: Diffuse extension or multifocal masses of tumor in the chest wall, with or without associated rib destruction Direct transdiaphragmatic extension of tumor to the peritoneum Direct extension of tumor to the contralateral pleura Direct extension of tumor to mediastinal organs Direct extension of tumor into the spine Tumor extending through to the internal surface of the pericardium with or without a pericardial effusion; or tumor involving the myocardium

Regional lymph nodes (N)

NX	Regional lymph nodes cannot be assessed
N0	No regional lymph node metastases
N1	Metastases in the ipsilateral bronchopulmonary or hilar lymph nodes
N2	Metastases in subcarinal or ipsilateral mediastinal lymph nodes, including ipsilateral internal mammary and peridiaphragmatic nodes
N3	Metastases in contralateral mediastinal, contralateral internal mammary, and ipsilateral or contralateral supraclavicular lymph nodes

Distant metastasis (M)

M0	No distant metastasis (no pathologic M0; use clinical M to complete stage group)
M1	Distant metastasis

Stage groupings

Stage I	T1	N0	M0
Stage IA	T1a	N0	M0
Stage IB	T1b	N0	M0
Stage II	T2	N0	M0
Stage III	T1, T2	N1	M0
	T1, T2	N2	M0
	T3	N0, N1, N2	M0
Stage IV	T4	Any N	M0
	Any T	N3	M0
	Any T	Any N	M1

From Edge SP, Byrd DR, Compton CC, et al (eds): AJCC Cancer Staging Manual, 7th ed. New York, Springer, 2010.

TABLE 4: Staging of mesothelioma according to Butchart

Stage	Description
I	Tumor confined within the "capsule" of the parietal pleura, ie, involving only the ipsilateral pleura, lungs, pericardium, and diaphragm
II	Tumor invading the chest wall or involving mediastinal structures, eg, the esophagus, heart, opposite pleura; lymph node involvement within the chest
III	Tumor penetrating the diaphragm to involve the peritoneum; involvement of the opposite pleura; lymph node involvement outside the chest
IV	Distant blood-borne metastases

Chemotherapy is commonly given either before or after surgical resection. In a further attempt to treat residual microscopic disease, intrapleural therapies such as heated chemotherapy or other treatments are being explored. Management of potential toxicities mandates that these treatments be performed at experienced center.

Chemotherapy

The benefit of chemotherapy for patients who have unresectable mesothelioma was clarified in a randomized trial. This study was a single-blind, multicenter, two-arm trial with cisplatin alone in the control arm and cisplatin combined with the multitargeted antifolate pemetrexed (Alimta) in the experimental arm. The study was based on the observation that pemetrexed produced a 16% objective response rate in previous phase II evaluation. In the randomized trial, patients treated with pemetrexed and cisplatin had an estimated median survival of 12.1 months, as compared with 9.3 months in those treated with cisplatin alone. On the basis of this improvement in survival, the combination of pemetrexed and cisplatin has received an FDA indication for the treatment of unresectable mesothelioma. The same combination is undergoing further evaluation in a neoadjuvant approach in patients with resectable disease.

THYMOMA

Thymoma is a rare mediastinal tumor that occurs mainly in the anterosuperior mediastinum.

EPIDEMIOLOGY

Gender

The tumor affects both sexes equally.

Age

Thymoma is most often seen in people in the fourth and fifth decades of life.

ETIOLOGY AND ASSOCIATED SYNDROMES

The etiology of thymoma is unknown, and the risk factors have not been identified. Thymoma is a tumor originating within the epithelial cells of the thymus. One-third to one-half of patients present with an asymptomatic anterior mediastinal mass, one-third present with local symptoms (eg, cough, chest pain, superior vena cava syndrome, and/or dysphagia), and one-third of cases are detected during the evaluation of myasthenia gravis. Distant metastases are distinctly uncommon at initial presentation of this tumor.

In addition to myasthenia gravis, which occurs in approximately 30% of patients with thymoma, a host of paraneoplastic syndromes have been seen in association with thymoma. These other syndromes, which occur in less than 5% of patients, include pure red cell aplasia, hypogammaglobulinemia, and a variety of other autoimmune disorders.

DIAGNOSIS

The most commonly described symptoms are pleuritic chest pain or discomfort, dry cough, and dyspnea. Physical examination may reveal adenopathy, wheezing, fever, superior vena cava syndrome, vocal cord paralysis, and other paraneoplastic syndromes.

Chest x-ray and CT scan

A chest x-ray provides an initial basis for diagnosis. The location, size, density, and presence of calcification within the mass can all be determined. Comparison of the film to previously obtained films is usually helpful.

Following identification of a mediastinal mass on conventional radiography, contrast-enhanced CT scanning should be performed. CT scanning can differentiate the cystic form from a solid lesion as well as the presence of fat, calcium, or fluid within the lesion. MRI is increasingly available for use in the evaluation of mediastinal pathology, but it is less frequently utilized than CT. MRI is superior to CT scanning in defining the relationship between mediastinal masses and vascular structures and is useful in the assessment of vascular invasion by the tumor.

Invasive diagnostic tests

CT-guided percutaneous needle biopsy specimens are obtained using fine-needle aspiration techniques and cytologic evaluation or with larger-core needle biopsy and histologic evaluation. Fine-needle specimens are usually adequate to distinguish carcinomatosis lesions, but core biopsies may be necessary to distinguish most mediastinal neoplasms. Immunohistochemical techniques and electron microscopy have greatly improved the ability to differentiate the cell of origin in mediastinal neoplasms. Most series reported diagnostic yields for percutaneous needle biopsy of 70% to 100%.

Mediastinoscopy

This is a relatively simple surgical procedure accomplished with the patient under general anesthesia. It is an adequate approach to the superior, middle, and upper posterior mediastinum, and most series report a diagnostic accuracy of 80% to 90%. Anterior mediastinotomy (Chamberlain approach) provides for direct biopsy of tissue and has a diagnostic yield of 95% to 100%. Thoracotomy is occasionally necessary to diagnose mediastinal neoplasms, but its indications have been largely supplanted by video-assisted thoracoscopic techniques, which yield an accuracy of 100%.

TABLE 5: Classification schemes for thymoma

WHO classification	Histiogenetic classification (Müller-Hermelink)
A	Medullary thymoma
AB	Mixed thymoma
B1	Predominantly cortical thymoma
B2	Cortical thymoma
B3	Well-differentiated thymic carcinoma
C	Thymic carcinoma
Epidermoid keratinizing carcinoma (squamous cell)	
Epidermoid nonkeratinizing carcinoma	
Lymphoepithelioma-like carcinoma	
Sarcomatoid carcinoma	
Basaloid carcinoma	
Mucoepidermoid carcinoma	
Undifferentiated carcinoma	

A = atrophic, similar to that of an adult thymus; B = bioactive; C = cancer (with obvious signs of cell mitoses)

The most common tumors in the differential diagnosis of an anterior mediastinal tumor are lymphomas and germ-cell tumors. Immunohistochemical markers are helpful to differentiate thymoma from tumors originating from other cell types.

PATHOLOGY

Two of the most common classification schemes for thymoma are listed in Table 5. Verley and Hollman propose a classification system based on tumor architecture, cellular differentiation, and predominant cell type. Bernatz et al describe a simpler classification by presenting thymoma based on the percentage of epithelial cells and lymphocytes. In both of these systems, thymoma with a predominance of epithelial cells is associated with a greater incidence of invasion and a subsequently worse prognosis.

STAGING AND PROGNOSIS

The staging system proposed by Masaoka et al has been widely adopted. Stage is an independent predictor of recurrence and long-term survival. The 5-year survival rates are 96% for stage I thymoma, 86% for stage II, 69% for stage III, and 50% for stage IV.

TREATMENT

Surgical treatment

All patients whose tumors are potentially resectable should undergo surgery. If the patient has evidence of myasthenia gravis, a preoperative consultation with a clinical neurologist should be considered. The incision of choice is almost always a median sternotomy, which is quick and easy to make and provides excellent exposure to the anterior mediastinum and neck. Although the surgeon is considered the best judge of a tumor's invasiveness, it is often difficult to grossly separate tumor invasion from tumor adherence to surrounding tissue. Experience with minimally invasive approaches (such as transcervical thymectomy) is growing; however, until longer term data become available, sternotomy should still be considered the standard surgical approach.

Complete resection of thymoma has been found to be the most significant predictor of long-term survival. Several studies have examined the extent of surgical resection on survival and disease-free survival rates. In 241 operative cases, Maggi and colleagues found an 82% overall survival rate in those whose tumors underwent complete resection and a 26% survival rate at 7 years in those undergoing biopsy alone. Other investigators reported similar results in surgical patients. Therefore, regardless of stage, tumor resectability is one of the important predictors of treatment outcome.

Radiation treatment

Thymomas are generally radiosensitive tumors, and the use of radiation therapy in their treatment is well established. It has been used to treat all stages of thymoma, either before or after surgical resection. General agreement exists regarding the postoperative treatment of invasive thymoma (stages II and III). The value of adjuvant radiation therapy for invasive thymomas is well documented and should be included in the treatment regimen regardless of the completeness of tumor resection.

TABLE 6: Common chemotherapy regimens for thymoma

Regimen	Dose and schedule
CAPPr	
Cyclophosphamide	500 mg/m² IV on day 1
Adriamycin (doxorubicin)	20 mg/m²/d infused continuously on days 1–3
Platinol (cisplatin)	30 mg/m²/d IV on days 1–3
Prednisone	100 mg/d PO on days 1–5
Repeat cycle every 3–4 weeks.	
Adapted from Shin DM, Walsh GL, Komaki R, et al: Ann Intern Med 129:100–104, 1998.	
Single agent	
Cisplatin	100 mg/m² IV on day 1
Appropriate IV prehydration, posthydration along with mannitol and electrolytes	
Repeat cycle every 3 weeks.	
Adapted from Bonomi PD, Finkelstein D, Aisner S, et al: Am J Clin Oncol 16:342–345, 1993.	
Ifosfamide	1.5 g/m² infused continuously on days 1–5
Mesna	Continuous infusion as appropriate
Repeat cycle every 3 weeks.	
Adapted from Highley MS, Underhill CR, Parnis FX, et al: J Clin Oncol 17:2737–2744, 1999.	

Table prepared by Ishmael Jaiyesimi, DO.

Chemotherapy

Chemotherapy has been used in the treatment of invasive thymomas with increasing frequency during the past decade (Table 6). The most active agents appear to be cisplatin, doxorubicin, ifosfamide, and corticosteroids. Combination chemotherapy has generally shown higher response rates and has been used in both neoadjuvant and adjuvant settings and in the treatment of metastatic or recurrent thymomas. CAP or CAPPr (cyclophosphamide, Adriamycin [doxorubicin], Platinol [cisplatin], and prednisone) regimens have been used in neoadjuvant and/or adjuvant settings. These regimens have also been used for recurrent thymoma.

UNRESECTABLE THYMOMA

Advanced-stage (III/IVA) thymomas are usually difficult to remove completely. Multidisciplinary approaches, including induction chemotherapy followed by surgical resection, postoperative radiation therapy, and consolidation chemotherapy, have been reported.

Induction chemotherapy consists of cyclophosphamide (500 mg/m^2 IV on day 1), doxorubicin (20 mg/m^2/d, continuous infusion, on days 1 to 3), cisplatin (30 mg/m^2/d IV on days 1 to 3), and prednisone (100 mg/d PO on days 1 to 5), repeated every 3 to 4 weeks for 3 courses. Twenty-two evaluable patients were consecutively treated from 1990 to 2000 in a prospective phase II study at M. D. Anderson Cancer Center. After induction chemotherapy, 17 of 22 patients (77%) had major responses, including three complete responses.

Twenty-one patients underwent surgical resection. All patients received postoperative radiation therapy and consolidation chemotherapy. With a median follow-up of 50.3 months, overall survival rates at 5 years and 7 years were 95% and 79%, respectively. The rate of disease progression-free survival was 77% at 5 and 7 years. The multidisciplinary approaches to unresectable thymoma appear to be promising.

SUGGESTED READING

ON SMALL-CELL LUNG CANCER

Blackhall FH, Shepherd FA: Small cell lung cancer and targeted therapies. Curr Opin Oncol 19:103–108, 2007.

De Ruysscher D, Pijls-Johannesma M, Bentzen SM, et al: Time between the first day of chemotherapy and the last day of chest radiation is the most important predictor of survival in limited-disease small-cell lung cancer. J Clin Oncol 24:1057–1063, 2006.

Fried DB, Morris DE, Poole C, et al: Systematic review evaluating the timing of thoracic radiation therapy in combined modality therapy for limited-stage small-cell lung cancer. J Clin Oncol 22:4837–4845, 2004.

Glisson BS: Recurrent small cell lung cancer: Update. Semin Oncol 30:72–78, 2003.

Lara PN Jr, Natale R, Crowley J, et al: Phase III trial of irinotecan/cisplatin compared with etoposide/cisplatin in extensive-stage small-cell lung cancer: Clinical and pharmacogenomic results from SWOG S0124. J Clin Oncol 27:2530–2535, 2009.

Movsas B, Moughan J, Komaki R, et al: Radiotherapy (RT) Patterns of Care Study (PCS) in lung carcinoma. J Clin Oncol 24:4553–4559, 2003.

O'Brien ME, Ciuleanu TE, Tsekov H, et al: Phase III trial comparing supportive care alone with supportive care with oral topotecan in patients with relapsed small-cell lung cancer. J Clin Oncol 24:5441–5447, 2006.

Slotman B, Faivre-Finn C, Kramer G, et al: Prophylactic cranial irradiation in extensive small-cell lung cancer. N Engl J Med 357:664–672, 2007.

ON MESOTHELIOMA

Flores RM, Pass HI, Seshan VE, et al: Extrapleural pneumonectomy versus pleurectomy/decortication in the surgical management of malignant pleural mesothelioma: Results in 663 patients. J Thorac Cardiovasc Surg 135:620–626, 2008.

Ray M, Kindler HL: Malignant pleural mesothelioma: An update on biomarkers and treatment. Chest 136:888–896, 2009.

Tilleman TR, Richards WG, Zellos L, et al: Extrapleural pneumonectomy followed by intracavitary intraoperative hyperthermic cisplatin with pharmacologic cytoprotection for treatment of malignant pleural mesothelioma: A phase II prospective study. J Thorac Cardiovasc Surg 138:405–411, 2009.

Vogelzang NJ, Rusthoven JJ, Symanowski J, et al: Phase III study of pemetrexed in combination with cisplatin versus cisplatin alone in patients with malignant pleural mesothelioma. J Clin Oncol 21:2636–2644, 2003.

ON THYMOMA

Huang J, Rizk NP, Travis WD, et al: Feasibility of multimodality therapy including extended resections in stage IVA thymoma. J Thorac Cardiovasc Surg 134:1477–1483, 2007.

Kim ES, Putnam JB, Komaki R, et al: A phase II study of a multidisciplinary approach with induction chemotherapy, followed by surgical resection, radiation therapy, and consolidation chemotherapy for unresectable malignant thymomas: Final report. Lung Cancer 44:369–379, 2004.

Abbreviations in this chapter

CALGB = Cancer and Leukemia Group B; ECOG = Eastern Cooperative Oncology Group; EORTC = European Organisation for Research and Treatment of Cancer; IMIG = International Mesothelioma Interest Group; JCOLCSG = Japanese Clinical Oncology Lung Cancer Study Group; RTOG = Radiation Therapy Oncology Group; SEER = Surveillance, Epidemiology, and End Results; SWOG = Southwest Oncology Group

CHAPTER 5

Breast cancer overview

Risk factors, screening, genetic testing, and prevention

Lori Jardines, MD, Sharad Goyal, MD, Paul Fisher, MD,
Jeffrey Weitzel, MD, Melanie Royce, MD, PhD, and Shari B. Goldfarb, MD

Breast cancer is the most common malignancy in women, accounting for 27% of all female cancers; it accounts for < 1% of all cancer cases in men. Breast cancer also is responsible for 15% of cancer deaths in women, making it the number-two cause of cancer death. An estimated 207,090 new breast cancer cases will be diagnosed in women and 1,970 new cases will be diagnosed in men in the United States in 2010, and 39,840 women and 390 men will die of this cancer. As of 2010, there are approximately 2.9 million breast cancer survivors in the United States.

This chapter provides an overview of breast cancer, with discussions of epidemiology, etiology and risk factors, genetic cancer risk assessment, signs and symptoms, screening and diagnosis, prevention (including lifestyle changes and chemoprevention), staging, and prognosis. The three chapters that follow focus on the management of stages 0 and I, stage II, and stages III and IV breast cancers.

EPIDEMIOLOGY

Gender

Breast cancer is relatively uncommon in men; the female-to-male ratio is approximately 100:1. The incidence of breast cancer in men has remained relatively stable over the past decades, except in Africa, where, for unclear reasons, the incidence is rising. *BRCA* mutations are associated with an increased risk for breast cancer in men.

The most common presentations of breast cancer in men are asymmetric gynecomastia or a palpable mass. All palpable masses in men should be carefully examined. Based upon the findings on physical examination, mammography and breast ultrasonography should be considered. Fine-needle aspiration (FNA) or core biopsy can be used to distinguish between gynecomastia and breast cancer. Core biopsy may be performed if the FNA is nondiagnostic.

TABLE 1: Survival of women with breast cancer, according to stage, without chemotherapy

Stage	Survival rate at 8 years (%)
I	90
II	70
III	40
IV	10

Age

The risk of developing breast cancer increases with age. The disease is uncommon in women younger than 40 years of age; only about 0.8% of breast cancers occur in women < 30 years old, and approximately 6.5% develop in women between 30 and 40 years old.

Race

Caucasian women have a higher overall rate of breast cancer than do African-American women; however, this difference is not apparent until age 50 and is marked only after menopause. In the United States, the incidence of breast cancer in Asian and Hispanic women is approximately half that in white women. Breast cancer risk is extremely low in Native-American women.

Geography

There is at least a fivefold variation in the incidence of breast cancer reported in different countries, although this difference appears to be narrowing. The incidence of breast cancer is significantly lower in Japan, Thailand, Nigeria, and India than in Denmark, the Netherlands, New Zealand, Switzerland, the United Kingdom, and the United States. Women living in North America have the highest rate of breast cancer in the world. It has been suggested that these trends in breast cancer incidence somehow may be related to dietary influences, particularly dietary fat consumption (see section on "Etiology and risk factors").

Socioeconomic status

The incidence of breast cancer is higher in women of higher socioeconomic background. This relationship is most likely related to lifestyle differences, such as age at first birth and dietary fat intake.

Disease site

The left breast is involved slightly more frequently than the right, and the most common locations of the disease are the upper outer quadrant and retroareolar region. The risk of contralateral breast cancer in women with a mutation of a breast cancer gene (*BRCA*) is approximately 40% at 10 years after the initial diagnosis of breast cancer. This risk is higher in *BRCA1* than *BRCA2* mutation carriers and in those first diagnosed at age < 50.

Risk for breast cancer is reduced in women who take tamoxifen. Bilateral salpingo-oophorectomy (BSO) also reduces breast cancer risk, especially when this procedure is performed in women younger than age 50. The protective effect of BSO is pronounced among women who develop breast cancer premenopausally.

Survival

Survival rates for patients with nonmetastatic breast cancer have improved in recent years (Table 1). These improvements may be secondary to advances in screening, adjuvant chemotherapy, and radiation therapy. The contribution of screening mammography to breast cancer–specific survival is variable, favoring a reduction in breast cancer mortality of up to 25% in some series. Its impact on overall survival is less certain.

ETIOLOGY AND RISK FACTORS

The development of breast cancer has been associated with numerous risk factors, including genetic, environmental, hormonal, and nutritional influences. Despite all of the available data on breast cancer risk factors, 75% of women with this cancer have no risk factors.

Genetic factors

Hereditary forms of breast cancer constitute only 5% to 10% of breast cancer cases overall. However, the magnitude of the probability that a woman will develop cancer if she inherits a highly penetrant cancer gene mutation justifies the intense interest in predictive testing. Commercial testing is available for several genes (*BRCA1*, *BRCA2*, tumor protein *p53* gene *[TP53]*) associated with a high risk for breast cancer development.

Elevated risk for breast cancer is also associated with mutations in the *PTEN* gene in Cowden's syndrome (described later). In addition, a modest increased risk (relative risk of RR = 3.9–6.4) may be seen in women who are heterozygous for a mutation in the *ATM* gene, ataxia telangiectasia mutated gene *(ATM)*, which is associated with the recessive disease ataxia-telangiectasia in the homozygous state. A moderately increased risk for breast cancer (2-fold for women and 10-fold for men) has also been associated with a variant (1100 delC) in the cell-cycle checkpoint kinase gene, *CHEK2*.

BRCA1 gene

The *BRCA1* gene is located on chromosome 17. This gene is extremely large and complex, and there are more than 1,000 different possible mutations. *BRCA1* mutations are inherited in an autosomal-dominant fashion and are associated with an increased risk for breast, ovarian, and, to a lesser degree, prostate cancers. A *BRCA1* mutation carrier has a 56% to 85% lifetime risk of developing breast cancer and a 15% to 45% lifetime risk of developing ovarian cancer.

BRCA2 gene

The *BRCA2* gene was localized to chromosome 13. *BRCA2* is approximately twice as large as *BRCA1* and is similarly complex.

Alterations in *BRCA2* have been associated with an increased incidence of breast cancer in both women (similar to *BRCA1*) and men (6% lifetime risk). *BRCA2* mutations are also associated with an increased risk for ovarian cancer, pancreatic cancer, prostate cancer, and melanoma. Together, mutations of *BRCA1* and *BRCA2* have been linked to most hereditary breast and ovarian cancer families and approximately half of hereditary breast cancer families.

The incidence of *BRCA* gene mutations in the general breast cancer population is unknown, since most of the data have come from studies of high-risk populations. In one population-based study of women with breast cancer, 9.4% of women < 35 years of age at the time of diagnosis and 12.0% of women < 45 years old who also had a first-degree relative with breast cancer had germline *BRCA1* or *BRCA2* mutations. However, a 40-year-old woman of Ashkenazi Jewish ancestry who has breast cancer has a 20% to 30% probability of bearing one of three founder *BRCA* gene mutations, based on data from high-risk clinics, testing vendors, and Israeli series.

Li-Fraumeni syndrome

This rare syndrome is characterized by premenopausal breast cancer in combination with childhood sarcoma, brain tumors, leukemia, and adrenocortical carcinoma. Tumors frequently occur in childhood and early adulthood and often present as multiple primaries in the same individual. Germline mutations in the *TP53* gene on chromosome 17p have been documented in persons with this syndrome. Inheritance is autosomal dominant, with a penetrance of at least 50% by age 50. Although the rarity of this syndrome, the diversity of tumor types, and the fact that the age of patients at risk spans from childhood to young adulthood makes coherent screening strategies beyond those for the early-onset breast cancer risk difficult to find, a recent pilot study with 18-fluorodeoxyglucose positron emission tomography/CT scanning was promising.

Gonzalez et al recently reported on the largest experience with clinical *TP53* testing published thus far. In all, 91 of 525 patients had a deleterious mutation. The investigators derived user-friendly mutation-probability tables based upon presenting features of individuals and families, with the highest yield noted among children with choroid plexus tumors. The discovery ot *TP53* mutations in *BRCA*-negative women diagnosed with breast cancer under 30 years old was cited in the 2009 NCCN guidelines *(Gonzalez KD et al: J Clin Oncol 27:1250–1256, 2009).*

Cowden's syndrome

This syndrome is inherited as an autosomal-dominant trait and is notable for a distinctive skin lesion (trichilemmoma) and mucocutaneous lesions. Patients with this uncommon syndrome have a high incidence of gastrointestinal polyps and thyroid disorders; lifetime estimates for breast cancer among women with this syndrome range from 25% to 50%. Germline mutations in the *PTEN* gene, located on chromosome 10q23, are responsible for this syndrome.

Family history

The overall RR of breast cancer in a woman with a positive family history in a first-degree relative (mother, daughter, or sister) is 1.7. Premenopausal onset of the disease in a first-degree relative is associated with a threefold increase in breast cancer risk, whereas postmenopausal diagnosis increases the RR by only 1.5. When the first-degree relative has bilateral disease, there is a fivefold increase in risk. The RR for a woman whose first-degree relative developed bilateral breast cancer prior to menopause is nearly 9.

Proliferative breast disease

The diagnosis of certain conditions on a breast biopsy is also associated with an increased risk for the subsequent development of invasive breast cancer. They include moderate or florid ductal hyperplasia and sclerosing adenosis, which pose only a slightly increased risk of breast cancer (1.5–2.0 times); atypical ductal or lobular hyperplasia, which moderately increases risk (4–5 times); and lobular carcinoma in situ (LCIS), which markedly increases risk (8–11 times; see more detailed discussion of LCIS in chapter 6). Patients who have a family history of breast cancer along with a personal history of atypical epithelial hyperplasia have an eightfold increase in breast cancer risk when compared with patients with a positive family history alone and an 11-fold increase in breast cancer risk when compared with patients who do not have atypical hyperplasia and have a negative family history.

Personal cancer history

A personal history of breast cancer is a significant risk factor for the subsequent development of a second, new primary breast cancer. This risk has been estimated to be as high as 1% per year from the time of diagnosis of an initial sporadic breast cancer. Women with *BRCA*-associated cancer have a 3% to 5% per year risk of contralateral breast cancer (cumulative lifetime risk of up to 64% in high-risk cohorts). Women with a history of endometrial, ovarian, or colon cancer also have a higher likelihood of developing breast cancer than do those with no history of these malignancies.

Menstrual and reproductive factors

Early onset of menarche (< 12 years old) has been associated with a modest increase in breast cancer risk (twofold or less). Women who undergo menopause before age 30 have a twofold reduction in breast cancer risk when compared with women who undergo menopause after age 55. A first full-term pregnancy before age 30 appears to have a protective effect against breast cancer, whereas a late first full-term pregnancy or nulliparity may be associated with a higher risk. There is also a suggestion that lactation protects against breast cancer development.

Radiation exposure

An increased rate of breast cancer has been observed in survivors of the atomic bomb explosions in Japan, with a peak latency period of 15 to 20 years. More recently, it has been noted that patients with Hodgkin lymphoma who are treated with mantle irradiation, particularly women who are younger than age 20 at the time of radiation therapy, have an increased incidence of breast cancer.

Exogenous hormone use

In regard to hormone replacement therapy (HRT) or postmenopausal hormone use, results from the WHI showed that the overall risks of estrogen plus progestin outweigh the benefits. This large randomized clinical trial sponsored by the NIH included more than 16,000 healthy women. Results from the WHI trial were published in 2002, after an average 5.6 years of follow-up, and included a 26% increase in risk of invasive breast cancer among women taking estrogen plus progestin, as compared with women taking placebo. In addition, in women taking these hormones, there were increased risks of heart disease, stroke, and blood clots.

The NIH stopped the estrogen-alone arm of the WHI trial in March 2004. No increase in breast cancer risk was observed in the estrogen-alone arm during the study period (7 years of follow-up). The NIH concluded that estrogen alone does not appear to increase or decrease a woman's risk of heart disease, although it does appear to increase her risk of stroke and decrease her risk of hip fracture.

Following the publication of the WHI trial results, the use of HRT in the United States declined by almost 40% from 2002 to 2003. During approximately the same period, there was a 6.7% decline in the age-adjusted incidence of breast cancer. Furthermore, the decrease was evident only among women 50 years of age and older and primarily among those with estrogen receptor–positive breast cancers.

Alcohol

Moderate alcohol intake (two or more drinks per day) appears to modestly increase breast cancer risk.

High-fat diet

Diets that are high in fat have been associated with an increased risk for breast cancer. Women who have diets high in animal fat from high-fat dairy foods have an increased risk of developing breast cancer. Whether the increase in breast cancer risk is associated with the fat content or an unknown carcinogen in these foods is unclear. There is no association between the consumption of red meat and an increased risk of breast cancer.

Obesity

Alterations in endogenous estrogen levels secondary to obesity may enhance breast cancer risk. Obesity appears to be a factor primarily in postmenopausal women.

In late 2007, the RRs of cancer incidence and mortality from the Million Women Study were reported. The study analyzed data on 1.2 million women in the UK (age from 1996–2001, 50–64 years) who were followed for an average of 5.4 years for cancer incidence and 7.0 years for cancer mortality. In all, 45,037 incident cancers and 17,203 deaths from the disease occurred during follow-up. An increased incidence of breast cancer with increasing body mass index (BMI) was noted. For breast cancer, the effect of BMI on risk differed significantly according to menopausal status (RR in postmenopausal women = 1.40). Calculations were adjusted for BMI, age, geographic region, socioeconomic status, age at first birth, parity, smoking status, alcohol use, physical activity, years since menopause, and use of HRT.

GENETIC CANCER RISK ASSESSMENT

Genetic testing clearly has the potential to benefit carefully selected and counseled families. Education and adequately trained health care professionals are key elements in the successful integration of genetic cancer risk assessment into clinical practice.

The genetic risk assessment process begins with an evaluation of perceived risk and the impact of cancer on the patient and family. This information forms the framework for counseling.

Comprehensive personal and family histories

Detailed information regarding personal, reproductive, and hormonal risk factors is noted. Family history, including age at disease onset, types of cancer, and current age or age at death, is obtained for all family members going back at least three generations.

Documentation of cancer cases

Documentation is crucial to accurate risk estimation. Pathology reports, medical record notes, and death certificates may all be used in determining the exact diagnosis.

Pedigree construction and evaluation

The family pedigree is then constructed and analyzed to determine whether a pattern of cancer in the family is consistent with genetic disease. Sometimes, small family structure or lack of information about the family limits assessment of a hereditary trait; other times, clues such as ancestry or early age at diagnosis influence risk assessment and the usefulness of genetic testing.

Individual risk assessment

Several models are used to estimate the likelihood that a detectable *BRCA1* or *BRCA2* mutation is responsible for the disease in the family. The *BRCA*PRO computer program is a cancer risk–assessment tool that uses a family history of breast or ovarian cancer in first- and second-degree relatives to calculate the probabilities that either

TABLE 2: Features indicating an increased likelihood of a BRCA mutation

Early-onset breast cancer, especially in the setting of a limited family structure
Ovarian cancer (with or without a family history of breast or ovarian cancer)
Breast and ovarian cancers in the same woman
Bilateral breast cancer
Ashkenazi Jewish heritage
Male breast cancer
ER, PR, and HER2 negative (“triple negative”) premenopausal breast cancer

ER = estrogen receptor; HER2 = human epidermal growth factor receptor type 2; PR = progesterone receptor a *BRCA1* or *BRCA2* mutation is responsible for the disease. It includes a Bayesian calculation (of conditional probability) to account for age-specific penetrance differences. If genetic testing is not performed or results are uninformative, the empiric breast cancer risk is estimated by the phenotype as well as the Claus model (derived from the Cancer and Hormone Study, which uses age at onset of breast cancer among first- and second-degree relatives) or Gail model. Personal and family characteristics that are associated with an increased likelihood of a *BRCA1* or *BRCA2* mutation are summarized in Table 2.

Education

Patients should be given information about the principles of genetics and hereditary cancer patterns and the application of genetic testing (appropriateness, limitations, advantages, and disadvantages).

Genetic counseling and testing

Informed consent is obtained before genetic testing is performed. For individuals who decide to undergo testing, a post-test counseling session is scheduled to disclose and explain the results in person.

Customized screening and prevention recommendations

Regardless of whether or not a woman undergoes genetic testing, a customized management plan is delineated, with the goal of preventing or detecting malignancy early, within the context of the patient's personal preferences and degree of risk (Table 3).

Laboratory methods

Several techniques/strategies for detecting mutations in cancer genes have been adopted by different researchers and commercial vendors.

Directed assays are available for specific founder or ancestral mutations that are common in a given population. Among Ashkenazi Jews, 1 in 40 individuals bears one of three founder mutations (185delAG and 5382insC in *BRCA1* and 6174delT in *BRCA2*); these mutations account for 25% of early-onset breast cancer in this population. Moreover, 95% of Ashkenazi Jews with a *BRCA* gene mutation will have one of the three founder mutations. However, complete gene sequencing can be performed if a patient does not test positive for a founder mutation.

The lifetime risk of breast cancer was 82% among founder mutation carriers in a large cohort of Jewish families identified via a New York breast cancer study. The lifetime risk of ovarian cancer was 54% for *BRCA1* and 23% for *BRCA2*, similar to the risk in multiplex families from the BCLC. However, a population-based study indicated a lifetime breast cancer risk of 40% to 73%.

Limitations

All of the approaches to detecting mutations have limitations. In general, discovery of an inactivating or "deleterious" mutation of either *BRCA1* or *BRCA2* indicates a high probability that a person will develop breast and/or ovarian cancer.

TABLE 3: Risk management options for BRCA mutation carriers[a]

Recommended for breast cancer detection

- Monthly self-examination of the breast beginning in late teen years
- Beginning at age 25 (or at least 10 years before the earliest onset cancer in the kindred):
  - Clinician breast examination every 6 months
  - Annual mammography
  - Consider annual breast MRI if there is significant mammographic density
  - Discussed as options:
    - Bilateral risk-reduction mastectomy (total or skin-sparing)
    - Participation in clinical trials for chemoprevention

Recommended for ovarian cancer detection or prevention

- Risk-reduction salpingo-oophorectomy recommended upon completion of childbearing
- Pelvic examination and Pap smear annually
- Considered optional:
  - Serum CA-125 every 6 months
  - Transvaginal ultrasonography every 6 months

[a] Also offered to women at increased risk because of a positive family history of hereditary breast and ovarian cancers but for whom genotypic information is not available.

One of the greatest challenges is the interpretation of missense mutations. These mutations are more likely to be significant if located in an evolutionarily conserved or functionally critical region of the protein. In the absence of a clear disease association, it is often difficult to exclude the possibility that a given missense alteration simply represents a rare polymorphism. Using advanced methods, a recent study was able to characterize 133/1,433 variants as likely polymorphisms and 43 as likely deleterious; the majority would still be designated as "genetic variants of uncertain significance."

Although less common, mutations in other genes besides *BRCA1* and *BRCA2* (eg, *CHEK2* and *TP53*) may predispose patients to breast cancer. Walsh et al demonstrated inherited genomic rearrangements of *BRCA1* and *BRCA2* in 35 of 300 (12%) sequence-negative, high-risk families. They also highlighted other single-gene breast cancer predisposition traits in a subset of families (eg, 14 with a *CHEK2* mutation and 3 with a *TP53* mutation). In part, this finding prompted accelerated implementation of a commercial screen.

Testing strategies

In general, testing should be initiated with the youngest affected individual in a given family. Even if one is convinced that a family has hereditary breast and ovarian cancers based on clinical criteria, there is only a 50% chance that an offspring or sibling of an affected patient will have inherited the deleterious allele. Therefore, only a positive test result (detection of a known or likely deleterious mutation) is truly informative.

Until the "familial mutation" is known, a negative test result could mean either that the unaffected person being tested did not inherit the cancer susceptibility mutation or that the person inherited the disease-associated gene, but the mutation was not detectable by the methods used.

In many cases, no affected family members are available for testing. In that case, one may proceed with genetic testing of an unaffected person, but only after that individual has been thoroughly counseled regarding its risks, benefits, and limitations.

Unless there is a suggestive family history, cancer susceptibility testing is not considered appropriate for screening unaffected individuals in the general population. However, it may be reasonable to test unaffected persons who are members of an ethnic group in which specific ancestral mutations are prevalent and whose family structure is limited (ie, the family is small, with few female relatives or no information due to premature death from noncancerous causes).

Impact of genetic cancer risk status on management

Data from the BCLC suggest that the cumulative risk of developing a second primary breast cancer is approximately 65% by age 70 among *BRCA* gene mutation carriers who have already had breast cancer. A large, retrospective cohort study of *BRCA* mutation carriers with a history of limited-stage breast cancer indicated up to a 40% risk of contralateral breast cancer at 10 years. A subsequent study of the same cohort noted almost a 13% risk for ovarian cancer in the same interval and that ovarian cancer was the cause of cancer death in 25% of stage I breast cancer patients with *BRCA* mutations.

Thus, knowledge of the genetic status of a woman affected with breast cancer might influence the initial surgical approach (eg, bilateral mastectomy might be recommended for a mutation carrier instead of a more conservative procedure). Moreover, since ovarian cancer risk may be markedly increased in women with *BRCA1* mutations (and to a lesser degree with *BRCA2* mutations), additional measures, such as surveillance for presymptomatic detection of early-stage tumors or consideration of oophorectomy, may be warranted.

According to data from *BRCA* mutated carriers who underwent risk-reduction salpingo-oophorectomy (RRSO), breast cancer risk is also decreased from bilateral oophorectomies.

Kauff et al reported their findings of a multicenter prospective analysis of RRSO to prevent *BRCA*-associated breast and ovarian cancers. During a median follow-up of 40 months, RRSO was associated with a 52% reduction in breast cancer risk and a 91% reduction in ovarian cancer risk, with the greatest risk reduction occurring in women with the *BRCA2* gene mutation. A total of 886 female *BRCA1* or *BRCA2* mutation carriers older than age 30 were enrolled from 1 of 11 study centers between 1994 and 2004. Women were treated with either ovarian surveillance (n = 325) or RRSO (n = 561). The investigators believe their results confirm that RRSO is highly protective against *BRCA*-associated breast and ovarian cancers.

Both retrospective and prospective data have demonstrated the efficacy (> 90% risk reduction) of bilateral mastectomy in women who are at high risk for the disease based upon *BRCA* genetic status. Women who opt for risk-reduction mastectomy should be offered reconstruction. Skin-sparing mastectomy may enhance the cosmetic results of reconstruction and should be discussed with the patient's surgeon. This procedure entails removing the breast tissue (including the nipple-areolar complex).

The efficacy of bilateral risk-reduction mastectomy has been confirmed in a large prospective study of 483 women with *BRCA* mutations. With a mean follow-up of 6.4 years, risk reduction mastectomy reduced the risk of breast cancer by 90% (95% in women who also underwent RRSO).

Data presented at ASCO in 2008 and 2009 suggested that a "synthetic lethality" strategy involving treatment with poly (ADP-ribose) polymerase (PARP) inhibitors is effective in women with BRCA-associated breast or ovarian cancer.

Rebbeck et al performed a meta-analysis of published studies of RRSO in *BRCA* mutation carriers and confirmed the magnitude of breast cancer risk reduction associated with the procedure. Critically, their findings firmly established a significant risk reduction of *BRCA1* carriers (HR = 0.49; 95% CI = 0.35–0.64), who are predisposed to ER-negative tumors in particular *(Rebbeck TR et al: J Natl Cancer Inst 101:80–87, 2009)*.

Potential benefits and risks of genetic testing

The ability to identify individuals at highest risk for cancer holds the promise of improved prevention and early detection of cancers. Patients who are not at high risk can be spared anxiety and the need for increased surveillance. Recent studies suggest a better emotional state among at-risk relatives who undergo testing than among those who choose not to know their status. The patient's perception of risk is often much higher than risk estimated by current models.

Potential risks

Potential medical, psychological, and socioeconomic risks must be addressed in the context of obtaining informed consent for genetic testing.

Concerns about insurance Fear about adverse effects of testing on insurability remains the premier concern among patients. Close behind that is concern about the cost of analyzing large complex genes ($3,600 for full sequencing of *BRCA1* and *BRCA2* and an additional $800 if the test for genomic rearrangements is ordered a la carte).

Legal and privacy issues The legal and privacy issues surrounding genetic testing are as complex as the testing technologies. Although several state laws regarding the privacy of medical information, genetic testing, and insurance and employment discrimination have been passed, they vary widely.

The 1996 Health Insurance Portability and Accountability Act (US public law 104-191), governing group medical plans, stipulates that genetic information may not be treated as a preexisting condition in the absence of a diagnosis of the condition related to such information. It further prohibits basing rules for eligibility or costs for coverage on genetic information. However, the law did not address genetic privacy issues and does not cover individual policies. Many states have laws addressing genetic discrimination, but concerns about gaps remained. Recent Federal legislation expanded protection against genetic discrimination to include individual policies.

Data from recent clinical trials suggested that poly (ADP-ribose) polymerase (PARP) inhibitors show promising antitumor effects as single agents in *BRCA*-associated breast and ovarian cancer *(Fong PC et al: N Engl J Med 361:1–12, 2009)*

The Genetic Information Nondiscrimination Act of 2008 (GINA) prohibits health insurers and employers from discriminating against individuals on the basis of genetic information.

Recommendations for genetic testing

Guidelines from ASCO recommend that cancer predisposition testing be offered only in the following situations: (1) if a person has a strong family history of cancer or early onset of disease; (2) if the test can be adequately interpreted; and (3) if the results will influence the medical management of the patient or family member.

NCCN practice guidelines for genetics/familial high-risk cancer screening are updated annually and published at www.nccn.org.

Weitzel et al characterized the impact of family structure on the prevalence of *BRCA* gene mutations among 306 women who developed breast cancer before the age of 50 years and who had no first- or second-degree relatives with breast or ovarian cancer. *BRCA* mutations were detected in 13.7% of women with limited family structure (ie, fewer than two first- or second-degree relatives surviving beyond age 45 years in either lineage) and 5.2% of those having adequate family structure. Family structure, therefore, apparently is a strong predictor of mutation status (odds ratio = 2.8; 95% confidence interval = 1.19–6.73, *P* = .019). Genetic testing guidelines may need to be more inclusive for single cases of breast cancer when family structure is limited.

ASCO recently presented an update of its policy statement regarding genetic testing to extend commentary on the lack of documented clinical utility of commercially available genomic tests relying on single nucleotide polymorphism markers with very modest relative risk for breast cancer *(Robson ME et al: J Clin Oncol 28:893–901, 2010)*

SIGNS AND SYMPTOMS

Mammographic findings

Increasing numbers of breast malignancies are being discovered in asymptomatic patients through the use of screening mammography. Mammographic features suggestive of malignancy include asymmetry, microcalcifications, a mass, or an architectural distortion.

When these features are identified on a screening mammogram (see Figures 1–5), they should, in most cases, be further evaluated with a diagnostic mammogram (and, in some cases, with a breast ultrasonographic image or, in highly selected cases, with MRI [Figure 6]) prior to determining the need for a tissue diagnosis. Often, pseudolesions, such as those caused by a summation artifact, dust on the mammographic cassettes, and dermal calcifications, are correctly identified in this manner. All mammographic lesions (and the examinations themselves) must be unambiguously categorized according to one of the six Breast Imaging Reporting Data System (BI-RAD) classifications developed by the ACR (Table 4).

Breast lump

When signs or symptoms are present, the most common presenting complaint is a lump within the breast. The incidence of this complaint can range from 65% to 76%, depending on the study.

Inflammatory breast cancer is particularly aggressive, although relatively uncommon, accounting for about 5% of all breast cancers. On breast palpation, there often is no definite mass, but the breast appears to be engorged with erythema, skin edema (peau d'orange), and skin ridging. A short trial of antibiotics or, on rare occasions, ultrasonography may be helpful in differentiating mastitis from inflammatory breast cancer.

Paget's disease

This condition has been associated with intraductal carcinoma involving the terminal ducts of the breasts and may have an associated invasive component. It presents as an eczematoid change in the nipple, a breast mass, or bloody nipple discharge. Cytology may be helpful in establishing the diagnosis; however, negative cytologic results should not preclude a biopsy.

Other local symptoms

Breast pain is the presenting symptom in ~5% of patients; breast enlargement, in 1%; skin or nipple retraction, in ~5%; nipple discharge, in ~2%; and nipple crusting or erosion, in 1%.

TABLE 4: BI-RAD classification of mammographic lesions

BI-RAD class	Description	Probability of malignancy (%)	Follow-up
0	Needs additional evaluation		Diagnostic mammogram, ultrasonographic image
1	Normal mammogram	0	Yearly screening
2	Benign lesion	0	Yearly screening
3	Probably benign lesion	< 2	Short interval follow-up
4[a]	Suspicious for malignancy	20	Biopsy
5	Highly suspicious for malignancy	90	Biopsy
6	Biopsy-proven malignancy	100	Treatment

BI-RAD = Breast Imaging Reporting Data System

[a] The ACR recommends that each site be divided into three subcategories: 4A, low suspicion; 4B, intermediate suspicion; and 4C, moderate concern but not classic for malignancy.

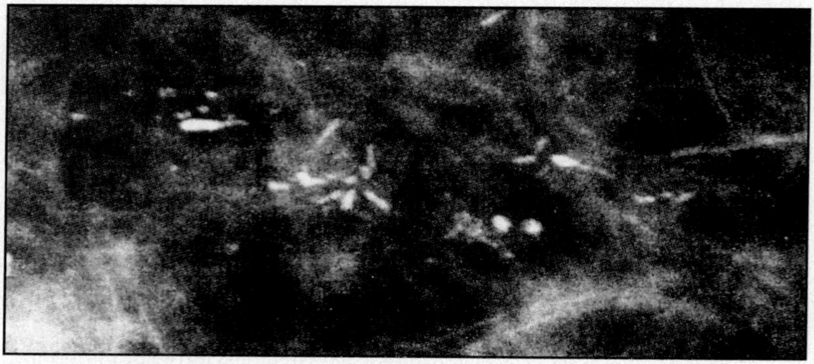

FIGURE 1: Malignant calcifications (comedocarcinoma) in a classic linear dot and dash configuration (BI-RAD 5 lesion). BI-RAD = Breast Imaging Reporting Data System.

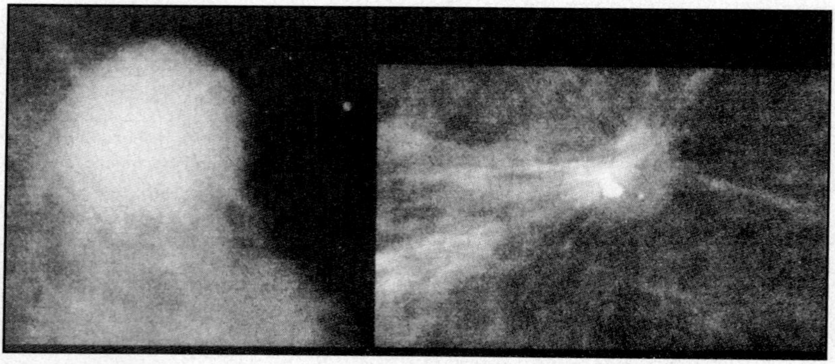

FIGURE 2: Left panel: A dense mass with partially unsharp margins (BI-RAD 4 lesion), which proved to be a fibroadenoma. Right panel: A small, spiculated mass (BI-RAD 5 lesion), which has engulfed a coarse, benign calcification. This lesion proved to be an invasive ductal carcinoma, not otherwise specified. BI-RAD = Breast Imaging Reporting Data System.

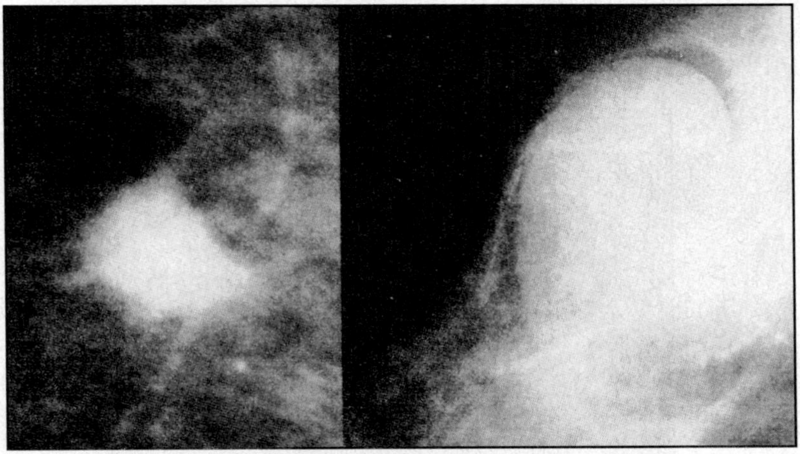

FIGURE 3: Left panel: This focal mass with truly nonsharp margins (BI-RAD 4 lesion) was diagnosed as a tubular carcinoma on stereotactic core biopsy. Right panel: A well-circumscribed lesion containing fat (BI-RAD 2 lesion), which is pathognomonic for a breast hamartoma (fibroadenolipoma). BI-RAD = Breast Imaging Reporting Data System.

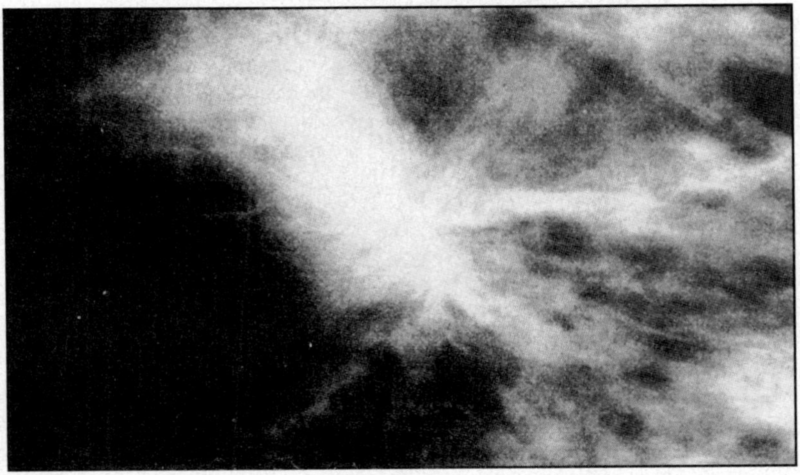

FIGURE 4: Focal architectural distortion may be difficult to see, but, if confirmed, it has the highest positive predictive value for breast carcinoma. This BI-RAD 4 lesion proved to be an invasive lobular carcinoma, which often has a subtle mammographic appearance. BI-RAD = Breast Imaging Reporting Data System.

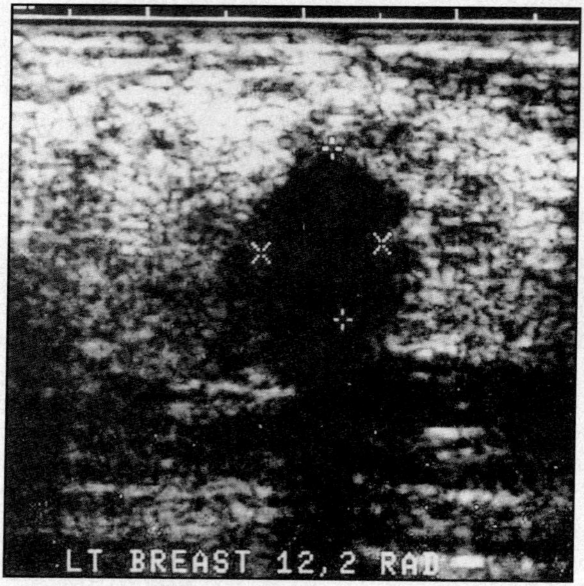

FIGURE 5: This breast ultrasonographic image demonstrates a hypoechoic, solid mass, which exhibits posterior shadowing and is taller than wide. This BI-RAD 4 lesion proved to be an invasive ductal carcinoma, not otherwise specified. BI-RAD = Breast Imaging Reporting Data System.

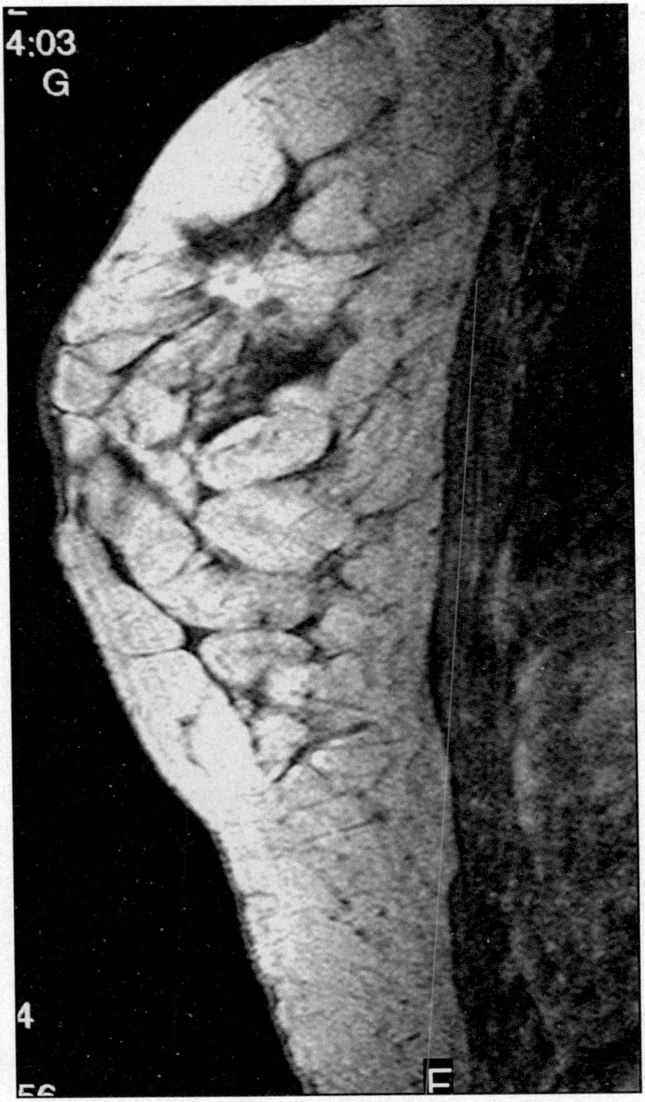

FIGURE 6: A 42-year-old woman presents with axillary adenopathy, which was positive on fine-needle aspiration. Results of a clinical breast exam, mammography, and ultrasonography were normal. A 7-mm enhancing cancer is clearly seen on this MRI of the breast.

SCREENING AND DIAGNOSIS

Screening

Breast self-examination

The role of breast self-examination is controversial. ACS recommends that beginning in their 20s, women should be instructed in the technique and informed about both the benefits and limitations of this screening tool. Other groups have suggested that routine breast self-examination may lead to more false-positive results and therefore more benign biopsies. One meta-analysis of 12 studies involving a total of 8,118 patients with breast cancer correlated the performance of breast self-examination with tumor size and regional lymph node status. Women who performed breast self-examination were more likely to have smaller tumors and less likely to have axillary node metastases than those who did not. A multicenter study from MSKCC and the University of Virginia attempted to measure the benefits and costs of adding clinical breast exams to yearly screening mammography. These exams detected an additional 14 breast cancers, or 0.02% of the 60,027 exams performed, and the cost for each additional cancer detected was $122,598. Based on this report, the benefit of clinical breast exams appear to be marginal.

A major problem with breast self-examination as a screening technique is that it is rarely performed well. Only 2% to 3% of women do an ideal examination a year after instruction has been provided.

Clinical breast examination

The American Cancer Society no longer recommends monthly self-breast examinations. However, all women should learn about the potential benefits, limitations, and harms (false positive results) of breast self-examinations. Women should receive instructions regarding proper technique for breast self-exams and then individually may choose to perform them monthly, occasionally, or never. Beginning at age 40, the clinical breast examination should be timed to occur near or prior to screening mammography. If the clinician detects an abnormality, the patient should then undergo diagnostic imaging rather than screening. Clinical breast examination should be performed and a complete breast history obtained when a woman presents for routine health care. The clinical examination should include inspection and palpation of the breast and regional lymph nodes. Between 14% and 21% of breast cancers are detected by clinical breast examination.

Mammography

Despite conflicting coverage in the lay press, the benefits of screening mammography have been well established by the findings of 11 large-scale evidence-based clinical trials. The ACS, the ACR, and the AMA have updated their guidelines since 1997 and recommend annual mammography beginning at age 40. The NCI also updated its guidelines in 1997, recommending that women undergo screening mammography every 1 to 2 years beginning in their 40s. The US Preventive Services Task Force (USPSTF) updated its guidelines and now recommends mammography every 1 to 2 years, alone or with clinical breast examination, for women aged 40 and older.

Screening mammography

Screening mammography is performed in the asymptomatic patient to detect an occult breast cancer. This contrasts with diagnostic mammography, which is performed in a patient with a breast abnormality (palpable mass, bloody nipple discharge, or some other clinical finding) to further identify the etiology of the problem.

Physical examination and mammography are complementary. Mammography has a sensitivity of 85% to 90% and, thus, would miss 10% to 15% of clinically evident tumors while detecting the majority of cases an average of 2 years prior to any perceptible clinical signs or symptoms.

Screening recommendations for average-risk patients No upper age limit has been suggested, and screening should continue in women who are in good health and would be candidates for breast cancer treatment. The previous recommendation for a "baseline" mammogram between the ages of 35 and 40 has been withdrawn. Thus, both the ACS and the NCCN recommend annual mammography starting at age 40 for women at average risk of breast cancer. The USPSTF currently recommends yearly screening mammograms starting at age 50.

Screening recommendations for high-risk patients Based on epidemiologic evidence that premenopausal familial breast cancer often presents at similar ages among affected family members, many breast imaging centers recommend that yearly screening for such high-risk individuals begin approximately 10 years prior to the youngest age at which a first-degree relative was diagnosed with breast cancer. For example, according to this algorithm, a woman whose mother developed breast cancer at age 45 could begin yearly screening at age 35, in addition to biannual clinical breast examinations. These commonly used screening algorithms are not based on formal studies but have arisen based on the natural history of the disease. They are, however, in keeping with the recommendations of the NCCN guidelines. Screening for women at genetic risk may begin at age 25. There are numerous studies supporting the use of breast MRI in women at genetic risk, all of which indicated that sensitivity is > 80%.

Digital mammography

Digital mammography was approved by the FDA in 2000 and is rapidly being adopted by leading breast cancer centers worldwide. Initial trials indicate a comparable sensitivity to film-based mammography, with the benefit of a reduced risk of women called back from screening for additional workup. The FDA also approved computer-aided detection systems for mammography beginning in 2001. Mammograms are scanned by a computer, and possible lesions are marked for further review by a radiologist. A number of studies have shown a reduced risk of "missed cancers" when computer-aided diagnosis is thus employed. Although some physicians are skeptical about the benefits of such computer-aided detection systems for mammography, many investigators in the field continue to support its use. For example, Lindfors et al published data showing that these systems increased the effectiveness of mammographic screening by 29%, with a comparable increase in screening cost.

Screening ultrasonography

Sensitivity of mammography is diminished when the breast tissue is dense. There have been recent reports in the literature concerning the role of screening breast ultrasonography in women with dense breasts on mammography and normal mammography and clinical breast examination. The results from a multicenter trial of leading breast imagers (ACRIN 6666) showed that the addition of ultrasound to mammography increased detection of breast cancer when compared with mammography alone among women at increased risk of breast cancer who also had dense breast tissue. However, there was also an increase in the number of benign biopsies.

Pending further investigation, screening ultrasonography of the breast is not sanctioned or approved, and, unlike high-risk MRI screening, it does not constitute standard of care. Screening breast ultrasound may have some value in high-risk women with dense breast tissue on mammography, however; it is currently available at some institutions and can be offered to women who meet the aforementioned criteria.

Magnetic resonance imaging

This diagnostic is a sensitive tool for detecting occult breast cancer foci. Due to its limited specificity and high cost, MRI is not likely to become a screening tool for average-risk women. However, the role of breast MRI screening for detecting breast cancer in very high risk women, such as carriers of a *BRCA* gene mutation, has now been well established. More controversial are guidelines from the ACS, which recommend that a screening breast MRI be performed in women having at least a 20% lifetime risk for breast cancer, including women having a history of radiotherapy when they were 10 to 30 years of age; or harboring a mutation of *BRCA1, BRCA2, TP53* or *PTEN*; or having a first-degree relative who harbors one of these mutations.

Several major studies have demonstrated the increased sensitivity of MRI for detecting cancers in women with inherited susceptibility to breast cancer compared with clinical breast examination, mammography, or ultrasonography. The sensitivity of breast MRI is > 75%; in contrast, the sensitivities of mammography and ultrasonography both are < 40%. The combined sensitivity of MRI plus mammography is about 95%, suggesting that it may be a viable strategy for screening young women at high risk for breast cancer.

Evaluation of a cystic mass

FNA

When a dominant breast mass is present and the history and physical examination suggest that it is a cyst, the mass can simply be aspirated with a fine needle. Aspiration of a simple benign breast cyst should yield nonbloody fluid and result in complete resolution of the lesion.

Ultrasonography

Ultrasound examination can also be used to determine whether a mass is solid or cystic and whether a cyst is simple, complicated, or complex. Simple cysts are anechoic and oval, with thin walls; if asymptomatic, a simple cyst may be treated as an incidental finding. Complicated cysts are similar, except that low-level echoes are present in the cyst lumen. In many instances, complicated cysts may be managed conservatively, unless a worrisome feature or history prompts aspiration. To evaluate complex masses (ie, previously turned complex cysts) that demonstrate a mixed cystic and solid lesion and that occasionally have thickened walls or septa, a biopsy (positive predictive value, 25%) is typically necessary.

Biopsy

A biopsy should be considered in the setting of an aspiration that is bloody or for a persistent solid component. Cytologic examination of the fluid is not routinely indicated, as the yield for positive cytology is so low. Cystic carcinoma accounts for < 1% of all breast cancers. However, an intraluminal solid mass is a worrisome sign suggesting (intra) cystic carcinoma and should be biopsied.

Evaluation of a solid mass

A solid, palpable mass can be evaluated in a variety of ways. The decision to observe a patient with a solid breast mass that appears to be benign should be made only after careful clinical and radiologic examinations. Either FNA for cytology or percutaneous core biopsy should also be performed.

Mammography

A mammogram is used to assess the radiologic characteristics of the mass and is important for the evaluation of the remainder of the ipsilateral breast as well as the contralateral breast.

FNA

This technique is a simple, easy-to-perform method for obtaining material for cytologic examination. The overall incidence of false-positive results ranges from 0% to 2.5% (0.7% when performed by experienced technicians), and the incidence of false-negative results varies from 3% to 27% (3% to 9% in experienced hands). Reasons for false-negative readings include less-than-optimal technique in preparing the cytologic material, a missed lesion on aspiration, tumor necrosis, and incorrect cytologic interpretation. FNA is limited in its ability to distinguish invasive from noninvasive cancers. For these reasons, the trend at leading breast centers has been to replace FNA with core biopsy.

Biopsy

In the past, an excisional biopsy of a small breast mass or an incisional biopsy of a larger breast mass was performed to establish a histologic diagnosis of breast cancer. Recently, excisional biopsies for diagnosis have been largely replaced by percutaneous procedures. For a suspected malignancy, core biopsy has become the preferred diagnostic tool. With a core biopsy, the surgeon can plan for the cancer surgery, allowing for definitive surgical management in a single procedure. Core biopsy is also more advantageous than an FNA because it allows evaluation of architectural and cellular characteristics.

Image-guided core biopsy

Ultrasound-guided core biopsies have been shown to offer increased targeting accuracy when compared with freehand core biopsy sampling. In certain limited clinical scenarios, use of vacuum-assisted, large-core needles may help reduce sampling error.

Evaluation of nonpalpable mammographic abnormalities

Excisional biopsy

Prior to 1991, almost all nonpalpable mammographic lesions were excised using surgical excision. This technique has become less prevalent with the availability of image-guided percutaneous biopsy techniques.

Stereotactic and ultrasonography-guided core biopsies

These methods have revolutionized the management of nonpalpable breast lesions, and, currently, the majority of biopsies can be performed percutaneously, which is quicker, less invasive, and less expensive than is excisional biopsy. Tissue acquisition is performed with automated core needles or directional vacuum-assisted biopsy probes. Guidance for percutaneous biopsy is usually provided by stereotaxis, ultrasonography, and, more recently, MRI.

Numerous studies comparing the sensitivity and specificity of stereotactic biopsy versus surgical biopsy have consistently found the two procedures to be statistically equivalent. The long-term false-negative rate for stereotactic biopsy is 1.4%, which equals best published results with surgical biopsy.

Up to 80% of patients with nonpalpable mammographic lesions are candidates for stereotactic core biopsy. Lesions near the chest wall or immediately behind the nipple often cannot be reached on the stereotactic table. Diffuse lesions, such as scattered calcifications or a large asymmetric density, are subject to undersampling with the percutaneous approaches. Some patients are unable to lie prone on the stereotactic table for the duration of the examination. Finally, stereotactic units and trained personnel are not universally available.

Ultrasonography-guided core biopsy is another accurate percutaneous technique, useful for lesions best imaged by ultrasonography. Since the biopsy gun is handheld and guided in real time by the ultrasound imager, its use is related to more variability in performance, depending on the experience and skill of the practitioner. The overall reported accuracy rate of ultrasonography-guided biopsy is comparable with rates achieved with stereotactic and surgical biopsies.

Ultrasonography-guided or stereotactic FNA

This biopsy option is somewhat less invasive than core biopsy, but FNA provides only cytologic (not histologic) pathology results. This technique can result in both false-positive and false-negative results, whereas a false-positive result has not been reported to date for core breast biopsies. FNA is most successful in centers that have an experienced cytopathologist, who, ideally, is available on-site to review smears for adequacy during FNA procedures.

Breast MRI

This modality is currently used to search for an occult primary tumor in the setting of known metastasis, evaluate the extent of disease in a biopsy-proven breast carcinoma (useful if breast conservation is being considered), and assess lesions in implant-augmented breasts. It is also useful for screening high-risk women, as described previously. Its role in screening women with dense breasts or for evaluating borderline lesions has not been established, and these indications typically are not reimbursable. Breast MRI has a high sensitivity, and clinical developments have improved its specificity. Breast MRI examinations have recently been facilitated by the development of computer-aided detection software, which can help to streamline the interpretation of these images and produce a more uniform result.

Breast surgeons are increasingly using breast MRI for surgical planning. In a study reported by Bedrosian et al (a retrospective review of 267 patients who had preoperative MRI prior to undergoing definitive surgery), preoperative breast MRI changed the planned surgical approach in 26% of cases, including 16.5% of cases of breast conservation switched to mastectomy. Imaging centers across the United States have a varying degree of expertise in performing, interpreting, and providing a standard reporting nomenclature for breast MRI. The ACR is currently developing an accreditation program in breast MRI to address this issue.

Ultrasonography

In investigating ultrasonographic features of solid masses that suggest benign or malignant disease, Stavros et al described such factors as sharp margins (benign) and taller-than-wide lesions (malignant). Although these features are useful for clinical decision-making, their utility in increasing the specificity of the breast lesion workup has not been verified.

Molecular breast imaging

Molecular breast imaging has demonstrated excellent specificity and sensitivity in new industry-sponsored trials using high-definition, breast-specific gamma cameras. Both technetium-based sestamibi scanning and breast-specific PET scanning have shown promise. However, their utility has not yet been demonstrated in large-scale clinical trials.

PREVENTION

Lifestyle changes

There is increasing evidence that lifestyle changes may alter an individual's breast cancer risk.

Physical activity

Exercise has been associated with a reduction in breast cancer risk. The benefit was greatest in younger, premenopausal women. The activity can be related to leisure or work-time activities.

Women who exercise 3.5 to 4.0 times per week may have a reduced incidence of breast cancer, when compared with women who do not exercise. The protective effect of exercise may be associated with a reduction in the frequency of ovulatory cycles and in circulating estrogen and progesterone levels.

Alcohol consumption

Numerous studies of the effects of alcohol consumption on breast cancer risk and the results of a cohort study addressing this issue have been published. When compared with nondrinkers, women who consumed 2.3 to 4.5 bottles of beer per day, 2.5 to 5.6 glasses of wine per day, or 2 to 4 shots of liquor per day had a 41% higher risk of developing invasive breast cancer. Some reports indicate that the consumption of a moderate amount of alcohol (red wine) may decrease the risk of breast cancer, although these results are not conclusive. The biologic basis for the association between alcohol consumption and an increased risk of breast cancer is unclear. It has been proposed that there is a positive correlation between alcohol and estrogen levels.

Alterations in diet and tobacco use

A reduced incidence of breast cancer has been observed in countries where the diet is typically low in fat. However, no reduction in breast cancer risk has been observed in the United States when women followed low-fat diets.

Prentice et al randomly assigned postmenopausal women without prior breast cancer to an intervention designed to reduce total daily fat consumption to a minimum of 20% or to no dietary intervention. They found no statistically significant reduction in invasive breast cancer risk over a period of approximately 8 years of follow-up. However, women consuming a high-fat diet at baseline showed a significant reduction in breast cancer risk ($P = .04$). The authors also noted an effect that varied by hormone receptor status of the tumor.

There appears to be an association between cigarette smoking and breast cancer risk. It is not clear whether the risk for breast cancer decreases when someone stops smoking.

Lactation

Although it has been suggested that lactation may protect against breast cancer, it is unclear whether lactation reduces breast cancer risk. A recent study failed to demonstrate any breast cancer risk reduction in women who breast-fed and showed no dose-response effect in women who breast-fed for longer periods.

Chemoprevention

The NIH and NCI have publicized the results of the NSABP BCPT. Women who had a risk of developing breast cancer equivalent to that of women 60 years of age qualified as participants in this double-blind, randomized trial. (For representative eligibility profiles, see Table 5.) A total of 13,388 women were randomized to receive tamoxifen or placebo.

Benefits of therapy The summary results indicated that tamoxifen prevented about half of both invasive and noninvasive breast cancers in all age groups. A secondary benefit of tamoxifen appeared to be a reduction in the incidence of hip fracture (Table 6). At present, no survival advantage has been shown for participants in this trial.

TABLE 5: Examples of eligible risk profiles used in the Breast Cancer Prevention Trial

Age (yr)	Risk profile
35	Two affected first-degree relatives plus personal history of biopsy
40	Two affected first-degree relatives plus no live births
45	Two affected first-degree relatives or one affected first-degree relative plus personal history of biopsy

Side effects Tamoxifen-treated women younger than age 50 had no apparent increase in side effects. However, women older than age 50 experienced serious side effects, including vascular events and endometrial cancer. Particularly worrisome was the increased incidence of endometrial cancer in the tamoxifen-treated patients (Table 6). In addition, a significant increase in pulmonary embolism and deep vein thrombosis was noted, especially in women older than age 50 (Table 6).

Current recommendations

Based on results of the BCPT, the FDA has approved tamoxifen for use in women at high risk (1.66% chance of getting breast cancer in the next 5 years, based on the Gail model) of breast cancer.

TABLE 6: Number of events among participants in the NSABP Breast Cancer Prevention Trial

Type of event	Placebo	Tamoxifen	Total
Invasive breast cancer	154 (5)[a]	85 (3)[a]	239 (8)[a]
Noninvasive breast cancer	59	31	90
Hip fracture	20	9	29
Colles' fracture	12	7	19
Spinal fracture	39	31	70
Endometrial cancer	14	33	47
All other invasive cancers	88	85	173
Fatal stroke	3	4	7
Nonfatal stroke	21	30	51
Transient ischemic attack	21	18	39
Fatal pulmonary embolism	0	2	2
Nonfatal pulmonary embolism	6	15	21
Deep vein thrombosis requiring hospitalization	3	3	6
Deep vein thrombosis not requiring hospitalization	16	27	43
Total	**456**	**380**	**836**

[a] Numbers in parentheses indicate the number of deaths due to breast cancer.

The NCI and NSABP are in the process of developing risk profiles based on age, number of affected first-degree relatives with breast cancer, number of prior breast biopsies, presence or absence of atypical hyperplasia or LCIS, age at menarche, and age at first live birth. These risk profiles may help guide women in making the decision as to whether or not to take tamoxifen.

An ASCO working group published an assessment of tamoxifen use in the setting of breast cancer risk reduction. All women older than 35 years of age with a Gail model risk of > 1.66% (or the risk equivalent to that of women 60 years of age) should be considered candidates for this treatment strategy. Comorbid conditions, such as a history of deep vein thrombosis, must be a part of the consent process and treatment decision.

Although the BCPT results establish tamoxifen as the standard of care for the primary chemoprevention of breast cancer in high-risk women, concern over the side effects of tamoxifen has prompted a continuing search for an agent that displays a more desirable efficacy/toxicity profile. Raloxifene (Evista), approved for the prevention of osteoporosis in postmenopausal women, and for the reduction in risk of invasive breast cancer in postmenopausal women with osteoporosis, displays antiestrogenic properties in the breast and endometrium and estrogenic effects in the bone, making it an attractive candidate for comparison with tamoxifen.

The CORE trial, a 4-year follow-up to the MORE trial that examined the effect of long-term therapy with raloxifene in postmenopausal women with breast cancer, found that daily intake of the agent reduced the risk of invasive breast cancer by 59%. Compared with placebo, the incidence of invasive estrogen receptor–positive breast cancer was also reduced in the raloxifene arm ($P < .001$). There was no statistically significant increased risk of blood clots in legs or lungs, between the raloxifene-treated and placebo groups. Long-term use of raloxifene did not increase the risk of uterine cancer, as does long-term use of tamoxifen.

The STAR trial (or NSABP P-2) began in July 1999 at almost 400 centers in North America. A total of 19,747 postmenopausal women, or women > 35 years old at increased risk of breast cancer by Gail criteria, were randomized to receive either tamoxifen (20 mg/d) or raloxifene (60 mg/d) for 5 years. Study endpoints included invasive and noninvasive breast cancers, cardiovascular disease, endometrial cancer, bone fractures, and vascular events.

There were 163 cases of invasive breast cancer in women assigned to tamoxifen and 168 of those assigned to raloxifene (incidence, 4.30 per 1,000 vs 4.41 per 1,000; risk ratio RR, 1.02; 95%, 0.82–1.28). There were fewer cases of noninvasive breast cancer in the tamoxifen group (57 cases) than in the raloxifene group (80 cases); (incidence, 1.51 vs 2.11 per 1,000; RR, 1.40; 95% CI, 0.98–2.00). There were 36 cases of uterine cancer with tamoxifen and 23 with raloxifene (RR, 0.62; 95% CI, 0.35–1.08). The risk of other cancers, fractures, ischemic heart disease, and stroke is similar for both drugs. There was no difference in the total number of deaths (101 for tamoxifen vs 96 for raloxifene) or in causes of death. The authors concluded that raloxifene is as effective as tamoxifen in reducing the risk of invasive breast cancer and has a lower risk of thromboembolic events and cataracts but a nonstatistically significant higher risk of noninvasive breast cancer.

STAGING AND PROGNOSIS

Vitamin D is a regulator of cellular growth and differentiation. In a prospective Canadian study, vitamin D levels in women newly diagnosed with breast cancer (T1-3, N0-1, M0) more than 10 years before the study began were assessed in archived blood samples taken after surgery and prior to systemic therapy (n = 512). Vitamin D deficiency was associated with an increased risk of distant recurrence (independent of age, BMI, insulin level, and T and N stage, and not significantly modified by ER status, or use of adjuvant chemotherapy or tamoxifen) and death, while patients with insufficient and sufficient vitamin D levels had similar outcomes. These early findings raise the question of whether vitamin D supplementation might improve breast cancer–specific survival *(Goodwin PJ et al: J Clin Oncol 26[15S]:511, 2008).*

Staging system

The most widely used system to stage breast cancer is the AJCC classification, which is based on tumor size, the status of regional lymph nodes, and the presence of distant metastasis (Table 7).

Clinical staging

Assessment of clinical stage is performed initially and is determined after the physical examination and appropriate radiologic studies have been performed.

Pathologic staging

Pathologic stage is determined following surgery for operable breast cancer. Pathologic tumor size may differ from clinical tumor size. In addition, axillary nodal metastases that were not clinically evident may be detected after pathologic examination. With the advent of powerful molecular techniques, isolated tumor cells (ITCs) can be identified in histologically negative nodes. In the current AJCC staging, pathologic staging of nodes for detection of ITCs was included to obtain more information and, it is hoped, gain insight into the biologic significance of these ITCs.

Prognostic factors

Numerous prognostic factors for breast cancer have been identified.

Lymph node status

Axillary nodal metastasis is the most important prognostic factor in patients with breast cancer. Survival was examined relative to the number of nodes involved and the location of nodes that contained metastatic deposits. For any given number of positive nodes, survival was independent of the level of involvement but was directly related to the number of involved nodes.

Overall, patients who have node-negative disease have a 10-year survival rate of 70% and a 5-year recurrence rate of 19%. As the number of positive nodes increases, so does the likelihood of relapse. Patients with > 10 positive lymph nodes have a recurrence rate of 72% to 82%. The majority of patients who develop recurrence after initial curative treatment of early-stage breast cancer will have distant metastases.

Hormone-receptor status

In general, hormone receptor–positive tumors have a more indolent course than do hormone receptor–negative tumors.

TABLE 7: TNM staging system for breast cancer

Primary tumor (T)

TX	Primary tumor cannot be assessed
T0	No evidence of primary tumor
Tis	DCIS
Tis	LCIS
Tis	Paget's disease of the nipple with no tumor
T1	Tumor ≤ 2 cm in greatest dimension
T1mic	Microinvasion ≤ 0.1 cm in greatest dimension
T1a	Tumor > 0.1 but not > 0.5 cm in greatest dimension
T1b	Tumor > 0.5 cm but not >1 cm in greatest dimension
T1c	Tumor > 1 cm but not > 2 cm in greatest dimension
T2	Tumor > 2 cm but not > 5 cm in greatest dimension
T3	Tumor > 5 cm in greatest dimension
T4	Tumor of any size, with direct extension to (a) the chest wall or (b) skin only, as described below
T4a	Extension to the chest wall, not including the pectoralis muscle
T4b	Edema (including peau d'orange) or ulceration of the skin of the breast or satellite skin nodules confined to the same breast
T4c	Both T4a and T4b
T4d	Inflammatory carcinoma

Note: Paget's disease associated with a tumor is classified according to the size of the tumor.

Regional lymph nodes (N)

NX	Regional lymph nodes cannot be assessed (eg, previously removed)
N0	No regional lymph node metastasis
N1	Metastasis in movable ipsilateral axillary lymph node(s); pathologic involvement of 1–3 axillary lymph nodes
N2	Metastasis in ipsilateral axillary lymph node(s) fixed or matted, or in clinically apparent[a] ipsilateral internal mammary nodes in the ***absence*** of clinically evident axillary lymph node metastasis; pathologic involvement of 4–9 axillary lymph nodes
N2a	Metastasis in ipsilateral axillary lymph nodes fixed to one another (matted) or to other structures
N2b	Metastasis only in clinically apparent[a] ipsilateral internal mammary nodes and in the ***absence*** of clinically evident axillary lymph node metastasis
N3	Metastasis in ipsilateral infraclavicular lymph node(s) with or without axillary lymph node involvement, or in clinically apparent[a] ipsilateral internal mammary lymph node(s) and in the presence of clinically evident axillary lymph node metastasis; or metastasis in ipsilateral supraclavicular lymph node(s) with or without axillary or internal mammary lymph node involvement; pathologic involvement of ≥ 10 axillary lymph nodes
N3a	Metastasis in ipsilateral infraclavicular lymph node(s) and axillary lymph node(s)
N3b	Metastasis in ipsilateral internal mammary lymph node(s) and axillary lymph node(s)
N3c	Metastasis in ipsilateral supraclavicular lymph node(s)

continued on following page

DCIS = ductal carcinoma in situ; LCIS = lobular carcinoma in situ

[a] "Clinically apparent" is defined as detected by imaging studies (excluding lymphoscintigraphy) or by clinical examination or grossly visible pathologically.

Pathologic classification (pN) ***(continued)***

pNX	Regional lymph nodes cannot be assessed (eg, previously removed)
pN0	No regional lymph node metastasis
pN0(I–)	No regional lymph node metastasis histologically; negative IHC
pN0(I+)	No regional lymph node metastasis histologically; positive IHC; no IHC cluster > 0.2 mm
pN0(mol–)	No regional lymph node metastasis histologically; negative molecular findings (RT-PCR)
pN0(mol+)	No regional lymph node metastasis histologically; positive molecular findings (RT-PCR)
pN1	Metastasis in 1–3 axillary lymph nodes, and/or internal mammary nodes with microscopic disease detected by SLN dissection but not clinically apparent
pN1mi	Micrometastasis (> 0.2 mm but ≤ 2.0 mm)
pN1a	Metastasis in 1–3 axillary lymph nodes
pN1b	Metastasis in internal mammary nodes with microscopic disease detected by SLN dissection but not clinically apparent
pN1c	Metastasis in 1–3 axillary lymph nodes and in internal mammary lymph nodes with microscopic disease detected by SLN dissection but not clinically apparent
pN2	Metastasis in 4–9 axillary lymph nodes, or in clinically apparent internal mammary lymph nodes in the absence of axillary lymph node metastasis to ipsilateral axillary lymph node(s) fixed to each other or other structures
pN2a	Metastasis in 4–9 axillary lymph nodes (≥ 1 tumor deposit > 2.0 mm)
pN2b	Metastasis in clinically apparent internal mammary lymph nodes in the absence of axillary lymph node metastasis
pN3	Metastasis in ≥ 10 axillary lymph nodes, or in infraclavicular lymph nodes, or in clinically apparent ipsilateral mammary lymph nodes(s) in the presence of ≥ 1 positive axillary lymph node(s); or in > 3 axillary lymph nodes with clinically negative microscopic metastasis in internal mammary lymph nodes; or in ipsilateral supraclavicular lymph nodes
pN3a	Metastasis in ≥ 10 axillary lymph nodes (at least 1 tumor deposit > 2.0 mm); or metastasis to the infraclavicular lymph nodes
pN3b	Metastasis in clinically apparent ipsilateral internal mammary lymph nodes in the presence of ≥ 1 positive axillary lymph node(s) in > 3 axillary lymph nodes and in internal mammary lymph nodes with microscopic disease detected by SLN dissection but not clinically apparent
pN3c	Metastasis in ipsilateral supraclavicular lymph nodes

Distant metastasis (M)

MX	Distant metastasis cannot be assessed
M0	No distant metastasis
cM0(I+)	No clinical or radiographic evidence of distant metastases; deposits of molecularly or microscopically detected tumor cells in blood, bone marrow, or other nonregional nodal tissue
M1	Distant metastasis

continued on following page

HC = immunohistochemistry; RT-PCR = reverse transcriptase-polymerase chain reaction; SLN = sentinel lymph node

TABLE 7: TNM staging system for breast cancer *(continued)*

Stage grouping

Stage 0	Tis	N0	M0
Stage IA	T1[b]	N0	M0
Stage IB	T0	N1mic	M0
	T1[b]	N1mic	M0
Stage IIA	T0–1	N1	M0
	T2	N0	M0
Stage IIB	T2	N1	M0
	T3	N0	M0
Stage IIIA	T0–3	N2	M0
	T3	N1–2	M0
Stage IIIB	T4	N0–2	M0
Stage IIIC	Any T	N3	M0
Stage IV	Any T	Any N	M1

[b] T1 includes T1mic

From: Edge SB, Byrd DR, Compton CC, et al (eds): AJCC Cancer Staging Manual, 7th ed. New York, Springer, 2010.

Other factors

Other considerations used to predict outcome are tumor size, histologic grade, lymphovascular permeation, S-phase fraction, and ploidy. Well differentiated breast cancers have a better prognosis than moderately or poorly differentiated cancers. Likewise smaller tumors are more favorable than larger ones and the absence of lymphovascular invasion is better than its presence.

More recently, molecular prognostic factors have been evaluated to determine their utility in predicting outcome. They include the growth factor receptors (epidermal growth factor receptor and human epidermal growth factor receptor type 2 [HER2]), tumor suppressor genes (*TP53*), proteolytic enzymes that may be associated with invasion of disease and metastasis (cathepsin D), and metastasis suppressor genes (*NME1*). Of these molecular markers, HER2 is probably the most widely studied in breast cancer to date.

All breast cancers should be evaluated by immunohistochemistry (IHC) staining for estrogen and progesterone receptor status and HER2 overexpression. The presence of the estrogen (ER) and/or the progesterone receptor (PR) imparts a more favorable prognosis. In addition, these receptors are predictive of response to hormonal therapy. A HER-2 IHC score of 0–1+ is considered negative, 2+ is equivocal, and 3+ is positive. Equivocal HER2-positive tumors undergo fluorescence in situ hybridization (FISH) analysis for evaluation of *HER2* gene amplification. HER2 amplification of 2.0 or greater is considered positive. HER2 is also referred to as HER2/*neu* or ErbB2. It is a 185-kd transmembrane tyrosine kinase that regulates cell growth, survival, migration, differentiation, and adhesion. Overexpression of HER2 leads to dimerization of the receptors, which causes activation of the tyrosine kinase. HER2 overexpression is seen in approximately 20 to 30% of all breast cancers and was traditionally considered a more aggressive and a less favorable disease with reduced disease-free and overall survival. However, the development of biologic agents such as trastuzumab (Herceptin) has revolutionized the treatment of this type of breast cancer.

SUGGESTED READING

ON RISK FACTORS AND GENETIC CANCER RISK ASSESSMENT

Daly MB, Axilbund JE, Buys S: Genetic/Familial high-risk assessment: Breast and ovarian. J Natl Compr Canc Netw 8:562–594, 2010.

John EM, Miron A, Gong G, et al: Prevalence of pathogenic *BRCA1* mutation carriers in 5 US racial/ethnic groups. JAMA 298:2869–2876, 2007.

Ravdin PM, Cronin KA, Howlader N, et al: The decrease in breast-cancer incidence in 2003 in the United States. N Engl J Med 356:1670–1674, 2007.

Walsh T, Casadei S, Coats KH, et al: Spectrum of mutations in *BRCA1*, *BRCA2*, CHEK2, and *TP53* in families at high risk of breast cancer. JAMA 295:1379–1388, 2006.

ON SCREENING AND DIAGNOSIS

Feigin KN, Keating DM, Telford PM, et al: Clinical breast examination in a comprehensive breast cancer screening program: Contribution and cost. Radiology 240:650–655, 2006.

Hollingsworth AB, Stough RG: Breast MRI screening for high risk patients. Semin Breast Dis 11:67–75, 2008.

Lindfors KK, McGahan MC, Rosenquist CJ, et al: Computer-aided detection of breast cancer: A cost-effectiveness study. Radiology 239:710–717, 2006.

Saslow D, Boetes C, Burke W, et al: American Cancer Society guidelines for breast screening with MRI as an adjunct to mammography. CA Cancer J Clin 57:75–89, 2007.

Schnall MD, Blume J, Bluemke DA, et al: MRI detection of distinct incidental cancer in women with primary breast cancer studied in IBMC 6883. J Surg Oncol 92:32–38, 2005.

ON PREVENTION

Anderson GL, Judd HL, Kaunitz AM, et al: Effects of estrogen plus progestin on gynecologic cancers and associated diagnostic procedures. The Women's Health Initiative Randomized Trial. JAMA 290:1739–1748, 2003.

Prentice RL, Caan B, Chlebowski RT, et al: Low-fat dietary pattern and risk of invasive breast cancer: The Women's Health Initiative Randomized Controlled Dietary Modification trial. JAMA 295:629–642, 2006.

Vogel VG, Costantino JP, Wickerham DL, et al: National Surgical Adjuvant Breast and Bowel Project (NSABP): Effects of tamoxifen vs raloxifene on the risk of developing invasive breast cancer and other disease outcomes: The NSABP Study of Tamoxifen and Raloxifene (STAR) P-2 trial. JAMA 295:2727–2741, 2006.

Weitzel JN, Buys SS, Sherman WH, et al: Reduced mammographic density with use of a gonadotropin-releasing hormone agonist-based chemoprevention regimen in *BRCA1* carriers. Clin Cancer Res 13:654–658, 2007.

Abbreviations in this chapter

ACR = American College of Radiology; ACRIN = ACR Imaging Network; ACS = American Cancer Society; AMA=American Medical Association; AJCC = American Joint Committee on Cancer; ASCO = American Society of Clinical Oncology; BCLC = Breast Cancer Linkage Consortium; BCPT = Breast Cancer Prevention Trial; CORE = Continuing Outcomes Relevant to Evista; FDA = US Food and Drug Administration; MORE = Multiple Outcomes of Raloxifene; MSKCC = Memorial Sloan-Kettering Cancer Center; NCCN = National Comprehensive Cancer Network; NCI = National Cancer Institute; NIH = National Institutes of Health; NSABP = National Surgical Adjuvant Breast and Bowel Project; STAR = Study of Tamoxifen and Raloxifene; USPSTF = US Preventive Services Task Force; WHI = Women's Health Initiative

CHAPTER 6

Stages 0 and I breast cancer

Lori Jardines, MD, Sharad Goyal, MD, Melanie Royce, MD, PhD, and Shari B. Goldfarb, MD

This chapter focuses on the diagnosis and management of early-stage breast cancer, ie, stages 0 and I disease. This is an important area, since more noninvasive and small breast cancers are being diagnosed due to the increasing use of screening mammography. Treatment of these malignancies will continue to evolve as the results of clinical trials lead to further refinements in therapy.

STAGE 0 BREAST CANCER

Stage 0 breast cancer includes noninvasive breast cancer—lobular carcinoma in situ (LCIS) and ductal carcinoma in situ (DCIS)—as well as Paget's disease of the nipple when there is no associated invasive disease.

LOBULAR CARCINOMA IN SITU

LCIS is nonpalpable, produces no consistent mammographic changes, and is often an incidental finding seen on a breast biopsy performed for another reason. The biologic behavior of LCIS continues to be an issue of debate. Most clinicians agree that it is a marker for increased risk for all types of breast cancer (both noninvasive and invasive).

Epidemiology and etiology

The incidence of LCIS has doubled over the past 25 years and is now 2.8 per 100,000 women. In the past, the peak incidence of LCIS was in women in their 40s. Over the past 3 decades, the peak incidence has increased to individuals in their 50s. The incidence of LCIS decreases in women who are in their 60s to 80s. The age of peak incidence of LCIS may be related to the use of hormone replacement therapy (HRT). It is also possible that the use of HRT prevents the usual regression of LCIS normally seen at the time of menopause.

Signs and symptoms

LCIS is nonpalpable and has no consistent features on breast imaging. Most often, LCIS is found in association with a separate mammographic abnormality or palpable mass.

Risk of invasive cancer

Approximately 20% to 25% of women will develop invasive cancer within 15 years after the diagnosis of LCIS. More often, the invasive cancer is ductal in origin, and both breasts are at risk. At this point, there are no reliable molecular markers to determine which patients with LCIS will progress to invasive cancer.

Just as the incidence of LCIS has increased, there has also been an associated increase in the incidence of cases of infiltrating lobular carcinoma in postmenopausal women. The increase in invasive lobular carcinoma peaks in women in their 70s.

Pathology

LCIS appears to arise from the terminal duct-lobular apparatus, and the disease tends to be multifocal, multicentric, and bilateral. Subsequently, other types of LCIS have also been described. One of these, pleomorphic LCIS, tends to be associated with infiltrating lobular carcinoma, and its cytologic features are similar to those of intermediate- or high-grade DCIS. Pleomorphic LCIS may be more aggressive, and more likely to progress to invasion than is classic LCIS.

Treatment options

The management of LCIS is continuing to evolve, since the disease appears to be heterogeneous. Presently, treatment options include close follow-up, participation in a chemoprevention trial, use of tamoxifen, or bilateral prophylactic total mastectomy with or without reconstruction. At present, the decision for a given treatment will depend upon the patient's individual risk profile for DCIS or invasive breast cancer after careful counseling. In the future, treatment decisions may be based upon an analysis of a series of molecular markers, which can separate those patients with a low risk for invasion from those who are at high risk for disease progression.

DUCTAL CARCINOMA IN SITU

DCIS is being encountered more frequently with the expanded use of screening mammography. In 2010, an estimated 54,010 new cases of in situ breast cancer are expected to occur among women. Of these, approximately 85% will be DCIS. In some institutions, DCIS accounts for 25% to 50% of all breast cancers.

Epidemiology

DCIS, like invasive ductal carcinoma, occurs more frequently in women, although it accounts for approximately 5% of all male breast cancers. The average age at diagnosis of DCIS is 54 to 56 years, which is approximately a decade later than the age at presentation for LCIS.

Signs and symptoms

The clinical signs and symptoms of DCIS include a mass, breast pain, or bloody nipple discharge. On mammography, the disease most often appears as microcalcifications. Because these microcalcifications are nonpalpable and are not always associated with a mass, DCIS is often discovered with mammography alone. Approximately 5% of patients who present with pathologic nipple discharge will have underlying breast cancer, and many of them will have DCIS alone.

> A cohort of patients with DCIS (n = 321) and DCIS with microinvasion (n = 72) were identified after being treated with lumpectomy and radiation. Of 42 patients with DCIS with microinvasion who underwent axillary dissection, 1 (2.3%) had pathologic involvement; none of 58 patients with DCIS who underwent axillary resection had such involvement. The authors concluded that the natural history of DCIS with microinvasion resembles DCIS alone, and patients with this condition may not require axillary evaluation *(Parikh RR et al: ASTRO Breast Cancer Symposium [abstract S1083], September 5–7, 2008).*

Kuhl et al investigated the sensitivity of mammography versus MRI in detecting DCIS and compared the biological profiles of abnormalities detected by each method. Over a 5-year study period, 198 women had a pathologic diagnosis of pure DCIS without associated invasive breast cancer or microinvasion. In all, 167 of these women underwent both imaging tests preoperatively; 93 (56%) of these cases were diagnosed by mammography, and 153 (92%) were diagnosed by MRI ($P < .001$). The sensitivity of mammography decreased with nuclear grade; it was highest in patients with low-grade DCIS and lowest in cases of high-grade DCIS. The sensitivity of MRI was superior to that of mammography across all DCIS subtypes. In addition, sensitivity increased with nuclear grade of DCIS; it was lowest in low-grade cases (80%) and highest in high-grade cases (98%), independent of presence or absence of necrosis.

Risk of invasive cancer

The risk of developing an invasive carcinoma following a biopsy-proven diagnosis of DCIS is between 25% and 50%. Virtually all invasive cancers that follow DCIS are ductal and ipsilateral and generally present in the same quadrant within 10 years of the DCIS diagnosis. For these reasons, DCIS is considered a more ominous lesion than LCIS (which is considered a marker for risk) and appears to be a more direct precursor of invasive cancer.

Pathology

A variety of histologic patterns are seen with DCIS (eg, solid, cribriform, papillary). Some researchers have divided DCIS into two subgroups: comedo and noncomedo types. As compared with the noncomedo subtypes, the comedo variant has a higher proliferative rate, overexpression of *v-erb-b2* erythroblastic leukemia viral oncogene homolog 2, neuro/glioblastoma-derived oncogene homolog (avian; *ErbB2*), also known as human epidermal growth factor receptor 2 (HER2/*neu*), and a higher incidence of local recurrence and microinvasion. DCIS is less likely to be bilateral and has approximately a 30% incidence of multicentricity.

TREATMENT OF NONINVASIVE BREAST CARCINOMA

Ductal carcinoma in situ

Breast-conserving surgery

Breast-conserving surgery, followed by radiation therapy to the intact breast, is now considered the standard treatment of DCIS. Because the incidence of positive lymph nodes after axillary lymph node dissection for DCIS is ~1% to 2%, axillary dissection is not indicated in most instances.

The most important factor in determining local tumor control within the breast is margin status. A surgical margin of 1 mm has been associated with a 43% chance of having residual disease at the time of reexcision. When a surgical margin of 10 mm can be obtained, there is an extremely low rate of recurrence (4%). A 10-mm surgical margin may not be practical, however, when trying to provide a good cosmetic outcome. When breast-conserving therapy is used alone (without irradiation), a margin of at least 10 mm is required, and the tumor should be small (< 1 cm) and a noncomedo type. Although a wide margin is always desirable, narrower margins are acceptable for DCIS when radiation therapy is used after lumpectomy.

Sentinel node biopsy

The sentinel lymph node is the first node in the draining lymphatic basin that receives primary lymph flow. The technique of sampling the first draining lymph node was initially described in the management of patients with melanoma to determine who would benefit from regional lymph node dissection and was performed using a vital blue dye. This same technique has been used in patients with breast cancer, and sentinel lymph node biopsy represents a minimally invasive way to determine whether the axilla is involved with disease. The precise methods for identifying the sentinel lymph node (filtered vs unfiltered technetium-99m sulfur colloid and/or blue dye) and assessing the node (hematoxylin and eosin staining vs immunohistochemistry [IHC] vs polymerase chain reaction [PCR]) are being studied.

When blue dye is used, it can be injected into the breast parenchyma at the primary tumor or subareolar site. The radioactive tracer can be injected subdermally or intraparenchymally at the site of the primary tumor or in the subareolar location. The site and technique of injection will be based upon individual patient factors, including the type and location of the previous breast biopsy.

When lymphatic mapping and sentinel lymph node biopsy are performed, a blue vital dye and/or a radioactive tracer (generally technetium-labeled sulfur colloid) can be used. When a radiotracer is used, lymphoscintigraphy can also be performed to aid in locating the sentinel node. When a sentinel node biopsy is performed using blue dye, the axillary surgery should be performed carefully to avoid disrupting the blue-stained afferent lymphatic channels. When a radioisotope is used, a hand-held gamma counter is used to locate the sentinel node.

Axillary lymph node dissection is not routinely recommended for patients with DCIS. Recently, however, investigators have used sentinel lymph node biopsy to determine whether individuals with DCIS may harbor occult nodal metastases. Current studies have identified metastatic disease to the axillary nodes in up to 12% of patients who have undergone sentinel lymph node biopsy. Despite this relatively high percentage of positive sentinel nodes, recurrence in the nodal basins is rare (about 2%). Based on this and recent work, there is no indication for routine sentinel lymph node biopsy in patients with DCIS.

Factors associated with an increased risk of axillary metastasis with a diagnosis of DCIS are extensive DCIS requiring mastectomy, suspicion of microinvasion, DCIS associated with a palpable mass, and evidence of lymphovascular permeation or invasion seen on review of the slides. These factors likely are associated with a preoperatively nondiagnosed invasive component. However, for patients diagnosed with DCIS who are scheduled for mastectomy, sentinel lymph node sampling, prior to mastectomy, is a reasonable practice. In the event that an occult invasive cancer within the mastectomy is found, a negative sentinel node would be reassuring and perhaps would make it possible to avoid follow-up axillary dissection.

Patients whose sentinel node biopsy is negative do not require a complete node dissection, because the risk of an axillary recurrence is extremely low. Many institutions are using IHC in the evaluation of the sentinel node. When there is no evidence of metastatic disease by routine hematoxylin and eosin staining and the node is IHC-negative, the node is considered pN0(i–). When the routine staining is negative, isolated tumor cells are seen on IHC, alone and no tumor cluster is greater than 0.2 mm, the node is staged as pN0(i+). The majority of the data suggest that there is no effect on survival, the patient is considered node-negative, and a complete axillary node dissection is not warranted. Some authors suggest, however, that the presence of isolated tumor cells on sentinel node biopsy has been associated with the presence of additional disease within the remaining axillary nodes and a decreased survival when an axillary node dissection was not performed. Additional studies will be necessary to resolve this conflict. If the focus of metastatic disease is > 0.2 mm but < 2 mm, the node is staged as pN1mi. In this instance, consideration should be given to a complete axillary node dissection or the administration of axillary radiation. The likelihood that additional nodal disease will be identified in the axilla increases with the size of the primary tumor.

Axillary node dissection following sentinel node biopsy is discussed further in chapter 7, "Stage II breast cancer."

Adjuvant radiation therapy

Retrospective series have analyzed data on patients with DCIS, as well as subsets of patients with early invasive cancer, treated with conservative surgery alone, omitting radiation therapy to the intact breast. In addition, several prospective, randomized trials have attempted to address this issue of omission of breast irradiation for both invasive cancer and DCIS. It is clear from all of these series that omission of breast irradiation results in a significantly higher ipsilateral breast tumor recurrence rate but that it has not, as yet, had an impact on overall survival.

Two large, prospective, randomized trials have demonstrated a significant reduction in local relapse with the use of postlumpectomy irradiation in treatment of DCIS. In the NSABP B-17, the local recurrence rate at 8 years was reduced from 27% to 12% with postlumpectomy irradiation.

Goyal and others evaluated toxicity and cosmetic results in 1,440 patients ≥ 40 years of age with early-stage breast cancer who were given high-dose-rate brachytherapy using the MammoSite device as sole locoregional treatment. At 36-month follow-up, there was a 27% rate of seroma, a 9.5% rate of breast infection, and a 2.1% rate of fat necrosis. On multivariate analysis, only skin spacing and presence of a breast infection predicted for cosmetic outcomes. At 3 years, 93% of patients experienced a good/ excellent cosmetic outcome *(Goyal S et al: Ann Surg Oncol 16:2450–2458, 2009).*

Similar results have been reported by a European cooperative group study of 1,010 women with DCIS randomly assigned to receive either 50 Gy of radiotherapy to the whole breast over 5 weeks or no further treatment. With a median follow-up of 4.25 years, the 4-year local relapse-free rate was 91% in the radiotherapy arm versus 84% in the observation arm. Hazard ratios (HRs) with postexcision radiotherapy were 0.62 for all local relapses, 0.65 for DCIS recurrences, and 0.60 for noninvasive recurrences.

Both trials showed that radiotherapy reduces the risk of both noninvasive and invasive recurrences. Identification of a subgroup of patients who did not benefit from post-lumpectomy irradiation has not as yet been clearly defined.

The VNPI, based on tumor size, grade, presence of necrosis, and width of the excision margin, is an algorithm commonly used to predict local recurrence after breast-conserving surgery for DCIS. In some series, VNPI lacked discriminatory power for guiding further patient management. In studies performed by this group, the width of the excision margin apparently was the most important predictor of local recurrence after breast-conserving surgery for DCIS.

One study demonstrated acceptable local control in patients with DCIS treated by excision alone, provided that wide negative margins were obtained. In this retrospective series of 469 patients, radiation therapy did not lower the local recurrence rate in patients with wide (≥ 10 mm) negative margins but did produce a significant benefit in patients with close (≤ 1 mm) margins. The authors concluded that radiation therapy is unlikely to benefit patients with wide negative margins and small tumors. However, adjuvant radiotherapy was omitted in a single-arm, prospective study of patients with grade 1 or 2 DCIS having a mammographic extent < 2.5 cm and treated with wide excision with final margins ≥ 1 cm. This trial was closed early, because the number of local recurrences met the predetermined stopping rules. The 5-year rate of ipsilateral breast tumor recurrence was 12%. Thus, the benefit of radiotherapy is still seen in traditionally low-risk patients.

Although there may be some patients for whom wide excision alone is appropriate therapy, no specific subgroup has been identified consistently in the available literature. Clearly, the omission of radiation therapy in subsets of patients remains a controversial issue worthy of further investigation. It is hoped that ongoing randomized studies will help to resolve some of the conflicts generated by selective, retrospective studies.

Two trials have addressed the need for postlumpectomy radiation therapy in older women with breast cancer. Both studies randomized patients, following lumpectomy and adjuvant hormonal therapy, to receive radiotherapy or observation. Both studies confirmed statistically significant improvements in local control with radiation therapy, and local relapse rates were acceptable in carefully selected patients. The authors concluded that selected elderly patients may be treated with hormonal therapy alone (without radiotherapy) following breast-conserving therapy.

Hughes et al published a prospective, nonrandomized study on behalf of the Eastern Cooperative Oncology Group (E5194) which tried to determine the risk of ipsilateral breast events in patients with ductal carcinoma in situ (DCIS) treated with local excision without irradiation. Patients with either low- or intermediate-grade DCIS measuring 2.5 cm or smaller, or high-grade DCIS measuring 1 cm or smaller who had microscopic margin widths of 3 mm or wider and no residual calcifications on postoperative mammograms were eligible. With a median follow-up of 6.2 years, the 5-year rate of ipsilateral breast events in the 565 eligible patients in the low/intermediate grade stratum was 6.1% (95% CI, 4.1% to 8.2%). With a median follow-up of 6.7 years, this incidence for the 105 eligible patients in the high-grade stratum was 15.3% *(Hughes L et al: J Clin Oncol 27: 5319–5324, 2009).*

Adjuvant trastuzumab therapy

Overexpression of *HER2/neu/ErbB2* is seen in more than 50% of cases of DCIS. It has been associated with high-risk disease (young age, estrogen receptor–negative status, high nuclear grade). The NSABP has opened a clinical trial in which patients with DCIS who are ErbB2-positive will undergo a wide excision with negative surgical margins. Patients will be stratified for menopausal status, need for hormone therapy, and nuclear grade. They will then be randomized to receive whole breast irradiation alone versus whole breast irradiation and two doses of trastuzumab (Herceptin) at weeks 1 and 4. Patients who are estrogen- and/or progesterone-positive should receive 5 years of hormone therapy. The goal of the study is to determine whether the addition of trastuzumab can prevent an ipsilateral breast tumor recurrence.

Adjuvant tamoxifen therapy

Adjuvant chemotherapy is not routinely employed for patients with DCIS. In NSABP B-24, 1,804 women with DCIS treated with lumpectomy and irradiation were randomly assigned to receive placebo or tamoxifen. At a median follow-up of 74 months, women in the tamoxifen group had fewer breast cancer events than did those in the placebo group (8.2% vs 13.4%; $P = .0009$). Tamoxifen decreased the incidence of both ipsilateral and contralateral events. The risk of ipsilateral invasive cancers was reduced by tamoxifen, regardless of the presence or absence of comedonecrosis or margin involvement.

In a more recent analysis of NSABP B-24, the benefit from tamoxifen was derived exclusively from patients with hormone receptor–positive disease. The pros and cons of tamoxifen should be discussed for the prevention of secondary breast cancers in women at high risk for breast cancer, such as women diagnosed with DCIS.

Wapnir et al analyzed data from 2,615 women with primary DCIS who participated in the NSABP B-17 and B-24 trials for ipsilateral breast tumor recurrence; patients were followed for a median of > 12 years. Ipsilateral breast tumor recurrence was a first failure in 465 patients (243 invasive, 222 noninvasive). The 12-year cumulative incidence of all such recurrences was 32.9% for lumpectomy only, 15.8% for lumpectomy with whole-breast irradiation, and 12.5% for lumpectomy with whole-breast irradiation plus tamoxifen. Radiotherapy significantly reduced invasive ipsilateral breast tumor recurrence. Tamoxifen conferred additional benefit on reducing invasive recurrences of this type. Women with invasive ipisilateral breast tumor recurrences had a twofold greater mortality risk relative to those who did not; the effect was greater for patients who underwent lumpectomy followed by whole-breast radiotherapy than for those who underwent only lumpectomy. Overall mortality was low and primarily due to development of ipsilateral breast tumor recurrence. The investigators concluded that occurrence of an invasive ipsilateral breast tumor recurrence after DCIS, and particularly after radiotherapy, confers increased risk for subsequent mortality, as seen after an invasive index tumor.

For nearly two decades there has been controversy as to the role of radiation therapy in women over the age of 70 years with small breast cancers. The CALGB 9343 trial enrolled women over age 70 with clinically node-negative disease, who had undergone lumpectomy with a clear margin (1-cm negative margin), had a tumor size of 2 cm or less, and were ER-positive or of indeterminate status. These women were randomized to either tamoxifen or tamoxifen plus radiation. The 631 eligible patients were followed for a median of 12 years.

Radiation therapy was found to have an impact on breast tumor recurrence, with six events occurring in the 317 women who received tamoxifen plus radiation, compared with 27 events that occurred in 319 women (2% vs 9%, $P < .0001$). However, there were no benefits in terms of ultimate mastectomy (2% with radiation vs 4% without, $P = .1779$), axillary recurrence (0% with vs 3% without radiation), the frequency of second primary cancers (12% vs 9%, $P = .7268$), or overall survival at 10 years (33% of patients in each treatment arm had died at 10 years, $P = .845$). To date, approximately 50% of the women are still alive, 3% have died from breast cancer, and 46% have died due to other causes. It is notable that approximately 50% of women who were over 70 years of age upon enrollment in this study are still alive 12 years later. The investigators concluded that in older women the benefits of radiation after lumpectomy are small and that omitting radiation in women over 70 years of age with clinical stage I breast cancer is a reasonable alternative.

STAGE I BREAST CANCER

Stage I breast cancer ranges from microinvasive tumors (≤ 0.1 cm) to tumors ≤ 2 cm without evidence of spread to the regional lymph nodes or with only limited nodal involvement (N1mi).

PATHOLOGY OF INVASIVE BREAST CANCER

Ductal carcinoma

Most cases of invasive carcinomas of the breast are ductal in origin. Of the different histologic subtypes of ductal carcinoma that have been described, tubular, medullary, mucinous (colloid), and papillary subtypes have been associated with a favorable outcome.

Lobular carcinoma

Approximately 5% to 10% of invasive breast cancers are lobular in origin. This histology has been associated with synchronous and metachronous contralateral primary tumors in as many as 30% of cases.

TREATMENT

Surgical and radiation treatments

Multiple studies have demonstrated that patients with stage I breast cancer who are treated with either breast-conserving therapy (lumpectomy and radiation therapy) or modified radical mastectomy have similar disease-free and overall survival rates.

Breast-conserving therapy

Extent of local surgery The optimal extent of local surgery has yet to be determined and, in the literature, has ranged from excisional biopsy to quadrantectomy. A consensus statement on breast-conserving therapy issued by the NCI recommended that the breast cancer be completely excised with negative surgical margins.

The extent of axillary surgery also continues to evolve. In recent years, patients with early-stage breast cancer who have clinically node-negative disease have the option to undergo sentinel lymph node biopsy rather than axillary node dissection. The present standard of care for patients with a positive sentinel node is complete nodal dissection. A study is under way to determine whether patients with a positive sentinel node require further axillary surgery.

Patient selection Specific guidelines must be followed when selecting patients for breast conservation. Patients may be considered unacceptable candidates for conservative surgery and radiation therapy either because the risk of breast recurrence following the conservative approach is significant enough to warrant mastectomy or the likelihood of an unacceptable cosmetic result is high. Some patients who are candidates for breast conservation can undergo breast MRI to identify sites of additional disease within the breast that may preclude breast-conserving treatment, although this is not a standard for evaluation. Contraindications to breast-conserving surgery are listed in Table 1.

TABLE 1: Contraindications to breast conservation

Absolute contraindications	Relative contraindications
Multicentric disease[a]	Tumor size vs breast size
Diffuse malignant microcalcifications	Tumor location
Pregnancy	Collagen vascular disease (excluding rheumatoid arthritis)
Persistently positive surgical margins	
Previous breast or mantle irradiation	

[a] If a satisfactory cosmetic outcome is anticipated, multicentric disease is considered to be a relative contraindication.

Risk factors for ipsilateral recurrence For patients undergoing conservative surgery followed by radiation therapy to the intact breast, the risk of ipsilateral breast tumor recurrence has been reported to range from 0.5% to 2.0% per year, with long-term failure rates varying from 7% to 20%. Risk factors for ipsilateral breast tumor recurrence include, but are not limited to, young age (< 35 to 40 years), an extensive intraductal component, major lymphocytic stromal reaction, peritumoral invasion, presence of tumor necrosis, and positive resection margins. After a wide excision has been performed, the specimen should be oriented and inked; the pathologist may then ink each margin a different color. If a positive surgical margin is present, the color-coded system will guide the reexcision to obtain negative surgical margins with the removal of the least amount of breast tissue possible.

Earlier studies demonstrated that an extensive intraductal component was a risk factor for local relapse. However, in subsequent reports, when negative surgical margins were achieved, patients with an extensive intraductal component could be safely treated with breast conservation. Although it is desirable to achieve negative surgical margins, the available data do not preclude the use of conservative treatment, provided that adequate radiation doses (> 6,000 cGy) to the tumor bed are employed. The role of the remaining risk factors previously cited in predicting recurrence is unclear, and patients should not be denied breast conservation because of their presence.

Cosmetic considerations include primary tumor size and location, overall breast size, total body weight, and a history of preexisting collagen vascular disease.

Tumor size and breast size are important in determining whether the patient will have an acceptable cosmetic outcome after surgical resection. Patients with large tumors with respect to breast size may consider neoadjuvant chemotherapy to reduce the size of the primary tumor and allow breast preservation. (See chapter 8 for discussion of neoadjuvant chemotherapy.)

Obese women with large, pendulous breasts may experience marked fibrosis and retraction of the irradiated breast, making a good to excellent cosmetic outcome less likely. Techniques of brachytherapy may prove beneficial for these women. Such women also could undergo bilateral reduction mammoplasty after the wide excision of the primary tumor site has been completed. The partial mastectomy specimen should be evaluated by the pathologist to ensure adequate resection margins. Radiopaque clips can be left to mark and identify the primary tumor site for the radiation oncologist. The follow-up mammograms will be more difficult to interpret due to scarring and radiotherapy effect.

Patients with collagen vascular disease may develop more severe reactions following radiation therapy. Although initial anecdotal reports demonstrated higher complication rates in patients with collagen vascular disease, a case-controlled study of patients with early-stage breast cancer showed higher complication rates only in those patients with scleroderma. Other case-controlled studies have also failed to demonstrate significantly higher complication rates in patients with collagen vascular disease undergoing radiation therapy. It appears that most patients without active significant collagen vascular diseases may be candidates for breast-conserving surgery and irradiation, although this approach remains controversial.

In some instances, it is necessary to excise skin to obtain a negative surgical margin. This does not necessarily preclude the patient from undergoing breast-conserving therapy and does not mean the patient should have a poor cosmetic outcome. When skin must be removed to obtain a negative surgical margin, complex skin closures, such as V-Y advancement flaps or Z-plasties, can be utilized to enhance cosmesis.

Patients with centrally located tumors Traditionally, patients who have centrally located tumors requiring excision of the nipple-areolar complex have not been offered the option of breast conservation. However, the cosmetic result achieved after local tumor excision that includes the nipple-areolar complex may not differ significantly from that obtained following mastectomy and reconstruction.

Furthermore, conservatively treated patients with subareolar lesions do not necessarily need to have the nipple-areolar complex sacrificed, as long as negative surgical margins can be achieved. However, if the complex is not removed, the remaining breast tissue and overlying skin remain sensate. Recent studies also indicate that the incidence of local recurrence is not increased when primary tumors in this location are treated conservatively.

Genetically predisposed breast cancer patients For women harboring germline mutations in *BRCA1* or *BRCA2*, there are limited data regarding long-term outcome. To date, studies have shown acceptable local control rates in the short term and increased but acceptable rates of acute, subacute, and chronic normal tissue reactions with lumpectomy followed by radiation therapy. Women with germline *BRCA1* and *BRCA2* mutations, however, are at high risk for second primary tumors in the contralateral breast.

A study from Yale University demonstrated high rates of second primary tumors in the ipsilateral breast. This study suggested that if breast-conserving therapy is chosen, some prophylactic measures, such as selective estrogen receptor modulators or oophorectomy, might be considered to reduce the risk of second primary tumors in the ipsilateral or contralateral breast. Other studies also indicated a trend toward higher rates of late local relapses in *BRCA* carriers. Further studies are clearly warranted to assess the long-term risks and benefits of breast-conserving strategies in women harboring mutations in *BRCA1* and *BRCA2*.

Role of axillary lymph node dissection The role of axillary lymph node dissection in the management of breast cancer has been questioned, particularly when a patient with a clinically negative axilla is undergoing breast-conserving therapy. In most instances, the breast surgery is performed with the patient under local anesthesia and sedation on an outpatient basis. When axillary lymph node dissection is added, the surgery is performed with the patient under general anesthesia.

It has also been suggested that if the status of the nodes will not alter therapy, the dissection is unnecessary, and the axilla can be treated with irradiation. On the other hand, if axillary lymph node staging is not performed, the patient will not be accurately staged, and important prognostic information will be unavailable.

Patients who may not be candidates for sentinel node biopsy are women who are pregnant or breast-feeding or who have had prior irradiation. A prior excisional biopsy does not preclude the use of lymphatic mapping and sentinel node biopsy. It has been suggested that sentinel node biopsy accurately evaluates the axilla, even in patients with tumors > 5 cm and in those who have been treated with neoadjuvant chemotherapy.

Once the sentinel node(s) have been identified, they can be sent to pathology for frozen section or touch-prep analysis.

Sensitivity and specificity In breast cancer, lymphatic mapping has been performed using a vital blue dye and/or lymphoscintigraphy. The success rate for identifying the sentinel node may be increased when these techniques are used in combination. The ability to identify the sentinel node can reach as high as 97% when blue dye and technetium-99m sulfur colloid are used together. When blue dye is used alone, the success rate is 83%, and when technetium-99m sulfur colloid is used alone, the success rate is 94%.

Results from a multi-institution practice have demonstrated that sentinel lymph node biopsy using dual-agent injection provides optimal sensitivity. In the study, 806 patients were enrolled by 99 surgeons for sentinel lymph node biopsy by single-agent (blue dye alone or radioactive colloid alone) or dual-agent injection at the discretion of the surgeons. All patients underwent complete level I/II dissection following the sentinel procedure. There were no significant differences in the identification of a sentinel node among patients who underwent single- compared with dual-agent injection. However, the false-negative rate was 11.8% for single-agent versus 5.8% for dual-agent injections ($P = .05$).

A series of 793 invasive breast cancer patients treated with lumpectomy and radiation therapy were stratified based on receptor status: patients in the luminal A group were estrogen receptor– or progesterone receptor–positive and ErbB2-negative; those in the luminal B group were estrogen receptor–, progesterone receptor–, and ErbB2-positive; those in the ErbB2 group were estrogen receptor– and progesterone receptor–negative and ErbB2-positive; and the basal group was estrogen receptor–, progesterone receptor–, and ErbB2-negative. Over a median follow-up of 70 months, the 5-year rate of ipsilateral breast tumor recurrence was 1.8% for the luminal A group, 1.5% for the luminal B group, 8.4% for ErbB2 group, and 7.5% for basal subtypes. These results may be useful in counseling patients about their outcomes after breast-conserving therapy *(Nguyen PL et al: J Clin Oncol 26:2373–2378, 2008).*

The sensitivity and specificity of sentinel lymph node biopsy are high, and the likelihood of a false-negative result is extremely low. False-negative rates vary among series, ranging from 0% to 11%. In one series, in 18% of the cases for which the frozen-section evaluation of the node was negative, the final pathologic evaluation revealed metastatic disease, and the patient ultimately required lymph node dissection. This potential result can be distressing to patients; however, they should be informed of this possibility at the time of the procedure.

Patients whose sentinel node biopsy is normal do not require a complete node dissection, because the risk of an axillary recurrence is extremely low. Many institutions are using IHC to evaluate the sentinel node. When there is no evidence of metastatic disease by routine hematoxylin and eosin staining and the node is IHC–, the node is considered pN0 (i–). When there are isolated tumor cells seen but no cluster is greater than 0.2 mm, the node is staged as pN0 (i+), and the patient does not require a complete node dissection. If the focus of metastatic disease in the node is > 0.2 mm but < 2 mm, the node is staged as pN1mi. In this instance, consideration should be given to performing a complete axillary node dissection or administering axillary radiation therapy, unless the patient is participating in a clinical trial. The likelihood that nonsentinel lymph nodes will also contain metastatic disease increases as the size of the primary tumor increases.

Radiation therapy after breast-conserving surgery

Based on the results of a number of retrospective single-institution experiences, as well as several prospective randomized clinical trials, breast-conserving surgery followed by radiation therapy to the intact breast is now considered a standard treatment for the majority of patients with stage I or II invasive breast cancer. A meta-analysis demonstrated a substantially reduced local relapse rate and a small but statistically significant decrease in breast cancer mortality with use of radiation following breast-conserving surgery.

Radiation dose and protocol Radiation therapy after breast-conserving surgery should employ careful treatment planning techniques that minimize treatment of the underlying heart and lungs. To achieve the optimal cosmetic result, efforts should be made to obtain a homogeneous dose distribution throughout the breast. Doses of 180 to 200 cGy/d to the intact breast, to a total dose of 4,500 to 5,000 cGy, are considered standard.

Additional irradiation to the tumor bed is often administered. Although the necessity of a boost to the tumor bed has been questioned, at least two randomized clinical trials have demonstrated a small but statistically significant reduction in ipsilateral breast tumor relapses with the use of a radiation boost to the tumor bed following whole-breast irradiation of 50 Gy. In one of these trials, involving more than 5,000 women randomized to receive either a 16-Gy boost to the tumor bed or not, a 4% absolute reduction in local relapse was seen with the use of the radiation boost (6.2% vs 10.2% at 10 years). This effect was particularly evident in patients younger than age 50. The boost is directed at the original tumor bed with either electron-beam irradiation or an interstitial implant, to bring the total dose to 50 to 66 Gy.

Regional nodal irradiation For patients who undergo axillary dissection and are found to have negative nodes, regional nodal irradiation is no longer routinely employed. For patients with positive nodes, radiation therapy to the supraclavicular fossa and/or internal mammary chain may be considered on an individualized basis (see chapter 7).

Whelan et al updated the 15-year Canadian experience with hypofractioned whole-breast radiotherapy. Women with invasive breast cancer who had undergone breast conserving surgery were randomized to receive whole-breast irradiation either at a standard dose of 50.0 Gy in 25 fractions (the control group) or at a dose of 42.5 Gy in 16 fractions. The risk of local recurrence at 10 years was 6.7% among the 612 women assigned to standard irradiation as compared with 6.2% among the 622 women assigned to the hypofractioned regimen. They concluded that 10 years after treatment, accelerated hypofractionated whole-breast irradiation was not inferior to standard radiation treatment (*Whelan TJ et al: N Engl J Med 362:513–520, 2010*).

A novel phase I trial investigating concurrent chemotherapy with APBI enrolled 27 patients with T1–2, N0–1 breast cancer to APBI (40.5 Gy in 15 fractions) concurrent with dose-dense AC (60 mg/m² of doxorubicin IV and 600 mg/m² of cyclophosphamide IV every 14 days with growth factor support). The authors reported that concurrent chemoradiotherapy was feasible with no skin toxicity of grade 2 or greater *(Zellars RC et al: J Clin Oncol 27: 2816–2822, 2009).*

Accelerated whole breast irradiation In contrast to conventional assumptions, the fractionation sensitivity for breast tumors may be much lower than expected; this allows for increasing the daily dose of radiation and shortening the overall treatment time. Based on this information, the Royal Marsden Hospital and the Gloucestershire Oncology Centre collaborated in a randomized clinical trial to evaluate the relative toxicity and efficacy of different whole-breast fractionation schemes. A total of 1,410 women were randomized to one of three arms: 50 Gy in 25 fractions over 5 weeks; 39 Gy in 13 fractions (3.0 Gy/fx) over 5 weeks; 42.9 Gy in 13 fractions (3.3 Gy/fx) over 5 weeks. The primary and secondary endpoints were late breast changes and local control. The 39 Gy arm was less likely to develop late radiation change compared to both 42.9 Gy and 50 Gy, but also had worse local control than the 42.9 Gy arm. Interestingly, the 42.9 Gy arm was not significantly different from the 50 Gy arm for both development of any late radiation change and local control. The Canadian NCI randomized 1,234 patients (1993–1996) with T1 and T2 tumors with negative margins and pathologically negative nodes (on level 1 and 2 dissection) to: 50 Gy in 25 fractions (2 Gy/fx) over 35 days or 42.5 Gy in 16 fractions (2.66 Gy/fx) over 22 days. With a median follow-up of 69 months, local recurrence-free survival (LFS) was equal (97.2% vs 96.8%), and there was no difference in OS and DFS. Cosmesis was identical with excellent or good scores at 3 and 5 years in 77% of patients in both groups. Toxicities were also comparable. A major limitation of the Canadian study is the lack of a lumpectomy boost, which significantly improves local control. The patients eligible for the study had low risk for disease recurrence, limiting the general scope of the results.

Accelerated partial breast irradiation There have been several reports demonstrating promising results with the use of partial breast irradiation, a potentially more convenient option for patients than the extended course of postoperative radiotherapy.

Additional options are now available to shorten the radiotherapy treatment time to 1 to 5 days (accelerated) and to focus an increased dose of radiation on just the breast tissue around the excision cavity (partial breast). Current accelerated partial breast irradiation (APBI) approaches include interstitial brachytherapy, intracavitary (balloon) brachytherapy, and accelerated external beam (three-dimensional conformal) radiotherapy. Intraoperative radiotherapy is even shorter, with the entire treatment given as a single dose delivered immediately after surgery. Each approach has benefits and limitations.

Ongoing randomized trials will shape how APBI is utilized in routine clinical practice. Some of the more important outcomes from these trials will be local toxicity, local and regional recurrence, and overall survival. If APBI is ultimately demonstrated to be as safe and effective as whole-breast radiotherapy, breast conservation may become an even more appealing choice, and the overall impact of treatment may be further reduced for certain women with newly diagnosed breast cancer.

Mastectomy options

There are data accruing in the literature to suggest that nipple-sparing mastectomy is oncologically safe and can be utilized in select cases of skin-sparing mastectomy. This surgical procedure can be considered in patients who will be undergoing mastectomy and will be undergoing immediate reconstruction. During the course of the surgery, the retroareolar tissue is removed and sent for frozen section analysis. If the tissue sent for frozen section is negative, the nipple-areolar complex (NAC) can be spared. If the final pathology is positive, the NAC can be removed at a subsequent surgery. Factors associated with tumor extension to the NAC are subareolar tumor location, multicentricity, tumor size, and nodal positivity. The rate of complications may be higher with this technique due to partial loss of the NAC caused by impaired blood supply.

Medical treatment

Medical management of local disease depends on clinical and pathologic staging. Systemic therapy is indicated only for invasive (infiltrating) breast cancers.

In the past, systemic therapy was not offered to patients with stage I disease (tumors up to 2.0 cm). However, adjuvant chemotherapy and hormonal therapy have been shown to improve disease-free and overall survival in selected patients with node-negative disease.

The sequence of systemic therapy and radiation therapy for patients treated with breast-conserving therapy has been the subject of considerable debate. Although concurrent CMF (cyclophosphamide, methotrexate, fluorouracil [5-FU]) and radiation therapy have been used with acceptable toxicity, the concurrent use of chemoradiation therapy has fallen out of favor due to reports of enhanced toxicities. Delaying chemotherapy for 6 to 8 weeks of radiation therapy does not appear to negatively impact systemic disease or survival. Recent studies do not demonstrate a compromise in local control if radiation is delayed until chemotherapy is complete. Currently, the majority of patients receiving chemotherapy and radiation therapy are treated with chemotherapy prior to radiation therapy.

For patients receiving tamoxifen or other hormonal agents, there had been considerable controversy regarding whether the hormonal agents should be administered during or after radiation therapy. Theoretically, tamoxifen may place cells in a resting state, making them less radiosensitive. Three retrospective studies, conducted independently but published together, reached a similar conclusion: The timing of therapy had no impact on local relapse rates. Additionally, no significant difference was found in time to any event, metastasis, or death whether subsequent therapy was radiotherapy first or chemotherapy first among patients with breast conservation.

Treatment regimens

Multiagent therapy with CMF, CMFP (CMF and prednisone), MFL (sequential methotrexate and 5-FU), AC (Adriamycin [doxorubicin] and cyclophosphamide),

TABLE 2: Adjuvant chemotherapy regimens for node-negative breast cancer

Regimen	Dose and frequency
MF	
Methotrexate	100 mg/m^2 IV on days 1 and 8
Fluorouracil (5-FU)	600 mg/m^2 IV on days 1 and 8 (1 h after methotrexate)
Folinic acid	10 mg/m^2 PO q6h × 6 doses (24 h after methotrexate)
Repeat every 4 weeks for 12 cycles.	
CMF	
(Bonadonna regimen [classical])	
Cyclophosphamide	100 mg/m^2 PO on days 1–14
Methotrexate	40 mg/m^2 IV on days 1 and 8
5-FU	600 mg/m^2 IV on days 1 and 8
Repeat every 28 days for 6 cycles	
(Bonadonna regimen [modified])	
Cyclophosphamide	600 mg/m^2 IV on day 1
Methotrexate	40 mg/m^2 IV on day 1
5-FU	600 mg/m^2 IV on day 1 and 8
Repeat every 3 weeks for 9 cycles.	
CMFP	
Cyclophosphamide	100 mg/m^2 PO on days 1–14
Methotrexate	40 mg/m^2 IV on days 1 and 8
5-FU	600 mg/m^2 IV on days 1 and 8
Prednisone	40 mg/m^2 PO on days 1 and 14
Repeat every 4 weeks for 6 cycles.	
FAC	
5-FU	500 mg/m^2 IV on days 1 and 4 or 8
Adriamycin (doxorubicin)	50 mg/m^2 IV by continuous 72-h infusion on days 1–3 (or 50 mg/m^2 on day 1)
Cyclophosphamide	500 mg/m^2 IV on day 1
Repeat at 21-day intervals if hematologic recovery occurs for 6 cycles.	
CAF	
Cyclophosphamide	600 mg/m^2 IV on day 1
Adriamycin (doxorubicin)	60 mg/m^2 IV on day 1
5-FU	600 mg/m^2 IV on day 1
Repeat every 21-28 days.	
FEC	
5-FU	500 mg/m^2 IV on day 1
Epirubicin	100 mg/m^2 IV on day 1
Cyclophosphamide	500 mg/m^2 IV on day 1
Repeat every 21 days.	
AC	
Adriamycin (doxorubicin)	60 mg/m^2 IV on day 1
Cyclophosphamide	600 mg/m^2 IV on day 1
Repeat every 21-28 days depending on hematologic recovery for 4 cycles.	
TC	
Docetaxel (Taxotere)	75 mg/m^2 IV on day 1
Cyclophosphamide	600 mg/m^2 IV over 30–60 min on day 1
Repeat every 21 days for 4 cycles.	

IMPORTANT: For patients aged 60 years and older, in the Bonnadonna regimen methotrexate is given at the lower dose of 30 mg/m^2 and the 5-FU dose is reduced to 400 mg/m^2.

and taxanes (paclitaxel, docetaxel [Taxotere]) has been used in patients with node-negative disease (Table 2). Hormonal therapy with tamoxifen (20 mg PO every day for 5 years) has been shown to be of value in both pre- and postmenopausal women with hormone receptor–positive breast cancer. (See chapter 7 for further discussion about tamoxifen and the ATAC trial, as well as for adjuvant chemotherapy regimens for node-positive breast cancer.)

Node-negative tumors < 1.0 cm Patients who have the lowest risk of recurrence are least likely to benefit from systemic treatment when the risks of treatment are considered. None of the reported trials in node-negative breast cancer included women with tumors < 1.0 cm, and, because of the low risk of recurrence (≤ 10%) in this group, systemic adjuvant therapy is not used routinely. Recent results from the NSABP in this group of patients are provocative in suggesting a potential benefit from systemic therapy.

In the Oncotype Dx validation study, the likelihood of distant recurrence in tamoxifen-treated patients with node-negative, estrogen receptor–positive breast cancer was tested using a reverse transcriptase (RT)-PCR assay of 21 prospectively selected genes (16 cancer-related genes and 5 reference genes) in paraffin-embedded tumor tissue. The levels of expression of the 21 genes were used in a prospectively defined algorithm to calculate a recurrence score and to determine a risk group for each patient.

The proportions of patients categorized as having a low, intermediate, or high risk by the RT-PCR assay were 51%, 22%, and 27%, respectively. The Kaplan-Meier estimates of the rates of distant recurrence at 10 years in the low-, intermediate-, and high-risk groups were 6.8%, 14.3%, and 30.5%, respectively. The rate in the low-risk group was significantly lower than that in the high-risk group ($P < .001$). In a multivariate Cox model, the recurrence score provided significant predictive power that was independent of age and tumor size ($P < .001$). The recurrence score was also predictive of overall survival ($P < .001$) and could be used as a continuous function to predict distant recurrence in individual patients.

The Oncotype Dx test has changed the treatment of breast cancer. It has shown that patients with low recurrence scores do not derive benefit from chemotherapy in addition to hormonal therapy, and therefore chemotherapy is omitted from their systemic therapy. Likewise, it showed patients with high risk-recurrence scores derive the most benefit from chemotherapy in addition to hormonal therapy, and therefore these patients are treated with chemotherapy followed by endocrine therapy. At this time, it is unclear whether patients with intermediate risk-recurrence scores benefit from chemotherapy in addition to endocrine therapy, but a large national trial is ongoing to answer this question.

It is important that the patient receive radiation therapy in a timely manner, however; irradiation should *not* be delayed for 3 to 4 months while Oncotype Dx test results are awaited.

Node-negative tumors ≥ 1.0 cm The selection of a specific treatment program and the characteristics that predict risk of recurrence and death in women with node-negative breast cancer require further delineation and clarification in clinical trials. At present, women with tumors ≥ 1.0 cm who have poor histologic or nuclear differentiation, negative estrogen receptors, a high-risk Oncotype Dx recurrence score, a high S-phase percentage, or a high Ki-67 level can be considered appropriate candidates for adjuvant systemic therapy.

An update of the NSABP B-20 trial indicated a significant advantage in the estrogen receptor–positive, node-negative population when chemotherapy with CMF or sequential MF is added to tamoxifen in the adjuvant setting. Patients receiving CMF plus tamoxifen appeared to derive the greatest benefit. Benefits with respect to both disease-free and overall survival have been reported for patients given chemotherapy and tamoxifen.

Chemotherapy and ovarian function suppression are both effective adjuvant therapies for patients with early-stage breast cancer. The efficacy of their sequential combination was investigated by the IBCSG Trial VIII. This study randomized more than 1,000 pre- and perimenopausal women with lymph node-negative breast cancer to receive either goserelin (Zoladex) for 24 months (n = 346), 6 courses of "classic" CMF chemotherapy (n = 360), or 6 courses of classic CMF followed by 18 months of goserelin (CMF then goserelin; n = 357). The primary outcome was disease-free survival.

In this study, patients with estrogen receptor-negative tumors achieved better 5-year disease-free survival rates if they received CMF (84% and 88% for CMF and CMF then goserelin, respectively) than if they received goserelin alone (73%). However, for patients with estrogen receptor-positive disease, chemotherapy alone and goserelin alone provided similar outcomes (81% 5-year disease-free survival rates for both treatment groups), whereas sequential therapy provided a statistically nonsignificant improvement compared with either modality alone.

Kwan et al assessed the association of alcohol consumption on breast cancer prognosis in the Life After Cancer Epidemiology (LACE) study. A total of 1,897 study participants were included in the study; all met the following criteria: 1) they were between 18 and 70 years of age; 2) they had a diagnosis of early-stage primary breast cancer and had completed their breast cancer treatment except for adjuvant hormonal therapy; and 3) they were free of recurrence and had no history of other cancers in the 5 years prior to enrollment. Alcohol consumption was assessed on average 2 years after breast cancer diagnosis. Fifty-one percent of the participants were considered drinkers (> 0.5 g/d of alcohol), and the majority drank wine (89%). With a median follow-up of 7.4 years, participants who consumed ≥ 6.0 grams of alcohol per day were found to have an increased risk of breast cancer recurrence (hazard ratio [HR], 1.35; 95% CI, 1.00–1.83) and risk of death from breast cancer (HR, 1.51; 95% CI, 1.00–2.29) as compared to nondrinkers. Furthermore, the increased risk of recurrence appeared to be greater among postmenopausal (HR, 1.51; 95% CI, 1.05–2.19) and overweight and obese women (HR, 1.60; 95% CI, 1.08–2.38). However, there was no association found with all-cause death and there appeared to be a reduction in risk of non–breast cancer death. The investigators concluded that regular alcohol consumption of four or more alcoholic drinks per week after a breast cancer diagnosis may increase the risk of breast cancer recurrence as well as death from breast cancer among women previously diagnosed with early-stage breast cancer, especially among postmenopausal overweight/obese women, but has no apparent impact on overall risk of death. In addition, cardioprotective effects on non–breast cancer death were suggested *(Kwan ML et al: J Clin Oncol Aug 30, 2010 [Epub ahead of print])*.

FOLLOW-UP OF LONG-TERM SURVIVORS

There is no consensus among oncologists as to the optimal follow-up routine for long-term breast cancer survivors. Based on guidelines from the NCCN, patients with stage 0 breast cancer should undergo a medical history and physical examination every 6 months for 5 years and then annually thereafter; mammography should be performed every year. Patients with stage I breast cancer should undergo a medical history and physical examination every 4 to 6 months for 5 years and then annually thereafter. In stage I patients, mammography should be performed every 6 months in the ipsilateral breast after radiation therapy following breast-conserving surgery. Thereafter, it can be done annually. If mastectomy was performed, mammography should be performed annually in the contralateral breast. Women receiving tamoxifen should undergo pelvic examination every 12 months if the uterus is present. All other follow-up evaluations are dictated by the development of symptoms.

LIFESTYLE MODIFICATIONS

The Women's Intervention Nutrition Study tested the effect of a dietary intervention in women with resected, early-stage breast cancer receiving conventional cancer management. Interim results showed that reduced dietary fat intake, with modest influence on body weight, may improve relapse-free survival. In all, 2,437 women were randomly assigned to a dietary intervention (n = 975) or a control (n = 1,462) group. After a median follow-up of 60 months, dietary fat intake was lower in the intervention group than in the control group (fat grams/day at 12 months, 33.3 vs 51.3, respectively), corresponding to a statistically significant ($P = .005$), 6-pound-lower mean body weight in the intervention group. A total of 277 relapse events (local, regional, distant, or ipsilateral breast cancer recurrence or new contralateral breast cancer) have been reported in the dietary group (9.8%) and in the control group (12.4%). The HR of relapse events in the intervention group compared with the control group was 0.76.

SUGGESTED READING

Chlebowski RT, Blackburn GL, Thomson CA, et al: Dietary fat reduction and breast cancer outcome: Interim efficacy results from the Women's Intervention Nutrition Study. J Natl Cancer Inst 98:1767–1776, 2006.

Fyles AW, McCready DR, Manchul LA, et al: Tamoxifen with or without breast irradiation in women 50 years of age or older with early breast cancer. N Engl J Med 351:963–970, 2004.

Hughes KS, Schnaper LA, Berry D, et al: Cancer and Leukemia Group B; Radiation Therapy Oncology Group; Eastern Cooperative Oncology Group: Lumpectomy plus tamoxifen with or without irradiation in women 70 years of age or older with early breast cancer. N Engl J Med 351:971–977, 2004.

Hughes KS, Schnaper LA, Cirrincione C, et al: Lumpectomy plus tamoxifen with or without irradiation in women age 70 or older with early breast cancer. J Clin Oncol 28(7S):507, 2010.

King TA, Fey JV, Van Zee KJ, et al: A prospective analysis of the effect of blue-dye volume on sentinel lymph node mapping success and incidence of allergic reaction in patients with breast cancer. Ann Surg Oncol 11:535–541, 2004.

Kuhl CK, Schradking S, Bieling HB, et al: MRI for diagnosis of pure ductal carcinoma in situ: a prospective observational study. Lancet 370:485–492, 2007.

Paik S, Shak S, Tang G, et al: A multigene assay to predict recurrence of tamoxifen-treated, node-negative breast cancer. N Engl J Med 351:2817–2826, 2004.

Vinh-Hung V, Verschraegen C: Breast-conserving surgery with or without radiotherapy: Pooled-analysis for risks of ipsilateral breast tumor recurrence and mortality. J Natl Cancer Inst 96:115–121, 2004.

Abbreviations in this chapter

ATAC = Arimidex and Tamoxifen Alone or in Combination; IBCSG = International Breast Cancer Study Group; NCCN = National Comprehensive Cancer Network; NCI = National Cancer Institute; NSABP = National Surgical Adjuvant Breast and Bowel Project; SSO = Society of Surgical Oncology; VNPI = Van Nuys Prognostic Index

CHAPTER 7

Stage II breast cancer

Lori Jardines, MD, Sharad Goyal, MD, Melanie Royce, MD, PhD, and Shari B. Goldfarb, MD

This chapter focuses on the treatment of stage II breast cancer, which encompasses primary tumors > 2 cm in greatest dimension that involve ipsilateral axillary lymph nodes as well as tumors up to 5 cm without nodal involvement.

Stage II breast cancer is further subdivided into stages IIA and IIB. Patients classified as having stage IIA breast cancer include those with T0–1, N1, and T2, N0 disease. Stage IIB breast cancer includes patients with T2, N1, and T3, N0 disease. Therefore, this patient population is more heterogeneous than are the populations with stages 0 and I disease. The pretreatment evaluation and type of treatment offered to patients with stage II breast cancer are based on tumor size, nodal status, status of receptors for estrogen and *v-erb-b2* erythroblastic leukemia viral oncogene homolog 2, neuro/glioblastoma-derived oncogene homolog (avian; *ErbB2*), also known as human epidermal growth factor receptor type 2 (HER2/*neu*), and Oncotype Dx recurrence score.

TREATMENT

SURGICAL AND RADIATION TREATMENT

Multiple studies have demonstrated that patients with stage II breast cancer who are treated with either breast-conservation therapy (lumpectomy and radiation therapy) or modified radical mastectomy have similar disease-free and overall survival rates.

Breast-conservation therapy

The optimal extent of local surgery has yet to be determined and, in the literature, has ranged from excisional biopsy to quadrantectomy. A consensus statement issued by the NCI recommended that the breast cancer be completely excised with negative surgical margins and that a level I–II axillary lymph node dissection be performed. Patients should subsequently be treated with adjuvant breast irradiation.

Patients with tumors > 4 to 5 cm may not be optimal candidates for breast conservation due to the risk of significant residual tumor burden and the potential for a poor cosmetic result following lumpectomy (or partial mastectomy). Neoadjuvant chemotherapy, typically used for locally advanced breast cancer, is increasingly used in earlier stage, operable breast cancers to reduce the size of the primary tumor and allow for breast-conserving therapy.

In a study of more than 300 patients treated with neoadjuvant chemotherapy at the M. D. Anderson Cancer Center, promising results were reported. At a median follow-up of 60 months, the 5-year actuarial rates of ipsilateral breast tumor recurrence-free and locoregional recurrence-free survival were 95% and 91%, respectively. The authors concluded that breast-conservation therapy after neoadjuvant chemotherapy results in acceptably low rates of recurrence-free survival in appropriately selected patients, even those with T3 or T4 disease. Advanced nodal involvement at diagnosis, residual tumor larger than 2 cm, multifocal residual disease, and lymphovascular space invasion predict higher rates of recurrence.

In some patients, preoperative chemotherapy produces a sufficient reduction in tumor size that allows patients to receive breast-conserving therapy. The NSABP B-18 trial showed that preoperative doxorubicin-based chemotherapy decreases tumor size by > 50% in approximately 90% of operable breast cancers, resulting in a greater frequency of lumpectomy.

In a subsequent trial, NSABP B-27, women with invasive breast cancer were randomized to receive 4 cycles of preoperative AC (Adriamycin [doxorubicin] and cyclophosphamide) chemotherapy followed by surgery or 4 cycles of preoperative AC followed by 4 cycles of docetaxel (Taxotere) followed by surgery or 4 cycles of preoperative AC followed by surgery followed by 4 cycles of postoperative docetaxel. A higher rate of complete pathologic response was seen at surgery in patients treated with AC followed by docetaxel versus AC alone. There were no significant differences in disease-free and overall survival between the treatment groups. However, those who had a complete pathologic response in the breast had significant improvement in disease-free (hazard ratio [HR] = 0.45; $P < .0001$) and overall survival (HR = 0.33; $P < .0001$) when compared with those with residual disease after preoperative chemotherapy. Since preoperative chemotherapy does not have a negative impact on survival, the preoperative approach is a reasonable option and has gained favor among many patients.

Preoperative chemotherapy had an ability to convert patients requiring mastectomy to candidates for breast-conserving surgery. However, there was an increase in local recurrence in the "converted" group compared with those deemed eligibile initially for breast-conserving surgery.

Patients undergoing sentinel lymph node biopsy

The timing of sentinel node biopsy in patients undergoing preoperative chemotherapy is controversial. Preoperative chemotherapy can sterilize the axillary nodes and lead to errors in determining nodal involvement. Formal studies are currently ongoing to determine whether sentinel node biopsy can be safely performed after the patient has completed neoadjuvant chemotherapy. American College of Surgeons Oncology Group (ACOSOG) Z7015 is an on going trial posing precisely this question.

A prospective study designed to determine the survival impact of micrometastases in the sentinel nodes of patients with invasive breast cancer included 790 patients who underwent sentinel node biopsy. The investigators found no significant difference in 8-year disease-free or overall survival among patients with micrometastatic tumor deposits in sentinel nodes defined as being pN0(i+) or pN1mic when compared with patients having negative sentinel nodes. The true significance of these micrometastatic deposits is still unclear, but it may help to better define groups of patients who should receive maximum adjuvant medical or surgical therapy or who could avoid additional therapy.

Although helpful in prognosis and treatment planning, completion axillary dissection after a positive sentinel node biopsy may not be required for small tumors and in the absence of lymphovascular invasion. Factors affecting the rate of positive nonsentinel nodes and the necessity of axillary dissection following a positive sentinel lymph node resection were evaluated in NSABP B-32. Women with operable invasive breast cancer and clinically negative nodes were randomized to undergo sentinel node resection with immediate conventional axillary dissection (group 1) or without axillary dissection (group 2). Patients in group 2 who had positive sentinel nodes underwent axillary dissection. Data from 1,166 patients with positive sentinel nodes that were available for multivariate analysis (595 from group 1; 571 from group 2) indicated that a significantly higher percentage of patients in group 2 had positive nonsentinel nodes than did those in group 1 (41.5% vs 35.5%; $P = .032$). Clinical tumor size was a significant predictor for positive nonsentinel nodes ($P = .0010$). Percentages of patients having positive nonsentinel nodes were significantly increased by the number of positive sentinel nodes, and lymphovascular invasion was a significant predictor for positive nonsentinel nodes. The percentages of patients with positive nonsentinel nodes significantly decreased with increases in the number of hot spots identified and the number of sentinel nodes removed.

The Z0011 trial is a randomized, multicenter trial of axillary node dissection enrolling women with clinical T1 or T2 N0 M0 breast cancer who have a positive sentinel node. It was designed to enroll 1,900 patients and to be a noninferiority trial to detect a less than 3% survival. Patients were treated with lumpectomy with whole breast irradiation and adjuvant systemic therapy. A total of 891 patients who were sentinel node–positive were randomized to axillary node dissection (ALND, ITT n = 420) or sentinel node dissection alone (SNLD, ITT n = 436). At a median follow-up of 6.3 years, locoregional recurrences were uncommon, occurring in 4.1% of ALND and 2.8% of SLND patients (*P* = .11). Regional recurrence occurred in only 0.7% of the entire study population (ALND 0.5%, SLND 0.9%). Local breast recurrence occurred in 3.6% of ALND and 1.8% of SLND patients. Only age (≤ 50 years) and higher Bloom-Richardson scores were associated with locoregional recurrence by multivariate analysis. Neither the number of positive sentinel nodes, the size of the sentinel node metastasis, nor the number of lymph nodes removed was associated with locoregional recurrence. A drawback of this study is its early closure and accrual of less than one-half of the targeted enrollment population (*Giuliano AE et al: J Clin Oncol 28[7s]: abstract CRA506, 2010*).

Radiation therapy after breast-conserving surgery

For patients with stages I and II breast cancer, radiation therapy following lumpectomy remains an acceptable standard of care. Randomized trials as well as single-institution experiences have consistently demonstrated a significant reduction in local relapse rates for radiotherapy following breast-conserving surgery. Furthermore, small but significant differences in distant metastasis and disease-free survival have been observed in randomized trials comparing lumpectomy alone with lumpectomy and radiation therapy for patients with invasive breast cancer.

An EBCTCG meta-analysis that included over 7,300 women from 10 trials who were treated with breast-conserving surgery and randomized to receive observation or radiation showed a highly significant benefit for radiation therapy. There was a threefold reduction in local relapse with radiation, with a 5-year local relapse risk of 7% in those allocated to radiation as compared with 26% in the nonirradiated cohorts. The 15-year risk of death from breast cancer was 30.5% among those allocated to radiotherapy and 35.9% among those who were not.

Based on the results of a number of retrospective, single-institution experiences as well as several prospective, randomized clinical trials, breast-conserving surgery followed by radiation therapy to the intact breast is now considered standard treatment for the majority of patients with stage II invasive breast cancer.

Radiation dose and protocol

Radiation dose to the intact breast follows the same guidelines used in patients with stages 0 and I disease, described in chapter 6.

Regional nodal irradiation

For patients who undergo axillary lymph node dissection and are found to have negative lymph nodes, regional nodal irradiation is no longer employed routinely. For patients with positive lymph nodes, radiation therapy to the supraclavicular fossa and/or internal mammary chain may be considered on an individualized basis.

Regional nodal irradiation should be administered using careful treatment planning techniques to minimize the dose delivered to the underlying heart and lungs. Prophylactic nodal irradiation to doses of 4,500 to 5,000 cGy results in a high rate of regional nodal control and may improve disease-free survival in subsets of patients.

Given the widespread use of systemic therapy for patients with either node-negative or node-positive disease, the role of axillary dissection has recently come into question. In patients with clinically negative axillae who do not undergo axillary dissection, radiation therapy to the supraclavicular and axillary regions at the time of breast irradiation results in a high rate (> 95%) of regional nodal control with minimal morbidity.

Radiation therapy after mastectomy

Available data suggest that in patients with positive postmastectomy margins, chest wall fixation, primary tumors > 5 cm, or involvement of four or more lymph nodes at the time of mastectomy, the risk of locoregional failure remains significantly high enough for postmastectomy radiation therapy to be considered.

Several prospective, randomized trials have evaluated the role of postmastectomy radiotherapy in addition to chemotherapy. Most of these trials have been limited to patients with pathologic stage II disease or with T3 or T4 primary lesions. All of these trials have shown an improvement in locoregional control with the addition of adjuvant irradiation, and several recent trials have demonstrated a disease-free and overall survival advantage in selected patients. Clinical practice guidelines developed by the ASCO support the routine use of postmastectomy radiation therapy for women with stage III or T3 disease or who have four or more involved axillary lymph nodes.

The EBCTCG meta-analysis included 8,500 women who primarily had node-positive disease and were treated with mastectomy and axillary clearance. Patients were randomized to receive postmastectomy radiation versus no postmastectomy radiation. The 5-year risk of local relapse was significantly lower in the radiation group (6%) than in those randomized to no radiation (23%). Radiotherapy produced similar proportional reductions in local recurrence, regardless of patient age or tumor characteristics. The 15-year breast cancer mortality risk was also markedly lower in the radiation patients (54.7%) than in those receiving no radiation (61.2%; $P = .0002$). The 5-year risk of local recurrence in patients with one to three positive nodes who received radiation therapy was 4% as compared with 16% in controls. In patients with four or more nodes, the 5-year risk of local recurrence was 12% in the radiation group and 26% in the control group.

Most ongoing trials evaluating dose-intensive chemotherapy, with or without bone marrow or stem-cell transplantation, routinely include postmastectomy radiation therapy to the chest wall and/or regional lymph nodes to minimize locoregional recurrence.

Current recommendations

There is no clearly defined role for postmastectomy irradiation in patients with small (T1 or T2) primary tumors and negative nodes.

For patients with four or more positive lymph nodes, with or without a large primary tumor, postmastectomy radiation therapy should be considered to lower the rate of local relapse and improve disease-free survival. For patients with young age, T1 or T2 tumors, one to three positive nodes, poorly differentiated subtypes, or lymphovascular invasion, postmastectomy radiation therapy may have a benefit with respect to disease-free and overall survival. However, controversies and uncertainties regarding this issue remain, and individualized decision-making based on the patient's overall condition and specific risk factors is reasonable.

For nearly two decades there has been controversy as to the role of radiation therapy in women over the age of 70 with small breast cancer. The CALGB 9343 trial enrolled women over the age of 70 years with clinically node-negative disease, who had undergone lumpectomy with a clear margin (1 cm negative margin), had a tumor size of 2 cm or less, and were ER-positive or indeterminate. These women were randomized to either tamoxifen or tamoxifen plus radiation. The 631 eligible patients were followed for a median of 12 years. Radiation therapy was found to have an impact on breast tumor recurrence, with 6 events occurring in the 317 women who received tamoxifen plus radiation, compared with 27 events that occurred in 319 women (2% vs 9%, $P < .0001$). However, there were no benefits in terms of ultimate mastectomy (2% with radiation vs 4% without, $P = .1779$), axillary recurrence (0% with vs 3% without radiation), the frequency of second primary cancers (12% vs 9%, $P = .7268$), or overall survival at 10 years (33% of patients in each treatment arm had died at 10 years, $P = .845$). To date, approximately 50% of the women are still alive, 3% have died due to breast cancer, and 46% have died due to other causes. It is notable that approximately 50% of women who were over 70 years of age upon enrollment in this study are still alive 12 years later. The investigators concluded that in older women the benefits of radiation after lumpectomy are small and that omitting radiation in women over 70 years of age with clinical stage I breast cancer is a reasonable alternative *(Hughes KS et al: J Clin Oncol 28[7s]: abstract 507, 2010).*

Minimizing pulmonary and cardiac toxicities

Early trials employing postmastectomy radiation therapy showed that the modest improvement in breast cancer mortality was offset by an excess risk of cardiovascular deaths, presumably due to the radiation treatment techniques used, that resulted in delivery of relatively high radiation doses to the heart. Recent trials employing more modern radiation therapy techniques have *not* demonstrated an excess of cardiac morbidity and, hence, have shown a slight improvement in overall survival due to a decrease in breast cancer deaths. Thus, in any patient being considered for postmastectomy radiation therapy, efforts should be made to treat the areas at risk while minimizing the dose to the underlying heart and lungs.

Radiation dose and protocol

The available literature suggests that doses of 4,500 to 5,000 cGy should be sufficient to control subclinical microscopic disease in the postmastectomy setting. Electron-beam boosts to areas of positive margins and/or gross residual disease reaching doses ~6,000 cGy and delivered, may be considered.

In patients who have undergone axillary lymph node dissection, even in those with multiple positive nodes, treatment of the axillae does not appear to be necessary in the absence of gross residual disease. Treatment of the supraclavicular and/or internal mammary chain should employ techniques and field arrangements that minimize overlap between adjacent fields and decrease the dose to underlying cardiac and pulmonary structures.

MEDICAL TREATMENT

Medical management of local disease depends on clinical and pathologic staging. Systemic therapy is indicated only for invasive (infiltrating) breast cancers.

A discussion of the sequencing of chemotherapy and irradiation and hormonal therapy with irradiation is provided in chapter 6.

Treatment regimens

Systemic adjuvant therapy has been shown to decrease the risk of recurrence and in some cases also the risk of death. Systemic therapy may be divided into chemotherapy and endocrine (hormonal) therapy. Chemotherapy often involves use of combination regimens, given for 4 to 8 cycles. It is most often delivered after primary surgery for breast cancer and before radiation therapy for those who are candidates for irradiation.

A study comparing two decision aids found that the 21-gene assay (Oncotype Dx) was more accurate than were the classic clinicopathologic features and therapy utilized in Adjuvant! Online in predicting recurrence among 465 women with hormone receptor–positive operable breast cancer and zero to three positive axillary nodes who were treated with chemohormonal therapy. Recurrence Score (RS) highly significantly predicted recurrence of both node-negative and node-positive disease ($P < .001$) when adjusted for other clinical variables. RS also was more accurate than were clinical variables at predicting recurrence when integrated by an algorithm modeled after Adjuvant! that was adjusted to 5-year outcomes. The 5-year recurrence rate was 5% or less for the 46% of patients with a low RS (< 18). The investigators concluded that the 21-gene assay may be used to select low-risk versus high-risk patients for specific chemotherapy regimens and clinical trials.

Chemotherapy

Multiagent therapy with CMF (cyclophosphamide, methotrexate, and fluorouracil [5-FU]), CMFP (cyclophosphamide, methotrexate, 5-FU, and prednisone), AC, and MF (sequential methotrexate and 5-FU) has been used in patients with node-negative disease (see Table 2 in Chapter 6).

For node-positive disease, systemic chemotherapy has changed over the past few decades. Anthracycline-containing regimens have been shown to be of greater benefit than nonanthracycline-containing regimens (eg, CMF). Epirubicin (Ellence) was approved by the FDA for use in combination with CEF (cyclophosphamide and 5-FU) for the adjuvant treatment of patients with node-positive breast cancer following resection of the primary tumor.

In a pivotal trial conducted by the NCIC, premenopausal women with node-positive breast cancer were randomly allocated to receive either CEF or CMF, administered monthly for 6 months. With a median follow-up of 59 months, the 5-year relapse-free survival rates were 53% and 63% (P = .009), and 5-year survival rates were 70% and 77% for CEF and CMF, respectively (P = .03).

Several trials have also shown the benefit of incorporating taxanes (paclitaxel and docetaxel [Taxotere]) in the adjuvant treatment of node-positive breast cancer, and these drugs are now routinely used in this setting. Taxanes can either be given in combination with an anthracycline or sequentially, either before or after an anthracycline. They can also be given in combination with other drugs such as cyclophosphamide.

A multicenter study designed to prospectively examine whether RS affects physician and patient adjuvant treatment selection and satisfaction indicates that the RS assay impacts medical oncologist adjuvant treatment recommendations, patient treatment choice, and patient anxiety. Seventeen medical oncologists at one community practice and three academic practices consecutively enrolled 89 assessable patients. Before and after obtaining the 21-gene RS assay, medical oncologists stated their adjuvant treatment recommendation and confidence in it. Patients indicated their treatment choice pre- and post-RS assay as well. The medical oncologist treatment recommendation changed for 28 patients (31%); 24 patients (27%) changed their treatment decision. The largest change after the RS results was conversion from the medical oncologist's pretest recommendation for chemotherapy plus hormonal therapy (CHT) to post-test recommendation for hormone therapy (HT) alone (20 cases [22.5%]). Nine patients (10.1%) changed their treatment decision from CHT to HT. The RS results increased medical oncologist confidence in their treatment recommendation in 68 cases (76%). Patient anxiety and decisional conflict were significantly lower after RS results *(Lo SS et al: J Clin Oncol 28:1671–1676, 2010).*

The E1199 trial compared paclitaxel with docetaxel and therapeutic schedules (ie, every 3 weeks vs weekly) in the adjuvant therapy of operable breast cancer. In all, 4,950 eligible patients with lymph node–positive or high-risk (tumor > 2 cm), node-negative breast cancer received 4 cycles of AC and then were randomized to receive IV paclitaxel or docetaxel given at 3-week intervals for 4 cycles or at 1-week intervals for 12 cycles. Study investigators concluded that weekly paclitaxel given after standard adjuvant AC improved disease-free and overall survival in women with breast cancer. As compared with standard therapy (ie, paclitaxel given every 3 weeks), the odds ratio (OR) for disease-free survival was 1.27 among those receiving weekly paclitaxel (P = .006), 1.23 among those receiving docetaxel every 3 weeks (P = .02), and 1.09 among those receiving weekly docetaxel (P = .29), with an OR > 1 favoring the groups receiving experimental therapy. Weekly paclitaxel was also associated with improved overall survival (OR = 1.32; P = .01). An exploratory analysis of a subgroup of patients with ErbB2-negative tumors found similar improvements in disease-free and overall survival with weekly paclitaxel, regardless of hormone-receptor expression. Grade 2, 3, or 4 neuropathy was more frequent with use of weekly paclitaxel (27%) than with paclitaxel given every 3 weeks (20%).

The BCIRG compared TAC (Taxotere [docetaxel], Adriamycin [doxorubicin], and cyclophosphamide) with the FAC regimen (5-FU, Adriamycin [doxorubicin], and cyclophosphamide) in 1,480 women with node-positive breast cancer (BCIRG 001/TAX 316). At a median follow-up of 55 months, the estimated 5-year disease-free survival was 75% for patients treated with TAC versus 68% for those treated with FAC. This represents a statistically significant reduction in the risk of relapse of 28% (P = .001). Furthermore, treatment with TAC resulted in a statistically significant reduction in the risk of death (30%; P = .008). Although there was more febrile neutropenia with TAC, it was ameliorated with growth factor support.

In the CALGB trial 9344, 3,121 women with operable, node-positive breast cancer were randomized to receive three different doses of doxorubicin with a standard dose of cyclophosphamide followed by either no further therapy or 4 cycles of paclitaxel (175 mg/m^2). This study did not show any substantial benefit from dose escalation of doxorubicin. However, the addition of 4 cycles of paclitaxel improved disease-free and overall survival. At 5 years, the disease-free survival was 65% for the AC-treated cohort and 70% for the AC plus paclitaxel treatment group, and overall survival was 77% and 80%, respectively. An unplanned subset analysis showed that the majority of the benefit was seen in those with estrogen receptor–negative tumors. Tamoxifen was given to 94% of patients with hormone receptor–positive tumors. Toxicity was modest with the addition of 4 cycles of paclitaxel.

Jones et al previously reported that 4 cycles of TC improved overall survival when compared with 4 cycles of AC in early breast cancer. Updated results of this study as well as the impact of age, hormone receptor status, and ErbB2 status on outcome and toxicity were published. Of note, 16% of patients in this trial were > 65 years. The median age in women under the age of 65 was 50 years (range, 27–64 years) and for women over age 65 was 69 years (range, 65–77). Baseline characteristics in the two age subgroups generally were well matched, except that older women tended to have more lymph-node involvement. At a median of 7 years follow-up, the difference in disease-free survival between the TC and AC groups was significant (81% vs 75%, respectively; P = .033; HR = 0.74; 95% confidence interval [CI], 0.56–0.98), as was the difference in overall survival (87% vs 82%; P = .032; HR = 0.69; 95% CI = 0.50–0.97). The TC regimen was superior in both older and younger patients. Older women experienced more febrile neutropenia with TC and more anemia with AC. However, studies comparing TC to an anthracycline-and-taxane containing regimen (ie, TAC) are ongoing.

In NSABP B-28, the addition of paclitaxel (225 mg/m^2) did not initially result in improvement of either disease-free or overall survival. However, with longer follow-up (median: 67 months), improvement in disease-free survival in favor of AC followed by paclitaxel has emerged.

From 1996 to 2005, ATLAS randomized 11,500 women (59% estrogen receptor–positive, 41% untested) who had completed ~5 years of adjuvant tamoxifen to 5 more years of tamoxifen versus stopping. Less than 1% of patients had switched to any other adjuvant hormonal therapy in the trial treatment period. At a mean follow-up of 4.2 years, the annual recurrence rate in each treatment group was approximately constant during and after the 5-year trial treatment period. Approximately 1,500 recurrences have been reported. A total of ~1,300 occurred during years 5–9, but only ~200 occurred during years 10–14. Overall, the recurrence rate was significantly lower among those allocated to continue tamoxifen. There was no significant heterogeneity in the recurrence rate reduction with respect to estrogen receptor status, time period, age, or nodal status at diagnosis. Breast cancer mortality and overall mortality were lower among those allocated to continue tamoxifen, but were not statistically significant. Further follow-up is needed to reliably assess the longer-term effects on recurrence and the net effects on mortality *(Peto R et al: SABCS abstract 48, 2007).*

Dose-dense treatment CALGB 9741 tested two novel concepts: dose density and sequential therapy. A total of 2,005 women with operable, node-positive breast cancer were randomly assigned to receive one of the following regimens: (1) sequential Adriamycin (A) for 4 doses followed by Taxol (paclitaxel; T) for 4 doses followed by cyclophosphamide (C) for 4 doses, with doses every 3 weeks; (2) sequential A for 4 doses followed by T for 4 doses followed by C for 4 doses, every 2 weeks with filgrastim (Neupogen); (3) concurrent AC for 4 doses followed by T for 4 doses, every 3 weeks; or (4) concurrent AC for 4 doses followed by T for 4 doses, every 2 weeks with filgrastim. At a median follow-up of 36 months, there was an improvement in disease-free (risk ratio [RR] = 0.74; P = .010) and overall survival (RR = 0.69; P = .013) in favor of dose density. Four-year disease-free survival was 82% for the dose-dense regimens and 75% for the others. There was no difference in disease-free or overall survival between the concurrent (dose-dense) and sequential schedules. Severe neutropenia was less frequent in patients who received the dose-dense treatments with granulocyte colony stimulating factor (GCSF) support. Therefore, the trial demonstrated that administering chemotherapy sequentially is as effective as concurrent administration, but outcomes are improved with dose-dense regimens (administered every 2 weeks).

The dosages, schedules, and frequencies of chemotherapy regimens used for node-positive breast cancer are detailed in Table 1. Other regimens also used in node-negative (Chapter 6) and/or metastatic disease (Chapter 8) are listed in their respective chapters.

Recommendations All patients with stage II breast cancer should be considered for systemic adjuvant therapy. Adjuvant chemotherapy in node-positive breast cancer improves disease-free and overall survival by 24% and 15%, respectively. Risk reductions for multiagent chemotherapy are proportionately the same in patients with node-negative and node-positive disease.

TABLE 1: Adjuvant chemotherapy regimens in node-positive breast cancer

Regimen	Dose and frequency
TAC	
Taxotere (docetaxel)	75 mg/m² IV on day 1
Adriamycin (doxorubicin)	50 mg/m² IV on day 1
Cyclophosphamide	500 mg/m² IV on day 1
Repeat every 21 days for 6 cycles.	
Martin M et al: Eur J Cancer 2(suppl):70, 2004.	
AC ⟶ T (conventional regimen)	
Adriamycin (doxorubicin) Cyclophosphamide	60 mg/m² IV on day 1 600 mg/m² IV on day 1 × 4 cycles
followed by	
Taxol (paclitaxel)	175 mg/m² IV by 3-h infusion every 3 weeks × 4 cycles
Dose-dense (concurrent regimen)*	
Adriamycin (doxorubicin) Cyclophosphamide	60 mg/m² IV on day 1 every 2 weeks 600 mg/m² IV on day 1 every 2 weeks × 4 cycles
followed by	
Taxol (paclitaxel)	175 mg/m² IV by 3-h infusion every 2 weeks × 4 cycles
*Severe neutropenia was less frequent in patients who received the dose dense treatments with granulocyte colony stimulating factor support.	
Dose-dense (sequential regimen)	
Adriamycin (doxorubicin)	60 mg/m² IV on day 1 every 2 weeks × 4 cycles
followed by	
Taxol (paclitaxel)	175 mg/m² IV by 3-h infusion every 2 weeks × 4 cycles
followed by	
Cyclophosphamide	600 mg/m² IV on day 1 every 2 weeks × 4 cycles
Citron M et al: J Clin Oncol 21:1431–1439, 2003.	
A-CMF	
Adriamycin (doxorubicin)	75 mg/m² IV on day 1
Repeat every 3 weeks for 4 courses.	
Cyclophosphamide	600 mg/m² IV on day 1
Methotrexate	40 mg/m² IV on days 1 and 8
Fluorouracil	600 mg/m² on day 1
Repeat every 3 weeks for 8 courses.	
Buzzoni R et al: J Clin Oncol 9:2134–2140, 1991.	

Regimen	Dose and frequency
AC ⟶ T + trastuzumab	
Adriamycin (doxorubicin)	60 mg/m^2 IV on day 1
Cyclophosphamide	600 mg/m^2 IV over 30 minutes on day 1
Repeat every 21 days for 4 cycles.	
followed by	
Taxol (paclitaxel)	175 mg/m^2 IV by 3-h infusion on day 1
Repeat every 21 days for 4 cycles.	
NOTE: All patients should receive dexamethasone (20 mg orally) 12 and 6 hours before paclitaxel, diphenhydramine (50 mg IV), and ranitidine (50 mg IV) 30 to 60 minutes before paclitaxel.	
or	
Taxol (paclitaxel)	80 mg/m^2 IV over 1 hour weekly for 12 doses
NOTE: All patients should receive dexamethasone (20 mg orally) 12 and 6 hours before the first dose of paclitaxel. If no hypersensitivity reaction occurs, convert to dexamethasone (10 mg IV), completed 30 minutes before each subsequent paclitaxel administration (dexamethasone may be tapered during the 12 weeks of paclitaxel).	
along with	
Trastuzumab	4 mg/kg IV, loading dose over 90 minutes on day 1 of the first paclitaxel dose (On the weeks paclitaxel is given, trastuzumab is given after paclitaxel.) 2 mg/kg IV, maintenance dose over 30 minutes every week for 51 weeks starting on day 8
Romond E et al: N Engl J Med 353:1673–1684, 2005.	
AC-TH	
Adriamycin (doxorubicin)	60 mg/m^2 every 3 weeks for 4 cycles and
Cyclophosphamide	600 mg/m^2 every 3 weeks for 4 cycles
Taxotere (docetaxel)	100 mg/m^2 every 3 weeks for 4 cycles
Herceptin	weekly (initial dose of 4 mg/kg)
followed by	11 weekly doses of 2 mg/kg concurrently with docetaxel
and then	every 3 weeks as monotherapy (14 doses of 6 mg/kg) for a total of 52 weeks of therapy
Slamon et al, SABCS, 2007.	
TCH	
Taxotere (docetaxel)	75 mg/m^2 and
Carboplatin	(at a target AUC of 6 mg/mL/min as a 30- to 60-minute infusion) every 3 weeks for 6 cycles
Herceptin	weekly (initial dose of 4 mg/kg)
followed by	17 weekly doses of 2 mg/kg concurrently with docetaxel and carboplatin
and then	every 3 weeks as monotherapy (12 doses of 6 mg/kg) for a total of 52 weeks of therapy
Slamon et al, SABCS, 2007.	

Chemotherapy for women 50 years of age and older is similar to that for younger women. However, multiagent chemotherapy affords the greatest benefit in women younger than age 50 with respect to reductions in the risk of recurrence and death from breast cancer. For instance, CMF or AC chemotherapy improves disease-free survival in women aged 50 to 69 by 18%, versus 33% for women younger than age 50. Limited data are available from randomized trials regarding women aged 70 and older. However, in the absence of comorbidity, such as heart, renal, or liver disease, systemic adjuvant therapy can be offered to women > 70 years old.

Endocrine therapy

The EBCTCG overview analyses demonstrated a significant advantage with the addition of tamoxifen (20 mg/d oral) for 5 years to the adjuvant therapy regimen of women with estrogen receptor–positive breast cancer regardless of age. Treatment with tamoxifen reduced the risk of death by 14% in women younger than age 50 and by 27% in those 50 years of age and older. Long-term follow-up from the NSABP conclusively demonstrates that there is no benefit to continuing tamoxifen therapy beyond 5 years. However, results from much larger studies have recently reported that a longer duration of tamoxifen may be more beneficial than 5 years of therapy.

Premenopausal women

Approximately 60% of premenopausal women with primary breast cancer have estrogen receptor–positive tumors. For this group of patients, the benefit of adjuvant endocrine therapy, either tamoxifen or ovarian ablation, was established in the EBCTCG overview. For premenopausal women, however, the long-term morbidity associated with permanent ovarian suppression may be significant. Ovarian suppression with luteinizing hormone-releasing hormone (LHRH) analogs offers an alternative to permanent ovarian ablation, which is potentially reversible on cessation of therapy.

The ZEBRA trial is a randomized study which is directly comparing goserelin (Zoladex) monotherapy with CMF in premenopausal women 50 years of age and younger with node-positive, stage II breast cancer. The study included 1,614 patients: 797 randomized to receive goserelin and 817 to receive CMF. Estrogen receptor status was known for 92.5% of patients and 80% had estrogen receptor–positive tumors.

At a median follow-up of 6 years, the estrogen receptor–positive patients treated with goserelin fared comparably to those who received CMF in terms of disease-free survival (HR = 1.01; $P = .94$) and overall survival (HR = 0.99; $P = .92$). Not surprisingly, CMF was superior to goserelin in patients with estrogen receptor–negative tumors. The onset of amenorrhea occurred on average 6 months sooner with goserelin than with CMF. More than 95% of patients on goserelin were amenorrheic versus 59% of patients receiving CMF. Reversibility of amenorrhea was greater for goserelin. One year after cessation of goserelin treatment, 23% remained amenorrheic versus 77% of CMF recipients.

Several studies have compared adjuvant chemotherapy with combined endocrine therapies, consisting of tamoxifen for 5 years and an LHRH agonist for 2 to 3 years, in premenopausal women. Overall, combination endocrine treatment yielded better results than did chemotherapy alone. Whether a strategy of combined endocrine therapy is better than tamoxifen alone, either with or without chemotherapy, in premenopausal patients with hormone receptor–positive tumors is the subject of several ongoing clinical trials.

In the SOFT trial, following adjuvant chemotherapy, tamoxifen alone is being compared with tamoxifen plus ovarian function suppression/ablation versus ovarian function suppression plus an aromatase inhibitor (exemestane [Aromasin]). The role of ovarian suppression and aromatase inhibitors in this setting is being further investigated by the TEXT study, which is comparing ovarian suppression with the LHRH analog triptorelin (Trelstar) plus tamoxifen versus triptorelin plus exemestane.

Whether combined endocrine therapies alone may be sufficient to achieve excellent outcomes without chemotherapy was investigated in the PERCHE trial. Chemotherapy use was determined by randomization; unfortunately, the trial closed due to inadequate accrual. In the TEXT clinical trial, where chemotherapy use was chosen by the physician, lymph node status was the predominant determinant of chemotherapy use (88% of node positive–treated vs 46% of node negative). Geography, patient age, and tumor size and grade were also determinants, but degree of receptor positivity and ErbB2 status were not. Currently, almost all premenopausal women with lymph node–positive, hormone receptor–positive breast cancer receive chemotherapy.

In premenopausal women with early breast cancer, addition of zoledronic acid to adjuvant endocrine therapy significantly improved clinical outcomes beyond endocrine therapy alone. In ABCSG-12, a phase III randomized study of 1,800 premenopausal women with stage I-II disease undergoing ovarian suppression with goserelin, therapy with tamoxifen or anastrozole plus zoledronic acid reduced the risk of disease-free survival events by 36% and relapse-free survival by 35% vs endocrine therapy alone ($P = .011$ and .015, respectively). At 5-year follow-up, disease-free survival was 98.2%. Investigators concluded that some premenopausal women with early breast cancer may achieve a strong treatment benefit without receiving chemotherapy.

Postmenopausal women

For many years, tamoxifen has been the gold standard adjuvant endocrine therapy for postmenopausal women with hormone receptor–positive tumors. However, after third-generation aromatase inhibitors (AI) demonstrated superior activity in metastatic breast cancer, large randomized clinical trials were initiated in patients with early-stage breast cancer to evaluate these drugs compared with tamoxifen, in combination with tamoxifen, and sequentially with tamoxifen.

The ATAC trial was the first large, randomized trial demonstrating the superiority of an aromatase inhibitor over tamoxifen in the adjuvant treatment of postmenopausal women with hormone receptor–positive breast cancer. After the initial ATAC analyses, the combination arm was closed because of low efficacy.

ATAC has shown that anastrozole (Arimidex; n = 3,125) is significantly more effective than tamoxifen (n = 3,116) in preventing recurrences and is better tolerated but associated with a higher risk of fractures on treatment. After treatment completion, fractures and serious adverse events continued to be collected in a blinded fashion.

At a median follow-up of 100 months, the ATAC trial showed significant improvement for anastrozole compared with tamoxifen for disease-free survival, time to recurrence, time to distant recurrence, and contralateral breast cancer.

Exploratory analysis from the ATAC Trial investigated the impact of BMI on recurrence and the relative benefit of anastrozole versus tamoxifen according to baseline BMI. Overall, women with a high BMI (> 35 kg/m^2) at baseline had more recurrences than women with a low BMI (< 23 kg/m^2; adjusted hazard ratio [HR] = 1.39; 95% CI = 1.06–1.82; *P* [heterogeneity] = .03) and significantly more distant recurrences (adjusted HR = 1.46; 95% confidence interval [CI] = 1.07–1.61; *P* [heterogeneity] = .01). The relative benefit of anastrozole versus tamoxifen was nonsignificantly better in thin women compared with overweight women. Recurrence rates were lower for anastrozole than tamoxifen for all BMI quintiles. These results confirm the poorer prognosis of obese women with early-stage breast cancer and suggest that the relative efficacy of anastrozole compared with tamoxifen is greater in thin postmenopausal women. Requiring independent confirmation is the concept that higher doses or more complete inhibitors might be more effective in overweight women *(Sestak I et al: J Clin Oncol 28:3411-3415, 2010).*

In the hormone receptor–positive population, the results follow: disease-free survival (HR = 0.85; 95% CI = 0.76–0.94; *P* = .003), time to recurrence (HR = 0.76; 95% CI = 0.67–0.87; *P* = .0001); time to distant recurrence (HR = 0.84; 95% CI = 0.72–0.97; *P* = .022); and incidence of new contralateral breast cancer (HR = 0.6; 95% CI = 0.42–0.85; *P* = .004). Absolute differences for anastrozole and tamoxifen increased over time, and hazard rates remained lower on anastrozole compared with tamoxifen after treatment completion. Breast cancer deaths were nonsignificantly fewer with anastrozole than with tamoxifen (351 vs 380 intent-to-treat; 246 vs 268 hormone receptor–positive), but there was no difference in overall survival (HR = 0.97, hormone receptor–positive). After treatment completion, fracture rates for anastrozole and tamoxifen were similar, and safety benefits were maintained. Myocardial infarction rates among patients were identical to those on or off treatment, and endometrial cancer rates remained lower for anastrozole than for tamoxifen off treatment. No new safety concerns were seen. These data confirm the long-term superior efficacy and safety of anastrozole over tamoxifen as initial adjuvant therapy for postmenopausal women with hormone-sensitive early breast cancer.

The use of an aromatase inhibitor as upfront adjuvant endocrine therapy for postmenopausal women with hormone receptor–positive breast cancer was confirmed in the BIG 1-98 trial. This study compared letrozole (Femara) with tamoxifen for 5 years as adjuvant endocrine therapy for this patient population. At a median follow-up time of 51 months for the monotherapy (non-crossover) arms, 352 disease-free survival events among 2,463 women receiving letrozole and 418 events among 2,459 women receiving tamoxifen were observed. This reflected an 18% reduction in the risk of an event (HR = 0.82; 95% CI = 0.71–0.95; *P* = .007). No predefined subsets showed differential benefit. Adverse events were similar to those noted in previous reports, with patients on tamoxifen experiencing more thromboembolic events, endometrial pathology, hot flashes, night sweats, and vaginal bleeding and those on letrozole experiencing more bone fractures, arthralgia, low-grade hypercholesterolemia, and cardiovascular events other than ischemia and cardiac failure. The present updated analysis yielded results similar to those from the previous primary analysis but more directly comparable with results from other trials of continuous therapy using a single endocrine agent. The BIG I-98 trial was later modified to include a crossover for both agents.

At a median follow-up of 71 months after randomization in the BIG 1-98 study, the letrozole monotherapy arm was compared with the sequential-therapy arms. In terms of disease-free survival, there was no difference between the letrozole monotherapy, tamoxifen sequenced to letrozole, or letrozole followed by tamoxifen arms. The letrozole followed by tamoxifen arm had an HR = 0.96, with 99% CI = 0.76–1.21, and the tamoxifen followed by letrozole arm had an HR = 1.05, with 99% CI = 0.84–1.32.

Other randomized trials have investigated the use of an aromatase inhibitor after tamoxifen. Two sequential strategies after tamoxifen were studied: (1) a switch to an aromatase inhibitor after 2 or 3 years of tamoxifen to complete a 5-year course of endocrine therapy, or (2) a switch to an aromatase inhibitor after 5 years of tamoxifen to complete 10 years of endocrine therapy, also called extended adjuvant therapy. With either strategy, the use of an aromatase inhibitor after tamoxifen provided significant reduction in events (recurrence, contralateral breast cancer, or death).

In the IES, 4,742 patients who had received 2 to 3 years of tamoxifen were randomized to receive either additional tamoxifen or a switch to exemestane to complete a 5-year course of endocrine therapy. After a median follow-up of 55.7 months, 809 events contributing to the analysis of disease-free survival had been reported (354 exemestane, 455 tamoxifen); an unadjusted HR of 0.76 (95% CI = 0.66–0.88; *P* = .0001) was in favor of exemestane, with an absolute benefit of 3.3% (95% CI = 1.6–4.9) by the end of treatment (ie, 2.5 years after randomization). A total of 222 deaths occurred in the exemestane group compared with 261 deaths in the tamoxifen group, with an unadjusted HR of 0.85 (95% CI = 0.71–1.02; *P* = .08) in the intent-to-treat group. When 122 patients with estrogen receptor–negative disease were excluded, the HR was 0.83 (0.69–1.00; *P* = .05). Results suggest that early improvements in disease-free survival noted in patients who switch to exemestane after 2 to 3 years on tamoxifen persist after treatment and translate into a modest improvement in overall survival.

Severe toxic events of exemestane were rare, and toxicity profiles were generally similar to those previously reported for aromatase inhibitors. Patients who received exemestane reported fewer venous thromboembolic events than did those on tamoxifen. No other statistically significant differences in reported cardiovascular events (excluding venous thromboembolic events) were noted either on treatment or including the post-treatment period. Myocardial infarctions were rare and occurred in 31 (1.3%) exemestane-treated patients as compared with 19 (0.8%) tamoxifen-treated patients (*P* = .08). Any effect of treatment on the risk of myocardial infarction seemed largely restricted to patients with a history of hypertension. Musculoskeletal pain, carpal tunnel syndrome, joint stiffness, paraesthesia, and arthralgia were reported more frequently in patients who switched to exemestane than in those who remained on tamoxifen. These effects emerged during the on-treatment period. In total, fractures occurred in 277 patients, but hip, spine, and wrist fractures were few. Including on-treatment and post-treatment follow-up, other types of fractures were more common in patients who switched to exemestane than in those on tamoxifen. Fewer clinically serious gynecologic events were reported in patients who switched to exemestane than in those on tamoxifen in the on-treatment period and throughout follow-up. The number of endometrial cancers did not differ significantly between the groups.

> **G**oss et al reported on a subset of women in the MA17 trial who were premenopausal at initial diagnosis and in whom subsequent menopause, prior to randomization, may have influenced their outcome on extended adjuvant letrozole. Women randomized to MA17 were divided into two groups: (1) premenopausal: women < 50 years of age who underwent bilateral oophorectomy when tamoxifen treatment was started or women < 50 years of age at the start of tamoxifen treatment who became amenorrheic during adjuvant chemotherapy or tamoxifen treatment; and (2) postmenopausal. Disease-free survival (DFS) from time of randomization for women in these two groups was compared; 889 women were identified as premenopausal and 4,277 as postmenopausal. The interaction between treatment and menopausal status was statistically significant for DFS (*P* = .02), indicating that women diagnosed with premenopausal breast cancer had significantly greater benefit (HR = 0.25; 95% CI = 0.12–0.51) with letrozole treatment in terms of DFS than those with postmenopausal status (HR = 0.69; 95% CI = 0.52–0.91). Letrozole was well tolerated in premenopausal women. These data indicate that women who are premenopausal at diagnosis but become postmenopausal any time before or during adjuvant tamoxifen should be considered for extended adjuvant therapy with letrozole *(Goss PE et al: SABCS abstract 13, 2009).*

Three other randomized trials showed a benefit to switching to anastrozole after 2 to 3 years of tamoxifen treatment versus continued tamoxifen for a total of 5 years. The ITA trial, with 448 patients enrolled and a median follow-up of 36 months, showed significant benefits in event-free (HR = 0.35; 95% CI = 0.20–0.63; *P* = .0002) recurrence-free survival (HR = 0.35; 95% CI = 0.18–0.68; *P* = .001) in the women switched to anastrozole. There were 19 total events in the tamoxifen group (n = 225) and 10 in the anastrozole group (n = 223). The 3-year difference in recurrence-free survival was 5.8% (95% CI = 5.2–6.4). Significantly longer locoregional recurrence-free survival (HR = 0.15; 95% CI = 0.03–0.65; *P* = .003) was noted for the anastrozole group. The difference in distant recurrence-free survival approached statistical significance (HR = 0.49; 95% CI = 0.22–1.05; *P* = .06).

A combined analysis of the ABCSG Trial 8 and ARNO 95 Trial, with 3,224 patients and a median follow-up of 28 months, investigated a similar strategy. It showed that sequential endocrine therapy with tamoxifen for 2 years followed by anastrozole for 3 years was superior to 5 years of tamoxifen in terms of event-free (HR = 0.6; 95% CI = 0.44–0.81; *P* = .0009) and distant recurrence-free survival (HR = 0.61; 95% CI = 0.42–0.87; *P* = .0067). No statistically significant difference in overall survival has emerged at this point (*P* = .16). Updated results from the ARNO 95 trial recently were reported, indicating that switching to anastrozole resulted in a significant reduction in the risk of disease recurrence (HR = 0.66; 95% CI = 0.44–1.00; *P* = .049) and improved overall survival (HR = 0.53; 95% CI = 0.28–0.99; *P* = .045) compared with continuing on tamoxifen. The overall safety profile for anastrozole was consistent with previous reports, and no new safety issues were identified.

In the MA-17 trial, 5,187 postmenopausal women who had taken tamoxifen for 5 years were randomly assigned to receive either letrozole or placebo for an additional 5 years. At a median follow-up of 30 months, an updated analysis of the MA.17 was performed. It confirmed the results of the first interim analysis. There continued to be an improvement in disease-free survival [HR = 0.58; 95% CI = 0.45–0.76; 2*P* < .001], and distant disease-free survival seen with letrozole [HR = 0.60; 95% CI = 0.43–0.84; P = .002]. The improvement in recurrence rate did not translate into a significant difference in overall survival. However, in a preplanned subset analysis of lymph node–positive patients, there was a statistically significant improvement in overall survival [HR = 0.61; 95% CI = 0.38–0.98; P = .04]. After the first interim analysis, the independent data and safety monitoring committee recommended termination of the trial, since letrozole therapy after the completion of standard tamoxifen treatment significantly improved disease-free survival. Toxicities associated with letrozole were similar to those seen with aromatase inhibitors in other trials.

Bone effects

The third-generation aromatase inhibitors have been shown to reduce bone mineral density (BMD) when compared with tamoxifen in the advanced adjuvant and neoadjuvant settings in women with early breast cancer. Five-year results from the ATAC trial showed that patients treated with anastrozole had an annual decline in lumbar BMD of 2% during the first 2 years of treatment and of 1% in years 3 to 5.

The bone subprotocol of IBIS-II assessed changes in the BMD in postmenopausal women aged 40 to 70 years with a high risk of breast cancer who received anastrozole or placebo for 5 years. To date, of the 1,540 women in the prevention study, 613 women have taken part in the bone subprotocol of the study. Of the 250 women whose lumbar spine and femoral neck BMD has been assessed at baseline and 1 year by dual-energy x-ray absorptiometry (DEXA) scans, 162 with normal BMD received only monitoring without bisphosphonate treatment, 59 osteopenic women were further randomized to receive either risedronate (Actonel) or placebo, and 29 osteoporotic women received treatment with risedronate. Data from this trial confirm the BMD losses observed with third-generation aromatase inhibitors in breast cancer patients, but it is also reassuring that BMD loss can be controlled if women receive DEXA scans at baseline and bisphosphonate treatment as needed along with aromatase inhibitors.

ABCSG-12 is a randomized, open-label, phase III, four-arm trial comparing tamoxifen (20 mg/d orally) and goserelin (3.6 mg every 28 days SC) with or without zoledronic acid (Zometa; 4 mg IV every 6 months) versus anastrozole (1 mg/d PO) and goserelin with or without zoledronic acid for 3 years in premenopausal women with endocrine-responsive breast cancer. The median patient age at diagnosis was 44 years. In a BMD subprotocol, patients underwent serial BMD measurements at 0, 6, 12, 24, 36, and 60 months. Of 1,801 patients in the trial, 404 were prospectively included in a bone substudy. A total of 201 patients received adjuvant zoledronic acid together with their endocrine treatment, whereas 203 patients did not. After 3 years of treatment, patients who did not receive zoledronic acid showed a BMD loss of 11.3% as compared with baseline ($P < .0001$). Bone loss was more pronounced if anastrozole was used in combination with goserelin as compared with tamoxifen (−13.6% vs −9%). At 60 months of follow-up (ie, 2 years after the completion of treatment), patients without zoledronic acid still showed impaired BMD as compared to baseline (−6.8%; P = .0005). In contrast, patients who had not used zoledronic acid showed unchanged BMD at 36 months (+.3%; P = .85) and increased BMD at 60 months (+3.9%; P = .02).

The Z-FAST study evaluated the efficacy and safety of zoledronic acid in preventing aromatase inhibitor-associated bone loss in postmenopausal women with early breast cancer who were receiving adjuvant letrozole therapy. A total of 602 patients with hormone receptor–positive early breast cancer starting letrozole were randomized to upfront zoledronic acid versus delayed zoledronic acid. The delayed group received zoledronic acid when either the post-baseline T-score decreased to below –2 or a clinical fracture occurred. All patients were treated with calcium and vitamin D.

The Z-FAST trial showed that the overall difference in the percentage change in BMD between the upfront and delayed zoledronic acid treatment groups, at both lumbar spine and total hip, progressively increased from baseline through 36 months. Therefore, administering zoledronic acid every 6 months for up to 36 months is effective in preventing bone loss associated with adjuvant aromatase inhibitor therapy in postmenopausal women with early breast cancer. At 36 months, the upfront zoledronic acid group (n = 189) showed a mean increase of 3.72% in lumbar spine BMD, whereas the delayed group (n = 188) showed a mean decrease of 2.95%, resulting in an absolute difference of 6.7% ($P < .001$). The upfront group (n = 189) showed a mean increase of 1.66% in total hip BMD, whereas the delayed group (n = 187) showed a mean decrease of 3.51%, resulting in an absolute difference of 5.2% ($P < .001$). The study was not designed to detect a significant difference in the fracture rate between treatment arms. Zoledronic acid was safe and well tolerated; no serious renal adverse events and no confirmed osteonecrosis of the jaw cases were reported.

Recommendations

Guidelines from ASCO and the NCCN highlight the appropriate use of aromatase inhibitors in postmenopausal women with hormone receptor–positive breast cancer. Aromatase inhibitors have a significant role in reduction of recurrence in early-stage breast cancer and should be included as part of the adjuvant endocrine therapy for postmenopausal women with hormone receptor–positive disease. Using an aromatase inhibitor as upfront therapy or switching at some point after 2 to 3 years of tamoxifen is an acceptable strategy. Since the risk of breast cancer recurrence after completion of adjuvant endocrine therapy remains substantial, extended therapy with an aromatase inhibitor is another viable strategy for patients who are completing 5 years of tamoxifen.

Several questions on the optimal use of aromatase inhibitors remain, and we must await completion of ongoing trials and/or development of new trials for answers. For instance, neither the optimal timing nor the duration of aromatase inhibitor therapy has been established, and the role of biomarkers in selecting optimal endocrine therapy remains controversial. Furthermore, long-term effects of aromatase therapy, including osteoporosis, have not yet been well characterized.

Treatment of ErbB2-positive tumors

ErbB2-expressing breast cancers have been shown to have a worse outcome than their ErbB2-negative counterpart. Studies have demonstrated significant benefit from the addition of trastuzumab to chemotherapy for both early-stage and metastatic breast cancer. In women with surgically resected breast cancer that overexpresses HER2, trastuzumab combined with chemotherapy improves disease-free and overall survival. Trastuzumab treatment decreases the risk of death by one-third ($P = .015$) in HER2-positive breast cancer. Cardiac toxicity is a potential side effect of trastuzumab therapy and is more prevalent in patients previously treated with doxorubicin. Trastuzumab should not be administered concurrently with doxorubicin because of an increased risk of cardiac toxicity. New York Heart Association Class III or IV congestive heart failure or death from cardiac causes at 3 years was seen in 4.1% of patients treated with doxorubicin and trastuzumab in the B-31 trial and 2.9% of patients in the N9831 trial.

Four major trials of trastuzumab in the adjuvant setting have been published. The NSABP B-31 and the NCCTG 9831 were jointly analyzed to include a total of 3,351 ErbB2-positive patients, with a median follow-up of 2.0 years (2.4 years in trial B-31 and 1.5 years in trial N9831). Both trials included two similar treatment arms: adjuvant chemotherapy with AC followed by paclitaxel with or without weekly trastuzumab for 1 year. Although there were differences between the two studies, including a third treatment arm in N9831 sequencing trastuzumab after paclitaxel that was not included in the joint analysis, the common question addressed was the effect of adding trastuzumab to AC followed by paclitaxel.

There were 261 events in the control group and 133 events in the trastuzumab group. The HR for a first event in the trastuzumab group, as compared with the control group, was 0.48 (95% CI = 0.39–0.59; $P < .0001$). The percentages of patients alive and disease-free at 3 years were 75.4% in the control group and 87.1% in the trastuzumab group (absolute difference: 11.8%; 95% CI = 8.1–15.4). At 4 years, the respective percentages were 67.1% and 85.3% (absolute difference: 18.2%; 95% CI = 12.7–23.7). Distant metastases were reported in 193 patients in the control group and 96 in the trastuzumab group. The HR for a first distant recurrence was 0.47 in the trastuzumab group as compared with the control group (95% CI = 0.37–0.61; $P < .0001$). At 3 years, 90.4% of women in the trastuzumab group were free of distant recurrence, as compared with 81.5% of women in the control group (absolute difference: 8.8%; 95% CI = 5.5–12.1); the respective rates at 4 years were 89.7% and 73.7% (absolute difference: 15.9%; 95% CI = 11.1–20.8). Both disease-free and overall survival were highly statistically significant for the trastuzumab-treated cohort.

Furthermore, there is an overall survival benefit to the addition of trastuzumab to chemotherapy. There were 62 deaths in the trastuzumab group, as compared with 92 deaths in the control group (HR = 0.67; 95% CI = 0.48–0.93; $P = .015$). The absolute survival rate at 3 years was 94.3% in the trastuzumab group and 91.7% in the control group (absolute difference: 2.5%; 95% CI = 0.1–5.0); at 4 years, the respective rates were 86.6% and 91% (absolute difference: 4.8%; 95% CI = 0.6–9.0). The principal adverse event associated with trastuzumab therapy among patients with prior exposure to anthracyclines is cardiac dysfunction.

In trial B-31, for patients initiated on trastuzumab therapy, the cumulative incidence of NYHA class III or IV congestive heart failure or death from cardiac causes at 3 years was 0.8% in the control group (4 patients had congestive heart failure, and 1 died of cardiac causes) and 4.1% in the trastuzumab group (31 patients had congestive heart failure). Of the 31 women in the trastuzumab group who had congestive heart failure, 27 have been followed for at least 6 months after the onset of heart failure,

The incidence of cardiac adverse events was investigated in patients with early breast cancer in the HERA trial who were treated with 1 year of trastuzumab after completion of (neo) adjuvant chemotherapy. There were 1,698 patients randomly assigned to observation and 1,703 randomly assigned to 1 year of trastuzumab treatment; 94.1% of patients had been treated with anthracyclines. The incidence of cardiac endpoints remains low even after longer-term follow-up. The incidence of discontinuation of trastuzumab because of cardiac disorders was 5.1%. At a median follow-up of 3.6 years, the incidence of cardiac endpoints remained low, though it was higher in the trastuzumab group than in the observation group (severe CHF, 0.8% vs 0.0%; confirmed significant LVEF decreases, 3.6% vs 0.6%). In the trastuzumab group, 59 of 73 patients with a cardiac endpoint reached acute recovery; of these 59 patients, 52 were considered by the cardiac advisory board to have a favorable outcome from the cardiac endpoint. The cumulative incidence of any type of cardiac endpoint increases during the scheduled treatment period of 1 year, but it remains relatively constant thereafter *(Procter M et al: J Clin Oncol 28:3422–3428, 2010).*

and only 1 reported persistent symptoms of heart failure at the most recent follow-up visit.

During treatment with paclitaxel alone or with trastuzumab, there was little imbalance between treatment groups in the incidence of any toxicity except for a higher incidence of left ventricular dysfunction in the trastuzumab group. Since the dramatic results are changing the way breast cancer is treated and many clinicians have adopted the use of trastuzumab for similar groups of patients, the same monitoring used in these trials can be adopted in clinical practice to minimize cardiac toxicity. Additional toxicities were rare cases of interstitial pneumonitis, some of which appeared to be related to trastuzumab therapy. In trial B-31, four patients in the trastuzumab group had interstitial pneumonitis, one of whom died. In the N9831 trial, five patients in the trastuzumab group had grade 3+ pneumonitis or pulmonary infiltrates, one of whom died.

The international HERA trial had a different design and assessed ErbB2-positive patients who received a variety of chemotherapeutic regimens, randomized to either observation versus 1 or 2 years of every-3-week trastuzumab. Results were reported for only the 1 year of trastuzumab versus the observation arm, which included 5,081 patients with 1-year medical follow-up. Similar to the previously mentioned joint analysis, reduction in observed events (ie, recurrence of breast cancer, contralateral breast cancer, second nonbreast malignant disease, or death) were noted for women who received trastuzumab. The unadjusted HR for an event in the trastuzumab group, as compared with the observation group, was 0.54 (95% CI = 0.43–0.67; $P < .0001$) in favor of trastuzumab. This represents an absolute benefit in terms of disease-free survival at 2 years of 8.4%. Overall survival in the two groups was not significantly different (29 deaths with trastuzumab vs 37 with observation). Severe cardiotoxicity developed in 0.5% of the women who were treated with trastuzumab.

The BCIRG 006 study evaluated the benefit of adjuvant trastuzumab (H) in 3,222 patients with ErbB2-positive breast cancer. Unique to this study was a nonanthracycline-containing regimen, which was expected to minimize the cardiotoxicity seen with trastuzumab following anthracycline-based chemotherapy. There were

From May 2000 to April 2005 in the NCCTG N9831 trial, a total of 2,448 eligible women were enrolled for the comparison between Arm A: AC→T (n = 1,087) versus Arm B: AC→T→H (n = 1,097). Median follow-up was 5.5 years, with 386 events. Addition of trastuzumab sequentially to AC→T significantly improved disease-free survival (DFS), univariately (HR [Arm B/Arm A] = 0.70; 95% CI = 0.57–0.86, log rank *P* = .0005), and after adjusting for age, tumor size, number of positive nodes, and ER (PPH: HRadj = 0.67; 95% CI = 0.55–0.82). The 5-year DFS was increased from 72% with AC→T to 80% with AC→T →H. From May 2000 to April 2005, a total of 1,903 eligible women were enrolled for the Arm B (n = 954) versus Arm C: AC→T+H→H (n = 949) comparison; median follow-up is 5.3 years, with 312 events. The log-rank *P* value testing whether DFS differs with respect to starting time of trastuzumab was 0.019 (not crossing prespecified OFB for statistical significance). After adjusting for tumor size, number of positive nodes, and ER, HRadj (Arm C/Arm B) = 0.75 (95% CI = 0.60–0.94). The 5-year DFS was increased from 80% with AC→T→H to 84% for AC→T+H→H. In summary, DFS is significantly improved with the addition of 52 weeks of H (sequentially or concurrently) to AC→T. There is a statistically significant 33% reduction in the risk of an event with the sequential addition of H following AC→T. There is a strong trend for a 25% reduction in the risk of an event with starting H concurrently with T relative to sequentially after T. Therefore, based on a positive risk/benefit ratio, the investigators recommend that trastuzumab be incorporated in a concurrent fashion with T chemotherapy *(Perez EA et al: SABCS abstract 80, 2009).*

three treatment arms: (1) AC followed by T; (2) AC followed by TH (docetaxel + trastuzumab); or (3) TCH (docetaxel, carboplatin, trastuzumab).

For the second interim analysis, there were 192, 128, and 142 events in the three arms, respectively. The HR for disease-free survival for AC followed by TH vs AC followed by T was 0.61 (95% CI = 0.48–0.76; *P* < .0001); for TCH vs AC followed by T, it was 0.67 (95% CI = 0.54–0.83; *P* = .0003). The absolute disease-free survival benefits (from years 2 to 4) for AC followed by TH vs AC followed by T and for TCH vs AC followed by T were 6% and 5%, respectively. There was no statistically significant difference in disease-free survival between the two trastuzumab-containing arms. The HR for overall survival for AC followed by TH as compared with AC followed by T was 0.59 (95% CI = 0.42–0.85; *P* = .004), whereas that for TCH vs AC followed by T was 0.66 (95% CI = 0.47–0.93; *P* = .017). There was a statistically significant higher incidence of cardiac events in the arm using AC followed by TH (20 grade 3/4 events); this was not found in the arm using TCH (four grade 3/4 events) when compared with the group using AC followed by T (five grade 3/4 events). There was also a statistically significant higher incidence of asymptomatic declines in left ventricular ejection fraction with AC followed by TH in comparison with AC followed by T or TCH. Furthermore, four leukemias were seen in the anthacycline-based arms versus 0 in the TCH arm. Thus, the investigators concluded that in light of similar efficacy, global safety appears to favor the use of TCH.

There are unresolved questions about the adjuvant use of trastuzumab, including sequential versus concurrent use with chemotherapy, the optimal duration, and whether anthracyclines can be omitted. Furthermore, the long-term safety of trastuzumab in this setting remains to be determined.

Toxic effects of medical therapy

Chemotherapy

The most frequent acute toxicities are nausea/vomiting, alopecia, and hematologic side effects such as leukopenia and thrombocytopenia. Neutropenia, with its risk of infection, is a potentially life-threatening complication that requires prompt medical attention and broad-spectrum antibiotics until hematologic recovery occurs.

Other toxicities may include transient or permanent amenorrhea, infertility, early menopause, neuropathy, leukemia, allergic reactions, cystitis, stomatitis, and nail/skin changes. Amenorrhea is drug- and dose-related and is often permanent in women older than age 40. Recent evidence demonstrates that chemotherapy-induced ovarian failure in the adjuvant chemotherapy setting is associated with a high risk of rapid bone demineralization in the first 6 to 12 months after treatment. Thus, premenopausal women undergoing adjuvant chemotherapy must be closely evaluated to prevent the development of early osteoporosis. Cardiac failure, although rare, is potentially life-threatening and may be irreversible.

Endocrine therapy

Toxicities with tamoxifen or aromatase inhibitors include hot flashes, menstrual irregularities, vaginal discharge (tamoxifen), vaginal dryness (AIs), and weight gain. Thrombophlebitis and endometrial hyperplasia are more common with tamoxifen. Arthralgias, osteoporosis, and fractures are more common with aromatase inhibitors, although the incidence of hip fractures is low.

FOLLOW-UP OF LONG-TERM SURVIVORS

There is no consensus among oncologists as to the appropriate and optimal follow-up routine for long-term breast cancer survivors. Recommendations for follow-up testing vary. The vast majority of relapses, both locoregional and distant, occur within the first 3 years. Surveillance is most intensive in the initial 5 years; thereafter, the frequency of follow-up visits and testing is reduced (Table 2).

RECOMMENDATIONS

History and physical examination

Surveillance methods include a detailed history and physical examination at each office visit. They are performed every 4 to 6 months for 5 years after completion of initial therapy, then annually thereafter. Patients at higher risk of recurrence or complications of treatment may require surveillance at shorter intervals. Patients who have been treated by mastectomy can be seen in the office annually after they have been disease- free for 5 years. Patients who were treated with breast-conserving surgery and radiotherapy can be followed at 6-month intervals until they have been disease-free for 6 to 8 years and then annually.

Approximately 71% of breast cancer recurrences are detected by the patients themselves, and they will report a change in their symptoms when questioned carefully. In patients who are asymptomatic, physical examination will detect a recurrence in

TABLE 2: Follow-up recommendations for asymptomatic long-term breast cancer survivors as per NCCN guidelines

Intervention*	Year 1	Year 2	Years 3–5	Year 6+
History and physical exam	Every 4 mo	Every 4 mo	Every 6 mo	Annually
Mammography	Annually (or 6 mo after post BCS irradiation)	Annually	Annually	Annually
Chest x-ray	NRR	NRR	NRR	NRR
Pelvic exam[a]	Annually	Annually	Annually	Annually
Bone density[b]	Every 1 to 2 yr	Every 1 to 2 yr	Every 1 to 2 yr	Every 1 to 2 yr

NCCN = National Comprehensive Cancer Network; NRR = not routinely recommended; BCS = breast-conserving surgery

[a] For patients with an intact uterus on tamoxifen

[b] For patients at risk for osteoporosis

*Bone scan, liver function tests, and tumor markers are not routinely recommended and are performed only if clinically indicated.

another 15%. Therefore, a patient's complaint on history or a new finding on physical examination will lead to the detection of 86% of all recurrences.

Mammography

Mammography should be performed annually in all patients who have been treated for breast cancer. For patients who have undergone breast-conserving surgery, the first follow-up mammogram should be performed approximately 6 months after completion of radiation therapy. The risk of developing contralateral breast cancer is approximately 0.5% to 1.0% per year. In addition, approximately one-third of ipsilateral breast tumor recurrences in patients who have been treated by conservation surgery and radiotherapy are detected by mammography alone. As the time interval between the initial therapy and follow-up mammography increases, so does the likelihood that local breast recurrence will develop elsewhere in the breast rather than at the site of the initial primary lesion.

Chest x-ray

Routine chest radiographs detect between 2.3% and 19.5% of recurrences in asymptomatic patients and may be indicated on an annual basis.

Liver function tests

Liver function tests detect recurrences in relatively few asymptomatic patients, and their routine use has been questioned. However, these tests are relatively inexpensive, and it may not be unreasonable to obtain them annually.

Tumor markers

There is no evidence that tumor markers, such as carcinoembryonic assay, CA-15-3, and CA-57-29, provide an advantage in survival or palliation of recurrent disease in asymptomatic patients. Therefore, the use of tumor markers to follow long-term breast cancer survivors is not recommended.

Bone scans

Postoperative bone scans are also not recommended in asymptomatic patients. In the NSABP B-09 trial, in which bone scans were regularly performed, occult disease was identified in only 0.4% of patients.

Liver and brain imaging

Imaging studies of the liver and brain are not indicated in asymptomatic patients. Position emission tomography scans are not routinely recommended. Their utility is primarily as an adjunct study, often to establish the extent of metastatic disease.

Pelvic examinations

Women with intact uteri who are taking tamoxifen should have yearly pelvic examinations because of their risk of tamoxifen-associated endometrial carcinoma, especially among postmenopausal women. The vast majority of women with tamoxifen-associated uterine carcinoma have early vaginal spotting, and any vaginal spotting should prompt rapid evaluation. However, since neither endometrial biopsy nor ultrasonography has demonstrated utility as a screening test in any population of women, routine use of these tests in asymptomatic women is not recommended.

Bone density

Premenopausal women who become permanently amenorrheic from adjuvant chemotherapy and postmenopausal women who are treated with an aromatase inhibitor are at increased risk for bone fracture from osteopenia/osteoporosis. These patients should undergo monitoring of bone health every 1 to 2 years.

SUGGESTED READING

Clarke M, Collins R, Darby S, et al: Effects of radiotherapy and of differences in the extent of surgery for early breast cancer on local recurrence and 15-year survival: An overview of the randomised trials. Lancet 366:2087–2106, 2005.

Coates AS, Keshaviah A, Thurlimann B, et al: Five years of letrozole compared with tamoxifen as initial adjuvant therapy for postmenopausal women with endocrine-responsive early breast cancer: Update of study BIG 1-98. J Clin Oncol 25:486–492, 2007.

Coombes RC, Kilburn LS, Snowdon CF, et al: Survival and safety of exemestane versus tamoxifen after 2–3 years' tamoxifen treatment (Intergroup Exemestane Study): A randomised controlled trial. Lancet 369:559–570, 2007.

Gnant M, Mlineritsch B, Schippinger W, et al: Endocrine therapy plus zoledronic acid in premenopausal breast cancer. N Engl J Med 360:679–691, 2009.

Goldstein LJ, Gray R, Badve S, et al: Prognostic utility of the 21-gene assay in hormone receptor–positive operable breast cancer compared with classical clinicopathologic features. J Clin Oncol 26:4063–4061, 2008.

Goss PE, Ingle JN, Pater JL, et al: Late extended adjuvant treatment with letrozole improves outcome in women with early-stage breast cancer who complete 5 years of tamoxifen. J Clin Oncol 26:1948–1955, 2008.

Jones S, Holmes FA, O'Shaughnessy J, et al: Docetaxel with cyclophosphamide is associated with an overall survival benefit compared with doxorubicin and cyclophosphamide: 7-year follow-up of US Oncology Research Trial 9735. J Clin Oncol 27:1177–8311, 2009.

Kaufmann M, Jonat W, Hilfrich J, et al: Improved overall survival in postmenopausal women with early breast cancer after anastrozole initiated after treatment with tamoxifen compared with continued tamoxifen: The ARNO 95 Study. J Clin Oncol 25:2664–2670, 2007.

Martin M, Pienkowski T, Mackey J, et al: Breast Cancer International Research Group 001 Investigators: Adjuvant docetaxel for node-positive breast cancer. N Engl J Med 352:2302–2313, 2005.

Piccart-Gebhart MJ, Procter M, Leyland-Jones B, et al: Herceptin Adjuvant (HERA) Trial Study Team: Trastuzumab after adjuvant chemotherapy in HER2-positive breast cancer. N Engl J Med 353:1659–1672, 2005.

Pierce LJ, Hutchins LF, Green SR, et al: Sequencing of tamoxifen and radiotherapy after breast-conserving surgery in early-stage breast cancer. J Clin Oncol 23:24–29, 2005.

Romond EH, Perez EA, Bryant J, et al: Trastuzumab plus adjuvant chemotherapy for operable HER2-positive breast cancer. N Engl J Med 353:1673–1684, 2005.

Sparano JA, Wang M, Martino S, et al: Weekly paclitaxel in the adjuvant treatment of breast cancer. N Engl J Med 358:1663–1671, 2008.

Winer EP, Hudis C, Burstein HJ, et al: American Society of Clinical Oncology technology assessment on the use of aromatase inhibitors as adjuvant therapy for postmenopausal women with hormone receptor-positive breast cancer: Status report. J Clin Oncol 23:619–629, 2005.

Abbreviations in this chapter

ABCSG = Austrian Breast and Colorectal Cancer Study Group; ARNO = Arimidex–Nolvadex; ASCO = American Society of Clinical Oncology; ATAC = Arimidex, Tamoxifen, Alone or in Combination; ATLAS = Adjuvant Tamoxifen: Longer Against Shorter; BCIRG = Breast Cancer International Research Group; BIG = Breast International Group; CALGB = Cancer and Leukemia Group B; EBCTCG = Early Breast Cancer Trialists Collaborative Group; FDA = US Food and Drug Administration; HERA = Herceptin Adjuvant; IBIS-II = International Breast Cancer Intervention Study-II; IES = Intergroup Exemestane Study; ITA = Italian Tamoxifen Arimidex; NCCN = National Comprehensive Cancer Network; NCCTG = North Central Cancer Treatment Group; NCI = National Cancer Institute; NCIC = National Cancer Institute of Canada; NSABP = National Surgical Adjuvant Breast and Bowel Project; NYHA = New York Heart Association; PERCHE = Premenopausal Endocrine Responsive Chemotherapy; SOFT = Suppression of Ovarian Function Trial; TEXT = Tamoxifen and Exemestane Trial; ZEBRA = Zoladex Early Breast Cancer Research Association; Z-FAST = Zometa–Femara Adjuvant Synergy Trial

CHAPTER 8

Stages III and IV breast cancer

Lori Jardines, MD, Sharad Goyal, MD, Melanie Royce, MD, PhD, Ishmael Jaiyesimi, DO, and Shari B. Goldfarb, MD

This chapter addresses the diagnosis and management of locally advanced, locally recurrent, and metastatic breast cancer, that is, stages III and IV disease.

Approximately 20% to 25% of patients present with locally advanced breast cancer. Inflammatory breast cancer is a particularly aggressive form of breast cancer that falls under the heading of locally advanced disease and accounts for 1% to 3% of all breast cancers.

Locoregional recurrence of breast cancer remains a major oncologic problem. Rates of locoregional recurrence may vary from < 10% to > 50%, depending on initial disease stage and treatment.

Metastatic disease is found at presentation in 5% to 10% of patients with breast cancer. The most common sites of distant metastasis are the lungs, liver, lymph nodes, and bone.

The optimal therapy for stage III breast cancer continues to change. The use of neoadjuvant chemotherapy has been effective in downstaging locally advanced breast cancer prior to surgical intervention. The optimal neoadjuvant chemotherapeutic regimens continue to evolve, and studies are currently being performed to evaluate new agents and delivery methods.

DIAGNOSIS

LOCALLY ADVANCED DISEASE

Patients with locally advanced breast cancer do not have distant metastatic disease; they are categorized in this group based on tumor size and/or nodal status. Such patients often present with a large breast mass or axillary nodal disease that is easily palpable on physical examination. In some instances, the breast is diffusely infiltrated with disease, and no dominant mass is evident.

Patients with inflammatory breast cancer often present with erythema and edema of the skin of the breast (peau d'orange); they may not have a discrete mass within the breast. These patients often are treated with antibiotics unsuccessfully for presumed mastitis before they are diagnosed with breast cancer.

Mammography

Mammography is beneficial in determining the local extent of disease in the ipsilateral breast, and in studying the contralateral breast.

Fine-needle aspiration (FNA) or biopsy

In the locally advanced setting, although breast cancer can be confirmed by either FNA cytology or core biopsy, the latter is preferred. Core biopsy provides more sufficient tissue to perform the wide variety of marker analyses. When suspecting inflammatory breast carcinoma, a skin biopsy is also recommended to ascertain the presence of dermal lymphatic invasion.

Search for metastasis

The presence of distant metastatic disease should be ruled out by physical examination, chest x-ray, bone scan, and CT of the chest, abdomen, and pelvis. [18] Fluorodeoxyglucose-positron emission tomography (FDG-PET) has moderate accuracy for detecting axillary metastasis. It is highly predictive for nodal tumor involvement when multiple intense foci of tracer uptake are identified, but it fails to detect small nodal metastasis. However, the addition of FDG-PET to the standard workup of patients with locally advanced breast cancer may lead to the detection of unexpected distant metastases. Abnormal PET findings should be confirmed to prevent patients from being denied appropriate treatment.

LOCOREGIONAL RECURRENCE

Biopsy or FNA

Locoregional recurrence of breast cancer can be diagnosed by surgical biopsy or FNA cytology. The biopsy specimen should be sent for hormone-receptor studies, and testing for HER2/*neu* overexpression, since since these biomarkers are not always concordant between the primary tumor and recurrence. Discrepancy rates ranging from 17% to 55% have been reported. When the suspected recurrent disease is not extensive, the biopsy procedure of choice is a negative margin excisional biopsy. For an extensive recurrence, an incisional biopsy can be used.

Search for distant metastasis

Prior to beginning a treatment regimen for a patient with locoregional recurrence, an evaluation for distant metastasis should be performed, since the findings may alter the treatment plan.

DISTANT METASTASIS FROM THE BREASTS

Metastatic breast cancer may be manifested by bone pain, shortness of breath secondary to a pleural effusion or lymphangitic spread, pleural or pulmonary nodules, or neurologic deficits secondary to spinal cord compression or brain metastases. In some instances, metastatic disease is identified after abnormalities are found on routine laboratory or radiologic studies.

Assessment of disease extent

It is important to assess the extent of disease using radiography, CT, and radionuclide scanning. Organ functional impairment may be determined by blood tests (liver/renal/hematologic) or may require cardiac and pulmonary function testing. A biopsy should be highly encouraged to confirm the diagnosis of metastatic disease; this is especially important when only a single distant lesion is identified.

METASTASIS TO THE BREASTS

The most common source of metastatic disease to the breasts is a contralateral breast primary. Metastasis from a nonbreast primary is rare, representing < 1.5% of all breast malignancies. Some malignancies that can metastasize to the breast include non-Hodgkin lymphoma, leukemias, melanoma, lung cancer (particularly small-cell lung cancer), gynecologic cancers, soft-tissue sarcomas, and gastrointestinal (GI) adenocarcinomas. Metastasis to the breasts from a nonbreast primary is more common in younger women. The average age at diagnosis ranges from the late 30s to 40s. Treatment depends on the status and location of the primary site.

Mammographic findings

Mammography in patients with metastatic disease to the breasts most commonly reveals a single lesion or multiple masses with distinct or semidiscrete borders. Less common mammographic findings include skin thickening or axillary adenopathy.

FNA or biopsy

FNA cytology has been extremely useful in establishing the diagnosis when the metastatic disease has cytologic features that are not consistent with a breast primary. When cytology is not helpful, core biopsy or even open biopsy may be necessary to distinguish primary breast cancer from metastatic disease.

TREATMENT

LOCALLY ADVANCED DISEASE

The optimal treatment for patients with locally advanced breast cancer has yet to be defined due to the heterogeneity of this group. There are approximately 40 different substage possibilities with the different combinations of tumor size and nodal status. Between 66% and 90% of patients with stage III breast cancer will have positive lymph nodes at the time of axillary dissection, and approximately 50% of patients will have four or more positive nodes.

Patients with locally advanced breast cancer have disease-free survival rates ranging from 0% to 60%, depending on tumor characteristics and nodal status. In general, the most frequent type of treatment failure is due to distant metastases, and the majority of them appear within 2 years of diagnosis. With the increased utilization of multimodality therapy, including chemotherapy, radiation therapy, and surgery, survival for this patient population has improved significantly.

TABLE 1: Doses and schedules of chemotherapy agents commonly used in patients with metastatic breast cancer

Drug/combination	Dose and schedule
FAC	
5-FU	500 mg/m² IV on days 1 and 8
Adriamycin (doxorubicin)	50 mg/m² IV on day 1
Cyclophosphamide	500 mg/m² IV on day 1
Repeat cycle every 3-4 weeks.	
TAC	
Taxotere (docetaxel)	75 mg/m² IV on day 1
Adriamycin (doxorubicin)	50 mg/m² IV on day 1
Cyclophosphamide	500 mg/m² IV on day 1
Repeat cycle every 21 days.	
FEC	
5-FU	500 mg/m² IV on day 1
Epirubicin	75 mg/m² IV on day 1
Cyclophosphamide	500 mg/m² IV on day 1
Repeat cycle every 21 days.	
Note: An absolute granulocyte count < 1,500/µL and/or platelet count < 100,000/µL on day 21 will cause a treatment delay of at least 1 week. Treatment wil be terminated if hematologic recovery takes more than 3 weeks.	
Paclitaxel	175 mg/m² by 3-h IV infusion every 3 weeks or 80 – 100 mg/m²/week
Docetaxel	60 – 100 mg/m² by 1-h IV infusion every 3 weeks or 40 mg/m²/week
Repeat if hematologic recovery has occurred (ie, absolute granulocyte count ≥ 1,500/µL and platelet count ≥ 100,000/µL).	
Capecitabine	1,000 – 1,250 mg/m² PO BID (divided dose, am and pm) for 14 days, followed by 1 week rest
Repeat cycle every 21 days.	
Capecitabine + docetaxel	
Capecitabine	2,000 – 2,500 mg/m² PO BID (divided dose, am and pm) for 14 days, followed by 1 week rest
Docetaxel	75 mg/m² IV infusion over 1 hour
Repeat cycle every 3 weeks.	
Vinorelbine + trastuzumab	
Vinorelbine	25 mg/m² IV on day 1 every week
Trastuzumab	4 mg/kg IV loading dose, then 2 mg/kg IV every week
Lapatinib and trastuzumab for ErbB2-overexpressing metastatic breast cancer	
Lapatinib	1,000 mg/d PO daily
Trastuzumab	4 mg/kg IV loading dose, then 2 mg/kg IV every week or 8 mg/kg IV loading dose, then 6 mg/kg IV every 3 weeks
Lapatinib and pazopanib for ErbB2-overexpressing metastatic breast cancer	
Lapatinib	1,000 mg/d PO
Pazopanib	400 mg/d PO

Drug/combination	Dose and schedule
Docetaxel or paclitaxel + carboplatin + trastuzumab (every-3-week dosing)	
Docetaxel	75 mg/m² IV on day 1 every 21 days *or*
Paclitaxel	175 mg/m² IV on day 1 every 21 days *plus*
Carboplatin	AUC of 5 – 6 on day 1 every 21 days *plus*
Trastuzumab	4 mg/kg IV loading dose on day 1, followed by 2 mg/kg weekly
Note: Patients must be premedicated with dexamethasone prior to docetaxel.	
Trastuzumab	4 mg/kg IV loading dose, then 2 mg/kg weekly or 8 mg/kg IV loading dose, then 6 mg/kg every 3 weeks
Paclitaxel or docetaxel + carboplatin + trastuzumab (weekly dosing)	
Paclitaxel	80 mg/m² IV on day 1 every week *or*
Docetaxel	35 mg/m² IV on day 1 every week *plus*
Carboplatin	AUC of 2 IV on day 1 every week *plus*
Trastuzumab	4 mg/kg IV loading dose, then 2 mg/kg every week
Gemcitabine + paclitaxel	
Gemcitabine	1,250 mg/m² IV on days 1 and 8 (as a 30-minute infusion) every 21 days (on day 1, given following paclitaxel)
Paclitaxel	175 mg/m² IV on day 1 (over 3 hours) every 21 days
Note: Standard paclitaxel premedications should be given.	
Pegylated doxorubicin (Doxil)	30 to 50 mg/m² IV on day 1 every 21 to 28 days
Nab-paclitaxel (Abraxane)	260 mg/m² IV on day 1 every 2 weeks 3 weeks or 100 to 150 mg/m2 on day 1, 8, and 15 IV followed by 1 week rest
Ixabepilone plus capecitabine	
Ixabepilone	40 mg IV over 3 hours on day 1 of 21-day cycle
Capecitabine	2,000 mg/m² orally (divided doses, BID) on days 1 to 14 followed by 1 week rest
Lapatinib plus capecitabine	
Lapatinib	1,250 mg/d PO
Capecitabine	2,000 mg/m²/PO (divided doses, BID) days 1 – 14, followed by 1 week rest
Repeat cycle every 21 days.	
Paclitaxel plus bevacizumab	
Paclitaxel	90 mg/m² IVPB on days 1, 8, and 15 of a 28-day schedule
Bevacizumab	10 mg/kg IV on day 1 and on day 15 of a 28-day schedule

AUC = area under the curve; IVPB = intravenous piggyback

Neoadjuvant systemic therapy

Neoadjuvant chemotherapy is administered prior to surgery and has the same impact on disease-free and overall survival as adjuvant chemotherapy. Neoadjuvant therapy with cytotoxic drugs permits in vivo chemosensitivity testing, can downstage locally advanced disease and render it operable, and may allow breast-conservation surgery to be performed. Preoperative chemotherapy requires a coordinated multidisciplinary approach to plan for surgical and radiation therapy. A multimodality treatment approach can provide improved control of locoregional and systemic disease. When neoadjuvant therapy is used, accurate pathologic staging is not possible. The majority of patients receiving neoadjuvant chemotherapy and treated with either breast conservation or mastectomy will require radiation therapy following surgery.

Active regimens

Preoperative chemotherapy regimens reported to result in high clinical response rates include anthracycline-containing regimens followed by a taxane (or vice versa). The most common anthracycline-containing regimens used are CAF (cyclophosphamide, doxorubicin [Adriamycin], and fluorouracil [5-FU]), FAC (5-FU, Adriamycin, and cyclophosphamide), or FEC (5-FU, epirubicin, cyclophosphamide); while the most common taxane regimens used are either weekly paclitaxel or every-3-week docetaxel (Table 1). Administration of TAC (docetaxel [Taxotere], Adriamycin [doxorubicin] and cyclophosphamide) or AT or may produce equivalently high response rates. Although not yet definitive, recent data indicate that enhancing dose density may increase the pathologic complete response rate for women with locally advanced disease. The doses of these combination chemotherapy regimens are given in Table 1, chapter 7.

There seems to be no difference in survival in women with locally advanced disease who receive chemotherapy before or after surgery. Neoadjuvant chemotherapy results in complete clinical response rates ranging from 20% to 53% and partial response rates (≥ 50% reduction in bidimensionally measurable disease) ranging from 37% to 50%, with total response rates ranging from 80% to 90%. Patients with large lesions are more likely to have partial responses. Pathologic complete responses (pCRs) do occur and are more likely to be seen in patients with smaller tumors that are triple negative or overexpress HER2/*neu*. A pCR in the primary tumor is often predictive of a complete axillary lymph node response. Patients with locally advanced breast cancer who have a pCR in the breast and axillary nodes have a significantly improved disease-free survival compared with those who have less than a pCR. However, a pCR does not eliminate the risk for recurrence.

Patients should be followed carefully while receiving neoadjuvant systemic therapy to determine treatment response. In addition to clinical examination, it may also be helpful to document photographically the response of ulcerated, erythematous, indurated skin lesions. Physical examination, mammography, and breast ultrasonography are best for assessing primary tumor response, whereas physical examination and ultrasonography are used to evaluate regional nodal involvement.

The role of MRI in evaluating response to preoperative chemotherapy is still evolving. Dynamic contrast-enhanced MRI performed at baseline, during chemotherapy, and before surgery has yielded more than 90% diagnostic accuracy in identifying tumors achieving a pCR and can potentially provide functional parameters that may help to optimize neoadjuvant chemotherapy strategies. However, despite its high sensitivity, a large number of patients still may have either false-negative or false-positive results on MRI scanning.

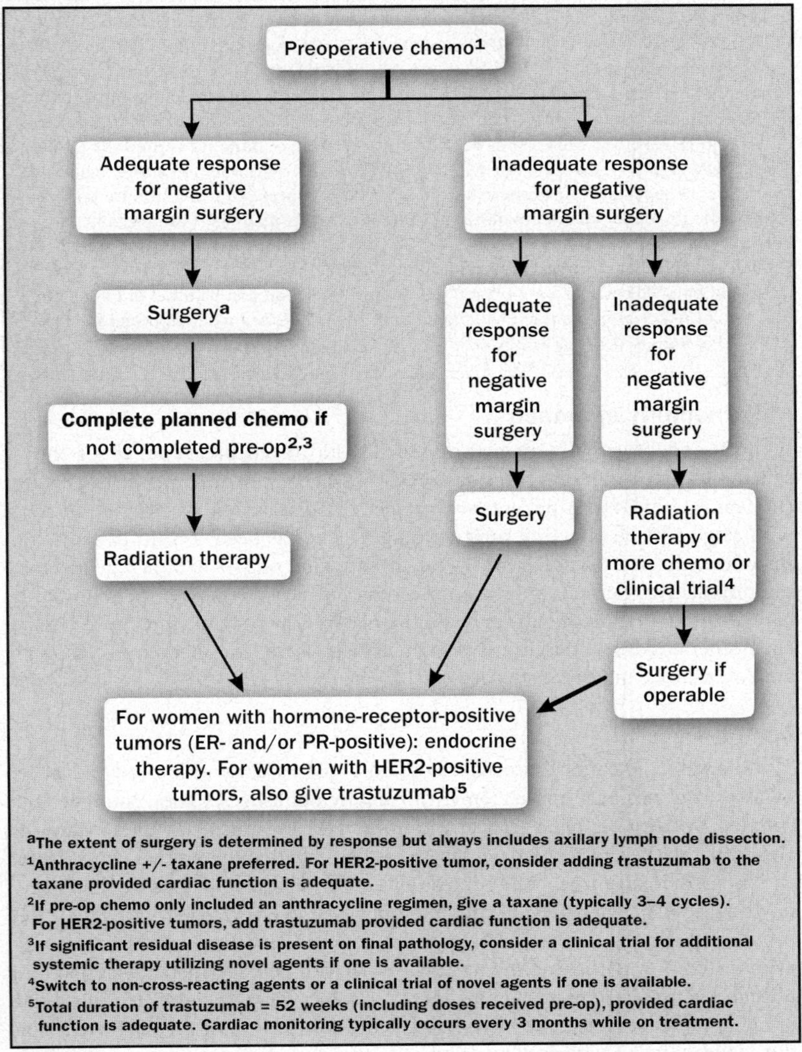

[a]The extent of surgery is determined by response but always includes axillary lymph node dissection.

[1]Anthracycline +/- taxane preferred. For HER2-positive tumor, consider adding trastuzumab to the taxane provided cardiac function is adequate.

[2]If pre-op chemo only included an anthracycline regimen, give a taxane (typically 3–4 cycles). For HER2-positive tumors, add trastuzumab provided cardiac function is adequate.

[3]If significant residual disease is present on final pathology, consider a clinical trial for additional systemic therapy utilizing novel agents if one is available.

[4]Switch to non-cross-reacting agents or a clinical trial of novel agents if one is available.

[5]Total duration of trastuzumab = 52 weeks (including doses received pre-op), provided cardiac function is adequate. Cardiac monitoring typically occurs every 3 months while on treatment.

FIGURE 1: Multimodality approach to locally advanced breast cancer FAC = 5-FU, Adriamycin, and cyclophosphamide; ER = estrogen receptor; PR = progesterone receptor.

Response to neoadjuvant chemotherapy has been shown to be prognostic in breast cancer. In order to improve the prognostic information that can be obtained from evaluating pathologic response after neoadjuvant chemotherapy, Symmans et al developed the residual cancer burden (RCB) method of measuring residual disease. Pathologic slides and reports from 382 patients were reviewed in two different treatment cohorts: paclitaxel followed by FAC (n = 241) and FAC alone (n = 141). RCB was calculated as a continuous index combining pathologic measurements of primary tumor (size and cellularity) and nodal metastases (number and size) for prediction of distant relapse-free survival (DRFS) in multivariate Cox regression analyses. RCB was independently prognostic in a multivariate model that included age, pretreatment clinical stage, hormone receptor status, hormone therapy, and pathologic response (pathologic complete response [pCR] versus residual disease [RD]; hazard ratio = 2.50; 95% CI = 1.70 to 3.69; *P* < .001). Minimal RD (RCB-I) in 17% of patients carried the same prognosis as pCR (RCB-0). Extensive RD (RCB-III) in 13% of patients was associated with poor prognosis, regardless of hormone receptor status, adjuvant hormone therapy, or pathologic stage of residual disease. The generalizability of RCB for prognosis of distant relapse was confirmed in the FAC-treated validation cohort. The investigators concluded that RCB determined from routine pathologic materials represented the distribution of RD, was a significant predictor of DRFS, and can be used to define categories of near-complete response and chemotherapy resistance (*Symmans WF et al: J Clin Oncol 25:4414–4422, 2007*).

Multimodality approach

A multimodality treatment plan for locally advanced breast cancer is shown schematically in Figure 1. This approach has been shown to result in a 5-year survival rate of 84% in patients with stage IIIA disease and a 44% rate in those with stage IIIB disease. The most striking benefit has been seen in patients with inflammatory breast cancer, with 5-year survival rates of 35% to 50% reported for a multimodality treatment approach including primary chemotherapy followed by surgery and radiation therapy and additional adjuvant systemic therapy. The same chemotherapy drugs, doses, and schedules used for single-modality therapy are employed in the multimodality approach.

Surgery

Traditionally, the surgical procedure of choice for patients with locally advanced breast cancer has been mastectomy. In recently published studies, some patients with locally advanced breast cancer who responded to treatment with neoadjuvant chemotherapy became candidates for breast-conservation therapy and were treated with limited breast surgery and adjuvant breast irradiation. Patients who have been downstaged using neoadjuvant chemotherapy should be evaluated carefully before proceeding with conservative treatment. It may be helpful to mark the site of the primary tumor with the placement of a clip during the course of percutaneous biopsy prior to beginning adjuvant therapy. There can sometimes be a complete clinical and/or radiographic response after neoadjuvant chemotherapy or hormonal therapy, and this may facilitate a wide local incision.

The role of sentinel node biopsy in the treatment of breast cancer after neoadjuvant chemotherapy has yet to be defined. Pathologically positive axillary lymph nodes can be sterilized when neoadjuvant chemotherapy is utilized. There are other biologic concerns with sentinel node biopsy after neoadjuvant chemotherapy. The lymphatics may undergo fibrosis or may become obstructed by cellular debris, making the mapping procedure unreliable, with false-negative rates of up to 25%. The rate of conversion from positive to negative nodes can be enhanced when 4 cycles of a doxorubicin-based regimen are followed by 4 cycles of paclitaxel (Taxol) or docetaxel (Taxotere). Sentinel lymph node biopsy will only be accurate if all the metastatic deposits within the axilla respond in a similar fashion to chemotherapy. Preliminary data from the NSABP B-27 trial demonstrated an 11% false-negative rate in women who underwent sentinel node biopsy after receiving 4 cycles of doxorubicin and cyclophosphamide followed by 4 cycles of docetaxel. However, patients with clinically positive nodes prior to neoadjuvant chemotherapy should have a full lymph node dissection.

Radiation therapy

Radiotherapy remains an integral component of the management of patients with locally advanced breast cancer. For patients with operable breast cancer undergoing mastectomy, radiation therapy to the chest wall and/or regional lymph nodes (to a total dose of 5,000–6,000 cGy) is usually employed, as discussed in chapter 7. Randomized trials suggest that postmastectomy patients with any number of positive nodes derive a disease-free and/or overall survival benefit from postmastectomy irradiation.

In a retrospective review, over 500 patients on six prospective trials treated with neoadjuvant chemotherapy, mastectomy, and radiation were compared with 134 patients treated with the same chemotherapy and mastectomy, but no radiation. Despite the more unfavorable characteristics, the radiated patients had a lower rate of local-regional relapse than did the unirradiated group (11% vs 22%). Patients who presented with clinically advanced stage III or IV disease but subsequently achieved a pathologic complete response to neoadjuvant chemotherapy still had a high rate of locoregional response, which was significantly reduced with radiation (10-year rates: 33% vs 3%; $P = .006$). Radiation improved cause-specific survival in the subsets of patients with stage IIIB disease, clinical T4 tumors, and ≥ 4 positive nodes. The authors concluded that radiation should be considered for these patients regardless of their response to initial chemotherapy.

Available data do not suggest a problem in delaying radiation therapy until the completion of systemic chemotherapy. Even in patients undergoing high-dose chemotherapy with autologous bone marrow or stem-cell transplantation, irradiation is generally indicated following mastectomy for patients with locally advanced disease (primary tumors ≥ 5 cm and/or ≥ four positive axillary nodes).

For patients whose disease is considered to be inoperable, radiation therapy may be integrated into the management plan prior to surgery.

High-dose chemotherapy

To date, available clinical trials investigating the role of adjuvant high-dose chemotherapy (HDC) with autologous stem cell transplant in breast cancer have not shown superiority in disease-free or overall survival over conventional adjuvant chemotherapy. Furthermore, in some HDC trials, study design, power, and strategy have been questioned. Thus, currently HDC cannot be recommended for patients with primary or metastatic breast cancer outside the context of a clinical trial.

LOCOREGIONAL RECURRENCE AFTER EARLY-STAGE OR EARLY INVASIVE BREAST CANCER

When a patient develops a local failure after breast-conservation treatment for early invasive cancer or ductal carcinoma in situ (DCIS), it is generally in the region of the initial primary tumor. The risk of ipsilateral breast tumor recurrence after conservative treatment in patients with early invasive cancer ranges from 0.5% to 2.0% per year, with long-term local failure rates that plateau at 15% to 20%. Local failure rates after wide excision alone for DCIS vary from 10% to 63%, as compared with rates between 7% and 21% after wide excision plus radiation therapy. Most patients whose disease recurs after conservative treatment for DCIS can be treated with salvage mastectomy. In one study, 14% of patients who developed local recurrence had synchronous distant metastatic disease.

The optimal treatment of a local or regional recurrence after mastectomy has yet to be defined. Locoregional recurrences are associated with initial nodal status and primary tumor size. Appropriate treatment may result in long-term control of locoregional disease. In many instances, these patients develop simultaneous distant metastasis, or distant disease develops some time after the locoregional recurrence manifests itself.

Recurrence of invasive cancer after breast conservation

After wide excision and breast irradiation

For patients with early invasive cancer who have undergone conservative surgery followed by irradiation and whose cancer recurs in the ipsilateral breast, salvage mastectomy is the most common treatment modality. The same is true for ipsilateral recurrence (of invasive or in situ disease) after conservative treatment for DCIS, when there is no evidence of distant metastatic disease.

Some studies with limited follow-up have reported acceptable results with repeated wide local excision for ipsilateral breast tumor relapses following conservative surgery and radiation therapy. Selection criteria for this approach are unclear, however, and use of this salvage procedure remains controversial. Although the use of limited-field reirradiation has been reported, selection criteria for this management option and long-term follow-up data are lacking.

After wide excision alone

In patients initially treated with wide local excision alone who sustain an ipsilateral breast tumor recurrence, small series with limited follow-up suggest that wide local excision followed by radiation therapy to the intact breast at the time of local recurrence may be a reasonable treatment alternative. In this situation, standard radiation doses would be employed.

Recurrent disease in the chest wall after mastectomy

When possible, disease recurring in the chest wall or axillary nodes should be resected and radiation therapy should be considered to aid in local control. Patients should be also evaluated for adjuvant chemotherapy.

Radiation treatment techniques are generally similar to those employed for patients treated with standard postmastectomy irradiation and consist of photon- and/or electron-beam arrangements directed at the chest wall and adjacent lymph node regions. Treatment planning should strive for homogeneous dose distributions to the target areas while minimizing the dose to the underlying cardiac and pulmonary structures.

Radiation dose and protocol

Conventional fractionation of 180 to 200 cGy/d to the area of locoregional recurrence and immediately adjacent areas at risk, to a total dose of 4,500 to 5,000 cGy, is indicated. A boost to the area of recurrence or gross residual disease, to a dose of approximately 6,000 cGy, results in acceptable long-term locoregional control.

Radical chest wall resection

A select group of patients with local chest wall recurrence secondary to breast cancer may be candidates for a radical chest wall resection, which may include resection of skin, soft tissue, and bone. Flap coverage or prosthetic chest wall reconstruction is required. Appropriate candidates would include patients who do not have distant metastases and who have persistent or recurrent chest wall disease after chest wall irradiation and those who present with a chest wall recurrence after a long disease-free interval.

Adjuvant systemic therapy

Ipsilateral breast tumor recurrence

Limited data support the use of adjuvant systemic therapy at the time of ipsilateral breast tumor recurrence. Retrospective studies have suggested a 20% to 50% risk of systemic metastases in patients who sustain an ipsilateral breast tumor recurrence. A study conducted at Yale University found that ipsilateral breast tumor recurrence was a significant predictor of distant metastases, particularly among women who relapsed within 4 years of the original diagnosis; these women had a rate of distant metastasis of approximately 50%. Similar findings were noted by the NSABP investigators.

These data suggest that women whose tumors recur in the ipsilateral breast within the first few years following the original diagnosis may be considered for adjuvant systemic therapy. Given the lack of prospective, randomized data, specific treatment recommendations for these women remain highly individualized.

Regional nodal recurrence and postmastectomy recurrence in the chest wall

Although there are limited data addressing the use of adjuvant systemic therapy at the time of locoregional relapse following mastectomy, given the high rate of systemic metastasis in this population, these patients may be considered for adjuvant systemic therapy. A randomized trial demonstrated a disease-free survival benefit with the use of adjuvant tamoxifen following radiation therapy at the time of postmastectomy recurrence in the chest wall in patients with estrogen receptor–positive tumors. The 5-year disease-free survival was increased from 36% to 59%, and the median disease-free survival was prolonged by > 4.5 years.

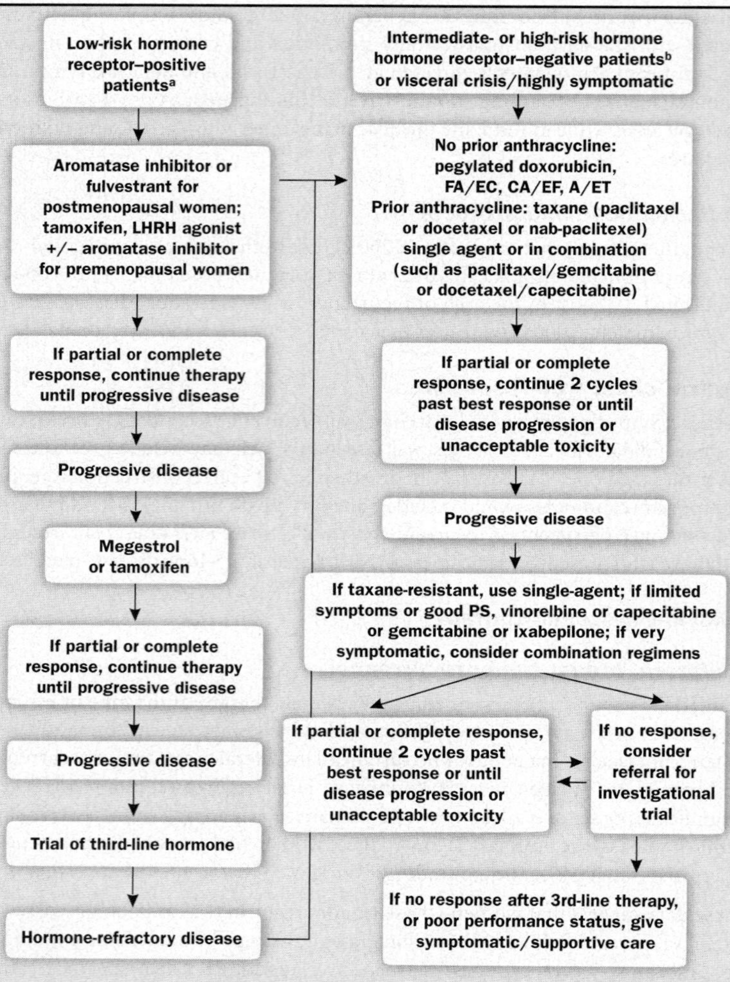

[a]Low-risk patients include those with a long disease-free interval, tumors that are positive for hormone receptors (estrogen and progesterone), or bone-only disease, as well as those without extensive visceral involvement.

[b]Intermediate- or high-risk patients include those with rapidly progressive disease, visceral involvement, hormone-refractory disease, or tumors that are negative for hormone receptors.

Patients with HER2-positive tumors: Add anti-HER2 therapy to chemotherapy (see Table 1 for acceptable regimens). Patients who have not received trastuzumab in the adjuvant setting typically get trastuzumab regimen as their 1st-line and lapatinib regimen as their 2nd-line anti-HER2 therapy, respectively, usually in combination with chemotherapy. Alternatively, patients may participate in a clinical trial of novel anti-HER2 therapies.

Patients with triple-negative (ER-, PR-, HER2-) tumors, especially *BRCA* mutation carriers, may consider novel agents such as PARP inhibitors, typically in combination with chemotherapy.

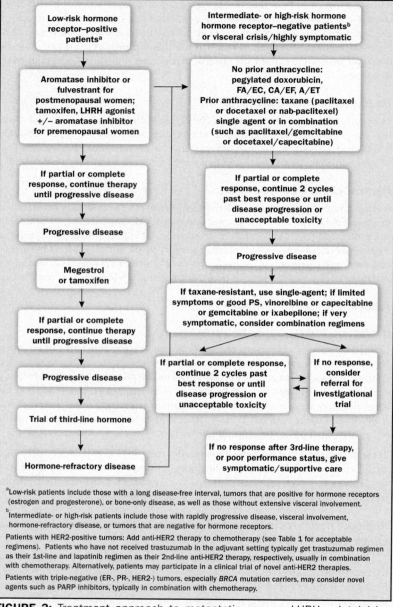

FIGURE 2: Treatment approach to metastatic cancer; LHRH = luteinizing hormone releasing hormone; FA = fluorouracil (5-FU) and Adriamycin (doxorubicin); EC = epirubicin and cyclophosphamide; CA = cyclophosphamide and Adriamycin (doxorubicin); EF = epirubicin and fluorouracil; A = adriamycin; ET = epirubicin and Taxol (paclitaxel).

Patients with estrogen receptor–negative tumors and aggressive locoregional recurrences may also be considered for systemic cytotoxic chemotherapy, given their relatively poor prognosis and the high rate of metastasis.

METASTATIC BREAST CANCER

Patients with metastatic cancer can be divided into two groups: those with stage IV disease at presentation and those who develop metastases after primary treatment. Biopsy is recommended for pathologic confirmation of presumed metastatic breast cancer. The management of stage IV disease depends on the site and extent of metastases, comorbid conditions, and clinical tumor characteristics.

Patients with delayed metastatic disease can be divided into two groups, that is, so-called low risk and intermediate or high risk, based on the biologic aggressiveness of the disease. As shown schematically in Figure 2, the management approach to these two groups differs.

Low-risk patients

The low-risk group includes patients who develop metastatic disease after a long disease-free interval (ie, a long disease-free interval from primary breast cancer diagnosis to presentation with metastasis), those whose tumors are positive for hormone receptors (estrogen and progesterone), those with bone-only disease, and those without extensive visceral organ involvement.

Hormone therapy

Low-risk patients who have hormone receptor–positive (ie, estrogen receptor–positive and/or progesterone receptor–positive) tumors should be treated with a trial of hormone therapy. Ovarian suppression, with either an LHRH agonist or bilateral oophorectomy, is an effective modality of hormone therapy in premenopausal women.

First-line hormonal therapy consists of an aromatase inhibitor or tamoxifen, with careful serial assessment of clinical and disease responses.

Hormone therapy may be associated with a "flare" response, a temporary worsening of signs and symptoms of disease within the first few weeks of treatment. This response generally means clinical benefit will follow.

If the tumor initially responds to first-line hormone therapy and then progresses, a second hormonal manipulation is warranted. Various hormonal agents are available (Table 2). They may be used sequentially and may provide disease palliation for prolonged periods of time in some patients.

Second-line hormonal agents The choice of second-line endocrine therapy depends on the front-line endocrine agent used. Typically, if tamoxifen was used, the second-line agent includes an aromatase inhibitor or fulvestrant (Faslodex) for postmenopausal women. For premenopausal women, the choice may be megestrol or induction of menopause with an LHRH (luteinizing hormone-releasing hormone) agonist with or without an aromatase inhibitor. If aromatase inhibitors were used as front-line agents for postmenopausal women, second-line options can be to change to another class of aromatase inhibitor, to fulvestrant, or to tamoxifen.

TABLE 2: Doses and schedules of hormonal agents commonly used in patients with metastatic breast cancer

Agent	Dose and schedule
Postmenopausal	
Tamoxifen	20 mg PO every day
or	
Toremifene (Fareston)	60 mg PO every day
Anastrozole	1 mg PO every day
or	
Letrozole	2.5 mg PO every day
or	
Exemestane	25 mg PO every day
Fulvestrant[a]	500 mg IM every month (A loading dose during the first month of therapy may be considered)
Megestrol	40 mg PO 4 times a day
Fluoxymesterone	10 mg PO 3 times a day
Aminoglutethimide	250 mg PO 4 times a day
Premenopausal	
Tamoxifen	20 mg PO every day
Luteinizing hormone-releasing hormone analogues	
Leuprolide	7.5 mg IM depot every 28 days 22.5 mg IM every 3 months 30 mg IM every 4 months
Goserelin	3.6 mg SC depot every 28 days 10.8 mg SC every 3 months
Megestrol	40 mg PO 4 times a day
Fluoxymesterone	10 mg PO 3 times a day

[a] The loading dose of fulvestrant is typically twice the maintenance dose at 500 mg given q2wks × 2.

EFECT was a randomized, double-blind, placebo-controlled, multicenter trial comparing the efficacy and tolerability of fulvestrant versus exemestane (Aromasin) in postmenopausal women with hormone receptor–positive advanced breast cancer following nonsteroidal aromatase inhibitor therapy. This was the first phase III trial to specifically evaluate endocrine therapeutic options following disease progression/recurrence occurring during nonsteroidal aromatase inhibitor therapy. A fulvestrant loading-dose regimen was utilized (via intramuscular injection): 500 mg on day 0, followed by 250 mg on days 14 and 28, and every 28 ± 3 days, thereafter. Exemestane was given as 25 mg capsule PO once daily. Treatment was administered until disease progression or death, or withdrawal for any other reason. This trial includes 693 women, ~60% of whom have received at least two prior endocrine therapies.

The FACT and CONFIRM trials investigated the role of endocrine therapy with fulvestrant in metastatic breast cancer. FACT was a multinational trial that enrolled women with ER(+) metastatic/recurrent breast cancer in the first-line setting. Patients were randomized to either anastrozole at 1-mg orally each day (control arm) or anastrozole plus fulvestrant at 500 mg on day 0, at 250 mg on days 14 and 28, and monthly thereafter. The primary endpoint was time to progression (TTP); 258 women were enrolled in the fulvestrant plus anastrozole group and 256 were in the anastrozole-alone group. The study found no significant differences between the treatment groups with respect to the number or percentage with progression or the median TTP or overall survival (37.8 months vs 38.2 months, respectively; hazard ratio [HR] = 1.00; 95% CI = 0.76–1.32; *P* = 1.00). Receptor status, visceral involvement, age, and measurable disease were not associated with a greater benefit with combination therapy *(Bergh J et al: SABCS 2009, abstract 23)*. CONFIRM (COmparisoN of Faslodex In Recurrent or Metastatic breast cancer) is a randomized, double-blind, parallel-group, multicenter, phase III trial in postmenopausal women with HER-positive advanced disease. Patients were randomized to fulvestrant at 500 mg IM (two injections, 250-mg each) on days 1, 14, and 28, and every 28 days thereafter versus fulvestrant at 250 mg IM plus placebo IM on days 1 and 28 and every 28 days thereafter (two injections per visit), with two placebo injections on day 14 (control arm). The ITT analysis showed that the percentages with progression were similar between the dosage groups (82% vs 85.8%), with a median TTP of 6.5 months with the 500-mg dose versus 5.5 months in those given the 250-mg dose (HR = 0.80; 95% CI = 0.68–0.94; *P* = .006). Median TTP was higher with the 500-mg dose; however, there were no significant differences between the groups in the secondary endpoints. The investigators are performing an exploratory substudy to identify cohorts with different levels of responsiveness to fulvestrant dose escalation *(Di Leo A et al: SABCS 2009, abstract 25)*. Clinical efficacies in premenopausal MBC patients with combined letrozole and goserelin therapy were comparable to those in postmenopausal patients treated with letrozole alone. In a study of 73 patients with hormone-responsive MBC, 35 premenopausal patients received goserelin (3.6-mg subcutaneously every 28 days) plus letrozole (2.5-mg orally daily), and 38 postmenopausal patients received letrozole alone as their first-line endocrine therapy in a metastatic setting. Baseline characteristics were similar in the two groups, except for a younger age (median, 41 vs 53.5 years; *P* < .001) and a shorter disease-free interval (median, 1.8 vs 3.3 years; *P* = .03) in the premenopausal group. Clinical benefit rates were comparable between the two groups (77% vs 74%; P = .77). At the median follow-up of 27.4 months, there was no statistical difference in the median TTP between the two groups (9.5 months [95% CI = 6.4–12.1 months] vs 8.9 months [95% CI = 6.4–13.3 months]). In patients who did not receive bisphosphonate, letrozole with or without goserelin caused a greater loss of bone mineral density at 6 months compared with that of patients receiving bisphosphonate treatment (premenopausal group, −16.7% vs 53.9%, *P* = .002; and postmenopausal group, −13.3% vs 17.4%, *P* = .04 at the lumbar spine). Although letrozole +/− goserelin resulted in a modest increase in bone resorption, concurrent treatment with bisphosphonate could prevent bone loss at 6 months *(Park IH et al: J Clin Oncol 28:2705–2711, 2010)*.

In the primary analysis (median follow-up of 13 months), the median time to disease progression was 3.7 months in both the fulvestrant and exemestane groups (HR = 0.963; 95% confidence interval [CI] = 0.819–1.133; *P* = .06531). Objective response and clinical benefit rates were also similar between groups, although the median duration of response (n = 38; from randomization: 13.5 months vs 9.8 months) and clinical benefit (n = 172; 9.3 months vs 8.3 months) appeared slightly longer in patients receiving fulvestrant. Overall survival data were immature at the time of the primary analysis. However, in a recent update with a median follow-up of 20.9 months, 209 patients (59.5%) in the fulvestrant group and 197 patients (57.9%) in the exemestane group had died. Median overall survival was not significantly different between treatments (24.3 months vs 23.1 months in the fulvestrant and exemestane groups, respectively [HR = 1.012; 95% CI = 0.833–1.229; *P* = .9072]).

The most commonly used second-line hormonal agents had been progestational drugs, such as megestrol. Recent randomized trials have indicated that that fulvestrant or the aromatase inhibitors, such as anastrozole (Arimidex), letrozole (Femara) and exemestane (Aromasin), are equally effective for palliation of metastatic disease, have less toxicity, and may provide a survival advantage compared with megestrol. Therefore, they are the drugs of choice for second-line therapy following tamoxifen administration. Tamoxifen may also be considered as second-line therapy for patients initially treated with an aromatase inhibitor.

Hormonal therapy continues until evidence of disease progression or drug-related toxicity precludes further therapy with the same agent. If a partial or complete response to the first hormonal treatment is documented at the time of disease progression, a second hormonal agent may provide further palliation of symptoms and avoid the initiation of systemic chemotherapy. However, subsequent hormonal responses tend to be of shorter duration, and, ultimately, the disease will become refractory to hormonal treatment.

Cytotoxic agents

Hormone-refractory disease should be treated with systemic cytotoxic therapy. Often sequential single-agent treatment regimens are administered. Patients should stay on each therapy until they either have progression of disease or too much toxicity from it. Chemotherapeutic doses and schedules, including those for combination regimens commonly used for metastatic breast cancer, are outlined in Table 1. (For a more detailed discussion of these agents, see section on "Intermediate- or high-risk patients.")

A prospective, multicenter study assessed the role of circulating tumor cells in predicting survival in 177 metastatic breast cancer patients before the start of a new treatment. Patients with levels of circulating tumor cells > 5/7.5 mL of whole blood had a shorter median progression-free survival (2.7 vs 7.0 months; *P* < .001) and shorter overall survival (10.1 vs > 18 months; *P* < .001) than did those with < 5 circulating tumor cells per 7.5 mL of whole blood. Of all the variables in the statistical model, the levels of circulating tumor cells at baseline and at the first follow-up visit were the most significant predictors of progression-free and overall survival in this group of patients.

Intermediate- or high-risk patients

Intermediate- or high-risk patients include those with rapidly progressive disease or visceral involvement and those with disease shown to be refractory to hormonal manipulation by a prior therapeutic trial.

Anthracycline-containing combinations

Regimens containing an anthracycline, such as FAC (see Table 1), are preferred for these patients. However, newer combinations of doxorubicin and a taxane are gaining favor for use in patients who have not received > 450 mg/m^2 of an anthracycline and whose relapse has occurred more than 12 months after the completion of adjuvant therapy.

Single agents

Many single cytotoxic drugs have shown some activity in metastatic breast cancer. They include paclitaxel, ixabepilone, capecitabine (Xeloda), vinorelbine, and gemcitabine (Gemzar) (see Table 1), as well as vinblastine, mitomycin, and thiotepa.

Paclitaxel

One of the most active agents is paclitaxel. It has demonstrated antitumor activity in patients with anthracycline-resistant disease and in those who have received three or more prior chemotherapy regimens for metastatic disease.

High-dose paclitaxel (250 mg/m^2 over 3 hours) has not been shown to be superior to 175 mg/m^2 over 3 hours. The higher dose regimen is associated with greater hematologic and neurologic toxicities.

Nab-paclitaxel

In a clinical trial, the tumor response rate was nearly double for patients who received nanoparticle albumin-bound paclitaxel (nab-paclitaxel or Abraxane) compared with those who received solvent-based paclitaxel. The proposed mechanism of delivery of this nab-driven chemotherapy is thought to be by targeting an albumin-specific (Gp60) receptor-mediated transcytosis path through the cell wall of proliferating tumor cells, using caveolin-1 activated caveolar transport. Once in the stromal microenvironment, the albumin-bound drug may be preferentially localized by SPARC, a protein secreted into the stroma by tumor cells. The resulting collapse of stroma surrounding the tumor cell may thus enhance the delivery of the nab-chemotherapeutic to the intracellular core of the tumor cell itself. Another advantage of nab-paclitaxel is its ease of use. Since it does not contain solvents like Cremophor, it eliminates the need for premedication with steroids or antihistamines for hypersensitivity reactions caused by these solvents. Furthermore, in contrast to solvent-based paclitaxel which require up to 3 hours for IV administration, nab-paclitaxel can be administered in 30 minutes.

Docetaxel

Approved by the FDA for anthracycline-resistant locally advanced or metastatic breast cancer, docetaxel has demonstrated overall response rates of 41% in patients with doxorubicin-resistant disease. It has been shown to be superior to mitomycin/vinblastine in patients whose disease progressed after an anthracycline-based chemotherapy regimen.

The recommended starting dose of docetaxel—100 mg/m^2 as a 1-hour IV infusion—requires premedication with dexamethasone to avoid fluid retention and the capillary leak syndrome. The usual regimen of dexamethasone is 8 mg twice daily for a total of 3 days, beginning 24 hours prior to the administration of docetaxel.

Although 100 mg/m^2 is the dose of docetaxel approved by the FDA, many recent trials have demonstrated a high rate of grade 4 hematologic toxicity at this dose level; a dose of 60 to 70 mg/m^2 may achieve equivalent therapeutic benefit with improved safety. As with paclitaxel, the docetaxel dosage must be modified in patients who have hepatic impairment, manifested by elevated transaminase or alkaline phosphatase levels.

To determine whether weekly infusion of paclitaxel improves response rates versus the standard 3-hour infusion, 577 patients with metastatic breast cancer who had received one or two prior regimens were randomized to receive standard (175 mg/m^2) or weekly (80 mg/m^2) paclitaxel. Weekly paclitaxel was shown to be superior with respect to response rate (40% vs 28%; $P = .017$), time to disease progression (9 months vs 5 months; $P = .0008$), and overall survival (24 months vs 16 months). The authors concluded that weekly paclitaxel is superior to standard paclitaxel in the management of metastatic breast cancer.

When trastuzumab (Herceptin) became standard therapy for ErbB2-positive tumors, all patients with ErbB2-positive disease received trastuzumab, whereas patients with ErbB2-negative disease were randomized to receive either the addition of trastuzumab or not. The addition of trastuzumab did not improve any of these endpoints in patients with ErbB2-negative disease. Weekly paclitaxel caused more grade 3 sensory/motor neuropathy and less grade 3 granulocytopenia.

Capecitabine

An orally active fluorinated pyrimidine carbonate, capecitabine has a substantial antitumor effect in patients whose disease has recurred or progressed after prior anthracycline or taxane therapy. Prolonged survival, limited toxicity, and response in visceral as well as soft-tissue disease add to the benefit of capecitabine. Toxicities include diarrhea, stomatitis, and hand-foot syndrome.

In 2008, Dr. O'Shaughnessy reported on a phase III clinical trial of lapatinib versus lapatinib plus trastuzumab (ASCO 2008, abstract 1015). This study included 296 metastatic breast cancer (MBC) patients with HER2-positive tumors who experienced disease progression after treatment with an anthracycline, a taxane, and trastuzumab. The average patient had received four or five prior regimens. The median time from the last trastuzumab treatment was 1 month. Patients were randomized to oral lapatinib (1,500 mg/d) or to lapatinib (1,000 mg/d) plus weekly trastuzumab. After at least 4 weeks of single-agent treatment, patients could cross over to combination treatment, which 52% of the control arm did. An updated report of the study was presented at the 2009 SABCS by Dr. Blackwell. In the updated intention-to-treat analysis, median OS was 14 months with lapatinib plus trastuzumab compared with 9.5 months with lapatinib alone, for a 26% reduction in risk of death ($P = .026$). One-year OS was 56% vs 41%. Baseline factors shown to predict better outcomes included good performance status, nonvisceral metastatic sites, fewer than three metastatic sites, and longer time from initial diagnosis to randomization. After adjustments for these significant baseline covariates, the OS benefit was still robust, with a 29% reduction in risk ($P = .016$). The majority of adverse events were grade 1 or 2, and the only grade 3 or 4 event with 5% or greater incidence was diarrhea, seen in 8% of patients on the combination treatment and in 7% treated with the single agent *(Blackwell K et al: SABCS 2009, abstract 61).*

Ixabepilone

Ixabepilone (Ixempra) was approved for the treatment of advanced breast cancer after failure of an anthracycline and a taxane, either as monotherapy or in combination with capecitabine. Its approval was based upon the results of two pivotal trials. One phase II study evaluated the efficacy and safety of ixabepilone in patients with metastatic breast cancer resistant to an anthracycline, a taxane, and capecitabine. Patients were heavily pretreated: 88% of the 126 patients had received at least two lines of prior chemotherapy in the metastatic setting. Ixabepilone (40 mg/m^2) was administered as a 3-hour IV infusion on day 1 of a 21-day cycle. The primary endpoint was objective response rate, assessed by an independent radiology facility (IRF). A total of 113 patients were assessable for response; the IRF-assessed overall response rate was 11.5% (95% CI = 6.3%–18.9%). Fifty percent of patients achieved stable disease; 14.3% achieved stable disease for longer than 6 months. The median duration of response and progression-free survival were 5.7 and 3.1 months, respectively. The median overall survival was 8.6 months. Grade 3/4 treatment-related events included peripheral sensory neuropathy (14%), fatigue/asthenia (13%), myalgia (8%), and stomatitis/mucositis (6%). Resolution of grade 3/4 peripheral sensory neuropathy occurred after a median of 5.4 weeks.

The AVADO trial involved approximately 750 ErbB2-negative patients with locally recurrent or metastatic breast cancer to assess first-line docetaxel (Taxotere) with or without bevacizumab (Avastin) at either its standard dose (15 mg/kg every 3 weeks) or at half the standard dose. Patient characteristics were similar between AVADO and E2100, the trial that led to FDA approval of Avastin as front-line treatment for metastatic disease in early 2008. In AVADO, patients did not have to receive chemotherapy until progression, and docetaxel could be discontinued after 6 or 9 cycles of chemotherapy while continuing treatment with bevacizumab (or placebo). Patients in both bevacizumab arms had a prolonged time to progression (TTP) vs those receiving chemotherapy alone (HR = 0.72 – 0.79; *P* < .05), but the improvements were modest vs E2100: Median TTP was increased from 8 months with docetaxel alone to 8.7 and 8.8 months with addition of the half-dose and standard dose of bevacizumab, respectively. Response rates with docetaxel alone vs half-dose and standard-dose bevacizumab were 44%, 55%, and 63%, respectively, and 1-year survival rates were 73%, 78%, and 83% *(Miles D et al: J Clin Oncol 26[15S]:abstract LBA101, 2008).*

The second study was a randomized, phase III trial evaluating the efficacy and safety of ixabepilone used in combination with capecitabine. This trial included 752 patients who were previously treated with anthracyclines and taxanes and whose tumors had demonstrated prior resistance to these therapies. Ixabepilone plus capecitabine prolonged progression-free survival relative to capecitabine (median, 5.8 months vs 4.2 months), with a 25% reduction in the estimated risk of disease progression (HR = 0.75; 95% CI = 0.64–0.88; *P* = .0003). The objective response rate was also increased (35% vs 14%, respectively; *P* < .0001). Grade 3/4 treatment-related sensory neuropathy (21% vs 0%), fatigue (9% vs 3%), and neutropenia (68% vs 11%) were more frequent with combination therapy, as was the rate of death as a result of toxicity (3% vs 1%, with patients with liver dysfunction [≥ grade 2 liver function tests] at greater risk). Capecitabine-related toxicities were similar for both treatment groups.

At the 32nd CTRC-AACR San Antonio Breast Cancer Symposium, researchers reported on the largest study to date of two targeted agents—lapatinib and trastuzumab—in ErbB2-positive metastatic breast cancer. Two hundred ninety-six women who had been heavily pretreated with anthracyclines and taxanes (median of six prior chemotherapy regimens), and had progressed on prior trastuzumab were randomized to either lapatinib only (L; 1,500 mg daily dose) or to trastuzumab (T; 4 mg/kg loading dose then 2 mg/kg weekly) plus lapatinib (L + T; 1,000 mg daily dose of lapatinib). There were 148 patients in each group. Fifty-two percent (52%) of women in the lapatinib arm crossed over at the time of progression of disease. Median progression-free survival was 8.1 weeks with L vs 12 weeks with L + T (hazard ratio [HR], 0.73, $P = .008$). Median overall survival time was 9.5 months with L vs 14 months weeks with L + T (HR, 0.74, $P = .026$). Both regimens were well tolerated; asymptomatic decline in left ventricular ejection fraction (> 20% and below the lower limit of normal) occurred in 3% of patients in the L arm and in 10% of patients in L + T arm. There was one death due to cardiac toxicity in the L + T arm. Investigation of the role of combined anti-ErbB2 therapy, with chemotherapy, in less heavily pretreated patients with early-stage disease is ongoing in the ALTTO study *(Blackwell K et al: SABCS 2009, abstract 61)*.

Key enzymes involved in the DNA repair pathway are PARP-1 and PARP-2—two of a number of members of the PARP family of nuclear enzymes. The presence of PARP renders the cells repairable and therefore contributes to their survival. Inhibition of PARP would result in unrepairable damage and cell death. In the cancer cells of mutation carriers, all BRCA-1 or BRCA-2 function is absent, and when PARP-1 is inhibited, cancer cells are unable to repair DNA damage by homologous recombination or base-excision repair, and cell death results.

A number of PARP inhibitors are currently in various stages of development. Olaparib and iniparib are in phase II/III studies as combination therapy. BSI-201, AG014699, and Veliparib (ABT-888) are in phase I/II investigations as combination therapy. At the 2009 ASCO meeting, Dr. O'Shaughnessy and colleagues presented their preliminary findings of a phase II trial of BSI-201 administered in combination with gemcitabine/carboplatin in patients with triple-negative metastatic breast cancer (ASCO 2009, abstract 3). In this trial, patients were randomized to a 21-day cycle of gemcitabine at 1,000 mg/m^2 IV plus carboplatin (AUC 2) on days 1 and 8 vs the same regimen plus BSI-201 5.6 mg/kg IV biweekly on days 1, 4, 8, and 11. Median PFS in those given BSI-201 with chemotherapy was 6.9 months vs 3.3 months for chemotherapy alone (HR = 0.342; 95% CI = 0.200–0.584; $P < .0001$). Median OS with the BSI-201 plus chemo combination was 9.2 months vs 5.7 months for chemo alone (HR = 0.348; 95% CI = 0.189–0.649; $P = .0005$).

Alterations in the PI3K pathway include deregulation of *PTEN*, or PI3K pathway mutations or hyperactivation. Everolimus (Afinitor) is an oral inhibitor of the mammalian target of rapamycin (mTOR), which is activated downstream of PI3K. Everolimus has been reported to enhance activity, reverse resistance to trastuzumab, and provide synergistic activity with paclitaxel. At the 2010 ASCO meeting, several presentations were related to the use of everolimus in combination with trastuzumab and/or other agents in patients with HER2-positive/overexpressing metastatic breast

Eribulin is a synthetic analog of halichondrin B. It binds to a unique site on tubulin and suppresses microtubule polymerization, sequesters tubulin into nonfunctional aggregates, and creates irreversible mitotic block. An open-label, phase III, randomized multicenter trial of eribulin in women with locally recurrent or metastatic breast cancer who had received two to five prior chemotherapy regimens (73% of patients had received prior capecitabine) was recently reported (EMBRACE). The primary endpoint was OS with PFS, with objective response rate and safety as secondary endpoints. Women were randomized in a 2:1 ratio to eribulin at 1.4 mg/m2, infused as a 2- to 5-minute IV on days 1 and 8 of a 21-day cycle, or to the treatment of physician's choice. The treatment of physician's choice could be any cytotoxic, hormonal, or biological monotherapy, or supportive care only. A total of 762 patients were enrolled: 508 to eribulin and 254 to physician's choice. The median number of prior chemotherapy regimens was four in each treatment arm. Disease characteristics were also similar, with approximately 67% being ER-positive. In the physician's choice arm, 96% received chemotherapy, with a wide range of agents being used. OS was significantly longer with eribulin versus physician's choice, with a hazard ratio (HR) = 0.81 (95% CI = 0.66–0.99; *P* = .041 by stratified log-rank test). In those given eribulin, median survival was 13.12 months, with 53.9% having a 1-year survival. Median survival was 10.65 months in the physician's choice treatment arm, with 43.7% having a 1-year survival. Median PFS for eribulin was 3.7 versus 2.2 months for physician's choice (HR = 0.87; 95% CI = 0.7–1.05; *P* = .14). A significant benefit was observed in the ORR, with 22.6% versus 16.8% of women having a clinical benefit rate (CR + PR +SD for at least 6 months). The overall incidence of adverse events was similar between the treatment arms: 98.8% and 93.1%, as were serious adverse events and those leading to treatment interruption, discontinuation, dose reduction, or dose delay *(Twelves C et al: J Clin Oncol 28[7s] abstract CRA1004, 2010).*

cancer. In a phase II study, the efficacy and safety of everolimus in combination with trastuzumab plus paclitaxel was assessed in 37 evaluable patients with trastuzumab and taxane-resistant HER2-positive MBC. Patients received everolimus 10 mg daily, trastuzumab 4 mg/kg IV loading dose then 2 mg/kg weekly, and paclitaxel 80 mg/m^2 IV on days 1, 8, and 15, every 4 weeks. Of 25 efficacy-evaluable patients, 20% (n = 5) had a confirmed partial response, 56% (n = 14) had stable disease and 24% (n = 6) had progressive disease. Grade 3/4 neutropenia occurred in 32% (n = 12), with one case of febrile neutropenia, grade 3 stomatitis in 13% (n = 5), and grade 3 asthenia/fatigue in 5% (n = 2).

New approaches

Multiple new approaches to treating metastatic breast cancer are being explored. Weekly schedules of the various taxanes (paclitaxel, nab-paclitaxel and docetaxel) have been reported to produce high response rates and lower toxicity than have 3-week schedules. Combinations of doxorubicin with paclitaxel or docetaxel have also shown substantial antitumor activity, as have combinations of capecitabine and docetaxel, carboplatin and paclitaxel, and gemcitabine and cisplatin. These newer combinations need to be compared with standard AC or FAC (CAF) regimens in phase III trials. Recent studies also suggest that sequential weekly chemotherapy may be as effective as more intensive combinations with respect to overall survival in patients with metastatic breast cancer.

Monoclonal antibodies and other targeted agents

Trastuzumab

Trastuzumab (Herceptin) is a humanized monoclonal antibody that selectively binds to the extracellular domain of the human epidermal growth factor type 2 (HER2) receptor. In women with surgically resected breast cancer that overexpresses HER2, trastuzumab combined with chemotherapy improves disease-free and overall survival. Trastuzumab treatment decreases the risk of death by one-third ($P = .015$) in HER2-positive breast cancer. Trastuzumab is approved for use as a single agent in second- and third-line therapy for metastatic breast cancer and in combination with paclitaxel as first-line therapy in this setting. A randomized trial consisting of 469 women showed that the combination of trastuzumab with chemotherapy yielded a 45% overall response rate, as compared with a 29% rate with chemotherapy alone—a 55% increase. The addition of trastuzumab had the greatest impact on response when combined with paclitaxel. Among the study group as a whole, 79% of women treated with trastuzumab chemotherapy were alive at 1 year, as compared with 68% of those given chemotherapy alone.

An update of these data has shown a superior median overall survival with chemotherapy plus trastuzumab compared with chemotherapy alone (25.4 months vs 20.9 months). The survival advantage was seen with both AC plus trastuzumab and paclitaxel plus the monoclonal antibody.

In another single-arm trial involving 222 women who had not responded to prior chemotherapy, trastuzumab shrunk tumors by 50% in 14% of women, with a median duration of response of 9 months. Overall, trastuzumab was well tolerated in both trials. Due to an increased risk of cardiac dysfunction observed in women treated with trastuzumab plus an anthracycline, trastuzumab should not be used in combination with this drug class outside of a clinical trial.

It is important to point out that trastuzumab also produces cardiac toxicity when administered by itself, particularly in patients who have had extensive prior exposure to an anthracycline. Finally, essentially all of the clinical benefit of trastuzumab (alone or in combination) is confined to patients whose breast cancer expresses high (3+ by IHC or amplified by FISH) levels of the ErbB2 oncoprotein.

One study explored the relationship between circulating ErbB2 extracellular domain (ECD) and tissue ErbB2 status and examined its predictive value in a cohort of metastatic breast cancer patients treated with weekly trastuzumab and paclitaxel. A retrospective analysis of patients treated on a previous trial evaluated the associations between pretreatment serum ErbB2 ECD and tissue ErbB2 status and the change in serum ErbB2 ECD after 12 weeks of therapy and response. Stored serum samples were available for 55 of 95 patients (58%). A statistically significant association was found between ErbB2 status and baseline serum ErbB2 ECD level. Patients whose ECD normalized after 12 weeks of therapy had a higher response proportion than did those with persistently high ECD levels (68% vs 15%; $P = .005$). A relative decline of more than 55% from baseline ErbB2 ECD predicted response to trastuzumab-based therapy.

Treatment of HER2/*neu*-overexpressing breast cancer is currently a very active area of research in both the neoadjuvant/adjuvant and metastatic setting, with many active drugs being studied.

Three randomized trials, E2100, AVADO, and RIBBON-1, have demonstrated significantly improved progression-free survival (PFS) with bevacizumab in combination with other chemotherapy agents and administered as first-line treatment in patients with metastatic breast cancer (MBC). At the 2010 ASCO meeting, Dr. O'Shaughnessy presented findings of a pooled analysis of the overall survival data from these three trials. In the pooled analysis of demographic and disease-related characteristics, patients treated with bevacizumab were of a similar age (56 years) to those who were not (55 years), with approximately 25% in each arm having triple-negative disease, and a similar disease-free interval (37 vs 39 months) and percentage with three or more metastatic sites (41% vs 38%). PFS was greater with bevacizumab-containing treatment in the pooled analysis (median of 9.2 vs 6.7 months, hazard ratio [HR] = 0.64; 95% CI = 0.57–0.71; *P* < .001). PFS was greater regardless of age, hormone receptor status, or disease-free interval. Across the studies, the HRs ranged from 0.48 to 0.69, with *P* values of .0003 or less. In each of the three trials, overall survival (OS) was a secondary endpoint measure. In the individual studies, the median OS follow-up ranged from 23 to 35 months. In the pooled analysis of OS, bevacizumab-treated patients had a median OS of 26.7 months, compared with 26.4 months in those who did not receive bevacizumab (HR = 0.97; 95% CI = 0.86–1.08). One-year survival rates of 82% and 77% were seen in bevacizumab-treated versus non–bevacizumab-treated patients, respectively. There was a 17% increase in the objective response rate with bevacizumab-containing regimens. The investigators concluded that patients with adverse prognostic features do benefit from the addition of bevacizumab, as do those with more indolent disease *(O'Shaughnessy J et al: J Clin Oncol 28[7s]: abstract 1005, 2010)*. The RIBBON-2 trial, which evaluated the combination of bevacizumab with various chemotherapy agents in the treatment of MBC as second-line therapy, found that the combination consistently demonstrated improved PFS. Brufsky and colleagues examined various subgroups of the RIBBON-2 participants to assess the consistency of the benefits on PFS. The hazard ratios of PFS consistently favored the bevacizumab-plus-chemotherapy arm over the placebo-plus-chemotherapy arm when data were pooled across all chemotherapy cohorts. Investigators concluded that bevacizumab combined with standard chemotherapies provides PFS benefits to HER2-negative MBC patients *(Brufsky A et al: J Clin Oncol 28[7s]: abstract 1021, 2010)*.

Lapatinib

Lapatanib (Tykerb) is a potent and specific reversible oral small molecule dual tyrosine kinase inhibitor of both human epidermal growth factor receptor type 2 (HER2) and epidermal growth factor receptor (EGFR). It is active in combination with capecitabine (Xeloda) in women with ErbB2-positive metastatic breast cancer. Women with ErbB2-positive, locally advanced, or metastatic breast cancer that had progressed after treatment with regimens that included an anthracycline, a taxane, and trastuzumab were randomly assigned to receive either lapatinib (at a dose of 1,250 mg/d continuously) plus capecitabine (at a dose of 2,000 mg/m^2 of body surface area) on days 1 through 14 of a 21-day cycle or monotherapy with capecitabine alone (at a dose of 2,500 mg/m^2 on days 1 through 14 of a 21-day cycle).

The interim analysis of time to disease progression met specified criteria for early reporting on the basis of superiority in the combination-therapy group. The HR for the independently assessed time to disease progression was 0.49 (95% CI = 0.34–0.71; *P* < .001), with 49 events in the combination-therapy group and 72 events in the monotherapy group. The median time to disease progression was 8.4 months in the combination-therapy group as compared with 4.4 months in the monotherapy group.

This improvement was achieved without an increase in serious toxic effects or symptomatic cardiac events. In March 2007, lapatinib in combination with capecitabine was approved by the FDA for treatment of women with ErbB2-positive advanced breast cancer that has progressed after treatment with trastuzumab.

Bevacizumab

Bevacizumab (Avastin) is a recombinant humanized monoclonal antibody that targets VEGF and is the first antiangiogenic agent to demonstrate benefit in women with HER2-negative advanced breast cancer.

The first large, open-label, randomized phase III trial evaluated the efficacy and safety of capecitabine (Xeloda) alone versus capecitabine in combination with bevacizumab in 462 women with metastatic breast cancer.Bevacizumab in combination with capecitabine did not significantly improve PFS (4.86 vs 4.17 months, hazard ratio [HR] = 0.98; 95% CI = 0.77–1.25; *P* = .857). There was also no difference in overall survival. However, the addition of bevacizumab to capecitabine improved the response rate from 9.1% to 19.8% (*P* = .001). The bevacizumab combination arm was well tolerated and did not worsen capecitabine-related toxicity such as diarrhea and hand-foot syndrome. Bevacizumab-related toxicities included hypertension (grade 3: 17.9% vs 0.5% for single-agent capecitabine), thromboembolic events (grades 2–4: 6.9% vs 5.6%), proteinuria (grades 1–4: 22.3% vs 7.4%), and minor bleeding (grade 1 or 2 epistaxis). Two patients treated with bevacizumab developed grade 3 proteinuria and, consequently, their therapy was discontinued. Nine patients developed grade 3/4 CHF or cardiomyopathy: seven in the combination arm (3.1%) and two in the single-agent capecitabine arm (0.9%). Serious hemorrhage and thromboembolic events were uncommon and did not differ between treatment arms. In this heavily pretreated patient population, the activity of bevacizumab was obscured. It was hypothesized that advanced stages of breast cancer may have redundant angiogenic pathways, making the inhibition of a single receptor pathway inadequate for significant clinical benefit.

In order to maximize antiangiogenic inhibition, the Eastern Cooperative Oncology Group (ECOG) performed a large, open-label phase III trial with weekly paclitaxel and bevacizumab. In ECOG 2100, a total of 722 patients were randomized to weekly paclitaxel, with or without bevacizumab as first-line therapy for locally advanced or metastatic breast cancer. The addition of bevacizumab to paclitaxel significantly improved the progression-free survival (PFS) time to 11.8 months, compared with 5.9 months in the paclitaxel-only arm (*P* < .001). A higher overall response rate of 36.9% was seen in the combination arm, compared with 21.2% in the single-agent arm (*P* < .001). Despite the improved PFS and overall response rate,there was no difference in median overall survival between the two treatment arms. Toxicities associated with the bevacizumab combination included hypertension, proteinuria, and neuropathy.

Two additional phase III studies investigated the role of bevacizumab in the first-line treatment of advanced breast cancer in combination with chemotherapy. The AVADO trial tested docetaxel in combination with either placebo or bevacizumab at 7.5 or 15 mg/m^2 given every 21 days in HER2-negative breast cancer. The RIBBON-1 trial investigated several chemotherapies (ie, anthracyclines, taxanes, and capecitabine) in combination with placebo versus bevacizumab at 15 mg/m^2 given every 3 weeks. Both trials demonstrated a modest but statistically significant improvement in PFS with the addition of bevacizumab. However, no statistically significant improvement in overall survival was seen; neither study was powered for an overall survival endpoint. RIBBON-2 tested the role of bevacizumab in the second-line treatment of metastatic breast cancer and was very similar in design to RIBBON-1 except that additional chemotherapies (eg, gemcitabine, vinorelbine) were permissible. Similar to the first-line setting, the addition of bevacizumab to chemotherapy statistically improved PFS (7.2 months vs 5.1 months) and response rates but not OS. PFS results were consistent across each chemotherapy cohort with the exception of the small vinorelbine subgroup of 76 patients. In summary, bevacizumab plus chemotherapy improves response rates and prolongs PFS when used as first- and second-line therapy for advanced breast cancer but it has not yet been shown to improve overall survival.

Adjunctive bisphosphonate therapy

Zoledronic acid (marketed in the US as Zometa) is an intravenously administered bisphosphonate that reduces skeletal-related events including pain and risk of fracture in women with breast cancer metastatic to bone. In addition, zoledronic acid treats hypercalcemia of malignancy. Multiple published reports have now confirmed the benefit of bisphosphonates as an adjunct to treatment of patients with bone metastasis. Use of these agents results in a significant reduction in skeleton-related events, including pathologic fracture, bone pain, and the need for radiation therapy to bone. Zoledronic acid and pamidronate (Aredia) are both available in IV formulations in the United States. An oral bisphosphonate used for this indication, ibandronate (Boniva), is also available in the US.

Patients with breast carcinoma who had all types of bone metastases (osteolytic, mixed, or osteoblastic) were randomized to receive treatment with either 4 or 8 mg of zoledronic acid as a 15-minute infusion or 90 mg of pamidronate as a 2-hour infusion every 3 to 4 weeks for 12 months. The proportion of patients who had a skeleton-related event (defined as a pathologic fracture, spinal cord compression, radiotherapy, or surgery to bone) was comparable between treatment groups (approximately 45%). However, among patients who had breast carcinoma with at least one osteolytic lesion, treatment with 4 mg of zoledronic acid was more effective than was 90 mg of pamidronate in reducing skeletal complications.

The most commonly reported adverse events for both zoledronic acid and pamidronate, which are more common and dramatic at the time of the first infusion, can include fatigue, muscle aches, bone pain, nausea, vomiting, fever, and/or swelling in the feet or legs. Rarely, zoledronic acid has been associated with osteonecrosis of the jaw. The 4-mg dose of zoledronic acid results in elevated serum creatinine levels in about 7.7% of patients, versus 6.0% with pamidronate. A larger proportion of patients had elevated serum creatinine levels with 8-mg of zoledronic acid; therefore, this dose is not recommended. Symptomatic hypocalcemia, although relatively rare, requires frequent monitoring of calcium and phosphate levels during treatment.

Denosumab, a fully human monoclonal antibody, inhibits RANKL, a key mediator of osteoclast activity. Primary results from a recently completed randomized pivotal study demonstrated that denosumab was superior to zoledronic acid (ZA) in delaying and preventing skeletal-related events (SREs) in breast cancer patients with bone metastases (BM). Patients with breast cancer and BM (N = 2,046) who had not been treated with intravenous (IV) bisphosphonates were randomized 1:1 to receive either subcutaneous (SC) denosumab at 120 mg and IV placebo, or SC placebo and IV ZA at 4 mg every 4 weeks. The primary endpoint was time to first on-study skeletal-related events (SREs). As previously reported, denosumab was superior to ZA in significantly delaying the time to first on-study SRE (hazard ratio [HR] = 0.82; 95% confidence interval [CI] = 0.71– 0.95; *P* < .0001 noninferiority; *P* = .01 superiority) and the time to first and subsequent on-study SRE (rate ratio 0.77; 95%CI = 0.66–0.89; *P* = .001). Denosumab also significantly delayed the time to first radiation to bone (HR = 0.74; 95% CI = 0.59–0.94; *P* = .01) and the time to first on-study SRE or hypercalcemia of malignancy (HCM) (HR = 0.82; 95% CI = 0.70–0.95; *P* = .007) compared with ZA. Denosumab reduced the mean skeletal morbidity rate (SMR) compared with ZA (0.45 vs 0.58, respectively; *P* = .004). The total number of SREs was 491 events for denosumab and 623 events for ZA. At the primary data analysis cut-off date (study duration: 34 months), the proportion of patients (95% CI) experiencing at least one on-study SRE was lower in the denosumab arm (30.7% [27.9%, 33.5%]) than the ZA arm (36.5% [33.5%, 39.4%]). The investigators concluded that denosumab was more efficacious than ZA in delaying time to first radiation to bone and first on-study SRE or HCM and in reducing SMR and the proportion of patients with an SRE. Overall, the incidence of adverse events (AEs) and serious AEs was consistent with what has been previously reported for these two agents *(Stopeck A et al: SABCS 2009, abstract 22).*

Radiation therapy

Irradiation remains an integral component of the management of metastatic breast carcinoma. Although bone metastases are the most commonly treated metastatic sites in patients with breast cancer, brain metastases, spinal cord compression, choroidal metastases, endobronchial lung metastases, and metastatic lesions in other visceral sites can be effectively palliated with irradiation.

Radiation dose and schedule

Depending on the disease site and volume of the radiation field, fractionation schedules ranging from 20 Gy in 5 fractions to 30 Gy in 10 fractions are used most commonly. In some situations, more protracted courses using lower daily doses may be indicated.

Bone metastasis

For patients with widespread bone metastasis, hemibody irradiation (6–7 Gy in one fraction to the upper body or 8 Gy to the lower body) has been shown to be effective. Strontium-89 chloride (Metastron) and other systemic radionuclides also provide effective palliation for widespread bone disease.

Brain metastasis

Patients who develop metastasis to the brain generally have poor outcomes. Nonetheless, radiation therapy can often be helpful in palliating their symptoms and may help control disease for some time. In one randomized trial, patients with one to three newly diagnosed brain metastases (breast as well as other sites) were randomly allocated to receive either whole-brain radiation therapy (WBRT, 164 patients) or WBRT followed by a stereotactic radiosurgery boost (167 patients). Univariate analysis showed that there was a survival advantage in the WBRT and surgery group for patients with a single brain metastasis (median survival: 6.5 months vs 4.9 months; $P = .0393$). Patients in the stereotactic surgery group were more likely to have a stable or improved Karnofsky performance status score at 6 months' follow-up than were patients allocated to WBRT alone (43% vs 27%, respectively; $P = .03$).

Surgery

There are selected indications for surgical intervention in patients with metastatic breast cancer, and the role of surgery at this point is generally palliative. Most commonly, palliative surgery is offered to patients with brain metastases, spinal cord compression, fractures, or symptomatic pleural or pericardial effusions not controlled by other means. It is also used for GI complications stemming from metastatic deposits. The curative benefit of surgery in the treatment of metastatic disease to the lungs or liver is not proven, but in highly selected cases surgery may be beneficial.

Locoregional therapy of the primary tumor in patients with distant metastases

Approximately 5%–10% of patients with newly diagnosed breast cancer will have distant metastatic disease at the time of presentation. Recent data suggest that survival may be improved if the disease is controlled locally and regionally. The treatment offered may be surgical resection, radiotherapy, or both.

Le Scodan and others retrospectively reviewed data on 581 patients who had synchronous metastases at diagnosis. In all, 320 patients received locoregional therapy (LRT), with 249 given exclusive locoregional radiotherapy (LRR), 41 given surgery of the primary tumor with adjuvant LRR, and 31 given surgery alone. No LRT was given to 262 patients. The 3-year survival rate was 43.4% in patients who were treated with LRT and 26.7% in those who were not ($P = .00002$).

Spinal cord compression

Patients with spinal cord compression who have progressive symptoms during irradiation, disease recurrence after irradiation, spinal instability, or who require diagnosis are candidates for surgery.

Solitary brain metastasis

Patients with a long disease-free interval and solitary brain metastasis may be candidates for resection. Evidence suggests an improved disease-free survival, overall survival, and quality of life in this subset of patients when treated with surgery combined with postoperative cranial irradiation, as compared with radiation therapy alone.

Gamma- and Cyber-knife radiosurgery is increasingly used to manage brain metastases. In some instances, these modalities have been used in patients who have multiple metastatic brain lesions or in patients who had previously received conventional treatment modalities for brain metastases, including whole-brain irradiation. No radiation-induced dementia and a remarkably low incidence of local failure were reported with these treatments. Although local control of brain metastasis was an issue in the past, these treatment modalities are shifting the question of survival to that of systemic control.

Chest wall resection

It is extremely rare for a patient with distant metastatic disease to be a candidate for chest wall resection; however, patients with symptomatic recurrence of disease in the chest wall who have limited distant disease and a life expectancy of > 12 months may be appropriate candidates.

Liver metastasis

Patients with metastatic disease to the liver often have a poor prognosis. Although rarely indicated, patients with single metastases or a prolonged disease-free or disease-stable interval may be candidates for resection to completely remove the metastatic lesion.

Follow-up of long-term survivors

For recommendations on the type and timing of follow-up evaluations, see chapter 7.

SUGGESTED READING

Adam R, Aloia T, Krissat J, et al: Is liver resection justified for patients with hepatic metastases from breast cancer? Ann Surg 244:897–908, 2006.

Brufsky A, Bondarenko IN, Smirnov V, et al: RIBBON-2: A randomized, double-blind, placebo-controlled, phase III trial evaluating the efficacy and safety of bevacizumab In combination with chemotherapy for second-line treatment of HER2-negative metastatic breast cancer. Cancer Res 69(suppl): abstract 42, 2009.

Chia S, Gradishar W, Mauriac L, et al: Double-blind, randomized placebo controlled trial of fulvestrant compared with exemestane after prior nonsteroidal aromatase inhibitor therapy in postmenopausal women with hormone receptor-positive, advanced breast cancer: results from EFECT. J Clin Oncol 26:1664–1670, 2008.

Dalenc F, Campone P, Hupperets R, et al: Everolimus in combination with weekly paclitaxel and trastuzumab in patients (pts) with prior resistance to trastuzumab and taxanes: A multicenter phase II clinical trial. J Clin Oncol 28[15S]: abstract 1013, 2010.

García-Mata J, García-Palomo A, Calvo L, et al: Phase II study of dose-dense doxorubicin and docetaxel as neoadjunvant chemotherapy with G-CSF support in patients with large or locally advanced breast cancer. Clin Transl Oncol 10:739–744, 2008.

Geyer CE, Forster J, Lindquist D, et al: Lapatinib plus capecitabine for HER2-positive advanced breast cancer. N Engl J Med 355:2733–2743, 2006.

Geyer CE, Martin A, Newstat B, et al: Lapatinb plus capecitabine in HER2+ advanced breast cancer: Genomic and updated effiacy data. J Clin Oncol 25[18S]:1035, 2007.

Le Scodan R, Stevens D, Brain E, et al: Breast cancer with synchronous metastases: Survival impact of exclusive logoregional radiotherapy. J Clin Oncol 27:1375–1381, 2009.

Miles D, Chan A, Romeiu G, et al: A randomized, double-blind study of bevacizumab in combination with docetaxel as first-line treatment of patients with HER2-negative locally recurrent or metastatic breast cancer: Efficacy and safety. J Clin Oncol 26(suppl); abstract LBA1011, 2008.

Miller K, Wang M, Gralow J, et al: Paclitaxel plus bevacizumab versus paclitaxel alone for metastatic breast cancer. N Engl J Med 357:2666–2676, 2007.

O'Shaughnessy JA, Brufsky A: RiBBON 1 and RiBBON 2: Phase III trials of bevacizumab with standard chemotherapy for metastatic breast cancer. Clinical Breast Cancer 8:370–373, 2008.

Perez EA, Lerzo G, Pivot X, et al: Efficacy and safety of ixabepilone (BMS-247550) in a phase II study of patients with advanced breast cancer resistant to an anthracycline, a taxane, and capecitabine. J Clin Oncol 25:3407–3414, 2007.

Sledge G, Miller K, Moisa C, et al: Safety and efficacy of capecitabine (C) plus bevacizumab (B) as first-line in metastatic breast cancer. J Clin Oncol 25:[18S]:1013, 2007.

Thomas ES, Gomez HL, Li RK, et al: Ixabepilone plus capecitabine for metastatic breast cancer progressing after anthracycline and taxane treatment. J Clin Oncol 25:5210–5217, 2007.

Abbreviations in this chapter

ALTTO = Adjuvant L and/or T Treatment Optimization; ASCO = American Society of Clinical Oncology; AVADO = Avastin and Docetaxel; ECOG = Eastern Cooperative Oncology Group; EFECT = Evaluation of Faslodex versus Exemestane Clinical Trial; FDA = US Food and Drug Administration; NSABP = National Surgical Adjuvant Breast and Bowel Project; RIBBON = Regimens in Bevacizumab for Breast Oncology

CHAPTER 9

Esophageal cancer

Jimmy J. Hwang, MD, Rajesh V. Iyer, MD, and Michael Mulligan, MD

Although still relatively uncommon in Western countries, esophageal cancer is fatal in the vast majority of cases. In the United States, an estimated 16,640 new cases will be diagnosed in the year 2010, and 14,500 deaths will result from the disease. This high percentage of deaths rivals that of pancreatic cancer and is more than four times that of rectal cancer.

The esophagus extends from the cricopharyngeal sphincter to the gastroesophageal (GE) junction and is commonly divided into the cervical, upper to mid-thoracic, and thoracic portions. This can be important, as histology and optimal treatment approaches may vary considerably based on the site of the cancer. It may not be possible to determine the site of origin if the cancer involves the GE junction itself.

EPIDEMIOLOGY

Gender Esophageal cancer is seven times more common and slightly more lethal in men than in women.

Age Adenocarcinoma of the esophagus (now more common in the United States than the squamous cell type) has a median age at diagnosis of 69 years. The incidence of squamous cell cancer of the esophagus increases with age as well and peaks in the seventh decade of life.

Race The incidence of squamous cell esophageal cancer is three times higher in blacks than in whites, whereas adenocarcinomas are more common in white men.

Geography Evidence of an association between environment and diet and esophageal cancer comes from the profound differences in incidence observed in various parts of the world. Esophageal cancer occurs at a rate 20 to 30 times higher in China than in the United States. An esophageal "cancer belt" extends from northeast China to the Middle East.

Survival Although the overall outlook for patients diagnosed with esophageal cancer has improved in the past 30 years, most patients still present with advanced disease, and their survival remains poor. One-third to one-half of patients treated with either chemoradiation therapy or chemoradiation therapy plus surgery are alive at 2 years, without recurrence of esophageal cancer.

Disease site The rate of cancer of the distal esophagus is about equal to that of the more proximal two-thirds. In general, squamous cell carcinoma is found in the body of the esophagus, whereas adenocarcinoma predominates in lesions closer to the GE junction.

ETIOLOGY AND RISK FACTORS

Cigarettes and alcohol Squamous cell carcinomas of the esophagus have been associated with cigarette smoking and/or excessive alcohol intake. Furthermore, cigarette smoking and alcohol appear to act synergistically, producing high relative risks in heavy users of tobacco and alcohol. Esophageal adenocarcinoma is increased twofold in smokers.

Diet High-fat, low-protein, and low-calorie diets have been shown to increase the risk of esophageal cancer. Exposure to nitrosamines has been proposed as a factor in the development of both squamous cell carcinoma and adenocarcinoma of the esophagus.

Barrett's esophagus and other factors Gastroesophageal reflux disease (GERD) and Barrett's esophagus (adenomatous metaplasia of the distal esophagus) have been linked to adenocarcinoma of the esophagus. Tylosis, Plummer-Vinson syndrome, history of head and neck cancer, and achalasia have also been associated with a higher-than-normal risk of developing squamous cell cancer of the esophagus.

ESOPHAGEAL

SIGNS AND SYMPTOMS

Because symptoms do not alert the patient until the disease is advanced, few esophageal cancers are diagnosed at an early stage.

Dysphagia The most common presenting complaint is dysphagia, which generally is not noted until the esophageal lumen is narrowed to one-half to one-third of normal, due to its elasticity.

Weight loss is common and has a significant role in prognosis (> 10% of total body weight as poor prognosis).

Cough that is induced by swallowing is suggestive of local extension into the trachea with resultant tracheoesophageal fistula.

Odynophagia and pain Pain with swallowing (odynophagia) is an ominous sign. Patients who describe pain radiating to the back may well have extra-esophageal spread. Supraclavicular or cervical nodal metastases may be appreciated on examination.

Hoarseness may be a sign of recurrent laryngeal nerve involvement due to extra-esophageal spread.

Metastatic disease may present as malignant pleural effusion or ascites. Bone metastasis can be identified by pain involving the affected site or by associated hypercalcemia. The most common metastatic sites are retroperitoneal or celiac lymph nodes.

The American College of Surgeons conducted a study utilizing its national cancer database to assess the presentation, stage distribution, and treatment of patients diagnosed with esophageal cancer between 1994 and 1997 (n = 5,044). The most common presenting symptoms were dysphagia (74.0%), weight loss (57.3%), reflux (20.5%), odynophagia (16.6%), and dyspnea (12.1%). The American College of Surgeons Database finds 50% of patients present with tumors in the lower third of the esophagus; 42% have adenocarcinoma histology, and 52% have squamous histology. Barrett's esophagus was found in 39% of those patients with adenocarcinoma.

Patients undergoing initial surgical resection had the following stage distribution: stages I (13.3%), II (34.7%), III (35.7%), and IV (12.3%).

DIAGNOSIS

In Western countries, the diagnosis of esophageal cancer is generally made by endoscopic biopsy of the esophagus. In the Far East, cytologic evaluation is frequently utilized.

Endoscopic ultrasonography (EUS) is extremely accurate (> 90%) in establishing the depth of tumor invasion (T stage) but less accurate (70%–80%) in determining nodal involvement (N stage) unless combined with fine-needle aspiration (FNA) of the involved nodes (93% accuracy) when nodes greater than 5 mm are biopsied. The addition of FNA increases the sensitivity from 63% to 93% and the specificity from 81% to 100%. EUS is not reliable in determining the extent of response to neoadjuvant treatment.

Endoscopy and barium x-rays Endoscopy allows for direct visualization of abnormalities and directed biopsies. Barium x-rays are less invasive and provide a good assessment of the extent of esophageal disease.

Bronchoscopy should be performed to detect tracheal invasion in all cases of esophageal cancer except adenocarcinoma of the distal third of the esophagus.

CT scan Once a diagnosis has been established and careful physical examination and routine blood tests have been performed, a CT scan of the chest, abdomen, and pelvis should be obtained to help assess tumor extent, nodal involvement, and metastatic disease.

PET A prospective trial designed to evaluate the utility of PET vs CT and EUS was performed by obtaining these studies in 48 consecutive patients prior to esophagectomy. PET achieved a 57% sensitivity, a 97% specificity, and an 86% accuracy compared with CT, which was 99% sensitive, 18% specific, and 78% accurate. In terms of nodal staging, PET was correct in 83% of cases, as compared with 60% of cases for CT and 58% for EUS ($P = .006$). This analysis suggests the improved accuracy of PET in the staging work up of patients with esophageal cancer.

Numerous studies report the accuracy of PET scanning in determining the presence of metastatic disease, with sensitivity approaching 90% and specificity over 90%.

As PET becomes more widely available, its use will probably become an important part of the preoperative evaluation of these patients. In a prospective trial of 39 patients with esophageal cancer, PET detected additional sites of metastatic disease at the initial evaluation when compared with conventional imaging. After induction therapy, PET did not add to the estimation of locoregional resectability and did not detect new distant metastases. However, this study suggested that changes in ([^{18}fluorodeoxyglucose]) FDG-PET following induction therapy may predict disease-free and overall survival after induction therapy and resection in patients with esophageal cancer. A large prospective national trial will evaluate the use of PET in the treatment of esophageal cancer.

Bone scan A bone scan should be obtained if the patient has bone pain or an elevated alkaline phosphatase level.

Thoracoscopy/laparoscopy Investigators have begun to examine the role of surgical staging prior to definitive therapy. These procedures are designed to allow pathologic review of regional lymph nodes and the accurate assessment of extra-esophageal tumor spread by direct visualization. A multi-institution trial (CALGB 9380) found these procedures to be feasible in over 70% of patients; they resulted in the upstaging of patients in 38% of cases reviewed. Further investigations need to be completed to determine the appropriate use of these tools in treatment algorithms for patients with esophageal cancer.

Warning Staging studies should be performed in a sequential manner. Invasive, lower yield, and less accurate studies and procedures should only be undertaken if management would change on the basis of specific findings.

SCREENING AND SURVEILLANCE

HIGH-RISK PATIENTS

Adenocarcinoma The role of screening patients with GERD and surveillance of patients with Barrett's esophagus by upper GI endoscopy remains under investigation. In 833 patients studied by endoscopy, there was a 13% incidence of intestinal metaplasia (Barrett's esophagus). Dysplasia or cancer was seen in 31% of patients with long-segment Barrett's esophagus, in 10% of short-segment Barrett's esophagus, and in 6% of GE-junction intestinal metaplasia.

Squamous cell carcinoma Mass screening in the high-risk areas of China and Japan is considered appropriate.

PATHOLOGY

The potential importance of the differences in histology on disease prognosis, and therefore treatment, which has been clinically recognized for several years, has resulted in differences in staging, based on histology in the seventh edition of the *AJCC Cancer Staging Manual.*

Adenocarcinoma The incidence of esophageal adenocarcinoma involving the GE junction has risen 4% to 10% per year since 1976 in the United States and Europe. As a result, adenocarcinoma is now the predominant histologic subtype of esophageal cancer. The distal one-third of the esophagus is the site of origin of most adenocarcinomas.

Squamous cell carcinomas occur most often in the proximal two-thirds of the esophagus. Squamous cell carcinoma is still the most prevalent histologic subtype worldwide.

Other tumor types Other, less frequently seen histologic subtypes include mucoepidermoid carcinoma, small-cell carcinoma, sarcoma, adenoid cystic leiomyosarcoma, and primary lymphoma of the esophagus. Occasionally, metastatic disease from another site may present as a mass in the esophagus or a mass pressing on the esophagus.

Metastatic spread The most common sites of metastatic disease are the regional lymph nodes, lungs, liver, bone, adrenal glands, and diaphragm. Adenocarcinoma can also metastasize to the brain.

STAGING AND PROGNOSIS

Based on data demonstrating that the depth of penetration has important prognostic significance, the American Joint Committee on Cancer (AJCC) TNM staging system for esophageal cancer was changed from a clinical one (1983) to a pathologic one in 2002. The seventh edition of the AJCC Cancer Staging Manual became available in January 2010, and staging updates for esophageal cancer are listed in Table 1. Both the clinical and pathologic staging systems are shown in Table 1, as patients may be cured without an operation. Although pathologic information obtained from an esophagectomy specimen is of prognostic importance, postoperative therapy to improve prognosis has not been rigorously tested. Moreover, recurrence rates for stages I (30%) and II (70%) cancers suggest early systemic spread undetected by current noninvasive staging.

TABLE 1: 1983 and 2010 AJCC TNM staging systems for esophageal cancer

1983 Classification (clinical)		2010 Classification (pathologic)	
Primary tumor (T)			
Tis	Carcinoma in situ	TX	Primary tumor cannot be assessed
T1	Tumor involves ≤ 5 cm of esophageal length, produces no obstruction, and has no circumferential involvement	T0	No evidence of primary tumor
		Tis	High-grade dysplasia[a]
T2	Tumor involves > 5 cm of esophageal length, causes obstruction, or involves the circumference of the esophagus	T1	Tumor invades lamina propria, muscularis mucosae, or submucosa
		T1a	Tumor invades lamina propria or muscularis mucosae
T3	Extraesophageal spread	T1b	Tumor invades submucosa
		T2	Tumor invades muscularis propria
		T3	Tumor invades adventitia
		T4	Tumor invades adjacent structures
		T4a	Resectable tumor invading pleura, pericardium, or diaphragm
		T4b	Unresectable tumor invading other adjacent structures, such as aorta, vertebral body, trachea, etc.
Regional lymph nodes (N)			
NX	Regional nodes cannot be assessed	NX	Regional nodes cannot be assessed
N0	No nodal metastases	N0	No regional nodal metastases
N1	Unilateral, mobile, regional nodal metastases (if clinically evaluable)	N1	Regional lymph node metastases involving 1 to 2 nodes
N2	Bilateral, mobile, regional nodal metastases (if clinically evaluable)	N2	Regional lymph node metastases involving 3 to 6 nodes
N3	Fixed nodes	N3	Regional lymph node metastases involving 7 or more nodes
Distant metastases (M)			
M0	No distant metastases	M0	No distant metastases
M1	Distant metastases	M1	Distant metastases

continued

TABLE 1: 1983 and 2010 AJCC TNM staging systems for esophageal cancer, *continued*

Pathologic stage grouping, AJCC 2010
Squamous cell carcinoma[b]

GROUP	T	N	M	Grade	Tumor Location[c]
Stage 0	Tis (HGD)	N0	M0	1	Any
Stage IA	T1	N0	M0	1, X	Any
Stage IB	T1	N0	M0	2–3	Any
	T2–3	N0	M0	1, X	Lower, X
Stage IIA	T2–3	N0	M0	1, X	Upper, middle
	T2–3	N0	M0	2–3	Lower, X
Stage IIB	T2–3	N0	M0	2–3	Upper, middle
	T1–2	N1	M0	Any	Any
Stage IIIA	T1–2	N2	M0	Any	Any
	T3	N1	M0	Any	Any
	T4a	N0	M0	Any	Any
Stage IIIB	T3	N2	M0	Any	Any
Stage IIIC	T4a	N1–2	M0	Any	Any
	T4b	Any N	M0	Any	Any
	Any T	N3	M0	Any	Any
Stage IV	Any T	Any N	M1	Any	Any

[a] High-grade dysplasia includes all non-invasive neoplastic epithelium that was formerly called carcinoma in situ, a diagnosis that is no longer used for columnar mucosae anywhere in the gastrointestinal tract.
[b] Squamous cell carcinoma or mixed histology including a squamous component or normal esophageal squamous (NOS) cells.
[c] Location of the primary cancer site is defined by the position of the upper (proximal) edge of the tumor in the esophagus.

TABLE 2: Treatment options and survival by stage in esophageal cancer

Stage[a]		Standard treatment	5-Year survival rate (%)
Stage 0	(Tis N0 M0)	Surgery	> 90
Stage I	(T1 N0 M0)	Surgery	> 70
Stage IIA	(T2–3 N0 M0)	Surgery, chemoradiation therapy, or combination	15–30
Stage IIB	(T2–3 N0 M0 or T1–2 N1 M0)	Surgery, chemoradiation therapy, or combination	10–30
Stage III	(T1–2 N2 M0; T3 N1 M0; or T4 Any N M0)	Chemoradiation therapy with or without surgery	10–25
Stage IV	(Any T Any N M1)	Radiation therapy ± intraluminal intubation and dilation ± chemotherapy	Rare

[a] According to the AJCC TNM system definitions (see Table 1)
Note: Surgical results are based on the pathologic staging system, whereas patients treated with combined-modality therapy or neoadjuvant chemoradiation therapy are clinically staged.

Pathologic information obtained from an esophagectomy specimen is of significant prognostic importance. Immunohistochemical analysis of the initial biopsy specimen may also have prognostic relevance. Clinical staging has been shown to be of prognostic importance, particularly in patients managed with primary radiotherapy or chemoradiation therapy.

Histology and grade Neither histology nor grade has been shown to be of prognostic importance in esophageal carcinoma.

Other prognostic factors Patient age, performance status, and degree of weight loss are of prognostic importance. The prognostic implications of tumor-suppressor genes and oncogenes are an area of active investigation.

TREATMENT

Treatment options for the various disease stages are given in Table 2, along with 5-year survival rates.

TREATMENT OF LOCALIZED DISEASE

Only 40% to 60% of patients with esophageal cancer present with clinically localized disease. The National Comprehensive Cancer Network (NCCN) guidelines state that patients with clinically localized disease may be treated with resection or chemotherapy plus irradiation (Tables 3 and 4). The overall 5-year survival rates for either surgery alone or combined chemotherapy and irradiation appear equivalent.

Chemoradiation therapy as primary management of localized or locoregionally confined esophageal cancer has been shown to be superior to irradiation alone. A series of randomized trials have demonstrated that adjuvant postoperative chemoradiation therapy does not offer a survival advantage to patients with esophageal cancer. Adequate patient selection, tumor staging, and treatment standardization will be required before the optimal therapeutic modalities in these patients will be determined.

Surgery

Preoperative medical evaluation helps determine the patient's risk of developing postoperative complications and mortality. In addition to the staging and nutritional status, it should include an evaluation of the pulmonary, cardiac, renal, and hepatic functions.

Extent of surgical resection The extent of resection depends on the location of the primary tumor, histology of the tumor, and nature of the procedure (palliative vs curative). A retrospective study has reported that superficial mucosal lesions may be treated via endoscopic mucosal resection, but those patients with submucosal invasion require esophagectomy. Indeed, the line between diagnostic and therapeutic endoscopic procedures has become somewhat blurred in the setting of esophageal disease, in particular in the management of Barrett's disease. Thus, there are studies ongoing about the efficacy of endoscopic mucosal resection, potentially followed by radiation with or without chemotherapy in the setting of early stage, minimally invasive esophageal cancer, especially in patients who are poor candidates for more

TABLE 3: Chemotherapy regimens for esophageal carcinoma

Drug/combination	Dose and schedule
Cisplatin/fluorouracil/radiation therapy	
Cisplatin	75 mg/m² IV on day 1 of weeks 1, 5, 8, and 11
Fluorouracil	1 g/m²/d IV infused continuously on days 1–4 of weeks 1, 5, 8, and 11
Radiation therapy	200 cGy/d 5 days per week (total regional treatment, 3,000 cGy), followed by a 2,000-cGy boost field (total, 5,000 cGy) in 5 weeks
Give chemotherapy concurrently with radiation therapy.	
Adapted from Herskovic A, Martz K, al-Sarraf M, et al: N Engl J Med 326:1593–1598, 1992.	
FOLFOX4/radiation therapy	
Oxaliplatin	85 mg/m² IV on day 1
Leucovorin	200 mg/m² IVPB on day 1
followed by	
Fluorouracil	400 mg/m² IV bolus and
Fluorouracil	600 mg/m², 22-hour continuous infusion on days 1 to 2
Repeat cycle every 2 weeks × 6 with radiation therapy.	
Adenis A, Etienne P, Michel P, et al: 2007 Gastrointestinal Cancers symposium [abstract 42].	
Irinotecan /cisplatin	
Irinotecan	65 mg/m² IVPB every week × 4 weeks
Cisplatin	30 mg/m² IVPB every week × 4 weeks
followed by 2 weeks rest and recycled every 6 weeks	
Ilson DH, Saltz L, Enzinger P, et al: J Clin Oncol 17:3270–3275, 1999.	

IVPB = intravenous piggyback

Table prepared by Ishmael Jaiyesimi, DO.

invasive esophagectomies. However, at this time, the role of such procedures in the treatment of most patients with esophageal cancer, in comparison to more established therapies such as esophagectomy, radiation, and chemotherapy is uncertain.

For tumors of the intrathoracic esophagus (squamous cell carcinomas) and tumors with extensive Barrett's esophagus (adenocarcinomas), it is necessary to perform a total esophagectomy with cervical anastomosis to achieve a complete resection. For distal lesions of the abdominal esophagus (adenocarcinomas) and cardia, it is often possible to perform an intrathoracic esophageal anastomosis above the azygos vein, although many surgeons would prefer to perform a total esophagectomy.

The resected esophagus may be replaced with tubularized stomach in patients with tumors of the intrathoracic esophagus or with a colon interposition in patients with tumors involving the proximal stomach, because such involvement makes this organ unsuitable for esophageal reconstruction. The esophageal replacement is usually brought up through the posterior mediastinum, although the retrosternal route is often used in palliative procedures.

TABLE 4: Postoperative chemoradiation therapy for gastric/esophageal cancer

Dose/combination	Dose and schedule
Adjuvant fluorouracil/leucovorin/radiation therapy for gastric and gastroesophageal junction adenocarcinoma	
Fluorouracil	425 mg/m² IV on days 1–5
Leucovorin	20 mg/m² IV on days 1–5 immediately before fluorouracil for 1 cycle then 3–4 weeks later
followed by	
Radiation therapy	4,500 cGy (180 cGy a day) given concurrently with
Fluorouracil	400 mg/m² IV on days 1–4 and on the last 3 days of radiation therapy
Leucovorin	20 mg/m² IV on days 1–4 and on the last 3 days of radiation therapy
One month after completion of radiation therapy:	
Fluorouracil	425 mg/m² IV on days 1–5
Leucovorin	20 mg/m² IV on days 1–5 immediately before fluorouracil
Repeat cycle every 28 days for 2 cycles.	

Adapted from Macdonald JS, Smalley S, Benedetti J, et al: Proc Am Soc Clin Oncol 19:1, 2000.

Table prepared by Ishmael Jaiyesimi, DO.

Patient selection The indications for esophagectomy in esophageal cancer vary from center to center within the United States.

Clearly, patients with distant metastases, evidence of nodal metastases in more than one nodal basin, or tumor extension outside the esophagus (airway, mediastinum, vocal cord paralysis) are candidates for palliative therapy. Patients with disease limited to the esophagus and no evidence of nodal metastases (stages I and IIA) may be treated with esophagectomy, although these patients can also be considered for definitive treatment with chemoradiation therapy.

Method of resection Considerable controversy also exists among surgeons regarding the method of resection. To date, two randomized studies have compared transhiatal esophagectomy (without thoracotomy) with the Ivor-Lewis (transthoracic) esophagectomy (with thoracotomy). These studies failed to show differences between the two procedures with regard to operative morbidity and mortality. In a randomized trial of 220 patients treated with either a transthoracic or transhiatal esophageal resection, there was a trend toward an improvement in 5-year survival. A meta-analysis failed to show differences in 5-year survival rates. Over the past 5 years, successful attempts have been made to use minimally invasive approaches to esophageal cancer with thoracoscopy and laparoscopy. Although those studies have shown a decrease in morbidity and the minimally invasive approach appears to be oncologically sound from the point of view of resection margins, the number of nodes resected is still not comparable to that of the standard transthoracic approach.

The need for pyloric drainage (pyloroplasty) following esophagectomy is another area of debate. A meta-analysis of nine randomized trials that included 553 patients showed a trend favoring pyloric drainage in improving gastric emptying and nutritional status, whereas bile reflux was better in the nondrainage group. The gastric emptying time evaluated by scintigraphy was twice as long in the nondrainage group as in the pyloric drainage groups.

Lymphadenectomy Considerable controversy exists regarding the need for radical lymphadenectomy in esophageal disease. Much of the controversy is due to the fact that different diseases are being compared.

Japanese series include mostly patients with squamous cell carcinomas of the intrathoracic esophagus, with 80% of the tumors located in the proximal and middle sections of the esophagus. Americans report combined series, with at least 40% to 50% of patients with adenocarcinomas of the distal esophagus. Skinner and DeMeester favor en bloc esophagectomy with radical (mediastinal and abdominal) lymphadenectomy, based on 5-year survival rates of 40% to 50% in patients with stage II disease, as compared with rates of 14% to 22% in historic controls.

In a retrospective study, Akiyama found a 28% incidence of cervical node metastases in patients with squamous cell carcinomas located in the middle and distal portions of the esophagus, as opposed to 46% in those with tumors of the proximal third. Overall survival at 5 years was significantly better in patients who underwent extended lymphadenectomy (three fields) than in those who had conventional lymphadenectomy (two fields); this finding was true in patients with negative nodes (84% and 55%, respectively) and in those with positive nodes (43% and 28%, respectively). Extended lymphadenectomy afforded no survival advantage in patients with tumors in the distal third of the esophagus.

In a study of 1,000 patients with esophagogastric junction adenocarcinomas, the tumors were classified according to the location of the center of the tumor mass in adenocarcinomas of the distal esophagus, cardia, and subcardia. The tumors located in the cardia and subcardia regions spread primarily to the paragastric and left gastric vessel nodes and did not benefit from extended esophagectomy. Kato et al have studied the use of sentinel node mapping to improve the sensitivity of lymphadenectomy.

Preoperative chemotherapy

The frequency of metastatic disease as the cause of death in patients with esophageal cancer has resulted in exploration of the early application of systemic therapy for esophageal cancer. The first of the two large studies was intergroup study 113. A total of 440 patients were treated with surgical resection alone or preceded by 3 cycles of cisplatin and fluorouracil (5-FU). Objective responses were reported in only 19% of patients receiving chemotherapy. No difference in resectability, operative mortality, median survival (14.9 months with chemotherapy vs 16.1 months with surgery alone), or 2-year survival (35% vs 37%) was reported.

However, the Medical Research Council evaluated 802 patients with resectable esophageal cancer in a similar study. Patients randomized to receive chemotherapy were administered 2 cycles of cisplatin (80 mg/m^2) and 5-FU

(1 g/m²/d as a continuous infusion for 4 days). Microscopically complete resection was performed more frequently in patients receiving chemotherapy, with no difference found in postoperative complications or mortality. Moreover, patients receiving neoadjuvant chemotherapy had significantly longer median (16.8 months vs 13.3 months) and 2-year survival (43% vs 34%) than patients treated with surgery alone. With a median follow up of 6 years, the updated results of this study continued to demonstrate a significant difference in overall survival at 5 years: 23% in patients who received preoperative chemotherapy, vs 17%, and this benefit was present in both histologies. The reasons for the differences in the outcomes are unclear but may be related to the chemotherapy regimen and schedule employed in the intergroup study, patient population, or study design. As a result, the role of neoadjuvant chemotherapy remains in question but is promising, especially with the potentially more efficacious newer generation of chemotherapy agents.

Polee et al have evaluated a biweekly combination of cisplatin and paclitaxel in this setting in a phase II study, with promising results. Objective responses occurred in 59% of 49 patients. No patients had progressive disease. Although 71% of patients had severe neutropenia, it was often asymptomatic. Forty-seven patients underwent resection subsequently. Complete pathologic responses occurred in 14% of patients. The median survival of patients in this study was 20 months, but it was 32 months in patients who had disease responsive to chemotherapy. The 3-year survival rate was 32%.

Given the uncertainty about the efficacy of preoperative chemotherapy and chemoradiation therapy, some investigators have administered preoperative chemotherapy, followed by chemoradiation therapy, then surgery. The true utility of this approach will need to be defined by randomized studies, but clearly, it is feasible, without a significant increase in toxicity or operative morbidity. Interestingly, these reports have also demonstrated that most patients had significant improvement or resolution of dysphagia with the induction chemotherapy alone.

Adjuvant/postoperative chemotherapy

As the most common source of treatment failure in patients with esophageal cancer who have undergone surgical resection, postoperative chemotherapy has also undergone limited investigation. The JCOG Group has compared preoperative and postoperative chemotherapy in 330 patients with stage II or III esophageal squamous cell carcinomas. Patients received 2 courses of either preoperative or postoperative chemotherapy with cisplatin/5-FU. The patients who received preoperative chemotherapy demonstrated a significant improvement in progression–free survival (2.9 years, vs 2.0 years). Thus, the investigators determined that preoperative therapy would be the new standard therapy.

Radiotherapy

Although radiotherapy alone is inferior to chemoradiation therapy in the management of locoregionally confined esophageal cancer, it may offer palliation to patients with advanced local disease too frail for chemotherapy.

Preoperative radiotherapy has been shown to be of little value in converting unresectable cancers into resectable ones or in improving survival. However, it decreases the incidence of locoregional tumor recurrence.

Stahl et al updated an earlier publication of a randomized trial comparing preoperative chemotherapy with chemoradiotherapy in 126 patients with T3-4NX adenocarcinoma of the lower esophagus/gastric cardia. Again, pathologic complete response was higher (15.6% vs 2%) and 3-year survival was trending toward improvement (47% vs 28%) in those patients receiving preoperative chemoradiotherapy *(Stahl M et al: J Clin Oncol 27:851–856, 2009).*

Postoperative radiotherapy (usually to 50 or 60 Gy) can decrease locoregional failure following curative resection but has no effect on survival.

Brachytherapy Intraluminal isotope radiotherapy (intracavitary brachytherapy) allows high doses of radiation to be delivered to a small volume of tissue. Retrospective studies suggest that a brachytherapy boost may result in improved rates of local tumor control and survival over external-beam radiotherapy alone. This technique can be associated with a high rate of morbidity if not used carefully.

A multi-institution prospective trial was conducted by the Radiation Therapy Oncology Group (RTOG) to determine the feasibility and toxicity of chemotherapy, external-beam irradiation, and esophageal brachytherapy in potentially curable patients with esophageal cancer. Nearly 70% of patients were able to complete external-beam irradiation, brachytherapy, and at least 2 cycles of 5-FU/cisplatin. The median survival was 11 months, and the 1-year survival was 49%. Because of the 12% incidence of fistula formation, the investigators urged caution in the routine application of brachytherapy as part of a definitive treatment plan.

Chemoradiation therapy

Preoperative chemoradiation therapy Initial trials of preoperative chemoradiation therapy reported unacceptably high operative mortality (~26%). Subsequent trials reported operative mortality of 4% to 11%, median survival as long as 29 months, and 5-year survival rates as high as 34%. In general, 25% to 30% of patients have no residual tumor in the resected specimen, and this group tends to have a higher survival rate than those who have a residual tumor discovered by the pathologist.

The superiority of preoperative chemoradiation therapy over surgery alone in esophageal adenocarcinoma has been investigated in several prospective trials. The first trial included 113 patients with adenocarcinoma of the esophagus. These patients were randomized to receive either preoperative chemoradiation therapy (2 courses of 5-FU and cisplatin given concurrently with 40 Gy of radiotherapy in 15 fractions) or surgery alone. Median survival was statistically superior in the combined-modality arm than in the surgery-alone arm (16 months vs 11 months). Rates of 3-year survival again statistically favored the combined-modality arm (32% vs 6%). Although toxicity was not severe, the short survival in the surgery control arm has minimized the impact of these results in the United States.

More recently, Dutch investigators studied radiation with weekly (for 5 weeks) carboplatin (AUC 2), with paclitaxel (50 mg/m^2). Most of the 363 patients enrolled in this study, all of whom had potentially resectable disease at the time of enrollment, had adenocarcinoma. The addition of neoadjuvant chemoradiation increased the likelihood of a complete (R0) resection (from 64.9% to 92.3% with neoadjuvant chemoradiation) and survival, both median (from 26 months vs 49 months with neoadjuvant therapy), and at 3 years (48% vs 59% with neoadjuvant therapy). There was no significant difference in operative morbidity or mortality reported.

A meta-analysis of randomized trials comparing neoadjuvant chemoradiation therapy followed by surgery with surgery alone found that neoadjuvant concurrent chemoradiation therapy improved 3-year survival (odds ratio, 0.66) compared with surgery alone, with a nonsignificant trend toward increased treatment mortality with neoadjuvant chemoradiation.

Newer chemotherapy agents are active and may improve outcome over these older trials. A phase II trial of 129 patients employed paclitaxel/carboplatin/5-FU with 45 Gy of radiation therapy followed by esophagectomy. A pathologic complete response was seen in 38% of patients, with a median survival of 22 months and a 3-year survival of 41%.

Another phase II trial from the University of Michigan administered paclitaxel/cisplatin with 45 Gy of radiation therapy twice daily (1.5 Gy bid). In this study, 19% of patients exhibited a pathologic complete response, with a 24-month median survival and a 3-year survival of 34%. A phase II trial from Memorial Sloan-Kettering Cancer Center combined cisplatin and irinotecan with 50.4 Gy of radiation therapy followed by surgery. Twenty-five percent of patients had a pathologic complete response. Ongoing studies by the RTOG are employing these newer chemotherapy agents.

Primary chemoradiation therapy Patients with locally advanced esophageal cancer (T1–4 N0–1 M0) may be cured with definitive chemoradiation therapy. Randomized trials have demonstrated a survival advantage for chemoradiation therapy over radiotherapy alone in the treatment of esophageal cancer. In an RTOG randomized trial involving 129 patients with esophageal cancer, irradiation (50 Gy) with concurrent cisplatin and 5-FU provided a significant survival advantage (27% vs 0% at 5 years) and improved local tumor control over radiation therapy alone (64 Gy). Median survival also was significantly better in the combined-therapy arm than in the irradiation arm (14.1 months vs 9.3 months).

Bedenne et al presented a randomized trial of preoperative chemoradiation therapy vs chemoradiation therapy alone, in which there was no difference in median or 2-year overall survival rates. A randomized intergroup trial was designed to investigate the role of high-dose irradiation in conjunction with systemic therapy. This study compared doses of 50.4 Gy with 64.8 Gy. Both treatment arms of the study administered concurrent 5-FU and cisplatin. This trial was stopped after an interim analysis revealed no statistically significant difference in survival between the two groups. The authors concluded that higher dose radiation therapy did not offer any survival benefit over the 50.4-Gy dose.

Patient selection Patients with disease involving the mid to proximal esophagus are excellent candidates for definitive chemoradiation therapy because resection in this area can be associated with greater morbidity than resection of more distal tumors.

Most of the trials demonstrating the efficacy of chemoradiation therapy have had a high proportion of patients with squamous cell cancers. Chemoradiation therapy has thus become standard treatment of locoregionally confined squamous cell cancer of the esophagus. It is essential that chemotherapy be given concurrently with irradiation when this approach is chosen as primary treatment for esophageal cancer. A typical regimen is 50 to 60 Gy over 5 to 6 weeks, with cisplatin (75 mg/m^2) and 5-FU (1 g/m^2/24 hours for 4 days) on weeks 1, 5, 8, and 11.

The literature also supports offering primary surgery, preoperative chemoradiation therapy, or primary chemoradiation therapy with surgical salvage if necessary to patients with adenocarcinoma. Entering these patients on protocols will allow us to further define standard treatment.

Sequential preoperative chemotherapy and radiation therapy Only modest benefits have been found with preoperative chemoradiation therapy to date, with systemic failure continuing to be an important problem. Thus, sequential therapy with chemotherapy followed by chemoradiation therapy has been explored.

Ajani et al reported a series of 43 patients who received 12 weeks of cisplatin and irinotecan followed by weekly paclitaxel with infusional 5-FU and concurrent radiation therapy (4,500 cGy) and then esophagectomy. Therapy was well tolerated, with no deaths from chemotherapy or chemoradiation therapy, and an operative mortality rate of 5%. Cisplatin and irinotecan induced responses in 37% of patients, and 91% of patients underwent complete resection. Pathologic complete responses occurred in 26% of patients, and some tumor shrinkage was noted in 63% of patients. With a median follow-up of more than 30 months, the median progression-free survival was 10.2 months, the median survival was 22.1 months, and the 2-year survival was 42%. The patients who had a pathologic response to therapy had significantly better outcomes than the rest of the study population. However, systemic recurrences remained a prominent cause of failure, with five patients experiencing recurrence first in the brain and an additional five patients, in the liver.

Esophagectomy following induction chemotherapy and chemoradiation therapy Controversy exists regarding the need for esophagectomy following chemoradiation therapy. Although previously described studies randomized patients to receive surgery with or without preoperative chemoradiation therapy, Stahl et al randomized patients to receive chemoradiation therapy with or without surgery. Also, all 172 patients in the study underwent initial induction chemotherapy (bolus 5-FU, leucovorin, etoposide, and cisplatin for 3 cycles). Those randomized to receive preoperative chemoradiation therapy received cisplatin/etoposide with 40 Gy of radiation, followed by surgery 3 to 4 weeks later. Those randomized to receive definitive chemoradiation therapy received cisplatin/etoposide with 65 Gy of radiation.

After a 6-year median follow-up, the local progression-free survival favored the group undergoing surgery (64% vs 41%). However, the treatment-related mortality was higher in those patients undergoing surgery (13% vs 4%), and so overall survival was statistically equivalent (at 3 years, 31% vs 24%). Since induction chemotherapy was used in all patients, these results should not be extrapolated to indicate the value of esophagectomy following chemoradiotherapy alone.

The incidence of residual disease in patients who have a complete clinical response to chemoradiation therapy is 40% to 50%, and those patients who have a pathologic complete response to chemoradiation therapy have the best survival rates with surgery.

Treatment in elderly patients Since more patients are being diagnosed with esophageal cancer at older ages, research is ongoing as how best to treat elderly patients. Retrospective studies from Nallapareddy et al have found chemoradiaton therapy is tolerable in elderly patients, whereas Rice et al have found a trimodality approach of chemoradiation therapy followed by surgery is also tolerable in the elderly. Close monitoring for toxicities such as dehydration, nutritional concerns, anemia, and postoperative arrhythmia was recommended in these two studies.

TREATMENT OF ADVANCED DISEASE

The goal of esophageal cancer treatment is generally palliative for patients with bulky or extensive retroperitoneal lymph nodes or distant metastatic disease. Therapeutic approaches should temper treatment-related morbidity with the overall dismal outlook. Most data relating to the treatment of unresectable and metastatic esophageal cancer are often derived from clinical trials in which patients with esophageal and gastric and gastroesophageal carcinomas are enrolled. Similarly patients in such studies may have either squamous cell carcinomas or adenocarcinomas. However, although subset analysis of data suggests a similar survival outcome in both histologic subsets, it is possible that there is a difference in response rates, by histology.

Local treatment In patients with a good performance status, the combination of 5-FU/mitomycin, or 5-FU/cisplatin, and radiotherapy (50 Gy) results in a median survival of 7 months to 9 months. This regimen usually renders patients free of dysphagia until death.

Photodynamic therapy (PDT) Porfimer (Photofrin) and an argon-pumped dye laser can provide effective palliation of dysphagia in patients with esophageal cancer. A prospective, randomized multicenter trial comparing PDT with neodymium/yttrium-aluminum-garnet (Nd:YAG) laser therapy in 236 patients with advanced esophageal cancer found that improvement of dysphagia was equivalent with the two treatments.

A review of 119 patients treated with endoluminal palliation reported a significant improvement in dysphagia scores and an increased ability to relieve stenosis caused by tumor when PDT was used in conjunction with laser therapy and irradiation.

Other approaches include external-beam radiotherapy with or without an intracavitary brachytherapy boost, simple dilatation, placement of stents, and laser recannulization of the esophageal lumen.

Palliative resection for esophageal cancer is rarely warranted, although it does provide relief from dysphagia in some patients.

Chemotherapy Phase I and II studies have demonstrated moderate response rates to taxanes in esophageal cancer. Taxanes in combination with platinum compounds and fluoropyrimidines are being tested in regimens with irradiation.

Although chemotherapy alone may produce an occasional long-term remission, there is no standard regimen for patients with metastatic cancer. Patients with advanced disease should be encouraged to participate in well-designed trials exploring novel agents and chemotherapy combinations.

CHEMOTHERAPY IN ADVANCED ESOPHAGEAL CANCER

In Britain, the ECF regimen, a combination of epirubicin (50 mg/m^2) and cisplatin (60 mg/m^2), both repeated every 21 days, with continuous infusion of 5-FU (200 mg/m^2/d), is considered to be a standard regimen for advanced esophagogastric cancers. However, in the remainder of the world, there is no regimen that is considered to be the standard treatment of metastatic esophageal cancer. Difficulties in determining optimal therapy for this disease include the possible differences between esophageal squamous cell cancers and adenocarcinomas. Moreover, most of the available data regarding the treatment of metastatic esophageal cancer are derived from studies in which most patients had gastric cancer or from small phase II studies.

Although the regimen has been fairly well tolerated, infusional 5-FU has rendered the combination unpopular in other countries. Several phase III studies have been performed and consistently demonstrated objective responses in about 40% of patients, with a median survival of 9 months and a 1-year survival of 36% to 40%. The main severe toxicities of this regimen are neutropenia, in about one-third of patients (32%–36%), lethargy (18%), and nausea and vomiting (11%–17%). The REAL-2 study evaluated 1,002 patients (60% esophageal or GE junction cancer) with advanced esophagogastric cancers. They were randomly assigned to receive epirubicin (50 mg/m^2 every 21 days) with either cisplatin (60 mg/m^2) or oxaliplatin (Eloxatin; 130 mg/m^2) every 21 days, and either infusional 5-FU (200 mg/m^2/d) or capecitabine (Xeloda; 625 mg/m^2 twice daily). In this study, the outcomes were similar in the resultant treatment groups, with median survivals around 10 months and 1-year survivals between 39% and 45%. Indeed, the single best-performing arm was EOX (epirubicin, oxaliplatin, Xeloda [capecitabine]), with a median survival of 11.2 months and a 1-year survival of 46.8%, although these results were not significantly superior to the other arms.

With the advent of many new chemotherapeutic agents (the taxoids, paclitaxel and docetaxel [Taxotere], irinotecan, and gemcitabine [Gemzar]) with varying mechanisms of activity, further studies have been conducted, and each of these drugs has demonstrated activity, with responses achieved in approximately 15% to 30% of patients.

However, the primary route of investigation for these new agents has been in combination with cisplatin and/or 5-FU. The results available to date suggest promising activity, with response rates often around 50% in phase II studies. Irinotecan (65 mg/m^2) and cisplatin (30 mg/m^2) administered weekly for 4 weeks every 6 weeks have also been active, with responses in 20 of 35 patients (57%) and an impressive median survival of 14.6 months. A Korean phase II study did not confirm these results but did suggest the combination was active, with a response rate of 31% of 32 patients, and a median survival of 9.6 months.

Following the example of the combination of irinotecan and 5-FU/leucovorin in colon cancer, the investigators have explored a modification of that schedule, with therapy administered for 2 weeks, with cycles repeated every 3 weeks. This simple modification has been investigated in 27 patients and was well tolerated, with severe neutropenia in 18% of patients and severe diarrhea in 11% of patients.

Paclitaxel (180 mg/m^2 over 3 hours) and cisplatin (60 mg/m^2 over 3 hours) adminis-

TABLE 5: Combination chemotherapy in advanced disease

Agents	Response rate (%)	Survival
Cisplatin/fluorouracil	19–40	Median = 7 months, 1 year = 27%
Cisplatin/paclitaxel	37–43	Median = 6–9 months
Cisplatin/gemcitabine	38–47	Median = 7–10 months
Cisplatin/irinotecan	30–57	Median = 9.6–14.6 months
Cisplatin/vinorelbine	33	Median = 6.8 months
Cisplatin/etoposide	45–48	Median = 8–10 months, 1 year = 26%–41%
Epirubicin/cisplatin/ fluorouracil	40–42	Median = 9 months, 1 year = 36%–40%
Cisplatin/fluorouracil/ paclitaxel	48	Median = 10.8 months, 1 year = 38%
Carboplatin/paclitaxel	45–50	Median = 9–11 months, 1 year = 43%–46%

tered every 14 days have been extensively evaluated in Europe. They were reported to produce objective responses in 43% of 51 patients, including two complete responses, and 43% of patients were alive 1 year after initiation of therapy (Table 5).

Because of the toxic and logistic difficulties of using cisplatin, carboplatin has become a popular chemotherapeutic drug. Several studies of carboplatin with paclitaxel in esophageal cancer have been undertaken. El-Rayes et al administered carboplatin (at an area under the concentration-time curve [AUC] of 5) with paclitaxel (200 mg/m^2 over 3 hours) every 3 weeks in 33 chemotherapy-naive patients. Objective responses were reported in 45% of patients, with a median survival of 9 months and 1-year and 2-year survival rates of 43% and 17% respectively.

Polee et al explored a weekly schedule of these drugs in a phase I study. With therapy administered for 3 consecutive weeks, followed by a 1-week break, a dose of carboplatin (at AUC 4) with paclitaxel (100 mg/m^2) was recommended for further investigation. Responses were noted in half of the 40 patients, with a median survival of 11 months and a 1-year survival of 46%. Both of these combinations were well tolerated, with the primary toxicity of myelosuppression.

Lorenzen et al treated 24 patients with esophageal and esophagogastric carcinomas and measurable disease with docetaxel (75 mg/m^2 IV) and capecitabine (1,000 mg/m^2 orally twice daily from days 1–14), with cycles repeated every 3 weeks. Only seven of the patients had adenocarcinomas, and eight had received prior chemotherapy. This combination had interesting antitumor activity, with objective responses in 11 patients (46%), including 56% of previously untreated patients and 2 of 8 patients who had received prior chemotherapy. Although patient numbers were small, there was no clear difference in response rates by histology. The therapy was reported to be fairly well tolerated overall, although dose reductions were necessary in 41% of patients. The main grade 3 and 4 toxicities were neutropenia (42% of patients, including two patients with neutropenic fever), diarrhea and neuropathy (13% of patients each), and hand-foot syndrome in 29% of patients.

The combination of docetaxel, cisplatin, and infusional 5-FU (DCF) has been approved by the US FDA for the treatment of metastatic gastric and GE junction adenocarcinomas. The activity of this regimen in esophageal cancers is unclear. Chiarion-Sileni et al reported a study that provides some insight into the potential activity of this regimen. They studied a modification of the DCF regimen, with cisplatin (75 mg/m^2) and docetaxel (60 mg/m^2) given on day 1 and 5-FU (750 mg/m^2/d) given on days 2 to 5 every 21 days for 3 cycles in patients with locally advanced esophageal cancer. This regimen was followed by radiation therapy with concurrent carboplatin. The response rate to chemotherapy alone with this regimen was 48% in 37 patients, suggesting that this combination is active in esophageal cancers as well.

Another response to the toxicity of the DCF regimen has been the elimination of the fluorouracil, and exploration of cisplatin and docetaxel alone. Kim et al evaluated this combination, with a dose of 70 mg/m^2 of each agent, administered every 21 days in 39 Korean patients with squamous cell carcinomas of the esophagus. They reported a 33% response rate, which included three complete responses (7.7%), and a median survival time of 8.3 months. The regimen was reported as well tolerated, with about one-third of patients experiencing grade 3 or 4 neutropenia.

The antimetabolite gemcitabine has also been evaluated in combination with cisplatin in esophageal cancer. A SWOG study, reported by Urba et al, combined 1,000 mg/m^2 of gemcitabine on days 1, 8, and 15 with 100 mg/m^2 of cisplatin on day 15 in 64 patients. Approximately one-quarter of these patients had received prior chemotherapy. Therapy was well tolerated, with severe neutropenia occurring in 31% of patients. The median survival of patients treated on this study was 7.3 months, and the 1-year survival rate was 20%. However, the heterogeneity of the patient population makes the efficacy of the therapy somewhat difficult to assess.

Oxaliplatin may also have a role in the treatment of esophageal cancer, both as a radiosensitizer and an agent in advanced disease. Mauer and colleagues reported the results of treatment with oxaliplatin, 5-FU, and leucovorin according to the FOLFOX4 schedule (oxaliplatin, 85 mg/m^2 on day 1; leucovorin, 500 mg/m^2 over 2 hours on days 1 and 2; and 5-FU, 400 mg/m^2 bolus, then 600 mg/m^2 over 22 hours on days 1 and 2, repeated every 14 days). Of 35 patients who were treated, objective responses were noted in 40%. The median survival rate was 7.1 months, the 1-year survival rate was 31%, and the 2-year survival rate was 11%. The median progression-free survival was 4.6 months. Although differences in patient populations were noted, these results are similar to those of other reported combinations.

The combination of oxaliplatin (130 mg/m^2 on day 1) with capecitabine (1,000 mg/m^2 twice daily on days 1 to 14) repeated every 21 days has also been studied in esophageal cancer. Thirty-eight percent of the 51 treated patients had objective responses, with a median survival of 8 months and a 1-year survival rate of 26%. This study was conducted in the Netherlands, and the tolerability and efficacy of this regimen in American patients remain to be determined.

The primary toxicity of these regimens is severe neutropenia, occurring in about 40% to 70% of patients. Severe diarrhea, nausea, and vomiting occur in ~10% to 15% of patients in many studies. Fatigue and asthenia also were significant side effects with both therapies.

With improving toxicity profiles and modest improvements in therapeutic outcomes, second-line therapy for advanced esophageal cancer is also increasingly being explored. Muro et al treated 28 Japanese patients with squamous cell carcinoma of the esophagus with docetaxel (70 mg/m^2) every 3 weeks; these patients had previously received cisplatin and 5-FU. As expected, severe neutropenia was the dominant toxicity (88%, including nine episodes of febrile neutropenia), with severe anorexia, fatigue, and anemia also reported. Objective responses were noted in 16% of these patients.

More recently, the CALGB performed a randomized phase II study combining cetuximab with several other typical chemotherapy regimens, including ECF, cisplatin/irinotecan, and FOLFOX, in patients with metastastic esophageal and gastroesophageal junction cancers. Each arm included about 80 patients, and each regimen resulted in response rates of 58%, 38%, and 51% respectively, and median survivals of 8 to 10 months. Each arm surpassed the prespecified endpoint suggesting enough promise to further explore in phase III studies. Again, however, the number of patients treated was too low to consider any of the regimens to be a standard at this time.

In addition, Lordick et al determined that irinotecan (55 mg/m^2) and docetaxel (25 mg/m^2) given on days 1, 8, and 15, with cycles repeated every 28 days, were tolerable, with severe asthenia in 21% of 24 patients and severe diarrhea in 13%. However, only three partial responses (13%) and eight patients with stable disease were noted, with a resultant median survival of 26 weeks. Although these studies suggest the feasibility of second-line cytotoxic chemotherapy in esophageal cancer, the significant toxicity and limited objective response rate warrant its use only with caution and preferably on a clinical study.

Oral tyrosine kinase inhibitors of the epidermal growth factor receptor (EGFR) have also been investigated in esophageal cancer. Gefitinib (Iressa), at a daily dose of 500 mg, as second-line therapy in patients with esophageal adenocarcinomas was evaluated by Ferry et al. It produced partial responses in 11% of 27 patients, and an additional 7 patients had stable disease. In patients with esophageal cancer that had previously been treated with platinum-based chemotherapy, Janmaat et al treated 37 patients with the same regimen. They reported a confirmed response in only 1 patient, and stable disease in another 10, although 18% of patients were free of disease progression at 6 months, suggesting that some patients indeed experience disease control and benefit from this therapy. However, Radovich et al reported only 1 response in 23 patients treated with erlotinib (Tarceva; 150 mg daily). The toxicities were as expected, including rash, diarrhea, vomiting, and elevation in transaminase levels. As with lung and colon cancers, the optimal population for treatment with these targeted agents remains to be defined.

The other class of agents that target the EGFR pathway, monoclonal antibodies such as cetuximab, has provided mixed results in patients with esophageal cancer. For example, a German study of cisplatin/5-FU with or without cetuximab (Erbitux) as initial therapy in patients with metastatic esophageal squamous cell cancers with

EGFR expression by immunohistochemistry suggested an improvement in patient outcomes. Sixty-two patients were randomized in a non-blinded fashion on the study, and crossover to cetuximab with cisplatin/5-FU was allowed in the patients who received initial cisplatin/5-FU alone. The response rates were similar (33% with cetuximab, vs 30%) in the two arms, but patients who received the additional cetuximab had a superior disease-control rate (75% vs 57%), median time to disease progression (5.9 months vs 3.6 months), and median overall survival (9.5 months vs 5.5 months). Moreover, of the five patients who crossed-over to second-line cetuximab, two had partial responses (one with single-agent therapy), and one had stable disease. However, given the sample size, and the unblinded nature of the study, with crossover, caution must be exercised when interpreting these results.

The SWOG studied cetuximab as a single agent as second-line therapy for metastatic esophageal adenocarcinoma. Of the 55 eligible and evaluable patients, only 1 had a partial response (2%), and 6 (11%) had stable disease. The median progression-free survival was 1.8 months, the median survival was 4.0 months, and the 6-month survival rate was 36%. The authors concluded that although the drug was well tolerated as single-agent therapy it did not meet its primary endpoint, and so could not be recommended as second-line therapy in esophageal cancer. The discordant results represented in these studies, between histologies and drugs, may reflect the differing biologies of esophageal adenocarcinomas and squamous cell carcinomas. Alternatively, they may reflect alterations in cancers after undergoing chemotherapy.

In addition to flavopiridol and the EGFR antagonists, it is anticipated that other targeted therapies, such as vascular endothelial growth factor antagonists, will be evaluated in this disease. Such avenues of exploration, in addition to early diagnosis and therapy for early-stage disease, are the most likely path toward significant improvements in therapy for esophageal cancer.

SUGGESTED READING

Bedenne L, Michel P, Bouche O, et al: Chemoradiation followed by surgery compared with chemoradiation alone in squamous cancer of the esophagus: FFCD 9102. J Clin Oncol 25:1160–1168, 2007.

Chiarion-Sileni V, Corti L, Ruol A, et al: Phase II trial of docetaxel, cisplatin and fluorouracil followed by carboplatin and radiation in locally advanced oesophageal cancer. Br J Cancer 96:432–438, 2007.

Cunningham D, Starling N, Rao S, et al: Capecitabine and oxaliplatin for advanced esophagogastric cancer. N Engl J Med 358:36–46, 2008.

Enzinger PC, Burtness B, Hollis D, et al: CALGB 80403/ECOG 1206: A randomized phase II study of three standard chemotherapy regimens (ECF, IC, FOLFOX) plus cetuximab in metastatic esophageal and GE junction cancer. J Clin Oncol 28:4006, 2010.

Ferry DR, Anderson M, Beddard K, et al: A phase II study of gefitinib monotherapy in advanced esophageal adenocarcinoma: Evidence of gene expression, cellular, and clinical response. Clin Cancer Res 13:5869–5875, 2007.

Gold PJ, Goldman B, Iqbal S, et al: Cetuximab as second-line therapy in patients with metastatic esophageal cancer: A phase II Southwest Oncology Group Study. J Clin Oncol 26:abstract 4536, 2008.

Igaki H, Kato H, Ando N, et al: A randomized trial of postoperative adjuvant chemotherapy with cisplatin and 5-fluorouracil versus neoadjuvant chemotherapy for clinical stage II/III squamous cell carcinoma of the thoracic esophagus (JCOG 9907). J Clin Oncol 26:abstract 4510, 2008.

Janmaat ML, Gallegos-Ruiz MI, Rodriguez JA, et al: Predictive factors for outcome in a phase II study of gefitinib in second-line treatment of advanced esophageal cancer patients. J Clin Oncol 24:1612–1619, 2006.

Jemal A, Siegel R, Xu J, et al: Cancer statistics, 2010. CA Cancer J Clin 60:277–300, 2010.

Kim JY, Do YR, Park KU, et al: A multi-center phase II study of docetaxel plus cisplatin as first-line therapy in patients with metastatic squamous cell esophageal cancer. Cancer Chemother Pharmacol 66:31–36, 2010.

Lee DH, Kim HT, Han JY, et al: A phase II trial of modified weekly irinotecan and cisplatin for chemotherapy-naive patients with metastatic or recurrent squamous cell carcinoma of the esophagus. Cancer Chemother Pharmacol 61:83–88, 2008.

Lordick F, Lorenzen S, Al-Batran S, et al: Cetuximab and cisplatin/5-FU (CF) versus CF in first-line metastatic squamous cell carcinoma of the esophagus (MESCC): A randomized phase II study of the Arbeitsgemeinschaft Internistische Onkologie (AIO). J Clin Oncol 26:abstract 4546, 2008.

Lorenzen S, Duyster J, Lersch C, et al: Capecitabine plus docetaxel every 3 weeks in first- and second-line metastastic oesophageal cancer: Final results of a phase II trial. Br J Cancer 92:2129–2133, 2005.

Lorenzen S, Schuster T, Porschen R, et al: Cetuximab plus cisplatin-5-fluorouracil versus cisplatin-5-fluorouracil alone in first-line metastatic squamous cell carcinoma of the esophagus: A randomized phase II study of the Arbeitsgemeinschaft Internistische Onkologie. Ann Oncol 20:1667–1673, 2009.

Mauer AM, Kraut EH, Krauss SA, et al: Phase II trial of oxaliplatin, leucovorin, and fluorouracil in patients with advanced carcincoma of the esophagus. Ann Oncol 16:1320–1325, 2005.

Santharalingam M, Moughan J, Coia LR, et al: Outcome results of the 1996–1999 patterns of care survey of the national practice for patients receiving radiation therapy for carcinoma of the esophagus. J Clin Oncol 23:2325–2331, 2005.

Stahl M, Stuschke M, Lehmann N, et al: Chemoradiation with and without surgery in patients with locally advanced squamous cell carcinoma of the esophagus. J Clin Oncol 23:2310–2317, 2005.

Van Cutsem E, Moiseyenko VM, Tjulandin S, et al: Phase III study of docetaxel and cisplatin plus fluorouracil compared with cisplatin and fluorouracil as first-line therapy for advanced gastric cancer: A report of the V325 Study Group. J Clin Oncol 24:4991–4997, 2006.

van der Gaast A, van Hagen P, Hulshof M, et al: Effect of preoperative concurrent chemoradiotherapy on survival of patients with resectable esophageal or esophagogastric junction cancer: Results from a multicenter randomized phase III study. J Clin Oncol 28:4004, 2010.

van Meerten E, Eskens FA, van Gameren EC, et al: First-line treatment with oxaliplatin and capecitabine in patients with advanced or metastatic oesophageal cancer: A phase II study. Br J Cancer 96:1348–1352, 2007.

Abbreviations in this chapter

CALGB = Cancer and Leukemia Group B; JCOG = Japanese Cooperative Oncology Group; SWOG = Southwest Oncology Group

In first-line metastatic NSCLC and first- and second-line MCRC

To reach beyond convention...

Think beyond the tumor

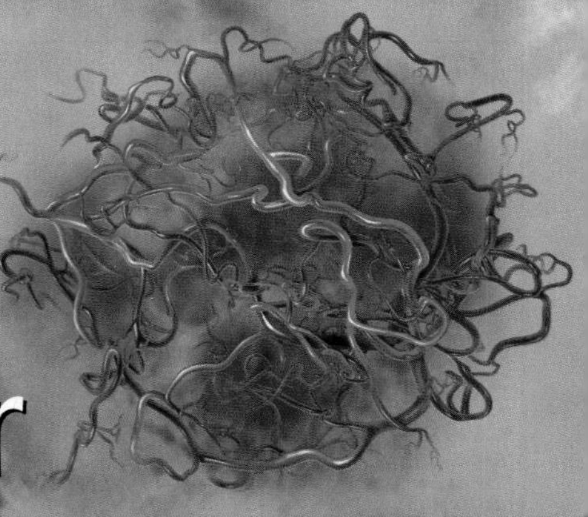

Indications

Avastin is indicated for the first-line treatment of unresectable, locally advanced, recurrent or metastatic non–squamous non–small cell lung cancer in combination with carboplatin and paclitaxel.

Avastin is indicated for the first- or second-line treatment of patients with metastatic carcinoma of the colon or rectum in combination with intravenous 5-fluorouracil–based chemotherapy.

Boxed WARNINGS and additional important safety information

- **Gastrointestinal (GI) perforation:** Serious and sometimes fatal GI perforation occurs at a higher incidence in Avastin-treated patients compared to controls. The incidences of GI perforation ranged from 0.3% to 2.4% across clinical studies. Discontinue Avastin in patients with GI perforation
- **Surgery and wound healing complications:** The incidence of wound healing and surgical complications, including serious and fatal complications, is increased in Avastin-treated patients. Do not initiate Avastin for at least 28 days after surgery and until the surgical wound is fully healed. The appropriate interval between termination of Avastin and subsequent elective surgery required to reduce the risks of impaired wound healing/wound dehiscence has not been determined. Discontinue Avastin at least 28 days prior to elective surgery and in patients with wound dehiscence requiring medical intervention
- **Hemorrhage:** Severe or fatal hemorrhage, including hemoptysis, GI bleeding, hematemesis, central nervous system hemorrhage, epistaxis, and vaginal bleeding, occurred up to 5-fold more frequently in patients receiving Avastin. Across indications, the incidence of grade ≥3 hemorrhagic events among patients receiving Avastin ranged from 1.2% to 4.6%. Do not administer Avastin to patients with serious hemorrhage or recent hemoptysis (≥1/2 tsp of red blood). Discontinue Avastin in patients with serious hemorrhage (ie, requiring medical intervention)
- Additional serious and sometimes fatal adverse events for which the incidence was increased in the Avastin-treated arm vs control included non-GI fistula formation (≤0.3%), arterial thromboembolic events (grade ≥3, 2.4%), and proteinuria including nephrotic syndrome (<1%). Additional serious adverse events for which the incidence was increased in the Avastin-treated arm vs control included hypertension (grade 3–4, 5%–18%) and reversible posterior leukoencephalopathy syndrome (RPLS) (<0.1%). Infusion reactions with the first dose of Avastin were uncommon (<3%), and severe reactions occurred in 0.2% of patients
- The most common adverse reactions observed in Avastin patients at a rate >10% and at least twice the control arm rate were epistaxis, headache, hypertension, rhinitis, proteinuria, taste alteration, dry skin, rectal hemorrhage, lacrimation disorder, back pain, and exfoliative dermatitis. Across all studies, Avastin was discontinued in 8.4% to 21% of patients because of adverse reactions
- Based on animal data, Avastin may cause fetal harm and may impair fertility. Advise patients of the potential risk to the fetus during and following Avastin and the need to continue adequate contraception for at least 6 months following the last dose of Avastin. For nursing mothers, discontinue nursing or Avastin, taking into account the importance of Avastin to the mother

Please see following brief summary of Prescribing Information, including **Boxed WARNINGS**, for additional important safety information.

Genentech
A Member of the Roche Group

AVASTIN®
bevacizumab
Reach beyond convention

 www.avastin.com

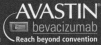

Solution for intravenous infusion
Initial U.S. Approval: 2004

WARNING: GASTROINTESTINAL PERFORATIONS, SURGERY AND WOUND HEALING COMPLICATIONS, and HEMORRHAGE

Gastrointestinal Perforations

The incidence of gastrointestinal perforation, some fatal, in Avastin-treated patients ranges from 0.3 to 2.4%. Discontinue Avastin in patients with gastrointestinal perforation. *[See Dosage and Administration (2.4), Warnings and Precautions (5.1).]*

Surgery and Wound Healing Complications

The incidence of wound healing and surgical complications, including serious and fatal complications, is increased in Avastin-treated patients. Discontinue Avastin in patients with wound dehiscence. The appropriate interval between termination of Avastin and subsequent elective surgery required to reduce the risks of impaired wound healing/wound dehiscence has not been determined. Discontinue at least 28 days prior to elective surgery. Do not initiate Avastin for at least 28 days after surgery and until the surgical wound is fully healed. *[See Dosage and Administration (2.4), Warnings and Precautions (5.2), and Adverse Reactions (6.1).]*

Hemorrhage

Severe or fatal hemorrhage, including hemoptysis, gastrointestinal bleeding, central nervous systems (CNS) hemorrhage, epistaxis, and vaginal bleeding occurred up to five-fold more frequently in patients receiving Avastin. Do not administer Avastin to patients with serious hemorrhage or recent hemoptysis. *[See Dosage and Administration (2.4), Warnings and Precautions (5.3), and Adverse Reactions (6.1).]*

1 INDICATIONS AND USAGE

1.1 Metastatic Colorectal Cancer (mCRC)

Avastin is indicated for the first- or second-line treatment of patients with metastatic carcinoma of the colon or rectum in combination with intravenous 5-fluorouracil–based chemotherapy.

1.2 Non-Squamous Non–Small Cell Lung Cancer (NSCLC)

Avastin is indicated for the first-line treatment of unresectable, locally advanced, recurrent or metastatic non–squamous non–small cell lung cancer in combination with carboplatin and paclitaxel.

1.3 Metastatic Breast Cancer (MBC)

Avastin is indicated for the treatment of patients who have not received chemotherapy for metastatic HER2-negative breast cancer in combination with paclitaxel.

The effectiveness of Avastin in MBC is based on an improvement in progression free survival. There are no data demonstrating an improvement in disease-related symptoms or increased survival with Avastin. *[See Clinical Studies (14.3).]*

Avastin is not indicated for patients with breast cancer that has progressed following anthracycline and taxane chemotherapy administered for metastatic disease.

1.4 Glioblastoma

Avastin is indicated for the treatment of glioblastoma with progressive disease following prior therapy as a single agent.

The effectiveness of Avastin in glioblastoma is based on an improvement in objective response rate. There are no data demonstrating an improvement in disease-related symptoms or increased survival with Avastin. *[See Clinical Studies (14.4).]*

1.5 Metastatic Renal Cell Carcinoma (mRCC)

Avastin is indicated for the treatment of metastatic renal cell carcinoma in combination with interferon alfa.

4 CONTRAINDICATIONS

None.

5 WARNINGS AND PRECAUTIONS

5.1 Gastrointestinal Perforations

Serious and sometimes fatal gastrointestinal perforation occurs at a higher incidence in Avastin treated patients compared to controls. The incidence of gastrointestinal perforation ranged from 0.3 to 2.4% across clinical studies. *[See Adverse Reactions (6.1).]*

The typical presentation may include abdominal pain, nausea, emesis, constipation, and fever. Perforation can be complicated by intra-abdominal abscess and fistula formation. The majority of cases occurred within the first 50 days of initiation of Avastin.

Discontinue Avastin in patients with gastrointestinal perforation. *[See Boxed Warning, Dosage and Administration (2.4).]*

5.2 Surgery and Wound Healing Complications

Avastin impairs wound healing in animal models. *[See Nonclinical Toxicology (13.2).]* In clinical trials, administration of Avastin was not allowed until at least 28 days after surgery. In a controlled clinical trial, the incidence of wound healing complications, including serious and fatal complications, in patients with mCRC who underwent surgery during the course of Avastin treatment was 15% and in patients who did not receive Avastin, was 4%. *[See Adverse Reactions (6.1).]*

Avastin should not be initiated for at least 28 days following surgery and until the surgical wound is fully healed. Discontinue Avastin in patients with wound healing complications requiring medical intervention.

The appropriate interval between the last dose of Avastin and elective surgery is unknown; however, the half-life of Avastin is estimated to be 20 days. Suspend Avastin for at least 28 days prior to elective surgery. Do not administer Avastin until the wound is fully healed. *[See Boxed Warning, Dosage and Administration (2.4).]*

5.3 Hemorrhage

Avastin can result in two distinct patterns of bleeding: minor hemorrhage, most commonly Grade 1 epistaxis; and serious, and in some cases fatal, hemorrhagic events. Severe or fatal hemorrhage, including hemoptysis, gastrointestinal bleeding, hematemesis, CNS hemorrhage, epistaxis, and vaginal bleeding occurred up to five-fold more frequently in patients receiving Avastin compared to patients receiving only chemotherapy. Across indications, the incidence of Grade ≥ 3 hemorrhagic events among patients receiving Avastin ranged from 1.2 to 4.6%. *[See Adverse Reactions (6.1).]*

Serious or fatal pulmonary hemorrhage occurred in four of 13 (31%) patients with squamous cell histology and two of 53 (4%) patients with non-squamous non-small cell lung cancer receiving Avastin and chemotherapy compared to none of the 32 (0%) patients receiving chemotherapy alone.

In clinical studies in non–small cell lung cancer where patients with CNS metastases who completed radiation and surgery more than 4 weeks prior to the start of Avastin were evaluated with serial CNS imaging, symptomatic Grade 2 CNS hemorrhage was documented in one of 83 Avastin-treated patients (rate 1.2%, 95% CI 0.06%–5.93%).

Intracranial hemorrhage occurred in 8 of 163 patients with previously treated glioblastoma; two patients had Grade 3–4 hemorrhage.

Do not administer Avastin to patients with recent history of hemoptysis of ≥1/2 teaspoon of red blood. Discontinue Avastin in patients with hemorrhage. *[See Boxed Warning, Dosage and Administration (2.4).]*

5.4 Non-Gastrointestinal Fistula Formation

Serious and sometimes fatal non-gastrointestinal fistula formation involving tracheo-esophageal, bronchopleural, biliary, vaginal, renal and bladder sites occurs at a higher incidence in Avastin-treated patients compared to controls. The incidence of non-gastrointestinal perforation was ≤0.3% in clinical studies. Most events occurred within the first 6 months of Avastin therapy.

Discontinue Avastin in patients with fistula formation involving an internal organ. *[See Dosage and Administration (2.4).]*

5.5 Arterial Thromboembolic Events

Serious, sometimes fatal, arterial thromboembolic events (ATE) including cerebral infarction, transient ischemic attacks, myocardial infarction, angina, and a variety of other ATE occurred at a higher incidence in patients receiving Avastin compared to those in the control arm. Across indications, the incidence of Grade ≥ 3 ATE in the Avastin containing arms was 2.4% compared to 0.7% in the control arms. Among patients receiving Avastin in combination with chemotherapy, the risk of developing ATE during therapy was increased in patients with a history of arterial thromboembolism, or age greater than 65 years. *[See Use in Specific Populations (8.5).]*

The safety of resumption of Avastin therapy after resolution of an ATE has not been studied. Discontinue Avastin in patients who experience a severe ATE. *[See Dosage and Administration (2.4).]*

5.6 Hypertension

The incidence of severe hypertension is increased in patients receiving Avastin as compared to controls. Across clinical studies the incidence of Grade 3 or 4 hypertension ranged from 5-18%.

Monitor blood pressure every two to three weeks during treatment with Avastin. Treat with appropriate anti-hypertensive therapy and monitor blood pressure regularly. Continue to monitor blood pressure at regular intervals in patients with Avastin-induced or -exacerbated hypertension after discontinuation of Avastin.

Temporarily suspend Avastin in patients with severe hypertension that is not controlled with medical management. Discontinue Avastin in patients with hypertensive crisis or hypertensive encephalopathy. *[See Dosage and Administration (2.4).]*

5.7 Reversible Posterior Leukoencephalopathy Syndrome (RPLS)

RPLS has been reported with an incidence of <0.1% in clinical studies. The onset of symptoms occurred from 16 hours to 1 year after initiation of Avastin. RPLS is a neurological disorder which can present with headache, seizure, lethargy, confusion, blindness and other visual and neurologic disturbances. Mild to severe hypertension may be present. Magnetic resonance imaging (MRI) is necessary to confirm the diagnosis of RPLS.

Discontinue Avastin in patients developing RPLS. Symptoms usually resolve or improve within days, although some patients have experienced ongoing neurologic sequelae. The safety of reinitiating Avastin therapy in patients previously experiencing RPLS is not known. *[See Dosage and Administration (2.4).]*

5.8 Proteinuria

The incidence and severity of proteinuria is increased in patients receiving Avastin as compared to controls. Nephrotic syndrome occurred in < 1% of patients receiving Avastin in clinical trials, in some instances with fatal outcome. *[See Adverse Reactions (6.1).]* In a published case series, kidney biopsy of six patients with proteinuria showed findings consistent with thrombotic microangiopathy.

Monitor proteinuria by dipstick urine analysis for the development or worsening of proteinuria with serial urinalyses during Avastin therapy. Patients with a 2 + or greater urine dipstick reading should undergo further assessment with a 24-hour urine collection.

Suspend Avastin administration for ≥ 2 grams of proteinuria/24 hours and resume when proteinuria is <2 gm/24 hours. Discontinue Avastin in patients with nephrotic syndrome. Data from a postmarketing safety study showed poor correlation between UPCR (Urine Protein/Creatinine Ratio) and 24 hour urine protein (Pearson Correlation 0.39 (95% CI 0.17, 0.57). *[See Use in Specific Populations (8.5).]* The safety of continued Avastin treatment in patients with moderate to severe proteinuria has not been evaluated. *[See Dosage and Administration (2.4).]*

5.9 Infusion Reactions

Infusion reactions reported in the clinical trials and post-marketing experience include hypertension, hypertensive crises associated with neurologic signs and symptoms, wheezing, oxygen desaturation, Grade 3 hypersensitivity, chest pain, headaches, rigors, and diaphoresis. In clinical studies, infusion reactions with the first dose of Avastin were uncommon (< 3%) and severe reactions occurred in 0.2% of patients.

Stop infusion if a severe infusion reaction occurs and administer appropriate medical therapy. *[See Dosage and Administration (2.4).]*

6 ADVERSE REACTIONS

The following serious adverse reactions are discussed in greater detail in other sections of the label:

- Gastrointestinal Perforations *[See Boxed Warning, Dosage and Administration (2.4), Warnings and Precautions (5.1).]*
- Surgery and Wound Healing Complications *[See Boxed Warning, Dosage and Administration (2.4), Warnings and Precautions (5.2).]*
- Hemorrhage *[See Boxed Warning, Dosage and Administration (2.4), Warnings and Precautions (5.3).]*
- Non-Gastrointestinal Fistula Formation *[See Dosage and Administration (2.4), Warnings and Precautions (5.4).]*
- Arterial Thromboembolic Events *[See Dosage and Administration (2.4), Warnings and Precautions (5.5).]*
- Hypertensive Crisis *[See Dosage and Administration (2.4), Warnings and Precautions (5.6).]*
- Reversible Posterior Leukoencephalopathy Syndrome *[See Dosage and Administration (2.4), Warnings and Precautions (5.7).]*
- Proteinuria *[See Dosage and Administration (2.4), Warnings and Precautions (5.8).]*

The most common adverse reactions observed in Avastin patients at a rate > 10% and at least twice the control arm rate, are epistaxis, headache, hypertension, rhinitis, proteinuria, taste alteration, dry skin, rectal hemorrhage, lacrimation disorder, back pain and exfoliative dermatitis.

Across all studies, Avastin was discontinued in 8.4 to 21% of patients because of adverse reactions.

6.1 Clinical Trial Experience

Because clinical trials are conducted under widely varying conditions, adverse reaction rates observed in the clinical trials of a drug cannot be directly compared to rates in the clinical trials of another drug and may not reflect the rates observed in practice.

The data below reflect exposure to Avastin in 2661 patients with mCRC, non-squamous NSCLC, MBC, glioblastoma, or mRCC in controlled (Studies 1, 2, 4, 5, 6 and 9) or uncontrolled, single arm (Study 7) trials treated at the recommended dose and schedule for a median of 8 to 16 doses of Avastin. *[See Clinical Studies (14).]* The population was aged 21-88 years (median 59), 46.0% male and 84.1% white. The population included 1089 first- and second-line mCRC patients who received a median of 11 doses of Avastin, 480 first-line metastatic NSCLC patients who received a median of 8 doses of Avastin, 592 MBC patients who had not received chemotherapy for metastatic disease received a median of 8 doses of Avastin, 163 glioblastoma patients who received a median of 9 doses of Avastin, and 337 mRCC patients who received a median of 16 doses of Avastin.

Surgery and Wound Healing Complications

The incidence of post-operative wound healing and/or bleeding complications was increased in patients with mCRC receiving Avastin as compared to patients receiving only chemotherapy. Among patients requiring surgery on or within 60 days of receiving study treatment, wound healing and/or bleeding complications occurred in 15% (6/39) of patients receiving bolus-IFL plus Avastin as compared to 4% (1/25) of patients who received bolus-IFL alone.

In Study 7, events of post-operative wound healing complications (craniotomy site wound dehiscence and cerebrospinal fluid leak) occurred in patients with previously treated glioblastoma: 3/84 patients in the Avastin alone arm and 1/79 patients in the Avastin plus irinotecan arm. *[See Boxed Warning, Dosage and Administration (2.4), Warnings and Precautions (5.2).]*

Hemorrhage

The incidence of epistaxis was higher (35% vs. 10%) in patients with mCRC receiving bolus-IFL plus Avastin compared with patients receiving bolus-IFL plus placebo. All but one of these events were Grade 1 in severity and resolved without medical intervention. Grade 1 or 2 hemorrhagic events were more frequent in patients receiving bolus-IFL plus Avastin when compared to those receiving bolus-IFL plus placebo and included gastrointestinal hemorrhage (24% vs. 6%), minor gum bleeding (2% vs. 0), and vaginal hemorrhage (4% vs. 2%). *[See Boxed Warning, Dosage and Administration (2.4), Warnings and Precautions (5.3).]*

Venous Thromboembolic Events

The incidence of Grade 3–4 venous thromboembolic events was higher in patients with mCRC or NSCLC receiving Avastin with chemotherapy as compared to those receiving chemotherapy alone. The risk of developing a second subsequent thromboembolic event in mCRC patients receiving Avastin and chemotherapy was increased compared to patients receiving chemotherapy alone. In Study 1, 53 patients (14%) on the bolus-IFL plus Avastin arm and 30 patients (8%) on the bolus-IFL plus placebo arm received full dose warfarin following a venous thromboembolic event. Among these patients, an additional thromboembolic event occurred in 21% (11/53) of patients receiving bolus-IFL plus Avastin and 3% (1/30) of patients receiving bolus-IFL alone.

The overall incidence of Grade 3–4 venous thromboembolic events in Study 1 was 15.1% in patients receiving bolus-IFL plus Avastin and 13.6% in patients receiving bolus-IFL plus placebo. In Study 1, the incidence of the following Grade 3–4 venous thromboembolic events was higher in patients receiving bolus-IFL plus Avastin as compared to patients receiving bolus-IFL plus placebo: deep venous thrombosis (34 vs. 19 patients) and intra-abdominal venous thrombosis (10 vs. 5 patients).

Neutropenia and Infection

The incidences of neutropenia and febrile neutropenia are increased in patients receiving Avastin plus chemotherapy compared to chemotherapy alone. In Study 1, the incidence of Grade 3 or 4 neutropenia was increased in mCRC patients receiving IFL plus Avastin (21%) compared to patients receiving IFL alone (14%). In Study 4, the incidence of Grade 4 neutropenia was increased in NSCLC patients receiving paclitaxel/carboplatin (PC) plus Avastin (26.2%) compared with patients receiving PC alone (17.2%). Febrile neutropenia was also increased (5.4% for PC plus Avastin vs. 1.8% for PC alone). There were 19 (4.5%) infections with Grade 3 or 4 neutropenia in the PC plus Avastin arm of which 3 were fatal compared to 9 (2%) neutropenic infections in patients receiving PC alone, of which none were fatal. During the first 6 cycles of treatment, the incidence of serious infections including pneumonia, febrile neutropenia, catheter infections and wound infections was increased in the PC plus Avastin arm [58 patients (13.6%)] compared to the PC alone arm [29 patients (6.6%)].

In Study 7, one fatal event of neutropenic infection occurred in a patient with previously treated glioblastoma receiving Avastin alone. The incidence of any grade of infection in patients receiving Avastin alone was 55% and the incidence of Grade 3-5 infection was 10%.

Proteinuria

Grade 3-4 proteinuria ranged from 0.7 to 7.4% in Studies 1, 2, 4 and 9. The overall incidence of proteinuria (all grades) was only adequately assessed in Study 9, in which the incidence was 20%. Median onset of proteinuria was 5.6 months (range 15 days to 37 months) after initiation of Avastin. Median time to resolution was 6.1 months (95% CI 2.8 months, 11.3 months). Proteinuria did not resolve in 40% of patients after median follow up of 11.2 months and required permanent discontinuation of Avastin in 30% of the patients who developed proteinuria (Study 9). *[See Warnings and Precautions (5.8).]*

Congestive Heart Failure

The incidence of Grade ≥ 3 left ventricular dysfunction was 1.0% in patients receiving Avastin compared to 0.6% in the control arm across indications. In patients with MBC, the incidence of Grade 3-4 congestive heart failure (CHF) was increased in patients in the Avastin plus paclitaxel arm (2.2%) as compared to the control arm (0.3%). Among patients receiving prior anthracyclines for MBC, the rate of CHF was 3.8% for patients receiving Avastin as compared to 0.6% for patients receiving paclitaxel alone. The safety of continuation or resumption of Avastin in patients with cardiac dysfunction has not been studied.

Metastatic Colorectal Cancer (mCRC)

The data in Table 1 and Table 2 were obtained in Study 1, a randomized, double-blind, controlled trial comparing chemotherapy plus Avastin with chemotherapy plus placebo. Avastin was administered at 5 mg/kg every 2 weeks.

All Grade 3–4 adverse events and selected Grade 1–2 adverse events (hypertension, proteinuria, thromboembolic events) were collected in the entire study population. Severe and life-threatening (Grade 3–4) adverse events, which occurred at a higher incidence (≥ 2%) in patients receiving bolus-IFL plus Avastin as compared to bolus-IFL plus placebo, are presented in Table 1.

Table 1
NCI-CTC Grade 3–4 Adverse Events in Study 1
(Occurring at Higher Incidence [≥ 2%] Avastin vs. Control)

	Arm 1 IFL + Placebo (n = 396)	Arm 2 IFL + Avastin (n = 392)
NCI-CTC Grade 3-4 Events	74%	87%
Body as a Whole		
Asthenia	7%	10%
Abdominal Pain	5%	8%
Pain	5%	8%
Cardiovascular		
Hypertension	2%	12%
Deep Vein Thrombosis	5%	9%
Intra-Abdominal Thrombosis	1%	3%
Syncope	1%	3%
Digestive		
Diarrhea	25%	34%
Constipation	2%	4%
Hemic/Lymphatic		
Leukopenia	31%	37%
Neutropenia[a]	14%	21%

[a]Central laboratories were collected on Days 1 and 21 of each cycle. Neutrophil counts are available in 303 patients in Arm 1 and 276 in Arm 2.

Grade 1–4 adverse events which occurred at a higher incidence (≥ 5%) in patients receiving bolus-IFL plus Avastin as compared to the bolus-IFL plus placebo arm are presented in Table 2. Grade 1–4 adverse events were collected for the first approximately 100 patients in each of the three treatment arms who were enrolled until enrollment in Arm 3 (5-FU/LV + Avastin) was discontinued.

Table 2
NCI-CTC Grade 1-4 Adverse Events in Study 1
(Occurring at Higher Incidence [≥ 5%] in IFL + Avastin vs. IFL)

	Arm 1 IFL + Placebo (n = 98)	Arm 2 IFL + Avastin (n = 102)	Arm 3 5-FU/LV + Avastin (n = 109)
Body as a Whole			
Pain	55%	61%	62%
Abdominal Pain	55%	61%	50%
Headache	19%	26%	26%
Cardiovascular			
Hypertension	14%	23%	34%
Hypotension	7%	15%	7%
Deep Vein Thrombosis	3%	9%	6%
Digestive			
Vomiting	47%	52%	47%
Anorexia	30%	43%	35%
Constipation	29%	40%	29%
Stomatitis	18%	32%	30%
Dyspepsia	15%	24%	17%
GI Hemorrhage	6%	24%	19%
Weight Loss	10%	15%	16%
Dry Mouth	2%	7%	4%
Colitis	1%	6%	1%
Hemic/Lymphatic			
Thrombocytopenia	0%	5%	5%
Nervous			
Dizziness	20%	26%	19%
Respiratory			
Upper Respiratory Infection	39%	47%	40%
Epistaxis	10%	35%	32%
Dyspnea	15%	26%	25%
Voice Alteration	2%	9%	6%
Skin/Appendages			
Alopecia	26%	32%	6%
Skin Ulcer	1%	6%	6%
Special Senses			
Taste Disorder	9%	14%	21%
Urogenital			
Proteinuria	24%	36%	36%

Avastin in Combination with FOLFOX4 in Second-line mCRC

Only Grade 3-5 non-hematologic and Grade 4–5 hematologic adverse events related to treatment were collected in Study 2. The most frequent adverse events (selected Grade 3–5 non-hematologic and Grade 4–5 hematologic adverse events) occurring at a higher incidence (≥ 2%) in 287 patients receiving FOLFOX4 plus Avastin compared to 285 patients receiving FOLFOX4 alone were fatigue (19% vs. 13%), diarrhea (18% vs. 13%), sensory neuropathy (17% vs. 9%), nausea (12% vs. 5%), vomiting (11% vs. 4%), dehydration (10% vs. 5%), hypertension (9% vs. 2%), abdominal pain (8% vs. 5%), hemorrhage (5% vs. 1%), other neurological (5% vs. 3%), ileus (4% vs. 1%) and headache (3% vs. 0%). These data are likely to under-estimate the true adverse event rates due to the reporting mechanisms used in Study 2.

Unresectable Non-Squamous Non-Small Cell Lung Cancer (NSCLC)

Only Grade 3-5 non-hematologic and Grade 4-5 hematologic adverse events were collected in Study 4. Grade 3–5 non-hematologic and Grade 4–5 hematologic adverse events (occurring at a higher incidence (≥2%) in 427 patients receiving PC plus Avastin compared with 441 patients receiving PC alone were neutropenia (27% vs. 17%), fatigue (16% vs. 13%), hypertension (8% vs. 0.7%), infection without neutropenia (7% vs. 3%), venous thrombus/embolism (5% vs. 3%), febrile neutropenia (5% vs. 2%), pneumonitis/pulmonary infiltrates (5% vs. 3%), infection with Grade 3 or 4 neutropenia (4% vs. 2%), hyponatremia (4% vs. 1%), headache (3% vs. 1%) and proteinuria (3% vs. 0%).

Metastatic Breast Cancer (MBC)

Only Grade 3–5 non-hematologic and Grade 4–5 hematologic adverse events were collected in Study 5. Grade 3–4 adverse events occurring at a higher incidence (≥2%) in 363 patients receiving paclitaxel plus Avastin compared with 348 patients receiving paclitaxel alone were sensory neuropathy (24% vs. 18%), hypertension (16% vs. 1%), fatigue (11% vs. 5%), infection without neutropenia (9% vs. 5%), neutrophils (6% vs. 3%), vomiting (6% vs. 2%), diarrhea (5% vs. 1%), bone pain (4% vs. 2%), headache (4% vs. 1%), nausea (4% vs. 1%), cerebrovascular ischemia (3% vs. 0%), dehydration (3% vs. 1%), infection with unknown ANC (3% vs. 0.3%), rash/desquamation (3% vs. 0.3%) and proteinuria (3% vs. 0%).

Sensory neuropathy, hypertension, and fatigue were reported at a ≥ 5% higher absolute incidence in the paclitaxel plus Avastin arm compared with the paclitaxel alone arm.

Fatal adverse reactions occurred in 6/363 (1.7%) of patients who received paclitaxel plus Avastin. Causes of death were gastrointestinal perforation (2), myocardial infarction (2), diarrhea/abdominal, and pain/weakness/hypotension (2).

Avastin is not approved for use in combination with capecitabine or for use in second or third line treatment of MBC. The data below are presented to provide information on the overall safety profile of Avastin in women with breast cancer since Study 6 is the only randomized, controlled study in which all adverse events were collected for all patients. All patients in Study 6 received prior anthracycline and taxane therapy in the adjuvant setting or for metastatic disease. Grade 1– 4 events which occurred at a higher incidence (≥5%) in patients receiving capecitabine plus Avastin compared to the capecitabine alone arm are presented in Table 3.

Table 3
NCI-CTC Grade 1–4 Adverse Events in Study 6 (Occurring at Higher Incidence [≥5%] in Capecitabine + Avastin vs. Capecitabine Alone)

	Capecitabine (n = 215)	Capecitabine + Avastin (n = 229)
Body as a Whole		
Asthenia	47%	57%
Headache	13%	33%
Pain	25%	31%
Cardiovascular		
Hypertension	2%	24%
Digestive		
Stomatitis	19%	25%
Metabolic/Nutrition		
Weight loss	4%	9%
Musculoskeletal		
Myalgia	8%	14%
Respiratory		
Dyspnea	18%	27%
Epistaxis	1%	16%
Skin/Appendages		
Exfoliative dermatitis	75%	84%
Urogenital		
Albuminuria	7%	22%

Glioblastoma

All adverse events were collected in 163 patients enrolled in Study 7 who either received Avastin alone or Avastin plus irinotecan. All patients received prior radiotherapy and temozolomide. Avastin was administered at 10 mg/kg every 2 weeks alone or in combination with irinotecan. Avastin was discontinued due to adverse events in 4.8% of patients treated with Avastin alone.

In patients receiving Avastin alone (N=84), the most frequently reported adverse events of any grade were infection (55%), fatigue (45%), headache (37%), hypertension (30%), epistaxis (19%) and diarrhea (21%). Of these, the incidence of Grade ≥3 adverse events was infection (10%), fatigue (4%), headache (4%), hypertension (8%) and diarrhea (1%). Two deaths on study were possibly related to Avastin: one retroperitoneal hemorrhage and one neutropenic infection.

In patients receiving Avastin alone or Avastin plus irinotecan (N=163), the incidence of Avastin-related adverse events (Grade 1– 4) were bleeding/hemorrhage (40%), epistaxis (26%), CNS hemorrhage (5%), hypertension (32%), venous thromboembolic event (8%), arterial thromboembolic event (6%), wound-healing complications (6%), proteinuria (4%), gastrointestinal perforation (2%), and RPLS (1%). The incidence of Grade 3–5 events in these 163 patients were bleeding/hemorrhage (2%), CNS hemorrhage (1%), hypertension (5%), venous thromboembolic event (7%), arterial thromboembolic event (3%), wound-healing complications (3%), proteinuria (1%), and gastrointestinal perforation (2%).

Metastatic Renal Cell Carcinoma (mRCC)

All grade adverse events were collected in Study 9. Grade 3–5 adverse events occurring at a higher incidence (≥ 2%) in 337 patients receiving interferon alfa (IFN-α) plus Avastin compared to 304 patients receiving IFN-α plus placebo arm were fatigue (13% vs. 8%), asthenia (10% vs. 7%), proteinuria (7% vs. 0%), hypertension (6% vs. 1%; including hypertension and hypertensive crisis), and hemorrhage (3% vs. 0.3%; including epistaxis, small intestinal hemorrhage, aneurysm ruptured, gastric ulcer hemorrhage, gingival bleeding, haemoptysis, hemorrhage intracranial, large intestinal hemorrhage, respiratory tract hemorrhage, and traumatic hematoma).

Grade 1–5 adverse events occurring at a higher incidence (≥ 5%) in patients receiving IFN-α plus Avastin compared to the IFN-α plus placebo arm are presented in Table 4.

Table 4
NCI-CTC Grades 1–5 Adverse Events in Study 9
(Occuring at Higher Incidence [≥ 5%] in IFN-α + Avastin vs. IFN-α + Placebo)

System Organ Class/ Preferred term*	IFN-α + Placebo (n = 304)	IFN-α + Avastin (n = 337)
Gastrointestinal disorders		
Diarrhea	16%	21%
General disorders and administration site conditions		
Fatigue	27%	33%
Investigations		
Weight decreased	15%	20%
Metabolism and nutrition disorders		
Anorexia	31%	36%
Musculoskeletal and connective tissue disorders		
Myalgia	14%	19%
Back pain	6%	12%
Nervous system disorders		
Headache	16%	24%
Renal and urinary disorders		
Proteinuria	3%	20%
Respiratory, thoracic and mediastinal disorders		
Epistaxis	4%	27%
Dysphonia	0%	5%
Vascular disorders		
Hypertension	9%	28%

*Adverse events were encoded using MedDRA, Version 10.1.

The following adverse events were reported at a 5-fold greater incidence in the IFN-α plus Avastin arm compared to IFN-α alone and not represented in Table 4: gingival bleeding (13 patients vs. 1 patient); rhinitis (9 vs.0); blurred vision (8 vs. 0); gingivitis (8 vs. 1); gastroesophageal reflux disease (8 vs.1); tinnitus (7 vs. 1); tooth abscess (7 vs.0); mouth ulceration (6 vs. 0); acne (5 vs. 0); deafness (5 vs. 0); gastritis (5 vs. 0); gingival pain (5 vs. 0) and pulmonary embolism (5 vs. 1).

6.2 Immunogenicity

As with all therapeutic proteins, there is a potential for immunogenicity. The incidence of antibody development in patients receiving Avastin has not been adequately determined because the assay sensitivity was inadequate to reliably detect lower titers. Enzyme-linked immunosorbent assays (ELISAs) were performed on sera from approximately 500 patients treated with Avastin, primarily in combination with chemotherapy. High titer human anti-Avastin antibodies were not detected.

Immunogenicity data are highly dependent on the sensitivity and specificity of the assay. Additionally, the observed incidence of antibody positivity in an assay may be influenced by several factors, including sample handling, timing of sample collection, concomitant medications, and underlying disease. For these reasons, comparison of the incidence of antibodies to Avastin with the incidence of antibodies to other products may be misleading.

6.3 Postmarketing Experience

The following adverse reactions have been identified during post-approval use of Avastin. Because these reactions are reported voluntarily from a population of uncertain size, it is not always possible to reliably estimate their frequency or establish a causal relationship to drug exposure.

Body as a Whole: Polyserositis
Cardiovascular: Pulmonary hypertension, RPLS
Digestive: Intestinal necrosis, mesenteric venous occlusion, anastomotic ulceration
Hemic and lymphatic: Pancytopenia
Renal: Renal thrombotic microangiopathy (manifested as severe proteinuria)
Respiratory: Nasal septum perforation, dysphonia

7 DRUG INTERACTIONS

A drug interaction study was performed in which irinotecan was administered as part of the FOLFIRI regimen with or without Avastin. The results demonstrated no significant effect of bevacizumab on the pharmacokinetics of irinotecan or its active metabolite SN38.

In a randomized study in 99 patients with NSCLC, based on limited data, there did not appear to be a difference in the mean exposure of either carboplatin or paclitaxel when each was administered alone or in combination with Avastin. However, 3 of the 8 patients receiving Avastin plus paclitaxel/carboplatin had substantially lower paclitaxel exposure after four cycles of treatment (at Day 63) than those at Day 0, while patients receiving paclitaxel/carboplatin without Avastin had a greater paclitaxel exposure at Day 63 than at Day 0.

In Study 9, there was no difference in the mean exposure of interferon alfa administered in combination with Avastin when compared to interferon alfa alone.

8 USE IN SPECIFIC POPULATIONS

8.1 Pregnancy

Pregnancy Category C

There *are no studies of bevacizumab in pregnant women. Reproduction studies in rabbits treated with approximately 1 to 12 times the recommended human dose of bevacizumab resulted in teratogenicity, including an increased incidence of specific gross and skeletal fetal alterations. Adverse fetal outcomes were observed at all doses tested. Other observed effects included decreases in maternal and fetal body weights and an increased number of fetal resorptions.* [See Nonclinical Toxicology (13.3).]

Human IgG is known to cross the placental barrier; therefore, bevacizumab may be transmitted from the mother to the developing fetus, and has the potential to cause fetal harm when administered to pregnant women. Because of the observed teratogenic effects of known inhibitors of angiogenesis in humans, bevacizumab should be used during pregnancy only if the potential benefit to the pregnant woman justifies the potential risk to the fetus.

8.3 Nursing Mothers

It is not known whether Avastin is secreted in human milk, but human IgG is excreted in human milk. Published data suggest that breast milk antibodies do not enter the neonatal and infant circulation in substantial amounts. Because many drugs are secreted in human milk and because of the potential for serious adverse reactions in nursing infants from bevacizumab, a decision should be made whether to discontinue nursing or discontinue drug, taking into account the half-life of the bevacizumab (approximately 20 days [range 11–50 days]) and the importance of the drug to the mother. *[See Clinical Pharmacology (12.3).]*

8.4 Pediatric Use

The safety, effectiveness and pharmacokinetic profile of Avastin in pediatric patients have not been established.

Juvenile cynomolgus monkeys with open growth plates exhibited physeal dysplasia following 4 to 26 weeks exposure at 0.4 to 20 times the recommended human dose (based on mg/kg and exposure). The incidence and severity of physeal dysplasia were dose-related and were partially reversible upon cessation of treatment.

8.5 Geriatric Use

In Study 1, severe adverse events that occurred at a higher incidence (≥ 2%) in patients aged ≥65 years as compared to younger patients were asthenia, sepsis, deep thrombophlebitis, hypertension, hypotension, myocardial infarction, congestive heart failure, diarrhea, constipation, anorexia, leukopenia, anemia, dehydration, hypokalemia, and hyponatremia. The effect of Avastin on overall survival was similar in elderly patients as compared to younger patients.

In Study 2, patients aged ≥ 65 years receiving Avastin plus FOLFOX4 had a greater relative risk as compared to younger patients for the following adverse events: nausea, emesis, ileus, and fatigue.

In Study 4, patients aged ≥ 65 years receiving carboplatin, paclitaxel, and Avastin had a greater relative risk for proteinuria as compared to younger patients. *[See Warnings and Precautions (5.8).]*

In Study 5, there were insufficient numbers of patients ≥ 65 years old to determine whether the overall adverse events profile was different in the elderly as compared with younger patients.

Of the 742 patients enrolled in Genentech-sponsored clinical studies in which all adverse events were captured, 212 (29%) were age 65 or older and 43 (6%) were age 75 or older. Adverse events of any severity that occurred at a higher incidence in the elderly as compared to younger patients, in addition to those described above, were dyspepsia, gastrointestinal hemorrhage, edema, epistaxis, increased cough, and voice alteration.

In an exploratory, pooled analysis of 1745 patients treated in five randomized, controlled studies, there were 618 (35%) patients aged ≥65 years and 1127 patients <65 years of age. The overall incidence of arterial thromboembolic events was increased in all patients receiving Avastin with chemotherapy as compared to those receiving chemotherapy alone, regardless of age. However, the increase in arterial thromboembolic events incidence was greater in patients aged ≥ 65 years (8.5% vs. 2.9%) as compared to those < 65 years (2.1% vs. 1.4%). *[See Warnings and Precautions (5.5).]*

10 OVERDOSAGE

The highest dose tested in humans (20 mg/kg IV) was associated with headache in nine of 16 patients and with severe headache in three of 16 patients.

Genentech
BIO ONCOLOGY™

Manufactured by:
Genentech, Inc.
1 DNA Way
South San Francisco, CA
94080-4990

7453214
4835706
Initial U.S.Approval: February 2004
Code Revision Date: July 2009

CHAPTER 10

Gastric cancer

Charles D. Blanke, MD, Deborah Citrin, MD,
and Roderich E. Schwarz, MD, PhD

Gastric cancer is more common than esophageal cancer in Western countries but is less fatal. More than 21,000 new cases of gastric cancer will be diagnosed in the United States in the year 2010, with 10,750 deaths expected. Worldwide, approximately 930,000 individuals develop gastric cancer annually, accounting for greater than 10% of neoplastic deaths. The incidence and mortality of gastric cancer have been declining in most developed countries, including the United States; the age-adjusted risk (world estimate) fell 5% from 1985 to 1990.

Gastric cancer is defined as any malignant tumor arising from the region extending between the gastroesophageal (GE) junction and the pylorus. It may not be possible to determine the site of origin if the cancer involves the GE junction itself, a situation that has become more common in recent years.

GASTRIC

Epidemiology

Gender Gastric cancer occurs more frequently in men, with a male-to-female ratio of 2.3:1.0; mortality is approximately doubled in men.

Age The incidence of gastric cancer increases with age. In the United States, most cases occur between the ages of 65 and 74 years, with a median age of 70 for males and 74 for females.

Race Gastric cancer occurs more frequently in American blacks and Asians vs whites; in black males, it tends to occur at a younger age (68 years).

Geography Evidence of an association between environment and diet and gastric cancer comes from the profound differences in incidence seen in various parts of the world. While relatively rare in North America and many European nations, gastric cancer is still common in Japan, the former Soviet Union, and parts of Central America and South America.

Survival Most patients still present with advanced disease, and their survival remains poor. From 1999 to 2006, only 23% of patients with gastric cancer presented with localized disease. The relative 5-year survival rate for gastric cancer of all stages is 26%.

Incidence Significant increases in age-adjusted incidence rates for tumors arising in the gastric cardia have been seen in males. Rates for other gastric adenocarcinomas either have not significantly changed (black males) or have declined (white males). Overall, rates of gastric adenocarcinoma have fallen for men and women between 1975 and 2007.

Etiology, risk factors, and prevention

Diet and environment Studies of immigrants have demonstrated that high-risk populations (eg, Koreans) have a dramatic decrease in the risk of gastric carcinoma when they migrate to the West and change their dietary habits. Low consumption of vegetables and fruits and high intake of salts, nitrates, and smoked or pickled foods have been associated with an increased risk of gastric carcinoma. Conversely, the increasing availability of refrigerated foods has contributed to the decline in incidence rates. Recent laboratory data from Japan suggest that oolong tea may contain a substance that can kill stomach cancer cells.

Occupational exposure in coal mining and processing of nickel, rubber, and timber has been reported to increase the risk of gastric carcinoma. Cigarette smoking may also increase the risk, though alcohol exposure does not have a clear relation to risk of gastric cancer.

Intestinal metaplasia, a premalignant lesion, is common in locations where gastric cancer is common and is seen in 80% of resected gastric specimens in Japan.

Individuals with blood group A may have a greater risk of gastric carcinoma than individuals with other blood groups. The risk appears to be for the infiltrative type of gastric carcinoma (rather than the exophytic type).

Gastric resection Although reports have suggested that patients undergoing gastric resection for benign disease (usually peptic ulcer disease) are at increased risk of subsequently developing gastric cancer, this association has not been definitely proven. Gastric resection may result in increased gastric pH and subsequent intestinal metaplasia in affected patients.

Pernicious anemia Although it has been widely reported that pernicious anemia is associated with the subsequent development of gastric carcinoma, this relationship also has been questioned.

Genetic abnormalities The genetic abnormalities associated with gastric cancer are still poorly understood. Abnormalities of the tumor-suppressor gene *TP53* (alias *p53*) are found in over 60% of gastric cancer patients, and the adenomatous polyposis coli (*APC*) gene in over 50%. The significance of these findings is not clear at present.

Overexpression, amplification, and/or mutations of oncogenes c-Ki-*ras*, HER2/*neu* (aka c-*erb*-b2), and c-*myc* most likely play a role in the development of some gastric neoplasms. A high S-phase fraction has been associated with an increased risk of relapse as well.

Gastric cancer may be part of several inherited cancer syndromes, including familial adenomatous polyposis, hereditary non-polyposis colorectal cancer, and Peutz-Jeghers Syndrome. Hereditary diffuse gastric cancer occurs due to mutations in the E-cadherin (*CDH1*) gene. Studies of prophylactic gastrectomy in carriers demonstrate high rates of occult cancers, approximating 80%.

Carriers of mismatch repair gene mutations have an increased risk for developing gastric cancer.

Family history Family members of a patient with gastric cancer have a twofold to threefold higher risk of stomach cancer than the general population.

Prevention Recent studies strongly implicate cyclo-oxygenase 2 (COX-2) in the development of many human cancers, including gastric cancer. Potential mechanisms of oncogenesis include stimulation of tumor angiogenesis, inhibition of apoptosis, immune suppression, and enhancement of invasive potential. Furthermore, COX-2 inhibitors have been shown to decrease the size of gastric adenomas in mice. This information strongly suggests that COX-2 inhibitors may play a role in the prevention, and even treatment, of GI tumors. However, trials with COX-2 inhibitors in other advanced GI malignancies, such as colon cancer, have not been positive, so patients should not be treated with these agents outside the setting of a clinical trial.

Helicobacter pylori, which colonizes approximately half of the world's population, is associated with gastric lymphomas and adenocarcinomas. The overall risk of developing malignancy in the presence of infection is low; however, more than 40% to 50% of gastric cancers are linked with *H pylori*. The bacterium has been designated a class I carcinogen. Antibiotics alone can cure localized, node-negative MALT (mucosa-associated lymphoid tissue) lymphomas in about 50% of patients. With regard to gastric adenocarcinoma, *H pylori* infection is associated with a 2.8-fold increase in the relative risk of the disease compared with uninfected controls. Data from Japan and China suggest that *H pylori* infection can lead to chronic atrophic gastritis. This condition appears to be a major risk factor for gastric cancer. Eradication of *H pylori* should thus decrease the incidence of gastric cancer by preventing it, and pilot trials assessing this strategy have been undertaken in Central and South America.

Signs and symptoms

Most gastric cancers are diagnosed at an advanced stage. Presenting signs and symptoms are often nonspecific and typically include pain, weight loss, vomiting, and anorexia.

Hematemesis is present in 10% to 15% of patients.

Physical findings Peritoneal implants to the pelvis may be palpable on rectal examination (Blumer's shelf). Extension of disease to the liver may be appreciated as hepatomegaly on physical examination. Nodal metastases can be found in the supraclavicular fossa (Virchow's node), axilla, or umbilical region. Ascites can accompany advanced intraperitoneal spread of disease.

Screening and diagnosis

Routine screening for gastric cancer is generally not performed in Western countries because the disease is so uncommon. However, screening appears more effective in high-incidence areas. Mass screening, as has been practiced in Japan since the 1960s, has probably contributed to the 2.5-fold improvement in long-term survival compared with Western countries, though differences in surgical technique and biology may also play a role.

Endoscopy and barium x-rays The diagnosis of gastric cancer in a patient presenting with any constellation of the symptoms previously described revolves around the use of upper endoscopy or double-contrast barium x-rays. The advantage of endoscopy is that it allows for direct visualization of abnormalities and directed biopsies. Barium x-rays do not facilitate biopsies but are less invasive and may provide information regarding motility.

CT scan Once a diagnosis has been established and careful physical examination and routine blood tests have been performed, a CT scan of the chest, abdomen, and pelvis should be obtained to help assess tumor extent, nodal involvement, and metastatic disease. CT may demonstrate an intraluminal mass arising from the gastric wall or focal or diffuse gastric wall thickening. It is not useful in determining the depth of tumor penetration unless the carcinoma has extended through the entire gastric wall. Direct extension of the gastric tumor to the liver, spleen, or pancreas can be visualized on CT, as can metastatic involvement of celiac, retrocrural, retroperitoneal, and porta hepatis nodes. Ascites, intraperitoneal seeding, and distant metastases (liver, lungs, bone) can also be detected.

Endoscopic ultrasonography (EUS) is a staging technique that complements information gained by CT. Specifically, depth of tumor invasion, including invasion of nearby organs, can be assessed more accurately by EUS than by CT. Furthermore, perigastric regional nodes are more accurately evaluated by EUS, whereas regional nodes farther from the primary tumor are more accurately evaluated by CT. Specific ultrasonographic features may aid in the diagnosis and staging of patients with gastric lymphomas.

Laparoscopy Laparoscopy is particularly suited to detect small-volume visceral and peritoneal metastases missed on a CT scan. It should be performed prior to curative-intent locoregional therapy or preoperative chemoradiation therapy.

Bone scan A bone scan should be obtained if the patient has bony pain or an elevated alkaline phosphatase level.

PET scan PET scanning may be used to show distant, metastatic disease and may also be helpful in assessing response to neoadjuvant therapy. In the latter setting, PET response correlates with better survival. As many as 40% of gastric cancers may not be detected by PET and this modality may not be optimal for staging tumors of mucinous histology. It does not have an established role in routine preoperative imaging of potentially resectable patients.

Pathology

Adenocarcinoma is the predominant form of gastric cancer, accounting for approximately 95% of cases. Histologically, adenocarcinomas are classified as intestinal or diffuse; mixed types occur but are rare. Intestinal-type cancers are characterized by cohesive cells that form glandlike structures and are often preceded by intestinal metaplasia. Diffuse-type cancers are composed of infiltrating gastric mucous cells that infrequently form masses or ulcers.

Primary lymphoma of the stomach is increasing in frequency and, occasionally, may be difficult to distinguish from adenocarcinoma.

Stromal tumors GI stromal tumors (GISTs) are mesenchymal tumors of the GI tract, most commonly arising from the stomach. These tumors share an ancestor with, or arise from, the interstitial cells of Cajal (the pacemaker cells of the gut). GISTs commonly express KIT (CD117), but this is not required for diagnosis. Most GISTs have mutations in either the *KIT* or *PDGFR* (platelet-derived growth factor receptor) genes.

Other histologic types Infrequently, other histologic types are found in the stomach, such as squamous cell carcinomas, small-cell carcinomas, and carcinoid tumors.

Metastatic spread of disease from primaries in other organs (eg, breast cancer and malignant melanoma) is also seen occasionally.

Gastric carcinomas spread by direct extension (lesser and greater omentum, liver and diaphragm, spleen, pancreas, transverse colon); regional and distant nodal metastases; hematogenous metastases (liver, lungs, bone, brain); and peritoneal metastases. Multicentricity characterizes up to 20% of gastric cancers. In younger women, the ovaries are at risk (Krukenberg tumors).

Staging and prognosis

At present, epithelial gastric cancers are most commonly staged by the TNM system (Table 1). Stromal tumors, lymphomas, carcinoids, and sarcomas are not covered by these TNM criteria. The most recent update of the TNM does include a system encompassing GISTs.

A more detailed Japanese staging system has been shown to have prognostic importance in gastric cancer. However, these results have not yet been duplicated in the United States, and this system is not widely used around the world. Resected GISTs can be assigned a numeric risk of recurrence based on tumor size, mitotic rate, and location of the primary.

Prognostic factors Aneuploidy may predict a poor prognosis in patients with adenocarcinoma of the distal stomach. High plasma levels of vascular endothelial growth factor (VEGF) and the presence of carcinoembryonic antigen (CEA) in peritoneal washings predict poor survival in surgically resected patients. As with colorectal cancer, intratumoral levels of dihydropyrimidine dehydrogenase (DPD) may be prognostic of gastric cancer; low levels appear to predict better response to fluorouracil (5-FU)–based chemotherapy and longer survival. The prognostic implications of tumor-suppressor genes and oncogenes are an area of active investigation. Patients with cancers of the diffuse type fare worse than those with intestinal-type lesions.

It has long been known that survival rates for patients with gastric cancers are higher in Asian nations than in the United States, but it was not clear whether this represented results from superior surgical techniques or racial differences in underlying biology. Recent analysis of outcomes in Asian-Americans versus white patients suggests true differences exist in tumor biology, though the specifics have not yet been identified.

TABLE 1: TNM staging system for gastric cancer

Primary tumor (T)	
TX	Primary tumor cannot be assessed
T0	No evidence of primary tumor
Tis	Carcinoma *in situ*: intraepithelial tumor without invasion of the lamina propria
T1	Tumor invades the lamina propria, muscularis mucosae
T1a	Tumor invades the lamina propria or or muscularis mucosae
T1b	Tumor invades submucosa
T2	Tumor invades muscularis propria[a]
T3	Tumor penetrates subserosal connective tissue without invasion of visceral peritoneum or adjacent structures[a,b,c]
T4	Tumor invades serosa (visceral peritoneum) or adjacent structures[a,b,c]
T4a	Tumor invades serosa (visceral peritoneum)
T4b	Tumor invades adjacent structures
Regional lymph nodes (N)	
NX	Regional lymph node(s) cannot be assessed
N0	No regional lymph node metastasis
N1	Metastasis in 1–2 regional lymph nodes
N2	Metastasis in 3–6 regional lymph nodes
N3	Metastasis in 7 or more regional lymph nodes
N3a	Metastasis in 7–15 regional lymph nodes
N3b	Metastasis in 16 or more regional lymph nodes
Distant metastasis (M)	
MX	Distant metastasis cannot be assessed
M0	No distant metastasis
M1	Distant metastasis
Stage grouping	
See Table 2	

From Edge SB, Byrd DR, Compton CC, et al (eds): AJCC Cancer Staging Manual, 7th ed. New York, Springer, 2010.

[a] A tumor may penetrate the muscularis propria with extension into the gastrocolic or gastrohepatic ligaments, or into the greater or lesser omentum, without perforation of the visceral peritoneum covering these structures. In this case, the tumor is classified T3. If there is perforation of the visceral peritoneum covering the gastric ligaments or the omentum, the tumor should be classified T4.

[b] The adjacent structures of the stomach include the spleen, transverse colon, liver, diaphragm, pancreas, abdominal wall, adrenal gland, kidney, small intestine, and retroperitoneum.

[c] Intramural extension to the duodenum or esophagus is classified by the depth of the greatest invasion in any of these sites, including the stomach.

TABLE 2: Treatment and survival by stage in patients with gastric carcinoma

Stage			Treatment	5-Year overall survival rate[a] (%)
Stage 0 (in situ)			Surgery	> 90%
Tis	N0	M0		
Stage IA			Surgery	70.8%
T1	N0	M0		
Stage IB			Surgery + CT or CRT	57.4%
T2	N0	M0		
T1	N1	M0		
Stage IIA			Surgery + CT or CRT	45.5%
T3	N0	M0		
T2	N1	M0		
T1	N2	M0		
Stage IIB			Surgery + CT or CRT	32.8%
T4a	N0	M0		
T3	N1	M0		
T2	N2	M0		
T1	N3	M0		
Stage IIIA			Surgery + CT or CRT	19.8% (distal tumors)
T4a	N1	M0		
T3	N2	M0		
T2	N3	M0		
Stage IIIB			Same as for stage IIIA Consider preoperative CRT	14%
T4b	N0	M0		
T4b	N1	M0		
T4a	N2	M0		
T3	N3	M0		
Stage IIIC				9.2%
T4b	N1	M0		
T4b	N3	M0		
T4a	N3	M0		
Stage IV			Palliative chemotherapy, radiation therapy, and/or surgery, neoadjuvant CRT	4%
Any T	Any	M1		

Sources of data: American College of Surgeons Commission on Cancer and American Cancer Society

[a] Some American centers are reporting superior 5-year survival rates to those presented here. Confirmation of these results on a national level may be forthcoming.

CRT = chemoradiation therapy

CT = chemotherapy

Treatment

PRIMARY TREATMENT OF LOCALIZED DISEASE

Management of gastric cancer relies primarily on surgical resection of the involved stomach, with reconstruction to preserve intestinal continuity, as resection provides the only chance for cure. Radiotherapy and chemotherapy now have better defined roles as adjuncts to surgery and in patients with unresectable tumors. Perioperative chemotherapy and chemoradiation therapy remain active areas of current investigation.

A phase III trial recently evaluated the morbididty and mortality of laparoscopic vs open gastrectomy for gastric cancer. An interim report of the KLASS trial found no significant differences in rates of post-operative complications or mortaility between the two approaches *(Kim HH et al: Ann Surg 251:417–420, 2010)*.

Surgery

The objectives of operative treatment for potentially curable gastric cancers are confirmation of resectability, performance of a complete resection, facilitation of appropriate pathologic staging, and reestablishment of GI continuity and function.

Confirmation of resectability Laparoscopy has emerged as an excellent tool to assess the extent of disease and resectability before the surgeon performs an open laparotomy. Laparoscopy adds to the accuracy of preoperative imaging primarily in cases of peritoneal spread or small liver metastases. As a result, morbidity, hospital stay, and costs have been reduced significantly in patients with unresectable lesions. In addition, peritoneal washings can be obtained.

Extent of resection The extent of gastric resection depends on the site and extent of the primary cancer. Subtotal gastrectomy is preferred over total gastrectomy, because it leads to comparable survival but lower morbidity. A 5-cm margin of normal stomach appears to be sufficient in proximal and distal resections. For lesions of the GE junction or the proximal third of the stomach, proximal subtotal gastrectomy can be performed. If total gastrectomy is necessary, transection of the distal esophagus and proximal duodenum is required, and omentectomy is performed. In Japan, there is a growing experience with more limited resections of early-stage gastric cancer. This trend includes endoscopic mucosal resection (EMR) of nonulcerated T1 N0 lesions and pylorus-preserving gastrectomy. Laparoscopic resections are also being performed more frequently.

An update of the randomized Dutch D1D2 trial has demonstrated a significant advantage to D2 dissection at 15 years in terms of deaths from gastric cancer (37% after D2, 48% after D1 dissection, $P = .01$ *(Songun I et al: Lancet Oncol 11:439–449, 2010)*. Interestingly, the beneficial D2 dissection impact on local recurrence and survival does not seem to be enhanced by chemoradiotherapy, whereas CRT appears to improve both categories after mere D1 dissections *(Dikken JL et al: J Clin Oncol 28:2430–2436, 2010)*.

Extent of lymphadenectomy The extent of lymph node resection, including the number removed at the time of gastrectomy, continues to be controversial. Preferably, lymphadenectomy includes the lymphatic chains along the celiac, left gastric, splenic, and hepatic arteries, which allows for more precise lymph node staging. The exact level designation of lymph nodes varies with the site and intragastric location of the primary tumor. To support current TNM staging criteria, 16 or more lymph nodes should be obtained at minimum and examined for an accurate N classification. Removal of lymph nodes immediately adjacent to the stomach (paracardial, paragastric at the lesser or greater curvature, parapyloric) has been termed D1 dissection. A more extensive D2 dissection would also remove retroperitoneal "second echelon" lymph nodes along the celiac trunk, left gastric artery, hepatic artery, splenic artery, and splenic hilus.

Improved long-term survival rates for Japanese patients had been attributed to the extended lymphadenectomies routinely performed in this country. Because the improvement in survival after gastrectomy during recent decades was usually associated with the performance of extended lymph node dissections (D2 dissections or greater), this practice appeared to be sensible if performed with acceptable complication rates. Retrospective data had shown that D2 lymphadenectomy is safe and does not increase morbidity.

Initial data in two European randomized trials showed no significant differences in overall long-term survival between D1 and D2 dissection groups. Both studies found higher postoperative morbidity and mortality in the D2 (extended) group, largely due to a higher rate of splenectomy and/or partial pancreatectomy performed with those dissections. A recent 15-year update of the Dutch trial showed a significant long-term survival advantage was conferred by D2 dissection in female patients who underwent curative resection (35% vs 21%, $P = .03$) and in patients with stage II (33% vs 15%, $P = .03$) or N2 diseases (19% vs 0%, $P = .07$). Of note, while chemotherapy did not appear to improve the local-recurrence and survival benefit of D2 dissection, CRT does appear to improve local recurrence and survival following D1 dissections. Gastrectomy with extended lymphadenectomy should primarily be performed in specialized centers by experienced surgeons, and splenectomy and pancreatectomy should be avoided; for adequate staging, at least 15 lymph nodes should be removed and analyzed. Recent population data reviews have linked higher total lymph node numbers (up to 40) to superior survival.

Reconstruction methods After distal gastrectomy, Billroth I gastroduodenostomy or, more commonly, Billroth II gastrojejunostomy methods are acceptable for reconstruction. Reflux esophagitis is a common problem when the gastric reservoir is too small. After total or subtotal gastrectomy, a Roux-en-Y esophagojejunostomy is usually performed.

Resection of extragastric organs may be required to control T4 disease. Such a resection can be associated with long-term survival. Splenectomy should be avoided unless it is indicated by direct tumor extension, because it significantly increases the rate of complications.

NEOADJUVANT THERAPY

Prompted by the promising results and acceptable toxicity of preoperative (neoadjuvant) chemoradiation therapy in other parts of the GI tract (eg, esophagus, rectum), there is growing interest in neoadjuvant therapy for gastric cancer. Neoadjuvant treatment may be performed in an attempt to convert an initially unresectable cancer to resectable status (so-called conversion therapy), or it may be used in advanced but resectable disease felt to be at high risk for recurrence, following surgery alone.

The MAGIC trial investigated perioperative treatment with epirubicin, cisplatin, and 5-fluorouracil versus surgery alone, demonstrating improvements in progression-free and overall survival rates with the addition of chemotherapy. In resectable patients, perioperative chemotherapy added to surgery is now a standard of care in many parts of the world.

ADJUVANT THERAPY

The 5-year survival rate after "curative resection" for gastric cancer is only between 30% and 40% (Table 2). Treatment failure stems from a combination of local or regional recurrence and distant metastases. Investigators have studied adjuvant therapy in the hope of improving treatment results. A North American Intergroup trial randomizing resected patients (stages IB–IV[M0]) to receive chemoradiation therapy or observation showed significant improvement in median disease-free (median 19 vs 30 months) and overall (26 vs 35 months) survival with adjuvant therapy, and the use of postoperative chemoradiation therapy, usually with continuous infusion of 5-FU, is the standard of care in the United States. Population studies have suggested that adjuvant therapy is underutilized in the United States.

Radiotherapy

Radiotherapy can decrease the rate of locoregional failure but has not been shown to improve survival as a single postoperative modality. Postoperative radiotherapy may be appropriate in patients who are not candidates for chemotherapy.

Chemotherapy

Chemotherapy alone as a surgical adjunct does not have a defined role in the United States. Individual randomized trials of chemotherapy plus surgery vs resection alone have showed no definite survival advantage, with the possible exception of patients with widespread nodal involvement and older patients who may do better with chemotherapy. Meta-analyses of postoperative chemotherapy plus surgery vs resection alone have tended to show minor reductions in death rates, but no specific regimen can be recommended. Alternative chemotherapy delivery methods such as intraperitoneal chemotherapy have been evaluated in phase III trials with promising results and are an area of future study.

Neoadjuvant chemoradiation has also been explored as a way to improve tolerability of chemoradiation and to improve resectability and pathologic response rates compared with chemotherapy. A phase III randomized trial suggested that neoadjuvant chemotherapy and radiation provides superior pathologic outcomes compared with neoadjuvant chemotherapy. A trend toward improved survival with chemotherapy and radiation was seen.

Chemoradiation therapy

Patients with T3–T4 any N M0 tumors are at highest risk of locoregional recurrence after potentially curative surgery (surgery in which all macroscopic tumor has been resected with no evidence of metastatic disease) for gastric cancer. Even patients with node-negative disease (T3 N0) have a gastric cancer-related mortality of about 50% within 5 years. Mortality is significantly worse in patients with node-positive disease or in those with incomplete (R1, R2) resection.

New radiation delivery and verification methods are being explored as a method to reduce the toxicity and improve the accuracy of treatments that include radiation. Additional studies of organ motion and newer intensity-modulated radiation therapy approaches have been reported. A recent series reported on 27 patients treated with 3DRT with 5-FU and leucovorin compared with 33 patients treated with IMRT and capecitabine and oxaliplatin. IMRT treatment led to a higher rate of treatment completion and less rise in serum creatinine at follow-up. An improvement in survival was also seen, but because the chemotherapy regimens were different, firm conclusions cannot be drawn. Combined adjuvant radiochemotherapy with IMRT/XELOX improves outcome with low renal toxicity in gastric cancer *(Boda-Heggemann J et al: Int J Radiat Oncol Biol Phys 75:1187–1195, 2009).*

In the North American Intergroup trial mentioned in the section on "Adjuvant therapy," patients were randomized to receive chemoradiation therapy or observation following resection of stages IB–IV (M0) adenocarcinoma of the stomach. Chemoradiation therapy following resection of these high-risk patients significantly improved both disease-free and overall survival rates. Because of the apparent benefit of reducing locoregional recurrences, but not distant recurrences, it is possible that more routine use of D2 lymphadenectomy may modify this recommendation in the future. D2 lymphadenectomy was performed in only 10% of the patients in this trial. Subgroup analysis revealed that outcome did not differ based upon the type of lymphadenectomy ($P = .80$). Still, since only a small percentage of patients underwent the recommended D2 dissection, further research is necessary before firm conclusions can be made in this area. A 10-year update of this trial was recently presented at the 2009 American Society of Clinical Oncology meeting. Patients who were offered chemoradiation continued to enjoy improved survival (HR = 1.32) and disease-free survival (HR = 1.51).

Despite this trial, significant controversy regarding the need for adjuvant treatment persists and is perhaps growing. Many studies support the contention that aggressive, formal D2 resection may obviate the need for adjuvant treatment in many cases. Other studies and subgroup analyses support the recommendations for adjuvant treatment as concluded in the North American trial. These conflicting results, as well as distinct differences in results between Eastern and Western nations, suggest that this issue may take many years to resolve. In the interim, it is appropriate to recommend adjuvant chemoradiotherapy to those patients in North America who undergo initial gastrectomy.

A recent retrospective study from Korea evaluated chemoradiation compared with observation in patients who underwent a D2 dissection. Overall survival in this series

The American College of Surgical Oncologists Z9001 randomized trial of 1 year of imatinib mesylate or placebo following resection of intermediate- or high-risk GISTs was updated at the 2010 ASCO meeting. Relapse-free survival (RFS) on both arms was worse, with high mitotic rate, larger tumor size, and tumors originating in the small bowel. On the placebo arm, *KIT* mutation in exon 11 was prognostic for worse RFS; patients with rectal primaries receiving imatinib also had poorer outcomes. Interestingly only 1 event occurred among patients harboring the *PDGFR* D842V mutation, believed to be imatinib-resistant. Thus, tumor pathology and mutational status were both prognostic and predictive of RFS after surgical resection of GIST *(Corless CL et al: J Clin Oncol 28[15s]: abstract 10006, 2010).*

was higher for patients who received adjuvant therapy, suggesting that a D2 dissection does not preclude the need for adjuvant therapy.

Imatinib mesylate (Gleevec) given for 1 year or longer now represents standard of care in the postoperative setting, for selected GIST patients.

Unresectable tumors

Patients with unresectable gastric cancers and no evidence of metastatic disease can be expected to survive approximately 6 months without any treatment.

Palliative resection Palliative resection, bypass, and/or stenting may be appropriate for some patients with obstructive lesions. Palliative resection may also be suitable for patients with bleeding gastric cancers that are not resectable for cure. Generally, resection appears to offer better palliative results than bypass.

Radiotherapy Radiation therapy alone can provide palliation in patients with bleeding or obstruction who are not operative candidates. Radiotherapy may convert unresectable cancers to resectable tumors.

Chemoradiation therapy Patients with locally advanced disease may be appropriately treated with chemoradiation therapy. This approach can provide relatively long-lasting palliation and may render some unresectable cancers resectable. Older studies have shown that postoperative chemoradiation therapy can reduce relapse rates and prolong survival in patients with incompletely resected stomach cancer.

MEDICAL TREATMENT OF ADVANCED GASTRIC CANCER

When possible, all newly diagnosed patients with disseminated gastric cancer should be considered candidates for clinical trials, and those with good performance status should be offered systemic therapy. Even though cure is not expected with chemotherapy, such treatment may provide palliation in selected patients and sometimes durable remissions. Several randomized chemotherapy trials have suggested improvement in survival and probably quality of life vs best supportive care alone across first and second lines of therapy.

Single-agent therapy

Several agents have established activity in gastric cancer: 5-FU, platinums (cisplatin, oxaliplatin [Eloxatin], and carboplatin), mitomycin, etoposide, some anthracyclines (doxorubicin and epirubicin), taxanes (paclitaxel and docetaxel [Taxotere]), irinotecan, antimetabolites (pemetrexed [Alimta], methotrexate,

TABLE 3: Chemotherapy regimens for gastric cancer

Drug/combination	Dose and schedule
ECF	
Epirubicin	50 mg/m^2 IV on day 1
Cisplatin	60 mg/m^2 IV on day 1
Repeat the cycle every 3 weeks to a maximum of 8 cycles.	
5-FU	200 mg/m^2/d as a continuous IV infusion for up to 6 months
Webb A, Cunningham D, Scarffe HJ, et al: J Clin Oncol 15:261–267, 1997.	
Roth AD, Fazio N, Stupp R, et al: J Clin Oncol 25:3217–3223, 2007.	
Epirubicin, oxaliplatin, capecitabine (EOX)	
Epirubicin	50 mg/m^2 on day 1
Oxaliplatin	130 mg/m^2 on day 1
Capecitabine	625 mg/m^2 BID on days 1–21
Repeat the cycle every 3 weeks to a maximum of 8 cycles.	
Cunningham D, Starling N, Rao S, et al: N Engl J Med 358:36–46, 2008.	
Docetaxel plus cisplatin and 5-FU (DCF)	
Docetaxel	75 mg/m^2 IVPB on day 1
Cisplatin	75 mg/m^2 IVPB on day 1
5-FU	750 mg/m^2/d continuous IV infusion on days 1 to 5
Repeat the cycle every 3 weeks.	
Ajani JA, Moiseyenko VM, Tjulandin S, et al: J Clin Oncol 25:3210–3216, 2007.	

IVPB = intravenous piggyback
Table prepared in part by Ishmael Jaiyesimi, DO.

trimetrexate (Neutrexin), and oral fluoropyrimidines (uracil and tegafur [UFT], S-1, capecitabine [Xeloda]). 5-FU and cisplatin have been used most commonly. The responses seen with single-agent chemotherapy have been traditionally partial and mostly short-lived, with little, if any, impact on overall survival.

Novel agents recently tested in patients with advanced gastric cancer include the epidermal growth factor receptor inhibitors cetuximab (Erbitux) and panitumumab (Vectibix), the VEGF inhibitor bevacizumab (Avastin), and the mTOR inhibitor everolimus (Afinitor). Additionally, trastuzumab (Herceptin), a monoclonal antibody against HER2, improves survival when added to platinum- or fluoropyrimidine-based chemotherapy, in patients whose tumors overexpress HER2. Bevacizumab appears promising when given with chemotherapy.

Combination chemotherapy

Response rates are consistently higher when combination chemotherapy regimens are used in gastric cancer. Combination therapy has been generally preferred over single

> **C**hemotherapy works modestly well in advanced gastric cancer, but only one biologic agent, trastuzumab, has appeared effective to date. Kang and associates presented AVAGAST, a randomized double-blind, placebo-controlled study of first-line chemotherapy with or without bevacizumab, in patients with incurable disease: 774 patients from 17 countries were enrolled and given capecitabine (or 5-FU)/cisplatin plus or minus the biologic. Investigators were looking for an improvement in overall survival (OS) from 10 to 12.8 months. The addition of bevacizumab did result in statistically significant improvements in the overall response rate and progression-free survival (the latter from 5.3 to 6.7 months), but it did not meet its primary objective. OS was 10.1 months for patients given placebo and 12.1 months for those getting the antiangiogenic agent (*P* = .1002). The trial reported interesting overall regional survival differences in efficacy for chemobiologic therapy (Americans did worst), and pre-planned biomarker analysis is awaited *(Kang Y et al: J Clin Oncol 28[18S]:abstract 4007, 2010).*

agents, though it remains unclear whether doublets or triplets represent ideal therapy (Table 3).

In the 1980s, the combination of 5-FU, doxorubicin, and mitomycin (FAM) was considered the standard regimen in the treatment of advanced gastric cancer. However, the NCCTG randomly compared this regimen with 5-FU plus doxorubicin and single-agent 5-FU and found no difference in survival among the patients treated with the three regimens.

Several different regimens, including FAMTX (5-FU, doxorubicin, and methotrexate) and ELF (etoposide, leucovorin, and 5-FU), have been tested. Most regimens show markedly better response rates and longer survival in early trials than in phase III studies. No combination has been confirmed as superior. However, ECF (epirubicin, cisplatin, 5-FU) approaches standard of care in Canada and in some parts of Europe. This regimen has proved superior to FAMTX in terms of objective response rate and survival and superior to the mitomycin, cisplatin, 5-FU (MCF) regimen in terms of toxicity. A combination of docetaxel, cisplatin, and 5-FU was shown to offer superior survival rates vs cisplatin and 5-FU; however, grade 3/4 toxic events occurred in 81% of patients treated with triple therapy. Modifications of this regimen have been proposed. The search for the optimal combination regimen continues, with the promising newer agents usually being introduced in combination regimens.

Newer agents with somewhat similar mechanisms of action to those of classic drugs have been tried in patients with advanced gastric cancer. Oxaliplatin (Eloxatin)- and cisplatin-containing regimens have been compared, with the former being less toxic and perhaps more efficacious. Additionally, regimens substituting oral capecitabine for IV 5-FU are popular because of ease of administration and fewer catheter-related complications. S-1 is another version of an oral fluoropyrimidine. Phase III studies of S-1 have been promising in regard to reduction of toxicity, but efficacy has not been superior. S-1 plus cisplatin improved survival for patients with advanced incurable gastric cancer patients vs S-1 alone in the Japanese SPIRITS trial. Likewise, no standard second-line therapy for advanced gastric cancer patients exists. Taxanes and the topoisomerase-1 inhibitor irinotecan have shown some activity in this setting.

Gastric cancer patients should be encouraged to participate in well-designed clinical trials. Outside experimental regimens, the recommended therapy for patients with good performance status is a 5-FU or platinum-based regimen.

SUGGESTED READING

Blanke CD, Demetri GD, von Mehren M, et al: Long-term results from a randomized phase II trial of standard-versus higher-dose imatinib mesylate for patients with unresectable or metastatic gastrointestinal stromal tumors expressing KIT. J Clin Oncol 26:620–625, 2008.

Blanke CD, Rankin C, Demetri GD, et al: Phase III randomized, intergroup trial assessing imatinib mesylate at two dose levels in patients with unresectable or metastatic gastrointestinal stromal tumors expressing the kit receptor tyrosine kinase: S0033. J Clin Oncol 26:626–632, 2008.

Cunningham D, Starling N, Rao S, et al: Capecitabine and oxaliplatin for advanced esophagogastric cancer. N Engl J Med 358:36–46, 2008.

Dematteo RP, Ballman KV, Antonescu CR, et al: Adjuvant imatinib mesylate after resection of localised, primary gastrointestinal stromal tumour: A randomised, double-blind, placebo-controlled trial. Lancet 373:1097–1104, 2009.

Dikken JL, Jansen EP, Cats A, et al: Impact of the extent of surgery and postoperative chemoradiotherapy on recurrence patterns in gastric cancer. J Clin Oncol 28:2430–2436, 2010.

Heinrich MC, Owzar K, Corless CL, et al: Correlation of kinase genotype and clinical outcome in the North American Intergroup Phase III Trial of imatinib mesylate for treatment of advanced gastrointestinal stromal tumor: CALGB 150105 Study by Cancer and Leukemia Group B and Southwest Oncology Group. J Clin Oncol 26:5360–5367, 2008.

Kozak KR, Moody JS: The survival impact of the intergroup 0116 trial on patients with gastric cancer. Int J Radiat Oncol Biol Phys 72:517–521, 2008.

Kim W, Song KY, Lee HJ, et al: The impact of comorbidity on surgical outcomes in laparoscopy-assisted distal gastrectomy: A retrospective analysis of multicenter results. Ann Surg 248:793–799, 2008.

Okines AF, Norman AR, McCloud P: Meta-analysis of the REAL-2 and ML17032 trials: Evaluating capecitabine-based combination chemotherapy and infused 5-fluorouracil-based combination chemotherapy for the treatment of advanced oesophago-gastric cancer. Ann Oncol 20:1529–1534, 2009.

Songun I, Putter H, Kranenbarg EM, et al: Surgical treatment of gastric cancer: 15-year follow-up results of the randomised nationwide Dutch D1D2 trial. Lancet Oncol 11:439–449, 2010.

Stahl M, Walz MK, Stuschke M, et al: Phase III comparison of preoperative chemotherapy compared with chemoradiotherapy in patients with locally advanced adenocarcinoma of the esophagogastric junction. J Clin Oncol 27:851–856, 2009.

Abbreviations in this chapter

MAGIC = Medical Research Council Adjuvant Gastric Infusional Chemotherapy; NCCTG = North Central Cancer Treatment Group

CHAPTER 11

Pancreatic, neuroendocrine GI, and adrenal cancers

Al B. Benson III, MD, Robert J. Myerson, MD, PhD, and Aaron R. Sasson, MD

PANCREATIC CANCER

Pancreatic cancer is the fifth leading cause of cancer death in the United States. In the year 2010, an estimated 43,140 new cases are expected to be diagnosed, and 36,800 deaths are expected to occur.

INCIDENCE AND EPIDEMIOLOGY

Gender

The incidence of pancreatic cancer is slightly higher in males than in females. These gender differences are most prominent among younger individuals.

Age

The peak incidence of pancreatic carcinoma occurs in the seventh decade of life. Two-thirds of new cases occur in people > 65 years old.

Race

The incidence of pancreatic cancer is higher in the black population, with an excess risk of 40% to 50% over that in whites. Perhaps more importantly, black males probably have the highest risk of pancreatic cancer worldwide.

Survival

Cancer of the pancreas is a highly lethal disease, with ductal adenocarcinoma being the most common histologic type. The overall 5-year survival has not improved in the last 30 years and remains < 5%. Median survival is approximately 6 months for patients with metastatic disease and 10 months for patients with locally advanced disease. Approximately 50% of patients diagnosed with pancreatic adenocarcinoma have clinically apparent metastatic disease, with only a minority (10%–20%) of patients being considered resectable. There have been some increases in 5-year survival following a curative resection (21%–25%); however, 50% of patients will die of recurrent tumor within 2 years.

Several epidemiologic studies have demonstrated worrisome projections regarding pancreatic cancer. A recent analysis of the SEER database has demonstrated a marked increase in the number of cancer cases over the next 20 years. This is attributed to the increasing number of adults over the age of 65 years. The authors estimated that there will be a 55% increase in the number of pancreatic cancer cases over the next 20 years, giving it the fourth highest incidence, preceded by cancers of the stomach and liver, and multiple myeloma *(Smith BD et al: J Clin Oncol 27:2758–2765, 2009).*

In the past, surgical resection has been associated with a high morbidity and mortality. Over the last 20 years, however, there have been marked improvements in outcomes following resection. Several single-institution series have reported mortality rates of < 3% following resection. Factors that appear to be important in predicting long-term survival following resection include clear surgical margins, small tumor size (< 2 cm), negative lymph nodes, and reduced perioperative morbidity.

Adenocarcinoma of the pancreas, the most common histologic type, has a median survival of 9 to 12 months and an overall 5-year survival rate of 3% for all stages. At the time of diagnosis, over 50% of patients with pancreatic adenocarcinoma have clinically apparent metastatic disease. Among patients whose disease is considered to be resectable, 50% will die of a recurrent tumor within 2 years.

ETIOLOGY AND RISK FACTORS

The specific risk factors for pancreatic cancer are not as striking as those for other gastrointestinal (GI) malignancies, such as esophageal and gastric carcinomas. There does, however, appear to be a significant relationship between pancreatic cancer and environmental carcinogens.

Cigarette smoking

Cigarette smoke is one of the carcinogens directly linked to the causation of pancreatic malignancies. Heavy cigarette smokers have at least a twofold greater risk of developing pancreatic carcinoma than nonsmokers. In Japan, cigarette smoking carries an even greater risk, which can be as much as 10-fold in men smoking one to two packs of cigarettes daily.

N-nitroso compounds

These compounds, found particularly in processed meat products, reliably induce pancreatic cancer in a variety of laboratory animals. No study has directly linked dietary carcinogens to pancreatic cancers in humans.

Caffeine

The contribution of caffeine consumption to the development of pancreatic carcinoma is controversial. A case-controlled study showed a correlation between caffeine consumption and pancreatic cancer. However, other studies have been unable to confirm this relationship.

Alcohol

A clear-cut relationship between alcohol use and pancreatic carcinoma has not been shown.

Diabetes

Hyperglycemia does not seem to be a risk factor for pancreatic cancer. However, 10% of all patients with pancreatic carcinoma present with new-onset diabetes.

A report by the American Institute for Cancer Research estimated that 28% of pancreatic cancers can be attributable to obesity. As the obesity health problem in the United States worsens, this percentage may increase in the future *(WCRF/AICR report, Policy and Action for Cancer Prevention, 2009).*

Genetic factors

Cancer of the pancreas is a genetic disease. To date, more than 80% of resected pancreatic cancers have been found to harbor activating point mutations in *KRAS*. In addition, the tumor-suppressor genes *CDKN2A, TP53,* and *DPC4* are all frequently inactivated in this cancer.

Research is also focusing on aberrantly methylated genes in pancreatic cancer using methylation-specific polymerase chain reaction and the identification of microRNAs as targets for detection strategies.

Familial pancreatic carcinoma has been associated with the following genetic syndromes: hereditary pancreatitis, ataxia-telangiectasia, hereditary nonpolyposis colorectal cancer, familial atypical mole melanoma syndrome, Peutz-Jeghers syndrome, and familial breast cancer. Families with *CDKN2A* germline mutations may be at higher risk of developing pancreatic cancer than those without these mutations.

SIGNS AND SYMPTOMS

The initial clinical features of pancreatic carcinoma include anorexia, weight loss, abdominal discomfort or pain, and new-onset diabetes mellitus or thrombophlebitis. The vague nature of these complaints may delay diagnosis for several months.

Pain

Specific symptoms usually relate to localized invasion of peripancreatic structures. The most common symptom is back pain, which stems from tumor invasion of the splanchnic plexus and retroperitoneum or pancreatitis. This pain is described as severe, gnawing, and radiating to the middle of the back. Pain can also be epigastric or in the right upper quadrant if bile duct obstruction is present.

Jaundice

In a majority of cases, patients also may present with jaundice. Painless or, sometimes, painful jaundice occurs when lesions involve the intrapancreatic bile duct.

GI symptoms

Tumor invasion of the duodenum or gastric outlet may give rise to nausea or vomiting as a presenting symptom. This symptom is rare early in the course of the disease. Changes in bowel habits related to pancreatic insufficiency may also be present, along with associated steatorrhea.

Glucose intolerance

Recent onset of glucose intolerance associated with GI symptoms in an elderly patient should alert physicians to the possibility of pancreatic carcinoma.

A palpable gallbladder

When it occurs without cholecystitis or cholangitis, a palpable gallbladder suggests malignant obstruction of the common bile duct until proven otherwise. This so-called Courvoisier's sign is present in about 25% of all patients with pancreatic cancer.

Other physical findings include Trousseau's syndrome (migratory superficial phlebitis), ascites, Virchow's node (left supraclavicular lymph node), or a periumbilical mass (Sister Mary Joseph's node).

SCREENING AND DIAGNOSIS

Early diagnosis of pancreatic carcinoma is difficult but essential if surgical resection and cure are to be improved. Defining early lesions at a resectable stage remains a diagnostic challenge. To date, leading medical organizations have not recommended routine screening of asymptomatic individuals for pancreatic cancer.

Serum markers

The use of serologic tumor markers, such as CA19-9, for pancreatic carcinoma was originally thought to be appropriate as a screening tool. However, since the prevalence of pancreatic carcinoma in the general population is extremely low (0.01%), many false-positive screening results are generated. Also, the sensitivity of CA19-9 is not high (20%) in stage I cancers. Nevertheless, CA19-9 may be a useful marker for diagnosing patients at high risk who have appropriate symptoms; such individuals include smokers, recent-onset diabetics, those with familial pancreatic cancer, or those with unexplained weight loss or diarrhea. This marker correlates with tumor burden and is useful in following disease and in assessing the adequacy of resection or therapy. CA19-9 should be interpreted with caution in patients who have jaundice, as it is falsely elevated in such patients. Furthermore, 5% to 15% of the population are unable to synthesize CA19-9; in such patients, levels of this marker would be falsely low, even in the presence of extensive tumor burden.

No currently available serum marker is sufficiently accurate to be considered reliable for screening asymptomatic patients.

Laparoscopy

This diagnostic tool is useful for staging patients with pancreatic carcinoma and for formulating treatment plans. Approximately 10% to 15% of patients thought to have resectable disease are found to have distant metastases at laparoscopy. The false-negative rate of laparoscopy is < 10%. The strongest indications for laparoscopy are locally advanced disease and tumors of the body and tail of the pancreas.

Peritoneal cytology

This technique currently is being investigated as an adjunct in staging of pancreatic carcinoma. Cytology is positive in 5% to 10% of patients who are thought to have localized disease. There are anecdotal cases of long-term survival after resection in which positive cytology of peritoneal washings was noted, but the clinical/prognostic value of this test is not yet known. However, there is increasing evidence that the presence of positive peritoneal cytology is a marker of advanced disease, and curative resection is extremely unlikely.

Imaging techniques

Imaging for pancreatic carcinoma is best performed with conventional ultrasonography and CT.

Ultrasonography

The limit of sonographic resolution for early pancreatic carcinoma is a diameter of 1.0 to 1.5 cm. A mass located in the pancreatic head will produce dilatation of the common bile duct and pancreatic duct. The actual sensitivity of ultrasonography in the diagnosis of pancreatic carcinoma is ~70%.

CT

This diagnostic tool provides better definition of the tumor and surrounding structures than does ultrasonography and is operator-independent. CT correctly predicts unresectable tumors in 85% of patients and resectable tumors in 70% of patients. Findings of tumor unresectability on CT scanning include distant lymphadenopathy, encasement or occlusion of the superior mesenteric artery (SMA) or celiac artery, occlusion of the portal vein or superior mesenteric vein (SMV), and distant metastases. Spiral CT increases the accuracy of detecting pancreatic carcinoma in general and vessel encasement in particular. This technique permits rapid data acquisition and computer-generated three-dimensional (3D) images of the mesenteric arterial and venous tributaries in any plane. Spiral CT is quicker and less expensive than angiography and uses less contrast medium.

PET

The use of positron emission tomography with ^{18}fluorodeoxyglucose (FDG-PET) in the evaluation of patients with pancreatic cancer is expanding. A recent study of 126 patients with focal, malignant, or benign pancreatic lesions showed high sensitivity of FDG-PET for detection of small pancreatic neoplasms. Lack of focal glucose uptake excludes pancreatic neoplasms (sensitivity, 85.4%; specificity, 60.9%).

Magnetic resonance imaging (MRI)

At present, MRI is not as accurate as CT in diagnosing and staging pancreatic carcinoma. MRI may be as useful as CT in staging and can provide magnetic resonance angiography and magnetic resonance cholangiopancreatography (MRC) images if needed. As yet, MRC is not a standard test for the diagnosis of pancreatic carcinoma, but it may become helpful in the future.

Endoscopic ultrasonography (EUS)

This test is a newer modality for the diagnosis of pancreatic carcinoma, and offers an overall diagnostic accuracy rate of approximately 85% to 90%. For the assessment of regional lymph node metastases, the accuracy of EUS is 50% to 70%. This technique is also important in the evaluation of portal vein/SMV involvement by tumor. EUS-guided fine-needle cytology of periampullary tumors may yield new information with respect to the diagnosis of pancreatic cancer. Further, this technique may pose less risk of spreading cells by needle tracking than does percutaneous biopsy. However, in patients with clinical suspicion of pancreatic cancer and a high-quality CT scan indicating resectability, routine EUS is not indicated.

TABLE 1: TNM staging of pancreatic tumors

Primary tumor (T)	
TX	Primary tumor cannot be assessed
T0	No evidence of a primary tumor
Tis	Carcinoma in situ[a]
T1	Tumor limited to the pancreas, ≤ 2 cm in diameter
T2	Tumor limited to the pancreas, > 2 cm in diameter
T3	Tumor extends beyond the pancreas but without involvement of the celiac axis or the superior mesenteric artery
T4	Tumor involves the celiac axis or the superior mesenteric artery (unresectable primary tumor)
Regional lymph nodes (N)	
NX	Regional lymph nodes cannot be assessed
N0	No regional lymph node(s) metastasis
N1	Regional lymph node(s) metastasis
Distant metastasis (M)	
M0	No distant metastasis (no pathologic M0; use clinical M to complete stage group)
M1	Distant metastasis

Stage grouping			
Stage 0	Tis	N0	M0
Stage IA	T1	N0	M0
Stage IB	T2	N0	M0
Stage IIA	T3	N0	M0
Stage IIB	T1–3	N1	M0
Stage III	T4	Any N	M0
Stage IV	Any T	Any N	M1

[a] This also includes the "PanINIII" classification

From Edge SP, Byrd DR, Compton CC, et al (eds): AJCC Cancer Staging Manual, 7th ed. New York, Springer, 2010.

In a comparison of EUS and spiral CT, both techniques showed comparable efficacy in detecting tumor involvement of lymph nodes and the SMVs and portal veins. However, EUS is less helpful in the evaluation of the SMA.

Recently, some investigators have expressed interest in using EUS to screen high-risk patients, individuals with defined genetic syndromes, and those with a strong family history of pancreatic cancer for evidence of the disease. In a recent study of 78 high-risk patients, screening showed neoplastic changes in 10% of the subjects. However, the challenge of EUS is the current inability to detect malignant precursor lesions, known as PanIN (pancreatic intraepithelial neoplasia).

Endoscopic retrograde cholangiopancreatography (ERCP)

This technique may someday be supplanted as a diagnostic tool by EUS, although ERCP presently is used in many clinics. Also, if a patient presents with jaundice and the CT scan reveals dilatation of the common bile duct without an obvious mass,

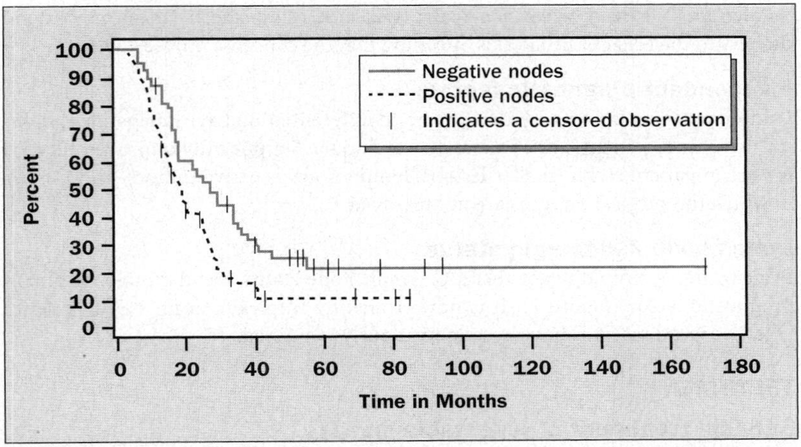

FIGURE 1: Actuarial survival as a function of regional lymph node status in patients with pancreatic cancer.

ERCP may be complementary to spiral CT. ERCP findings of pancreatic cancer include an abrupt or tapered cutoff of either or both the main pancreatic and common bile ducts.

PATHOLOGY

Adenocarcinoma

This type of tumor, arising from the exocrine gland ductal system, is the most common type of pancreatic cancer, accounting for 95% of all cases. Two-thirds of these cancers originate in the pancreatic head, and the remainder arise in the body or tail. Most ductal carcinomas are mucin-producing tumors and usually are associated with a dense desmoplastic reaction.

Although most pancreatic adenocarcinomas arise from the ductal epithelium, pancreatic acinar carcinomas and cancers arising from mucinous cystic neoplasms are also found.

Multicentricity, which is usually microscopic, is not unusual.

Metastatic spread Perineural invasion occurs in the majority of patients with pancreatic carcinoma. In addition, pancreatitis distal to and surrounding the tumor is usually present. Most patients present with lymph node metastases in the region of the pancreaticoduodenal drainage basins. The subpyloric and inferior pancreatic head, SMA, and para-aortic lymph node groups also may be involved. Distant metastatic spread most commonly involves the liver and peritoneal surfaces.

STAGING AND PROGNOSIS

Pancreatic adenocarcinoma is staged according to local spread of disease, nodal status, and distant metastatic involvement using the AJCC TNM system (Table 1). The T staging of the primary tumor includes an analysis of direct extension of disease to the duodenum, bile duct, or peripancreatic tissues. A T4 advanced cancer may extend directly to the SMA or celiac axis, meaning that the cancer is unresectable.

Independent prognostic factors

Lymph node metastases and tumor size and differentiation have independent prognostic value in patients with pancreatic carcinoma. Significantly improved survival is seen in patients with smaller lesions, lymph node-negative tumors, and tumors in which the surgical margins are not involved.

Lymph node and margin status

Prior to the age of adjuvant therapy, lymph node status was the most dominant prognostic factor (Figure 1). It is now rivaled by surgical margin status in series where surgical margins have been meticulously examined.

TREATMENT

Surgical treatment of resectable disease

The rate of resection for curative intent ranges from 10% to > 75%, with the higher percentage resulting from both a more aggressive approach and better preoperative staging for resectability. Also, there is growing evidence that patients with potentially resectable pancreatic cancer have a shorter hospital stay, reduced surgical mortality, and an overall better outcome if the surgery is performed at "high-volume" medical centers staffed by experienced surgeons (approximately 16 operable cases per year).

Extended resections may include portal or superior mesenteric vessels, the colon, the adrenal glands, or the stomach. If resection of adjacent organs or tissues results in the conversion of a positive to a negative resection margin, it is of great potential benefit to the patient. With regard to the extent of lymph node dissection, several recent, prospective, randomized studies have shown an increase in postoperative morbidity, but with no improvement in overall survival in patients undergoing an extended lymph node dissection.

Determination of resectability

The initial approach to surgery for pancreatic carcinoma includes a determination of resectability. This determination should be first made preoperatively with high-quality CT or MRI and, perhaps, EUS. Operative determination of resectability includes careful examination of the liver, porta hepatis, and portal and superior mesenteric vessels. The head of the pancreas and uncinate process are mobilized by an extensive Kocher maneuver to evaluate the head of the pancreas. The SMA is palpated, and its relationship to the tumor is assessed. The hepatic artery and celiac trunk are examined to make certain there is no vascular encasement.

Currently, pancreatic lesions may be classified as resectable, borderline resectable, and unresectable. Indicators of borderline resectable tumors include impingement or abutment on the SMV/portal vein, short segment venous occlusion with a suitable proximal and distal vein for reconstruction, minimal involvement of the gastroduodenal artery and hepatic artery, and < 180° involvement of the SMA. Criteria for unresectability include detection of distant metastases and circumferential involvement of the SMA, hepatic artery, or celiac artery.

Operative intervention

Intraoperative biopsy Most patients with resectable periampullary tumors can successfully undergo pancreaticoduodenectomy without an intraoperative biopsy. A time-consuming frozen section interpretation may not be informative, and histologic confirmation may be impossible with small lesions associated with peritumoral pancreatitis. Most large series of pancreaticoduodenectomy for carcinoma include resections of benign pathology based on clinical judgment. A negative fine-needle cytology should not deter an experienced surgeon from proceeding with resection. In patients without a histologic diagnosis, however, a biopsy is warranted in patients deemed to be unresectable while undergoing an attempt at resection.

Whipple vs pylorus-preserving procedure If the tumor is deemed to be resectable, a standard pancreaticoduodenectomy (Whipple procedure) or pylorus-preserving Whipple procedure (PPW) is performed. The PPW theoretically eliminates the nutritional problems caused by a reduced gastric reservoir and gastric dumping, but this finding has not been shown to alter long-term nutritional status. If there is any doubt about cancer proximity or blood supply to the pylorus, an antrectomy should be performed. If the tumor approaches the pylorus or involves the subpyloric nodes, classic antrectomy is preferred. Recent prospective randomized studies have shown there to be no significant difference between pylorus-preserving and standard Whipple resection.

Reconstruction technique The most common reconstruction technique after a Whipple resection requires a single retrocolic jejunal loop to complete the pancreaticojejunostomy, which is followed by a cholangiojejunostomy and gastrojejunostomy. A duct-mucosal anastomosis is preferred to the pancreaticojejunostomy. Pancreaticogastrostomy is also an effective and safe means of creating the anastomosis.

Postoperative complications Operative mortality of pancreaticoduodenectomy is currently < 6% in major surgical centers. The leading causes of postoperative mortality include postoperative sepsis, hemorrhage, and cardiovascular events. Most of the septic complications arise from pancreaticojejunostomy leaks.

In many series, early delayed gastric emptying is the leading cause of morbidity for pylorus-preserving procedures. The number-two cause of morbidity, seen in 5% to 15% of all patients, is a leak or fistula from the pancreatic anastomosis. Today, with appropriate drainage and nutritional support, more than 95% of pancreatic fistulas will heal using conservative measures.

An analysis of 200 patients who underwent resection of pancreatic adenocarcinoma in the era prior to adjuvant therapy found that the most important factors influencing long-term survival were the diameter of the primary tumor, status of the resected lymph nodes, and status of the resected margins. Patients with tumors < 3 cm in diameter had significantly longer median survival and 5-year survival rates (21 months and 28%, respectively) than those with tumors ≥ 3 cm (11.5 months and 15%). Patients with no lymph node involvement had a 5-year survival rate of 36%, as compared with < 5% for those with positive nodes. Patients who underwent resections with negative margins had a 5-year survival rate of 26%, versus 8% for those with positive margins. The type of resection (pylorus-preserving vs standard Whipple procedure) did not influence survival.

Body and tail tumors Tumors in the body and tail of the pancreas are typically larger than tumors in the head of the pancreas and are often metastatic upon presentation. For those patients who are surgical candidates, resection employs a distal pancreatectomy with concomitant splenectomy. Due to the large size of these tumors, removal may require resection of adjacent organs. Of note, the rate of pancreatic leaks following distal pancreatectomy is approximately 30% to 40%, although, with appropriate treatment, they resolve using conservative measures.

Surgical palliation

Surgical palliation is also considered in patients undergoing exploration with curative intent. Jaundice, gastric obstruction, and pain may be alleviated by surgical palliation.

Biliary tract obstruction

Either a choledochojejunostomy or cholecystojejunostomy can be used to bypass the biliary obstruction. Recurrent jaundice and cholangitis are less likely to develop when the common duct is used for decompression. Nonoperative means of biliary decompression can often be accomplished with endoscopically placed expandable metallic stents.

Duodenal obstruction

Although duodenal obstruction is rare as a presenting symptom, duodenal involvement may occur eventually in 25% of patients. Some investigators believe that prophylactic bypasses are safe and should be performed in all patients. One phase III trial supports prophylactic bypass, but the subject remains controversial.

Pain relief

Severe back pain may be an incapacitating symptom. Pain relief may be achieved by chemoablation of the celiac plexus or by alcohol injection, which may be performed intraoperatively, percutaneously, or endoscopically. An intraoperative injection of 25 mL of ethanol (95%) on both sides of the celiac axis will ablate tumor pain. (For further discussion of these techniques, see chapter 34 on "Pain Management.")

Neoadjuvant and adjuvant therapies

Radiation therapy

Even with apparently adequate surgical resection, pancreatic cancer has a high risk of locoregional recurrence. Moreover, most lesions are unresectable, even when there is no apparent distant metastatic disease. Thus, there is a theoretical rationale for the adjunctive use of radiation therapy, either before or after surgery, in almost all patients. Preoperative (neoadjuvant) radiation therapy may help render locally advanced lesions resectable with negative margins (R0 resection). Postoperative (adjuvant) radiation therapy may help eliminate suspected residual microscopic disease in the tumor bed and/or regional lymphatics. Alternative radiation techniques, including intensity-modulated radiotherapy (IMRT) and 3D conformal radiation therapy, are being explored.

With an effective chemotherapeutic agent, there is greater potential for adequate locoregional cytotoxicity—as well as control of subclinical distant disease—than could be obtained with limited doses of adjuvant radiation therapy alone.

Preoperative chemoradiation therapy Several single-institution studies have evaluated the role of preoperative irradiation in conjunction with fluorouracil (5-FU)- and gemcitabine (Gemzar)-based chemotherapy. In these studies, 60% to 80% of the lesions were completely resected 1.0 to 1.5 months after the completion of chemoradiotherapy. Median survival has ranged from 16 to 36 months, but no phase III trials have been conducted to evaluate preoperative therapy versus postoperative sequencing.

Preoperative radiation therapy, to 4,500 to 5,000 cGy, in conjunction with chemotherapy should be considered for patients with pancreatic adenocarcinoma who are medically fit but who have marginally resectable disease. There are research initiatives to further address the role of neoadjuvant chemotherapy. For example, phase II studies explore high-dose gemcitabine and high-dose gemcitabine and cisplatin with short-term radiation therapy for locally advanced cancer. Other neoadjuvant strategies include the addition of oxaliplatin (Eloxatin), bevacizumab (Avastin), cetuximab (Erbitux), or erlotinib (Tarceva) to gemcitabine/irradiation combinations.

Postoperative chemoradiation therapy The role of radiotherapy in the adjuvant setting has been called into question by several European trials. Criticism of these studies includes lack of radiotherapy quality control and suboptimal chemotherapy and radiotherapy schedules in the arms that included radiotherapy. In addition, for most GI sites, the preferred sequencing of modalities has been to give several months of full-dose multidrug chemotherapy before proceeding to radiotherapy with concurrent chemotherapy, a sequencing that was not used in the European trials.

A recently activated clinical trial conducted by the EORTC, RTOG, and SWOG addresses all of these criticisms. Postoperative care for patients with cancer of the pancreatic head will be double-randomized, with all patients receiving six cycles of gemcitabine. The first randomization will be to receive or not receive concurrent erlotinib with gemcitabine. The second randomization will be whether to administer either no further therapy or radiotherapy (50.4 Gy/28 fractions) with concurrent infusional fluorouracil or equivalent capecitabine (Xeloda). All radiotherapy treatment plans will be centrally reviewed in advance of treatment. Thus, this trial is evaluating the contribution of postoperative radiotherapy using standard-of-care techniques with proactive quality control.

The ACOSOG Z05031 trial was a phase II trial that tested a regimen of radiation therapy, cisplatin, interferon-alfa, and 5-FU in patients with resected pancreatic cancer. The trial demonstrated a median survival of 27.1 months, which was the longest survival reported with use of adjuvant therapy in a cooperative group trial. However, use of this regimen was associated with significant toxicity, and only 56% of patients completed the entire treatment course.

In addition, the GI Intergroup has completed a randomized phase II trial to explore new combinations incorporating the monoclonal antibodies bevacizumab and cetuximab, each given with gemcitabine; irradiation is given with oral capecitabine. The preliminary results suggest no added benefit with the addition of either bevacizumab or cetuximab.

Postoperative chemotherapy

A German randomized phase III trial including 368 patients with resected pancreatic cancer compared postoperative gemcitabine given for 6 months with observation. Disease-free survival was significantly superior for patients receiving postoperative gemcitabine (13.4 months vs 6.9 months; $P < .001$), including for patients with either R0 or R1 resection. Overall survival, however, was not significantly different between the gemcitabine and control groups (22.1 months vs 20.2 months; $P = .06$). In an updated analysis, the benefits of gemcitabine as compared with observation remained. Despite an improvement in median survival of only 2 months noted among treated patients (22.8 months vs 20.2 months; $P = .005$), a 5-year survival of 21% in the treatment arm versus 9% in the observation arm was reported.

The results of ESPAC 3, a multicenter trial comparing adjuvant 5-FU/leucovorin versus gemcitabine in patients with a resected pancreatic adenocarcinoma, was presented at the American Society of Clinical Oncology (ASCO) 2009 meeting. Following R0/R1 resection, patients were randomized to 5-FU (425 mg/m^2) bolus on days 1–5 every 28 days versus gemcitabine (1,000 mg/m^2) given intravenously on days 1, 8, and 15 every 4 weeks. Both regimens were continued for 6 months. A total of 1,088 patients were randomized. After a minimum follow-up of 2 years, median survival for the 5-FU/leucovorin group was 23 months, compared with 23.6 months for the gemcitabine group. There was no statistical significance between the two study arms.

These two studies confirm the benefit of adjuvant chemotherapy following surgical resection. In the US, adjuvant radiation therapy is frequently utilized but its role is currently being studied.

Locally advanced but potentially resectable lesions

These lesions comprise 10% to 15% of cases presenting to physicians. Data from phase II preoperative chemoradiotherapy trials indicate that trimodality therapy is crucial for margin-free resection and long-term survival. A meta-analysis from the ESPAC1 trial showed that chemotherapy alone is ineffective for patients who have had resection for microscopic disease at a margin (R1), thus adding further support to both chemotherapy and radiation therapy for these borderline resectable patients. The investigators will be mounting a trial with preoperative capecitabine, bevacizumab, and radiation therapy for these patients.

Treatment of unresectable lesions

Irradiation

Radiation therapy can prolong and/or improve quality of life in some patients with unresectable adenocarcinoma of the pancreas. It is better combined with chemotherapy. Long-term survival is, unfortunately, highly unusual.

Chemoradiation

The addition of chemotherapy to radiation therapy has been shown to improve the survival of patients with unresectable pancreatic adenocarcinoma, with moderate doses of radiation only slightly less effective than higher doses. In a GITSG trial of unresectable disease, moderate-dose radiation (4,000 cGy) with 5-FU chemotherapy significantly improved survival, as compared with higher doses of radiation (6,000 cGy) and no chemotherapy (median survival, 9.6 vs 5.2 months). The GITSG has also compared chemotherapy plus irradiation with chemotherapy alone and demonstrated a significant improvement with combined-modality therapy (median survival, 42 vs 32 weeks).

A systematic review of 11 trials including 794 patients with locally advanced pancreatic cancer using radiation/combined-modality therapy showed a survival benefit for chemoradiation over irradiation alone, but there was not a significant advantage for chemoradiation followed by chemotherapy compared with chemotherapy alone.

The ECOG conducted a randomized, prospective trial in patients with locally advanced, unresectable, nonmetastatic pancreatic adenocarcinoma. Patients were randomized to receive either gemcitabine monotherapy or radiation therapy given concurrently with and followed by gemcitabine. The overall survival was 11 months in the combination-therapy group and 9.2 months in the chemotherapy-only group ($P = .034$). Despite the statistical significance of these findings, this trial was plagued by poor accrual and was terminated early.

Based on these data, except in a protocol setting, the palliative management of a patient with unresectable pancreatic adenocarcinoma who has significant local symptoms should probably consist of moderate doses of radiation (4,000–5,000 cGy) in conjunction with 5-FU–based chemotherapy. As in adjuvant treatment, carefully shaped portals approximately 12 × 12 cm should be used. Many practitioners would favor several months of gemcitabine-based chemotherapy before proceeding to radiotherapy and 5-FU for patients experiencing no substantial local symptoms. This allows early delivery of optimal chemotherapy and spares the patient destined to rapid dissemination of disease from the morbidity associated with use of 5-FU plus radiotherapy.

Approaches under investigation At present, clinical investigators are exploring a variety of chemoradiation therapy approaches. Trials with combined gemcitabine and irradiation are of particular interest due to the activity of this drug in pancreatic cancer and the fact that it is a potent radiosensitizer. The benefit of irradiation for patients with locally advanced disease, however, remains a research question because of toxicity concerns and the relatively brief survival rates.

Objective response by size criteria is difficult to achieve with radiotherapy. This may be due to the substantial sclerotic component associated with pancreatic adenocarcinomas rather than true radiation resistance. Regardless, until it becomes possible to achieve a high incidence of objective clinical responses, it will be difficult to persuade surgeons to attempt resections after chemoradiotherapy for unequivocal clinical T4 lesions. Recent results reported from the University of Michigan and Rush University Medical Center are of particular interest in this regard. The Michigan group has a long interest in concurrent radiotherapy and gemcitabine because of the drug's radiosensitizing properties. Previous work from the group suggested that normal tissue tolerance limits the ability to give full doses of both radiotherapy and gemcitabine concurrently. However, in their most recent work, these investigators have taken advantage of technical developments in radiation oncology by using IMRT, breath-holding techniques to limit respiratory excursion, and online daily setup verification to treat macroscopic disease with tight planning target volumes. Radiation doses were successfully escalated from 50 to 60 Gy in 25 fractions over 5 weeks with gemcitabine (1,000 mg/m^2 over 100 minutes) given on weeks 1, 2, 4 and 5. Objective responses were seen in 52% of 27 cases, with a mean overall survival of 23 months, including two cases converted to resectable with minimal residual disease at surgery.

The dose of gemcitabine that can be given concurrently with irradiation depends on the volume and dose of radiation. If full doses of gemcitabine (1,000 mg/m^2/wk) are given concurrently with irradiation, the dose of radiation must be markedly reduced to avoid unacceptable GI toxicity.

Treatment of metastatic adenocarcinoma

Pancreatic adenocarcinoma is still one of the most frustrating, resistant solid neoplasms to treat, and therapy for metastatic disease remains palliative. Few agents have demonstrated activity in > 10% of patients diagnosed with this disease. Moreover, most of the reported series have been small, and not all encouraging results have been duplicated.

Chemotherapy

As metastatic pancreatic carcinoma is incurable, the anticipated risks of chemotherapy, which are often substantial, must be balanced against the gains that may be achieved; unfortunately, these are few. Patients who are debilitated due to their underlying or comorbid disease should not be offered chemotherapy, as their likelihood of deriving any benefit is exceedingly slim. However, patients who desire therapy and who, while symptomatic, still have a good performance status may be offered "standard" chemotherapy (Table 2), or, if possible, they should be encouraged to participate in a clinical trial.

5-FU Historically, single-agent 5-FU has been associated with a response rate of 25% in pancreatic cancer. The use of 5-FU, doxorubicin, and mitomycin (FAM) and 5-FU plus doxorubicin offer no advantage over 5-FU alone. 5-FU plus leucovorin appears to be ineffective.

Gemcitabine is indicated for the treatment of locally advanced or metastatic pancreatic adenocarcinoma. Gemcitabine was compared with 5-FU in a group of 126 previously untreated patients and showed a small, but statistically significant, improvement in response rate. Median survival in the gemcitabine group was 5.7 months, with 18% of patients alive at 12 months, as compared with 4.4 months in the group receiving 5-FU, with 2% of patients alive at 12 months. Perhaps more importantly, clinical benefit response (a composite measurement of pain, performance status, and weight) occurred in 23.8% of the gemcitabine-treated group, as compared with 4.8% of the 5-FU–treated group. Due to its palliative potential, gemcitabine has become the standard of care for patients with unresectable pancreatic adenocarcinoma.

Combination therapy There have been a number of attempts to improve the therapeutic outcome for patients with metastatic pancreatic cancer by comparing promising combinations of agents in randomized clinical trials. Unfortunately, the results have been disappointing. The ECOG compared gemcitabine with or without 5-FU, demonstrating a median survival of 5.4 months for gemcitabine versus 6.7 months for the combination; however, this difference was not statistically significant. Another trial explored the addition of irinotecan to gemcitabine. There was no

TABLE 2: Chemotherapy regimens for pancreatic cancer

Drug/combination	Dose and schedule
Infusional 5-FU with radiation therapy	
Concurrent radiation therapy and chemotherapy phase:	
5-FU	150–250 mg/m²/day, infused over 24 hours/day during radiation therapy
Radiation therapy	Median dose of 4,500 cGy/25 fractions (range, 4,000 cGy/20 fractions to 5,040 cGy/28 fractions)
Fisher B, et al: Int J Radiat Oncol Biol Phys 45:291-295, 1999.	
Single-agent regimen	
Gemcitabine	1,000 mg/m² IV infused over 30 minutes once a week for 7 weeks, followed by a 1-week rest period
Subsequent cycles once a week for 3 consecutive weeks of every 4 weeks	
Burris HA, et al: J Clin Oncol 15:2403–2413, 1997.	
Erlotinib plus gemcitabine	
Erlotinib	100 mg PO daily
Gemcitabine	1,000 mg/m² IV infused over 30 minutes once a week for 7 weeks, followed by a 1-week rest period
Subsequent cycles once a week for 3 consecutive weeks of every 4 weeks	
Moore MJ, et al: J Clin Oncol 23(16S): abstract 1, 2005.	
Gemcitabine adjuvantly in resected pancreatic carcinoma	
Gemcitabine	1,000 mg/m² IV over 30 minutes on days 1, 8, and 15 every 4 weeks for 6 cycles
Neuhaus P, et al: J Clin Oncol 26(15S): abstract LBA450, 2008.	

5-FU = fluorouracil; IV = intravenous; PO = orally. Table prepared by Ishmael Jaiyesimi, DO.

survival benefit when this regimen was compared with gemcitabine alone, although the combination did increase the tumor response rate (16.1% vs 4.4%; $P < .001$).

A meta-analysis of 15 randomized trials showed a significant survival benefit for patients with advanced pancreatic cancer and a good performance status who received gemcitabine either with a platinum analog (hazard ratio [HR]: 0.85; $P = .01$) or a fluoropyrimidine (HR: 0.9; $P = .03$).

Preliminary results from a randomized phase II trial comparing FOLFIRINOX–(5-FU/leucovorin, irinotecan, and oxaliplatin) versus gemcitabine for 88 patients with metastatic pancreatic cancer showed response rates of 38.7% versus 11.7%, respectively, with a median duration of response of 6.3 months versus 4.6 months. Results of a phase III trial are pending.

A phase III study of 565 patients compared gemcitabine with the combination of gemcitabine plus the multitargeted antifolate pemetrexed (Alimta) and demonstrated a significant response benefit with the combination (14.8% vs 7.1%;

A European randomized trial of 319 patients with advanced pancreatic cancer compared capecitabine plus gemcitabine with gemcitabine alone and showed no difference in overall survival (8.4 vs 7.2 months; *P* = .234). The combination showed improved median overall survival in good performance status patients (10.1 vs 7.4 months; *P* = .014; *Herrmann R et al: J Clin Oncol 25:2212–2217, 2007).*

P = .004). However, overall and progression-free survival rates were comparable. There was increased hematologic toxicity with the combination.

Three Intergroup metastatic pancreatic cancer trials have been reported. ECOG completed a trial of gemcitabine vs fixed-rate infusion gemcitabine vs fixed-rate gemcitabine plus oxaliplatin, accruing 832 patients. At a median follow-up of 12.2 months, neither of the two investigational regimens was significantly better than standard gemcitabine (both groups only had approximately 1 month longer median survival). CALGB compared bevacizumab plus gemcitabine vs gemcitabine alone, finding no difference between the regimens. SWOG evaluated gemcitabine with or without cetuximab. The study reported no difference in outcome.

The NCIC has presented a randomized phase III study comparing gemcitabine with or without erlotinib in 530 patients with metastatic pancreatic cancer. The combination produced improvement in both overall (6.24 vs 5.91 months; hazard ratio [HR]:0.82; *P* = .038) and progression-free survival (HR:0.77; *P* = .007). As with other epidermal growth factor receptor–targeted agents, skin rash was associated with response. Diarrhea was increased with the combination.

Agents with marginal activity include mitomycin, doxorubicin, ifosfamide, streptozocin (Zanosar), and docetaxel (Taxotere). To date, monoclonal antibody therapy and hormonal manipulation have been ineffective.

In a phase III trial, 607 patients with metastatic pancreatic cancer were given gemcitabine and erlotinib with either bevacizumab or placebo. Patients receiving bevacizumab had significantly longer progression-free survival, but their improvement in overall survival was not significant *(Van Cutsem E et al: J Clin Oncol 27:2231–2237, 2009).* In the CONKO 003 trial, 168 patients who progressed after gemcitabine therapy received 5-FU and leucovorin with or without oxaliplatin. The study demonstrated a significant advantage in progression-free survival favoring patients receiving oxaliplatin *(Pelzer U et al: J Clin Oncol 26[15S]: abstract 4508, 2008).*

Novel approaches A progressively better understanding of the molecular biology of pancreatic cancer has revealed numerous new therapeutic targets. Some agents currently being studied include vaccines and dasatinib (Sprycel), an inhibitor of multiple tyrosine kinases. In addition, EndoTAG-1, a cationic liposomal paclitaxel agent, has shown early promise when combined with gemcitabine.

PANCREATIC CYSTIC NEOPLASMS

Pancreatic cystic neoplasms comprise a variety of neoplasms with a wide range of malignant potential. These neoplasms are divided into serous cystadenomas, mucinous cystadenomas, and intraductal papillary mucinous neoplasms (IPMN). The latter two mucinous neoplasms do carry a malignant potential. These cysts typically require differentiation from inflammatory pseudocysts. The correct diagnosis is paramount to institute appropriate therapy.

Differentiating these cystic neoplasms from a pseudocyst is often based on a patient's prior history of pancreatitis and risk factors for pancreatitis. Radiographically, the stigmata of pancreatitis such as diffuse calcifications or inflammatory changes surrounding the pancreas may often help in distinguishing pseudocyst from a cystic neoplasm.

Distinguishing serous cyst adenomas from mucinous neoplasms (mucinous adenomas or IPMN) is also important as serous cystadenomas do not have any significant malignant potential. Radiographically, serous cystadenomas occasionally have a starburst appearance with a centrally located scar; this scar is present in approximately 30% of the patients when evaluated with a CT scan. Mucinous cystadenomas often typically have multiple cystic areas with intracystic septae and may occasionally have peripheral calcifications. Furthermore, they occur almost exclusively in females. IPMN are associated with a connection to the pancreatic duct either via endoscopic retrograde cholangiopancreatography or magnetic resonance cholangiopancreatography. This distinguishes IPMN from mucinous cystic neoplasms.

Further evaluation of cystic neoplasms often includes endoscopic ultrasound with fine needle aspiration. Analysis of cystic fluid can help in obtaining a correct diagnosis. Cyst fluid CEA has been shown to be the most accurate for differentiating mucinous cystic neoplasms. Whereas a high CEA level (ie, greater than 182 ng/mL) is more indicative of a mucinous cystic neoplasm, a very low cystic fluid CEA is more indicative of a serous cystadenoma.

Occasionally it requires a combination of tests to help in distinguishing inflammatory pseudocysts from cystic neoplasm. A multidisciplinary approach incorporating gastroenterologists, surgeons, and radiologists is often required.

With regard to treatment, resection is typically indicated for symptomatic cystic neoplasms. Most authorities agree that mucinous cystic neoplasms greater than 3 cm should also be considered for resection in the appropriate medically fit patient.

PANCREATIC ENDOCRINE TUMORS (PETs)

PETs cover a spectrum of neoplasms. Many, although not all, of these tumors originate from the pancreatic islets of Langerhans.

PETs are not rare. Autopsy studies have documented an incidence as high as 1.5%. Most of these lesions are clinically silent.

Approximately 20% of patients with Zollinger-Ellison syndrome (ZES) develop the syndrome in the setting of the multiple endocrine neoplasia type 1 (MEN-1) syndrome. MEN-1 is inherited as an autosomal-dominant trait and is characterized by tumors of multiple endocrine organs, including the pituitary, pancreas, and parathyroid. The gene for MEN-1, which has been localized to the long arm of chromosome 11, has been identified and named *MENIN*.

The normal islet contains α, β, γ cells and enterochromaffin cells, which primarily secrete glucagon, insulin, somatostatin, and serotonin, respectively. All of these hormones may be secreted in excess by PETs. Other hormones that may be secreted by these tumors include vasoactive intestinal peptide (VIP), gastrin, pancreatic polypeptide (PP), and calcitonin. The aggressiveness of a PET in terms of its metastatic potential appears to be due to the cell of origin.

TYPES OF TUMORS

Insulinomas

These are beta-cell tumors of the pancreatic islets that produce insulin. Four-fifths of insulinomas occur as a solitary lesion, and < 10% of these tumors demonstrate malignant potential (in terms of invasiveness or the development of metastases). In patients with the MEN-1 syndrome, insulinomas are multicentric (10% of patients). In addition, a small group of insulinomas are associated with diffuse islet-cell hyperplasia or nesidioblastosis.

Gastrinomas

These tumors are gastrin-secreting tumors associated with the ZES. These tumors can be either sporadic or familial. Sporadic gastrinomas do not have associated endocrinopathies, whereas hereditary gastrinomas occur in patients with MEN-1 syndrome. Patients with the sporadic form of ZES may have single or multiple gastrinomas. This finding contrasts with patients with hereditary MEN-1 PETs, who generally have a more diffuse tumor process within the pancreas.

It is known that 80% to 90% of gastrinomas are located within the "gastrinoma triangle," defined as the junction of (1) the cystic and common duct, (2) the second and third portions of the duodenum, and (3) the neck and body of the pancreas. Although tumors most characteristically are located within the pancreas, a significant percentage of patients with ZES demonstrate primary tumors of the duodenal wall. Extrapancreatic and extraintestinal locations occur in approximately 10% of patients.

More than 90% of gastrinomas are malignant. The spectrum of clinical disease progression includes localized tumors, regional lymph node metastases, and widespread metastatic disease.

Other types

Approximately three-quarters of VIPomas and approximately half of all glucagonomas and somatostatinomas are malignant.

Nonfunctional tumors

Although many PETs cause considerable morbidity due to the inappropriately elevated levels of the hormones that they secrete, even "nonfunctional" PETs, such as those without an associated demonstrable hormone-related syndrome (ie, as PPomas, neurotensinomas, and nonsecretory PETs), may be aggressive. Nonfunctional tumors account for up to 30% of all PETs. Two-thirds of these nonfunctional tumors will demonstrate metastatic lesions at some point during the patient's lifetime.

SIGNS AND SYMPTOMS

The symptom complex that is observed depends on which hormone or hormones are secreted in excess.

Insulinomas

These are associated with symptoms of recurrent hypoglycemia. Diagnosis of these tumors is made by the demonstration of inappropriately elevated levels of insulin, proinsulin, and C peptide at the time of hypoglycemia and an elevated insulin-glucose ratio (> 0.3).

Gastrinomas

Symptoms of gastrinoma-ZES are due to the effect of elevated levels of circulating gastrin. Ulceration of the upper GI tract is seen in > 90% of patients. Diarrhea is the second most common symptom. Approximately 25% of gastrinomas occur in the context of MEN-1 and are associated with parathyroid hyperplasia and hypercalcemia.

The diagnosis of ZES is established by the demonstration of hypergastrinemia (fasting serum gastrin concentration > 1,000 pg/mL) and gastric acid hypersecretion in a patient with ulcerative disease. Medications used for acid suppression could falsely elevate gastrin levels and should be discontinued prior to testing.

VIPomas

An excess of VIP causes a profuse, watery diarrhea, hypokalemia, hypophosphatemia, and hypochlorhydria, referred to as WDHA syndrome.

Glucagonomas

These tumors are associated with a rash (described as a necrotizing migratory erythema), glossitis, cheilosis, constipation and ileus, venous thrombosis, and hyperglycemia. Not all of these manifestations are secondary to elevated glucagon levels alone. The etiology of these signs and symptoms remains unknown, but some patients respond to supplemental zinc and amino acid infusions.

Somatostatinomas

These tumors are rare and are associated with elevated blood glucose levels, achlorhydria, cholelithiasis, and diarrhea.

TUMOR LOCALIZATION

Insulinomas

Ultrasonography, CT, MRI, and selective arteriography with portal vein sampling have been utilized for the preoperative localization of insulinomas. The sensitivity of these preoperative imaging tests ranges from approximately 30% to 60%. This is because 40% of insulinomas measure ≤ 1 cm and two-thirds of these tumors are < 1.5 cm in size.

Because the success of preoperative localization tests is disappointing, and 90% of these tumors will be found and successfully resected by an experienced endocrine surgeon, there is a general trend toward performing fewer tests. Some centers utilize preoperative ultrasonography if the patient has not undergone prior pancreatic surgery. Other centers still routinely employ portal vein catheterization and angiography. Most centers with EUS availability use the modality as a standard diagnostic tool for these tumors.

More recently, intraoperative sonography has been shown to aid the surgeon. In one series, 84% of tumors not localized preoperatively were correctly located by surgical exploration and intraoperative sonography. Many lesions not discovered by surgical palpation may be found by this technique. At present, there is much less reliance on blind distal resection than was previously advocated. Obviously, the technique of intraoperative ultrasonography may not be as helpful in the MEN-1 syndrome, in which multiple small insulinomas may be found.

Gastrinomas

CT, ultrasonography, selective abdominal angiography, selective venous sampling of gastrin, intraoperative ultrasonography, EUS, and intraoperative endoscopy have all been reported to be useful in localizing gastrinomas. More recently, somatostatin receptor scintigraphy (SRS) has become a valuable tool for PET localization; several studies have suggested greater sensitivity and specificity with SRS than with other diagnostic tests.

TREATMENT

Surgery for insulinomas

For larger insulinomas in the body or tail of the pancreas, a distal pancreatectomy may be preferable to enucleation. For tumors in the head of the pancreas, enucleation of the tumor is usually possible. Patients with MEN-1 or islet-cell hyperplasia may benefit from an 80% distal pancreatectomy. If the insulinoma is not found at surgery, a blind pancreatectomy is not warranted. Further imaging and venous sampling studies may reveal the exact location of the tumor.

A surgical cure results in normal values on subsequent provocative testing, during which blood insulin and glucose concentrations are measured simultaneously. Some insulinoma recurrences actually represent persistent disease after incomplete tumor excisions or overlooked secondary multiple tumors.

Surgery for gastrinoma-ZES

The ideal treatment of gastrinoma-ZES is surgical excision of the gastrinoma. However, this approach is possible in only 20% of patients, most of whom have a sporadic tumor. With the development of effective antisecretory agents and preoperative localization with octreotide scanning, the majority of patients demonstrating widespread metastatic disease can be identified and spared surgical exploration. In addition, some series report that patients with nonmetastatic sporadic gastrinoma may have a higher incidence of extrapancreatic sites than was previously thought. One series has reported that two-thirds of gastrinomas are extrapancreatic.

Patients with sporadic gastrinoma

All patients with sporadic gastrinoma should undergo localization studies and be considered for exploratory laparotomy, with the goal of potential cure of ZES. Recent evidence suggests that resection of primary gastrinoma decreases the incidence of liver metastases and ZES. Overall, surgery produces complete remission in approximately 60% of patients with sporadic ZES, and subsequent survival is excellent.

Patients with ZES and MEN-1

Some experts believe that surgery should not be used in the management of patients with MEN-1 and ZES. Instead, they recommend treatment with antisecretory medications. This approach is somewhat controversial, as some authors believe that all patients without demonstrated liver metastases should undergo surgery to remove duodenal and pancreatic gastrinomas.

Moreover, since many patients with ZES and MEN-1 die of metastatic gastrinoma at a young age, a surgical approach may be warranted. Surgery should be performed only if imaging studies localize the tumor. Although radical surgery may not provide a cure, removal of large tumors may decrease metastatic potential and increase survival.

Surgical procedure

During surgery, the entire pancreas should be mobilized and scanned ultrasonographically to permit a thorough examination of the pancreatic head, duodenum, stomach, mesentery, liver, and splenic hilum. Intraoperative endoscopy with transillumination of the bowel wall may also be useful in identifying duodenal lesions. In general, enucleation is the treatment of choice, except for lesions within the duodenal wall, which may require pancreaticoduodenectomy. If no tumor is found, blind distal pancreatectomy should be avoided, since 90% of gastrinomas are located within the gastrinoma triangle. (This triangle is formed by the angles at the junction between the cystic and common bile ducts, the junction between the second and third parts of the duodenum, and the junction between the head and neck of the pancreas.)

Surgical resection of liver metastases is controversial. However, several authors have demonstrated meaningful survival in patients with small, isolated lesions. The use of ablative procedures, with open, laparoscopic, or percutaneous techniques, can reduce the neurohormonal tumor burden.

Radiation therapy for PETs

Adjuvant therapy

The role of adjuvant radiation therapy for PETs of the pancreas is unclear. Because of the rarity of these lesions and their often indolent behavior, the role of this therapy will probably never be demonstrated. However, postoperative irradiation can be considered for patients with positive nodes or microscopically close margins. Concurrent chemotherapy with such agents as 5-FU and/or streptozocin also can be considered. Radiation doses are the same as those used in adjuvant treatment of pancreatic cancer.

Palliative therapy

Anecdotal reports indicate that pancreatic PETs may respond to palliative doses of irradiation. Long-term control of unresectable disease has been reported.

Chemotherapy for PETs

PETs are more sensitive to chemotherapy than are carcinoid tumors.

Single agents

Agents that have demonstrated antitumor activity include recombinant human interferon alfa-2a and alfa-2b (Roferon-A, Intron A, respectively), 5-FU, doxorubicin, dacarbazine, and streptozocin.

A randomized, phase III trial of sunitinib compared with placebo for advanced pancreatic neuroendocrine tumors reported a significant improvement in PFS favoring sunitinib (11.4 months vs 5.5 months, respectively; *P* = .0001; *Raymond E et al: 2010 Gastrointestinal Cancers Symposium, January 22–24, 2010; Orlando, Florida; abstract 127*).

Combination regimens

Combination chemotherapy is often more effective than is monotherapy. For example, in an ECOG study involving the treatment of patients with PETs, the combination of 5-FU and streptozocin demonstrated a higher response rate than did use of streptozocin alone (63% vs 36%), as well as a better complete response rate (33% vs 12%) and median survival duration (26.0 vs 16.5 months). Therapy with doxorubicin plus streptozocin was superior to therapy with both 5-FU plus streptozocin and single-agent chlorozotocin in terms of response and survival and is the combination most widely used in the United States. Etoposide combined with cisplatin is active in poorly differentiated neuroendocrine malignancies but is marginally effective in well-differentiated lesions.

New agents

Antiangiogenic approaches and the recognition of other potential biologic targets have contributed to the development of a number of early-phase clinical trials incorporating bevacizumab with temozolomide (Temodar) and with 5-FU, leucovorin, and oxaliplatin (FOLFOX) chemotherapy, temozolomide with capecitabine, sunitinib (Sutent), sorafenib (Nexavar), vatalanib, imatinib (Gleevec), thalidomide (Thalomid), temsirolimus (Torisel), and everolimus (Afinitor). Phase III trials are evaluating sunitinib and everolimus.

Treatment of symptoms

Octreotide

Octreotide (Sandostatin) is often successful in palliating the symptoms of patients with PETs, although this success depends somewhat on the cell type. For example, insulinomas are marginally responsive to octreotide, but gastrinomas and VIPomas often respond. However, when compared with carcinoid tumors, the median duration of response of PETs to octreotide is significantly shorter (~10 weeks).

SEER data between 1973 and 1999 suggest an increasing median survival of patients with metastatic carinoid tumors since the era of octreotide treatment.

As discussed more fully in the section on carcinoid tumors, a promising experimental approach for patients whose tumors express somatostatin receptors is the use of octreotide conjugated to a therapeutic radioisotope.

Other agents

Omeprazole (Prilosec), an inhibitor of the function of the parietal cell hydrogen pump, is more effective than histamine type 2 (H_2) -receptor antagonists in blocking gastric acid production and is useful in the symptomatic management of gastrinomas.

Other agents available for symptomatic treatment of insulinomas include diazoxide (Hyperstat), an insulin-release inhibitor, and, more recently, glucagon delivered by continuous infusion through a portable pump. Both of these agents are used in conjunction with frequent high-carbohydrate meals.

Patients with the glucagonoma syndrome are treated symptomatically with insulin, high-protein meals, supplemental zinc, amino acid infusions, and anticoagulants.

Bisphosphonate therapy should be considered for patients with bone metastases.

Hepatic arterial embolization

Hepatic arterial embolization, given with chemotherapy (chemoembolization) or without, is an alternative palliative therapy for patients with either carcinoid tumors or a PET who have predominant liver metastases or symptoms. Embolization is best reserved for patients with < 75% tumor involvement of the liver, bilirubin level < 2 mg/dL, and an ECOG performance status of ≤ 2. In addition, a patent portal vein is required for this procedure.

Other liver-directed therapeutic strategies include radiofrequency ablation (RFA) for select patients and clinical trials investigating the role of ^{90}yttrium microspheres.

CARCINOID TUMORS OF THE GI TRACT

Carcinoid tumors typically arise from components derived from the primitive gut, lungs, and, rarely, the gonads. Approximately 85% of all carcinoids originate from the gut, predominantly the appendix, followed by the small bowel and rectum.

These tumors have the propensity to cause considerable morbidity by virtue of creating a syndrome of hormonal excess. For example, although the majority of carcinoids are hormonally inert, these neoplasms may produce excessive amounts of serotonin (from dietary tryptophan), prostaglandins, kinins (secondary to kallikrein release), and a variety of other hormones, which may account for the "carcinoid syndrome." SEER data suggest an increase in the incidence of carcinoid tumors between 1973 and 1990.

SIGNS AND SYMPTOMS

Flushing

The most common sign of the carcinoid syndrome is flushing, which is often triggered by alcohol, catecholamines, or emotional stress. It ranges in severity from a minor annoyance to profound vasodilatation with near syncope and hypotension.

Diarrhea

Diarrhea is also common and is due to GI hypermotility. It usually occurs after meals and is rarely voluminous, bulky, or foul-smelling.

Abdominal cramps

Diarrhea may be associated with crampy pain, although other etiologies for the pain must be considered, including bowel obstruction due to tumor or mesenteric fibrosis.

Bronchospasm

Patients may also develop bronchospasm, which may be mediated by histamine. This problem is often associated with flushing, although it is less common.

> A single-arm study of ^{90}yttrium-edotreotide administered to 90 symptomatic patients with carcinoid tumor refractory to octreotide resulted in stable disease or response for 74% of patients *(Bushnell JL Jr et al: J Clin Oncol 28:1652–1659, 2010)*.

The PROMID Study Group reported data from a prospective, randomized trial of patients with well differentiated midgut carcinoid. Eighty-five treatment-naive patients were randomized to 30 mg/month of long-acting octreotide or placebo. Treatment was given for 18 months or until tumor progression or death. The median time to tumor progression was significantly longer in the treatment arm (14.3 months) than in the placebo group (6 months; $P < .000072$). More than two-thirds of patients using octreotide and one-third of those given placebo had stable disease. Median overall survival had not been reached in the octreotide arm *(Rinke A et al: J Clin Oncol 27:4656–4663, 2009).*

Valvular heart disease

A late finding is right-sided valvular heart disease, although left-sided lesions may be noted occasionally. The fibrous deposits may lead to tricuspid insufficiency and/or pulmonary stenosis. Valve replacement is rarely necessary, however.

Symptom triad

If there is sufficient shunting of dietary tryptophan from niacin to serotonin synthesis, patients may develop diarrhea, dermatitis, and dementia. However, this symptom triad is rare if patients maintain adequate intake of a balanced diet.

DIAGNOSIS

Diagnostic studies include CT/MRI of the abdomen and a 24-hour urine test for 5-hydroxyindoleacetic acid. Some radiologists prefer to obtain a triple-phase CT scan of the liver to detect these highly vascular liver metastases.

Octreotide scanning

^{111}Indium octreotide scintigraphy (OctreoScan) has a higher sensitivity for detecting pancreatic tumors and is superior to CT or MRI for detecting metastatic disease, particularly extrahepatic disease. One study suggests that ^{111}indium octreotide scintigraphy can reduce costs by avoiding unnecessary surgeries. Also, a positive scan may predict which patients may benefit from treatment with somatostatin analogs (eg, octreotide). Initial studies with a new peptide tracer, ^{111}indium 1,4,7,10-tetraazacyclododecane-N,N,N',N'-tetraacetic acid-lanreotide, suggest high tumor uptake and a more favorable dosimetry than is seen with ^{111}indium diethylene triamine pentaacetic acid-D-[Phe1]-octreotide.

STAGING AND PROGNOSIS

Staging

Neuroendocrine tumors are staged according to local spread of disease, nodal status, and distant metastatic involvement, using the AJCC TNM system (Table 3).

The site of tumor origin is potentially prognostic, as most appendiceal carcinoids (75%) are < 1 cm when found and are usually cured by resection. Similarly, rectal carcinoids are usually small and completely resectable for cure.

In contrast, small bowel carcinoids tend to present at a more advanced stage, and approximately one third have multicentric primary lesions. However, if the disease is completely resectable, patients have a 20-year survival rate of 80%; patients with unresectable intra-abdominal or hepatic metastases have median survival durations of 5 and 3 years, respectively.

TABLE 3: TNM staging of neuroendocrine tumors

Primary tumor (T)

Stomach

TX	Primary tumor cannot be assessed
T0	No evidence of primary tumor
Tis	Carcinoma in situ/dysplasia (tumor size < 0.5 mm), confined to mucosa
T1	Tumor invades lamina propria or submucosa and ≤ 1 cm in size
T2	Tumor invades muscularis propria or > 1 cm in size
T3	Tumor penetrates subserosa
T4	Tumor invades visceral peritoneum (serosa) or other organs or adjacent structures
	(For any T, add [m] for multiple tumors)

Duodenum/ampulla/jejunum/ileum

TX	Primary tumor cannot be assessed
T0	No evidence of primary tumor
T1	Tumor invades lamina propria or submucosa and ≤ 1 cm in size[a] (small intestinal tumors); tumor ≤ 1 cm in size (ampullary tumors)
T2	Tumor invades muscularis propria or > 1 cm in size (small intestinal tumors); tumor > 1 cm in size (ampullary tumors)
T3	Tumor invades through the muscularis propria into subserosal tissue without penetration of overlying serosa (jejunal or ileal tumors) or invades the pancreas or retroperitoneum (ampullary or duodenal tumors) or into nonperitonealized tissues
T4	Tumor invades visceral peritoneum (serosa) or other organs
	(For any T, add [m] for multiple tumors)

Colon or rectum

TX	Primary tumor cannot be assessed
T0	No evidence of primary tumor
T1	Tumor invades lamina propria or submucosa and ≤ 2 cm in size
T1a	Tumor size < 1 cm in greatest dimension
T1b	Tumor size 1–2 cm in greatest dimension
T2	Tumor invades muscularis propria or > 2 cm in size with invasion of lamina propria or submucosa
T3	Tumor invades through the muscularis propria into the subserosa or into nonperitonealized pericolic or perirectal tissues
T4	Tumor invades the peritoneum or other organs
	(For any T, add [m] for multiple tumors)

Regional lymph nodes (N)

Stomach/duodenum/ampulla/jejunum/ileum/colon/rectum

NX	Regional lymph nodes cannot be assessed
N0	No regional lymph node metastasis
N1	Regional lymph node metastasis

Distant metastasis (M)

Stomach/duodenum/ampulla/jejunum/ileum/colon/rectum

M0	No distant metastasis (no pathologic M0; use clinical M to complete stage group)
M1	Distant metastasis

Stage grouping

Stage 0	Tis[b]	N0	M0
Stage I	T1	N0	M0
Stage IIA	T2	N0	M0
Stage IIB	T3	N0	M0
Stage IIIA	T4	N0	M0
Stage IIIB	Any T	N1	M0
Stage IV	Any T	Any N	M1

[a] Tumor limited to ampulla of Vater for ampullary gangliocytic paraganglioma;

[b] Tis applies only to the stomach.

From Edge SP, Byrd DR, Compton CC, et al (eds): AJCC Cancer Staging Manual, 7th ed. New York, Springer, 2010.

Gastric carcinoids Types I and II are often multifocal, associated with an elevated gastrin level, and relatively indolent, whereas type III gastric carcinoids are solitary, have a normal gastrin level, and have a more aggressive clinical course.

TREATMENT

The management of carcinoid tumors focuses not only on treating bulky disease, as with other solid malignancies, but also on treating the complications of hormonal excess.

Treatment of bulky disease

Surgery

Appendiceal carcinoids For tumors that are found incidentally in the appendix and that are probably between 1 and 2 cm, appendectomy is the treatment of choice. For tumors > 2 cm, a right hemicolectomy and lymph node dissection are appropriate.

Small intestines and rectal carcinoids should be resected with a wedge lymphadenectomy to evaluate nodal disease. Small distal rectal tumors (< 2 cm) can undergo local excision via transanal techniques. Duodenal lesions should be locally excised if they are small (< 2 cm), with radical resection reserved for larger tumors.

Tumor debulking Liver resection or ablation of liver metastases with cryotherapy or radiofrequency techniques is useful in patients with limited extrahepatic disease and/or symptomatic carcinoid syndrome. Tumor debulking can protect liver functional reserve and improve quality of life.

Liver transplantation may be of benefit in selected patients without extrahepatic disease whose cancer progresses after other therapeutic interventions.

Preoperative and intraoperative considerations

All patients with metastatic, hormonally active carcinoid tumors require echochardiogram prior to any surgical intervention to evaluate for valvular disease. Furthermore, patients will require preoperative treatment with octreotide either subcutaneously or intravenously. Administration of intravenous octreotide is the preferred method of managing carcinoid crisis.

Radiation

Carcinoid tumors are responsive to radiation therapy and frequently are well palliated with this modality. Overall, treatment with higher radiation doses (29–52 Gy) has been associated with higher response rates (40%–50%) than has treatment with lower doses (10%).

Chemotherapy

Since carcinoid tumors tend to be resistant to most chemotherapeutic agents, there are no standard regimens for the treatment of unresectable tumors.

Single agents Agents that have reported activity include 5-FU, doxorubicin, and recombinant human interferon alfa-2a and alfa-2b. However, the response rate with these agents is in the range of 10% to 20%, the response duration is < 6 months, and complete remission is rare.

Combination regimens Combination chemotherapy regimens represent little improvement over single-agent therapy, with response rates ranging from 25% to 35%, response durations < 9 months, and rare complete remissions.

New agents Antiangiogenic approaches and the recognition of other potential biologic targets have contributed to the development of a number of early-phase clinical trials incorporating bevacizumab with temozolomide and with FOLFOX chemotherapy, temozolomide and capecitabine, sunitinib, sorafenib, vatalanib, imatinib, thalidomide, temsirolimus, and everolimus. Phase III trials are planned or ongoing to further evaluate sunitinib and everolimus. The SWOG is currently coordinating an Intergroup randomized phase III trial comparing depot octreotide (Sandostatin LAR) plus interferon alfa-2b versus depot octreotide plus bevacizumab in advanced, poor-prognosis carcinoid patients.

Management of poorly differentiated (high-grade or anaplastic) neuroendocrine tumors and metastatic disease and postresection therapy of isolated resectable disease consists of the same systemic treatment as that used for small-cell lung cancer.

Treatment of symptoms

Somatostatin analogs

Octreotide The most active agent is the somatostatin analog octreotide. Even though native somatostatin is effective in controlling many symptoms, due to its short half-life (< 2 minutes), this agent would have to be administered via continuous infusion to be clinically useful. However, octreotide may be administered subcutaneously every 8 to 12 hours, facilitating outpatient therapy. The initial dose of octreotide is 100 to 600 μg/d in two to four divided doses, although the effective dose varies between patients and must be titrated to the individual patient's symptoms.

Octreotide not only is useful in managing the chronic problems of the carcinoid syndrome, but it also is effective in treating carcinoid crisis (volume-resistant hypotension), which may be precipitated by surgery or effective antitumor treatment.

Octreotide is well tolerated, although chronic treatment may be associated with cholelithiasis, increased fecal fat excretion, fluid retention, nausea, and glucose intolerance. Occasional objective antitumor responses have been observed in patients who have received octreotide; the median duration of symptomatic improvement is 1 year. One report evaluating the cost-effectiveness of octreotide suggested that it may double survival time. Other somatostatin analogs, including lanreotide and vapreotide, are under investigation. A sustained-release formulation of lanreotide (Somatuline Depot) is specifically indicated for the long-term treatment of acromegalic patients who have responded inadequately to surgery and/or radiotherapy or for whom surgery and/or radiotherapy is not an option.

Depot octreotide This long-acting somatostatin analog allows for monthly dosing, avoiding the need for three daily injections. This relatively new agent improves quality of life while apparently maintaining the same activity seen with daily octreotide. The usual monthly dose is 20 or 30 mg.

Patients who demonstrate disease resistance with somatostatin analog treatment alone may benefit from combination therapy with interferon-alfa and this somatostatin analog.

Radiolabeled somatostatin analogs A promising experimental treatment approach involves the use of octreotide or other somatostatin analogs conjugated to radioisotopes (eg, ^{111}indium or ^{90}yttrium) in patients whose tumors express somatostatin receptors (eg, those with a positive OctreoScan result). This approach allows targeted in situ radiotherapy by taking advantage of internalization of the radioligand into the cell to produce DNA damage and cell death, with little effect on normal tissue. Initial reports have shown favorable results with this technique.

Other agents

Other agents that have been used for symptomatic management include histamine type 1 (H_1)- and H_2-receptor antagonists, methoxamine (Vasoxyl), cyproheptadine, and diphenoxylate with atropine. The symptom complex of diarrhea, dermatitis, and dementia may be prevented or treated with supplemental niacin.

Bisphosphonate therapy should be considered for patients with bone metastases.

Hepatic arterial embolization

Hepatic arterial embolization with such agents as Ivalon or Gelfoam, with or without chemotherapy (chemoembolization), is an option for patients with either a carcinoid tumor or an islet-cell carcinoma who have predominant liver metastases or who are symptomatic. These lesions often are hypervascular, and, thus, peripheral hepatic embolization may provide symptomatic relief in some patients. It is unclear whether this therapy has any effect on patient survival.

Other liver-directed therapeutic strategies include RFA for select patients and, as is being investigated in clinical trials, the possible use of ^{90}yttrium microspheres.

ADRENOCORTICAL CARCINOMA

Adrenocortical carcinoma is a rare, highly malignant neoplasm that accounts for about 0.2% of cancer deaths. Long-term survival is dismal overall; the survival rate is 23% at 5 years and 10% at 10 years.

ETIOLOGY

The etiology of adrenocortical cancer is unknown, but some cases have occurred in families with a hereditary cancer syndrome (eg, multiple neoplasia type I, Li-Fraumeni syndrome, Beckwith-Wiedemann syndrome).

SIGNS AND SYMPTOMS

Approximately half of adrenocortical neoplasms produce hormonal and metabolic syndromes of hormone hypersecretion (such as Cushing's syndrome, virilizing or feminizing syndromes, and hyperaldosteronism). In children, Cushing's syndrome is rare but is often due to adrenal carcinoma. Mixed syndromes, such as Cushing's syndrome and virilization, strongly suggest adrenal carcinoma. The combination of hirsutism, acne, amenorrhea, and rapidly progressing Cushing's syndrome in a young female is a typical presentation. In men, estrogen-secreting tumors are associated with gynecomastia, breast tenderness, testicular atrophy, impotence, and decreased libido.

Often, the diagnosis of adrenocortical carcinoma is not evident until the discovery of metastases or until the primary tumor becomes large enough to produce abdominal symptoms. Smaller tumors may be discovered incidentally, when unrelated abdominal complaints are investigated radiographically.

STAGING AND TREATMENT

Adrenal gland tumors are staged according to local spread of disease, nodal status,and distant metastatic involvement, using the AJCC TNM system (Table 4).

Surgery

Complete surgical resection is the treatment of choice in patients with localized disease, as it offers the best chance of extending the disease-free interval and survival.

Although laparoscopic adrenalectomy is often utilized for adenomas, its role in the management of adrenocortical cancer is controversial. Recent data have shown worse outcomes following laparoscopic resections, compared with open resections. Any disruption of the tumor capsule can lead to peritoneal dissemination, and as such open technique is often utilized.

Following resection, the role of adjuvant therapy is unknown, with no prospective data available. A retrospective study suggests that adjuvant treatment with mitotane

TABLE 4: TNM staging of adrenal gland tumors

Primary tumor (T)			
Stomach			
TX	Primary tumor cannot be assessed		
T0	No evidence of primary tumor		
T1	Tumor ≤ 5 cm in greatest dimension, no extra-adrenal invasion		
T2	Tumor > 5 cm, no extra-adrenal invasion		
T3	Tumor of any size with local invasion, but not invading adjacent organs[a]		
T4	Tumor of any size with invasion of adjacent organs[a]		
Regional lymph nodes (N)			
NX	Regional lymph nodes cannot be assessed		
N0	No regional lymph node metastasis		
N1	Metastasis in regional lymph node(s)		
Distant metastasis (M)			
M0	No distant metastasis (no pathologic M0; use clinical M to complete stage group)		
M1	Distant metastasis		
Stage grouping			
Stage I	T1	N0	M0
Stage II	T2	N0	M0
Stage III	T1	N1	M0
	T2	N1	M0
	T3	N0	M0
Stage IV	T3	N1	M0
	T4	N0	M0
	T4	N1	M0
	Any T	Any N	M1

[a] Adjacent organs include the kidney, diaphragm, great vessels, pancreas, spleen, and liver.

From Edge SP, Byrd DR, Compton CC, et al (eds): AJCC Cancer Staging Manual, 7th ed. New York, Springer, 2010.

(Lysodren) improves recurrence-free survival. Owing to the study methodology, however, the conclusions are not universally accepted.

Medical therapy

Mitotane

This drug is one of only a few effective agents; it exerts a specific cytolytic effect on adrenocortical cells and has been used to treat unresectable or metastatic adrenocortical carcinoma. Only 15% to 30% of patients experience objective tumor regression, with a median duration of about 7 months. Mitotane is given at a dose of 4 to 8 g/day as tolerated, although the dose is variable.

Chemotherapy

Limited studies of combination chemotherapy regimens, including cisplatin/etoposide/mitotane, cisplatin/etoposide/doxorubicin/mitotane, and streptozocin/mitotane, have demonstrated responses of between 35% and 50%. The preferred treatment approach remains participation in a clinical trial, when available.

Controlling hormone hypersecretion

Hormone hypersecretion can be controlled medically, in most cases. Agents that are effective in reducing steroid production and in palliating associated clinical syndromes include the antifungal drug ketoconazole, 800 mg/day; aminoglutethimide (Cytadren), 1 to 2 g/day; and metyrapone (Metopirone), 1 to 4 g/day or higher as needed to control cortisol levels. These agents may be used alone or with mitotane.

PHEOCHROMOCYTOMA

Pheochromocytomas are catecholamine-secreting tumors that arise from chromaffin cells in the adrenal medulla or extra-adrenal sympathetic ganglia. These tumors constitute a surgically correctable cause of hypertension in 0.1% to 1.0% of hypertensive persons.

Only about 10% of pheochromocytomas are considered to be malignant. The vast majority (90%) of pheochromocytomas are found in the adrenal medulla, and 97% are located below the diaphragm. Approximately 10% each of pheochromocytomas are bilateral, malignant, multifocal, extra-adrenal, found in children, or associated with a familial syndrome.

Pheochromocytomas in patients with familial syndromes, such as MEN-2 and von Hippel-Lindau syndrome, are less likely to be malignant than are other adrenal lesions. In contrast, pheochromocytomas in patients with a family history of malignant pheochromocytoma are more apt to be malignant.

EPIDEMIOLOGY AND ETIOLOGY

Pheochromocytomas occur in all age groups, but the incidence peaks in the third to fifth decades of life. Most pheochromocytomas (90%) are sporadic. Approximately 10% of cases are inherited as an autosomal-dominant trait, either independently or as a part of the MEN-2 syndrome; bilateral tumors are more common in this setting.

Both MEN-2A and MEN-2B include medullary thyroid carcinoma and pheochromocytoma. MEN-2A includes hyperparathyroidism, whereas MEN-2B includes ganglioneuromas and marfanoid habitus. In MEN-2 families, pheochromocytoma occurs in 5.5% to 100% (mean, 40%), depending on the kindred studied. Bilateral medullary hyperplasia is almost always present. Pheochromocytomas are bilateral in 70% of cases and usually multicentric, but they are rarely extra-adrenal or malignant. Genetic testing is recommended for patients suspected of having MEN-2.

SIGNS AND SYMPTOMS

Patients can present with various symptoms, ranging from mild labile hypertension to hypertensive crisis, myocardial infarction, or cerebral vascular accident, all of which can result in sudden death. The classic pattern of paroxysmal hypertension occurs in 30% to 50% of cases; sustained hypertension may also occur and resembles essential hypertension. A characteristic presentation includes "spells" of paroxysmal headaches, pallor or flushing, tremors, apprehension, palpitations, hypertension, and diaphoresis.

DIAGNOSIS

The diagnosis of pheochromocytoma relies on an appropriate history and documentation of excessive catecholamine production.

Catecholamine measurements

Measurement of 24-hour urinary catecholamines and their metabolites, vanillylmandelic acid and metanephrine, is commonly used; the metanephrine level is considered to be the most specific single test. Serum catecholamine measurements are more susceptible to false elevations due to stress-related physiologic fluctuations. The evaluation of serum catecholamines after clonidine suppression, however, provides a useful diagnostic tool that is more convenient than urine collection. Dynamic provocative tests are rarely indicated. Recently, the measurement of plasma-free metanephrines has been shown to be an excellent test for excluding or confirming pheochromocytoma.

Radiologic studies

Almost all pheochromocytomas are localized in the abdomen, mostly in the adrenal medulla; other locations include the posterior mediastinum or any distribution of the sympathetic ganglia. After the diagnosis is established biochemically, radiologic methods may be needed for preoperative localization of the lesion; CT and MRI are most widely used. Iodine methyl-iodobenzyl guanidine (MIBG) and SRS provide a "functional" image; they are most helpful in the detection of occult contralateral or extra-adrenal lesions.

Differentiating benign from malignant tumors

The histologic differentiation between benign and malignant lesions is extremely difficult and often impossible to make; this distinction may require the development of lymph node, hepatic, bone, or other distant metastases. Recurrent symptoms of pheochromocytoma, often emerging many years after the original diagnosis, are suggestive of malignancy. Biochemical confirmation of recurrent catecholamine hypersecretion and localization of metastatic lesion(s) with ^{131}iodine–MIBG scan constitute diagnostic proof.

TREATMENT

Preoperative medical management

Phenoxybenzamine (Dibenzyline), an oral, long-acting, noncompetitive alpha-adrenoceptor blocker, is a widely used, very helpful first drug; it is given at a dose of 10–40 mg/day. Propranolol, a beta-blocker (20–80 mg/day), is usually added after a few days to prevent tachycardia or arrhythmia. The use of β-blockers alone is hazardous, because it may precipitate a paradoxical rise in blood pressure. The tyrosine hydroxylase inhibitor metyrosine (Demser) may be added in patients whose blood pressure is not well controlled with the combination of an alpha- and a beta-blocker.

Surgery

The principles of pheochromocytoma resection are complete tumor resection, avoidance of tumor seeding, and minimal tumor manipulation. Adrenalectomy can be performed by means of an open anterior transabdominal, open posterior retroperitoneal, laparoscopic lateral transabdominal, or laparoscopic posterior retroperitoneal approach. In the past, an open anterior approach was the standard, because it allowed for complete exploration and inspection for potential tumor foci. However, with the improved accuracy of preoperative imaging and increased experience with laparoscopic procedures, there is little need for exploration in areas in which a tumor has not been identified.

Except in tumors > 6 cm, the laparoscopic approach to pheochromocytoma is probably the technique of choice. In the absence of obvious local tumor invasion or metastatic disease, a laparoscopic procedure is acceptable to many experienced endocrine surgeons.

The most critical intraoperative aspect of surgery is control of blood pressure immediately after removal of the tumor, when all agonistic effects are abolished and the effects of alpha- and beta-blockers are still present. Close cooperation with the anesthesiologist to expand fluid volume and prepare the appropriate infusions of agonists to support vascular stability is critical.

Treatment of metastatic malignant pheochromocytoma

The treatment of choice for metastatic malignant pheochromocytoma remains problematic.

Medical and radiation therapy

Medical therapy with alpha- or beta-blockers, as well as metyrosine, is almost always required to maintain hemodynamic stability. Chemotherapy utilizing streptozocin-based regimens or the combination of cyclophosphamide, vincristine, and dacarbazine has yielded promising responses. Treatment with ^{131}iodine–MIBG or (in Europe) with radiolabeled somatostatin has met with only limited success; however, clinical trials continue to investigate these approaches. In most cases, uncontrolled catecholamine hypersecretion eventually escapes biochemical blockade, and fatal hypertensive crisis ensues.

Surgery

In those cases in which limited and resectable lesions can be identified, surgery can effect complete and lasting remission of the disease.

SUGGESTED READING

ON PANCREATIC CANCER

Ben-Josef E, Griffith K, Francis IR, et al: Phase I radiation dose-escalation trial of intensity-modulated radiotherapy (IMRT) with concurrent fixed dose-rate gemcitabine (FDR-G) for unresectable pancreatic cancer. J Clin Oncol 27(15s): abstract 4602, 2009.

Berger AC, Garcia M, Hoffman JP, et al: Postresection CA19-9 predicts overal survival in patients with pancreatic cancer treated with adjuvant chemoradiation: A prospective validation by RTOG 9704. J Clin Oncol 26:2918–5922, 2008.

Bilimoria KY, Bentrem DJ, Ko CY, et al: Multimodality therapy for pancreatic cancer in the US: Utilization, outcomes, and the effect of hospital volume. Cancer 110:1227–1234, 2007.

Colucci G, Labianca R, Di Costanzo F, et al: Randomized phase III trial of gemcitabine plus cisplatin compared with single-agent gemcitabine as first-line treatment of patients with advanced pancreatic cancer: The GIP-1 study. J Clin Oncol 28:1645–1641, 2010.

Cunningham D, Chau I, Stoken DD, et al: Phase III randomized comparison of gemcitabine versus gemcitabine plus capecitabine in patients with advanced pancreatic cancer. J Clin Oncol 27:5513–5518, 2009.

Herrmann R, Bodoky G, Ruhstaller T, et al: Gemcitabine plus capecitabine compared with gemcitabine alone in advanced pancreatic cancer: A randomized, multicenter, phase III trial of the Swiss Group for Clinical Cancer Research and the Central European Cooperative Oncology Group. J Clin Oncol 25:2212–2217, 2007.

Jemal A, Siegel R, Xu J, et al: Cancer statistics, 2010. CA Cancer J Clin 60:277–300, 2010.

Kindler HL, Niedzwiecki D, Hollis D, et al: A double-blind, placebo-controlled, randomized phase III trial of gemcitabine (G) plus bevacizumab (B) versus gemcitabine plus placebo (P) in patients (pts) with advanced pancreatic cancer (PC): A preliminary analysis of Cancer and Leukemia Group B (CALGB). J Clin Oncol 25(18S): abstract 4508, 2007.

Loehrer PJ Sr, Powell ME, Cardenes HR, et al: A randomized phase III study of gemcitabine in combination with radiation therapy versus gemcitabine alone in patients with localized, unresectable pancreatic cancer: E4201. J Clin Oncol 26(15S): abstract 4506, 2008.

Moore MJ, Goldstein D, Hamm J, et al: Erlotinib plus gemcitabine compared with gemcitabine alone in patients with advanced pancreatic cancer: A phase III trial of the National Cancer Institute of Canada Clinical Trials Group. J Clin Oncol 25:1960–1966, 2007.

Mulcahy MF: Adjuvant therapy for pancreas cancer: Advances and controversies. Semin Oncol 34:321–326, 2007.

Neoptolemos J, Büchler M, Stocken DD, et al: ESPAC-3(v2): A multicenter, international, open-label, randomized, controlled phase III trial of adjuvant 5-fluorouracil/folinic acid (5-FU/FA) versus gemcitabine (GEM) in patients with resected pancreatic ductal adenocarcinoma. J Clin Oncol 27(18S): abstract 4505, 2009.

Neuhaus P, Riess H, Post S, et al: CONKO-001: Final results of the randomized, prospective, multicenter phase III trial of adjuvant chemotherapy with gemcitabine versus observation in patients with resected pancreatic cancer (PC). J Clin Oncol 26(15S): abstract 4504, 2008.

Oettle H, Post S, Neuhaus P, et al: Adjuvant chemotherapy with gemcitabine vs observation in patients undergoing curative-intent resection of pancreatic cancer: A randomized controlled trial. JAMA 297:267–277, 2007.

Philip PA, Benedetti J, Fenoglio-Preiser C, et al: Phase III study of gemcitabine [G] plus cetuximab [C] versus gemcitabine in patients [pts] with locally advanced or metastatic pancreatic adenocarcinoma [PC]: SWOG S0205 study. J Clin Oncol 25(18S): abstract 4509, 2007.

Philip PA, Mooney M, Jaffe D, et al: Consensus report of the National Cancer Institute clinical trials planning meeting on pancreas cancer treatment. J Clin Oncol 27:5660–5669, 2009.

Poplin E, Feng Y, Berlin J, et al: Phase III, randomized study of gemcitabine and oxaliplatin versus gemcitabine (fixed-dose rate infusion) compared with gemcitabine (30-minute infusion) in patients with pancreatic carcinoma E6201: a trial of the Eastern Cooperative Oncology Group. J Clin Oncol 27:3778-3785, 2009.

Russo S, Butler J, Ove R, et al: Locally advanced pancreatic cancer: A review. Semin Oncol 34:327–334, 2007.

Sultana A, Tudur Smith C, Cunningham D, et al: Systematic review, including meta-analyses, on the management of locally advanced pancreatic cancer using radiation/combined modality therapy. Br J Cancer 96:1183–1190, 2007.

Terzolo M, Angeli A, Fassnacht M, et al: Adjuvant mitotane treatment for adrenocortical carcinoma. N Engl J Med 356:2372-2380, 2007.

Ujiki MB, Talamonti MS: Guidelines for the surgical management of pancreatic adenocarcinoma. Semin Oncol 34:311–320, 2007.

Wong GY, Schroeder DR, Carns PE, et al: Effect of neurolytic celiac plexus block on pain relief, quality of life, and survival in patients with unresectable pancreatic cancer: A randomized controlled trial. JAMA 3:1092–1099, 2004.

Ychou M, Desseigne F, Guimbaud R, et al: Randomized phase II trial comparing folfirinox (5FU/leucovorin [LV], irinotecan [I] and oxaliplatin [O]) vs gemcitabine (G) as first-line treatment for metastatic pancreatic adenocarcinoma (MPA): First results of the ACCORD 11 trial. J Clin Oncol 25(18S): abstract 4516, 2007.

ON NEUROENDOCRINE GI TUMORS

Cwikla JB, Sankowski A, Seklecka N, et al: Efficacy of radionuclide treatment DOTATATE Y-90 in patients with progressive metastatic gastroenteropancreatic neuroendocrine carcinomas (GEP-NETS): A phase II study. Ann Oncol 21:787–794, 2010.

Durán I, Salazar R, Casanovas O, et al: New drug development in digestive neuroendocrine tumors. Ann Oncol 18:1307–1313, 2007.

Faiss S, Pape UF, Bohmig M, et al: Prospective, randomized, multicenter trial on the antiproliferative effect of lanreotide, interferon alfa, and their combination for therapy of metastatic neuroendocrine gastroenteropancreatic tumors. The International Lanreotide and Interferon Alfa Study Group. J Clin Oncol 15:2689–2696, 2003.

Fazio N, Oberg K: Prospective, randomized, multicenter trial on the antiproliferative effect of lanreotide, interferon alfa, and their combination for therapy of metastatic neuroendocrine gastroenteropancreatic tumors. J Clin Oncol 22:573–574, 2004.

Ho AS, Picus J, Darcy MD, et al: Long-term outcome after chemoembolization and embolization of hepatic metastatic lesions from neuroendocrine tumors. AJR Am J Roentgenol 188:1201–1207, 2007.

Kwekkeboom DJ, Teunissen JJ, Bakker WH, et al: Radiolabeled somatostatin analog [177Lu-DOTA0,Tyr3]octreotate in patients with endocrine gastroenteropancreatic tumors. J Clin Oncol 23:2754–2762, 2005.

Mazzaglia PJ, Berber E, Milas M, et al: Laparoscopic radiofrequency ablation of neuroendocrine liver metastases: A 10-year experience evaluating predictors of survival. Surgery 142:10–19, 2007.

Musunuru S, Chen H, Rajpal S, et al: Metastatic neuroendocrine hepatic tumors: Resection improves survival. Arch Surg 141:1000–1004, 2006.

Oberg K, Kvols L, Caplin M, et al: Consensus report on the use of somatostatin analogs for the management of neuroendocrine tumors of the gastroenteropancreatic system. Ann Oncol 15:966–973, 2004.

Teh SH, Deveney C, Sheppard BC: Aggressive pancreatic resection for primary pancreatic neuroendocrine tumor: Is it justifiable? Am J Surg 193:610–613, 2007.

Yao JC, Hoff PM: Molecular targeted therapy for neuroendocrine tumors. Hematol Oncol Clin North Am 21:575–581, 2007.

ON ADRENAL NEOPLASMS

Jossart GH, Burpee SE, Gagner M: Surgery of the adrenal glands. Endocrinol Metab Clin North Am 29:57–68, 2000.

Kendrick ML, Lloyd R, Erickson L, et al: Adrenocortical carcinoma: Surgical progress or status quo? Arch Surg 136:543–549, 2001.

Libè R, Fratticci A, Bertherat J: Adrenocortical cancer: Pathophysiology and clinical management. Endocr Relat Cancer 14:13–28, 2007.

Terzolo M, Angeli A, Fassnacht M, et al: Adjuvant mitotane treatment for adrenocortical carcinoma. N Engl J Med 356:2372–2380, 2007.

Vassilopoulou-Sellin R, Schultz PN: Adrenocortical carcinoma: Clinical outcome at the end of the 20th century. Cancer 92:1113–1121, 2001.

Wajchenberg BL, Albergaria Pereira MA, Medonca BB, et al: Adrenocortical carcinoma: Clinical and laboratory observations. Cancer 88:711–736, 2000.

ON CARCINOIDS

Anthony LB, Kang T, Shyr T: Malignant carcinoid syndrome: Survival in the octreotide era. J Clin Oncol 23(suppl): abstract 4084, 2005.

Goede AC, Winslet MC: Surgery for carcinoid tumours of the lower gastrointestinal tract. Colorectal Dis 5:123–128, 2003.

Kolby L, Persson G, Franzen S, et al: Randomized clinical trial of the effect of interferon alpha on survival in patients with disseminated midgut carcinoid tumours. Br J Surg 90:687–693, 2003.

Krenning EP, de Jong M: Therapeutic use of radiolabelled peptides. Ann Oncol 11(suppl 3):267–271, 2000.

Modlin IM, Lye KD, Kidd M: A 5-decade analysis of 13,715 carcinoid tumors. Cancer 97:934–959, 2003.

Moller JE, Connolly HM, Rubin J, et al: Factors associated with progression of carcinoid heart disease. N Engl J Med 348:1005–1015, 2003.

Schell SR, Camp ER, Caridi JG, et al: Hepatic artery embolization for control of symptoms, octreotide requirements, and tumor progression in metastatic carcinoid tumors. J Gastrointest Surg 6:664–670, 2002.

van der Horst-Schrivers AN, Wymenga AN, de Vries EG: Carcinoid heart disease. N Engl J Med 348:2359–2361, 2003.

ON PHEOCHROMOCYTOMAS

Baghai M, Thompson GB, Young WF Jr, et al: Pheochromocytomas and paragangliomas in von Hippel-Lindau disease: A role for laparoscopic and cortical-sparing surgery. Arch Surg 137:682–689, 2002.

Goldstein RE, O'Neill JA Jr, Holcomb GW III, et al: Clinical experience over 48 years with pheochromocytoma. Ann Surg 229:755–764, 1999.

Lenders JW, Eisenhofer G, Mannelli M, et al: Phaeochromocytoma. Lancet 366:665–675, 2005.

Rose B, Matthay KK, Price D, et al: High-dose 131I-metaiodobenzylguanidine therapy for 12 patients with malignant pheochromocytoma. Cancer 98:239–248, 2003.

Safford SD, Coleman RE, Gockerman JP, et al: Iodine-131 metaiodobenzylguanidine is an effective treatment for malignant pheochromocytoma and paraganglioma. Surgery 134:956–962, 2003; discussion 962–963.

Scholz T, Eisenhofer G, Pacak K, et al: Clinical review: Current treatment of malignant pheochromocytoma. J Clin Endocrinol Metab 92:1217–1225, 2007.

Vaughan ED Jr: Diseases of the adrenal gland. Med Clin North Am 88:443–466, 2004.

Zendron L, Fehrenbach J, Taverna C, et al: Pitfalls in the diagnosis of phaeochromocytoma. Br Med J 13:629–630, 2004.

Abbreviations in this chapter

ACOSOG = American College of Surgeons Oncology Group; AICR = American Institute for Cancer Research; AJCC = American Joint Committee on Cancer; CALGB = Cancer and Leukemia Group B; CONKO = Charité Onkologie Clinical Studies in GI Cancer; ECOG = Eastern Cooperative Oncology Group; ESPAC = European Study Group for Pancreatic Cancer; EORTC = European Organisation for Research and Treatment of Cancer; GITSG = Gastrointestinal Tumor Study Group; NCIC = National Cancer Institute of Canada; PROMID = Placebo-controlled Prospective Randomized Study on the Antiproliferative Efficacy of Octreotide LAR in Patients with Metastatic Neuroendocrine Midgut Tumors; RTOG = Radiation Therapy Oncology Group; SEER = Surveillance, Epidemiology and End Results; SWOG = Southwestern Oncology Group; WCRF = World Cancer Research Fund

CHAPTER 12

Liver, gallbladder, and biliary tract cancers

Lawrence D. Wagman, MD, John M. Robertson, MD, Laura Raftery, MD, and Bert O'Neil, MD

HEPATOCELLULAR CANCER

Worldwide, hepatocellular carcinoma is the fifth most common malignancy and the third most common cause of cancer mortality. Most patients with hepatocellular carcinoma suffer from cirrhosis, primarily caused by alcoholism or chronic infection with hepatitis B virus (HBV) or hepatitis C virus (HCV); decades may pass between infection with viral hepatitis and development of this cancer. The approximately equal annual incidence and mortality of 1 million reported around the world stands as evidence of its lethality.

EPIDEMIOLOGY

Gender

Hepatocellular carcinoma is the most common tumor in males worldwide, with a male-to-female ratio of 5:1 in Asia and 2:1 in the United States.

Geography

Eighty percent of new hepatocellular cancer cases occur in developing countries, but the incidence of this cancer is also rising in developed countries. Modeling of the spread of HCV infection suggests that this number may continue to increase dramatically. In the United States, the incidence of hepatocellular carcinoma is 5 per 100,000, whereas in the Far East and sub-Saharan Africa, this neoplasm occurs at an incidence of 150 per 100,000 population and comprises almost 50% of all diagnosed tumors.

Age

The incidence of hepatocellular cancer increases with age. The mean age at diagnosis is 53 years in Asia and 67 years in the United States.

Race

From 2003 to 2005, the incidence of hepatocellular tumors in the United States was higher among Asian immigrants (12 per 100,000) and black individuals (7 per

100,000) than among white individuals (4 per 100,000). However, a study analyzing SEER data has shown that the incidence of hepatocellular carcinoma is rising in both white and black populations in the United States.

Survival

In patients who meet stringent criteria and undergo transplant, the 5-year survival is approximately 65% to 70%; the 5-year recurrence rate is less than 20%. The 5-year survival rate following liver resection (governed by a different set of operative criteria) is about equal to that following transplant. This result is in spite of a majority of patients experiencing metastases or a recurrence in the remaining part of the liver. Fewer than 20% of resected patients who have tumor recurrence are able to undergo transplant. Seventy-five percent of patients have unresectable disease that is diagnosed at an advanced stage. Median survival in these patients can range from months to years, depending upon the stage of disease, the biologic aggressiveness of the tumor, vascular invasion, and "background" liver function, among other important factors.

ETIOLOGY AND RISK FACTORS

Hepatitis B

The annual incidence of hepatocellular carcinoma in HBV carriers is 0.5% and in patients with known cirrhosis is 2.5%. In one study, the relative risk of hepatocellular carcinoma in HBV carriers was 100 in Asian patients, who likely acquired the virus at birth. The epidemiology of HBV infection is different in the Western world, where it is acquired later in life, and risk in white individuals appears to be related to inflammatory activity and cirrhosis.

In endemic areas of hepatitis B, approximately 90% of all patients with hepatocellular carcinoma are positive for hepatitis B surface antigen (HBsAg). The presence of the hepatitis B "e" antigen has been found to increase risk ninefold. An important reason to provide antiretroviral agents to patients with chronic HBV infection is the relationship between the risk of hepatocellular carcinoma development and absolute serum levels of HBV DNA. The most compelling epidemiologic evidence of a causal relationship between HBV infection and hepatocellular carcinoma is the observation of a significant decline in the incidence of childhood hepatocellular carcinoma after the introduction of a national immunization program in Taiwan. The hepatitis B "*X*" gene, which can interact with *p53*, has been a focus of study on the pathogenesis of hepatocellular carcinoma.

In a study following patients with chronic liver disease for development of hepatocellular carcinoma, 18,000 Chinese patients with chronic HBV infection were screened with α-fetoprotein determinations and liver ultrasonography every 6 months or received no screening for 5 years. The hepatocellular carcinoma mortality rate was 37% lower in the screened group than in the controls, and this outcome can be attributed to early-stage tumor detection and resection *(Zhang BH et al: J Cancer Res Clin Oncol 137:417–422, 2004).*

Hepatitis C

The risk of hepatocellular carcinoma in patients with chronic HCV infection and established cirrhosis is 2% to 8% per year. The molecular mechanisms of HCV infection and carcinogenesis are poorly understood, yet the disease is believed to occur in the context of chronic inflammation, which leads to fibrosis and cirrhosis. Unlike patients with HBV infection, patients with hepatocellular carcinoma infected with HCV usually have cirrhotic livers at diagnosis; this finding suggests an extended period of infection (or hepatic damage) before malignancy develops.

Alcohol

Patients with alcoholic cirrhosis are at risk for hepatocellular carcinoma, and the addition of HCV infection increases that risk dramatically. About 60 to 80 g of alcohol (equivalent to four to six beers) must be consumed daily over 5 to 10 years for a male to develop cirrhosis (odds ratio, 4). The interaction between alcohol consumption and HCV infection approximately doubles the odds ratio.

Other possible etiologies

These include aflatoxin, hemochromatosis, hepatic venous obstruction, Thorotrast (a contrast agent no longer used for radiologic procedures), androgens, estrogens, and α_1-antitrypsin deficiency. Emerging risk factors for hepatocellular carcinoma are obesity and nonalcoholic fatty liver disease. In a prospective, cohort study of patients with biopsy-proven nonalcoholic steatohepatitis, older age, and advanced fibrosis were risk factors for hepatocellular carcinoma.

Prevention

A large 5-year randomized study performed in China has confirmed that treatment of chronic HBV infection with the antiviral lamivudine (Epivir) not only decreases the risk of progression to cirrhosis of the liver but also decreases the rate of progression to hepatocellular cancer. Treated patients had a 3.9% risk of hepatocellular cancer over 5 years, compared with 7.4% for those in the placebo group (hazard ratio: 0.49; $P = .047$). It remains controversial whether antiviral therapy with ribavirin (Copegus, Rebetol) and interferon decreases the risk of hepatocellular carcinoma in cirrhotic patients with HCV infection who achieve a sustained virologic response. If there is any benefit to therapy in such cases, it appears to be small.

SIGNS AND SYMPTOMS

Nonspecific symptoms

Patients with hepatocellular cancer usually present with abdominal pain and other vague symptoms, including malaise, fever, chills, anorexia, weight loss, and jaundice.

Physical findings

An abdominal mass is noted on physical examination in one-third of patients with hepatocellular cancer. Less common findings include splenomegaly, ascites, abdominal tenderness, muscle wasting, and spider nevi. Up to 10% of patients may present with an acute abdomen due to a ruptured tumor.

SCREENING AND DIAGNOSIS

Presently, no organization recommends routine screening of average-risk, asymptomatic adults for liver, gallbladder, and biliary tract cancers.

α-Fetoprotein

This serum marker is produced by 70% of hepatocellular carcinomas. The normal range for this serum marker is 0 to 20 ng/mL, and a level > 200 ng/mL is essentially diagnostic for hepatocellular cancer in the absence of chronic, active hepatitis B infection. In the presence of active hepatitis B infection, the diagnostic cutoff is considered to be at least 1,000 ng/mL. In the setting of HCV infection, the cutoff for diagnosis of hepatocellular carcinoma has not been well studied. In hepatitis C, values > 200 ng/mL appear to be highly predictive of hepatocellular carcinoma. False-positive results may be due to acute or chronic hepatitis, germ-cell tumors, or pregnancy. In its guidelines for diagnosis of hepatic masses suspicious for hepatocellular carcinomas, the NCCN does not recommend biopsy for patients with an α-fetoprotein level > 400 ng/mL, except in the presence of HBsAg positivity. In that situation, a cutoff value of 4,000 ng/mL is recommended for biopsy.

Hepatitis B and C

Given the association between hepatitis B and C and hepatocellular cancer at the time of diagnosis of a hepatic mass, blood should be sent for hepatitis B and C antigen and antibody determinations.

Imaging

The initial diagnostic test in the symptomatic patient may be ultrasonography, as it is noninvasive and can detect lesions as small as 1 cm. Ultrasonographic findings should be followed up with more specific imaging.

Triple-phase, high-resolution CT and contrast-enhanced magnetic resonance imaging (MRI) are the primary imaging modalities used to diagnose and stage hepatocellular carcinoma. Typically, hepatocellular carcinoma is a hypervascular tumor with washout in the portal venous phase. Reports have documented a high number of false-positive results with CT angioportography (CTAP) and CT hepatic angiography (CTHA). CT scan predicts resectability in only 40% to 50% of cases and does not accurately determine the functional extent of cirrhosis. Major difficulties arise when the liver parenchyma is not homogeneous and the lesions are smaller than 1 cm. Use of positron emission tomography (PET) scanning is not defined in this disease, and the uptake of ^{18}F-fluorodeoxyglucose by hepatocellular tumors is variable.

Laparoscopy

This procedure is useful for the evaluation of small tumors, the extent of cirrhosis, peritoneal seeding, and the volume of noninvolved liver and, therefore, may be used prior to open laparotomy for resection. Laparoscopic or intraoperative ultrasonography should be used to confirm preoperative imaging tests. The laparoscopic results may change surgical management in up to one-third of selected patients.

High-risk patients

Individuals at high risk should be screened for hepatocellular carcinoma using ultrasonography and serum α-fetoprotein levels. Screening increases the proportion of cancers that are resectable. However, a study comparing 6-month and 12-month survival intervals in a cohort of HCV-infected patients with hemophilia showed no substantial benefit to more frequent screening.

PATHOLOGY

Three morphologic patterns of hepatocellular carcinoma have been described: nodular, diffuse, and massive. Diffuse and massive types account for > 90% of cases. The nodular type usually has multiple lesions in both lobes.

Histologic arrangements

Several histologic arrangements have been identified: trabecular, compact, pseudoglandular or acinar, clear cell, and a fibrolamellar variant, which is associated with a relatively favorable prognosis and a younger age at diagnosis. The fibrolamellar variant is more commonly resectable and is not usually associated with infection and cirrhosis.

STAGING AND PROGNOSIS

The staging system for hepatocellular cancer is based on the number and size of lesions and the presence or absence of vascular tumor invasion (Tables 1and 2). The Okuda staging system accounts for the degree of liver dysfunction and may better predict prognosis than the TNM staging system. However, the Okuda staging system does not adequately predict resectability and primarily predicts end-stage disease. Child-Pugh System and MELD (Model for End-Stage Liver Disease) scores measure liver function, and are not cancer staging systems. Because of the limited value of standard staging, the most important factors determining survival are technical resectability of lesions and the degree of dysfunction of the normal liver. Groups in Spain, Italy, and China have created prognostic indices that may prove useful for making treatment decisions. The Barcelona Clinic Liver Cancer staging system was designed to be a diagnostic and treatment strategy to compare tumor stage, liver function status, and performance status in its schema. Surgical resection is considered to be the best treatment for patients with solitary tumors and normal bilirubin levels who do not have portal hypertension. According to the Barcelona schema, patients may be considered for liver transplantation if the above criteria are not met or for ablation if the disease is at an early stage (solitary tumors < 5 cm or up to three nodules with no single nodule > 3 cm). Such patients will have a 5-year survival of 50% to 75%. Chemoembolization is appropriate for patients with intermediate-stage disease who are asymptomatic and have preserved liver function, with a bilirubin level < 3 mg/dL; their 3-year survival will be 50% or better. For patients with advanced disease, there are fewer established therapeutic options; enrollment in a research study may be the best of these alternatives.

Of the roughly 20% of patients who can undergo resection, factors associated with improved survival include curative resection, small tumor size, well-differenti-

TABLE 1: TNM staging of liver cancer

Primary tumor (T)			
TX	Primary tumor cannot be assessed		
T0	No evidence of primary tumor		
T1	Solitary tumor without vascular invasion		
T2	Solitary tumor with vascular invasion or multiple tumors (none > 5 cm)		
T3a	Multiple tumors > 5 cm		
T3b	Single tumor or multiple tumors of any size involving a major branch of the portal vein or hepatic vein		
T4	Tumor(s) with direct invasion of adjacent organs other than the gallbladder or perforation of the visceral peritoneum		
Regional lymph nodes (N)			
NX	Regional lymph nodes cannot be assessed		
N0	No regional lymph node metastasis		
N1	Regional lymph node metastasis		
Distant metastasis (M)			
M0	No distant metastasis		
M1	Distant metastasis		
Stage grouping			
Stage I	T1	N0	M0
Stage II	T2	N0	M0
Stage IIIA	T3a	N0	M0
Stage IIIB	T3b	N0	M0
Stage IIIC	T4	N0	M0
Stage IVA	Any T	N1	M0
Stage IVB	Any T	Any N	M1

From Edge SB, Byrd DR, Compton CC, et al (eds): AJCC Cancer Staging Manual, 7th ed. New York, Springer, 2010.

ated tumors, and normal performance status. Cirrhosis, nodal metastases, and an elevated prothrombin time are indicative of a poor prognosis, as are male sex, age > 50 years, poor performance status, duration of symptoms < 3 months, tumor rupture, aneuploidy, high DNA synthesis rate, hypocalcemia, vascular invasion, and a high serum α-fetoprotein level.

TREATMENT

Surgery

Surgery is the form of treatment that offers the greatest potential for cure, even though only a small minority of patients will actually be cured. Unfortunately, many patients whose disease is thought to be resectable are clinically understaged preoperatively.

Only stage I or II tumors have a significant likelihood of being resectable for cure. Resectability is limited by the functioning liver tissue at the completion of a negative margin operation. Therefore, even a large tumor may still be potentially resectable for

TABLE 2: TNM staging of intrahepatic bile duct cancer

Primary tumor (T)			
TX	Primary tumor cannot be assessed		
T0	No evidence of primary tumor		
Tis	Carcinoma in situ (intraductal tumor)		
T1	Solitary tumor without vascular invasion		
T2a	Solitary tumor with vascular invasion		
T2b	Multiple tumors, with or without vascular invasion		
T3	Tumor perforating the visceral peritoneum or involving the local extrahepatic structures by direct invasion		
T4	Tumor with periductal invasion		
Regional lymph nodes (N)			
NX	Regional lymph nodes cannot be assessed		
N0	No regional lymph node metastasis		
N1	Regional lymph node metastasis present		
Distant metastasis (M)			
M0	No distant metastasis		
M1	Distant metastasis		
Stage grouping			
Stage 0	Tis	N0	M0
Stage I	T1	N0	M0
Stage II	T2	N0	M0
Stage III	T3	N0	M0
Stage IVA	T4	N0	M0
	Any T	N1	M0
Stage IVB	Any T	Any N	M1

From Edge SB, Byrd DR, Compton CC, et al (eds): AJCC Cancer Staging Manual, 7th ed. New York, Springer, 2010.

cure. Moreover, contiguous involvement of large vessels (including the portal vein and inferior vena cava) or bile ducts does not automatically mitigate against a resection. Resection is contraindicated in patients with metastatic disease to non-portal nodes and in extrahepatic locations. The use of the Child-Pugh score and volumetric evaluation aids in assessment of resectability. For cirrhotic patients in whom less than 30%–35% of the liver remains at the completion of resection, operative treatment is contraindicated. Likewise, this is true for noncirrhotic patients in whom less than 25%–30% of the liver remains.

Bilobar disease may be addressed with formal resection, tumor ablation techniques (eg, cryoablation, radiofrequency ablation [RFA], and ethanol injection ablation), or a combination of the modalities.

Contraindications to resection

These include imminent clinical hepatic failure (jaundice in the absence of biliary obstruction), hypoalbuminemia, ascites, renal insufficiency, hypoglycemia,

TABLE 3: Child-Pugh score[a]

Measure	1 point	2 points	3 points
Bilirubin (mg/dL)	< 2	2–3	> 3
Albumin (g/dL)	> 3.5	2.8–3.5	< 2.8
Prothrombin time (seconds)	1–3	4–6	> 6
Ascites	None	Slight	Moderate
Encephalopathy (grade)	None	I–II	III–IV

[a] Grade A = 5–6 points; grade B = 7–9 points; grade C = 10–15 points.

Schwartz M, Roayaie S, Konstadoulakis M: Nat Clin Pract Oncol 4:424-432, 2007.

prolongation of the prothrombin and partial thromboplastin times, main portal vein involvement, extrahepatic metastatic disease, or other comorbid diseases that would preclude surgery of any kind.

Noncirrhotic versus cirrhotic patients

Resection should be performed in all noncirrhotic patients, when feasible. Resection of hepatocellular carcinoma in the presence of cirrhosis is more controversial due to its increased morbidity in this setting. Cirrhosis has been a major deterrent to resection in western nations. Resectability rates vary from 0% to 43% for cirrhotic patients, whereas up to 60% of patients without cirrhosis undergo resection. Use of the modified Child-Pugh classification of liver reserve (Table 3) may guide the surgeon in preoperative assessment of liver function status and may aid in the selection of operable patients.

When resection is performed in the presence of cirrhosis, Child-Pugh class A patients fare better than do Child-Pugh class B or C patients. Survival rates at 5 years following resection range from 4% to 36%, with noncirrhotic patients living longer than cirrhotic patients.

Transplantation

Owing to the risk of hepatic failure following resection in cirrhotic patients, transplantation has become an option for patients with hepatocellular cancer and cirrhosis. In a study of 181 patients with hepatocellular carcinoma, Starzl and Iwatsuki found similar overall 5-year survival rates in patients treated with transplantation vs resection (36% vs 33%). Survival rates were similar in the two groups when tumors were compared for TNM stage. However, survival was significantly improved in patients with concomitant cirrhosis if they were treated with transplantation. Tumor recurrence rates for stages II and III tumors were significantly lower after transplantation than after resection, but no differences were seen for stage IV tumors. Numerous additional studies have examined the relative value of transplantation, ablation, and resection. There is much debate over their interpretation.

Patients with cirrhosis and single tumors < 5 cm or multiple tumors (up to three with none > 3 cm) can be considered for transplantation. Larger tumors may be treated with resection when feasible. The University of California San Francisco has prepared "expanded criteria" for transplant eligibility. The use of transplantation is significantly limited by the scarcity and lack of immediate availability of donor organs. Recently, changes in the organ allocation system have decreased waiting times for patients with documented hepatocellular cancer.

Therapies for nonresectable hepatocellular carcinoma

Given the high risk of recurrence after resection, the multifocal nature of hepatocellular carcinoma, and its association with chronic liver disease, therapies for nonresectable disease can play an important role in management. A number of prognostic factors have been identified for patients with unresectable hepatocellular carcinoma. These factors, taken alone, can greatly affect survival rates, making cross-treatment comparisons more difficult because considerable selection bias may be present in any nonrandomized trial. Additionally, comparisons are difficult, as there are few randomized trials among the large number of non-resectional, liver-directed therapies currently available. It is worth noting that a number of these treatments do not have overlapping toxicities and that research into combinations is potentially worthwhile.

Ablation

Ablation techniques include RFA, cryotherapy, and injection of chemicals (eg, ethanol) directly into the tumor. RFA can be performed via laparotomy or percutaneously via CT or ultrasonographic guidance. It is best suited for lesions < 3 cm. The overall recurrence rate after ablation is > 70%. Some recurrence represents undertreatment of lesions, microscopic satellites that were not included in the ablation site, poor imaging due to technical issues, inexperience of the ablator, and selection of large tumors. Ablation is safe and effective for patients who cannot undergo resection or who need a bridge to transplant.

Intratumoral ethanol injection The direct injection of 95% ethanol into a neoplastic lesion causes cellular dehydration and coagulation necrosis. This procedure has been largely replaced by RFA, which in several clinical trials has shown efficacy superior to ethanol injection.

> **S**ide effects of RFA may include pleural effusions and peritoneal bleeding. In 1,000 patients treated with RFA for hepatocellular carcinoma, neoplastic seeding from percutaneous RFA occurred at a rate of 3.2% per patient or 1.8% per treatment. The patients underwent 1,845 RFA treatments for 3,837 nodules; 20% had nodules > 3 cm. The observation period was 5 to 64 months, and poor differentiation was the only risk factor for neoplastic seeding in multivariate analysis. Surrogate markers for poor differentiation were larger tumor size and elevated tumor marker levels. Other investigators have reported occurrences of "seeding" in as many as 12% and as few as 0.9% of patients undergoing RFA for hepatocellular carcinoma, with subcapsular tumor location being a risk factor *(Imamura J et al: Am J Gastroenterol 103:3057–3062, 2008).*

Cryotherapy and RFA

Cryotherapy and RFA techniques are suitable for treating localized disease. Cryotherapy has been used intraoperatively to ablate small, solitary tumors outside a planned resection (ie, in patients with bilobar disease). Cryotherapy must be performed using laparotomy, which limits its

The SHARP trial compared sorafenib (Nexavar: 400 mg PO bid) vs placebo in 600 patients with Child-Pugh class A liver disease. About one-third of patients had undergone embolization, and the disease progressed. In all, 70% of patients had portal vein thrombosis and/or metastatic lesions. In spite of a low radiographic response rate, median survival for the 300 patients given sorafenib was significantly better than that for the placebo group (10.7 vs 7.9 months; hazard ratio [HR], 0.69). This is the first well-powered trial to convincingly demonstrate a survival benefit with the use of a systemic agent for this disease. Sorafenib is the standard of care for hepatocellular carcinoma not amenable to locoregional therapy and the first FDA-approved agent for this indication. Studies using the drug with embolization are ongoing *(Llovet JM et al: N Engl J Med 359:378–390, 2008).*
In the Asia-Pacific Trial, 226 patients with Child-Pugh class A liver disease were randomized to receive sorafenib and placebo. These patients primarily had HBV infection; compared with the SHARP study patients, they had more local therapy before their entry into the trial and, as a whole, more advanced disease. Median survival was 6.5 months, compared with 4.2 months for sorafenib and placebo (HR, 0.68) *(Cheng AL et al: Lancet Oncol 10:25–34, 2009).* More data are needed to establish the role of sorafenib in treating Child-Pugh class B liver disease.

use in the palliative setting. RFA creates necrosis through the use of heated electrodes at the site of the tumor and has efficacy superior to that of ethanol injections for lesions > 2 cm.

Hepatic Transcatheter Embolization/ Transarterial Chemoembolization (TACE)

Normal hepatocytes receive most of their blood supply from the portal vein, whereas tumors create new blood vessels from branches of the hepatic arterial system. This target is exploited by embolization of the hepatic artery with any number of substances, resulting in radiographic responses in about 50% of patients and evidence of tumor liquefaction in over two-thirds of patients. At 2 years, the overall survival benefit from this procedure ranges from 20% to 60%. Embolization is accomplished by advancing a catheter within the tumor-feeding branch of the hepatic artery. Materials injected have included polyvinyl alcohol, iodized oil (Lipiodol), collagen, and autologous blood clot. If chemotherapy is given, it usually is suspended in iodized oil, which is retained in the tumor. Common chemotherapeutic agents used have included cisplatin and doxorubicin, which may produce systemic side effects. Postembolization syndrome, with fever, abdominal pain, and, occasionally, ileus, occurs in 50% of patients when a large volume of liver is treated. Complications include infection and abscess. As few complete responses are achieved, treatments may be repeated on the same tumor for better results. Due to risk of liver failure, chemoembolization may be contraindicated in patients with portal vein thrombosis and for most individuals with Child-Pugh B status. Patients with Child-Pugh C liver disease cannot receive chemoembolization due to risk of liver failure. One innovation in chemotherapy delivery during TACE is the use of drug-eluting beads (DEBs). These perforated beads allow for slow, localized release of chemotherapy after embolization. In a study by Varela et al, 27 patients with Child-Pugh class A liver disease and unresectable hepatocellular cancer underwent DEB-TACE. Pharmacokinetic samples were analyzed for doxorubicin, demonstrating lower systemic drug exposure than expected with conventional TACE. Two patients had abscesses, but the radiographic response rate was a promising 75%. Studies of this technology are now being planned and conducted at multiple sites.

The effect of TACE on survival remains controversial, with randomized studies returning mixed results. A randomized, controlled trial in Spain was stopped early due to a survival benefit. Meta-analysis of studies indicates a positive impact on overall survival.

> **Mature data on the use of ^{90}yttrium microspheres for hepatocellular carcinoma have been published. A total of 526 treatments were administered to 291 patients. The 30-day mortality rate was 3%, response rates (World Health Organization criteria) were 42%, and the median time to disease progression was 7.9 months. Patients with Child-Pugh A disease survived for a median of 17.2 months (*Salem R et al: Gastroenterology 138:52–64, 2010*).**

Radiation therapy

Adjuvant treatment There is no evidence that adjuvant radiation therapy can improve local or regional tumor control after adequate resection or ablation.

Unresectable disease Whole-liver radiation therapy can provide palliation in patients with unresectable tumors but is limited to a total dose of ≤ 30 Gy due to the risk of radiation-induced liver disease. Whole-liver irradiation has been combined with chemotherapy and TACE, with objective response rates of approximately 40% to 50% and median survival rates of about 18 months. Patients with tumor regrowth after chemoembolization may respond to radiotherapy.

Radiation therapy has also been delivered using ^{90}yttrium microspheres infused via the hepatic artery to carefully selected patients; response rates as high as 89% have been reported. One study reported that 56% of treated T3 tumors were downstaged to T2, which allowed subsequent liver-directed therapy or use as a bridge to transplant.

Three-dimensional conformal radiation therapy treatment planning can allow patients with nondiffuse disease to be safely irradiated to doses well above the whole-liver tolerance dose, with doses up to 90 Gy given safely to selected patients, a response rate of 40%, and a median survival of 15 months.

Multiple institutions have reported response rates as high as 90% with acceptable toxicity when conformal radiation therapy was combined with TACE. Good response and local tumor control rates have also been reported for proton, carbon ion, and stereotactic radiotherapy.

> **Sunitinib (Sutent), an oral inhibitor of multiple receptor tyrosine kinases, was tested in patients with hepatocellular carcinoma in a phase II trial. The median overall survival was almost 10 months. However, sunitinib was more difficult to tolerate than is sorafenib, and its use was related to more serious treatment-related adverse events (eg, grade 3/4 cytopenias, transaminitis, vasculitis). It also required monitoring of cardiac function (*Zhu AX et al: J Clin Oncol 26[15S]:4521, 2008*).**

Chemotherapy

Systemically administered chemotherapy The low response rates to chemotherapy are related to the role of the hepatocyte in detoxification. Hepatocytes also have high multidrug resistance expression. Furthermore, many patients with hepatocellular carcinoma have cirrhosis or hepatic dysfunction, which

TABLE 4: Systemic chemotherapy

	Year	Phase	Patients	Response rate (%)	Median survival (months)
Paclitaxel[a]	1998	II	20	0	3.0
Capecitabine[b]	2000	II	37	13	6.0
Irinotecan[c]	2001	II	14	7	8.2
Gemcitabine[d]	2002	II	30	0	6.9
Doxorubicin[e]	2005	III	94	11	6.8
Nolatrexed[f]	2007	III	222	1	5.6
Cisplatin/interferon alpha-2b/cisplatin/ 5-FU[e]	2005	III	94	21	8.7
Gemcitabine/ oxaliplatin[g]	2007	II	34	18	11.5
Capecitabine/ oxaliplatin[h]	2007	II	50	6	9.3
Capecitabine/ cisplatin[i]	2009	Cohort	178	20	10.5

5-FU = 5-fluorouracil

[a] Chao Y, Chan WK, Birkhofer MJ, et al: Br J Cancer 78:34–39, 1998.
[b] Loranzo RD, Patt YZ, Hassan MM, et al: Proc Am Soc Clin Oncol 19:1025, 2000.
[c] O'Reilly EM, Stuart KE, Sanz-Altamira PM, et al: Cancer 91:101–105, 2001.
[d] Fuchs CS, Clark JW, Ryan DP, et al: Cancer 94:3186–3191, 2002.
[e] Yeo W, Mok TS, Zee B, et al: J Natl Cancer Inst 97:1532–1538, 2005.
[f] Gish RG, Porta C, Lazar L, et al: J Clin Oncol 25:3069–3075, 2007.
[g] Louafi S, Bolge V, Ducreux M, et al: Cancer 109:1384–1390, 2007.
[h] Bolge V, Raoul JL, Pignon JP, et al: Br J Cancer 97:862–867, 2007.
[i] Shim JH, Park JW, Nam BH, et al: Cancer Chemother Pharmacol 63:459–467, 2009.

complicates the administration of chemotherapeutic agents that undergo hepatic metabolism. Agents with partial response rates near or above 10% include doxorubicin, 5-fluorouracil (5-FU), and cisplatin. Table 4 describes the results of studies testing various chemotherapeutic agents in patients with hepatocellular carcinoma.

Biologic therapy Inhibiting angiogenesis in hepatocellular carcinoma is based on several factors. Hepatocellular carcinoma is a vascular tumor; increased levels of vascular endothelial growth factor are found in hepatomas compared with normal hepatic tissue, and increased endothelial growth factor levels before resection of tumor or TACE are associated with early relapse, aggressive behavior, and poor prognosis. Other targets include EGFR (epidermal growth factor receptor, which is frequently expressed in hepatoma cells), the mitogen-activated protein kinase (MAPK) pathway, and the phosphatidylinositol 3-kinase/Akt/mammalian target of rapamycin (P13K/Akt/mTOR) pathway. Conventional markers of radiographic response are poorly related to tumor cell kill in hepatocellular carcinoma. More meaningful markers of therapeutic benefit may be time to disease progression, progression-free survival, and overall survival.

BILIARY TRACT CANCERS

Gallbladder carcinoma is diagnosed approximately 5,000 times a year in the UnitedStates, making it the most common biliary tract tumor and the fifth most common gastrointestinal tract cancer. Approximately 4,500 cases of bile duct tumors occur each year in the United States.

> **Erlotinib (Tarceva), an oral agent that inhibits the epidermal growth factor receptor (EGFR, HER1)-related tyrosine kinase enzyme, was evaluated for efficacy in hepatocellular carcinoma. A number of phase II trials examining agents targeting EGFR have been tested in patients with hepatocellular carcinoma, and they appear to have only modest activity. In two phase II studies with erlotinib, "disease control" was greater than 50% (response rate, > 10%), and median survival was 10 to 13 months. The combination of bevacizumab (Avastin) and erlotinib in a phase II study of 40 patients with Child-Pugh A or B liver disease that was not amenable to surgery or regional therapy resulted in a progression-free survival of 9 months and a median survival of 15.6 months, which compares favorably with sorafenib. Use of this regimen in the cirrhotic patient may be associated with bleeding and thrombosis *(Thomas MB et al: J Clin Oncol 27:843–850, 2009).***

EPIDEMIOLOGY

Gallbladder cancer

Gender

Women are more commonly afflicted with gallbladder cancer than are men, with a female-to-male ratio of 1.7:1.

Age

The median age at presentation of gallbladder cancer is 73 years.

Race

An incidence five to six times that of the general population is seen in southwestern Native Americans, Hispanics, and Alaskans.

Bile duct cancer

Gender

Bile duct tumors are found in an equal number of men and women.

Age

Extrahepatic bile duct tumors occur primarily in older individuals; the median age at diagnosis is 70 years.

ETIOLOGY AND RISK FACTORS

Gallbladder cancer

The risk of developing gallbladder cancer is higher in patients with cholelithiasis, calcified gallbladders, and in typhoid carriers. Gallstones are present in 70% or more of patients with gallbladder cancer and presumably cause chronic inflammation. The overall incidence of gallbladder cancer in individuals with cholelithiasis is 1% to 3% and in patients with so-called porcelain gallbladders, caused by chronic cholecystitis, 10% to > 50%. In patients having gallbladder polyps measuring > 1 cm, the risk of cancer is high.

Bile Duct Cancer

Primary sclerosing cholangitis (PSC)

Thirty percent of cholangiocarcinomas are diagnosed in patients with PSC with or without ulcerative colitis. The annual incidence of cholangiocarcinoma in patients with PSC is estimated at 1.5% per year; their lifetime risk of developing this malignancy is 10% to 15%. These patients have a highly abnormal biliary system, making diagnosis of cholangiocarcinoma difficult.

Ulcerative colitis

Patients with ulcerative colitis have an incidence of bile duct cancer that is 9 to 21 times higher than that of the general population. This risk does not decline after total colectomy for ulcerative colitis.

Other risk factors

Congenital anomalies of the pancreaticobiliary tree, parasitic infections, biliary papillomatosis, and Lynch syndrome are also associated with bile duct tumors. No association of bile duct cancer with calculi, infection, or chronic obstruction has been found.

SIGNS AND SYMPTOMS

Gallbladder cancer

Early and late disease

In the early stages, gallbladder cancer is usually asymptomatic. Later, symptoms similar to those of benign gallbladder disease arise; they include right upper quadrant pain, nausea, vomiting, fatty food intolerance, anorexia, jaundice, and weight loss. This nonspecificity of symptoms delays presentation for medical attention and contributes to the low curability of gallbladder cancer.

Physical findings

These may include tenderness, an abdominal mass, hepatomegaly, jaundice, fever, and ascites.

Bile duct cancer

Jaundice

This is the most frequent symptom found in patients with high bile duct tumors; it is present in up to 98% of such patients.

Nonspecific signs and symptoms

Patients who do not present with jaundice have vague complaints, including abdominal pain, weight loss, pruritus, fever, and an abdominal mass.

DIAGNOSIS

Gallbladder cancer

Gallbladder carcinomas are often diagnosed at an advanced stage, such that by the time symptoms have developed, most tumors are unresectable.

A retrospective review of 73 consecutively treated patients with an R0 resection of gallbladder cancer found that adjuvant chemoradiotherapy was a significant predictor of overall survival after adjusting for prognostic factors. This suggested that a benefit to postoperative therapy may exist, although it remains to be proven in phase III studies *(Gold DG et al: Int J Radiat Oncol Biol Phys 75:150–155, 2009).*

Laboratory values

Findings in patients with gallbladder carcinoma are nonspecific but may include anemia, leukocytosis, and an elevated bilirubin level.

Ultrasonography

This diagnostic study is useful for defining a thickened gallbladder wall and may show tumor extension into the liver. It is valuable in measuring the size of a polyp.

CT and MRI

CT is more helpful than ultrasonography in assessing adenopathy and spread of disease into the liver, porta hepatis, or adjacent structures. MRI may be used to evaluate intrahepatic spread.

Cholangiography

Endoscopic retrograde cholangiopancreatography (ERCP), transhepatic cholangiography (THC), or magnetic resonance cholangiography (MRC) may be useful in the presence of jaundice to determine the location of biliary obstruction and involvement of the liver.

Bile duct cancer

Cholangiocarcinoma may present earlier than gallbladder cancer by virtue of the development of biliary obstruction with jaundice, which may be painless. Tissue confirmation of suspected bile duct cancer can be difficult. The goals of the diagnostic evaluation include the determination of the level and extent of obstruction, the extent of local invasion of disease, and the identification of metastases.

Many patients with cholangiocarcinoma are thought to have metastatic adenocarcinoma of an unknown primary, although occasionally the metastatic lesion may produce biliary dilatation without the primary lesion itself being radiographically visualized. Recently, microarray-based technology for genetic analysis has become available to help characterize tumors that are difficult to identify.

Ultrasonography

It is generally accepted that ultrasonography should be the first imaging procedure in the evaluation of the jaundiced patient.

CT

This diagnostic modality is a complementary test to ultrasonography, but both tests are accurate for staging in only 50% of patients and for determining resectability in < 45% of patients.

Cholangiography

This diagnostic technique is essential to determine the location and nature of the obstruction. Percutaneous THC is used for proximal lesions, and ERCP is used for distal lesions. Magnetic resonance cholangiopancreatography (MRCP) may replace invasive studies in the near future. Histologic confirmation of tumor can be made in 45% to 85% of patients with the use of exfoliative or brush cytology during cholangiography.

PATHOLOGY

Gallbladder cancer

Histologic types

Over 85% of gallbladder neoplasms are adenocarcinomas, and the remaining 15% are squamous cell or mixed tumors.

Route of spread

The initial route of spread of gallbladder cancer is locoregional rather than distant. For patients undergoing resection for presumed high-risk gallbladder masses or preoperatively defined disease limited to the gallbladder, 25% of patients will have lymphatic involvement, and 70% will have direct extension of disease into the liver defined at operation.

Bile duct cancer

Adenocarcinoma

Morphologically, more than 90% of bile duct tumors are adenocarcinomas. Three macroscopic appearances have been identified. The papillary and nodular types occur more frequently in the distal bile duct, whereas the sclerosing type is found in the proximal bile duct. Patients with papillary lesions have the best prognosis. Immunohistochemical staining may be positive for cytokeratin 7 and 20.

Other histologic types

Unusual malignant diseases of the biliary tract include adenosquamous carcinoma, leiomyosarcoma, and mucoepidermoid carcinoma.

Route of spread

Most bile duct tumors grow slowly, spreading frequently by local extension and rarely by the hematogenous route. Nodal metastases are found in up to one-third of patients.

TABLE 5: TNM staging of gallbladder cancer

Primary tumor (T)			
TX		Primary tumor cannot be assessed	
T0		No evidence of primary tumor	
Tis		Carcinoma in situ	
T1		Tumor invades lamina propria or muscular layer	
	T1a	Tumor invades lamina propria	
	T1b	Tumor invades muscular layer	
T2		Tumor invades perimuscular connective tissue; no extension beyond serosa or into liver	
T3		Tumor perforates the serosa (visceral peritoneum) and/or directly invades the liver and/or one other adjacent organ or structure, such as the stomach, duodenum, colon, pancreas, omentum, or extrahepatic bile ducts	
T4		Tumor invades main portal vein or hepatic artery or invades two or more extrahepatic organs or structures	
Regional lymph nodes (N)			
NX		Regional lymph nodes cannot be assessed	
N0		No regional lymph node metastasis	
N1		Metastases to nodes along the cystic duct, common bile duct, hepatic artery, and/or portal vein	
N2		Metastases to periaortic, pericaval, superior mesentery artery and/or celiac artery lymph nodes	
Distant metastasis (M)			
M0		No distant metastasis	
M1		Distant metastasis	

Stage grouping			
Stage 0	Tis	N0	M0
Stage I	T1	N0	M0
Stage II	T2	N0	M0
Stage IIIA	T3	N0	M0
Stage IIIB	T1–3	N1	M0
Stage IVA	T4	N0–1	M0
Stage IVB	Any T	N2	M0
	Any T	Any N	M1

From Edge SB, Byrd DR, Compton CC, et al (eds): AJCC Cancer Staging Manual, 7th ed. New York, Springer, 2010.

STAGING AND PROGNOSIS

Gallbladder cancer

Gallbladder cancer is staged primarily at the time of surgery, and staging is determined by lymphatic involvement and extension of disease into adjacent structures (Table 5).

TABLE 6: Staging of perihilar bile duct tumors

Primary tumor (T)

TX	Primary tumor cannot be assessed
T0	No evidence of primary tumor
Tis	Carcinoma in situ
T1	Tumor confined to the bile duct, with extension up to the muscle layer or fibrous tissue
T2a	Tumor invades beyond the wall of the bile duct to surrounding adipose tissue
T2b	Tumor invades adjacent hepatic parenchyma
T3	Tumor invades unilateral branches of the portal vein or hepatic artery
T4	Tumor invades main portal vein or its branches bilaterally; or the common hepatic artery; or the second-order biliary radicals bilaterally; or unilateral second-order biliary radicals with contralateral portal vein or hepatic artery involvement

Regional lymph nodes (N)

NX	Regional lymph nodes cannot be assessed
N0	No regional lymph node metastasis
N1	Regional lymph node metastasis (including nodes along the cystic duct, common bile duct, hepatic artery, and portal vein)
N2	Metastasis to periaortic, pericaval, superior mesenteric artery, and/or celiac artery lymph nodes

Distant metastasis (M)

M0	No distant metastasis
M1	Distant metastasis

Stage grouping

Stage 0	Tis	N0	M0
Stage I	T1	N0	M0
Stage II	T2a–b	N0	M0
Stage IIIA	T3	N0	M0
Stage IIIB	T1–3	N1	M0
Stage IVA	T4	N0–1	M0
Stage IVB	Any T	N2	M0
	Any T	Any N	M1

From Edge SB, Byrd DR, Compton CC, et al (eds): AJCC Cancer Staging Manual, 7th ed. New York, Springer, 2010.

Stage

Survival of gallbladder carcinoma is directly related to disease stage. The 5-year survival rate is 83% for tumors that are confined to the gallbladder mucosa; this rate decreases to 33% if the tumor extends through the gallbladder. For patients who have involvement of the lymph nodes or metastatic disease, 5-year survival rates range from 0% to 15%.

TABLE 7: Staging of distal bile duct tumors

Primary tumor (T)			
TX	Primary tumor cannot be assessed		
T0	No evidence of primary tumor		
Tis	Carcinoma in situ		
T1	Tumor confined to the bile duct histologically		
T2	Tumor invades beyond the wall of the bile duct		
T3	Tumor invades the gallbladder, pancreas, duodenum or other adjacent organs without involvement of the celiac axis, or the superior mesenteric artery		
T4	Tumor involves the celiac axis, or the superior mesenteric artery		
Regional lymph nodes (N)			
NX	Regional lymph nodes cannot be assessed		
N0	No regional lymph node metastasis		
N1	Regional lymph node metastasis		
Distant metastasis (M)			
M0	No distant metastasis		
M1	Distant metastasis		
Stage grouping			
Stage 0	Tis	N0	M0
Stage IA	T1	N0	M0
Stage IB	T2	N0	M0
Stage IIA	T3	N0	M0
Stage IIB	T1	N1	M0
	T2	N1	M0
	T3	N1	M0
Stage III	T4	Any N	M0
Stage IV	Any T	Any N	M1

From Edge SB, Byrd DR, Compton CC, et al (eds): AJCC Cancer Staging Manual, 7th ed. New York, Springer, 2010.

Type of therapy

Median survival is also improved in patients who have undergone curative resection, as compared with those who have had palliative procedures or no surgery (17 months vs 6 and 3 months, respectively).

Bile duct cancer

Over 70% of patients with cholangiocarcinoma present with local extension, lymph node involvement, or distant spread of disease. The AJCC staging system for extrahepatic tumors is shown in Tables 6 and 7.

Stage

Survival for these patients is poor and is directly related to disease stage. Median survival time is 12 to 20 months for patients with disease limited to the bile ducts and ≤ 8 months when the disease has spread.

Tumor location

Survival is also related to tumor location, with patients who have distal lesions doing better than those with mid or proximal tumors.

Success of therapy

Curative resection and negative margins result in improved survival.

TREATMENT

In the absence of polyps identified ultrasonographically and confirmed by CT during the workup of suspected cholelithiasis, relatively few patients with gallbladder cancer are diagnosed prior to surgery. Only 1% to 2% of cholecystectomy specimens are found to contain malignancy.

Surgery for gallbladder cancer

Surgical management of gallbladder carcinoma is based on the local extension of the tumor. Surgery may be curative, but < 30% of patients are potentially resectable at time of diagnosis.

Early-stage disease

Tumors that invade the lamina propria may be treated by cholecystectomy only. This is usually the situation in a gallbladder cancer that is identified by the pathologist following a cholecystectomy for presumed stone disease. Laparoscopic cholecystectomy should not be performed if the diagnosis of gallbladder cancer is suspected preoperatively (eg, gallbladder polyp of greater than 1 centimeter on preoperative imaging, thickened gallbladder wall without a history of gallstones or cholecystitis). All suspected gallbladder cancers, as well as those documented intraoperatively and those for which the pathology on cholecystectomy identifies disease greater than T1a, should be treated with a formal resection.

> A phase II trial of sorafenib (Nexavar) in 46 patients with advanced cholangiocarcinoma showed disease control in 32% of patients; 54% treated for at least 12 weeks showed stable disease or partial response *(Dealis C et al: J Clin Oncol 26[15S]:4590, 2008)*. Another phase II study of cetuximab (Erbitux) plus gemcitabine (Gemzar) and oxaliplatin (Eloxatin) in patients with advanced or metastatic cholangiocarcinoma demonstrated an overall response rate of 58%. Six patients underwent curative resection after a major response (32%). One patient had a complete response, and six had stable disease *(Greunberger B et al: J Clin Oncol 269[15S], 2008)*.

The resection should include the gallbladder bed (segments IVb and V) and a portahepatic, paraduodenal, and gastrohepatic ligament lymphadenectomy, as well as a bile duct resection if the disease extends to the cystic duct.

Disease that involves the gallbladder node is particularly curable and should be resected. Nodal disease beyond the pericholedochal (porta hepatis) nodes defines the surgically incurable patient.

The usual pattern of spread is locoregional, although lymphangitic metastasis can be observed for T3 and T4 disease. Based on retrospective data, some surgeons will perform radical surgery in T3 and T4 disease with intent to cure.

Surgery for bile duct cancer

The rate of resectability is 15% to 20% for high bile duct tumors and up to 70% for distal lesions. Guidelines for surgery include the absence of retropancreatic and paraceliac nodal metastasis, noncontiguous liver metastasis, major vascular invasion, or extrahepatic invasion of adjacent organs. Some surgeons will attempt en bloc resection with vascular reconstruction.

A phase III trial evaluated overall survival in 410 patients with inoperable biliary tract cancer. Patients were randomized to gemcitabine (Gemzar) and cisplatin vs gemcitabine alone. Metastatic disease was present in 75% of patients and locally advanced disease was present in 25% of patients. Median overall survival was 11.7 months in the combined-treatment arm, compared with 8.2 months with gemcitabine. Patients treated with gemcitabine and cisplatin also had an improved progression-free survival time, 8.5 months vs 6.5 months, and similar toxicity compared with the single agents *(Valle JW et al: J Clin Oncol 27[15S]:abstract 4503, 2009).*

Assessing resectability

High-resolution CT or MRI with biliary reconstruction may be supplemented with hepatic arteriography, portal venography, or duplex imaging preoperatively to assess resectability.

Preoperative treatments

Preoperative stenting for patients with jaundice caused by obstruction is controversial. Many surgeons find that placement of a biliary stent may confound imaging and impede surgery. This must be weighed against the benefit of relieving an obstruction and improving surgical outcome. Three randomized trials have shown no benefit to preoperative decompression of the biliary tree in patients with obstructive jaundice. Some authors advocate the preoperative placement of biliary stents to facilitate dissection of the hilus. This procedure should be performed close to the planned resection to reduce the risk of cholangitis and maintain the duct at its maximally dilated size.

Proximal tumors

Local excision is often possible for proximal lesions. Hepatic resection is indicated for high bile duct tumors. Resection is not indicated in situations in which a clear surgical margin cannot be obtained.

Mid-ductal and distal tumors

Mid-ductal lesions can often be removed by resection of the bile duct with associated portal lymphadenectomy. Distal or mid-ductal lesions that cannot be locally excised should be removed by pancreaticoduodenectomy.

Reconstruction techniques

Biliary-enteric continuity is usually reconstructed with a Roux-en-Y anastomosis to the hilum for high lesions and in a standard drainage pattern following pancreaticoduodenectomy.

Liver transplantation

This procedure has been attempted for unresectable tumors, but early recurrence and poor survival have prevented the widespread application of this approach. Protocols for transplantation for patients with localized, unresectable disease who respond to neoadjuvant chemoradiation therapy are ongoing.

Surgical bypass

For patients found to have unresectable disease at surgical exploration, operative biliary bypass may be performed using a variety of techniques. Bypass results in excellent palliation and obviates the need for further intervention.

Adjuvant radiochemotherapy for gallbladder cancer

Because of the rarity of biliary cancers, there is a paucity of prospective data to guide our practices. In the United States, gallbladder cancer commonly is treated with 5-FU and radiation after resection. A randomized trial performed in Japan showed that treatment with 5-FU and mitomycin produced a survival benefit in patients with resected gallbladder cancers. These data came from a planned subset of a larger trial in which 112 patients with gallbladder cancer were randomized. At 5 years, 26% of chemotherapy-treated patients were alive, compared with 14% of those treated with surgery and observation alone. Based on these data, consideration of chemotherapy for these patients is warranted, but definitive conclusions require a larger randomized trial. Two analyses using the SEER database have concluded that adjuvant radiation therapy may have a survival benefit for node-positive gallbladder cancer. One of these studies also found a benefit for tumors that were T2+.

For advanced, unresectable gallbladder cancer, palliation of obstructive jaundice and pain should be the goal. Combined-modality chemoradiation therapy may benefit patients with advanced disease. Regarding chemotherapy, many regimens using oxaliplatin (Eloxatin), gemcitabine (Gemzar), as well as capecitabine (Xeloda) alone, or in combination with cisplatin have been tried. Modest response rates are the norm, and the indolence or aggressiveness of the tumor primarily influences survival.

Adjuvant chemoradiotherapy for cholangiocarcinoma

Delivery of adjuvant chemoradiotherapy is common for patients who have had margin-negative or microscopically positive margin resections, with observational series providing supporting evidence of improved outcomes. Chemoradiotherapy with infusional 5-FU or capecitabine is also given in the setting of positive regional lymph nodes.

Management of unresectable, locally advanced disease

The majority of patients present with unresectable disease, and palliative care is the goal of their management. Most of these patients experience a rapid decline in health. A few patients have disease that proves relatively indolent, and survival can be measured in years rather than months.

There is considerable experience using brachytherapy alone or combined with external-beam radiation therapy for unresectable bile duct tumors. Median survival ranges from 10 to 24 months, and 5-year survival rates are approximately 10% with these approaches. Cholangitis, however, may occur more frequently in people treated with brachytherapy.

Photodynamic therapy (PDT) in cholangiocarcinoma is an interesting option that may provide a significant survival benefit in addition to treating biliary stenosis and cholestasis and improving quality of life. A randomized trial of stenting alone vs with PDT found a significantly longer median survival and improved quality of life in the PDT group. Although it is unlikely that all of the tumor was treated with PDT, this study did show the importance of local tumor control and its association with quality of life. As previously discussed, another palliative option is use of ^{90}yttrium microspheres.

Chemotherapy

Biliary tract malignancies are uncommon cancers, and the numbers of clinical trials and of patients in those trials are limited. Generally speaking, responses to chemotherapy are infrequent and brief. However, newer drugs and drug combinations are better tolerated and stand to improve on past results.

5-FU

This drug has historically been the most active single agent, with single-agent response rates in the 10% to 20% range.

Capecitabine

This prodrug of 5-FU (see chapter 13, on "Colon, Rectal, and Anal Cancers") produced responses in 4 of 8 gallbladder cancers but in only 1 of 18 cholangiocarcinomas in a phase II study presented by Hassan et al from the M. D. Anderson Cancer Center.

Gemcitabine

Multiple studies have documented gemcitabine as an active agent, particularly in gallbladder cancer. Cisplatin and gemcitabine may be a synergistic doublet, with reported response rates for gallbladder cancer in the range of 30% to 50%.

Combination chemotherapy

Combined 5-FU and gemcitabine have modest activity in biliary malignancies. A group in Toronto published results of combination therapy with capecitabine and gemcitabine. The mix of cholangiocarcinoma and gallbladder cancer in the 45 patients studied was nearly 50:50. The overall response rate was 31%, and the median survival was a promising 14 months. This regimen is a reasonable alternative to gemcitabine and cisplatin for biliary tract neoplasms.

Hepatic arterial chemotherapy

There is limited experience with hepatic arterial chemotherapy for biliary tract neoplasms, but there are case reports of responses to floxuridine in the literature.

Treatment recommendations

In the absence of a clinical trial, patients should be offered gemcitabine and/or 5-FU (or capecitabine), with or without leucovorin. Other agents, such as doxorubicin or cisplatin, may be added, but, as noted, there is no unequivocal evidence that combination chemotherapy produces any substantial benefits in improving quality of life or survival.

SUGGESTED READING

ON HEPATOCELLULAR CARCINOMA

Cheng BQ, Jia CQ, Liu CT, et al: Chemoembolization combined with radiofrequency ablation for patients with hepatocellular carcinoma larger than 3 cm: A randomized controlled trial. JAMA 299:1669–1677, 2008.

Ghoori S, Schiavo M, Russo A, et al: First-line treatment for hepatocellular carcinoma: resection or transplantation? Transplant Proc 39:2271–2273, 2007.

Gupta S, Bent S, Kohlwes J: Test characteristics of alpha-fetoprotein for detecting hepatocellular carcinoma in patients with hepatitis C: A systematic review and critical analysis. Ann Intern Med 139:46–50, 2003.

Llovet J, Bruix J: Systematic review of randomized trials for unresectable hepatocellular carcinoma: Chemoembolization improves survival. Hepatology 37:429–442, 2003.

Mok TS, Yeo W, Yu S, et al: An intensive surveillance program detected a high incidence of hepatocellular carcinoma among hepatitis B virus carriers with abnormal alpha-fetoprotein levels or abdominal ultrasonography results. J Clin Oncol 23:8041–8047, 2005.

Nakayama H, Sugahara S, Tokita M, et al: Proton beam therapy for hepatocellular carcinoma: The University of Tsukuba experience. Cancer 115:5499–5506, 2009.

Salem R, Lewandowski RJ, Mulcahy MF, et al: Radioembolization for hepatocellular carcinoma using yttrium-90 microspheres: A comprehensive report of long-term outcomes. Gastroenterology 138:52–64, 2010.

Tse RV, Hawkins M, Lockwood G, et al: Phase I study of individualized stereotactic body radiotherapy for hepatocellular carcinoma and intrahepatic cholangiocarcinoma. J Clin Oncol 26:657–664, 2008.

Varela M, Real MI, Burrel M, et al: Chemoembolization of hepatocellular carcinoma with drug eluting beads: Efficacy and doxorubicin pharmacokinetics. J Hepatol 46:474-481, 2007.

Yao FY, Bass NM, Ascher NL, et al: Liver transplantation for hepatocellular carcinoma: Lessons from the first year under the Model of End-Stage Liver Disease (MELD) organ allocation policy. Liver Transpl 10:621–630, 2004.

Yeo W, Mok TS, Zee B, et al: A randomized phase III study of doxorubicin versus cisplatin/interferon alpha-2b/doxorubicin/fluorouracil (PIAF) combination chemotherapy for unresectable heaptocellular carcinoma. J Natl Cancer Inst 97:1532–1538, 2005.

ON GALLBLADDER TUMORS

Gold DG, Miller RC, Haddock MG, et al: Adjuvant therapy for gallbladder carcinoma: The Mayo Clinic experience. Int J Radiat Oncol Biol Phys 75:150–155, 2009.

Patt YZ, Hassan MM, Aguayo A, et al: Oral capecitabine for the treatment of hepatocellular carcinoma, cholangiocarcinoma, and gallbladder carcinoma. Cancer 101:578–586, 2004.

Takada T, Amano H, Yasuda H, et al: Is postoperative adjuvant chemotherapy useful for gallbladder carcinoma? A phase III multicenter prospective randomized controlled trial in patients with resected pancreaticobiliary carcinoma. Cancer 95:1685–1695, 2002.

Wang SJ, Fuller CD, Kim JS, et al: Prediction model for estimating the survival benefit of adjuvant radiotherapy for gallbladder cancer. J Clin Oncol 26:2112–2117, 2008.

ON BILE DUCT TUMORS

Alberts SR, Al-Khatib H, Mahoney MR, et al: Gemcitabine, 5-fluorouracil, and leucovorin in advanced biliary tract and gallbladder carcinoma: A North Central Cancer Treatment Group phase II trial. Cancer 103:111–118, 2005.

Cheng Q, Luo X, Zhang B, et al: Predictive factors for prognosis of hilar cholangiocarcinoma: Postresection radiotherapy improves survival. Eur J Surg Oncol 33:202–207, 2007.

Knox JJ, Hedley D, Oza A, et al: Combining gemcitabine and capecitabine in patients with advanced biliary cancer: A phase II trial. J Clin Oncol 23:2332–2338, 2005.

Rea DJ, Heimbach JK, Rosen CB, et al: Liver transplantation with neoadjuvant chemoradiation is more effective than resection for hilar cholangiocarcinoma. Ann Surg 242:451–461, 2005.

Abbreviations in this chapter

AJCC = American Joint Committee on Cancer; NCCN = National Comprehensive Cancer Network; NCI = National Cancer Institute; SEER = Surveillance, Epidemiology, and End Results; SHARP = Sorafenib Hepatocellular Carcinoma Assessment Randomized Protocol

CHAPTER 13

Colon, rectal, and anal cancers

Steven R. Alberts, MD, Deborah Citrin, MD,
and Miguel Rodriguez-Bigas, MD

COLORECTAL CANCER

Despite the existence of excellent screening and preventive strategies, colorectal carcinoma (CRC) remains a major public health problem in Western countries. ACS estimated that in 2010, 142,570 people will be diagnosed with CRC, and 51,370 will die of the disease. CRC is the third most common type of cancer in both sexes (after prostate and lung cancers in men and lung and breast cancers in women) and the second most common cause of cancer death in the United States.

About 72% of new CRCs arise in the colon, and the remaining 28% arise in the rectum. Rectal cancer is defined as cancer arising below the peritoneal reflection, up to approximately 12 to 15 cm from the anal verge.

The lifetime risk of being diagnosed with CRC in the United States is estimated to be 5.9% for men and 5.5% for women.

EPIDEMIOLOGY

Gender Overall, the incidence of CRC and mortality rates are higher in men than in women; tumors of the colon are slightly more frequent in women than in men (1.2:1), whereas rectal carcinomas are more common in men than in women (1.7:1).

Age The vast majority, 90%, of all new CRC cases occur in individuals older than age 50. In the United States, the median age at presentation is 72 years.

Race The incidence and mortality rates of CRC are highest among African-American men and women compared with white men and women (15% higher and 40% higher, respectively). The incidence rates among Asian Americans, Hispanics/Latinos, and American Indians/Alaskan natives are lower than those among whites.

Geography The incidence of CRC is higher in industrialized regions (the United States, Canada, the Scandinavian countries, northern and western Europe, New Zealand, Australia) and lower in Asia, Africa (among blacks), and South America (except Argentina and Uruguay).

TABLE 1: Five-year relative survival rates in colorectal cancer by stage at diagnosis (1995–2005)

Stage at diagnosis	5-year survival rate (%)
All stages	64
In early, localized stage	90
After spread to adjacent organs or lymph nodes	67
After spread to distant sites	10
Unstaged	35

Horner MJ et al: SEER Cancer Statistics Review 1975–2006. National Cancer Institute, Bethesda, MD. www.seer.cancer.gov/csr/1975_2006. Accessed May 29, 2010.

Survival Five-year survival rates (Table 1) for patients with CRC have improved in recent years. This fact may be due to wider surgical resections, modern anesthetic techniques, and improved supportive care. In addition, better preoperative staging and abdominal exploration reveal clinically occult disease and allow treatment to be delivered more accurately. Survival also has improved through the use of adjuvant chemotherapy for colon cancer and adjuvant chemoradiation therapy for rectal cancer. Mortality from CRC is decreasing, likely from earlier diagnosis and screening as well as improvements in treatment modalities.

ETIOLOGY AND RISK FACTORS

The specific causes of CRC are unknown, but environmental, nutritional, genetic, and familial factors, as well as preexisting diseases, have been found to be associated with this cancer. A summary of selected risk factors for CRC is shown in Table 2.

Environment Asians, Africans, and South Americans who emigrate from low-risk areas assume the colon cancer risk for their adopted country, suggesting the importance of environmental factors in CRC. Smoking and alcohol intake (four or more drinks per week) increase the risk of CRC.

Diet Diets rich in fat and cholesterol have been linked to an increased risk of colorectal tumors. Dietary fat causes endogenous production of secondary bile acids and neutral steroids and increases bacterial degradation and excretion of these acids and steroids, thereby promoting colonic carcinogenesis. Historically, diets rich in cereal fiber or bran and yellow and green vegetables are said to have protective effects, although studies have failed to prove a risk reduction with increasing dietary fiber intake. A protective role also has been ascribed to calcium salts and calcium-rich foods, because they decrease colon-cell turnover and reduce the cancer-promoting effects of bile acid and fatty acids.

Physical activity Several studies have reported a lower risk of CRC in individuals who participate in regular physical activity. High levels of physical activity may decrease the risk by as much as 50%. Being overweight or obese has been consistently associated with a higher risk of CRC.

TABLE 2: Summary of selected risk factors for colorectal cancer

Factor		Relative risk
Heredity and medical history		
Family history		
1 first-degree relative		2.2
> 1 first-degree relative		4
Relative with diagnosis before age 45		3.9
Inflammatory bowel disease		
Crohn's disease	colon	2.6
Ulcerative colitis	colon	2.8
Ulcerative colitis	rectum	1.9
Others		
Obesity (per 5-unit increase in BMI)		
Men	colon	1.3
	rectum	1.1
Women	colon	1.1
Alcohol consumption		1.1
Red meat consumption		1.3
Diabetes		1.3
Processed meat consumption		1.2

Source: Colorectal Cancer Facts and Figures, 2008–2010. Atlanta, American Cancer Society, 2010.
BMI = body mass index

Inflammatory bowel disease Patients with inflammatory bowel disease (ulcerative colitis, Crohn's disease) have a higher incidence of CRC. The risk of CRC in patients with ulcerative colitis is associated with the duration of active disease, extent of colitis, development of mucosal dysplasia, and duration of symptoms.

The risk of CRC increases exponentially with the duration of colitis, from approximately 3% in the first decade to 20% in the second decade to > 30% in the third decade. CRC risk also is increased in patients with Crohn's disease, although to a lesser extent.

Adenomatous polyps Colorectal tumors develop more often in patients with adenomatous polyps than in those without polyps. There is approximately a 5% probability that carcinoma will be present in an adenoma; the risk correlates with the histology and size of the polyp. The potential for malignant transformation is higher for villous and tubulovillous adenomas than for tubular adenomas. Adenomatous polyps < 1 cm have a slightly greater than 1% chance of being malignant, in comparison with adenomas > 2 cm, which have up to a 40% likelihood of malignant transformation.

Cancer history Patients with a history of CRC are at increased risk of a second primary colon cancer or other malignancy. The risk of a second CRC is higher if the first diagnosis was made prior to age 60.

Prior surgery Following ureterosigmoidostomy, an increased incidence of colon cancer at or near the suture line has been reported. Cholecystectomy also has been associated with colon cancer in some studies but not in others.

Prior radiation to the prostate has been associated with a 1.7 relative risk of rectal cancer compared with nonirradiated tissues. In this study, the effect was limited to the irradiated tissues only, not to the rest of the bowel.

Family history and genetic factors Individuals with a first-degree relative with the disease have an increased risk of developing CRC. Those with two or more relatives with the disease make up about 20% of all people with CRC. The risk of developing CRC is significantly increased in several forms of inherited susceptibility (Table 3). About 5% to 10% of all patients with CRC have an inherited susceptibility to the disease. The risks of developing CRC in the subgroups of familial or hereditary CRC vary from 15% in relatives of patients with CRC diagnosed before 45 years of age, through 20% for family members with two first-degree relatives with CRC, to approximately 70% to 95% in patients with familial adenomatous polyposis and hereditary nonpolyposis CRC (HNPCC).

Familial adenomatous polyposis (FAP) is inherited as an autosomal-dominant trait with variable penetrance. Patients characteristically develop pancolonic and rectal adenomatous polyps. Approximately 50% of patients with FAP will develop adenomas by 15 years of age, and 95% by age 35. Left untreated, 100% of patients with FAP will develop CRC, with an average age at diagnosis ranging from 34 to 43 years. Prophylactic surgery, either total colectomy with ileorectal anastomosis or restorative proctocolectomy with an ileal anal pouch anastomosis, performed in the mid to late teens, is the prophylactic procedure of choice in this group of patients. The familial adenomatous polyposis coli *(APC)* gene has been localized to chromosome 5q21. Currently, it is possible to detect mutations in the *APC* gene in up to 82% of families with FAP. The use of nonsteroidal anti-inflammatory drugs (NSAIDs) such as sulindac (Clinoril, nonspecific COX-1 [cyclo-oxygenase-1] and COX-2 inhibitor) and celecoxib (Celebrex, COX-2 inhibitor) has been shown to decrease the size and number of adenomas in FAP patients. However, these agents should not be a substitute for surgery. A small study also revealed that sulindac does not prevent adenomas in mutation carriers who had not yet developed adenomas.

HNPCC is transmitted as an autosomal-dominant trait. It is associated with germline mutations in DNA mismatch repair genes (*MSH2*, *MLH1*, *PMS2*, and *MSH6)*. The incidence of a mutated mismatch repair (*MMR*) gene is approximately 1 in 1,000 people. In 1990 and 1991, the Amsterdam criteria were proposed and published, respectively. These criteria were proposed to identify high-risk families suspected of having Lynch syndrome to further study and delineate the syndrome. In 1999, they were revised (Amsterdam II) to recognize extracolonic manifestations as part of the family history. The criteria include the following factors:

- three or more relatives with a histologically verified HNPCC-associated cancer (colorectal, endometrial, small bowel, ureter, or renal pelvis), one of whom is a first-degree relative of the other two (FAP should be excluded)
- CRC involving at least two generations
- one or more CRCs diagnosed before the age of 50.

TABLE 3: Hereditary polyposis syndromes

Adenomatous polyposis	
Familial adenomatous polyposis (FAP)	Characterized by hundreds or thousands of sessile or pedunculated polyps throughout the large intestine; histologic examination reveals microscopic adenomas; average age at onset of polyps, 15 years; at onset of symptoms, 33 years; at diagnosis, 36 years; at diagnosis of colon cancer in the era of endoscopic surveillance; if untreated, 42 years; extracolonic features include mandibular osteomas, upper GI polyps, and congenital hypertrophy of the retinal pigment epithelium. An attenuated form of FAP exists that is clinically characterized by the presence of tens or hundreds of polyps (predominantly right-sided).
MYH-associated polyposis (MAP)	This syndrome is characterized by multiple adenomas but usually less than 100. It is caused by biallelic mutations in the base excision repair gene *MYH* (MUTYH). It has been reported that 7% to 17% of patients with FAP phenotype and no *APC* gene mutation detected will have biallelic mutations in *MYH*. The onset of adenomas is between 35 and 45 years of age, and CRC usually occurs in the mid 50s. There are fewer extracolonic manifestations with MAP than with FAP. Some studies have reported a slightly increased risk of CRC in patients with monoallelic mutations in *MYH*, whereas it is elevated in patients with biallelic mutations.
Hamartomatous polyposis	
Peutz-Jeghers syndrome	In infancy and childhood, melanin deposits manifest as greenish-black to brown mucocutaneous pigmentation (which may fade at puberty) around the nose, lips, buccal mucosa, hands, and feet; polyps (most frequent in the small intestines; also found in the stomach and colon) are unique hamartomas with branching bands of smooth muscle surrounded by glandular epithelium; may produce acute and chronic GI bleeding, intestinal obstruction, or intussusception; 50% of patients develop cancer (median age at diagnosis, 50 years); ovarian cysts and unique ovarian sex-cord tumors reported (5% to 12% of female patients).
Juvenile polyposis	Three forms: familial juvenile polyposis coli (polyps limited to the colon), familial juvenile polyposis of the stomach, and generalized juvenile polyposis (polyps distributed throughout the GI tract); polyps are hamartomas covered by normal glandular epithelium, found mostly in the rectum in children and sometimes in adults; may produce GI bleeding, obstruction, or intussusception; mixed juvenile/adenomatous polyps or synchronous adenomatous polyps may lead to cancer, but gastric cancer has not been reported in patients with familial juvenile polyposis of the stomach.
Cowden's disease (multiple hamartoma syndrome)	Multiple hamartomatous tumors of ectodermal, mesodermal, and endodermal origin; mucocutaneous lesions are prominent and distinctive; also reported: breast lesions ranging from fibrocystic disease to cancer (50% of patients), thyroid abnormalities (10% to 15%), cutaneous lipomas, ovarian cysts, uterine leiomyomas, skeletal and developmental anomalies, and GI polyps; no associated risk of cancer in GI polyps; probably does not warrant clinical surveillance.

The majority of CRC tumors from HNPCC patients have microsatellite instability (MSI-H). The Bethesda guidelines were developed to test tumors from high-risk individuals for MSI-H to identify individuals at risk of HNPCC. These criteria are much less restrictive than the Amsterdam criteria and serve to help identify patients at risk of HNPCC who might benefit from further evaluation. They have been modified and include the following:

- CRC diagnosed in a patient who is younger than 50 years of age
- The presence of synchronous, metachronous CRC or other HNPCC-associated tumors regardless of age
- CRC with MSI-H histology diagnosed in a patient who is younger than 60 years of age
- CRC diagnosed in one or more first-degree relatives with an HNPCC-related tumor, with one of the cancers being diagnosed younger than age 50 years
- CRC diagnosed in two or more first- or second-degree relatives with HNPCC-related tumors regardless of age.

With newer molecular techniques, mutations in the DNA MMR genes, namely *MLH-1*, *MSH-2*, *MSH-6*, and on rare occasions *PMS-2*, have been found in as many as 90% of individuals meeting the original Amsterdam criteria, whereas detection of mutations has been lower using the other criteria or guidelines. Because MSI occurs in more than 90% of cases of CRC with Lynch syndrome compared with sporadic cases (in which it occurs in about 15% of colorectal tumors), MSI testing has been used to screen tumors prior to genetic testing. Immunohistochemistry (IHC) for DNA (*MMR*) has also been advocated for screening tumors prior to genetic testing. Both of these methods will not detect all tumors, but they are complementary. In addition to having MSI-H, *MSH-6* colorectal tumors may be MSI-L (microsatellite instability low) or MSS (stable).

CHEMOPREVENTION

Chemoprevention aims to block the action of carcinogens on cells before the development of cancer.

Controlled trials of vitamins C and E and calcium have produced mixed results. Clinical trials have shown that calcium supplementation modestly decreases the risk of colorectal adenomas.

NSAIDs inhibit colorectal carcinogenesis, possibly by reducing endogenous prostaglandin production through COX inhibition. Sulindac has induced regression of large bowel polyps in patients with FAP. Controlled studies have shown a reduction in the incidence of colorectal polyps with regular, long-term use of aspirin. HMG-CoA (hydroxymethyl glutaryl coenzyme A) reductase inhibitors may reduce the risk of CRC after extended treatment.

Women who use postmenopausal hormones appear to have a lower rate of CRC than do those who do not. Postmenopausal hormones may increase the risk of other types of cancer, however.

SIGNS AND SYMPTOMS

During the early stages of CRC, patients may be asymptomatic or complain of vague abdominal pain and flatulence, which may be attributed to gallbladder or peptic ulcer disease. Minor changes in bowel movements, with or without rectal bleeding, are also seen; they are frequently ignored and/or attributed to hemorrhoids or other benign disorders.

Cancers occurring in the left side of the colon generally cause constipation alternating with diarrhea; abdominal pain; and obstructive symptoms, such as nausea and vomiting.

Right-sided colon lesions produce vague, abdominal aching, unlike the colicky pain seen with obstructive left-sided lesions. Anemia resulting from chronic blood loss, weakness, weight loss, and/or an abdominal mass may also accompany carcinoma of the right side of the colon.

Patients with cancer of the rectum may present with a change in bowel movements; rectal fullness, urgency, or bleeding; and tenesmus.

SCREENING AND DIAGNOSIS

Fecal occult blood testing (FOBT) consists of guiac-based testing (gFOBT), which can be performed in the doctor's office, or a fecal immunohistochemical test (FIT), which is usually processed in clinical laboratories. The difference between these tests is based on the detected analyte. Blood in the stool detected by gFOBT depends on the reaction of a pseudoperoxidase with heme or hemoglobin, whereas FIT depends on the reaction with globin. These tests should collect two samples from three consecutive bowel movements. The majority of the adenomas and CRCs go undetected because they usually are not bleeding at the time of the test. Newer gFOBT and FIT appear to have a better sensitivity than older tests without sacrificing specificity.

Three large prospective randomized controlled clinical trials have demonstrated a 15% to 33% decrease in CRC mortality over an 8- to 13-year period of follow-up in those individuals randomized to undergo FOBT. A positive FOBT result should be followed by colonosocopy.

Stool DNA (sDNA) testing takes advantage of molecular changes or mutations that occur in the carcinogenesis of CRC. DNA shed in the stool is analyzed for molecular changes. Multiple targets, including mutations in *KRAS, p53, APC,* and *BAT 26* (which can be a surrogate marker for MSI), are analyzed. There are no data on the performance of sDNA for screening; however, the test has been shown to be able to detect both significant adenomas and CRCs.

Digital rectal examination should be an integral part of the physical examination. It can detect lesions up to 7 cm from the anal verge.

Sigmoidoscopy Flexible proctosigmoidoscopy is safe and more comfortable than examination using a rigid proctoscope. Almost 50% of all colorectal neoplasms are within the reach of a 60-cm sigmoidoscope. Even though flexible sigmoidoscopy visualizes only the distal portion of the colorectum, the identification of adenomas can lead to colonoscopy. When we add the percentage of colorectal neoplasms in the distal 60 cm of the colorectum to the percentage of patients with distal polyps leading to complete colonoscopy, 80% of those individuals with a significant neoplasm anywhere in the colorectum can be identified. Four prospective randomized controlled trials evaluating flexible sigmoidoscopy for screening have been conducted in the United States and Europe, but results are not yet available.

Colonoscopy (optical) provides information on the mucosa of the entire colon, and its sensitivity in detecting tumors is extremely high. Most physicians consider colonoscopy to be the best screening modality for CRC. Colonoscopy can be used to obtain biopsy specimens of adenomas and carcinomas and permits the excision of adenomatous polyps. For this reason, colonoscopy is the only screening modality ever shown to reduce the incidence of cancer in screened individuals. Colonoscopy is the best follow-up strategy for evaluating patients with a positive gFOBT and the best screening modality for high-risk patients.

Limitations of colonoscopy include its inability to detect some polyps and small lesions because of blind corners and mucosal folds and the fact that sometimes the cecum cannot be reached. A supplementary double-contrast barium enema may be needed if a colonoscopic exam fails to reach the cecum.

Colonoscopy (CT virtual) utilizes CT images that are reconstructed to visualize the colon. It requires a bowel preparation and adequate distention of the colon for success. There is no prospective randomized study demonstrating that colonoscopic CT reduces CRC mortality. However, a trial comparing optical colonoscopy with colonoscopic CT resulted in similar detection rates for advanced neoplasia.

Barium enemas can accurately detect CRC; however, the false-negative rate associated with double-contrast barium enemas ranges from 2% to 61% because of misinterpretation, poor preparation, and difficulties in detecting smaller lesions. A supplementary colonoscopy may be needed if a double-contrast barium enema does not adequately visualize the entire colon or to obtain histopathology or perform polypectomy in the event of abnormal findings. There is no role for single-contrast barium enema. If this modality is to be used, a well-conducted double-contrast barium enema needs to be performed.

Recommendations for average-risk individuals Adults at average risk should begin CRC screening at age 50. The ACS guidelines on screening and surveillance for the early detection of colorectal adenomatous polyps and cancer provide several options for screening average-risk individuals (Table 4).

The recommendations for screening and surveillance for high-risk individuals are illustrated in Table 5.

Treatment of endoscopically removed polyps Adenomatous colon polyps should be completely removed endoscopically to prevent progression to malignancy. Colon polyps with severe dysplasia or carcinoma in situ can also be managed with colonoscopic polypectomy as long as the entire polyp is removed. A malignant polyp is defined as one with cancer invading through the muscularis mucosa and into the submucosa (pT1).

Management of malignant polyps removed by colonoscopy is somewhat controversial. In general, malignant polyps can be removed colonoscopically as long as they can be removed with a confirmed negative margin and do not invade the submucosa

TABLE 4: American Cancer Society guidelines on screening and surveillance for the early detection of colorectal adenomas and cancer—Average risk

Test	Interval	Comment
gFOBT or FIT	Annual	Positive test should be followed by colonoscopy.
sDNA	Uncertain	Positive test should be followed by colonoscopy. If test is negative, testing interval is uncertain.
Flexible sigmoidoscopy (insertion to 40 cm or to the splenic flexure)	Every 5 years	Positive test should be followed by colonoscopy.
Colonoscopy	Every 10 years	Provides opportunity to visualize, sample, and/or remove significant lesions.
CTC	Every 5 years	If lesions > 6 mm, should be followed by colonoscopy. It may detect extracolonic abnormalities.
DCBE	Every 5 years	If lesions > 6 mm, should be followed by colonoscopy.

gFOBT = guaiac fecal occult blood test; FIT = fecal immunohistochemical test; sDNA = stool DNA testing; CTC = CT colonography; DCBE = double-contrast barium enema
Adapted from Levin B, Lieberman DA, McFarland B, et al: CA Cancer J Clin 58:130–160, 2008.

beneath the polyp stalk, do not have lymphovascular invasion, or are poorly differentiated. These characteristics increase the risk of nodal metastases.

Studies from Japan and the United States have correlated the incidence of lymph node metastases with the level of submucosal involvement. Individuals with cancer in polyps invading the upper third of the submucosa have a low risk of nodal metastases, whereas those invading the lower third have up to a 25% incidence of nodal metastases. Sessile polyps with submucosal invasion should probably be removed by colon resection. Each situation should be individualized according to the histology, prognostic factors, extent of submucosal invasion, and completeness of excision. The comorbidities and general health of the patient are also factors to consider.

Initial workup An initial diagnostic workup for patients suspected of having colorectal tumors should include a complete history and physical examination including a three-generation family history. It should also include:

- digital rectal examination and FOBT
- colonoscopy
- biopsy of any detected lesions.

Adequate staging prior to surgical intervention requires:

- chest x-ray
- CT scan of the abdomen and pelvis

TABLE 5: Joint guideline from the American Cancer Society, the US Multi-Society Task Force on CRC, and the American College of Radiology for screening and surveillance in high-risk individuals

Risk category	Age to begin	Practice[a] and comments
Increased risk based on history of polyps at prior colonoscopy		
Individuals with small rectal hyperplastic polyps		Same as average risk. Exception: individuals with hyperplastic polyposis syndrome who are at increased risk need more frequent intervals.
Individuals with 1 or 2 small adenomas and low-grade dysplasia	5 to 10 years after initial colonoscopy	Interval depends on clinical factors such as prior colonoscopic findings, family history, patient comfort, and physician judgment.
Individuals with 3 to 10 adenomas or 1 adenoma > 1 cm or any adenoma with villous features or high-grade dysplasia	3 years after initial polypectomy	Polypectomy must have been complete. If subsequent exam is normal or 1 to 2 TAs with LGD interval for subsequent exam, 5 years.
Individuals with > 10 adenomas in a single examination	< 3 years after initial polypectomy	Consider familial syndrome. May need genetic counseling.
Individuals with sessile adenomas excised in a piecemeal fashion	2 to 6 months to verify completeness	Completeness of removal based on pathologic and excision endoscopic assessment. Interval follow-up exam based on endoscopist's judgment.
Increased risk based on personal history of CRC		
Individuals with CRC	Should undergo preoperative colonoscopy. If not feasible, 3 to 6 months postoperatively if no unresectable metastases noted. Intraoperative colonoscopy an alternative.	Preferred in patients with non-obstructing tumors. CTC or DCBE can be utilized to evaluate the colon preoperatively in obstructing tumors.
Individuals 1 year after resection	1 year after surgery or 1 year following colonoscopy performed to clear the colon of synchronous disease	This is in addition to preoperative or perioperative colonoscopy. If 1 year, exam is normal, then at 3 years. If latter is normal, then every 5 years. Exam intervals can be shortened depending on findings. More frequent exams of the rectum to detect local recurrence may be considered.

continued

Increased risk based on family history		
CRC or adenomas in a first-degree family member at age < 60 years. or in > two first-degree family members at any age	Colonoscopy every 5 years, start at age 40 years or 10 years before the youngest relative diagnosed	
CRC or adenomas in a first-degree family member at age > 60 years or in two second-degree relatives diagnosed at any age	Surveillance at age 40 years	Intervals as for average risk. Individuals may choose any recommended form of screening and surveillance.
High risk		
Genetic diagnosis of FAP or suspected FAP without genetic testing confirmation	FSIG annually, colonoscopy if AAPC	Consider genetic counseling and testing if not already performed
Genetic or clinical diagnosis of HNPCC or Lynch syndrome or individuals at risk of HNPCC (first-degree relatives of affected)	Colonoscopy every 1 to 2 years. Begin at age 20 to 25 years or 10 years before earliest case in the immediate family.	Consider genetic counseling and testing if not already performed
IBD, ulcerative colitis, and Crohn's colitis	Colonoscopy and biopsies 8 years post diagnosis of pancolitis or 12 to 15 years after the onset of left-sided disease	Interval every 1 to 2 years, with biopsies evaluating for dysplasia

[a] Colonoscopy recommended for subsequent exams except for individuals with small rectal hyperplastic polyps, or individuals with a family history of CRC, or adenomatous polyps in a first-degree relative age > 60 or two second-degree relatives with CRC, where colonoscopy or any other screening option for average-risk individuals can be utilized. AAPC = attenuated adenomatous polyposis coli; CTC = CT colonography; DCBE = double-contrast barium enema; FAP = familial adenomatous polyposis; FSIG = flexible sigmoidoscopy; HNPCC = hereditary nonpolyposis CRC; IBD = inflammatory bowel disease; LGD = low-grade dysplasia; TA= tubular adenoma

Adapted from Levin B, Lieberman DA, McFarland B, et al: CA Cancer J Clin 58:130–160, 2008.

- endorectal ultrasonography or MRI to evaluate and appropriately stage a rectal cancer for potential neoadjuvant therapy
- CBC with platelet count
- liver and renal function tests
- urinalysis
- measurement of carcinoembryonic antigen (CEA) level. If CEA levels are elevated preoperatively, postoperative CEA levels should be monitored every 3 months for 3 years in patients with stage II or III CRC and every 6 to 12 months thereafter
- endoscopic ultrasonography (EUS) or MRI of the pelvis for rectal cancers.

In monitoring response to therapy for metastatic cancer, CEA levels should be measured every 1 to 8 months during active treatment.

TABLE 6: AJCC Staging for Cancer of the Colon and Rectum

TX	Primary tumor cannot be assessed
T0	No evidence of primary tumor
Tis	Carcinoma in situ: intraepithelial or invasion of lamina propria[a]
T1	Tumor invades submucosa
T2	Tumor invades muscularis propria
T3	Tumor invades through the muscularis propria into pericolorectal tissues
T4a	Tumor penetrates to the surface of the visceral peritoneum[b]
T4b	Tumor directly invades or is adherent to other organs or structures[b,c]

[a]*Note:* Tis includes cancer cells confined within the glandular basement membrane (intraepithelial) or mucosal lamina propria (intramucosal) with no extension through the muscularis mucosae into the submucosa.

[b]Tumor that is adherent to other organs or structures, grossly, is classified cT4b. However, if no tumor is present in the adhesion, microscopically, the classification should be pT1–4a depending on the anatomic depth of wall invasion. The V and L classifications should be used to identify the presence or absence of vascular or lymphatic invasion, whereas the PN site-specific factor should be used for perineural invasion.

[c]*Note:* Direct invasion in T4 includes invasion of other organs or other segments of the colorectum as a result of direct extension through the serosa, as confirmed on microscopic examination (for example, invasion of the sigmoid colon by a carcinoma of the cecum) or, for cancers in a retroperitoneal or subperitoneal location, direct invasion of other organs or structures by virtue of extension beyond the muscularis propia (ie, respectively, a tumor on the posterior wall of the descending colon invading the left kidney or lateral abdominal wall; or a mid or distal rectal cancer with invasion of prostate, seminal vesicles, cervix, or vagina).

NX	Regional lymph nodes cannot be assessed
N0	No regional lymph node metastasis
N1a	Metastasis in one regional lymph node
N1b	Metastasis in two to three regional lymph nodes
N1c	Tumor deposit(s) in the subserosa, mesentery, or nonperitonealized pericolic or perirectal tissues without regional nodal metastasis
N2a	Metastasis in four to six regional lymph nodes
N2b	Metastasis in seven or more regional lymph nodes

Note: A satellite peritumoral nodule in the pericolorectal adipose tissue of a primary carcinoma without histologic evidence of residual lymph node in the nodule may represent discontinuous spread, venous invasion with extravascular spread (V1/2), or a totally replaced lymph node (N1/2). Replaced nodes should be counted separately as positive nodes in the N category, whereas discontinuous spread or venous invasion should be classified and counted in the Site-Specific Factor Category Tumor Deposits (TD).

M0	No distant metastasis (no pathologic M0; use clinical M to complete stage group)
M1a	Metastasis confined to one organ or site (eg, liver, lung, ovary, nonregional node)
M1b	Metastases in more than one organ/site or the peritoneum

continued

TABLE 6: AJCC Staging for Cancer of the Colon and Rectum *continued*

Clinical staging			
0	Tis	N0	M0
I	T1	N0	M0
	T2	N0	M0
IIA	T3	N0	M0
IIB	T4a	N0	M0
IIC	T4b	N0	M0
IIIA	T1–T2	N1/N1c	M0
	T1	N2a	M0
IIIB	T3–T4a	N1/N1c	M0
	T2–T3	N2a	M0
	T1–T2	N2b	M0
IIIC	T4a	N2a	M0
	T3–T4a	N2b	M0
	T4b	N1–N2	M0
IVA	Any T	Any N	M1a
IVB	Any T	Any N	M1b
Pathologic staging			
0	Tis	N0	M0
I	T1	N0	M0
	T2	N0	M0
IIA	T3	N0	M0
IIB	T4a	N0	M0
IIC	T4b	N0	M0
IIIA	T1–T2	N1/N1c	M0
	T1	N2a	M0
IIIB	T3–T4a	N1/N1c	M0
	T2–T3	N2a	M0
	T1–T2	N2b	M0
IIIC	T4a	N2a	M0
	T3–T4a	N2b	M0
	T4b	N1–N2	M0
IVA	Any T	Any N	M1a
IVB	Any T	Any N	M1b

From: Edge SB, Byrd DR, Compton CC, et al (eds): AJCC Cancer Staging Manual, 7th ed. Springer, New York, 2010.

FDG-PET scanning FDG (^{18}F-fluorodeoxyglucose)-PET scanning has emerged as a highly sensitive study for the evaluation of patients who have metastatic disease. Although not usually recommended in the evaluation of early-stage primary disease, this modality can aid in the staging of recurrence.

PATHOLOGY

Adenocarcinomas constitute 90% to 95% of all large bowel neoplasms. These tumors consist of cuboidal or columnar epithelium with multiple degrees of differentiation and variable amounts of mucin.

Mucinous adenocarcinoma is a histologic variant characterized by huge amounts of extracellular mucus in the tumor and the tendency to spread within the peritoneum. Approximately 10% of colorectal adenocarcinomas are mucinous. It is more commonly seen in younger patients.

Signet-ring–cell carcinoma is an uncommon variant, comprising 1% of colorectal adenocarcinomas. These tumors contain large quantities of intracellular mucinous elements (causing the cytoplasm to displace the nucleus) and tend to involve the submucosa, making their detection difficult with conventional imaging techniques.

Other tumor types Squamous cell carcinomas, small-cell carcinomas, carcinoid tumors, and adenosquamous and undifferentiated carcinomas also have been found in the colon and rectum. Nonepithelial tumors, such as sarcomas and lymphomas, are exceedingly rare.

Metastatic spread CRC has a tendency toward local invasion by circumferential growth and for lymphatic, hematogeneous, transperitoneal, and perineural spread. Longitudinal spread is usually not extensive, with microscopic spread averaging only 1 to 2 cm from gross disease, but radial spread is common and depends on anatomic location.

The most common site of extralymphatic involvement is the liver, with the lungs the most frequently affected extra-abdominal organ. Other sites of hematogeneous spread include the bones, kidneys, adrenal glands, and brain, although metastases can spread to any organ.

STAGING AND PROGNOSIS

The TNM staging classification, which is based on the depth of tumor invasion in the intestinal wall, the number of regional lymph nodes involved, and the presence or absence of distant metastases, has largely replaced the older Dukes' classification scheme (Table 6).

Pathologic stage is the single most important prognostic factor following surgical resection of colorectal tumors. The prognosis for early stages (I and II) is favorable overall, in contrast to the prognosis for advanced stages (III and IV). However, there appears to be superior survival for patients with stage III disease whose disease is confined to the bowel wall (ie, ≤ T2, N+).

Histologic grade may be correlated with survival. Five-year survival rates of 56% to 100%, 33% to 80%, and 11% to 58% have been reported for grades 1, 2, and 3 colorectal tumors, respectively.

Other prognostic factors (such as age at diagnosis, presurgical CEA level, gender, presence and duration of symptoms, site of disease, histologic features, obstruction or perforation, perineural invasion, venous or lymphatic invasion, ploidy status, and S-phase fraction) have not consistently been correlated with overall disease recurrence and survival. Furthermore, the size of the primary lesion has had no influence on survival. Elevated expression of thymidylate synthase (TS) and allelic loss of chromosome 18 have been correlated with a poor prognosis. MSI status has been correlated as an independent prognostic factor for survival, favoring patients with unstable tumors (MSI-H).

TREATMENT

PRIMARY TREATMENT OF LOCALIZED DISEASE

Management of CRC relies primarily on resection of the bowel with the adjacent draining lymph nodes. The need for neoadjuvant or adjuvant chemotherapy, with or without concurrent irradiation, depends on tumor location (colon vs rectum) and stage of disease. In surgery for both colon and rectal cancers, if the tumor is attached to other organs, an en bloc resection of the primary tumor and adjacent organ(s) is indicated. If the adhesions are violated, there is an increase in local recurrence and a decrease in survival; thus, the potential cure for that patient will be compromised. Occasionally, neoadjuvant chemoradiation therapy will be indicated in colon tumors prior to surgical resection. In rectal cancer, preoperative (preferred) or postoperative chemoradiation is indicated for stages II and III disease.

Surgery

Colon The primary therapy for adenocarcinoma of the colon is surgical extirpation of the bowel segment containing the tumor, the adjacent mesentery, and draining lymph nodes. Based on studies that correlated the number of lymph nodes removed and survival, it is recommended that at least 12 lymph nodes be available for examination by a pathologist to confirm. Surgical resection can be performed by open or laparoscopic approach.

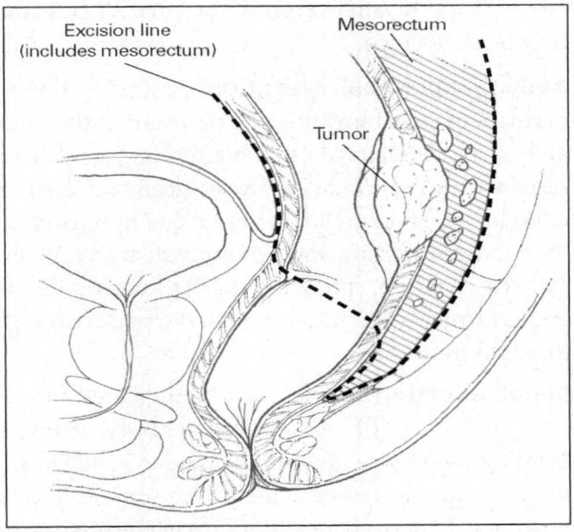

FIGURE 1: Mesorectal excision.

Adapted with permission from N Engl J Med 345:690–692, 2001.

The type of resection depends on the anatomic location of the tumor. Right, left, or transverse colectomy is the surgical treatment of choice in patients with right, left, or transverse colonic tumors, respectively. Tumors in the sigmoid colon may be treated with wide sigmoid resection. The length of colon resected depends largely on the requirement for wide mesenteric nodal clearance.

Rectum For rectal carcinoma, the distal surgical margin should be at least 2 cm, although some investigators have suggested that a smaller but still negative margin may be adequate. The resection should include the node-bearing mesorectum surrounding the rectum. This procedure, which is termed total mesorectal excision (TME), is accomplished using a sharp dissection technique (see Figure 1). Posteriorly, the mesorectal dissection is carried out along the presacral fascia. Anteriorly, the dissection follows the posterior vaginal wall in females or Denonvilliers' fascia in males, either of which may be resected in the presence of an anterior wall rectal cancer. The use of TME has been associated with a significant reduction in local recurrence rates for patients with rectal cancer.

Reported rates of local recurrence following TME for rectal cancer have generally been < 10%, compared with rates of recurrence up to 30% prior to the advent of TME. Selective use of radiation therapy can improve upon the results of TME alone.

Circumferential resection margin is an important predictor of local failure in patients with rectal cancer. A population-based review of 3,196 patients with rectal cancer found that local recurrence at 5 years was 23.7% with margins of 0–2 mm vs 8.9% with margins greater than 2 mm. Distant metastases and survival were also poorer for the group with smaller margins. Because only 10% of patients in this study received neoadjuvant therapy and patients who received postoperative radiation therapy were excluded, it is not clear whether these data can be extrapolated to patients treated with radiation therapy.

Sphincter-sparing approaches Technologies (eg, circular stapling devices) and the application of surgical techniques, such as coloanal anastomosis and creation of intestinal pouches, are employed to maintain anal sphincter function for tumors in the lower one-third of the rectum. If the tumor is located proximally between 6 and 15 cm from the anal verge, a low anterior resection with end-to-end anastomosis may be performed.

Abdominoperineal resection, removing the anus and sphincter muscle with permanent colostomy, may be necessary if the tumor is located in the distal rectum and other characteristics of the tumor (eg, bulky size, proximity to the sphincter musculature) preclude an oncologically adequate sphincter-sparing approach. An alternative procedure for distant rectal tumors is to resect the entire rectum, sparing the anoderm and anal sphincter musculature, and to perform a coloanal anastomosis. Either procedure, sphincter-sparing resection or abdominoperineal resection, can be performed with autonomic nerve preservation, minimizing bladder and sexual function morbidity.

Local excision alone may be indicated for selected patients who have small (< 3 to 4 cm), T1, well to moderately differentiated rectal cancers without histologic evidence of lymphovascular involvement, provided that a full-thickness negative margin can be achieved. In some series, transanal excision for these good histology T1 lesions results in excellent long-term control. However, some large studies with long-term follow-up demonstrated significant local recurrence rates, even with T1 lesions. For T2 or T3 tumors, the standard therapy remains a transabdominal resection because of the risk of mesorectal nodal spread. Preoperative transrectal ultrasonography is useful in defining lesions that can be resected by local excision alone. A trial sponsored by the CALGB demonstrated reasonable results for patients with T2 rectal cancer undergoing negative margin local excision followed by fluorouracil (5-FU) and external-beam radiation therapy (EBRT). The locoregional recurrence rate at 6 years was only 14%. A similar study conducted by ACOSOG but with neoadjuvant chemoradiation followed by local excision has been completed, but results are not yet available.

Laparoscopic colonic resection Multiple large randomized trials have established laparoscopic colonic resection as an oncologically acceptable method of treating cancer of the colon. Resection of rectal cancer using laparoscopic approaches has also been and is being evaluated in a number of randomized trials. Laparoscopy for rectal resection still requires confirmation as an oncologically equivalent procedure to open surgery. The potential advantages include a shorter hospital stay, reduced postoperative ileus, decreased time away from work, fewer adhesive complications, and a lower risk of hernia formation. The potential disadvantages compared with open transabdominal resection include longer operative time, higher operative costs, and technical considerations related to operative skill. Large randomized trials with long-term follow-up are still needed. Robotic surgery is also being evaluated in rectal cancer.

Patterns of failure

The natural history and patterns of failure following "curative" resection are different for colon and rectal carcinomas. Locoregional failure as the only or major site of recurrence is common in rectal cancer, whereas colon cancer tends to recur in the peritoneum, liver, and other distant sites, with a lower rate of local failure. As a result, local therapy, such as irradiation, may play a significant role in the treatment of rectal tumors but is not used routinely for colon cancers.

ADJUVANT THERAPY FOR COLON CANCER

Approximately 75% of all patients with CRC will present at a stage when all gross carcinoma can be surgically resected. Nevertheless, despite the high resectability rate, almost half of all patients with colorectal adenocarcinoma die of metastatic disease, primarily because of residual disease that is not apparent at the time of surgery. These individuals are candidates for adjuvant local or systemic therapies.

Systemic chemotherapy

Systemic combined chemotherapy is the principal adjuvant therapy for colon cancer (Table 7). The current standard for resected stage III colon cancer is a combination of 5-FU, leucovorin, and

> A phase III randomized trial of neoadjuvant radiation for T3–4, M0 rectal cancer compared outcomes when either capecitabine (Xeloda) or capecitabine and oxaliplatin (Eloxatin) was added to radiation therapy. With 598 patients randomized, this trial showed no significant benefit to the addition of oxaliplatin. The investigators concluded that oxaliplatin does not add meaningful benefit when added to capecitabine and radiation therapy *(Gérard JP et al: J Clin Oncol 28:1638–1644, 2010).*

TABLE 7: Adjuvant chemotherapy regimens for colorectal adenocarcinoma (nonmetastatic)

Drug/combination	Dose and schedule
Oxaliplatin/fluorouracil/leucovorin (FOLFOX4)	
Oxaliplatin	85 mg/m^2 IV piggyback over 2 hours on day 1 only
Leucovorin	200 mg/m^2/d over 2 hours on day 1 given simultaneously with oxaliplatin
Fluorouracil	400 mg/m^2 IV bolus over 2 to 4 minutes on days 1 and 2
Fluorouracil	600 mg/m^2 continuous infusion over 22 hours on days 1 and 2 every 14 days for 12 cycles
Andre T, Boni C, Mounedji-Boudiaf L, et al: N Engl J Med 350:2343–2351, 2004.	
FLOX	
Fluorouracil	500 mg/m^2 IV bolus weekly for 6 weeks
Leucovorin	500 mg/m^2 IV weekly for 6 weeks each 8-week cycle x 3
Oxaliplatin	85 mg/m^2 IV administered on weeks 1, 3, and 5 of each 8-week cycle x 3
Kuebler JP, Weiand HS, O'Connell MJ, et al: J Clin Oncol 25:2198–2204, 2007.	
Capecitabine	
Capecitabine	1,250 mg/m^2 twice daily on days 1–14 every 3 weeks for 24 weeks

Twelves C, Wong A, Nowacki MP, et al: N Engl J Med 352:2696–2704, 2005.

oxaliplatin (FOLFOX, FLOX). For patients in whom the use of oxaliplatin is thought to be contraindicated (eg, in the presence of a peripheral neuropathy), alternatives for adjuvant therapy include capecitabine (Xeloda) or 5-FU and leucovorin. The development of 5-FU–containing regimens is described in the section on treatment of advanced and metastatic CRC.

The use of chemotherapy for resected stage II colon cancer is of uncertain survival benefit. When determining the benefit of adjuvant therapy for this group of patients, several factors should be taken into consideration, including the number of lymph nodes analyzed after surgery, the prognostic features (T4 lesion, perforation, peritumoral lymphovascular invasion, poorly differentiated histology, MSI), anticipated life expectancy, and comorbid conditions.

FOLFOX, FLOX Oxaliplatin has been approved by the FDA for adjuvant therapy for resected stage III CRC. In a phase III trial for resected stages II and III colon cancer from Europe (MOSAIC), the use of FOLFOX4 compared with the same infusional regimen without oxaliplatin led to a higher 3-year disease-free survival rate (78% vs 73%) in those receiving FOLFOX. More recently, FOLFOX6 or a modified version of it (Table 8) has been used in clinical trials as well as in clinical practice. In a subgroup analysis, a significant disease-free survival benefit was seen for patients with stage III colon cancer and for patients with high-risk stage II colon cancer. A significant overall survival advantage was also seen for patients with stage III disease.

In a separate randomized phase III trial, conducted by the NSABP, for patients with resected stage II or III colon cancer, FLOX was compared with a weekly bolus of 5-FU and leucovorin. The 3-year disease-free survival benefit from FLOX was similar to that seen with FOLFOX4. Stages II and III disease were not evaluated separately.

Capecitabine is an oral fluorinated pyrimidine approved by the FDA for adjuvant therapy for patients with stage III colon cancer who have undergone complete resection of the primary tumor when treatment with fluoropyrimidine therapy alone is preferred. Capecitabine was not inferior to bolus 5-FU and low-dose leucovorin for disease-free survival, with a hazard ratio in the capecitabine group of 0.87 (95% CI = 0.75–1.00). Capecitabine is an alternative for patients who are unlikely to tolerate 5-FU, leucovorin, and oxaliplatin.

5-FU plus leucovorin Studies have demonstrated the benefits of 5-FU plus leucovorin in the adjuvant treatment of colon carcinomas. Acceptable adjuvant regimens of 5-FU plus leucovorin for colon cancer include both low-dose leucovorin and high-dose leucovorin regimens (Table 7).

> **Two recent phase III trials of adjuvant therapy for resected colon cancer assessed the potential added benefit of targeted therapy to mFOLFOX6. NSABP C-08 randomized patients with resected stage II or III colon cancer to 12 cycles of mFOLFOX6 alone or with bevacizumab. Bevacizumab was given for 6 months beyond mFOLFOX6. NCCTG N0147 randomized patients with resected stage III colon cancer to 12 cycles of mFOLFOX6 alone or with cetuximab. The final design of this trial only randomized patients with wild-type *KRAS* to one of the two treatment arms. Both trials failed to show benefit to the addition of a targeted therapy to mFOLFOX6 *(Wolmark N et al: J Clin Oncol 27:18s, abstract LBA4, 2009; Alberts SR et al: J Clin Oncol 28:18s, abstract CRA3507, 2010).***

Irinotecan Two phase III trials of FOLFIRI (5-FU, irinotecan, leucovorin) compared the same infusional regimen without irinotecan in either patients with resected stages II and III colon cancer (PETACC3) or high-risk stage III disease (ACCORD-2). They did not show a benefit to the use of irinotecan in the adjuvant setting. Given the results of these two studies, the use of irinotecan currently is not considered a primary option for patients with resected stage II or III colon cancer.

Radiation therapy

Postoperative irradiation to the tumor bed can be considered in patients with T4 (B3 or C3) tumors located in retroperitoneal portions of the colon, because more than 30% of these patients develop local recurrence. Retrospective studies suggest improved local tumor control with irradiation, particularly in patients with positive resection margins. If available, intraoperative radiotherapy may be considered for patients with T4 or recurrent cancers as an additional boost.

ADJUVANT THERAPY FOR RECTAL CANCER

Local recurrence alone or in combination with distant metastases occurs in up to 50% of patients with rectal carcinoma. Nodal metastases and deep bowel wall penetration are significant risk factors for locoregional failure.

TABLE 8: Chemotherapy for advanced disease

Drug/combination	Dose and schedule
Oxaliplatin/fluorouracil/leucovorin (FOLFOX6)	
Leucovorin	400 mg/m^2 IV infused over 2 hours on day 1
Oxaliplatin	100 mg/m^2 IV infused over 2 hours on day 1*
Fluorouracil	400 mg/m^2 IV bolus on day 1 then 1,200 mg/m^2/day for 2 days (total 2,400 mg/m^2 over 46–48 hours) continuous infusion
Repeat cycle every 2 weeks.	
* Modified FOLFOX6 uses 85 mg/m^2	
Maindrault-Goebel F, Louvet C, Andre T, et al: Eur J Cancer 35:1338–1342, 1999.	
Capecitabine/oxaliplatin (CAPOX)	
Oxaliplatin	130 mg/m^2 IV infused on day 1 only followed by
Capecitabine	1,000 mg/m^2 orally twice daily in the evening on day 1 to the morning of day 15
Repeat cycle every 3 weeks.	
Cassidy J, Tabernero J, Twelves C, et al: J Clin Oncol 22:2084–2091, 2004.	
Fluorouracil as an irradiation enhancer—bolus	
Leucovorin	20 mg/m^2 IV bolus on days 1–5, 29–33 immediately before fluorouracil
Fluorouracil	325 mg/m^2/day IV bolus on days 1–5, 29–33
Hyams DM, Mamounas EP, Petrelli N, et al: Dis Colon Rectum 40:131–139, 1997.	
Fluorouracil as an irradiation enhancer—continuous infusion	
Fluorouracil	225 mg/m^2/day IV continuous infusion during irradiation
O'Connell MJ, Martenson JA, Wieand HS, et al: N Engl J Med 331:502–507, 1994.	
Capecitabine as an irradiation enhancer	
Capecitabine	825 mg/m^2 twice daily during irradiation
Dupuis O, Vie B, Lledo G, et al: Oncology 73:169–176, 2007.	

continued

In the absence of nodal metastases, the rate of local recurrence may be as low as 5% to 10% for stage I rectal cancer and 15% to 30% for stage II tumors. In stage III disease, the incidence of pelvic failure increases to 50% or more. The use of TME significantly reduces this risk of local recurrence; however, local recurrence remains a concern in patients with stages II and III disease.

Local recurrence in the pelvis is complicated by involvement of contiguous organs, soft and bony tissues, and deep nodal disease. Presenting symptoms vary from vague pelvic fullness to sciatica related to mass effect in the fixed space of the bony pelvis and invasion of the sciatic nerve.

Because local recurrence in the absence of metastatic disease is more common in rectal cancer than in colon cancer, aggressive resections, such as pelvic exenteration (anterior and posterior), sacral resection, and wide soft-tissue and pelvic floor resection, have been employed to treat these recurrences. Modern techniques of pelvic

TABLE 8: Chemotherapy for advanced disease, *continued*

Irinotecan/fluorouracil/leucovorin (FOLFIRI)	
Leucovorin	400 mg/m² IV infused over 2 hours prior to fluorouracil on days 1 and 2
Irinotecan	180 mg/m² IV infused over 90 minutes on day 1
Fluorouracil	400 mg/m² IV bolus on day 1, then 600 mg/m² IV
Fluorouracil and leucovorin plus bevacizumab	
Leucovorin	500 mg/m² IV infused over 2 hours once a week for 6 weeks, then a 2-week rest period
Fluorouracil	500 mg/m² IV bolus slow push 1 hour after leucovorin infusion once a week for 6 weeks, then a 2-week rest period
Bevacizumab	5 mg/kg IV continuous infusion over 90 minutes every 2 weeks
Kabbinavar F, Hurwitz H, Fehrenbacher I, et al: J Clin Oncol 21:60–65, 2003.	
FOLFIRI with cetuximab in wild-type *KRAS*	
Irinotecan	180 mg/m² IV on day 1
Leucovorin	400 mg/m² on day 1
Fluorouracil	400 mg/m² bolus IV on day 1
Fluorouracil infusion	2.4 g/m² over 46 hours IV continuous infusion every 2 weeks
Cetuximab	400 mg/m² on day 1, then 250 mg/m²/week 4
Van Cutsem E, Lang I, D'haens G, et al: J Clin Oncol 26(18S):abstract 2, 2008.	
FOLFOX with cetuximab in wild-type *KRAS*	
Oxaliplatin	85 mg/m² IV over 2 hours on day 1
Fluorouracil bolus	400 mg/m² IV bolus over 2 to 4 minutes
Leucovorin	400 mg/m² IV on day 1
Fluorouracil	2,400 to 3,000 mg/m² IV continuous infusion over 46 hours
Repeat cycle every 2 weeks.	
Cetuximab	400 mg/m² IV on day 1, then 250 mg/m² IV once a week over 22 hours continuous infusion on days 1 and 2
Repeat cycle every 2 weeks.	
Bokeymeyer C, Bondarenko I, Hartmann JT, et al: J Clin Oncol 26(18s):abstract 4000, 2008. Andre T, Louvet C, Maindrault-Goebel F, et al: Eur J Cancer 35:1343–1347, 1999.	

floor reconstruction, creation of continent urinary diversion, and vaginal reconstruction may be required for functional recovery.

The findings of the NSABP R-02 trial indicated postoperative adjuvant chemotherapy resulted in survival rates similar to those of postoperative chemoradiation therapy but was associated with a significantly higher rate of locoregional failure.

Pre- or postoperative radiation therapy

Radiation therapy has been used to reduce the locoregional recurrence rate of rectal tumors. Preoperative radiation therapy has been demonstrated to reduce local tumor recurrence, even in patients undergoing TME surgery. However, with the exception

TABLE 9: Five-year overall survival in Patterns of Care Study (PCS) vs the National Cancer Data Base (NCDB), Gastro-intestinal Tumor Study Group (GITSG), and Mayo/North Central Cancer Treatment Group (Mayo/NCCTG) studies

Study		5-year survival	
Bimodality vs trimodality		**S + RT**	**S + RT + CT**
Stage II			
	PCS	61%	81%
	NCDB	55%	62%
Stage III			
	PCS	33%	65%
	NCDB	39%	42%
Postop CRT vs postop RT		**Postop RT**	**Postop CRT**
	GITSG (7175)	52%	59%
	Mayo/NCCTG (7945)	48%	57%
	PCS	50%	69%

S = surgery; RT = radiation therapy; CT = chemotherapy;
CRT = concurrent radiation therapy and chemotherapy
Adapted from Coia LR, Gunderson LL, Haller D, et al: Cancer 86:1952–1958, 1999.

of one study, preoperative therapy has not affected overall survival in patients with stage II or III rectal cancer. An improvement in local tumor control also has been observed with postoperative irradiation, but again with no benefit with regard to disease-free or overall survival. Preoperative radiation therapy reduced local recurrence rates when combined with TME (11.4% vs 5.8%; $P < .001$) in a Dutch phase III trial at a median follow-up of 4.8 years. In a French study of 762 patients, preoperative chemoradiation therapy compared with preoperative radiotherapy reduced local failure rates in patients with T3–T4 rectal cancers from 17% to 8%.

Chemoradiation therapy

Postoperative chemoradiation therapy Clinical trials of surgical adjuvant treatment indicate that postoperative radiation therapy with concurrent chemotherapy (chemoradiation therapy) is superior to postoperative radiation therapy alone or surgery alone. Postoperative chemoradiation therapy is a standard of care for patients with stage II or III rectal cancer based largely on the findings of the NCCTG and GITSG trials. A summary of the 5-year survival results of the Patterns of Care Study (PCS) of the American College of Radiology and the results of the National Cancer Data Base (NCDB), both of which are representative of American national averages, is shown in Table 9.

The most effective combination of drugs, optimal mode of administration, and sequence of irradiation and chemotherapy still need to be determined. Radiation doses of 45 to 55 Gy are recommended in combination with 5-FU–based chemotherapy. Postoperative bolus 5-FU administration with irradiation is inferior to protracted venous infusion, resulting in lower 3-year rates of both overall survival (68% vs 76%) and disease-free survival (56% vs 67%).

An adjuvant treatment combining chemotherapy and pelvic irradiation in patients with stage II or III rectal cancer used the following regimen: 5-FU, 500 mg/m^2/day administered as a rapid IV infusion on days 1 to 5 and 450 mg/m^2/day on days 134 to 138 and days 169 to 173. Patients received a protracted IV infusion of 5-FU, 225 mg/m^2/day, by portable ambulatory infusion pump during the entire period of pelvic irradiation. Pelvic radiation therapy began on day 64 with a multiple-field technique to the tumor bed and nodal groups. A total of 4,500 cGy in 180-cGy fractions was administered over a 5-week period. Patients received a minimal boost dose of 540 cGy to the entire tumor bed, adjacent nodes, and 2 cm of adjacent tissue. A second boost dose of 360 cGy was allowed in selected patients with excellent displacement of the small bowel.

Neoadjuvant therapy For rectal cancers approaching the anal sphincter, preoperative (neoadjuvant) irradiation or the combination of chemotherapy and irradiation will significantly reduce the size of the majority of tumors. This approach allows for sphincter-preserving surgery in many patients. In addition, the long-term morbidity of radiation therapy for rectal cancer may be reduced if it is administered prior to surgery. The use of preoperative chemotherapy and radiation therapy is particularly important for patients presenting with locally advanced, unresectable rectal cancer, as the disease of the majority will be rendered resectable following neoadjuvant therapy. One additional role of neoadjuvant therapy may be in facilitating transanal excision of T2 and T3 rectal cancers in poor-surgical-risk patients. A number of investigators have reported good results with transanal excision of T2 and T3 tumors following a complete response to neoadjuvant therapy. However, this approach cannot be considered the current standard of care.

Preoperative vs postoperative chemoradiation therapy Preoperative chemoradiation therapy is now preferred in most cases to postoperative adjuvant treatment, particularly in patients with T3 or T4 lesions. Such treatment may enhance resectability and may be associated with a lower frequency of complications compared with postoperative treatment. In a report of a randomized trial conducted by the GRCSG, Sauer et al found that compared with postoperative chemoradiotherapy, preoperative chemoradiotherapy significantly decreased local failure (6% vs 13%; $P = .006$) and sphincter preservation in low-lying tumors (39% vs 19%; $P < .004$). In addition, the incidence of chronic anastomotic stricture was also lowest in the preoperative chemoradiotherapy group (4% vs 12%; $P = .003$). These findings are consistent with those from another large multi-institutional phase III trial, which found that short-course preoperative radiation therapy improved local tumor control and disease-free survival compared with postoperative chemoradiation therapy. In the NSABP R-03 study that compared preoperative and postoperative chemoradiotherapy, patients treated with preoperative chemoradiotherapy had an improved 5-year disease-free survival (64.7% vs 53.4%). No patient with a pathologic complete response had a recurrence. Collectively, these trials suggest that for patients with indications for chemoradiotherapy, preoperative therapy is preferred.

Choice of chemotherapy during radiation therapy The optimal chemotherapy to use in combination with radiation remains an area of active research. Although most large randomized trials have used bolus or infusional 5-FU in combination with radiation, the availability of oral agents, such as capecitabine, has raised

In patients with metastatic colorectal cancer responding to FOLFOX, a break from chemotherapy was compared with maintenance chemotherapy (5-FU, leucovorin) in the randomized trial OPTIMOX2. Control of disease was significantly longer with maintenance chemotherapy than with a break from chemotherapy (13.1 vs 9.2 months; *Chibaudel B et al: J Clin Oncol 27:5757–5733, 2009).*

interest in combining capecitabine and radiation alone and with other chemotherapeutic agents. The NSABP R-04 is comparing capecitabine-containing regimens combined with radiation to infusional 5-FU regimens. A number of retrospective and phase II studies have suggested that the combination of capecitabine and radiation provides pathologic response rates similar to those observed with 5-FU and radiation.

A recent phase III trial of chemotherapy regimens during radiation suggested no benefit from a capecitabine and oxaliplatin regimen compared with capecitabine alone (see sidebar). Many studies are ongoing with combinations of capecitabine, oxaliplatin, and irinotecan during radiation therapy.

TREATMENT OF ADVANCED COLON CANCER

Local recurrences from colon cancers usually occur at the site of anastomosis, in the resection bed, or in the contiguous and retroperitoneal (para-aortic, paracaval) lymph nodes. Anastomotic recurrences diagnosed during surveillance in asymptomatic patients are the most curable, followed by local soft-tissue recurrences. Regional and retroperitoneal lymph node recurrences portend a poor prognosis and systemic disease.

Chemotherapy

The development of chemotherapy for advanced CRC has become an active field (Table 8). After decades of 5-FU–based treatment, and of little clinical gains, the arrival of new, effective agents has significantly changed the way this cancer is treated. Although 5-FU remains the backbone of most regimens, the new agents irinotecan and oxaliplatin have become an important part of front-line treatment of this disease in the United States and abroad. The recent development of molecular targeted agents has provided additional improvements in both response and survival for patients with CRC.

5-FU remains an important agent in the treatment of advanced CRC. Mainly in the past, 5-FU was administered as a bolus injection either weekly or daily for 5 days, every 4 to 5 weeks (Table 8). With these regimens, response rates have been approximately 10% to 15%. The development of permanent venous access devices and portable infusion pumps has permitted the prolonged infusion of 5-FU on an outpatient basis.

The pattern of 5-FU toxicity differs depending on whether it is administered as a bolus or a prolonged infusion than by other methods. Bolus administration has pronounced myelotoxic effects, whereas the dose-limiting toxic effects of prolonged-infusion 5-FU are mucositis and diarrhea. Palmar-plantar erythrodysesthesia (hand-foot syndrome) has been reported with prolonged infusions. Infusional 5-FU is now an important component of therapy when combined with either irinotecan or oxaliplatin.

Biochemical modulation of 5-FU Interest in the biochemical modulation of 5-FU by leucovorin is based on preclinical studies demonstrating that leucovorin raises the level of *N*5,*N*10-methylenetetrahydrofolate and, thus, forms a stable tertiary complex of TS, the folate coenzyme, and 5-FU (in the form of 5-fluorodeoxyuridine). The use of 5-FU with leucovorin results in higher response rates than 5-FU alone and may prolong survival.

The genes *KRAS* and to some degree *BRAF* have been associated with a lack of response to the EGF receptor inhibitors cetuximab (Erbitux) and panitumumab (Vectibix). There is increasing retrospective evidence to show that mutations in *KRAS* or *BRAF* may significantly shorten overall survival. However, these mutations do not preclude a potential benefit from chemotherapy *(Laurent-Puig P et al: J Clin Oncol 27:5924–5930, 2009; Richman SD et al: J Clin Oncol 27:5931–5937, 2009).*

Although there is no agreement as to the optimal dose of leucovorin, historically two dosing schedules (as shown in Table 7) have been used with either low-dose or high-dose leucovorin.

FOLFOX was approved by the FDA in 2004 as first-line therapy. Initial evidence of activity was demonstrated in patients with pretreated, 5-FU–resistant CRC (45% response rate). In subsequent trials, patients with untreated metastatic CRC receiving FOLFOX had response rates of over 50%. In addition, patients receiving oxaliplatin, infusional 5-FU, and leucovorin have achieved overall survival rates > 20 months in several reported trials. However, many of these patients have received second- and even third-line therapies at the time of disease progression, reducing the validity of survival evaluation. Currently, there are several accepted FOLFOX regimens in use, including FOLFOX4, FOLFOX6, modified FOLFOX6, and FOLFOX 7.

Oxaliplatin's toxicity profile includes nausea/vomiting and cumulative, reversible peripheral neuropathy. Patients may also develop a reversible, cold-induced, acute pharyngolaryngeal neuropathy. The OPTIMOX trials demonstrated that patients with either stable or responding metastatic CRC may benefit from an oxaliplatin-free interval with either no therapy or maintenance 5-FU and leucovorin followed by reintroduction of FOLFOX at the time of disease progression. The use of maintenance therapy compared with continued FOLFOX provided a comparable overall period of disease control. Maintenance therapy lessened the amount of oxaliplatin-induced neuropathy.

Irinotecan has significant clinical activity in patients with metastatic CRC whose disease has recurred or spread after standard chemotherapy. Its FDA approval was based on two phase III trials showing that irinotecan (350 mg/m^2 once every 3 weeks) significantly increased survival, compared with best supportive care and infusional 5-FU, respectively, in patients with recurrent or progressive cancer following first-line 5-FU therapy. Irinotecan increased the median survival by 27% and 41%, respectively, in the two trials. Irinotecan is active in patients whose disease progressed while receiving 5-FU. Reproducible 15% to 20% response rates in this patient population led to the approval of irinotecan for use in patients with 5-FU–refractory disease. The dosage schedules most commonly used are 125 mg/m^2 weekly for 4 weeks, followed by a 2-week rest period (United States) and 350 mg/m^2 every 3 weeks (Europe). The primary toxicities of irinotecan are diarrhea and neutropenia. Intensive loperamide is important in the management of the former complication. An initial 4-mg load-

The need for surgery, radiation, or intraluminal stenting of the primary tumor in patients presenting with synchronous metastatic colorectal cancer was assessed in patients from a prospective institutional database. All of the patients had received standard chemotherapy with or without bevacizumab (Avastin). Of 233 patients identified in the database, 217 (93%) never required any intervention for their primary tumor *(Poultsides GA et al: J Clin Oncol 27:3379–3384, 2009).*

ing dose is given at the first sign of diarrhea, followed by 2-mg doses every 2 hours until diarrhea abates for at least a 12-hour period.

Studies have shown that variation in the metabolism of irinotecan is associated with the pattern of allelic inheritance with the gene *UGT 1A1*. Although it is recommended that *UGT 1A1* testing be performed prior to the use of irinotecan, dose-modification recommendations, based on the pattern of alleles inherited, are not currently available. However, it is recommended that patients with the *UGT 1A1*28* pattern of inheritance should receive a reduced dose of irinotecan.

FOLFIRI Several randomized trials have shown improved response rates and overall survival when irinotecan is added to an infusional regimen of 5-FU and leucovorin compared with 5-FU and leucovorin alone. A bolus combination of irinotecan, 5-FU, and leucovorin (IFL) had also shown better response rates and overall survival but proved to be much more toxic. The use of IFL is no longer recommended.

In a phase III trial comparing the sequence of FOLFIRI followed by FOLFOX or the reverse sequence for patients with metastatic CRC, no difference in median survival was seen. Grade 3 or 4 mucositis, nausea, and vomiting occurred more frequently with FOLFIRI, whereas grade 3 or 4 neutropenia and neurosensory toxicity were more frequent with FOLFOX. Response rates were similar between the two groups. The results of this clinical trial and others stress the importance of using all available agents in the treatment of metastatic CRC, and the sequence of their use appears to be less important.

Capecitabine In a phase III trial of previously untreated patients with metastatic colon cancer, capecitabine produced higher response rates than did 5-FU and leucovorin. Overall survival and time to disease progression were similar (noninferior) to those with 5-FU and leucovorin. As established in European trials, the recommended dose of capecitabine is 2,500 mg/m^2 each day, given as a twice-daily dose, for 14 days followed by a 1-week rest period. However, most North American patients will not tolerate this dose of capecitabine and should instead receive 2,000 mg/m^2 each day, given as a twice-daily dose, for 14 days followed by a 1-week rest period. The side effects of capecitabine tend to be similar to those seen with prolonged infusion of 5-FU, with hand-foot syndrome being the most common.

Capecitabine and oxaliplatin may also provide significant benefit. Results of completed clinical trials with capecitabine and oxaliplatin are similar to those obtained with FOLFOX. This combination avoids the need for a central venous catheter.

Capecitabine and irinotecan may also be of benefit. This combination should be used with caution. Although some clinical trials have shown this combination to be tolerable and active, other trials of capecitabine and irinotecan have shown significant toxicity.

Molecular targeted agents

A variety of monoclonal antibodies and small molecules are being evaluated in clinical trials and preclinical studies. Three of these agents (bevacizumab [Avastin], cetuximab [Erbitux], and panitumumab [Vectibix]) have been approved by the FDA for use in CRC.

Bevacizumab is a humanized monoclonal antibody that binds circulating vascular endothelial growth factor (VEGF). When given with a 5-FU–containing regimen in several different trials as first-line therapy in patients with metastatic CRC, bevacizumab led to an improved outcome. The addition of bevacizumab to 5-FU and leucovorin resulted in significant improvement in progression-free survival. Even better results were seen with IFL, when the addition of bevacizumab to IFL resulted in significant improvement in overall survival and response rates. These studies led to approval by the FDA of bevacizumab. It is indicated for use in first-line therapy for metastatic CRC when combined with 5-FU–based chemotherapy, such as FOLFOX.

Cetuximab is a human/mouse chimeric antibody directed against the epithelial growth factor receptor (EGFR). In a randomized trial of patients with CRC refractory to irinotecan, patients were randomized to receive either cetuximab and irinotecan or cetuximab alone. The addition of cetuximab to irinotecan led to a significantly higher response rate compared with cetuximab alone. The median survival for those receiving cetuximab and irinotecan was also longer, though not significantly. Based on the results of this study, cetuximab was approved by the FDA for use in patients whose disease is refractory to irinotecan with tumors expressing EGFR. Data from a phase III trial in which cetuximab was evaluated in addition to FOLFIRI compared with FOLFIRI alone suggest that patients with tumors harboring mutant *KRAS* derived no benefit from the addition of cetuximab. A benefit in progression-free survival and response rates was seen with the addition of cetuximab in patients with wild-type *KRAS*.

Panitumumab is a monoclonal antibody that targets EGFR. In a pivotal phase III trial, 463 patients with metastatic CRC who had failed to respond to previous standard therapy were randomized between panitumumab (6 mg/kg every 2 weeks) plus best supportive care vs best supportive care alone. Patients in the panitumumab arm achieved a significantly improved time to disease progression (96 days vs 60 days) and objective response rate (8% vs 0%). On the basis of the results of this trial, the FDA approved panitumumab for the treatment of patients with CRC that has metastasized following standard chemotherapy.

Combination of targeted agents The successes observed with cetuximab and bevacizumab in combination with 5-FU–based chemotherapy have led to studies combining these agents with 5-FU–based chemotherapy in patients with metastatic CRC. Combined antibody therapy with bevacizumab and cetuximab, when added to chemotherapy, surprisingly has shown no benefit and in some cases resulted in significantly shorter progression-free survival and an inferior quality of life. Similarly, the addition of panitumumab and bevacizumab to chemotherapy results in increased toxicity and decreased progression-free survival when compared with chemotherapy and bevacizumab alone. Therefore, the combination of chemotherapy and bevacizumab with either cetuximab or panitumumab should not be used outside of a clinical trial.

Chemotherapy and surgery for stage IV CRC

For previously untreated patients with stage IV disease and limited organ involvement, such as liver-only metastases, in whom surgery is thought possible, consideration should be given to neoadjuvant chemotherapy followed by synchronous or staged partial colectomy and metastasectomy. The appropriate chemotherapy in this setting is uncertain. However, the use of FOLFOX or FOLFIRI is reasonable. The addition of bevacizumab may enhance the response. However, because of the potential risk for bleeding or other surgical complications, bevacizumab should be discontinued 6 to 8 weeks before surgery. In addition, because of liver-associated changes with oxaliplatin or irinotecan, after approximately 2 to 3 months of chemotherapy, it is preferable to proceed with surgery after about 3 months of chemotherapy. Additional chemotherapy can be given after recovery from surgery. Patients with the development of limited metastatic disease after surgery and adjuvant therapy for stages II to III disease may also obtain long-term benefit from further chemotherapy and surgery.

Metastasectomy

Metastases to the liver and lungs account for most cases of non-nodal systemic disease in CRC. Resection of metastases, or metastasectomy, has gained recognition as a viable treatment. Resection of liver metastases results in cure rates of 5% to 60%, depending on the number of metastases and the stage of disease. Resection of solitary metastases in patients with stage I or II disease results in a 5-year survival rate of ~40% to 60%.

Metastasectomy for liver metastases should only be considered when complete resection is feasible on the basis of anatomic grounds and when adequate hepatic function can be maintained. Debulking resections are generally not recommended. Patients who are initially unresectable can be considered for resection after neoadjuvant chemotherapy as long as all disease, including the primary tumor, can be resected. Hepatic resection is the treatment of choice for resectable liver metastases from CRC. Ablative techniques can be considered in amenable lesions where surgical resection is not feasible.

Metastasectomy for lung metastases can be considered for highly selected patients in whom complete resection is feasible with maintenance of adequate pulmonary function. Resectable extrapulmonary metastases, particularly liver metastases, do not preclude resection.

TREATMENT OF ADVANCED RECTAL CANCER

Radiation therapy

Radiation therapy is moderately effective in palliating the symptoms of advanced rectal cancer. Pain is decreased in 80% of irradiated patients, although only 20% report complete relief. Bleeding can be controlled in more than 70% of patients. Obstruction cannot be reliably relieved by irradiation, and diverting colostomy is recommended. Only 15% of patients with recurrent rectal cancers achieve local disease control with irradiation, and median survival is < 2 years.

Chemoradiation therapy may be useful to convert fixed unresectable lesions into resectable lesions. These regimens have generally used protracted infusions of 5-FU (200 to 250 mg/m^2/day) delivered via a portable infusion pump during pelvic radiation therapy (450 cGy over 5 weeks).

Intraoperative radiotherapy (localized irradiation given to the tumor or tumor bed at the time of resection) is under active investigation in advanced and locoregionally recurrent rectal cancers.

Laser photoablation

Laser photoablation is occasionally employed for temporary relief of obstructive rectal cancer in patients who are not surgical candidates because of the presence of distant metastases, surgical comorbidity, or extensive intra-abdominal disease.

Endoscopic stent placement

Endoscopic stents may have a place in patients with obstructing neoplasms. In this situation, the stent can serve as a bridge to relieve the obstruction before surgery and/or to allow for the administration of systemic therapy. The stent can migrate; thus, if there is response to therapy, the stent may dislodge and cause acute problems, such as perforation or pain. In some instances, the stent can also erode into adjacent structures, such as when radiation is utilized.

Follow-up of long-term survivors

Patients who have completed therapy for CRC require monitoring for potential treatment-related complications, recurrent disease, and new metachronous cancers. Specific follow-up recommendations for these patients are controversial. Guidelines for post-treatment surveillance/monitoring adopted by the NCCN are shown in Table 10.

TABLE 10: NCCN recommendations for post-treatment surveillance/monitoring[a]

- History and physical examination every 3 months for 2 years, then every 6 months for a total of 5 years
- CEA level evaluation every 3 months for 2 years, then every 6 months for years 2 to 5 for T2 or greater lesions
- Colonoscopy in 1 year, repeat in 1 year if results are abnormal or at least every 2 to 3 years if results are negative for polyps. If no preoperative colonoscopy has been performed due to an obstructing lesion, colonoscopy in 3 to 6 months
- Abdominal/pelvic CT scan in addition to chest x-ray or chest CT for patients with resected stage IV disease only: Every 6 months for 2 years, then every 6 to 12 months for a total of 5 years

[a] http://www.nccn.org
CEA = carcinoembryonic antigen

ANAL CANAL CARCINOMA

EPIDEMIOLOGY, ETIOLOGY, AND RISK FACTORS

In the United States, about 4,650 new cases of anal canal carcinoma are diagnosed each year. Overall, it is slightly more common in women than in men. More than 80% of anal canal tumors occur in individuals > 60 years of age. Epidemiologic studies suggest that receptive anal intercourse is strongly related to anal cancer.

The incidence rate of anal cancer for single men is reported to be six times that for married men. In people < 35 years old, anal carcinoma is more common in men than in women. A history of genital warts has been observed, suggesting that papillomavirus may be an etiologic factor.

DIAGNOSIS

The diagnosis of anal canal carcinoma is usually delayed because the symptoms (bleeding, pain, and sensation of mass) are so often attributed to benign anorectal disorders, such as hemorrhoids or anal fissures.

Evaluation should include a careful rectal examination, endoscopic examination with description of lesion size, and assessment of whether there is invasion of disease into adjacent organs (vagina, urethra, or bladder). Reexamination with the patient under general anesthesia may be necessary. A diagnostic incisional biopsy is required.

Pelvic CT is suggested to evaluate pelvic nodes. Although distant metastases are uncommon at diagnosis, a chest x-ray and liver function tests are recommended. Suspicious inguinal nodes discovered on physical examination must be assessed pathologically. The incidence of inguinal nodal metastases at diagnosis varies from 13% to 25%. The presence of perirectal, inguinal, and pelvic lymph node involvement correlates with tumor size and is unusual for tumors < 2 cm in diameter. Formal groin dissection is not advised; needle aspiration should be performed, with limited surgical biopsy if results of aspiration are inconclusive.

PATHOLOGY

Squamous cell carcinomas Most anal canal malignancies are squamous cell carcinomas. They have been classified as cloacogenic carcinomas, basaloid carcinomas, transitional cell carcinomas, or mucoepidermoid carcinomas. However, there is little difference in the natural history of these various types.

Unusual tumors arising in the anal canal include small-cell carcinomas, anal melanomas, and adenocarcinomas.

Small-cell carcinomas of the anal canal are aggressive neoplasms similar in natural history to bronchogenic small-cell carcinomas. If such a histology is identified, the clinician should be alerted to the possibility of early distant metastases, and treatment should include chemotherapeutic regimens used in bronchogenic small-cell carcinomas.

TABLE 11: TNM classification of anal canal tumors

Primary tumor (T)	
TX	Primary tumor cannot be assessed
T0	No evidence of primary tumor
Tis	Carcinoma in situ
T1	Tumor ≤ 2 cm in greatest dimension
T2	Tumor > 2 cm but not > 5 cm in greatest dimension
T3	Tumor > 5 cm in greatest dimension
T4	Tumor of any size that invades adjacent organs (eg, vagina, bladder, urethra, bladder)[a]
Regional lymph nodes (N)	
NX	Regional lymph nodes cannot be assessed
N0	No regional lymph node metastasis
N1	Metastasis in perirectal lymph node(s)
N2	Metastasis in unilateral internal iliac and/or inguinal lymph node(s)
N3	Metastasis in perirectal and inguinal lymph nodes and/or bilateral internal iliac and/or inguinal lymph nodes
Distant metastasis (M)	
MX	Distant metastasis cannot be assessed
M0	No distant metastasis
M1	Distant metastasis
Grade (G)	
GX	Grade of differentiation cannot be assessed
G1	Well differentiated
G2	Moderately differentiated
G3	Poorly differentiated
G4	Undifferentiated

Stage groupings			
Stage 0	Tis	N0	M0
Stage I	T1	N0	M0
Stage II	T2	N0	M0
	T3	N0	M0
Stage IIIA	T1–3	N1	M0
	T4	N0	M0
Stage IIIB	T4	N1	M0
	Any T	N2–3	M0
Stage IV	Any T	Any N	M1

[a] Direct invasion of the rectal wall, perirectal skin, subcutaneous tissue, or sphincter muscle(s) is not classified as T4.

From Greene FL, Page DL, Fleming ID, et al (eds): AJCC Cancer Staging Manual, 6th ed. New York, Springer-Verlag, 2002. In the 7th edition of the AJCC Cancer Staging Manual (2010), these definitions of TNM and the stage groupings have not changed.

Although advanced anal melanomas generally are associated with a dismal survival, prognosis may be related to the depth of disease penetration. Early anal melanomas < 2.0 mm in depth can be cured with wide excision. More advanced disease can be treated with local excision and EBRT, with excellent local tumor control. Abdominoperineal resection is indicated only rarely in the management of anal melanoma, because lesions large enough to require radical surgery are almost always associated with distant spread of disease.

Adenocarcinomas are uncommon cancers associated with a poor prognosis. Treatment should be aggressive and based on a multimodality approach. The rarity of this tumor precludes the development of specific clinical trials.

STAGING

The size of the primary tumor is the most important clinical predictor of survival for patients with anal carcinomas. Both the UICC and the AJCC have agreed on a unified staging system (Table 11). The TNM classification distinguishes between anal canal carcinoma and anal margin tumors, because the latter exhibit biologic behavior similar to that of other skin cancers and are staged as skin cancers.

Pathologic complete response to neoadjuvant therapy is known to predict improved disease control in patients with rectal cancer. A recently reported phase II trial evaluated concurrent infusional 5-FU and radiation prior to surgery vs the same regimen with two cycles of FOLFOX6 prior to surgery. Patients who received FOLFOX6 after 5-FU and radiotherapy had a pathologic complete response rate of 28%, compared with 21% in patients treated with 5-FU and radiotherapy. There was a 5% rate of grade 3 or higher toxicity during the FOLFOX6 treatment (*Garcia-Aguilar J et al: 2010 Gastrointestinal Cancers Symposium: abstract 421, 2010*). Other studies, such as the Lyon R90-01 trial, have suggested that longer durations between radiotherapy and surgery may increase pathologic downstaging without a detrimental effect or morbidity of surgery.

TREATMENT

Surgery

In selected individuals with small superficial T1 tumors, local excision has achieved adequate local tumor control and survival. However, most studies of local excision have been retrospective, with small numbers of patients. Prior to the advent of primary radiotherapy and combined-modality treatment (see later in this chapter), abdominoperineal resection was considered to be the conventional treatment for patients with invasive anal canal cancer. Unfortunately, even with radical surgical procedures, local recurrences are frequent. Currently, radical extirpative surgery is indicated only after the failure of combined-modality treatment. Salvage abdominoperineal resection for persistent or recurrent disease has resulted in a 5-year survival of up to 60%. In one series, patients presenting with lymphadenopathy at primary diagnosis and those who received less than 55 Gy at initial chemoradiation treatment had a worse prognosis.

Radiation therapy

Trials of primary EBRT in patients with anal canal carcinomas have used doses varying between 4,500 and 7,550 cGy. Local tumor control rates of 60% to 90%, with

TABLE 12: Chemotherapy regimen for anal canal cancer

Drug/combination	Dose and schedule
Fluorouracil/mitomycin/radiation therapy	
Fluorouracil	1 g/m^2/d IV infused continuously on days 1–4 and 29–32
Mitomycin	15 mg/m^2 IV on day 1
Irradiation	200 cGy/d for 5 days per week (total dose, 3,000 cGy)

Give chemotherapy concurrently with irradiation; start both modalities on the same day.

Leichman L, Nigro ND, Vaitkevicius VK, et al: Am J Med 78:211-215, 1985.
Table prepared by Ishmael Jaiyesimi, DO.

5-year survival rates of 32% to 90%, are similar to the results of surgical series when the trials are controlled for tumor size.

Interstitial radiation therapy alone has been used primarily in Europe for early-stage lesions. A relatively high radiation dose is delivered to a small volume. This modality carries a high potential for radiation necrosis and fails to incorporate the treatment of the inguinal nodes.

Combined-modality treatment

Chemotherapy given concurrently with irradiation is the preferred therapy for most patients with anal canal cancer (Table 12). Investigators from Wayne State University pioneered the use of simultaneous pelvic irradiation and chemotherapy in the treatment of patients with anal canal carcinomas. They demonstrated that the majority of such patients could be treated with this combination, obviating the need for an abdominoperineal resection. The original study design used 3,000 cGy over 3 weeks with 5-FU (1,000 mg/m^2/day) as a continuous infusion on days 1 to 4 and then repeated on days 29 to 32. Mitomycin, 15 mg/m^2, was administered as an IV bolus on day 1. A total of 4 to 6 weeks after the completion of therapy, patients had a deep muscle biopsy of the anal canal scar.

An updated analysis of this experience demonstrated that 38 of 45 patients (84%) were rendered disease-free after chemotherapy and irradiation. Individuals who had positive results on biopsy underwent an abdominoperineal resection.

Because of the success of this experience, other investigators have attempted to implement infusional 5-FU and mitomycin with irradiation as definitive therapy. Most studies have used similar schedules of 5-FU and mitomycin but have used higher doses of pelvic irradiation (4,500 to 5,700 cGy). Five-year survival rates > 70% have been reported.

A randomized trial from the RTOG showed that the use of mitomycin with irradiation and 5-FU increased complete tumor regression and improved colostomy-free survival over irradiation and 5-FU alone. At 4 years, the colostomy-free survival rate was higher in the mitomycin arm than in the 5-FU–alone arm (71% vs 59%), as was the disease-free survival rate (73% vs 51%).

Several investigators have compared the results of irradiation alone vs irradiation plus chemotherapy. The current standard chemotherapy regimen for concurrent

RTOG 0529 was a phase II trial that evaluated dose-painted IMRT with 5-FU and mitomycin in patients with T2–4N0–3M0 anal cancer. The dose of radiation was dependent on tumor and nodal stage. There was a reduction of grade 3 or higher gastrointestinal or genitourinary toxicities with IMRT compared with that observed on RTOG 9811, which utilized conventional radiation approaches. Real-time quality assurance resulted in modification of contours in 79%. Early clinical response rates were similar to those observed with conventional regimens *(Kachnic LA et al: 2010 Gastrointestinal Cancers Symposium: abstract 405, 2010)*. These data suggest IMRT with chemotherapy may be a suitable treatment for patients with anal carcinoma, but contouring is complicated for this indication, even when clearly defined in a clinical trial.

radiation is concurrent 5-FU and mitomycin. Intergroup RTOG 98-11 compared concurrent mitomycin and 5-FU with induction 5-FU and cisplatin with concurrent cisplatin, 5-FU, and mitomycin. The mitomycin-containing regimen resulted in a lower colostomy rate but greater hematologic toxicity. Cummings et al found that with identical irradiation doses and techniques, the local tumor control rate for cancers > 2 cm rose from 49% with radiation therapy alone to 85% when 5-FU and mitomycin were combined with irradiation. Papillon and Montbarbon found an increase in the rate of local tumor control with a combined-modality approach compared with pelvic irradiation alone (81% vs 66%). Two randomized studies have shown improved local tumor control with chemoradiation therapy over irradiation.

A complete response to combined chemotherapy and radiation therapy is expected in 80% to 90% of patients with anal cancer. It is important to evaluate the response of therapy with a careful examination of the anal canal after treatment. Anal canal cancers can continue to regress for up to 3 or more months after completion of treatment. For this reason, it is recommended that a biopsy be performed no sooner than 3 months after the completion of treatment, unless there is evidence of disease progression or other evidence to suggest early recurrence. If pathologic evidence of recurrence is diagnosed, abdominoperineal resection is expected to yield long-term disease control and survival in 40% to 60% of patients.

Toxicity from combined radiotherapy and chemotherapy for anal carcinoma is significant, with high rates of dermatitis (often requiring treatment breaks) and gastrointestinal toxicity. Treatment breaks may decrease the efficacy of radiation. Intensity-modulated radiotherapy (IMRT) can help reduce the radiation dose to normal structures, such as the bowel, skin, genitalia, and femurs.

Two recent trials have addressed the use of IMRT with concurrent chemotherapy to reduce these toxicities. These studies have suggested that local tumor control and survival may be improved with IMRT. Toxicity was markedly reduced with the IMRT approach. The RTOG has completed a trial of IMRT for anal cancer and has recently published contouring guidelines for radiation oncologists who use IMRT.

Chemotherapy

Reports of other chemotherapeutic agents in anal cancer have been relatively anecdotal, with limited phase II studies. Because of the activity of cisplatin in other squamous cell carcinomas, this agent has been employed as a single agent or combined with infusional 5-FU in advanced disease.

Novel chemoradiation regimens have been evaluated in the hope of providing improved tumor control rates in patients receiving combined chemotherapy and radiation. Recent studies have evaluated chemotherapy combinations including cetuximab with radiation. These early studies are promising in regard to tolerability and response rates. The combination of cetuximab, cisplatin, and 5-FU with radiation therapy is being tested by the AAMCTC and the ECOG.

Considerations for immunocompromised patients

Immunocompromised patients are at higher risk of developing anal carcinoma. Because these patients may also have increased toxicity with combined chemotherapy and radiation, careful delivery of combined therapy should include a consideration of chemotherapy dose modification. Several series have evaluated the ability of immunocompromised patients to tolerate definitive chemoradiotherapy for anal cancer. Some series suggest that a CD4+ cell count lower than 200 cells/μL in HIV-positive patients is associated with higher rates of toxicity. Recent studies have shown that the vast majority of immunocompromised patients can tolerate concurrent chemoradiotherapy, although dose adjustments may be required. The use of IMRT may benefit this patient subset.

SUGGESTED READING

ON COLORECTAL CARCINOMA

André T, Boni C, Navarro M, et al: Improved overall survival with oxaliplatin, fluorouracil, and leucovorin as adjuvant treatment in stage II or III colon cancer in the MOSAIC trial. J Clin Oncol 27:3109–3116, 2009.

Bernstein TE, Endreseth BH, Romundstad P, et al: Circumferential resection margin as a prognostic factor in rectal cancer. Br J Surg 96:1348–1357, 2009.

Braendengen M, Tveit KM, Berglund A, et al: Randomized phase III study comparing preoperative radiotherapy with chemoradiotherapy in nonresectable rectal cancer. J Clin Oncol 26:3687–3694, 2008.

Fazio VW, Zutshi M, Remzi FH, et al: A randomized multicenter trial to compare long-term functional outcome, quality of life, and complications of surgical procedures for low rectal cancers. Ann Surg 246:481–488, 2007.

Fleshman J, Sargent DJ, Green E, et al: Laparoscopic colectomy for cancer is not inferior to open surgery based on 5-year data from the COST Study Group trial. Ann Surg 246:655–662, 2007.

Greenberg JA, Shibata D, Herndon JE 2nd, et al: Local excision of distal rectal cancer: An update of cancer and leukemia group B 8984. Dis Colon Rectum 51:1185–1191, 2008.

Jayne DG, Guillou PJ, Thorpe H, et al: Randomized trial of laparoscopic-assisted resection of colorectal carcinoma: 3-year results of the UK MRC CLASICC Trial Group. J Clin Oncol 25:3061–3068, 2007.

Jemal A, Siegel R, Xu J, et al: Cancer statistics, 2010. CA Cancer J Clin 60:277-300, 2010.

Jimeno A, Messersmith WA, Hirsch FR, et al: KRAS mutations and sensitivity to epidermal growth factor response inhibitors in colorectal cancer: Practical application of patient selection. J Clin Oncol 27:1130–1136, 2009.

Kim DH, Pickhardt PJ, Taylor AJ, et al: CT colonography versus colonoscopy for the detection of advanced neoplasia. N Engl J Med 357:1403–1412, 2007.

Leung KL, Kwok SP, Lam SC, et al: Laparoscopic resection of rectosigmoid carcinoma: Prospective randomised trial. Lancet 363:1187–1192, 2004.

Levin B, Lieberman DA, McFarland B, et al: Screening and surveillance for the early detection of colorectal cancer and adenomatous polyps, 2008: A joint guideline from the American Cancer Society, the US Multi-Society Task Force on Colorectal Cancer, and the American College of Radiology. CA Cancer J Clin 58:130–160, 2008.

Olivatto LO, Araujo CM, Vilhena B, et al: Phase I study of cetuximab in combination with 5-FU, cisplatin, and radiotherapy in patients with locally advanced squamous cell anal canal carcinoma. 2010 Gastrointestinal Cancers Symposium: abstract 492, 2010.

Papamichael D, Audisio R, Horiot JC, et al: Treatment of the elderly colorectal cancer patient: SIOG expert recommendations. Ann Oncol 20:5–16, 2009.

Peeters KC, Marijnen CA, Nagtegaal ID, et al: The TME trial after a median follow-up of 6 years: Increased local control but no survival benefit in irradiated patients with resectable rectal carcinoma. Ann Surg 246:693–701, 2007.

Roh MS, Colangelo LH, O'Connell MJ, et al: Preoperative multimodality therapy improves disease-free survival in patients with carcinoma of the rectum: NSABP R-03. J Clin Oncol 27:5124–5130, 2009.

Sauer R, Becker H, Hohenberger W, et al: Preoperative versus postoperative chemoradiotherapy for rectal cancer. N Engl J Med 351:1731–1740, 2004.

Seburg-Montefiore D, Stephens RJ, Steele R, et al: Preoperative radiotherapy versus selective postoperative chemoradiotherapy in patients with rectal cancer (MRC CR07 and NCIC–CTG C016): A multicentre, randomised trial. Lancet 373:811–820, 2009.

Siena S, Sartore-Bianchi A, Di Nicolantonio F, et al: Biomarkers predicting clinical outcome of epidermal growth factor receptor-targeted therapy in metastatic colorectal cancer. J Natl Cancer Inst 101:1308–1324, 2009.

Sinicrope FA, Sargent DJ: Clinical implications of microsatellite instability in sporadic colon cancers. Curr Opin Oncol 21:369–373, 2009.

Tol J, Koopman M, Cats A, et al: Chemotherapy, bevacizumab, and cetuximab in metastatic colorectal cancer. N Engl J Med 360:563–572, 2009.

Van Cutsem E, Köhne CH, Hitre E, et al: Cetuximab and chemotherapy as initial treatment for metastatic colorectal cancer. N Engl J Med 360:1408–1417, 2009.

Van Cutsem E, Labianca R, Bodoky G, et al: Randomized phase III trial comparing biweekly infusional fluorouracil/leucovorin alone or with irinotecan in the adjuvant treatment of stage III colon cancer: PETACC-3. J Clin Oncol 27:3117–3125, 2009.

You YN, Baxter NN, Stewart A, Nelson H: Is the increasing rate of local excision for stage I rectal cancer in the United States justified? A nationwide cohort study from the National Cancer Database. Ann Surg 245:726–733, 2007.

ON ANAL CANAL CARCINOMA

Ajani JA, Winter KA, Gunderson LL, et al: Fluorouracil, mitomycin, and radiotherapy vs fluorouracil, cisplatin, and radiotherapy for carcinoma of the anal canal: A randomized controlled trial. JAMA 299;1914–1921, 2008.

Das P, Bhatia S, Eng C, et al: Predictors and patterns of recurrence after definitive chemoradiation for anal cancer. Int J Radiat Oncol Biol Phys 68:794–800, 2007.

Eng C, Crane CH, Rodriguez-Bigas MA: Should cisplatin be avoided in the treatment of locally advanced squamous cell carcinoma of the anal canal? Nat Clin Pract Gastroenterol Hepatol 6:16–17, 2009.

Ghouti L, Houvenaeghel G, Moutardier V, et al: Salvage abdominoperineal resection after failure of conservative treatment in anal epidermoid cancer. Dis Colon Rectum 48:16–22, 2005.

Mullen JT, Rodriguez-Bigas MA, Chang GJ, et al: Results of surgical salvage after failed chemoradiation therapy for epidermoid carcinoma of the anal canal. Ann Surg Oncol 14:478–483, 2007.

Podnos YD, Tsai NC, Smith D, et al: Factors affecting survival in patients with anal melanoma. Am Surg 72:917–920, 2006.

Salama JK, Mell LK, Schomas DA, et al: Concurrent chemotherapy and intensity-modulated radiation therapy for anal canal cancer patients: A multicenter experience. J Clin Oncol 25:4581–4586, 2007.

Vuong T, Kopek N, Ducruet T, et al: Conformal therapy improves the therapeutic index of patients with anal canal cancer treated with combined chemotherapy and external beam radiotherapy. Int J Radiat Oncol Biol Phys 67:1394–1400, 2007.

Abbreviations in this chapter

AAMCTC = AIDS Associated Malignancies Clinical Trials Consortium; ACOSOG = American College of Surgeons Oncology Group; ACS = American Cancer Society; AJCC = American Joint Committee on Cancer; CALGB = Cancer and Leukemia Group B; ECOG = Eastern Cooperative Oncology Group; GITSG = Gastrointestinal Tumor Study Group; GRCSG = German Rectal Cancer Study Group; NCCN = National Comprehensive Cancer Network; NCCTG = North Central Cancer Treatment Group; NSABP = National Surgical Adjuvant Breast and Bowel Project; RTOG = Radiation Therapy Oncology Group; UICC = International Union Against Cancer

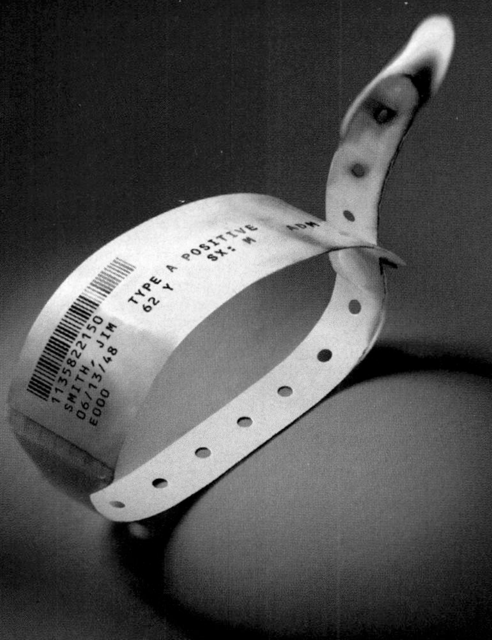

Help reduce the risk of infection in patients receiving moderate-risk* chemotherapy regimens

Act before febrile neutropenia strikes

Potential consequences of febrile neutropenia may be serious and can impact patient care

First- and every-cycle Neulasta® achieved:

- **94% reduction in febrile neutropenia (17% placebo vs 1% Neulasta®; $P < 0.001$).[1,2]**
- **93% reduction in febrile neutropenia–related hospitalization (14% placebo vs 1% Neulasta®; $P < 0.001$).[1,2]**
- **80% reduction in febrile neutropenia–related IV anti-infective use (10% placebo vs 2% Neulasta®; $P < 0.001$).[1,2]**

Neulasta® (pegfilgrastim) is indicated to decrease the incidence of infection, as manifested by febrile neutropenia, in patients with nonmyeloid malignancies receiving myelosuppressive anti-cancer drugs associated with a clinically significant incidence of febrile neutropenia.

Neulasta® is not indicated for the mobilization of peripheral blood progenitor cells for hematopoietic stem cell transplantation.

Important Safety Information

Do not administer Neulasta® to patients with a history of serious allergic reactions to pegfilgrastim or filgrastim.

Splenic rupture, including fatal cases, can occur following the administration of Neulasta®. Evaluate for an enlarged spleen or splenic rupture in patients who report left upper abdominal or shoulder pain after receiving Neulasta®.

Acute respiratory distress syndrome (ARDS) can occur in patients receiving Neulasta®. Evaluate patients who develop fever and lung infiltrates or respiratory distress after receiving Neulasta® for ARDS. Discontinue Neulasta® in patients with ARDS.

Serious allergic reactions, including anaphylaxis, can occur in patients receiving Neulasta®. The majority of reported events occurred upon initial exposure. Allergic reactions, including anaphylaxis, can recur within days after the discontinuation of initial anti-allergic treatment. Permanently discontinue Neulasta® in patients with serious allergic reactions.

Severe sickle cell crises can occur in patients with sickle cell disorders receiving Neulasta®. Severe and sometimes fatal sickle cell crises can occur in patients with sickle cell disorders receiving filgrastim, the parent compound of pegfilgrastim.

The granulocyte colony-stimulating factor (G-CSF) receptor, through which pegfilgrastim and filgrastim act, has been found on tumor cell lines. The possibility that pegfilgrastim acts as a growth factor for any tumor type, including myeloid malignancies and myelodysplasia, diseases for which pegfilgrastim is not approved, cannot be excluded.

Bone pain and pain in extremity occurred at a higher incidence in Neulasta®-treated patients as compared with placebo-treated patients.

Please see brief summary of Neulasta® Prescribing Information on adjacent pages.

***Regimens associated with ≥ 17% risk of febrile neutropenia.**

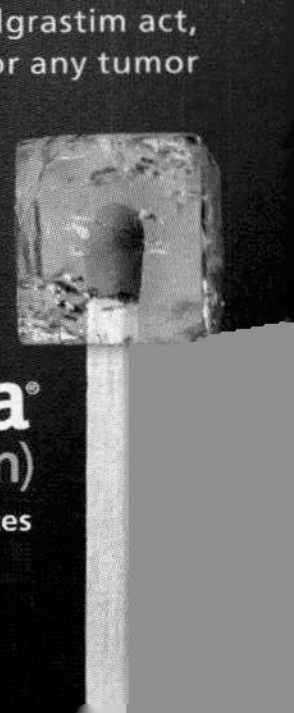

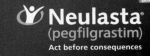

Neulasta®
(pegfilgrastim)
Act before consequences

References: 1. Vogel C, et al. *J Clin Oncol.* 2005;23:1178-1184. **2.** Neulasta® (pegfilgrastim) Prescribing Information. Thousand Oaks, Calif: Amgen.

in the 12–21 years age group (n = 13) and 47.9 (±22.5) mcg·hr/mL in the youngest age group (0–5 years, n = 11). The terminal elimination half-lives of the corresponding age groups were 20.2 (±11.3) hours, 21.2 (±16.0) hours and 30.1 (±38.2) hours, respectively. The most common adverse reaction was bone pain.

The 6 mg fixed dose single-use syringe formulation should not be used in infants, children, and smaller adolescents weighing less than 45 kg.

Geriatric Use

Of the 932 patients with cancer who received Neulasta in clinical studies, 139 (15%) were age 65 and over, and 18 (2%) were age 75 and over. No overall differences in safety or effectiveness were observed between patients age 65 and older and younger patients.

ADVERSE REACTIONS

(See **WARNINGS**, **Splenic Rupture**, **Acute Respiratory Distress Syndrome (ARDS)**, **Allergic Reactions**, and **Sickle Cell Disorders**.)

Clinical Trial Experience

Because clinical trials are conducted under widely varying conditions, adverse reaction rates observed in the clinical trials of Neulasta cannot be directly compared to rates in the clinical trials of other drugs and may not reflect the rates observed in practice. The adverse reaction information from clinical trials does, however, provide a basis for identifying the adverse events that appear to be related to Neulasta use and for approximating rates.

The data described below reflect exposure to Neulasta in 932 patients. Neulasta was studied in placebo- and active-controlled trials (n = 467, and n = 465, respectively). The population encompassed an age range of 21 to 88 years. Ninety-two percent of patients were female. The ethnicity of the patients was as follows: 75% Caucasian, 18% Hispanic, 5% Black, and 1% Asian. Patients with solid tumors (breast [n = 823], lung and thoracic tumors [n = 53]) or lymphoma (n = 56) received Neulasta after nonmyeloablative cytotoxic chemotherapy. Most patients received a single 100 mcg/kg (n = 259) or a single 6 mg (n = 546) dose per chemotherapy cycle over 4 cycles.

In the placebo-controlled trial, bone pain occurred at a higher incidence in Neulasta-treated patients as compared to placebo-treated patients. The incidence of other commonly reported adverse events were similar in the Neulasta- and placebo-treated patients, and were consistent with the underlying cancer diagnosis and its treatment with chemotherapy. The data in Table 1 reflect those adverse events occurring in at least 10% of patients treated with Neulasta in the placebo-controlled study.

Table 1. Adverse Events Occurring in ≥10%[a] of Patients in the Placebo-Controlled Study

Event	Neulasta (n = 467)	Placebo (n = 461)
Alopecia	48%	47%
Bone Pain[b]	31%	26%
Diarrhea	29%	28%
Pyrexia (not including febrile neutropenia)	23%	22%
Myalgia	21%	18%
Headache	16%	14%
Arthralgia	16%	13%
Vomiting	13%	11%
Asthenia	13%	11%
Peripheral Edema	12%	10%
Constipation	10%	6%

[a]*Events occurring in ≥ 10% of Neulasta-treated patients and at a higher incidence as compared to placebo-treated patients*

[b]*Bone pain is limited to the specified adverse event term "bone pain"*

In the active controlled studies, common adverse events occurred at similar rates and severities in both treatment arms (Neulasta, n = 465; Filgrastim, n = 331). These adverse experiences occurred at rates between 72% and 15% and included: nausea, fatigue, alopecia, diarrhea, vomiting, constipation, fever, anorexia, skeletal pain, headache, taste perversion, dyspepsia, myalgia, insomnia, abdominal pain, arthralgia, generalized weakness, peripheral edema, dizziness, granulocytopenia, stomatitis, mucositis, and neutropenic fever.

Bone Pain

The analysis of bone pain described below is based on a composite analysis using multiple, related, adverse event terms.

In the placebo-controlled study, the incidence of bone pain was 57% in Neulasta-treated patients compared to 50% in placebo-treated patients. Bone pain was generally reported to be of mild-to-moderate severity.

Among patients experiencing bone pain, approximately 37% of Neulasta-and 31% of placebo-treated patients utilized non-narcotic analgesics and 10% of Neulasta- and 9% of placebo-treated patients utilized narcotic analgesics.

In the active-controlled studies, the use of non-narcotic and narcotic analgesics in association with bone pain was similar between Neulasta-and Filgrastim-treated patients. No patient withdrew from study due to bone pain.

Laboratory Abnormalities

In clinical studies, leukocytosis (WBC counts > 100 x 10^9/L) was observed in less than 1% of 932 patients with nonmyeloid malignancies receiving Neulasta. Leukocytosis was not associated with any adverse effects.

Immunogenicity

As with all therapeutic proteins, there is a potential for immunogenicity. Binding antibodies to pegfilgrastim were detected using a BIAcore assay. The approximate limit of detection for this assay is 500 ng/mL. Pre-existing binding antibodies were detected in approximately 6% (51/849) of patients with metastatic breast cancer. Four of 521 pegfilgrastim-treated subjects who were negative at baseline developed binding antibodies to pegfilgrastim following treatment. None of these 4 patients had evidence of neutralizing antibodies detected using a cell-based bioassay.

The detection of antibody formation is highly dependent on the sensitivity and specificity of the assay, and the observed incidence of antibody positivity in an assay may be influenced by several factors, including sample handling, concomitant medications, and underlying disease. Therefore, comparison of the incidence of antibodies to Neulasta with the incidence of antibodies to other products may be misleading.

Cytopenias resulting from a neutralizing antibody response to exogenous growth factors have been reported on rare occasions in patients treated with other recombinant growth factors. There is a theoretical possibility that an antibody directed against pegfilgrastim may cross-react with endogenous G-CSF, resulting in immune-mediated neutropenia. This has not been observed in clinical studies of Neulasta.

Postmarketing Experience

The following adverse reactions have been identified during postapproval of Neulasta. Because these reactions are reported voluntarily from a population of uncertain size, it is not always possible to reliably estimate their frequency or establish a causal relationship to drug exposure.

- splenic rupture (see **WARNINGS: Splenic Rupture**)
- acute respiratory distress syndrome (ARDS) (see **WARNINGS: Acute Respiratory Distress Syndrome**)
- allergic reactions (including anaphylaxis, skin rash, urticaria, erythema/flushing) (see **WARNINGS: Allergic Reactions**)
- sickle cell crisis (see **WARNINGS: Sickle Cell Disorders**)
- injection site pain
- Sweet's syndrome (acute febrile dermatosis)

OVERDOSAGE

The maximum amount of Neulasta that can be safely administered in single or multiple doses has not been determined. Single subcutaneous doses of 300 mcg/kg have been administered to 8 healthy volunteers and 3 patients with non-small cell lung cancer without serious adverse effects. These patients experienced a mean maximum ANC of 55 x 10^9/L, with a corresponding mean maximum WBC of 67 x 10^9/L. The absolute maximum ANC observed was 96 x 10^9/L with a corresponding absolute maximum WBC observed of 120 x 10^9/L. The duration of leukocytosis ranged from 6 to 13 days. Leukapheresis should be considered in the management of symptomatic individuals.

DOSAGE AND ADMINISTRATION

The recommended dosage of Neulasta is a single subcutaneous injection of 6 mg administered once per chemotherapy cycle. Neulasta should not be administered in the period between 14 days before and 24 hours after administration of cytotoxic chemotherapy (see **PRECAUTIONS**).

The 6 mg fixed-dose formulation should not be used in infants, children, and smaller adolescents weighing less than 45 kg.

No dosing adjustment is necessary for renal dysfunction.

Neulasta should be visually inspected for discoloration and particulate matter before administration. Neulasta should not be administered if discoloration or particulates are observed.

Rx Only

This product, its production, and/or its use may be covered by one or more US Patents, including US Patent Nos. 5,824,784; 4,810,643; 4,999,291; 5,582,823; 5,580,755, as well as other patents or patents pending.

REFERENCE

*Heil G, Hoelzer D, Sanz MA, et al. A randomized, double-blind, placebo-controlled, phase III study of Filgrastim in remission induction and consolidation therapy for adults with de novo Acute Myeloid Leukemia. *Blood.* 1997;90:4710-4718.

v.10 Issue Date: 11/2008

AMGEN®

Manufactured by:
Amgen Manufacturing, Limited,
a subsidiary of Amgen Inc.
One Amgen Center Drive
Thousand Oaks, CA 91320-1799

CHAPTER 14

Prostate cancer

Judd W. Moul, MD, FACS, Andrew J. Armstrong, MD, ScM, and
Joseph Lattanzi, MD

PROSTATE

Prostate cancer is the most common non-skin cancer and the second leading cause of cancer mortality in American men. Despite the fact that this cancer will be diagnosed in an estimated 217,730 American men in the year 2010 and will lead to the death of approximately 32,030 men, there is no universally agreed-upon strategic plan for its diagnosis and management. The estimated number of deaths increased from last year. However, the death rate per 100,000 people declined 2.4% per year from 2000–2006, and the demoninator (aging population) grew, so the overall rate of death is lower.

EPIDEMIOLOGY

Age The risk of developing prostate cancer begins to increase at age 50 years in white men who have no family history of the disease and at age 40 years in black men and those who have a first-degree relative (father, brother) with prostate cancer. Risk increases with age, but, unlike other cancers, prostate cancer has no "peak" age or modal distribution. There has been a downward "age migration" in the PSA (prostate-specific antigen) era such that the median age at diagnosis is now approximately 60 years old.

Race The highest incidence of prostate cancer in the world is found in American black men, who have approximately a 9.8% lifetime risk of developing this cancer. This rate is slightly higher than the 8% lifetime risk for American white men. Black men have an incidence of prostate cancer that is 1.6 times that of white men.

The Japanese and mainland Chinese populations have the lowest rates of prostate cancer. Interestingly, although Japanese immigrants to the United States have a higher incidence of prostate cancer than Japanese people living in Japan, their rate is still about half that of American whites.

Socioeconomic status appears to be unrelated to the risk of prostate cancer, and the explanation for racial variability is unknown. However, an interplay of diet, hormonal factors, and genetics likely accounts for the variability.

Geography The incidence of prostate cancer is highest in Scandinavian countries (22 cases per 100,000 population) and lowest in Asia (5 per 100,000). Risk may be inversely related to ultraviolet light exposure, as the incidence increases the farther one lives from the equator. However, studies show extremely high rates of prostate cancer in populations of African heritage, such as Jamaicans.

ETIOLOGY AND RISK FACTORS

Family history Men who have a first-degree relative with prostate cancer have approximately a twofold increased risk of developing prostate cancer during their lifetime. An individual who has two first-degree relatives with prostate cancer has a ninefold increase in lifetime risk.

PROSTATE

True hereditary prostate cancer occurs in a small number of men and tends to develop at an early age (< 55 years old).

Dietary fat Although early studies suggested a link between dietary fat and prostate cancer risk, more recent studies have failed to confirm these observations. Thus, the relationship between dietary fat and prostate cancer risk remains unclear. Using animal models, one study pointed to high levels of simple carbohydrates being a culprit in promoting prostate cancer growth.

Studies indicate that progression of prostate cancer, which is likely to be more clinically relevant, has different risk factors from those associated with its initiation/incidence and that some of these risk factors are likely modifiable. Findings from the Health Professionals Follow-up study have, however, demonstrated different dietary risk factors for the incidence compared with progression of prostate cancer. For example, African-American race, a positive family history, low consumption of tomato products, and high consumption of alpha-linolenic acid have been associated with higher risks of incident prostate cancer. However, height, body mass index, low physical activity, smoking, low consumption of tomato sauce, high calcium and alpha-linolenic acid intake, African-American race, and positive family history have all been associated with more advanced cancer.

In addition, findings suggest that cruciferous or brassica family vegetables may reduce the risk of advanced prostate cancer. This family includes broccoli, cauliflower, cole slaw, and sauerkraut. Interestingly, the intake of brussels sprouts, spinach, and mustard greens did not appear to be protective, and the consumption of fruit was not associated with the incidence or progression of prostate cancer.

Vasectomy Several large epidemiologic studies suggest that vasectomy may increase the relative risk of prostate cancer by as much as 1.85. However, these same studies do not report an increased risk of dying from prostate cancer associated with vasectomy but do indicate a statistically increased risk of dying from lung cancer. These findings argue against an association between vasectomy and prostate cancer. Currently, this association is unproven and does not constitute grounds for fundamental changes in the use of vasectomy.

> Recent data are emerging about the potential role of a novel retrovirus, termed xenotropic murine leukemia virus–related virus (XMRV). Initial studies found that this virus expression in the prostate was linked only to patients with an uncommon predisposing genetic variant of hereditary prostate cancer due to deficiencies in interferon response (*RNASEL* polymorphism), but recent reports have identified viral DNA or protein in sporadic higher-grade tumors and have even linked detection of this virus (controversially) to chronic fatigue–like syndromes. Further validation of this work is required before a viral etiology to aggressive prostate cancer is established (*Schlaberg R et al: Proc Natl Acad Sci U S A 106:16351–16356, 2009*).

Sexual activity/sexually transmitted disease A large prospective study of more than 29,000 men demonstrated an association between high ejaculatory frequency (more than 21 ejaculations/month) and a decreased risk of prostate cancer, with a lifetime relative risk of 0.67. However, there may be several confounding factors associated with high sexual activity, such as differences in prostate cancer screening or lifestyle. There was no associated increased risk for men in the lowest ejaculatory frequency category.

Inflammation may underlie the findings associated with a relatively higher risk of prostate cancer in men seen in STD (sexually transmitted disease) clinics, but it may also be related to screening bias. Several cohort studies and one meta-analysis have demonstrated a protective role for the daily intake of aspirin and the risk of prostate cancer. In addition, the lipid-lowering and anti-inflammatory statin compounds have been associated with a reduction in the risk of high-grade tumors. These findings require prospective validation in randomized trials.

Prevention Active research on the chemoprevention of prostate cancer is ongoing. Two prospective randomized trials have demonstrated a 20% to 25% reduction in the risk of prostate cancer among men who were randomized to receive either finasteride or dutasteride (Avodart) daily vs those men on the placebo arm. Finasteride or dutasteride chemopreventive agents have not been universally accepted, however, because of concerns over the relative merits of prevention of low-grade disease, with little effect on high-grade tumors. In addition, concerns over side effects such as impotence, as well as reductions in PSA levels with these therapies that may make cancer detection more challenging, have limited the generalized use of these drugs and thus an individualized risk/benefit discussion about use of these agents as preventive measures is recommended. Finally, randomized trials using selenium and vitamin E have failed to demonstrate a benefit of these agents to reduce prostate cancer risk. Ongoing studies will examine vitamin D and omega-3 fatty acid supplementation as preventive strategies in cancer, including prostate cancer.

Andriole and colleagues recently reported on a long-term prostate cancer prevention study with dutasteride (Avodart, a dual 5-alpha-reductase inhibitor), in men with an elevated PSA level and a negative initial biopsy. They demonstrated a 22.8% relative risk reduction overall in prostate cancer incidence (5.1% absolute risk), although the for-cause rate of biopsies (ie, not protocol-specified) was not different between the two arms. There was an apparent greater reduction in this trial of low-grade (Gleason < 7) tumors, and no major effect in preventing higher-grade tumors, with a higher percentage of Gleason 8–10 tumors detected in the dutasteride arm in years 3 to 4. Dutasteride is known to reduce PSA levels by more than twofold, and its use in prevention should take into account consideration of risk and uncertainty around the benefits, appropriate surveillance strategies while on a dihydrotestosterone inhibitor, and side effects (including erectile/sexual dysfunction; *Andriole GL et al: N Engl J Med 362:1192–1202, 2010).*

SIGNS AND SYMPTOMS

Early-stage disease Men with organ-confined prostate cancer often are completely asymptomatic, given the predominant posterior peripheral zone location of prostate adenocarcinomas. Men with a large component of benign prostatic hyperplasia often present with bladder outlet obstruction unrelated to prostate cancer.

Locally advanced disease Bladder outlet obstruction is the most common sign of locally advanced prostate cancer. A few men with locally advanced disease present with hematuria, urinary tract infections, and irritative voiding symptoms secondary to bladder outlet obstruction.

Advanced disease Rarely, men with bulky lymph node metastasis may present with bilateral lower-extremity edema. Men with bony metastasis often present with bone pain and, uncommonly, with lower-extremity weakness or paralysis from spinal cord compression.

SCREENING AND DIAGNOSIS

Prostate cancer screening with PSA levels and digital rectal examination (DRE) has resulted in not only an increase in prostate cancer detection but also a stage shift. More cancers are now being detected at earlier stages, when they are potentially curable. Prior to screening efforts, most prostate cancers were detected when they produced local symptoms or distant metastases, at which point treatment for cure often was impossible.

DRE Prostate biopsy prompted by abnormal findings on DRE, such as nodularity or induration of the prostate, leads to a diagnosis of prostate cancer in only 15% to 25% of cases. This rate compares with a prostate cancer prevalence of < 5% among men of similar age without an abnormal DRE. Although neither accurate nor sensitive for prostate cancer detection, abnormal DRE is associated with a fivefold increased risk of cancer present at the time of screening.

PSA is a serine protease produced by the prostatic epithelium and secreted in the seminal fluid in large quantities. The level of PSA in serum is increased by inflammation of the prostate, urinary retention, prostatic infection, benign prostatic hyperplasia, prostate cancer, and prostatic manipulation. The optimal threshold to recommend prostatic biopsy has come under increasing scrutiny. The overall sensitivity for PSA levels is approximately 50% to 70% depending on the threshold used, but it is not as specific and does not allow for differentiation between indolent and aggressive disease.

Two large randomized multisite trials examined the role of PSA screening in US and European populations over time. In the PLCO trial, nearly 77,000 US men were randomized to annual PSA and DRE screening or to standard practice (which included PSA screening in men). After 7 years of follow-up, prostate cancer was more commonly detected in screened men, but fatal disease was not detectably different. In contrast, in the European study, named ERSPC, 182,000 men in various countries were assigned to PSA screening at various intervals or to no screening. Contamination seemed to be less common in the control group in this study, and at 9 years' median follow-up, a 20% reduction in prostate cancer mortality was noted. In this study, nearly twice as many screened men were diagnosed with prostate cancer. The number needed to screen in this study to save one prostate cancer death was 1,410, and the number needed to treat with local therapy was 48. Data from the PCPT illustrate that there is no "normal" level for PSA. Indeed, there is a continuum of risk that exists, even at low levels of PSA. For example, among men in the placebo arm of the study, 11% of men with a serum PSA level < 1 ng/mL had prostate cancer at the end-of-study biopsy. The proportion of men with prostate cancer rose to 30% among those with PSA levels between 3.1 and 4.0 ng/mL, which is still within the "normal" range. Furthermore, with a median follow-up of 9 years, the cancer-specific survival rate was improved by 20% in the screening group vs controls. However, they report an overdetection of small, nonlethal cancers.

Using a baseline PSA value to risk-stratify young men for their future risk of prostate cancer is increasingly recognized as clinically useful by both the NCCN and AUA guidelines. Tang et al studied over 9,500 men aged 50 or younger showing that a baseline PSA of 1.5 to 2.4 ng/mL increased the relative risk for prostate cancer by 9.3 for white men and 6-7-fold for black men. Overall, a PSA > 1.5 was a powerful predictor of subsequent prostate cancer *(Tang P et al: J Urol 183:946–950, 2010)*.

An additional potentially more worthwhile approach for PSA screening may be to use the rate of rise in PSA (PSA velocity) in combination with the absolute PSA value. This approach has been shown to be useful in the form of age-adjusted PSA velocity, but accepted guidelines are still controversial, and the independent predictive utility of this measure remains to be demonstrated.

Another commonly employed test for patients with a PSA level < 10 ng/mL is the percent-free PSA level. There is an inverse relationship between the percent-free PSA level and the risk of a cancer diagnosis. Most urologists utilize a cutoff of 10% to prompt a recommendation for a repeat biopsy. In men who have never had a prostate biopsy but who have a total PSA level > 4.0 ng/mL, a percent-free PSA less than 25% may suggest a 50% to 60% probability of prostate cancer. In men who have had a prior negative biopsy but who have a persistently elevated PSA level > 4.0 ng/mL, a percent-free PSA < 10% should prompt a repeat biopsy.

Current screening recommendations There remains significant controversy as to the wisdom and effectiveness of PSA screening for the general male population. This is exemplified in recent updates to both the AUA and ACS guidelines for 2010. The AUA took a more "proactive" stance by recommending that all men consider having a baseline PSA test at age 40. This guideline is useful to risk-stratify men to future testing frequency. If at age 40 the PSA level is less than 1.0 ng/mL, the man can be reassured that he is at low risk and will be asked to return at age 45 for retesting. However, men who have a baseline PSA level greater than or equal to 1.0 ng/mL are at greater future risk and need annual surveillance. For young men between age 40 and 49 (and perhaps 50 and 59), a PSA level that rises to 2.5 ng/mL or higher should prompt urologic referral for consideration of prostate biopsy. PSA velocity of 0.25 to 0.50 ng/mL/year also would prompt concern in younger men. At age 50, annual testing is recommended.

On the other hand, the ACS took a more cautious stance with its 2010 update. The ACS is now de-emphasizing mass screening programs, while emphasizing a discussion of the pros and cons of testing with PSA levels based on individualized risk. The NCCN has also adapted an individualized risk assessment and informed discussion with patients about the pros and cons of screening, to begin in the 40s for high-risk men, and at 50 for men of average risk. Readers should refer to acs.org or nccn.org for updates of these guidelines.

Using data from the Shared Equal Access Regional Cancer Hospital, the Duke Prostate Center, and Johns Hopkins Hospital, investigators concluded that higher body mass index was significantly associated with higher plasma volume and lower PSA concentrations in men undergoing radical prostatectomy. Hemodilution may therefore be responsible for the lower serum PSA concentrations among obese men with prostate cancer. While obese men may be less likely to be diagnosed with incident prostate cancer, they are, however, more likely to have aggressive disease at presentation, and more likely to suffer relapse and prostate cancer–specific mortality.

Biopsy When indicated, prostate biopsy is usually performed as an office procedure by transrectal ultrasonographic guidance using an automated 18-gauge biopsy gun. The procedure is performed with, at most, local anesthesia and carries a risk of significant infection of only 1 in 200 cases. Additional side effects of hematuria and hematochezia are common for 2 to 3 days following the biopsy. Hematospermia may last for up to 4 to 6 weeks. Since about the year 2000, prostate biopsy includes laterally directed extended core protocols employing 8 to 20 biopsy cores per procedure. Multiple studies have demonstrated that the addition of the lateral cores improves the accuracy of biopsy.

If the biopsy result is negative, these men are typically followed conservatively with serial PSA levels and DRE repeated annually. Repeat biopsy is performed only when PSA levels rise at abnormal rates (> 0.8 ng/mL/year) or if DRE findings show new nodularity or induration. Men in whom high-grade prostatic intraepithelial neoplasia or atypical small acinar proliferation (ASAP) found on biopsy usually should undergo repeat biopsy, since one-third to one-half will be found to have prostate cancer. Recently, the recommendation of repeat biopsy for PIN alone has been relaxed, such that repeat biopsy may not be recommended and a more personalized approach to follow-up is taken.

A new urine test called PCA-3, has become more widely available. This test, performed on voided urine after an "attentive" DRE, is based on reverse transcriptase–polymerase chain reaction assay for a prostate-specific gene (*DD3*). It is becoming useful not as a primary screening test, but to dictate the need for repeat prostate biopsy in men with persistently elevated PSA levels.

In addition, researchers at Johns Hopkins University have developed a blood-based test called EPCA-2, which detects a nuclear matrix protein linked to prostate cancer. Elevated levels of EPCA-2 were found to be more sensitive and specific for prostate cancer, even in men with normal PSA levels and benign prostatic hypertrophy, and predicted extracapsular disease as well. Further validation of this test in larger cohorts of screened men is necessary. Currently, this test is being further optimized and validated in a large series of patients. Additional studies are investigating the role of a novel fusion protein (TMPRSS2-ETS) commonly found in prostate tumors, both as a diagnostic and prognostic marker. This fusion gene is androgen regulated, directs oncogenic signals, and has been found in over 50% of localized prostate cancers. Other markers will need to be employed to detect the 50% of tumors that lack this fusion protein before this test is likely to be useful as a screening tool.

PATHOLOGY

Adenocarcinomas make up the vast majority of prostate carcinomas. A total of 70% of prostate adenocarcinomas occur in the peripheral zone, 20% in the transitional zone, and approximately 10% in the central zone.

Other tumor types are relatively rare and include ductal adenocarcinoma, which occurs in the major ducts and often projects into the urethra; and mucinous adenocarcinoma, which secretes abundant mucin and does not arise from the major ducts. Transitional carcinoma of the prostate occurs within the ducts and, to a lesser extent, in the prostatic acini. Typically, primary transitional carcinomas are aggressive cancers that have a poor prognosis. Similarly, neuroendocrine (small-cell) tumors are rare and aggressive, have a poor prognosis, and typically require aggressive surgical management. Other rare types include foamy carcinoma, mucinous adenocarcinoma, large-cell neuroendocrine tumors, and signet ring tumors.

Histologic grade The grading system developed by Gleason from data accumulated by the Veterans Administration Cooperative Urologic Research Group appears to provide the best prognostic information in addition to clinical stage and is the predominant grading system in widespread use.

Metastatic spread Adenocarcinoma of the prostate may spread locally through direct extension into periprostatic fat or via the ejaculatory ducts into seminal vesicles; lymphatically to regional lymph nodes, including the hypogastric and obturator lymph nodes; and hematogeneously to bone. The most common sites of bony metastases are the lumbosacral spine (probably related to venous drainage of the prostate through Batson's plexus) and the axial skeleton, but any bone, including the skull and ribs, can be involved. Rare sites of metastatic spread include the liver and lungs.

PROGNOSIS AND NATURAL HISTORY

Staging systems The most widely used and universally accepted staging system for prostate cancer is the TNM system (Table 1). In the TNM system, T1 and T2 tumors are confined to the gland, whereas T3 and T4 tumors have local extension.

In 2010, the AJCC updated prostate cancer staging recommendations in its 7th edition of the AJCC Cancer Staging Manual. These guidelines incorporate a more risk-based approach that utilizes the Gleason grading system and current PSA value in the staging system, which brings this system more in line with the risk-adapted approaches described in this chapter. Additionally, microscopic bladder neck invasion as a form of extracapsular extension was incorporated into T3 disease rather than as T4, given the more favorable outcomes of this subgroup of men. This scoring system is shown in Table 2. Use of either this staging system or the NCCN/D'Amico approach, or a nomogram-based risk assessment will provide a more accurate prognostic classification system for prostate cancer at initial diagnosis.

Risk-adapted staging The development of the "Partin Tables" in 1993 ushered in a new era of combining clinical stage, Gleason score, and PSA level to predict pathologic stage after radical prostatectomy. More recently, this has led to the D'Amico et al risk groupings for newly diagnosed men with clinically localized disease (Table 3). Patients are divided into three risk groups (low, intermediate, or high) of occult

TABLE 1: 2002 TNM staging system of prostate cancer

Localized disease	
T1a	Tumor incidental histologic finding in ≤ 5% of resected tissue; not palpable
T1b	Tumor incidental histologic finding in > 5% of resected tissue
T1c	Tumor identified by needle biopsy (eg, because of elevated PSA level)
T2a	Tumor involves one-half of one lobe or less
T2b	Tumor involves more than one-half of one lobe but not both lobes
T2c	Tumor involves both lobes
Local extension	
T3a	Extracapsular extension (unilateral or bilateral)
T3b	Tumor invades seminal vesicle(s)
T4	Bladder invasion, fixed to pelvic side wall, or invasion of adjacent structures
Metastatic disease	
N1	Positive regional lymph nodes
M1	Distant metastasis

PSA = prostate-specific antigen
Adapted from Greene FL, Page DL, Fleming ID, et al (eds): AJCC Cancer Staging Manual, 6th ed. New York, Springer-Verlag, 2002.

TABLE 2: TNM staging system of prostate cancer, 2010 updates[a]

Anatomic Stage/Prognostic Groups

GROUP	T	N	M	PSA	Gleason
Stage I	T1a–c	N0	M0	PSA < 10	Gleason ≤ 6
	T2a	N0	M0	PSA < 10	Gleason ≤ 6
	T1–2a	N0	M0	PSA X	Gleason X
Stage IIA	T1a–c	N0	M0	PSA < 20	Gleason 7
	T1a–c	N0	M0	PSA ≥ 10 < 20	Gleason ≤ 6
	T2a	N0	M0	PSA < 20	Gleason ≤ 7
	T2b	N0	M0	PSA < 20	Gleason ≤ 7
	T2b	N0	M0	PSA X	Gleason X
Stage IIB	T2c	N0	M0	Any PSA	Any Gleason
	T1–2	N0	M0	PSA ≥ 20	Any Gleason
	T1–2	N0	M0	Any PSA	Gleason ≥ 8
Stage III	T3a–b	N0	M0	Any PSA	Any Gleason
Stage IV	T4	N0	M0	Any PSA	Any Gleason
	Any T	N1	M0	Any PSA	Any Gleason
	Any T	Any N	M1	Any PSA	Any Gleason

From Edge SB, Byrd DR, Compton CC, et al (eds): AJCC Cancer Staging Manual, 7th ed. New York, Springer, 2010.
[a]When either PSA or Gleason is not available, grouping should be determined by T stage and/or either PSA or Gleason as available.

TABLE 3: D'Amico et al risk stratification for clinically localized prostate cancer

Low risk	Diagnostic PSA < 10.0 ng/mL *and* highest biopsy Gleason score ≤ 6 *and* clinical stage T1c or T2a
Intermediate risk	Diagnostic PSA ≥ 10 but < 20 ng/mL *or* highest biopsy Gleason score = 7 *or* clinical stage T2b
High risk	Diagnostic PSA ≥ 20 ng/mL *or* highest biopsy Gleason score ≥ 8 *or* clinical stage T2c/T3

PSA = prostate-specific antigen

micrometastases and relapse after initial local therapy. Although not perfect, this system is currently in widespread use and allows a framework for multimodal and multidisciplinary treatment strategies based on risk grouping. Kattan et al have developed preoperative and postoperative nomograms as clinical tools to predict the risk of recurrence after radical prostatectomy. Although these nomograms are imperfect, they may be useful for estimating risk and planning therapy as well as for stratifying and selecting patients for clinical trials. In addition, Stephenson et al have developed a fairly robust postsurgical nomogram of over 12,000 men that is able to predict with > 80% accuracy 15-year prostate cancer-specific mortality. In this model, Gleason sum, PSA level, and clinical stage were the most important factors in predicting long-term outcome, whereas body mass index and PSA velocity were not able to add to the predictive accuracy of the model.

According to the 2010 Guidelines, the NCCN defines as a "very low" risk group men with prostate cancer who have low volume using the Epstein criteria (T1c stage, Gleason < 7, PSA level < 10 ng/mL, fewer than three positive biopsy cores, < 50% cancer in each core, and PSA density < 0.15 ng/mL/g). These patients have a very low risk of prostate cancer death within 10 to 20 years and could be considered good candidates for active surveillance. These criteria are imperfect (eg, as discussed in a 2008 nomogram analysis reported in *Cancer* by FK Chun and colleagues), and current efforts to improve upon them using nomograms may better help to select men who can safely defer initial aggressive therapy.

Prognosis The optimal management of patients with prostate cancer varies widely and is highly dependent upon a patient's age, overall health, and tumor risk assessment. The natural history of the disease process can be heterogeneous, ranging from an incidental finding unlikely to result in cancer-specific mortality to very aggressive, resulting in early widespread metastatic disease and death. Therefore, treating physicians should carefully consider the value of curative therapy with potential toxicity in the context of a patient's comorbidities and life expectancy.

TABLE 4: Risk of dying of clinically localized prostate cancer without definitive locoregional therapy

	Age			
Gleason score	**55–59**	**60–64**	**65–69**	**70–74**
2–4	4%	5%	6%	7%
5	6%	8%	10%	11%
6	18%	23%	27%	30%
7	70%	62%	53%	42%
8–10	87%	81%	72%	60%

Adapted from Albertsen PC, Hanley JA, Fine J: JAMA 293:2095–2101, 2005.

Recent studies have incorporated baseline function into the quality-of-life assessment and outcomes associated with radical surgery or radiation therapy. This allows for a more precise and detailed individual assessment of the long-term urinary, sexual, and gastrointestinal side effects of local therapies *(Chen RC et al: J Clin Oncol 27:3916–3922, 2009).*

Among patients with clinically localized prostate cancer treated conservatively (observation or hormonal therapy alone), those with a low Gleason score (2–4) have a small risk of dying of their cancer within 15 years (4% to 7%). However, those with poorly differentiated tumors (Gleason score 8 to 10) have a greater risk of dying of prostate cancer than of any other cause, even when the cancer is diagnosed in the eighth decade of life. Indeed, a man diagnosed before the age of 60 with a clinically localized, Gleason score 8 to 10 prostate cancer has an 87% risk of dying of the disease within 15 years if untreated (Table 4).

D'Amico et al combined a number of national datasets to report 10-year cancer-specific mortality rates for men undergoing radical prostatectomy or external-beam radiotherapy (EBRT) by this risk grouping and age at diagnosis. These 10-year mortality graphs are useful to counsel contemporary-era men contemplating surgery or radiation therapy. Given recent advances in the treatment of metastatic disease, identifying men at high risk for metastatic disease following local therapy is important, as these agents are incorporated earlier in the disease course.

TREATMENT OF LOCALIZED PROSTATE CANCER

There are several treatment options for localized prostate cancer, including radical prostatectomy, EBRT, brachytherapy (interstitial radiation/seeds), and cryotherapy. Multiple treatment series with each modality have documented the validity of the risk-stratification model based on clinical palpation stage, Gleason score, and serum PSA level. More recently, it has been suggested that biopsy quantification may also be an important factor. Specifically, counting the number of involved needle biopsy cores or the percentage of each core involved by cancer may be prognostic. Low-risk patients experience a favorable 85% to 90% freedom from recurrence, compared with approximately 75% and 35% to 50% for the intermediate- and high-risk patients, respectively. Although no randomized studies have been performed, contemporary series, which stratify patients by the risk model, demonstrate remarkably similar outcomes independent of the treatment modality. For this reason, treatment recommendations should be individualized based on patient preference, life expectancy, and discussion of potential toxicities.

TREATMENT OF CLINICALLY LOCALIZED DISEASE (T1, T2)

Active Surveillance

Active surveillance in very low– to low-risk patients who have a limited life expectancy (< 10 to 15 years) also is emerging as an important initial treatment modality. Ongoing studies (CALGB/NCIC START study) are examining the necessity of immediate vs deferred active definitive therapy. However, at this time, the majority of men in the United States receive initial radical surgery or radiation as treatment of localized prostate cancer.

This is fast becoming an initial treatment selection of low and very low–risk men (Gleason score of 6 or less, low volume, PSA level < 10, ng/mL T1c disease). Most studies have suggested a less than 5% to 10% prostate cancer-specific mortality rate for men in this category who choose initial deferred therapy, particularly those men with slow PSA doubling times (< 3 years). In these men, nonprostate cancer–specific mortality far outweighs prostate cancer–specific mortality, illustrating the need to assess age, comorbidities, and life expectancy in the initial treatment decisions of a man with prostate cancer. Approximately 25% to 30% of men will progress during this period and require definitive therapy, and this time, it is not known whether deferred active therapy results in inferior outcomes for these men compared with immediate therapy.

Radical prostatectomy

Radical prostatectomy can be performed retropubically through a lower midline incision—an approach that may include pelvic lymph node dissection. Robotic-assisted laparoscopic prostatectomy (RALP) is now the most popular form of radical prostatectomy in the United States. Radical perineal prostatectomy is uncommon but remains a viable option.

Although the morbidity of radical prostatectomy was a major concern in the past, improvements were made during the 1980s. Among the various treatment options for prostate cancer, only radical prostatectomy has been demonstrated to confer a survival advantage over no treatment. After a median of 8.2 years of follow-up, Bill-Axelson and colleagues found a 35% reduction in the risk of death and of metastases among men randomized to undergo radical prostatectomy compared with those randomized to undergo watchful waiting. The benefits of surgery appear to plateau at 10 years. The hazards of anesthesia, risk of blood loss, and hospital stay have all been minimized. Nationwide, Medicare data suggest that surgical outcomes are significantly better at those centers performing > 40 prostatectomies per year than at other hospitals with a lower surgical volume.

Transfusion is usually unnecessary, and treatment-related mortality is < 0.05% at leading prostate cancer centers. The average hospital stay of a man undergoing radical prostatectomy is now approximately 1 to 2 days at leading referral centers in the United States; several institutions routinely discharge patients within 24 hours. Although urinary incontinence is common in the first few months after prostatectomy, most men recover urinary control; at some leading centers, 90% to 98% of men report few or no long-term urinary problems.

Nerve-sparing radical prostatectomy is appropriate for men with small-volume disease. It offers those men with good potency prior to surgery the probability of recovering that function following the operation. By permitting better visualization of Santorini's dorsal venous plexus, the apical prostate, the urethra, and the striated urethral sphincter, the nerve-sparing technique also reduces blood loss and improves recovery of urinary continence. In appropriately selected individuals, a nerve-sparing procedure confers no greater risk of prostate cancer recurrence after considering other relevant clinical information (PSA level, Gleason score, margin status, seminal vesicle involvement, and the presence of extraprostatic spread).

Referral centers have reported that 50% to 90% of patients who are fully potent prior to surgery recover erections following a nerve-sparing procedure, but the quality (rigidity and duration) of these recovered erections may be compromised compared with preoperative erections. Erection recovery rates can be higher than 80% in patients < 60 years of age and lower in older men. Potency may return anywhere from 2 to 24 months following surgery. Regardless of potency, sensation of the penis is not changed after this procedure, and men still experience orgasm. Nerve-sparing radical prostatectomy has not compromised cancer control outcomes in well-selected men with early-stage disease. Also, recent studies have suggested that early postoperative use of sildenafil, tadalafil (Cialis), vacuum erection device (VED), and/or intracavernosal injection (ICI) of vasoactive medications, such as papaverine, may facilitate the return of natural erections more quickly. Generally speaking, recovery of erectile function after radical prostatectomy is mediated by age (the younger, the better), pretreatment erectile function (the stronger, the better), and a nerve-sparing approach (bilateral is better than unilateral, which is better than none, which is better than wide dissection).

Robotic radical prostatectomy

A multi-institutional study of 431 men with pT3 prostate cancer were randomized to receive adjuvant radiation therapy or observation after prostatectomy. Patients who were given adjuvant radiation had a 28% and 29% lower risk of death and metastases, respectively *(Thompson IM et al: J Urol 181:956–962, 2009).*

Laparoscopic prostatectomy was initially described by Schuessler in 1997 but was abandoned because of its technical difficulty and long operative time with little apparent benefit over the conventional technique. A resurgence in the technique was prompted by improved instrumentation and refinements in the procedure itself, although the laparoscopically naive urologist must endure a substantial learning curve (with attendant perioperative morbidity) prior to meeting the outcome standards set by the open technique.

The RALP was developed to overcome some of the difficulties of the standard laparoscopic prostatectomy (eg, intracorporeal suturing). The robotic technique allows for three-dimensional (3D) visualization of the operative field and provides for a significantly wider range of movements intracorporeally than do standard laparoscopic instruments. This advance has prompted the assimilation of the technique into the armamentarium of many urologists.

Robot-assisted laparoscopic prostatectomy (RALP) has become very popular in the U.S. A recent systematic review by Murphy et al showed the learning curve to be steep and few published reports have reported outcomes in a standardized manner. The cost of the technology is substantial and little is known of the cost-effectiveness compared to the open technique (*Murphy DG et al: Eur Urol 57:735–745, 2010*).

Current evidence suggests that in experienced hands, the laparoscopic and robotic techniques have similar oncologic efficacy to that of the open procedure. However, the length of follow-up (usually < 24 months) in these studies is limited, suggesting that a measure of caution be taken when interpreting the results. Furthermore, recent studies suggest the learning curve is prolonged, with 200 to 250 cases necessary before results can be compared with those of experienced surgeons. Long-term effects of these modalities on sexual and urinary health (as measured by a psychometrically valid survey) have not been reported, and such data are critical in the context of the prostatectomy patient when evaluating technical results. Although vision with robotic prostatectomy is excellent, the current-generation robotic device does not allow tactile sensation for the operating surgeon. Furthermore, the vast majority of robotic prostatectomies are performed via a transabdominal approach, whereas the open retropubic approach avoids the peritoneal cavity.

Pelvic lymph node dissection Studies now indicate that regional pelvic lymph node dissection may not be necessary for patients with stage T1c disease if the total Gleason score is < 7 and the PSA level is < 10.0 ng/mL, ie, low-risk individuals. Selected intermediate-risk men may also not require this staging procedure, but in high-risk men, it is still considered imperative.

Neoadjuvant hormonal therapy

Approximately 15% to 35% of men who undergo radical prostatectomy for clinical stage T2 prostate cancer will be found to have pathologic T3 disease following surgery. This finding led some investigators to evaluate the efficacy of neoadjuvant androgen deprivation therapy in prospective clinical trials. Early data from these trials suggested that neoadjuvant hormonal therapy led to a reduction in positive surgical margins. However, these findings need to be considered in a technical context: Androgen deprivation therapy causes artifactual changes in prostate morphology that cause difficulties for the pathologic identification of prostate cancer foci.

Indeed, more recent data from prospective studies have shown no benefit of neoadjuvant therapy with regard to progression-free survival. At present, therefore, it appears that neoadjuvant hormonal therapy does not improve the curative potential of radical prostatectomy but instead is associated with morphologic alterations that complicate the prognostic utility of standard pathology. Neoadjuvant hormonal therapy is sometimes used for technical downsizing to facilitate surgical resectability. However, it is not routinely recommended to improve cancer control.

Adjuvant therapy post prostatectomy

The potential indications for adjuvant therapy following radical prostatectomy in patients with clinical T1 or T2 malignancy include pathologic evidence of T3 disease, positive nodes, a rising PSA level, and positive surgical margins, among others. Possible adjuvant treatments include radiation therapy and androgen deprivation either alone or in combination.

Radiation therapy Men with positive margins or pathologic T3 disease following radical prostatectomy are potential candidates for early adjuvant EBRT. Some controversy exists as to the efficacy of early postoperative therapy vs intervention once a biochemical failure has been documented in patients who achieve an undetectable PSA level following surgery.

Three randomized trials have been completed demonstrating a benefit to early adjuvant radiation therapy for men with positive margins, seminal vesicle invasion, or extracapsular extension. Typically, this treatment is offered after continence is restored to allow healing to take place after surgery. With a median follow-up of 12 years, the most mature study (SWOG 8794) by Thompson et al confirmed a significant improvement in the risk of metastasis (43% vs 54%) and overall survival (41% vs 52%) to adjuvant radiation. The largest trial, by Bolla et al (EORTC 22911), included 1,000 patients with T3 disease randomly assigned to 60 Gy vs observation. At 5 years, progression-free survival was significantly improved (74% vs 53%), with no demonstration of an overall survival benefit. A subsequent update suggested the benefit might be limited to patients with positive surgical margins. A German trial of nearly 400 patients also demonstrated a biochemical progression-free survival benefit (72% vs 54%) to early radiation therapy in this pT3 group. The benefit of therapy was observed with or without positive margins.

An alternate approach to early adjuvant radiation therapy is salvage radiation therapy for PSA recurrence. It remains unclear whether early salvage radiation based on PSA thresholds is inferior to the adjuvant approach but has the benefit of not treating all men with T3 disease with radiation. Of note, in the SWOG trial approximately one-third of patients initially assigned to observation ultimately received salvage radiation largely for PSA recurrence. In a retrospective analysis, there was a 5-year bNED (biochemical no evidence of disease, or undetectable PSA levels) advantage (77% vs 38%) to early vs salvage therapy. Based on this emerging evidence and a relatively low toxicity to radiation, the use of early adjuvant radiation in this high-risk group should be considered.

The use of salvage radiation after a PSA recurrence in the other patient groups should be based on the risk of having an isolated local/regional failure. Approximately 60% to 70% of patients with favorable disease after surgical failure (PSA level < 2.0 ng/mL, a slow PSA doubling time, and a long interval to failure after surgery) will experience durable disease-free survival after salvage radiotherapy, presumably due to a smaller tumor burden and a lower likelihood of occult metastatic disease.

Stephenson et al evaluated a large number of patients with salvage EBRT and persistent or increasing PSA levels after surgery from five American academic institutions. Forty-five percent of patients were free of disease at 4 years after salvage EBRT. Patients with no adverse risk features achieved a 4-year progression-free probability of 77%. The authors subsequently developed a nomogram based on established risk factors to more accurately identify patient-specific risks to assist in clinical decision-making. Patients who experience PSA failure after radical prostatectomy generally should be restaged with pelvic CT, bone scan, and DRE. Patients with no evidence of metastatic disease should be evaluated for radiotherapy.

Hormonal therapy Significant controversy exists within the academic community as to the timing of initiating androgen deprivation following radical prostatectomy. Clinical trials have documented a survival benefit only for those patients with nodal involvement.

Treatment recommendations for postprostatectomy recurrence

Following radical prostatectomy, it is expected that serial PSA levels will become undetectable. Any detectable PSA level (> 0.2 ng/mL) following surgery indicates possible recurrent disease and the need for restaging and possible salvage therapies, including radiation or hormonal therapy, experimental protocols, or observation. However, some patients can develop low levels of detectable PSA after prostatectomy without cancer recurrence, presumably due to small foci of benign prostate tissue in situ. Although there is concern for recurrence when the PSA level is > 0.2 ng/mL, most clinicians will wait until a PSA threshold > 0.4 ng/mL is reached to assume that the rise in PSA level represents meaningful recurrence.

Recent findings have suggested that tumor grade, time to PSA recurrence after surgery, and PSA doubling time predict the 5-, 10-, and 15-year risks of prostate cancer mortality and can help to guide the timing and need for androgen ablation. Although these findings do not prove that early androgen ablation is more beneficial than delayed androgen ablation based on a PSA threshold or development of metastatic disease, it does help to risk-stratify patients into those most likely to derive benefit from androgen ablation early. Moreover, men with a PSA doubling time of less than 15 months may be more likely to die of prostate cancer than of other competing causes, suggesting that these men should be evaluated in controlled trials of hormonal or novel therapeutic agents.

Definitive radiation therapy

EBRT utilizes high-energy photons to destroy cancer cells by damaging cellular DNA. Traditional EBRT utilized bony landmarks and standard-beam arrangements to deliver dose to the pelvic region. Technologic advances in treatment planning, driven by improved computing power and the incorporation of individualized patient anatomy, have led to dramatic improvements in treatment delivery.

3D conformal EBRT creates 3D representations of target structures (ie, the prostate) and designs highly tailored treatment portals utilizing various angles to create a volume of high radiation dose that conforms to the target shape. The anatomic information used to define the target is generally derived from CT images obtained while the patient is placed in an immobilization device in the precise treatment position. With the selective delivery of dose to the target and avoidance of the surrounding normal tissue, the therapeutic ratio is improved. This approach has permitted the use of doses far higher than tolerable with traditional therapy, with fewer bowel and bladder complications.

Treatment volumes in patients with low-risk disease are designed to encompass the prostate plus a margin for daily variations. Patients with a high risk for periprostatic extension and/or regional lymph node metastasis have historically received initial pelvic treatment of 45 to 50 Gy, followed by a coned-down boost to the prostate.

RTOG 9413 was designed to test the addition of whole pelvic radiation and the timing of androgen deprivation in the treatment of high-risk patients (lymph nod-positive potential > 15% or locally advanced [Gleason score ≥ 6 and > stage cT2c disease] cancers). At a median follow-up of 59.5 months, Roach et al noted an improved 4-year progression-free survival (60%) among those receiving whole pelvic radiotherapy in conjunction with neoadjuvant androgen deprivation, compared with other treatment arms (44% to 50%). In a subsequent update, the value of whole pelvic fields was limited to only patients receiving hormonal therapy, and the benefit became nonsignificant with a trend toward improved outcomes. Furthermore, a European randomized trial (GETUG-01) did not show a benefit to larger pelvic fields. Therefore, at this time, there is no consensus as to the use of whole pelvic or more limited prostate-only fields in the intermediate-/high-risk patient groups.

EBRT dose The previous standard radiation dose with conventional therapy was 70 Gy given over 7 weeks; however, more recent work has suggested a positive dose response, particularly in the intermediate- and high-risk patient populations. Multiple single-institution experiences have demonstrated that 3D conformal EBRT techniques with doses of 75 Gy and higher can be delivered with minimal toxicities.

A randomized trial from the M. D. Anderson Cancer Center compared 70 Gy given conventionally with 78 Gy delivered with a conformal boost. With a median follow-up of 8.7 years, it showed an advantage in freedom from failure for the higher-dose arm in patients with a PSA level > 10 ng/mL (78% vs 39%). Kupelian et al presented pooled data for nearly 5,000 patients from 9 institutions over a narrow time range (1994–1995) to remove treatment technique, stage migration, and lead-time bias. They demonstrated favorable biochemical control outcomes for doses higher than 72 Gy in all risk groups.

The RTOG has completed a dose-escalation trial to assess toxicity with 3D conformal EBRT. In this multi-institutional trial, 78 Gy (prescribed as a minimum to the tumor volume in 2-Gy fractions) was well tolerated, with only 3% of patients experiencing significant (grade 3+) acute gastrointestinal/genitourinary (GI/GU) morbidity and a 6% rate of significant late toxicity. A comparison trial is being conducted by the RTOG (P0126); it will accrue 1,520 cases and provide information regarding any beneficial effect on mortality with higher radiation doses. Although no standard exists, doses ≥ 75 Gy with 3D conformal EBRT techniques appear to be well tolerated and improve biochemical response rates.

Intensity-modulated radiation therapy (IMRT) is becoming a widely used treatment for prostate cancer. This refinement of conformal therapy employs high nonuniform beam intensity profiles and dynamic multileaf collimation to create even more conformal dose distributions. Further improving the therapeutic index compared with 3D conformal EBRT, IMRT is associated with reduced toxicity, permitting further dose escalations previously unattainable.

IMRT was pioneered in several major centers, and Memorial Sloan-Kettering Cancer Center has reported a series of 772 patients treated with doses between 81 and 86.4 Gy. With a median follow-up of 24 months, the side-effect profile was improved, despite these higher doses, with less than 1% of patients experiencing late grade 3+ GI/GU toxicity. The early PSA relapse-free survival rates for favorable-intermediate–and unfavorable-risk groups were 92%, 86%, and 81%, respectively. Although IMRT is quickly becoming the standard of care at most institutions, some caution should be exercised. The precision of dose delivery and the complexity of treatment planning demand a strong commitment by both physicians and physics personnel to ensure high-quality IMRT.

Proton therapy Technically a form of EBRT, proton therapy has been utilized in clinical practice for more than 10 years. It offers a potential advantage over photon-based IMRT by exploiting superior dose distributions of the Bragg peak effect. The routine implementation of this technology has been hampered by the staggering costs of building and maintaining a facility. The largest experience involving 1,277 patients at the Loma Linda proton facility was reported in 2004 and demonstrated "comparable control rates with minimal toxicity" compared with other local therapies. Although there are theoretical benefits and ongoing trials evaluating the possibility of further safe dose escalation with protons, to date there is little clinical evidence to support a significant benefit over IMRT. With several new centers now under construction or online, and a published economic evaluation questioning its cost-effectiveness, the future of eventual widespread application of proton therapy remains unclear.

Stereotactic body radiotherapy (SBRT) is being investigated as a method to treat early-stage prostate cancers. Utilizing several highly focused fractions, this method exploits the alpha/beta ratio typical of slowly growing malignancies. The technique, which employs high-dose (approximately 700 cGy) for several fractions (typically 5), can be delivered by several specialized methods, including linear accelerator-based models, tomotherapy, and CyberKnife. A recent preliminary experience (median follow-up of 33 months) from Stanford University in 40 patients demonstrated both the efficacy and safety of this approach utilizing the CyberKnife. This methodology represents a major paradigmatic shift; although patients are often intrigued by the convenience of a short course of therapy over the typical 8-week course of IMRT, it is critical to recognize that longer follow-up in a large patient population will be necessary to promote this as a standard technique.

Androgen ablation with EBRT Two potential benefits of the use of transient androgen ablation prior to EBRT have been identified. First, there may be some synergy between the apoptotic response induced by androgen deprivation and radiotherapy that may increase local tumor control.

Second, androgen deprivation results in an average 20% decrease in prostate volume. This volume reduction not only may reduce the number of target cells, and thereby improve tumor control, but also may shrink the prostate and, thus, diminish the volume of rectum and bladder irradiated during conformal therapy. Complete androgen blockade can be achieved with luteinizing hormone-releasing hormone (LHRH) agonists plus an oral antiandrogen or LHRH antagonist therapy.

The survival benefits of androgen suppression therapy (AST) for patients with intermediate-risk disease have been uncertain. A single-institution prospective trial by D'Amico et al randomized patients with a PSA level > 10 ng/mL, a Gleason score ≥ 7, or radiographic evidence of extraprostatic disease to receive EBRT (70 Gy) alone or the same EBRT with 6 months of AST. After a median follow-up of 4.5 years, patients treated with combined EBRT and AST were found to have improved progression-free, prostate cancer-specific, and overall survival ($P = .04$). Although hormone therapy for 3 years has been shown to be beneficial in locally advanced cases, this trial in men with more localized disease showed a benefit to a shorter duration of hormone therapy. However, it is not known whether high-dose radiotherapy will obviate the need for AST in this group of patients. The survival benefit in this study was largely confined to those men with few cardiovascular comorbidities, illustrating the importance of patient selection for AST.

Recent secondary findings from a large randomized study (RTOG 9202) suggest that men with high-grade tumors (Gleason score 8–10) and high-risk (T2c–T4) localized disease benefit from long-term androgen ablation (2 years) compared with short-term androgen ablation (4 months), based on improved prostate cancer-specific and overall survival. A caveat to these findings has been the increased incidence or acceleration of incident cardiovascular death in men older than 65 years of age starting androgen ablation compared with those men who did not receive androgen ablation. These findings suggest that cardiac evaluation should be considered in those men older than age 65 with cardiovascular risk factors prior to undergoing androgen ablation. RTOG 94-08 was presented at ASTRO in April 2010. This study examined a short course (4 months) of hormonal therapy with external radiotherapy (66.6 or 68.4 Gy) in 1,979 men. For intermediate-risk men, the 8-year survival rate was 66% in men who received radiation therapy alone and 72% in men who also received hormones. The hormonal therapy consisted of complete hormonal therapy, and there were no added benefits for hormones in low-risk men.

Interstitial radiotherapy In the 1970s, the use of permanently placed radioactive iodine implants produced initial results as good as those obtained with other available radiotherapy techniques and posed a small risk of impotence and other morbidity when compared with conventional EBRT and radical prostatectomy. However, ultimate control rates were unacceptable. The technique used (freehand placement of seeds during laparotomy) was found to distribute the radioactive seeds unevenly throughout the gland; cold regions may have contributed to the relatively poor outcome.

The advent of improved imaging and seed placement techniques coupled with better patient selection has resulted in vast improvements in cancer control. The perception of fewer side effects in a single outpatient treatment has also contributed to some popularity of this treatment modality. Transrectal ultrasonography is now utilized to guide seed placement from a transperineal approach, which has corrected the problem of poor seed placement in experienced hands. Two radioactive seed isotopes have been used: iodine (I-125), with a half-life of 60 days, and palladium (Pd-103), with a shorter half-life (17 days) and subsequent higher dose rate. The advantage of the brachytherapy technique is that substantial dose can be delivered to the prostate with minimal effect on the surrounding tissue.

Although concentrating dose with brachytherapy represents a potential advantage over EBRT, it also highlights the need for appropriate patient selection. Significant dose falloff 2 to 3 mm beyond placement of the seeds within the gland limits the application of seed monotherapy in patients with potential periprostatic or regional disease extension. Large studies from several leading institutions have now matured and confirm the long-term effectiveness and safety of this approach in low-risk populations. Favorable results have also been reported in selected intermediate-risk patients. Typical monotherapy doses of 145 Gy for I-131 and 125 Gy for Pd-103 are utilized. To date, the data do not support the use of either isotope over the other.

In addition to disease risk factors, certain patient selection factors are important in considering implants. A large prostate size (> 60 cc) may make the procedure more challenging, both from the perspective of increased prostate gland swelling due to the increased number of needles and the difficulty of the pubic bone obstructing needle placement. Patients with outlet obstruction symptoms IPSS (International Prostate Symptom Score) score > 15 have an increased risk of requiring catheterization following implantation. Patients who have undergone prior transurethral resection of prostate (TURP) have been reported to have an increased risk of incontinence; recognizing this risk and placing seeds farther from the defect may help to minimize this risk. Therefore, with proper counseling, patients with small TURP defects may still be considered implant candidates.

For patients with intermediate- or high-risk disease, implants may be combined with EBRT. There is sound logic in combining high-dose therapy to the prostate with an implant and moderate doses of EBRT to the regional tissues to sterilize micrometastatic disease. In this situation, an implant (110 Gy of I-131 or 100 Gy of Pd-104) usually either precedes or follows 20 to 45 Gy delivered to the pelvis. Some reports have suggested an increase in rectal toxicity with this approach; however, this is likely due to the poor quality of the implant. At least one study from a leading implant center suggested no significant increase in severe early or late GI/GU morbidity with combination therapy. The value of supplemental EBRT needs to be evaluated in comparison to full-dose EBRT in terms of long-term morbidity and cancer control.

High-dose–rate (HDR) devices Besides permanent implants, which deliver low-dose–rate (LDR) radiotherapy, brachytherapy for prostate cancer has been delivered using temporary high-dose–rate devices, usually in patients with locally advanced disease. In this technique, a high dose (minimum, approximately 5 Gy) is delivered to the prostate over ≤ 1 hour by remotely inserting a highly radioactive source into catheters placed into the prostate under ultrasonographic guidance while the patient is under anesthesia. Several treatments are given on separate occasions, and EBRT is used for approximately 5 weeks as well.

More reports are accumulating on the application of HDR brachytherapy to prostate cancer. Various dose-fractionation combinations of HDR with or without combined pelvic EBRT have been employed, with a dose-response relationship apparent in biochemical control. Although the follow-up is short and no prospective randomized trials evaluating this approach have yet been published, it appears that HDR prostate brachytherapy in combination with pelvic EBRT may be effective. The long-term consequences for normal tissue of delivering large doses per fraction using this technique are unclear.

Medications and devices to manage impotence after prostatectomy, EBRT, or brachytherapy

Treatment for postprostatectomy impotence includes the phosphodiesterase inhibitors sildenafil, vardenafil (Levitra), and tadalafil, prostaglandin E1, administered as a urethral suppository (Muse); intercavernosal injection (Caverject, Edex); or VEDs that are useful for improving erections in men who have poor erectile function after prostatectomy, radiation therapy, or brachytherapy. These therapies are effective in 15% to 40% of men with postprostatectomy impotence and in 50% to 75% of men with postradiotherapy erectile dysfunction. Insertion of a penile prosthesis is typically offered to patients only after unsuccessful trials with the previously mentioned less invasive interventions.

DETECTION AND TREATMENT OF RECURRENCE

Significance and definition of a rising PSA level post irradiation

The use of PSA levels following definitive therapy (either radiotherapy or radical prostatectomy) can detect early recurrences that may be amenable to salvage treatment. A rising PSA profile following radiotherapy is unequivocal evidence of the presence of a residual prostatic neoplasm. However, the definition of a rising PSA level after radiation therapy varies in the literature. A 1996 consensus conference recommended that PSA failure be considered to have occurred after three consecutive PSA level rises, with the rate of failure defined as halfway between the first rise and the previous PSA level. More recently, this definition has been replaced by an absolute PSA rise of 2 ng/mL above the posttreatment nadir PSA level.

Moreover, patients with a rising PSA level after irradiation may be a heterogeneous group, including patients with truly localized failure as well as those with metastatic disease. Also, certain patients will have a slowly rising PSA level after irradiation and may not require additional treatment. In patients who do not receive androgen ablation, the 5-year actuarial risk of distant metastasis from the time that the PSA level begins to rise is ~50%. A rapidly emerging key concept in rising PSA levels is PSA velocity, or more specifically PSA doubling time. Multiple recent studies have found that a PSA doubling time < 10 to 12 months predicts early clinical relapse if biochemical recurrence is untreated. In addition, recent studies have documented the real phenomenon of postradiotherapy PSA bounce, which is defined as a rise above the baseline PSA following the initiation of radiotherapy. This may occur in 20% to 40% of men depending on the threshold of PSA rise and is not known to have prognostic significance. Thus, PSA rises should be confirmed over time to ensure that they are durable rather than transient prior to initiating salvage systemic therapy.

Treatment recommendations for recurrence post irradiation

In general, men who have clear evidence of a rising PSA level 2 years after definitive radiotherapy for localized prostate cancer should be advised about the options of hormonal therapy (see section on "Treatment of locally advanced disease [T3, T4]"), salvage surgery, salvage cryotherapy, observation, or experimental therapy.

If patients have minimal comorbidity, good life expectancy, and only local evidence of disease recurrence, salvage surgery is an option but should be preceded by a bone scan, CT scan, cystoscopy, and extensive counseling because urinary difficulties after salvage prostatectomy are substantial and highly prevalent. Factors that determine success of salvage surgery after radiation therapy include low (< 4 to 10 ng/mL) preoperative PSA level, low pathologic stage (T3a or less), and prior type of radiation therapy (brachytherapy, IMRT being favorable). However, no randomized trials have been conducted in this setting to provide level I evidence favoring surgery over other modes of treatment.

TREATMENT OF LOCALLY ADVANCED DISEASE (T3, T4)

The treatment of patients with locally advanced prostate cancer is centered on a multimodality and multidisciplinary approach, including radiation therapy (EBRT with or without HDR interstitial therapy), androgen ablation plus EBRT, or radical prostatectomy with or without androgen deprivation.

EBRT with and without HDR interstitial therapy

For patients with locally extensive prostate cancer, local failure remains a potential problem after EBRT. This problem has prompted investigations into alternative means to intensify therapy.

One strategy has been to deliver large fractions of radiotherapy using HDR interstitial techniques in combination with EBRT. The large interstitial fractions, which may be on the order of 5 Gy, deliver a high dose to the prostate but spare normal tissues, due to the rapid dose falloff outside the implanted volume. Early experience with this strategy is encouraging, but long-term data on outcome, particularly in patients with locally extensive disease, and on morbidity are awaited.

Patients with locally advanced prostate cancer probably are not good candidates for permanent prostate implants. Patients with stage T3/T4 tumors are at high risk of gross extraprostatic involvement, and this localized therapy may not offer adequate dosimetric coverage of extraprostatic disease.

As mentioned in the previous section, there may be a synergistic effect between hormonal therapy given in conjunction with radiation therapy. In addition to enhancing apoptosis and producing local cytoreduction, the use of early androgen deprivation may possibly delay or even prevent the development of metastatic disease.

The current body of evidence from three large randomized trials (RTOG 92-02, RTOG 85-10, and EORTC 22863) suggests that immediate long-term androgen deprivation in conjunction with EBRT improves outcomes among men with locally advanced or high-risk (Gleason score ≥ 8) prostate cancer compared with radiation therapy alone. An analysis of RTOG 85-31 by Horwitz et al, which employed early indefinite androgen deprivation, demonstrated that patients with locally advanced disease (T3N0) had improved cause-specific failure and distant metastatic failure compared with EBRT alone. Furthermore, a comparison to RTOG 86-10, which studied similar patients treated with only 4 months of hormonal therapy, favored the long-term approach. The EORTC trial randomized 415 patients and demonstrated a 15% overall survival benefit to 3 years of combined therapy vs radiation therapy alone. Finally, recent randomized studies by Widmark et al and the National Cancer Institute of Canada have confirmed that external beam radiotherapy with 2–3 years of hormonal therapy is necessary for locally advanced or high-risk prostate cancer as compared to hormonal therapy alone, due to improvements in local control as well as systemic control, and this combination should be considered a standard initial therapy for high-risk men.

Radical prostatectomy with or without adjuvant therapy

Surgical monotherapy can be considered a reasonable option for patients with locally advanced prostate cancer. Stage T3 disease can be successfully treated with low morbidity and significant reductions in risk of local recurrence, with clinical overstaging (up to 26%) reported by Yamada et al. Well- and moderately differentiated cancers have cancer-specific survival rates of 76% at 10 years, comparable to those of other treatment modalities.

The Mayo Clinic has one of the largest radical prostatectomy series for T3 disease, consisting of more than 1,000 patients. In this population, of whom 34% received adjuvant therapy, 15-year cancer-specific survival and local recurrence rates were 77% and 21%, respectively. In an ECOG clinical trial, 98 men who were found to have nodal metastases following radical prostatectomy and pelvic lymphadenectomy were randomized to receive immediate androgen deprivation or be followed until clinical disease progression. At a median follow-up of 7 years, 18 of 51 men in the observation group had died, compared with only 4 of 47 in the treatment group ($P = .02$). In one interesting series, da Pozzo found that adjuvant radiation therapy with androgen deprivation therapy was associated with a survival benefit (biochemical and prostate cancer specific) in node-positive men treated with radical prostatectomy initially, even after adjustment for known confounders. This finding suggests that local tumor control may prevent distant failure in this disease.

Treatment of node-positive disease

Whether any local treatment adds to the overall survival duration in patients with known nodal involvement is debatable. Until recently, the standard of care had been to perform frozen-section pathologic analysis on pelvic lymph nodes at the time of radical prostatectomy, prior to removal of the prostate. If this analysis revealed micrometastases, radical prostatectomy was thought to be contraindicated. Although retrospective in nature, recent data from several American centers, including one large study from the Mayo Clinic, have reported a survival benefit in men who undergo radical prostatectomy despite the presence of micrometastases to regional pelvic lymph nodes. These men tend to do better and survive longer when started on early hormonal therapy, either with orchiectomy or an LHRH analog.

Radiation therapy There are also compelling data that long-term survival is achievable in these patients with combination radiation and hormonal therapy. Data from the M. D. Anderson Cancer Center indicate a benefit to pelvic/prostate radiation therapy plus immediate hormonal manipulation compared with hormones alone. A subset analysis of patients with node-positive disease from RTOG 85-31 revealed immediate hormonal therapy plus radiation therapy resulted in 5- and 9-year cause-specific survival rates of 84% and 76%, respectively. Therefore, aggressive locoregional therapy appears to be effective in this cohort of unfavorable patients.

TREATMENT OF ADVANCED SYSTEMIC DISEASE

Defining advanced disease

Metastatic prostate cancer This is a heterogeneous group of patients that ranges from those with pathologically detected locoregional nodal metastases at the time of radical prostatectomy to those with widespread systemic disease. The most common sites of metastatic disease are the bone and pelvic and abdominal lymph nodes. Other, less common sites include the liver and lungs. Complications of metastatic prostate cancer include pain, fatigue, skeletal fractures, spinal cord compression, urinary outlet obstruction, and failure to thrive. First-line hormonal therapy for men with metastatic prostate cancer delays these complications.

Rising PSA level A large series of more than 2,000 patients treated with radical prostatectomy at Johns Hopkins University demonstrated that approximately 17% of cases recurred, with only 5.8% being local disease. In the remaining patients, disease recurred initially with either a rise in PSA level alone (9.7%) or evidence of clinical metastases (1.7%).

Outcomes for men with only a rising PSA level can vary greatly. Time to PSA recurrence (< vs > 2 years), PSA doubling time (< vs > 9 months), and Gleason score (8–10 vs 5–7) are among the important factors for predicting the development of metastatic disease and survival. The major developments for hormonal therapy in advanced prostate cancer were achieved prior to routine PSA testing and were often complicated by problematic study design. There are no prospective data that confirm a benefit to early hormonal therapy for men with a rising PSA alone. However, for patients with a rising PSA level who are at high risk for the development of metastases, some physicians agree that early hormonal therapy is likely to benefit this group of patients as well as those with radiologic evidence of metastatic disease. Ongoing randomized phase III studies are also testing the role of docetaxel (Taxotere) with androgen deprivation therapy in this setting, but the role of chemotherapy in the nonmetastatic setting remains experimental.

First-line therapies for advanced disease

The standard first-line treatment of advanced prostate cancer, regardless of whether local treatment has been applied, is to ablate the action of androgens by medical or surgical means. For the majority of patients, androgen ablation can result in a decline in PSA level, palliation of disease-related symptoms, and regression of metastatic disease on imaging.

TABLE 5: Hormonal approaches to the treatment of advanced prostate cancer

Method	Mechanism of action	Side effects
Surgical castration	Removal of testicular androgens	Hot flashes (50%), psychological effects
Diethylstilbestrol (DES)	Inhibition of gonadotropin secretion	Gynecomastia, cardiovascular risks at high doses
LHRH analogs (agonists and antagonists) (goserelin, leuprolide, degarelix)	Inhibition of gonadotropin secretion	Hot flashes (50%), less gynecomastia than with DES, fatigue
Antiandrogens (bicalutamide, flutamide, nilutamide)	Blockade of binding of dihydrotestosterone to its receptor	Abnormal liver function studies, diarrhea (10%)
Ketoconazole	Adrenal androgen synthesis inhibitor, possible autocrine/paracrine androgen inhibition	LFT abnormalities, nausea, drug interactions
Glucocorticoids	Inhibition of androgen receptor activity, adrenal androgen synthesis inhibition, independent cytotoxic effects	Weight gain, immunosuppression, ulcers, bone density loss/fracture, hyperglycemia

LHRH = luteinizing hormone-releasing hormone; LFT = liver function test

Bilateral orchiectomy The advantages of orchiectomy over other means of castration include an immediate decline in testosterone levels and ease of compliance for patients. Given these advantages, however, many men still opt for medical castration, with the potential advantage of intermittent hormonal therapy. In addition, the psychological impact of orchiectomy can be significant. Nonetheless, bilateral orchiectomy may be appropriate and cost-effective for a select group of patients.

LHRH analogs LHRH agonists, such as leuprolide (Lupron, Eligard) and goserelin (Zoladex), interfere with the normal pulsatile secretion of LH from the pituitary gland, resulting in an eventual decline in serum testosterone levels. The effect is reversible with cessation of therapy. Because LH is initially increased with LHRH agonists, testosterone levels increase initially as well. This finding can result in a transient rise in PSA levels and potential growth of metastatic sites. Because of this initial "flare response" with LHRH agonists, consideration should be given to the administration of an antiandrogen prior to the LHRH, especially in patients who are at risk for complications from the disease (such as spinal cord compression, worsening pain, or urinary outlet obstruction; Table 5). Side effects of androgen-deprivation therapy include hot flashes, metabolic-type syndrome and weight gain, loss of libido, loss of peripheral hair growth, gynecomastia, an elevated risk of diabetes, loss of bone mineral density and an increased risk of fracture, and finally an increased risk of cardiovascular complications (including myocardial infarction, stroke, sudden cardiac death, deep vein thrombosis, and angina). The overall risk/benefit profile of androgen-deprivation therapy thus depends on an individual man's preexisting cardiovascular risk and comorbidities and should be individually tailored based on this risk assessment.

The flare phenomenon can also be avoided through the use of gonadotropin-releasing hormone (GnRH) antagonists. This class of drugs leads to immediate suppression of androgen production without the initial testosterone surge that results with GnRH agonist therapy. Abarelix (Plenaxis) is a GnRH antagonist that was approved in 2003. However, the manufacturer halted US sales to new patients in 2005. A second agent, degarelix (Firmagon), was approved by the FDA in December 2008. As a receptor antagonist, degarelix reversibly binds to the GnRH receptors in the pituitary gland, immediately suppressing the secretion of the LH, follicle-stimulating hormone (FSH), and, subsequently, testosterone levels. Currently available in a monthly formulation and not associated with anaphylaxis, degarelix is expected to be available in a 3-month depot formulation by 2011.

Antiandrogens Antiandrogens function to block the binding of dihydrotestosterone (DHT) to the androgen receptor, blocking the translocation of the DHT-androgen receptor complex into the nuclei of cells. There are two general classes: steroidal and nonsteroidal. Steroidal antiandrogens include cyproterone and megestrol. The most commonly used antiandrogens include the nonsteroidal agents flutamide, bicalutamide, and nilutamide. These agents differ slightly in their affinity for the androgen receptor and their side-effect profiles. For example, nilutamide has been associated with interstitial lung disease and visual adaptation (light-dark) disturbances, whereas flutamide is associated with diarrhea. Antiandrogens as a category have not been as highly associated with cardiovascular risk outcomes, but this may be due to the low numbers of patients treated with antiandrogen monotherapy. Consideration of prophylactic breast radiation prior to the use of prolonged antiandrogen monotherapy should be considered, given the high risk (> 50%) of developing gynecomastia. Tamoxifen has also been shown to prevent gynecomastia in these men but is associated with other adverse events such as deep vein thrombosis/pulmonary embolism.

Typically, antiandrogens are used in combination with surgical or medical castration. Some trials comparing antiandrogens alone with LHRH analogs have shown similar efficacy, but more recent trials in metastatic disease suggest that monotherapy with antiandrogens may be inferior in terms of time to disease progression and possibly survival. For example, a randomized trial of monotherapy with high-dose bicalutamide (150 mg daily) compared with flutamide plus goserelin demonstrated that patients treated with bicalutamide monotherapy had fewer side effects, such as loss of libido or erectile dysfunction, and trended toward improved quality of life. However, in patients with radiographic evidence of metastases, bicalutamide monotherapy was associated with a small 6-week decrease in survival (hazard ratio = 1.3). Despite this finding, for men who are intolerant to the side effects of LHRH analogs, monotherapy with antiandrogens can be considered after careful discussion with patients.

Antiandrogen monotherapy with flutamide or bicalutamide is also sometimes used to treat PSA recurrence. Used alone or in combination with a 5-alpha reductase inhibitor (finasteride or dutasteride), this approach is associated with fewer side effects than traditional AST, but the approch is not considered standard and its efficacy relative to primary gonadal suppression is not established. A significant downside is nipple tenderness or gynecomastia, but this "peripheral blockade" approach may preserve potency and libido. Prophylactic breast irradiation may prevent this complication.

CAB Complete androgen blockade, or CAB, refers to the elimination of testicular androgens in combination with blockade of adrenal androgens, generally with an LHRH analog and an antiandrogen agent. The use of CAB is somewhat controversial. Several randomized trials comparing LHRH agonists alone vs CAB have demonstrated a survival benefit with CAB. However, in one of the largest trials conducted by the United States Intergroup, more than 1,300 men were randomized to undergo orchiectomy vs orchiectomy plus flutamide. There was no significant advantage to CAB in terms of time to disease progression or overall survival. Some investigators believe that bicalutamide, a more potent agent, may be associated with greater survival when used as part of CAB. Recent meta-analyses suggest a small but incremental benefit of noncyproterone antiandrogens in combination with GnRH agonists in terms of overall survival (15% to 20% relative risk reduction). This finding led ASCO to advise an informed discussion of the risks and benefits of CAB.

Many investigators believe that the advantages observed in trials that include an LHRH antagonist exist because of the "flare phenomenon," which occurs with LHRH agonists alone and may be lost with a short period of treatment with antiandrogens during the expected flare period. ASCO has published guidelines for the initial management of androgen-sensitive (recurrent, metastatic) prostate cancer. Based on the literature, immediate androgen deprivation was associated with a moderate decrease in prostate cancer mortality and a moderate increase in other causes of mortality. Currently, there is no definitive evidence favoring the early initiation of androgen deprivation in this population.

Several phase III trials evaluating the role of intermittent androgen deprivation are ongoing. A phase III European trial investigating the use of intermittent hormone therapy in patients with locally advanced or metastatic prostate cancer has been reported. In this trial, 766 patients were registered, and 626 patients whose PSA level decreased to < 4 ng/mL or to 80% below the initial value after 3 months of induction treatment were randomized to receive continuous vs intermittent hormone therapy. The primary outcome of disease progression was not statistically different between groups. There was also no significant difference in overall survival. Among the 314 patients on intermittent therapy, 50% were off therapy for at least 52 weeks following initial LHRH induction. Patients whose PSA level dropped below 2 ng/mL spent a median of 82% of their time receiving no therapy (*Calais da Silva FE et al: Eur Urol 55:1269–1277, 2009*).

Diethylstilbestrol (DES) Estrogen administration, in the form of DES, also produces chemical castration. DES inhibits prostate growth, primarily through the inhibition of the hypothalamic-pituitary-gonadal axis, which blocks testicular synthesis of testosterone and thus lowers plasma testosterone levels. Since doses higher than 3 mg/d cause significant cardiovascular mortality, DES has fallen out of favor as a first-line therapy to induce castration.

Ketoconazole (Nizoral) Ketoconazole is an antifungal agent that can inhibit adrenal and testicular steroid synthesis at higher doses,

TABLE 6: The incidence of complications from advanced prostate cancer with immediate vs deferred androgen deprivation

Complication	Immediate	Deferred
Pathologic fracture	2.3%	4.5%
Spinal cord compression	2.0%	5.0%
Ureteral obstruction	7.0%	11.8%
Extraskeletal metastases	7.9%	11.8%

leading to a decline in adrenal and testicular androgens. It has the benefit of a rapid decline in testosterone, which can be useful for patients who present emergently with a complication of newly diagnosed advanced disease. Ketoconazole is started at a dose of 200 mg three times daily and is increased to a total dose of 400 mg three times daily. Ketoconazole is associated with significant side effects (such as fatigue, nausea, and vomiting) and drug interactions, however, and must be given with supplemental hydrocortisone to avoid symptoms of adrenal insufficiency. Because of the side effects, its use is more common in the second-line setting, where responses can be expected in 20% to 40% of patients following disease progression with CAB. There are current efforts under way to develop second-generation adrenal androgen synthesis inhibitors such as abiraterone acetate or TAK700, with or without prednisone before and after docetaxel. These agents can inhibit paracrine and autocrine androgen production, which may drive prostate tumor growth as well. Phase III studies have been completed or are under way for these compounds, and results are eagerly awaited.

Early vs late treatment Whether to treat patients early with hormonal therapy or wait until patients become symptomatic has been tested in a large European trial conducted by the MRC. Men were randomized to receive immediate hormonal therapy (orchiectomy or an LHRH analog) vs delayed therapy, which was initiated with symptomatic disease progression. Men who were treated with early therapy were less likely to experience urinary obstructive symptoms requiring intervention, pathologic fractures, and spinal cord compression than those treated in the delayed arm (Table 6). The survival benefit was less clear, however, because many of the men in the delayed arm died before they received any hormonal therapy. This study was also complicated by the initiation of PSA monitoring during the study period. Many patients and physicians currently are not comfortable delaying therapy until the onset of symptoms while the PSA level is rising; this fact limits the applicability of its findings in the modern era.

Other smaller trials have examined this issue as well. A Cochrane Database review was conducted in 2002; it demonstrated an increase in progression-free survival and a small, but significant, improvement in survival with early hormonal therapy. A randomized EORTC study (30891) of early vs deferred androgen deprivation therapy for men with localized prostate cancer not amenable to local treatment did not show a prostate cancer-specific survival advantage to the immediate use of androgen deprivation therapy in these men. Balancing comorbidity and the risk of cardiovascular complications is an important consideration in the timing of androgen deprivation therapy in this population, given the competing causes of mortality.

One setting in which early adjuvant hormonal therapy has been associated with a survival benefit is in the postprostatectomy setting in men found to have pathologic lymph node-positive disease. Messing and colleagues published an adjuvant study that evaluated immediate hormonal therapy vs delayed treatment upon detection of distant metastases or symptomatic recurrence in men who had undergone radical prostatectomy and lymph node dissection and were found to have nodal metastases. At a median follow-up of 11.9 years (range, 9.7–14.5 for surviving patients), men assigned immediate androgen deprivation therapy had a significant improvement in overall survival, prostate cancer-specific survival, and progression-free survival.

Immunotherapy There is currently level 1 evidence to support the use of sipuleucel-T (Provenge) immunotherapy vaccination as a therapy for men with presymptomatic metastatic castration-resistant prostate cancer, based on several phase II studies and one large phase III study. This phase III study (IMPACT trial) demonstrated a 4.1 to 5 month survival advantage over sham vaccination. Thus, autologous dendritic cell therapy vaccination (three infused doses over 4 weeks following initial leukapheresis), utilizing a prostatic acid phosphatase-GMCSF fusion protein to stimulate immune cells, has may become a standard of care prior to docetaxel in men with metastatic asymptomatic to minimally symptomatic castration-resistant prostate cancer. Men with pain requiring narcotics, with visceral metastases, and with a life expectancy under 6 months are not eligible for this therapy. Of note, vaccination did not lead to PSA declines, tumor responses, improved palliation, or delayed tumor progression by our current measures, and thus this therapy should be regarded as adjunctive to other current therapies that are more cytoreductive and palliative.

Intermittent androgen deprivation Androgen deprivation is associated with several short-term and long-term adverse effects. These side effects make treatment breaks provided by intermittent androgen deprivation an attractive option. Additionally, results from preclinical studies suggest that hormonal resistance may be delayed with intermittent androgen deprivation. These potential advantages have led to significant interest among patients and caregivers in intermittent androgen deprivation.

Over the past decade, several phase II studies of intermittent androgen deprivation have demonstrated feasibility and safety with suggestion of improved quality of life without negative effects on time to disease progression or survival. More recently, a phase III trial was reported. In this trial, patients randomized to the intermittent therapy arm were off therapy for a median of 52 weeks with no significant difference in time to disease progression or overall survival. The results of several ongoing phase III trials in metastatic disease and PSA-only relapse will better define the role of intermittent androgen deprivation. With the currently available information, intermittent androgen deprivation may be considered in most patient settings.

Treatment recommendations Just as for localized disease, initial treatment for advanced prostate cancer must be individualized. A patient who presents with a rising PSA level only after local treatment and a slow PSA doubling time, a prolonged time to PSA recurrence, and a low initial Gleason score may not require immediate therapy, especially if there are other more likely significant comorbidities. However, a patient with multiple metastatic sites will need immediate treatment, generally with orchiectomy, LHRH agonists or antagonists, or CAB initially followed by monotherapy with an LHRH analog, to prevent the sequelae of metastatic disease, such as fracture, spinal cord compression, and ureteral obstruction. Degarelix or ketoconazole may be considered as initial systemic therapies for patients presenting with spinal cord compression as the first sign of prostate cancer, as well as combined androgen blockage. Palliative radiation in this setting should also be considered. Given the overall limitations of hormone therapy, all appropriate patients should be offered access to clinical trials.

For patients with a rising PSA level who are at high risk for the development of metastases, a discussion regarding the potential advantages to early treatment and an explanation of the lack of randomized prospective data are warranted. Some investigators favor early treatment for these patients based on the data from the MRC trial and the Cochrane Database review, understanding that this information is extrapolated from data obtained prior to PSA testing and from patients with clinical and radiographic metastases.

Second-line hormonal therapies

It is important to realize that there has been a shift in terminology from "androgen-independent" or "hormone-refractory" prostate cancer to a newer term: castration-resistant prostate cancer. This change reflects an understanding that prostate cancer often remains dependent on androgenic signaling, even in the presence of castrate levels of testosterone. Tumors may produce their own androgens through autocrine signaling, amplify low levels of testosterone ligand signaling through androgen receptor (AR) mutations or duplications, and may have activation of the AR through other ligands. Thus, progression of disease despite castration does not necessarily imply resistance to all hormonal strategies, as exemplified by the response to anti-androgens, ketoconazole, and newer second-generation agents such as MDV3100 or abiraterone acetate. Thus, true hormone-refractory disease may refer to disease that has progressed despite therapies employing all known hormonal strategies.

Outcomes with initial androgen ablation can vary from responses that last from months to years; they also vary as a function of the Gleason grade, pretreatment PSA velocity, and extent of disease at the time of initiating treatment. Once PSA levels begin to rise with androgen ablation, the disease is often referred to as "hormone refractory." This term is actually a misnomer, because preclinical data suggest that tumors may become hypersensitive to androgens, resulting in worsened disease if androgen ablation is removed entirely. Moreover, many patients have disease that remains sensitive to further hormonal manipulations, such as second-line antiandrogens, steroids, or ketoconazole.

An example of this sensitivity to hormonal manipulation is exemplified in the anti-androgen withdrawal response. Up to one-third of patients with a rising PSA level while receiving treatment with an antiandrogen will have a decline in PSA level and or clinical regression with antiandrogen withdrawal. The mechanism of this response has not been fully elucidated but supports the hypothesis that the androgen receptor remains important in progressive disease.

TABLE 7: Phase III trials in the postdocetaxel castration-resistant prostate cancer setting

Trial	Experimental agent	Type of therapy	Status
Mitoxantrone/prednisone vs cabazitaxel/prednisone	Cabazitaxel	Antimicrotubule agent	Completed, positive
Palliative radiation ± ipilimumab	Ipilimumab	Immunomodulatory (CTLA-4 blockade)	Ongoing
MDV3100 vs placebo	MDV3100	Novel antiandrogen	Ongoing
Prednisone ± abiraterone acetate/placebo	Abiraterone acetate	Adrenal/autocrine androgen synthesis inhibitor	Completed
Prednisone ± sunitinib	Sunitinib	Oral VEGF/PDGF inhibitor	Ongoing

Although second-line hormonal therapy has demonstrated benefit in terms of PSA levels and response, there are no data to demonstrate a survival advantage with second-line hormonal therapy. Its role has further come into question with data that support the use of docetaxel chemotherapy for men with metastatic androgen-independent prostate cancer to improve survival. The survival advantage of docetaxel is not limited by the number of prior hormonal therapies. However, as exemplified by recent novel antiandrogens (MDV3100) and adrenal/autocrine synthesis-inhibiting agents (abiraterone acetate), men with castration-resistant disease remain sensitive to agents targeting the androgen receptor, and this remains a rich area of clinical investigation. In phase I/II trials, the novel oral antiandrogen MDV3100 demonstrated striking PSA declines (50% to 70% achieved a > 30% decline) and partial tumor responses both in the predocetaxel and postdocetaxel settings, with responses that were durable in many men over 6 months. The drug can prevent androgen-induced nuclear translocation and has shown tumoricidal activity even in bicalutamide-resistant model systems. Abiraterone acetate with prednisone has demonstrated similar outcomes in these settings as well, showing that hormonal sensitivity may remain even among docetaxel-resistant men. Phase III trials of these agents are completed or ongoing (Table 7).

For patients with a rising PSA level only, timing of chemotherapy is even less clear. The ECOG attempted a trial comparing ketoconazole/hydrocortisone with docetaxel in patients with a rising PSA level but no evidence of metastatic disease after hormonal therapy, but the trial was closed early due to lack of accrual. Ongoing randomized studies of androgen-deprivation therapy with and without chemotherapy should address this question within the coming few years. Until prospective data are available, physicians will need to counsel patients carefully on the different options and timing of those options available at the time of disease progression, including second-line hormonal manipulation, chemotherapy, and especially clinical trials.

TABLE 8: Standard chemotherapy regimens for prostate cancer

Drug/combination	Dose and schedule
Mitoxantrone/prednisone	
Mitoxantrone	12 mg/m^2 IV every 3 weeks
Prednisone	5 mg orally twice daily started on day 1
Repeat cycle every 21 days.	
Tannock IF, Osoba D, Stockler MR, et al: J Clin Oncol 14:1756–1764, 1996.	
Docetaxel/prednisone	
Docetaxel	75 mg/m^2 IV every 3 weeks
Prednisone	5 mg orally twice daily started on day 1

Note: Standard docetaxel premedication should be given prior to the administration of docetaxel. GnRH agonist or other forms of castration are continued through chemotherapy. General antiemetic prophylaxis with dexamethasone should be routinely considered.

Tannock IF, de Wit R, Berry WR, et al: N Engl J Med 351:1502–1512, 2004.

Table prepared by Ishmael Jaiyesimi, DO.

Chemotherapy for castration-resistant disease

Docetaxel The role of chemotherapy changed significantly in 2004 with the results of two large randomized trials demonstrating a survival benefit for men with castration-resistant metastatic prostate cancer treated with docetaxel-based chemotherapy (Table 8). Investigators from the SWOG 9916 trial randomized patients to receive mitoxantrone plus prednisone vs docetaxel (60 mg/m^2) plus estramustine (Emcyt) and dexamethasone every 3 weeks. Patients in the docetaxel arm had a significant improvement in survival by 2 to 3 months. Currently, estramustine is no longer being utilized in the front-line setting due to the 7% to 10% risk of arterial and venous thromboembolic events and the equivalent survival benefits seen with docetaxel alone compared with mitoxantrone.

A second international randomized phase III trial (TAX327) by Tannock et al showed a similar survival benefit of 3 months with docetaxel (75 mg/m^2) plus prednisone given every 3 weeks compared with mitoxantrone and prednisone. These trials were the first to demonstrate a survival benefit with chemotherapy in advanced prostate cancer and have sparked numerous studies involving docetaxel in combination with newer agents. Toxicities of docetaxel include myelosuppression and peripheral neuropathy, both of which can be dose-limiting. Additional toxicities include constipation, tearing due to docetaxel deposition in tear ducts, onycholysis, and fluid retention (peripheral or pulmonary edema, pleural effusion). Weekly docetaxel with prednisone (30 mg/m^2) for 5 of 6 weeks provided an intermediate level of control and survival that was not statistically different from that with mitoxantrone and prednisone, despite favorable PSA declines and tumor and pain responses. Weekly docetaxel is less well tolerated, and early treatment discontinuation likely limits this schedule's utility.

A recent 5-year update of this study has confirmed a 3-month survival advantage to every-3-week docetaxel in the overall study population. Additional benefits of docetaxel over mitoxantrone included superior PSA responses, pain and quality-of-life responses, greater durability of response, and improved radiographic responses. In addition, nearly 18% of men experienced normalized PSA levels with every-3-week docetaxel, as opposed to 8% of men treated with mitoxantrone. Men with normalized PSA levels lived on average 33 months, compared with 16 months among men without normalized PSA levels, nearly a twofold difference. Current studies indicate that a 30% or greater decline in the serum PSA level within 3 months of treatment initiation may be the best predictor of overall survival of all current surrogate markers in this disease and may be used to assist in prognostication after treatment initiation. Although not a credentialed surrogate for FDA approval, this level of decline was shown in both pivotal studies to be more predictive of survival than other metrics, including the traditional confirmed a 50% decline in PSA level and pain responses. The timing of docetaxel initiation is controversial, given its known toxicities and the many active hormonal and now immunologic therapies that can be administered prior to docetaxel. However, it has been demonstrated that the absolute survival advantage of docetaxel is greatest (3 to 4 months) in men with minimal symptoms, whereas men who have impaired performance status or pain due to cancer are not able to tolerate 10 full cycles well and often have a reduction in the overall survival benefit (1 to 2 month advantage). Thus, the early timely use of docetaxel in men with clear prostate cancer progression based on PSA or radiographic disease is warranted for palliation and prevention of pain onset as well as improved survival.

Several nomograms currently exist for men with metastatic castration-resistant prostate cancer that can predict overall survival (Halabi, MSKCC, Armstrong-TAX327). These studies indicate that the presence of visceral metastatic disease, anemia, performance status, PS level, PSA doubling time, PSA, elevated alkaline phosphatase, low albumin, Gleason score, the presence of significant pain, the type of progression and lactate dehydrogenase level are highly predictive of survival and can be used to inform on prognosis. In addition, circulatory tumor cells are FDA approved as prognostic markers of survival in men receiving docetaxel. These cells can be enumerated in 7.5 mL of whole blood either prior to systemic chemotherapy or while the patient is receiving chemotherapy, and the number of circulating tumor cells (CTCs) in whole blood correlates strongly with overall survival. Although CTCs are not credentialed at this time as surrogates and thus have not been used or studied to guide therapeutic choices in men with castration-resistant prostate cancer, the ability to detect and characterize these cells holds promise as a predictive and intermediate biomarker to aid in personalized medicine approaches. These cells can be further characterized in research settings for molecular profiling, indicating their potential to help guide systemic therapy in the future.

Mitoxantrone plus prednisone Mitoxantrone (12 mg/m^2) plus prednisone has been approved for use in advanced prostate cancer based on improvement in palliation of pain and quality of life over prednisone alone despite no improvement in overall survival. Toxicities of mitoxantrone include a cumulative cardiotoxicity, typically after 10 to 12 cycles of therapy. Thus pretreatment ejection fraction assessment is recommended in all men as well as serial ejection fraction assessments every 4 to

5 cycles or based on new onset of cardiac symptoms. Given the recent approval of cabazitaxel (Jevtana; see discussion later in this chapter), use of mitoxantrone has generally been limited to third-line therapy, or for palliative therapy in men who are not candidates for microtubule-targeting therapies because of neuropathy, for example.

Bisphosphonates Bone metastases from prostate cancer are associated with increased bone formation around tumor deposits, resulting in characteristic osteoblastic metastases. However, concomitant with the osteoblastic activity is a marked increase in bone resorption and osteolysis, which can be inhibited by bisphosphonates.

Studies of bisphosphonates in prostate cancer have demonstrated mixed results. A combined analysis of two multicentered randomized controlled trials comparing pamidronate with placebo in men with androgen-independent progressive prostate cancer demonstrated no benefit in terms of skeleton-related events or palliation of symptoms. A phase III trial with an oral bisphosphonate, clodronate, demonstrated no difference in either symptomatic bone metastases or prostate cancer-related deaths when compared with placebo.

A phase III trial demonstrated a reduction in skeleton-related events for men with castration-resistant metastatic prostate cancer with a more potent bisphosphonate, zoledronic acid (Zometa). However, it is important to note that this trial did not show an improvement in quality of life with zoledronic acid, nor did it demonstrate a reduction in the development of new metastases.

At this time, the recommendation for zoledronic acid in prostate cancer is limited to men with castration-resistant metastatic prostate cancer, pending ongoing randomized studies in the hormone-sensitive population. It is important to recognize the limitations of this therapy and to understand that there is no defined role for its use in men with androgen-dependent prostate cancer. Although these men are at higher risk for osteoporosis, less potent oral bisphosphonates may be a more reasonable approach, given the long-term side effects associated with zoledronic acid (renal insufficiency and osteonecrosis of the mandible).

Phase III results of several novel bone-targeting agents are awaited, notably denosumab, a RANKL antagonist, and toremifene (Fareston), a selective estrogen-receptor modifier. Both agents have demonstrated reductions in morphometric fractures, with few adverse effects in men with advanced recurrent prostate cancer. In addition, denosumab (Prolia) has recently shown an improvement in the prevention of skeleton-related events in men with metastatic castration-resistant prostate cancer as compared

A novel approach to the prevention of bone loss and skeletal events in recurrent prostate cancer involves the use of an inhibitor antibody to block RANKL (Receptor Activator for Nuclear Factor Ligand), a molecule involved in osteoclast-mediated bone resorption and remodeling. This antibody, termed denosumab, has demonstrated an ability to improve bone mineral density in men undergoing ADT, as well as an improved capability in preventing fracture and restoring bone density as compared to zoledronic acid in head-to-head studies. While osteonecrosis is also a side effect with this compound, its subcutaneous administration and lack of kidney toxicity may lead to a role for this agent as an alternative bone-health agent in prostate cancer, if approved by the FDA.

with zoledronic acid. If approved by the US FDA, denosumab may become a suitable bone-health agent that may be used as adjunctive treatment with hormonal therapy or chemotherapy. Further studies of the role of denosumab in the prevention of metastasis and hormone therapy–induced clinical fractures will help to guide the rational use of this agent, which is given by subcutaneous injection. Side effects of denosumab include osteonecrosis of the jaw, similar to that of zoledronic acid. Further evaluation of these agents on clinical fracture rates, safety, and other endpoints are awaited.

Second-line chemotherapy

In 2010, it was demonstrated that a novel synthetic taxane, cabazitaxel, demonstrated improved overall survival as compared with mitoxantrone in men with metastatic castration-resistant prostate cancer whose disease had progressed on docetaxel chemotherapy. The overall survival benefit was 2 months (from 12.7 to 15.1 months, HR 0.70, $P < .0001$), and improvements in PSA response, tumor response, and progression-free survival were notable. Each regimen was similarly palliative, but the duration of response favored cabazitaxel. Cabazitaxel is dosed at 25 mg/m^2 IV every 3 weeks with prednisone dosed at 5 mg orally twice daily. The risk of neutropenia and sepsis due to myelosuppression in this heavily pretreated group of men is high (7% to 8%) and prophylactic G-CSF should strongly be considered. Other toxicities include neuropathy, fatigue, diarrhea, nausea, and vomiting. Continuation of testosterone suppression was required. Cabazitaxel has demonstrated activity in docetaxel-resistant cell lines and was approved by the US FDA in 2010 for second-line treatment of men with chemorefractory castration-resistant prostate cancer.

Newer therapies

Several newer therapies for men with prostate cancer (some as single agents and some with chemotherapy) are under investigation. Since docetaxel is the only approved chemotherapy in the front-line setting to date associated with a survival advantage in patients with metastatic castrate-resistant prostate cancer, it has become the "backbone" upon which novel therapies and response modifiers are added in an attempt to improve patient outcomes. Recent reports demonstrated that the addition of bevacizumab (Avastin) to docetaxel did not improve overall survival in men with metastatic castration-resistant prostate cancer. Thus, docetaxel-prednisone remains the front-line treatment of choice for men with metastatic castration-resistant prostate cancer who have failed to respond to prior hormonal therapy.

Based on promising results in phase II testing, several phase III trials building upon docetaxel were opened (Table 9). Whether building upon docetaxel with targeted therapy will be of benefit is still unknown pending the results of the remaining phase III trials. Phase III trials of other therapies both before or after docetaxel, including novel agents targeting the androgen receptor (abiraterone acetate, MDV3100, TAK700 for example), are awaited. Table 7 presents ongoing phase III studies of novel agents in the postdocetaxel setting. Finally, many of these agents are being tested in men with asymptomatic CRPC or minimally symptomatic men with metastatic CRPC (ie the window prior to docetaxel use), with the aim of delaying chemotherapy use/need.

Table 9: Phase III docetaxel combination trials in castration-resistant metastatic prostate cancer

Trial	Experimental agent	Type of therapy	Phase	Status
Docetaxel/ prednisone ± bevacizumab	Bevacizumab	Antiangiogenesis	III	Negative
Docetaxel/ prednisone + aflibercept	Aflibercept (VEGF-trap)	Antiangiogeneis	III	Completed
Docetaxel/ prednisone ± atrasentan	Atrasentan	ET-A receptor antagonist	III	Ongoing
Docetaxel/ prednisone ± dasatinib	Dasatinib	Antimetastatic and bone-targeting agent (src kinase)	III	Ongoing
Docetaxel/ prednisone ± ZD4054	ZD4054 (zibotentan)	ET-A receptor antagonist	III	Ongoing
Docetaxel/ prednisone ± lenalidomide	Lenalidomide	Immunomodulatory agent	III	Ongoing

Sipuleucel-T vaccine was approved by the FDA for advanced prostate cancer in April 2010. In addition, current trials are investigating the use of systemic agents, including docetaxel, in locally advanced or PSA-recurrent disease, either prior to or adjuvant following surgery or radiation therapy. Accrual to these trials has been a priority (RTOG 0521 [now completed], VA 553, CALGB 90203), as they are investigating the role of systemic therapy to prevent disease recurrence, similar to the widely accepted use of systemic therapy for other tumor types such as breast and colorectal cancers. RTOG is exploring the role of docetaxel in addition to long-term androgen-deprivation therapy for men with locally advanced high-risk prostate cancer who have completed IMRT of the prostate. CALGB 90203 randomized high-risk men (Gleason score > 8 or nomogram-defined high risk) to immediate radical prostatectomy vs docetaxel for 6 cycles with androgen deprivation therapy followed by radical prostatectomy. The use of neoadjuvant or adjuvant docetaxel for high-risk men will be guided through evidence provided by these trials.

Recent guidelines by the PCWG2 have updated methods for categorizing disease states in men with castration-resistant prostate cancer (node only, PSA only, locally advanced, bone metastatic visceral disease). In addition, the requirements for confirmation bone scans and changes in the reporting and assessment of disease progression have been updated to be more consistent with our understanding of prostate cancer biology bone scan flares with effective therapy, and to prevent the unnecessary early abandonment of potentially active agents based on PSA changes alone. For example, healing of bone lesions may cause an apparent "worsening" of disease on bone scan despite declines in PSA levels and improvement in pain, likely due to osteoblastic activity in regressing tumors. Physicians are encouraged to evaluate these potential flare cases with a confirmatory bone scan 6 or more weeks later; if the patient develops no additional new lesions or disease progression, he should be maintained on therapy. Many older therapies may have been unnecessarily stopped prematurely due to this misclassification of bone scan progression using older criteria.

Radiation therapy for palliating bone metastasis

Radiotherapy is effective in controlling local pain associated with skeletal prostate metastasis. In general, a treatment regimen of 30 Gy over 10 treatments results in rapid and durable local symptom control and a reduced dependence on analgesics. Single-dose palliative radiation therapy may provide equal palliation as well.

For patients with more extensive bone involvement causing pain that may be difficult to address with localized EBRT, alternatives include wide-field irradiation (ie, hemibody irradiation) or systemic administration of radioactive bone-seeking isotopes that can deliver therapeutic doses to skeletal metastatic disease. Radioactive isotopes used in this fashion include strontium-89 chloride (Metastron) and samarium SM 153 lexidronam (Quadramet). An ongoing phase III study of radium-223 (alpharadin) will test whether this radioisotopic alpha emitter can improve overall survival and improve palliation compared with best supportive care in the postchemotherapy setting.

SUGGESTED READING

Andriole GL, Crawford ED, Grubb RL 3rd; PLCO Project Team: Mortality results from a randomized prostate-cancer screening trial. N Engl J Med 360:1351–1354, 2009.

Armstrong AJ, Garrett-Mayer E, de Wit R, et al: Prediction of survival following first-line chemotherapy in men with castration-resistant metastatic prostate cancer. Clin Cancer Res 16:203–211, 2010.

Armstrong AJ, Tannock IF, de Wit R, et al: The development of risk groups in men with metastatic castration-resistant prostate cancer based on risk factors for PSA decline and survival. Eur J Cancer 46:517–525, 2010.

Armstrong AJ, Garrett-Mayer ES, Yang YC, et al: A contemporary prognostic nomogram for men with hormone-refractory metastatic prostate cancer: A TAX327 study analysis. Clin Cancer Res 13:6396–6403, 2007.

Attard G, Reid AH, A'Hern R, et al: Selective inhibition of CYP17 with abiraterone acetate is highly active in the treatment of castration-resistant prostate cancer. J Clin Oncol 27:3732–3748, 2009.

Bañez LL, Hamilton RJ, Partin AW, et al: Obesity-related plasma hemodilution and PSA concentration among men with prostate cancer. JAMA 298:2275–2280, 2007.

Barry MJ: Screening for prostate cancer—The controversy that refuses to die. N Engl J Med 360:1351–1354, 2009.

D'Amico AV, Chen MH, Renshaw AA: Androgen suppression and radiation vs radiation alone for prostate cancer: A randomized trial. JAMA 299:289–295, 2008.

D'Amico AV, Denham JW, Crook J, et al: Influence of androgen suppression therapy for prostate cancer on the frequency and timing of fatal myocardial infarctions. J Clin Oncol 25:2420–2425, 2007.

de Bono JS, Scher HI, Montgomery RB, et al: Circulating tumor cells predict survival benefit from treatment in metastatic castration-resistant prostate cancer. Clin Cancer Res 14:6302–6309, 2008.

Droz JP, Balducci L, Bolla M, et al: Management of prostate cancer in older men: Recommendations of a working group of the International Society of Geriatric Oncology. BJU Int 106:462–469, 2010.

Freedland SJ, Humphreys EB, Mangold LA, et al: Death in patients with recurrent prostate cancer after radical prostatectomy: Prostate-specific antigen doubling time subgroups and their associated contributions to all-cause mortality. J Clin Oncol 25:1765–1771, 2007.

Freedland SJ, Mavropoulos J, Wang A, et al: Carbohydrate restriction, prostate cancer growth, and the insulin-like growth factor axis. Prostate 68:11–19, 2008.

Giovannucci E, Liu Y, Platz EA, et al: Risk factors for prostate cancer incidence and progression in the health professionals follow-up study. Int J Cancer 121:1571–1578, 2007.

Jemal A, Siegel R, Xu J, Ward E: Cancer statistics, 2010. CA Cancer J Clin 60:277–300, 2010.

Kawachi MH, Bahnson RR, Barry M, et al: NCCN clinical practice guidelines in oncology: Prostate cancer early detection. J Natl Comp Canc Netw 8:240–262, 2010.

Keating NL, O'Malley AJ, Freedland SJ, et al: Diabetes and cardiovascular disease during androgen deprivation therapy: Observational study of veterans with prostate cancer. J Natl Cancer Inst 102:39–46, 2010.

Kirsh VA, Peters U, Mayne ST, et al: Prospective study of fruit and vegetable intake and risk of prostate cancer. J Natl Cancer Inst 99:1200–1209, 2007.

Klotz L, Zhang L, Lam A, et al: Clinical results of long-term follow-up of a large, active surveillance cohort with localized prostate cancer. J Clin Oncol 28:126–131, 2010.

Loblaw DA, Virgo KS, Nam R, et al: Initial hormonal management of androgen-sensitive metastatic, recurrent, or progressive prostate cancer: 2006 update of an American Society of Clinical Oncology practice guideline. J Clin Oncol 25:1596–1605, 2007.

Lu-Yao GL, Albertsen PC, Moore DF, et al: Survival following primary androgen deprivation therapy among men with localized prostate cancer. JAMA 300:173–181, 2008.

Lu-Yao GL, Albertsen PC, Moore DF, et al: Outcomes of localized prostate cancer following conservative management. JAMA 302:1202–1209, 2009.

Messing EM, Manola J, Yao J, et al: Immediate versus deferred androgen deprivation treatment in patients with node-positive prostate cancer after radical prostatectomy and pelvic lymphadenectomy. Lancet Oncol 7:472–479, 2006.

Moul JW, Wu H, Sun L, et al: Early versus delayed hormonal therapy for prostate specific antigen only recurrence of prostate cancer after radical prostatectomy. J Urol 179(5 suppl):S53–S59, 2008.

Sanda MG, Dunn RL, Michalski J, et al: Quality of life and satisfaction with outcome among prostate-cancer survivors. N Engl J Med 358:1250–1261, 2008.

Scher HI, Halabi S, Tannock I, et al: Design and end points of clinical trials for patients with progressive prostate cancer and castrate levels of testosterone: Recommendations of the Prostate Cancer Clinical Trials Working Group. J Clin Oncol 26:1148–1159, 2008.

Schröder FH, Hugosson J, Roobol MJ, et al; ERSPC Investigators: Screening and prostate-cancer mortality in a randomized European study. N Engl J Med 360:1320–1328, 2009.

Schröder FH, Roach M 3rd, Scardino P: Clinical decisions: Management of prostate cancer. N Engl J Med 359:2605–2609, 2008.

Stephenson AJ, Kattan MW, Eastham JA, et al: Prostate cancer-specific mortality after radical prostatectomy for patients treated in the prostate-specific antigen era. J Clin Oncol 27:4300–4305, 2009.

Thompson IM, Ankerst DP, Chi C, et al: Assessing prostate cancer risk: Results from the Prostate Cancer Prevention Trial. J Natl Cancer Inst 98:529–534, 2006.

Thompson I, Thrasher JB, Aus G, et al: AUA Prostate Cancer Clinical Guideline Update Panel: Guideline for the management of clinically localized prostate cancer: 2007 update. J Urol 177:2106–2131, 2007.

Tran C, Ouk S, Clegg NJ, et al: Development of a second-generation antiandrogen for treatment of advanced prostate cancer. Science 324:787–790, 2009.

Trock BJ, Han M, Freedland SJ, et al: Prostate cancer-specific survival following salvage radiotherapy vs observation in men with biochemical recurrence after radical prostatectomy. JAMA 299:2760–2769, 2008.

Walsh PC, DeWeese TL, Eisenberger MA: Clinical practice: Localized prostate cancer. N Engl J Med 357:2696–2705, 2007.

Wong YN, Mitra N, Hudes G, et al: Survival associated with treatment vs observation of localized prostate cancer in elderly men. JAMA 296:2683–2693, 2006.

Zheng SL, Sun J, Wiklund F, et al: Cumulative association of five genetic variants with prostate cancer. N Engl J Med 358:910–919, 2008.

Abbreviations in this chapter

ACS = American Cancer Society; ASCO = American Society of Clinical Oncology; ASTRO = American Society for Therapeutic Radiology and Oncology; AUA = American Urological Association; CALGB = Cancer and Leukemia Group B; ECOG = Eastern Cooperative Oncology Group; EORTC = European Organisation for Research and Treatment of Cancer; ERSPC = European Randomized Screening Study for Prostate Cancer; MRC = Medical Research Council; MSKCC = Memorial Sloan-Kettering Cancer Center; NCCN = National Comprehensive Cancer Network; NCIC = National Cancer Institute of Canada; PCPT = Prostate Cancer Prevention Trial; PCWG = Prostate Cancer Working Group; PLCO = Prostate, Lung, Colorectal, and Ovarian Cancer Screening; RTOG = Radiation Therapy Oncology Group; SWOG = Southwest Oncology Group

CHAPTER 15

Testicular cancer

Patrick J. Loehrer, MD, Atreya Dash, MD,
Mark K. Buyyounouski, MD, MS, and Douglas Skarecky, BS

TESTICULAR

Testicular cancer, although an uncommon malignancy, is the most frequently occurring cancer in young men. In the year 2010, an estimated 8,480 cases of testicular cancer will have been diagnosed in the United States, with approximately 350 men succumbing to the disease. For unknown reasons, the incidence of this cancer has increased since the turn of the century, from 2 cases per 100,000 population in the 1930s, to 3.7 cases per 100,000 population from 1969 to 1971, to 5.4 cases per 100,000 population from 1995 to 1999. The greatest rise has been observed in Puerto Rico (1973 to 1997: 220%). This trend seems greatest for the development of seminoma.

Most testicular tumors are of germ-cell origin. These cancers are uniquely sensitive to chemotherapy and are considered the model for the treatment of solid tumors. Perhaps the most controversial area in the management of germ-cell tumors is the proper approach to early-stage disease (ie, surveillance vs primary retroperitoneal lymphadenectomy for nonseminomatous germ-cell tumors [NSGCTs] or radiation therapy for seminomas). In advanced disease, chemotherapy plays an essential role, but novel treatment regimens are currently being evaluated through multi-institutional clinical trials.

EPIDEMIOLOGY

Age

Testicular cancer can occur at any age, but it is most common between the ages of 15 and 35 years. There is a secondary peak in incidence after age 60. Seminoma is the most common histology in the older population, but it is rare in those younger than age 10. There is a slightly increased prevalence of testicular cancer among fathers and brothers of testicular cancer patients.

Race

Testicular cancer is rare among blacks (1.6/100,000 population), yet black men present with higher grade disease and have significantly worse survival at 5 and 10 years. The incidence of this cancer has increased in whites during the 20th century but has remained flat in blacks. Non-Hispanic white patients typically present with disease at early stages when compared with black, Native-American, Hawaiian, and Hispanic patients.

Table 1: Anticipated cure rates in patients with germ-cell tumors, according to disease stage

Stage	Incidence at presentation (%)	Cure rate (%)
I (testis alone)	40	100
II (extension to retroperitoneal lymph nodes)	40	98
III (disseminated disease)	20	80

Geography

Denmark has the highest incidence of testicular cancer; the Far East has the lowest incidence of this disease.

Primary site

Germ-cell tumors present most commonly in the testes (90%) and only infrequently in extragonadal sites (10%). The most common extragonadal sites (in decreasing order of frequency) are the retroperitoneum, mediastinum, and pineal gland. Many patients presumed to have a primary retroperitoneal germ-cell tumor may have an occult germ-cell tumor of the testicle. This possibility should be evaluated with testicular ultrasonography, especially when the retroperitoneal tumor is predominantly one-sided.

Survival

The 5-year survival rate for all patients with testicular cancer is ~95%. Cure rates are highest for early-stage disease, which is treated primarily with surgery or radiation therapy (early seminoma), and lower for advanced disease, for which chemotherapy is the primary therapy (Table 1).

ETIOLOGY AND RISK FACTORS

The specific cause of germ-cell tumors is unknown, but various factors have been associated with an increased risk of this malignancy.

Prior testicular cancer

Perhaps the strongest risk factor for germ-cell tumors is a history of testicular cancer. Approximately 1% to 2% of patients with testicular cancer will develop a second primary in the contralateral testis over time. This represents a 500-fold increase in incidence over that noted among the normal male population.

The risk of contralateral testicular cancer was studied in a large population-based cohort of men diagnosed with testicular cancer before the age of 55. For 29,515 cases reported from 1973 through 2001 to the NCI's SEER Program, the 15-year cumulative risk of developing metachronous contralateral testicular cancer was 1.9%, reaffirming the practice of not performing a biopsy on the contralateral testis at initial presentation.

Cryptorchidism

Patients with cryptorchidism have a four- to eightfold increased risk of developing germ-cell tumors when compared with their normal counterparts. Orchiopexy, even at an early age, appears to reduce the incidence of germ-cell tumor only slightly (if at all). For an undescended testis, the most common malignant histology is seminoma. For those undergoing early orchiopexy, the most common malignancy is nonseminoma. Of note, in ~10% of patients with cryptorchidism who develop germ-cell tumors, the cancer is found in the normally descended testis. Biopsies of nonenlarged cryptorchid testes demonstrate an increased incidence of intratubal germ-cell neoplasm, a presumed precursor lesion.

Wood and Elder conducted an extensive review of the data about cryptorchidism as it related to testicular cancer. The relative risk of testicular cancer in cryptorchidism is 2.75 to 8. A relative risk of 2 to 3 has been noted in patients who undergo orchiopexy by ages 10 to 12 years. Patients who undergo orchiopexy after age 12 or no orchiopexy are 2 to 6 times as likely to have testicular cancer *(Wood HM et al: J Urol 181:452–461, 2009).*

Genetics

Klinefelter syndrome (47XXY) is associated with a higher incidence of germ-cell tumors, particularly primary mediastinal germ-cell tumors. For first-degree relatives of individuals affected with 47XXY, approximately a 6- to 10-fold increased risk of germ-cell tumors has been observed. In addition, patients with Down syndrome have been reported to be at increased risk for germ-cell tumors. Also thought to be at greater risk are patients with testicular feminization, true hermaphrodism, persistent Müllerian syndrome, and cutaneous ichthyosis. In a genome-wide analysis of gene expression, *PEPP-2* (X-linked homeobox gene), otoancorin (*OTOA*), and a kinase anchor protein (*AKAP4*) represent three candidate genes for diagnostic and therapeutic targets in testicular cancer. The International Testicular Cancer Linkage Consortium has been genotyping families with multiple cases of testicular cancer and found regions on several chromosomes (3, 5, 12, 18) which are worthy of further investigation. Two new single-nucleotide polymorphism studies implicate *KITLG* (12p22) and *SPRY4* (5q31.3) as plausible gene loci.

Family history

Although familial testicular cancer has been observed, its incidence among first-degree relatives remains low. One investigator, however, reported a sixfold increased risk among male offspring of a patient with testicular cancer.

Environment

Numerous industrial occupations and drug exposures have been implicated in the development of testicular cancer. Although exposure to diethylstilbestrol (DES) in utero is associated with cryptorchidism, a direct association between DES and germ-cell neoplasm is weak at best.

Virtually all adult patients with germ-cell tumors have increased copies of isochromosome 12p, usually as i(12p). This is a useful marker in patients with undifferentiated tumors who fit the clinical profile of patients with germ-cell malignancy. In addition, mutations in v-kit Hardy-Zuckerman 4 feline sarcoma viral oncogene homolog (*KITi*) have also been observed in seminoma, especially in tumors of primary mediastinal origin. Two genome single-nucleotide polymorphism searches confirm a potential candidate in *KITLG* (12p22). The clinical significance of this observation is unknown.

Reports have suggested an increased risk of testicular cancer among individuals exposed to exogenous toxins, such as Agent Orange and solvents used to clean jets. One author has suggested that, based on epidemiologic evidence, exposure to ochratoxin A correlated with incidence data for testicular cancer.

Prior trauma, elevated scrotal temperature (secondary to the use of thermal underwear, jockey shorts, and electric blankets), and recurrent activities such as horseback riding and motorcycle riding do not appear to be related to the development of testicular cancer.

No supporting findings substantiate a viral etiology.

Fertility

An increased risk of infertility exists for men with unilateral testicular cancer successfully treated with orchiectomy. For example, 40% of patients have subnormal sperm counts, and, by 1 year, 25% continue to have subnormal sperm counts.

SIGNS AND SYMPTOMS

Local disease

Scrotal mass

The most common complaint of patients on presentation is a painless scrotal mass that, on physical examination, cannot be separated from the testis. This finding distinguishes the mass from epididymitis. Not infrequently, the mass may be painful and, thus, may mimic epididymitis or testicular torsion.

Hydrocele

Approximately 20% of patients with germ-cell tumors have an associated hydrocele.

Inguinal adenopathy

Patients generally do not have inguinal adenopathy in the absence of prior scrotal violation.

Other symptoms

They include low back pain (from retroperitoneal adenopathy) and gynecomastia (usually bilateral). In cases of massive retroperitoneal lymphadenopathy, abdominal pain, nausea, vomiting, and constipation may be reported.

Disseminated disease

Patients with disseminated germ-cell tumors usually present with symptoms from lymphatic or hematogeneous dissemination. Mediastinal adenopathy may be associated with chest pain or cough. Supraclavicular lymphadenopathy may also be present.

The cumulative 10-year risk of developing metachronous testicular cancer for patients with extragonadal germ-cell tumors is 10.3%. Patients with extragonadal tumors of the retroperitoneum and NSGCTs have a 14.3% 10-year risk for the development of metachronous testicular cancer. Some, however, may have previously undiagnosed occult testicular primary tumors.

Hematogeneous spread to the lungs may be associated with dyspnea, cough, or hemoptysis. Infrequently, patients with extensive disease may present with signs and symptoms of CNS metastases or bone pain from osseous metastases (most common in patients with seminoma).

Metastases to the liver are not uncommon and may manifest as fullness in the upper abdomen or vague abdominal discomfort. More likely, they will be identified on CT scan in an otherwise asymptomatic patient.

Primary mediastinal germ-cell tumors

Primary mediastinal germ-cell tumors are associated with several unique syndromes, including Klinefelter syndrome and acute megakaryocytic leukemia. In addition, mediastinal tumors have a great propensity for the development of non–germ-cell malignant histology as a major component of the tumor (eg, embryonal rhabdomyosarcoma, adenocarcinoma, and peripheral neuroectodermal tumor).

SCREENING AND DIAGNOSIS

Screening

Self-examination

Testicular self-examination is both simple to learn and safe to perform. The rarity of testicular cancer, however, calls into question the value of routine aggressive screening procedures.

Testicular biopsy

Testicular biopsy of a suspicious lesion is not recommended. Approximately 95% of patients with a mass within the testicle have a malignancy. Orchiectomy is the preferred treatment for patients with a testicular mass.

Carcinoma in situ (CIS) appears to be the precursor lesion for most testicular germ-cell tumors, except spermatocytic seminoma. Most patients harboring CIS can be expected to develop testicular cancer, but with a latency period of a decade or more. The incidence of CIS in infertile men is about 0.6%. In patients with prior testicular cancer, biopsy will reveal CIS in the contralateral testis at a rate of approximately 5% to 6%. Men with a history of cryptorchidism and presumed extragonadal germ-cell tumor are at greater risk for CIS. Some investigators suggest routine biopsy of the contralateral testis in men with CIS.

Diagnosis

Ultrasonography

Ultrasound can reliably identify masses within the testis. In virtually all patients, ultrasonography can distinguish a testicular lesion from an extratesticular mass and may detect lesions that are not palpable on physical examination. Ultrasonographic findings cannot consistently differentiate benign lesions from malignant tumors of the testis (95% of such masses are malignant). Most patients with testicular cancer, and especially those with seminoma, have lesions that are hypoechoic when compared with adjacent tissue. NSGCT, however, may cause mixed signals, including hyperechoic masses, which are commonly seen with teratoma.

Serum markers

Serum levels of β-subunit human chorionic gonadotropin (β-hCG) and α-fetoprotein (AFP) are elevated in approximately 80% to 85% of patients with extensive germ-cell tumors. Patients with pure seminoma may have elevated levels of β-hCG but not of AFP (a significantly elevated AFP level usually indicates the presence of NSGCT elements). False-positive β-hCG levels can be seen in patients who have hypogonadism (cross-reactivity with luteinizing hormone) or who use marijuana; AFP levels may be elevated in patients with liver dysfunction or hepatitis. Levels of actin-β-106/193/384 fragments in cell-free DNA levels were increased in patients with testicular cancer when compared with controls, with up to 87% sensitivity and 95% specificity. This analysis was predictive of stage III disease in seven patients. The high sensitivity of cell-free DNA could assist in the management of testicular cancer, especially when traditional serum markers are not elevated.

Inguinal orchiectomy

When a testicular mass is discovered, the patient should undergo an orchiectomy through an inguinal incision.

Trans-scrotal incisions or biopsies

These procedures should not be performed, as they may ultimately lead to aberrant lymphatic drainage from the tumor.

STAGING EVALUATION

The principal objective of the staging evaluation is to ascertain whether the patient has early-stage disease (which is amenable to local therapy) or disseminated disease (which requires chemotherapy).

Chest x-ray

A chest x-ray can determine whether or not a patient has gross supradiaphragmatic metastases, which would mandate initial chemotherapy.

Chest CT

In patients with a normal chest x-ray, chest CT is recommended in both patients with seminoma and those with NSGCT when abdominal adenopathy is found to rule out occult metastases within the lungs or mediastinum. If such metastases are present, the patient should be treated with primary chemotherapy.

Abdominopelvic CT

This test provides important information about the retroperitoneal lymph nodes. Usually, periaortic adenopathy is noted on the ipsilateral side of the primary tumor. Patients with primary retroperitoneal germ-cell tumors often show an enlarged retroperitoneal mass in the midline. Although hepatic metastases are infrequent, CT presently is the most viable method of determining these metastatic lesions.

Positron emission tomography (PET)

^{18}F-fluorodeoxyglucose (FDG) is emerging as a significant adjunct in staging and follow-up. Seminomas are FDG-avid. In some cases, nodal and extranodal metastases not appreciated on CT scans may be noted with FDG-PET. The optimal use of FDG-PET is in patients with residual masses following systemic therapy for pure seminoma. In such cases, the scans should be performed at least 3 to 4 weeks beyond the last course of chemotherapy. As teratoma is not PET-avid, its usefulness in NSGCTs is limited to patients with late recurrences manifested with marker-only disease.

Other scans

In the absence of symptoms or signs, a CT scan (or MRI) of the head and radionuclide bone scan are unnecessary. A lymphangiogram is rarely used today to identify microscopic nodal involvement in patients with stage I disease who choose to undergo surveillance. PET scans may be useful in patients with residual disease following chemotherapy for seminoma. If a PET scan is positive in such patients, surgical resection of the residual mass is indicated. Otherwise, the residual mass can be simply followed with periodic radiographic evaluation.

PATHOLOGY

Germ-cell tumors are classified into two broad histologic categories: seminoma and NSGCT. Patients with seminoma who have increased AFP levels or any focus of NSGCT components (including teratoma) are considered to have NSGCT.

Seminoma

Seminoma is the most common single histology, accounting for approximately 30% of all germ-cell tumors. Up to 10% of seminomas have focal syncytiotrophoblastic cells, which are believed to be the source of β-hCG in some cases. Elevated AFP levels connote NSGCT.

Spermatocytic seminoma

This is a rare subset of germ-cell tumors, often grows to a large size, occurs almost exclusively in men older than age 50, and rarely, if ever, metastasizes. Unlike classic seminoma, immunohistochemical staining is currently negative for placental-like alkaline phosphatase (PLAP). Other evidence suggests a different cell of origin for spermatocytic seminoma compared with other germ-cell tumors.

Nonseminomatous germ-cell tumors

Embryonal carcinoma

This lesion is composed of large pleomorphic cells with different architectural patterns. This tumor may be associated with an elevation in the serum levels of β-hCG and/or AFP.

Endodermal sinus tumor (yolk sac carcinoma)

This is the most common testicular tumor seen in infants and young children. Like embryonal carcinoma, the yolk sac tumor has a variety of architectural patterns. This tumor is associated with an elevated serum level of AFP.

Choriocarcinoma

As a pure entity, choriocarcinoma is one of the least common germ-cell tumors. These tumors have a great propensity for hematogeneous spread, often skipping the retroperitoneum. Choriocarcinoma is associated with an increased serum level of β-hCG.

Teratoma

The teratoma is a generally benign tumor with elements from each of the germ layers (ectoderm, mesoderm, and endoderm). Teratoma is uncommonly seen as the sole histology in primary tumors, but it is frequently associated with other histologic elements, including those previously mentioned. Of patients with residual disease following chemotherapy for NSGCT, about 45% have evidence of teratoma in resected specimens.

A subset of patients with immature teratoma that contains non–germ-cell histologies (eg, sarcoma, adenocarcinoma) has been reported. In contrast to most teratomas, these tumors may grow locally and can be lethal. In addition, late recurrences of both teratoma and carcinoma have been reported in patients with teratoma. Serum markers are normal in patients with pure teratoma.

PATTERN OF SPREAD

Testicular cancer spreads in a fairly predictable fashion: from the testicle to the retroperitoneal lymph nodes and, later, hematogeneously to the lungs or other visceral sites. Only 10% of patients present with hematogeneous metastases (usually in the lungs) in the absence of discernible retroperitoneal adenopathy.

STAGING SYSTEMS

Clinical staging systems (Royal Marsden and TNM systems) for testicular cancer are outlined in Table 2. These staging systems help define the population for appropriate primary therapy.

Table 2: Staging systems for testicular cancer

Royal Marsden system	TNM system[a]	Description
I	TX, N0, M0	Disease confined to the testis and peritesticular tissue
II	TX, N1 or N2a, M0	< 6 positive lymph nodes without extension into retroperitoneal fat; no node > 2 cm (infradiaphragmatic)
A < 2 cm B 2–5 cm C > 5–10 cm D > 10 cm		
	TX, N2b, M0	≥ 6 positive lymph nodes, well encapsulated and/or retroperitoneal fat extension; any node > 2 cm
	TX, N3, M0	Any node > 5 cm
III	TX, NX, M1	Supradiaphragmatic and infradiaphragmatic adenopathy (no extralymphatic metastasis)
IV		Disseminated disease (lungs, liver, bone)

[a] The definition of TNM for testicular cancer has not changed between the 6th and 7th editions of the AJCC Cancer Staging Manual.

Good-, intermediate-, and poor-risk subgroups

For patients with NSGCTs who are candidates for chemotherapy, other staging systems (such as those by Indiana University and MSKCC) were developed to segregate patients into good- and poor-risk categories. More recently, the IGCCCG formulated a classification that more clearly defines good-, intermediate-, and poor-risk disease (Table 3) and is currently being used to stratify patients for appropriate chemotherapy and in ongoing trials.

TREATMENT

Stage I or II disease

Surgery

Initial intervention for testicular cancer is radical inguinal orchiectomy. Orchiectomy may be deferred temporarily in patients with advanced-stage disease in whom the diagnosis of NSGCT can be made on clinical grounds (elevated markers). In such patients, an orchiectomy must be performed sooner or later, as there is incomplete penetration of chemotherapy into the testes.

Further therapy hinges on the pathologic diagnosis. In general, most clinical stage I tumors are typically followed with surveillance. Patients with pure seminomas (normal AFP level with or without an elevated β-hCG level) are treated with radiotherapy or chemotherapy, whereas most NSGCTs are treated with surgery and/or chemotherapy.

Table 3: IGCCCG criteria for good-, intermediate-, and poor-risk testicular cancer patients treated with chemotherapy

NONSEMINOMA

Good risk

All of the following:

- AFP < 1,000 ng/mL, β-hCG < 5,000 IU/L, and LDH < 1.5 × upper limit of normal
- Nonmediastinal primary
- No nonpulmonary visceral metastasis

Intermediate risk

All of the following:

- AFP = 1,000–10,000 ng/mL, β-hCG = 5,000–50,000 IU/L, or LDH = 1.5–10 × normal
- Nonmediastinal primary site
- No nonpulmonary visceral metastasis

Poor risk

Any of the following:

- AFP > 10,000 ng/mL, β-hCG > 50,000 IU/L, or LDH > 10 × normal
- Mediastinal primary site
- Nonpulmonary visceral metastasis

SEMINOMA

Good risk

- No nonpulmonary visceral metastasis

Intermediate risk

- Nonpulmonary visceral metastasis

IGCCCG = International Germ-Cell Cancer Collaborative Group; AFP = α-fetoprotein; hCG = human chorionic gonadotropin; LDH = lactate dehydrogenase

Inguinal orchiectomy In addition to removal of the testis, the spermatic cord is dissected high into the retroperitoneum. The vas deferens is isolated from the testicular vessels and ligated separately with a permanent suture. Also, the testicular vessels are freed from the peritoneum and carefully ligated with a permanent suture.

Retroperitoneal lymph node dissection (RLND) for NSGCTs For patients with NSGCTs and either no evidence or a small volume of disease on CT (stage I [N0] or stage II [N1, N2a, N2b] disease), RLND was generally indicated because it (1) accurately and definitively defines the presence or absence of retroperitoneal metastases and (2) removes the retroperitoneum as a site of recurrence, thus obviating the need for surveillance with CT. Today, most patients undergo surveillance or primary chemotherapy (see discussion later in this chapter).

RLND can be accomplished transperitoneally or retroperitoneally through a thoracoabdominal approach. The thoracoabdominal approach is more technically difficult but eliminates the risk of postoperative small-bowel obstruction and usually requires a shorter hospital stay.

Nerve-sparing surgery Regardless of the approach, urologic oncologists recommend a unilateral, nerve-sparing procedure. For right-sided tumors, the medial border of the template is the midpoint of the aorta, and, for left-sided tumors, the medial border is the midpoint of the inferior vena cava (IVC). The sympathetic trunks responsible for normal bladder neck closure during ejaculation course lateral to the aorta on the left side and behind the IVC on the right side. Below the inferior mesenteric artery, both sympathetic trunks send branches to the region anterior to the aorta. The branches coalesce and then pass to the bladder neck.

Critical aspects of nerve-sparing surgery include preservation of the ipsilateral sympathetic nerve trunk and bilateral preservation of branches below the level of the inferior mesenteric artery. In our experience and that of other authors, it is possible to maintain normal ejaculatory function in virtually all patients using this technique. With a template dissection, there is some risk of disease outside the template. Eggener et al at MSKCC have reported good recovery of ejaculation with bilateral dissection using a nerve-sparing approach.

Surveillance (NSGCTs)

In patients with clinical stage I disease (normal serum markers and normal CT scans of the chest and abdomen), surveillance is a reasonable option. In unselected patients with clinical stage I NSGCTs, the risk of recurrence is approximately 25%. Ideally, there should be an absence of vascular invasion and embryonal carcinoma predominance in the orchiectomy specimen. Thus, close follow-up with chest x-ray, analysis of serum markers (β-hCG and AFP), and physical exam should be performed (Table 4).

When followed up in this way, most patients will be detected with low-volume disease. If recurrence occurs, such cases should be curable with 3 cycles of BEP (bleomycin, 30 IU/wk × 9 wk; etoposide, 100 mg/m^2/d; and Platinol [cisplatin], 20 mg/m^2/d) or 4 cycles of EP (etoposide plus cisplatin at the same doses; see Table 5). If patients recur with higher-volume disease (ie, intermediate or poor prognosis), up to 50% may not be cured. Thus, diligent follow-up with a compliant patient is crucial.

Stage I disease: seminoma

Radiation therapy

Seminomas of the testes are exquisitely sensitive to irradiation. This characteristic, combined with their predictable lymphatic spread, makes these cancers amenable to radiotherapy. Since low radiation doses are used, acute and late side effects are few. Radiotherapy is not indicated in patients with NSGCT, except in the palliative setting.

Fields and doses The radiotherapy portals have traditionally included the retroperitoneal lymph nodes, which are the primary drainage of the testis, from T10 to L5 and the ipsilateral hemipelvis, including the inguinal scar. However, studies

TABLE 4: Follow-up schedule for germ-cell tumor

Surveillance	Chest X-ray	β-hCG/AFP	Chest CT	ABD/ Pelvic CT
Clinical stage I seminoma	q4mo, years 1–2	q4mo, years 1–2	—	q4mo, years 1–2
	q6mo, years 3–5	q6mo, years 3–5	—	q6mo, years 3–5
	After 5 years, annually	After 5 years, annually	—	As indicated
Clinical stage I NSGCT	q2mo, year 1	q2mo, year 1	—	q4mo, years 1–2
	q4mo, year 2	q4mo, year 2	—	q4mo, year 2
	q6mo, years 3–5	q6mo, years 3–5	—	q6mo, years 3–5
	After 5 years, annually	After 5 years, annually	—	As indicated
Following chemotherapy complete remission ± surgical RLND	q2mo, year 1	q2mo, year 1	—	q4mo, years 1 & 2[a]
	q4mo, year 2	q4mo, year 2	—	
	q6mo, years 3–5	q6mo, years 3–5	—	q6mo, years 3–5[a]
	After year 5, annually	After year 5, annually	—	As indicated
Following treatment for mediastinal or other GCT salvage	q2mo, year 1	q2mo, year 1	q4mo, years 1–2[a]	As indicated
	q4mo, year 2	q4mo, year 22	q6mo, years 3–5[a]	As indicated
	q6mo, years 3–5	q6mo, years 3–5	—	—
	After year 5, annually	After year 5, annually	—	As indicated

[a] For patients with resected teratoma only.

that reduced the size of the retroperitoneal field and omitted hemipelvis irradiation in selected patients (eg, those who have not undergone prior orchiopexy or other pelvic, inguinal, or scrotal surgery) favor smaller treatment volumes. A study by Fossa and colleagues randomized 478 men with stage I seminomas to receive irradiation of the para-aortics (T11 to L5) and ipsilateral hemipelvis vs irradiation of the para-aortics only. The actuarial rate of 3-year freedom from relapse was about 96% for both groups, although there were more pelvic relapses in patients given retroperitoneal radiation therapy only. Pelvic and/or inguinal failures occurred in < 5% of these patients. The few failures observed following radiotherapy most often occurred in the next echelon of lymph node drainage sites, such as the mediastinum or left supraclavicular fossa.

TABLE 5: Chemotherapy regimens for testicular cancer

Drug/combination	Dose and schedule
BEP	
Bleomycin	30 IU IV bolus on days 2, 9, and 16
Etoposide	100 mg/m² IV infused over 30 minutes on days 1–5
Platinol (cisplatin)	20 mg/m² IV infused over 15–30 minutes on days 1–5
Repeat cycle every 21 days for 3 or 4 cycles.	
NOTE: Treat patients every 21 days on schedule, regardless of the granulocyte count. Reduce etoposide dose by 20% in patients who previously received radiotherapy or had granulocytopenia with fever/sepsis during the previous cycle. Patients receiving 4 cycles of BEP should undergo pulmonary function tests at baseline and at 9 weeks.	
Williams SD, Birch R, Einhorn LH, et al: N Engl J Med 316:1435–1440, 1987	
EP	
Etoposide	100 mg/m² IV infused over 30 minutes on days 1–5
Platinol (cisplatin)	20 mg/m² IV infused over 15–30 minutes on days 1–5
Repeat cycle every 21 days for 4 cycles.	
NOTE: Treat patients every 21 days on schedule, regardless of the granulocyte count. Reduce etoposide dose by 20% in patients who previously received radiotherapy or had granulocytopenia with fever/sepsis during the previous cycle.	
de Wit R, Roberts JT, Wilkinson PM, et al: J Clin Oncol 19:1629–1640, 2001	
VIP	
VePesid (etoposide)	75 mg/m²/d IV on days 1–5
Ifosfamide	1.2 g/m²/d IV on days 1–5
Platinol (cisplatin)	20 mg/m²/d IV on days 1–5
Mesna	400 mg IV bolus prior to the first ifosfamide dose, then 1.2 g/m²/d IV infused continuously on days 1–5
Repeat cycle every 21 days for 4 cycles.	
Loehrer PJ, Lauer R, Roth BJ, et al: Ann Intern Med 109:540–546, 1988	
TIP (salvage therapy)	
Taxol (paclitaxel)	175 mg/m² on day 1
Ifosfamide	1 g/m² on days 1–5
Platinol (cisplatin)	20 mg/m² on days 1–5
Mesna	400 mg IV bolus prior to the first ifosfamide dose, then 1.2 g/m²/d IV infused continuously on days 1–5
Repeat cycle every 21 days for 4 cycles.	
Kondagunta GV, Bacik J, Donadio A, et al: J Clin Oncol 23:6549–6555, 2005; Mead GM, Cullen MH, Huddart R, et al: Br J Cancer 93:178–184, 2005	
VeIP (salvage therapy)	
Vinblastine	0.11 mg/kg/d on days 1 and 2
Ifosfamide	1.2 g/m²/d IV on days 1–5
Platinol (cisplatin)	20 mg/m²/d IV on days 1-5
Mesna	400 mg/m² IV bolus prior to first ifosfamide dose, then 1.2 g/m²/d IV infused continuously for 5 days
Repeat cycle every 21 days for 4 cycles.	
Loehrer PJ, Lauer R, Roth BJ, et al: Ann Intern Med 109:540–546, 1988; Miller KD, Loehrer PJ, Gonin R, et al: J Clin Oncol 15:1427–1431, 1997	

Table prepared by Ishmael Jaiyesimi, DO.

The smaller treatment volume reduces the dose to the remaining testicle and probably the risk of secondary malignancy. The ipsilateral hemipelvis is treated only when there is a history of ipsilateral inguinal surgery. Violation of the inguinal region can alter the testicular lymphatic drainage pathway to the para-aortic region. The hemiscrotum is often treated if the tumor penetrated the tunica albuginea, a trans-scrotal incision was performed, or orchiopexy was performed for cryptorchidism. However, this practice has been questioned, since the incidence of scrotal failure is low, even in the presence of these risk factors. In fact, some surgeons advocate the use of trans-scrotal exploration to rule out benign lesions.

Side effects The acute side effects of radiotherapy are limited to nausea, vomiting, and, infrequently, diarrhea, all of which usually can be readily controlled with medication. Long-term complications recently reported at the MDACC demonstrated increased mortality ratios for overall, cardiac-specific, and secondary cancer deaths for men treated with radiation therapy for seminoma between 1951 and 1999. No difference in mortality risk was noted in the first 15 years following treatment; however, over the entire period, the all-cause mortality risk was 1.59. The cardiac-specific mortality rate after 15 years was 1.61, and the secondary cancer mortality rate was 1.91.

Permanent infertility from scattered irradiation to the contralateral testis is uncommon, whereas prolonged aspermia for more than 1 year may occur, especially with irradiation of the hemiscrotum. Nevertheless, sperm banking is recommended for patients concerned about childbearing.

Follow-up Relapse following adjuvant radiotherapy occurs in 2% to 5% of patients, and the far majority of recurrences (approximately 90%) occur within the first 2 to 3 years after treatment. Recurrences are typically found in lymph nodes of the pelvis, abdomen, groin, mediastinum, supraclavicular fossa, and neck. Physical examination of these areas and CT evaluations of the abdomen and pelvis can aid with the detection of recurrence.

Owing to increasing concerns about late effects related to radiographic studies, two evidence-based studies have suggested fewer follow-up evaluations than have traditionally been performed. Follow-up with imaging studies two to three times a year during the first 3 to 4 years of follow-up has been suggested. The additional value of chest imaging and tumor markers (AFP, β-hCG, and lactate dehydrogenase [LDH]) has been questioned, because few recurrences are detected on the basis of these evaluations alone. However, these studies are routinely done, as solitary pulmonary recurrences can occur, and these tumor markers may also support the suspicion of recurrence indicated on physical examination or imaging. Chest x-ray is the preferred method for imaging the chest, because the radiation exposure is lower compared with CT. Late recurrences are well documented, and annual follow-up until at least year 6 has been suggested, a point in time at which the risk of recurrence falls below 0.3% per year.

Adjuvant radiotherapy vs surveillance vs chemotherapy Based on surveillance data, the overall incidence of disease failure without radiotherapy is 15% to 27% (median, 20%). Relapse rates with surveillance appear to be lowest in patients with primary tumors smaller than 4 cm and no evidence of rete testis involvement. Relapse rates following surveillance are highest, approximately 25% to 35%, for patients with both tumor size > 4 cm and rete testis invasion. A risk-adapted strategy that utilizes adjuvant treatment rather than surveillance for this group has been advocated by some clinicians, but it would result in overtreatment for at least 65% of men.

Follow-up in patients undergoing surveillance is rigorous and intended to identify disease before tumor is bulky or supradiaphragmatic requiring chemotherapy. Disease progression usually is not associated with symptoms until the tumor burden is large. Surveillance requires abdominopelvic CT scans and chest x-rays at 3- to 4-month intervals for 3 to 4 years and then annually for at least an additional 5 years. Late failures beyond 5 years have been observed. Salvage rates reported in patients who relapse while undergoing surveillance are approximately 90% initially, with ultimate salvage rates after relapse of 95%. Those patients who do develop recurrence may receive 4 cycles of EP or radiation.

Thus, in summary, various options exist for the primary treatment of clinical stage I seminoma, including radiation therapy and observation with monitoring of serum markers, CT, and chest x-ray. Primary chemotherapy has decreased the risk of recurrence comparable to radiation therapy, but it still requires abdominal CT imaging for follow-up because failures in the retroperitoneum are common. Risk-adapted therapy has not yet defined the optimal population for primary chemotherapy.

Stage II disease

Fields and doses The radiotherapy fields are similar to those used for stage I disease, except that they are widened to include any retroperitoneal or pelvic adenopathy with a 2- to 3-cm margin. In the past, mediastinal and supraclavicular treatment was standard in patients with stage II disease. However, data from several series revealed only a 3% rate of mediastinal/supraclavicular relapse. In addition, late cardiac toxicity has been reported. Although treatment to supradiaphragmatic sites has largely been abandoned in these cases, one report indicates that the rate of failure in the left supraclavicular fossa is higher than was previously believed. An analysis from another group indicates the opposite, however, that supradiaphragmatic radiotherapy for stage IIA-B seminoma is unnecessary. The overall actuarial rate of freedom from disease at 5 years for patients with retroperitoneal adenopathy < 2 cm (IIA) is 95%, 2 to 5 cm (IIB) is 90%, and > 5 and < 10 cm (IIC) is 85%.

Involved areas are usually treated with 30 to 36 Gy, and uninvolved areas are treated with 20 to 25 Gy. There is no evidence of a dose-response effect above 25 Gy for uninvolved areas and above 35 Gy for involved areas. Failures within the irradiated volume are anecdotal.

Chemotherapy

Stage I seminomas Several studies have evaluated the role of primary chemotherapy, typically carboplatin as adjuvant therapy, for clinical stage I seminoma. Single-cycle carboplatin has been studied as an alternative to adjuvant radiotherapy in a randomized trial conducted by the UKMRC/EORTC. At a median follow-up of 4 years, 3-year relapse-free survival rates were similar among the 1,477 randomized patients. However, first-echelon retroperitoneal nodal recurrences were more common in the chemotherapy group (74% vs 9%), raising concern regarding the efficacy of single-cycle carboplatin. Retroperitoneal nodal recurrences following radiotherapy are typically marginal misses at the edge of the treatment field.

Further questioning the role of single-cycle carboplatin in stage I disease, a pooled analysis of two randomized trials in advanced-stage disease demonstrated that single-agent carboplatin is inferior to cisplatin-based combination therapy. Phase II results evaluating 2 cycles of carboplatin (400 mg/m^2) for prophylactic treatment of stage I seminomas were more promising. However, acute toxicity (ie, the degree of lethargy and time missed from work) is unlikely to be less than that of a 2-week course of radiotherapy. A risk-adjusted method has also been evaluated, but thus far these chemotherapy options do not preclude the necessity for continued surveillance with computerized tomography. In summary, observation, radiation therapy, and chemotherapy can be considered options after careful, informed decision-making.

Stage I NSGCT Chemotherapy has been used in lieu of primary RLND and is the preferred choice when surveillance is not feasible.

> **Although most patients with stage I NSGCT are managed with surveillance or primary RLND, the success of chemotherapy prompted another approach. A trial conducted in Germany randomized patients with clinical stage I NSGCT to receive 1 cycle of BEP (n = 191) vs primary RLND (n = 191). Only 2 recurrences occurred with chemotherapy vs 15 with surgery *(Albers P et al: J Clin Oncol 26:2966–2972, 2008).***

Stage II seminomas Those with larger lymph node metastases are typically treated with platinum-based chemotherapy. Among patients who are candidates for radiotherapy, it is essential that renal function be preserved in case chemotherapy is necessary for salvage treatment. Recent preliminary evidence indicates that the 5-year freedom-from-failure rates may be improved to 97% by administration of neoadjuvant carboplatin combined with reduced-field radiotherapy. Alternatively, systemic therapy alone (BEP × 3 vs EP × 4) may be used in lieu of radiation therapy.

Stage II NSGCTs Over the past several years, the threshold for primary surgery in patients with stage II disease on CT scans has changed. At present, masses > 3 cm in greatest cross-sectional diameter or those with more extensive longitudinal lymphatic spread are generally handled primarily with chemotherapy. For patients with tumor sizes ≤ 3 cm, primary RLND is considered the standard approach. Up to 25% of patients with enlarged lymph nodes on CT scans will have pathologic stage I (false-positive) disease by RLND.

Adjuvant chemotherapy The risk of systemic recurrence is 5% to 10% in patients with pathologic stage I nonseminomas, 15% to 30% in those with completely resected stage IIA (N2a) disease, and 30% to 50% in those with stage IIB (N2b) disease. Recurrence usually occurs in the lungs within the first 24 months after surgery. The risk of retroperitoneal recurrence in patients with stage I, IIA, or IIB disease is < 1% after a properly performed RLND. Following RLND, patients with complete resection of stage II disease can be considered candidates for adjuvant chemotherapy.

The decision of whether or not to prescribe adjuvant therapy following lymph node dissection is somewhat arbitrary and often depends on the patient's social circumstances and likelihood of adhering to close follow-up. A patient with completely resected carcinoma who undergoes RLND has a 70% chance of cure; thus, the majority of patients will never need chemotherapy. However, these patients must be monitored carefully with chest x-rays and serum marker determinations every month for 1 year, every 2 months for an additional year, and then every 6 months for the next 3 years. (CT scanning is not performed routinely unless clinically indicated.) The 30% of patients followed in such a manner who do develop recurrence will present with a tumor of low volume (eg, small pulmonary metastases or elevated serum markers); nearly 100% of these patients should be cured with appropriate systemic therapy.

> **The quality of surveillance for stage I testicular cancer in the community was reported from private insurance claims between 2002 and 2007. Seven hundred men underwent radical orchicotomy and 279 were managed with surveillance. Compliance with surveillance follow-up protocols recommended by referral centers was poor. Nearly 30% of all surveillance patients received no abdominal imaging, chest imaging, or tumor marker tests within the first year of diagnosis *(Yu HY et al: J Clin Oncol 27:4327–4332, 2009).***

However, some patients with resected stage II disease elect to receive adjuvant chemotherapy to minimize the risk of cancer recurrence. For such therapy, 2 cycles of BEP (bleomycin, 30 IU/wk × 8; etoposide, 100 mg/m^2 on days 1 to 5 and 29 to 34; and cisplatin, 20 mg/m^2 on days 1 to 5 and 29 to 34) are recommended (Table 5). In a patient who agrees to close follow-up, the chance of dying of cancer should be negligible in either scenario. For patients who have persistently elevated or increasing serum markers following RLND or who have undergone incomplete lymph node dissection, 3 cycles of BEP are indicated.

In a study of 75 patients with stage I NSGCTs, compliance with clinical examinations was 61.5% in year 1 and 35.5% in year 2, whereas compliance with abdominal/pelvic CT was only 25.0% and 11.8% in years 1 and 2, respectively. Careful selection of highly motivated patients for surveillance is indicated.

Stage III disease

Seminomas

Chemotherapy is the treatment of choice for patients with stage III seminomas (see Table 5). The management of patients with bulky disease after chemotherapy (residual mass: > 3 cm) is somewhat controversial. Investigators at MSKCC suggested that such patients require consolidation with radiotherapy or surgical removal of radiographically evident disease. Data from the Royal Marsden Hospital and the Centre Léon Bérard reported a relapse rate of 10% to 15% in patients with residual masses with or without postchemotherapy surgery or radiotherapy, supporting the practice of observation in patients with residual masses following chemotherapy. FDG-PET may be helpful in the decision to treat residual masses > 3 cm but should be performed 4 to 6 weeks after the last course of chemotherapy.

NSGCTs

As mentioned previously, patients with NSGCTs being treated with chemotherapy can be classified as having good-, intermediate-, or poor-risk disease (see Table 3).

Good-risk disease Three cycles of BEP given every 3 weeks or, alternatively, 4 cycles of EP at the same dosages appear to yield equivalent results. More than 90% of good-risk patients should be cured with these therapies.

Two prospective randomized trials comparing cisplatin with carboplatin in good-risk patients with disseminated germ-cell tumors have demonstrated inferior results for carboplatin-containing regimens.

Postchemotherapy resection Patients having persistent radiographic disease with normal serum markers 4 to 6 weeks following chemotherapy for an NSGCT, should undergo surgical resection of the residual mass and bilateral template RLND when possible. In patients with a seminoma, a residual mass > 3 cm, and an abnormal PET scan, resection is also recommended.

Postresection chemotherapy Histologic examination of residual disease will reveal necrotic fibrous tissue in approximately 45% of such cases, benign teratoma in about 45%, and persistent carcinoma in about 10% to 15%. If persistent carcinoma is detected in the resected specimen, 2 additional cycles of EP should be administered. For patients with complete resection of mature and immature teratoma or necrosis, no additional therapy is needed.

Poor-risk disease A cohort of patients with disseminated germ-cell tumors presents with advanced or poor-risk disease. "Poor risk" has been variously defined (see Table 3) but represents a patient population with a cure rate of ≤ 50% with standard cisplatin-based combination chemotherapy. Irradiation is useful in the treatment of metastatic NSGCTs to the brain.

Chemotherapy During the past few years, several trials have evaluated a variety of combination regimens in patients with poor-risk disease (Table 5). They include the use of high-dose therapy, sequential therapy, and VIP (VePesid [etoposide], ifosfamide, and Platinol [cisplatin]). VIP appears to be therapeutically equivalent to BEP; however, for most patients with advanced disease, BEP is the preferred regimen, because it produces less myelosuppression. In patients with underlying pulmonary dysfunction, VIP is preferred.

In a study by Bhatia et al, 65 patients with recurrent testicular cancer were treated with tandem cycles of high-dose etoposide plus carboplatin followed by peripheral stem cell transplantation (SCT) as initial salvage therapy. With a median follow-up of 39 months, 37 patients (57%) remain continuously disease-free, with 3 additional patients (5%) disease-free with subsequent surgery. There was no treatment-related mortality.

A prospective Intergroup trial evaluating high-dose chemotherapy and SCT has been published. This trial comparing 4 cycles of BEP with 2 cycles of BEP followed by 2 tandem courses of high-dose chemotherapy plus SCT in previously untreated patients with poor-risk disease was recently completed. No difference in the outcome between the two arms was seen, but greater toxicity was seen in the high-dose arm. Thus 4 cycles of BEP remain the standard of care for poor-risk patients.

Postchemotherapy resection The ultimate goal of combination chemotherapy in these patients is the resolution of all radiographically visible disease and the normalization of tumor markers. If residual radiographic abnormalities persist in the lungs and/or abdomen, surgical resection of residual disease is indicated.

Postchemotherapy RLND must clear the region of residual disease. In general, postchemotherapy resections are extremely difficult, and incomplete resections are unacceptable. After the retroperitoneum is cleared of persistent radiographic disease, persistent pulmonary lesions are resected. In cases with residual disease in the retroperitoneum and thorax, RLND should be performed first. If necrosis is found, the disease within the chest can be observed. If teratoma or cancer is noted, the supradiaphragmatic disease should be resected.

A recent update to an Australian trial compared 3 vs 4 cycles of BEP given to patients with good-prognosis germ-cell tumors. At an 8-year follow-up, the survival benefit was maintained with the 3-cycle regimen *(Grimison PS et al: J Clin Oncol [15S]: abstract 6016, 2009).*

Complicating factors associated with postchemotherapy resection include the risk of oxygen toxicity secondary to bleomycin as well as intense fibrosis and adherence of residual disease to the aorta and other vital retroperitoneal organs. Inspired oxygen levels must remain below 35% to prevent bleomycin-related acute respiratory distress syndrome, which has a fatality rate ≥ 50%.

After successful resection, the only visible structures remaining should include the back muscles, nerves, anterior spinous ligament, aorta, IVC, renal vessels, kidneys, and ureters. Up to 20% of patients with advanced abdominal disease may require resection of a kidney or even the IVC. Operative mortality in centers with experience performing resection of these advanced-stage tumors should be < 2%. Although intraoperative, postoperative, and late complication rates were higher between groups receiving open primary or postchemotherapeutic RLND, they were not significantly different when the procedure was performed by fellowship-trained urologists. A more thorough RLND increases the 2-year relapse-free probability from 90% (10 nodes removed) to 97% (50 nodes removed).

Postresection chemotherapy As mentioned, 2 additional cycles of chemotherapy are indicated for patients with persistent viable carcinoma in the resected specimen. For patients with resected teratoma of nonviable necrotic tissue, no additional chemotherapy is warranted.

Refractory or recurrent disease

Surgery

Some patients with recurrent disease appear to have localized or minimally metastatic disease. In such cases, salvage surgery may achieve a durable complete remission. A 25% cure rate was seen in a select group of patients with elevated serum markers who underwent such surgery at Indiana University. These patients had completely resected viable carcinoma without chemotherapy following surgery.

Salvage chemotherapy

Approximately 20% to 30% of patients with disseminated germ-cell tumors do not attain complete remission with induction chemotherapy or relapse after such therapy. These patients may be candidates for salvage chemotherapy. Occasional patients may be erroneously classified as having recurrent disease based on false-positive markers or abnormal radiographic findings. Some of these false-positive results may be due to a growing teratoma; pseudonodules from bleomycin-induced pulmonary disease; or elevated markers from other causes, such as an elevated β-hCG level from marijuana usage, cross-reactivity with luteinizing hormone, or an elevated AFP level associated with hepatitis or liver dysfunction. Another cause of persistently elevated markers is a tumor sanctuary site (eg, in the testes or brain). Assuming that false disease progression has been ruled out, several approaches to salvage therapy can be used. When possible, autologous bone marrow transplant is preferred. It can achieve slightly more durable response rates than other options.

Ifosfamide is one of a few drugs (including etoposide, gemcitabine [Gemzar], and paclitaxel) that has clinical activity in patients with cisplatin-refractory disease. As second-line therapy, VeIP (vinblastine, 0.11 mg/kg on days 1 and 2 [total dose = .22 mg/kg]; plus ifosfamide, 1.2 g/m^2 [plus mesna (Mesnex)]; plus Platinol, 20 mg/m^2, both on days 1 to 5) produces durable complete remissions in ~30% of NSGCT patients and 50% of seminoma patients previously treated with BEP chemotherapy (Table 5). Toxicity, which is primarily hematologic, can be minimized with the use of a colony-stimulating growth factor.

Seminoma Patients with recurrent seminoma appear to be more sensitive to salvage therapy. In a study by Miller et al, 24 patients with seminoma were treated with VeIP as second-line therapy (following relapse after cisplatin-etoposide combination therapy). Of the 24 patients, 20 patients (83%) achieved a complete response, and 13 patients (54%) are long-term survivors, including 4 of 6 with extragonadal primary sites. Thus, initial salvage therapy in these patients should be VeIP rather than high-dose chemotherapy with bone marrow rescue.

High-dose chemotherapy with stem cell rescue High-dose chemotherapy with tandem courses of carboplatin and etoposide plus autologous stem cell rescue produces durable complete remission in 5% to 10% of patients whose disease is overtly refractory to cisplatin. When this approach is used in patients with recurrent, but not cisplatin-refractory, disease, improved response rates are observed; over 60% of all patients with recurrence of testicular cancer (excluding extragonadal recurrence) will be cured. Approximately 70% of patients treated with second-line therapy are curable with this approach.

A retrospective review by Einhorn et al evaluated 184 patients who had progressed on initial platinum-based therapy. They were treated with 2 consecutive courses of high-dose chemotherapy with carboplatin and etoposide followed by infusion of autologous peripheral-blood hematopoietic stem cells. Of the 135 patients who received this treatment as second-line therapy, 94 were disease-free; 22 of 49 patients who received this treatment as third-line therapy or later were disease-free, and 18 of 40 platinum-refractory patients were disease-free.

Other agents Few drugs besides etoposide and ifosfamide have activity in patients with cisplatin-refractory disease. Oral etoposide given according to a chronic schedule (50 mg/m^2/d for 21 days) has produced objective responses in ~20% of patients who were previously treated with IV etoposide. Paclitaxel has a similar response rate in minimally pretreated patients (< 6 cycles). Gemcitabine produces a response rate of approximately 15% in patients with cisplatin-refractory disease.

The ECOG conducted a phase II trial of gemcitabine (1,000 mg/m^2) plus paclitaxel (110 mg/m^2) given on days 1, 8, and 15 of a 4-week cycle for a maximum of 6 cycles in patients with recurrent germ-cell tumor not thought to be curable with standard chemotherapy or surgery. Of 28 evaluable patients, 6 responded, including 3 who had complete responses (2 of whom were free of disease at 15+ and 25+ months).

In a group of patients not considered to be curable with standard salvage chemotherapy, cisplatin plus epirubicin produced durable complete remissions in 7 of 30 patients.

SURVIVORSHIP ISSUES

Delayed toxicity from systemic therapy

Delayed toxicity from systemic therapy for germ-cell tumors has been well characterized. In the absence of signs and symptoms, specific monitoring for these late effects is not generally warranted. A number of late effects have been observed.

Fertility problems and fetal malformation

Fertility problems, manifested by azoospermia or oligospermia at or beyond 2 years, occur in 45% to 55% of treated patients. No increased risk of fetal malformation has been observed in the offspring of men previously treated with chemotherapy for testicular cancer.

Cardiovascular disease

The risk of hypertension or other cardiovascular disease may be increased in patients with testicular cancer who received chemotherapy, but this theory is controversial. The only exception is Raynaud's phenomenon, which occurs at a rate directly proportional to the number of cycles of cisplatin-based chemotherapy.

Renal and pulmonary toxicities

Although renal and pulmonary dysfunction can occur acutely during therapy, long-term consequences from therapy are uncommon.

Secondary malignancies

Perhaps of greatest concern is the development of secondary malignancies.

Late recurrence

The incidence of late recurrence is estimated at 3.2% in NSGCT and 1.4% in seminoma. These late recurrences typically occur beyond 5 years (longest: 32+ years) from primary therapy, frequently present with an elevated serum level of AFP, and are particularly resistant to salvage chemotherapy. Thus, surgical resection of disease is the primary treatment strategy.

> **I**n a study of 75 patients with late recurrence, the 5-year cancer-specific survival (CSS) was 79% vs 36% for men undergoing complete or incomplete surgical resection, respectively. The 5-year CSS for chemotherapy-naive patients was 93% compared with 49% for men having a history of chemotherapy in their initial management *(Sharp DS et al: J Clin Oncol 26:5624–5629, 2008).*

Testicular cancer

Approximately 1% to 2% of patients may develop a second primary testicular cancer. As such, several examinations should be part of every physical exam.

Other cancers

In a large series of 40,000 men by Travis et al, the relative risk for developing secondary tumors was 1.9 for 10-year survivors of testicular cancer and remained 1.7 for 35-year survivors. The greatest elevated risk was for cancers of the pleura, pancreas, bladder, and stomach. In another large retrospective analysis of 635 patients with extragonadal germ-cell tumors treated from 1975 to 1996, only an increased number of hematologic and skin malignancies were observed.

The contribution of chemotherapy and/or radiation therapy to the development of these other malignancies, as opposed to a natural propensity toward their development, is unknown. However, in several series, etoposide has been shown to pose an increased risk for the development of secondary leukemia (dose-related). At higher dosages (> 2 g/m^2 cumulative), etoposide has been associated with a greater incidence of acute leukemia. Very high dosages of etoposide with stem cell rescue do not appear to be linked to a higher risk than standard-dose chemotherapy. In one paper by Travis and colleagues, both increased dosages of radiation therapy and cisplatin were associated with an increased risk for acute leukemia. Although these risks are real, they still are low compared with the risk of death caused by testicular cancer. Nonetheless, indiscriminate use of chemotherapy for early-stage (stage I) disease should be tempered by the recognition of the long-term hazards of therapy.

Follow-up for relapse

Because the relapse rate for testicular cancer is low, patients with pathologically confirmed stage I NSGCTs require no further therapy, and follow-up can be accomplished easily with chest x-ray, tumor markers, and physical examination. Similarly, for patients who have stage II disease and receive adjuvant chemotherapy, the risk of relapse is low. For patients with either of these two clinical scenarios, follow-up tests (chest x-ray, serum markers) should be performed every 2 months for 1 year, every 4 months for the second year, every 6 months for years 3 through 5, and annually thereafter.

In patients with resected stage II NSGCTs who do not receive adjuvant chemotherapy, the follow-up tests are the same as those listed above. However, in these patients, follow-up tests are performed every month for 1 year, every 2 months for 2 years, every 6 months for years 3 through 5, and then annually.

SUGGESTED READING

Aparicio J, Germa JR, Garcia del Muro X, et al: Risk-adapted management for patients with clinical stage I seminoma: The Second Spanish Germ Cell Cancer Cooperative Group study. J Clin Oncol 23:8717–8723, 2005.

Bedano PM, Brames MJ, Williams SD, et al: Phase II study of cisplatin plus epirubicin salvage chemotherapy in refractory germ cell tumors. J Clin Oncol 24:5403–5407, 2006.

Buyyounouski MK: Surveillance for stage I seminoma: Better the devil you know than the devil you don't? Oncology (Williston Park) 23:762, 764, 2009.

Carver BS, Cronin AM, Eggener S, et al: The total number of retroperitoneal lymph nodes resected impacts the clinical outcome after chemotherapy for metastatic testicular cancer. Urology 75:1431–1435, 2010.

Chung PW, Warde PR, Panzarella T, et al: Appropriate radiation volume for stage IIA/B testicular seminoma. Int J Radiat Oncol Biol Phys 56:746–748, 2003.

Classen J, Schmidberger H, Meisner C, et al: Radiotherapy for stages IIA/B testicular seminoma: Final report of a prospective multicenter clinical trial. J Clin Oncol 21:1101–1106, 2003.

Classen J, Schmidberger H, Meisner C, et al: Para-aortic irradiation for stage I testicular seminoma: Results of a prospective study in 675 patients. A trial of the German testicular cancer study group (GTCSG). Br J Cancer 90:2305–2311, 2004.

Classen J, Souchon R, Hehr T, et al: Posttreatment surveillance after paraaortic radiotherapy for stage I seminoma: A systematic analysis. J Cancer Res Clin Oncol 136:227–232, 2010.

Corvin S, Sturm W, Schlatter E, et al: Laparoscopic retroperitoneal lymph-node dissection with the waterjet is technically feasible and safe in testis-cancer patients. J Endourol 19:823–826, 2005.

Daugaard G, Petersen PM, Rorth M: Surveillance in stage I testicular cancer. APMIS 111:76–83, 2003.

DeSantis M, Becherer A, Bokemeyer C, et al: 2-18Fluoro-deoxy-*D*-glucose positron emission tomography is a reliable predictor for viable tumor in postchemotherapy seminoma: An update of the prospective multicentric SEMPET trial. J Clin Oncol 22:1034–1039, 2004.

Einhorn LH, Williams SD, Chamness A, et al: High-dose chemotherapy and stem-cell rescue for metastatic germ-cell tumors. N Engl J Med 357:340–348, 2007.

Ellinger J, Wittkamp V, Albers P, et al: Cell-free circulating DNA: Diagnostic value in patients with testicular germ cell cancer. J Urol 181:363–371, 2009.

Hinton S, Catalano PJ, Einhorn LH, et al: Cisplatin, etoposide and either bleomycin or ifosfamide in the treatment of disseminated germ cell tumors. Cancer 97:1869–1875, 2003.

Hoffman KE, Chen MH, Punglia RS, et al: Influence of year of diagnosis, patient age, and sociodemographic status on recommending adjuvant radiation treatment for stage I testicular seminoma. J Clin Oncol 26:3937–3942, 2008.

Hofmann O, Caballero OL, Stevenson BJ, et al: Genome-wide analysis of cancer/testis gene expression. Proc Natl Acad Sci U.S.A 105:20422–20427, 2008.

Holmes L Jr, Escalante C, Garrison O, et al: Testicular cancer incidence trends in the USA (1974–2004): Plateau or shifting racial paradigm? Public Health 122:862–872, 2008.

Houck W, Abonour R, Vance G, et al: Secondary leukemias in refractory germ cell tumor patients undergoing autologous stem-cell transplantation using high-dose etoposide. J Clin Oncol 22:2155–2158, 2004.

Huyghe E, Matsuda T, Thonneau P: Increasing incidence of testicular cancer worldwide: A review. J Urol 170:5–11, 2003.

Jemal A, Siegel R, Xu J, et al: Cancer statistics, 2010. CA Cancer J Clin 60:277–300, 2010.

Jones WG, Fossa SD, Mead GM, et al: Randomized trial of 30 versus 20 Gy in the adjuvant treatment of stage I testicular seminoma: A report on Medical Research Council Trial TE18, European Organisation for the Research and Treatment of Cancer Trial 30942 (ISRCTN 18525328). J Clin Oncol 23:1200–1208, 2005.

Loehrer PJ, Bosl GJ: Carboplatin for stage I seminoma and the sword of Damocles. J Clin Oncol 23:8566–8569, 2005.

Martin JM, Panzarella T, Zwahlen DR, et al: Evidence-based guidelines for following stage 1 seminoma. Cancer 109:2248–2256, 2007.

Oliver RT, Mason MD, Mead GM, et al: Radiotherapy versus single-dose carboplatin in adjuvant treatment of stage I seminoma: A randomised trial. Lancet 366:293–300, 2005.

Rapley EA, Nathanson KL: Predisposition alleles for testicular germ cell tumour. Curr Opin Genet Dev 20:225–230, 2010.

Rapley EA, Turnbull C, Alocamp AA, et al: A genome-wide associaton study of testicular germ cell tumor. Nat Genet 41:807–810, 2009.

Rick O, Bokemeyer C, Weinknecht T, et al: Residual tumor resection after high-dose chemotherapy in patients with relapsed or refractory germ cell cancer. J Clin Oncol 22:3713–3719, 2004.

Sharp DS, Carver BS, Eggener SE, et al: Clinical outcome and predictors of survival in late relapse of germ cell tumor. J Clin Oncol 26:5524–5529, 2008.

Subramanian VS, Nguyen CT, Stephenson AJ, et al: Complications of open primary and post-chemotherapy retroperitoneal lymph node dissection for testicular cancer. Urol Oncol 28:504–509, 2010 [Epub ahead of print Dec 20, 2008].

Travis LB, Fossa SD, Schonfeld SJ, et al: Second cancers among 40,576 testicular cancer patients: Focus on long-term survivors. J Natl Cancer Inst 97:1354–1365, 2005.

Zagars GK, Ballo MT, Lee AK, et al: Mortality after cure of testicular seminoma. J Clin Oncol 22:640–647, 2004.

Abbreviations in this chapter

ECOG = Eastern Cooperative Oncology Group; IGCCCG = International Germ-Cell Cancer Collaborative Group; ITCLC = International Testicular Cancer Linkage Consortium; MDACC = The University of Texas M. D. Anderson Cancer Center; MSKCC = Memorial Sloan-Kettering Cancer Center; NCI = National Cancer Institute; SEER = Surveillance, Epidemiology and End Results; UKMRC/EORTC = United Kingdom Medical Research Council/European Organisation for Research and Treatment of Cancer

CHAPTER 16

Urothelial and kidney cancers

Mark Hurwitz, MD, Philippe E. Spiess, MD, Jorge A. Garcia, MD, and Louis L. Pisters, MD

UROTHELIAL CANCER

In the year 2010, an estimated 70,530 new cases of bladder cancer were diagnosed in the United States, and approximately 14,680 patients died of this disease.

Urothelial cancers encompass carcinomas of the bladder, ureters, and renal pelvis; these cancers occur at a ratio of 50:3:1, respectively. Cancer of the urothelium is a multifocal process. Patients with cancer of the upper urinary tract have a 30% to 50% chance of developing cancer of the bladder at some time in their lives. On the other hand, patients with bladder cancer have a 2% to 3% chance of developing cancer of the upper urinary tract. The incidence of renal pelvis tumors is decreasing.

EPIDEMIOLOGY

Gender

Urothelial cancers occur more commonly in men than in women (3:1) and have a peak incidence in the seventh decade of life.

Race

Cancers of the urothelial tract are also more common in whites than in blacks (2:1).

ETIOLOGY AND RISK FACTORS

Cigarette smoking

The major cause of urothelial cancer is cigarette smoking. A strong correlation exists between the duration and amount of cigarette smoking and cancers at all levels of the urothelial tract. This association holds for both transitional cell and squamous cell carcinomas.

Analgesic abuse

Abuse of compound analgesics, especially those containing phenacetin, has been associated with an increased risk of cancers of the urothelial tract. This risk appears to be greatest for the renal pelvis, and cancer at this site is usually preceded by renal papillary necrosis. The risk associated with analgesic abuse is seen after the consumption of excessive amounts (5 kg).

Chronic urinary tract inflammation

Chronic urinary tract inflammation also has been associated with urothelial cancers. Upper urinary tract stones are associated with renal pelvis cancers. Chronic bladder infections can predispose patients to cancer of the bladder, usually squamous cell cancer.

Occupational exposure

Occupational exposure to toxins has been associated with an increased risk of urothelial cancers. Workers exposed to arylamines in the organic chemical, rubber, and paint and dye industries have an increased risk of urothelial cancer similar to that originally reported for aniline dye workers.

Balkan nephropathy

An increased risk of cancer of the renal pelvis and ureters occurs in patients with Balkan nephropathy. This disorder is a familial nephropathy of unknown cause that results in progressive inflammation of the renal parenchyma, leading to renal failure and multifocal, superficial, low-grade cancers of the renal pelvis and ureters.

Genetic factors

There are reports of families (eg, Lynch syndrome) with a higher risk of urothelial carcinoma of the urothelium, but the genetic basis for this familial clustering remains undefined.

SIGNS AND SYMPTOMS

Hematuria

Blood in the urine is the most common symptom in patients presenting with urothelial tract cancer. It is most often painless, unless obstruction due to a clot or tumor and/or deeper levels of tumor invasion have already occurred.

Urinary voiding symptoms

Urinary voiding symptoms of urgency, frequency, and/or dysuria are also seen in patients with cancers of the bladder or ureters but are uncommon in patients with cancers of the renal pelvis.

Vesical irritation without hematuria

Vesical irritation without hematuria can be seen, especially in patients with carcinoma in situ of the urinary bladder.

Symptoms of advanced disease

Constitutional symptoms include night sweats, fever, weight loss, and anorexia. Pain can also be a symptom of more advanced disease, as is edema of the lower extremities secondary to lymphatic obstruction.

DIAGNOSIS

Initial workup

The initial evaluation of a patient suspected of having urothelial cancer consists of excretory urography (CT, MRI or IVP) followed by cystoscopy. Retrograde pyelography can better define the exact location of upper tract lesions. Definitive urethroscopic examination and biopsy can be accomplished utilizing rigid or flexible instrumentation.

At the time of cystoscopy, urine is obtained from both ureters for cytology, and brush biopsy is obtained from suspicious lesions of the ureter. Brush biopsies significantly increase the diagnostic yield over urine cytology alone. Also, at the time of cystoscopy, a bimanual examination is performed to determine whether a palpable mass is present and whether the bladder is mobile or fixed.

Evaluation of a primary bladder tumor

In addition to biopsy of suspicious lesions, evaluation of a bladder primary tumor includes biopsy of selected mucosal sites to detect possible concomitant carcinoma in situ. Biopsies of the primary lesion must include the muscularis propia to determine whether there is invasion of muscle by the overlying carcinoma. A repeat biopsy must be performed if no muscle was identified in the original specimen.

CT

For urothelial cancers of the upper tract or muscle invasive bladder cancers, a CT scan of the abdomen/pelvis is performed to detect local extension of the cancer, involvement of the abdominal/pelvic lymph nodes, or systemic metastases. The CT imaging usually consists of an abdominal/pelvic CT scan with contrast (usually with delayed images to assess the entire urinary tract).

Bone scan

For patients with bone pain or an elevated alkaline phosphatase level, a radioisotope bone scan is performed.

A chest x-ray

A chest x-ray completes the staging evaluation. Any suspicious findings in a chest-x-ray must be followed by a CT scan of the chest with contrast.

PATHOLOGY

Transitional cell carcinomas

These constitute 90% to 95% of urothelial tract cancers.

Squamous cell cancers

These malignancies account for 3% to 7% of urothelial carcinomas and are more common in the renal pelvis and ureters.

Adenocarcinomas

These tumors account for a small percentage (< 3%) of bladder malignancies and are predominantly located in the trigone region. Adenocarcinomas of the bladder that arise from the dome are thought to be urachal in origin.

Carcinoma in situ

In approximately 30% of newly diagnosed bladder cancers, there are multiple sites of bladder involvement, most commonly with carcinoma in situ. Although carcinoma in situ can occur without macroscopic cancer, it most commonly accompanies higher disease stages.

When carcinoma in situ is associated with superficial tumors, rates of recurrence and disease progression (development of muscle invasion) are higher (50%–80%) than when no such association is present (10%). Carcinoma in situ involving the bladder diffusely without an associated superficial tumor is also considered an aggressive disease. Most patients with this type of cancer will go on to develop muscle-invasive bladder cancers.

STAGING AND PROGNOSIS

Staging system

Urothelial tract cancers are staged according to the AJCC TNM classification system (Table 1). Superficial bladder cancer includes papillary tumors that involve only the mucosa (Ta) or submucosa (T1) and flat carcinoma in situ (Tis). The natural history of superficial bladder cancer is unpredictable, and recurrences are common. Most tumors recur within 6 to 12 months and are of the same stage and grade, but 10% to 15% of patients with superficial cancer will develop invasive or metastatic disease.

Prognostic factors

For carcinomas confined to the bladder, ureters, or renal pelvis, the most important prognostic factors are T stage and differentiation pattern. The impact of associated carcinoma in situ on Ta and T1 lesions was discussed previously (see section on "Pathology"). Less-differentiated Ta–T1 lesions also are associated with higher recurrence and disease progression rates. Patients with well-differentiated Ta lesions without carcinoma in situ have a 95% survival rate, whereas those with high-grade T1 lesions have a 10-year survival rate of 50%. The presence of lymphovascular invasion or micropapillary features within the surgical specimen appears to be independently associated with overall survival, cause-specific survival, as well as local and distant recurrence in patients with node-negative bladder cancer at the time of cystectomy. As such, the presence of lymphovascular invasion and micropapillary features should be included in the pathologic assessment of bladder cancer.

Muscle invasive carcinoma carries a 5-year survival rate of 20% to 50%. When regional lymph nodes are involved, the 5-year survival rate is 0% to 30%. For patients with unresectable or metastatic bladder cancer, Karnofsky performance status < 80% and visceral disease (lung, liver, or bone) have also been shown to predict survival.

TABLE 1: TNM staging of urothelial tract cancers

Primary tumor (T)			
TX		Primary tumor cannot be assessed	
T0		No evidence of primary tumor	
Ta		Noninvasive papillary tumor	
Tis		Carcinoma in situ: "flat tumor"	
T1		Tumor invades subepithelial connective tissue (lamina propria)	
T2		Tumor invades muscularis propria	
	pT2a	Tumor invades superficial muscularis propria (inner half)	
	pT2b	Tumor invades deep muscularis propria (outer half)	
T3		Tumor invades perivesical tissue	
	pT3a	Microscopically	
	pT3b	Macroscopically (extravesical mass)	
T4		Tumor invades any of the following: prostatic stroma, seminal vesicles, uterus, vagina, pelvic wall, abdominal wall	
	T4a	Tumor invades prostatic stroma, uterus, vagina	
	T4b	Tumor invades pelvic wall, abdominal wall	
Regional lymph nodes (N)			
NX		Lymph nodes cannot be assessed	
N0		No lymph node involvement	
N1		Single regional lymph node metastasis in the true pelvis (hypogastric, obturator, external iliac, or presacral lymph node)	
N2		Multiple regional lymph node metastasis in the true pelvis (hypogastric, obturator, external iliac, or presacral lymph node)	
N3		Lymph node metastasis to the common iliac lymph nodes	
Distant metastasis (M)			
M0		No distant metastasis	
M1		Distant metastasis	

Stage grouping

Stage 0a	Ta	N0	M0
Stage 0is	Tis	N0	M0
Stage I	T1	N0	M0
Stage II	T2a	N0	M0
	T2b	N0	M0
Stage III	T3a	N0	M0
	T3b	N0	M0
	T4a	N0	M0
Stage IV	T4b	N0	M0
	Any T	N1–N3	M0
	Any T	Any N	M1

From Edge SB, Byrd DR, Compton CC, et al (eds): AJCC Cancer Staging Manual, 7th ed. New York, Springer, 2010.

> **A** retrospective series of patients with no viable tumor at the time of radical cystectomy (pT0) would suggest that up to 9% of these patients may develop a recurrence following surgery. On multivariate analysis, the presence of lymphovascular invasion and concomitant carcinoma in situ on the transurethral bladder tumor resection specimen predicted poorer overall and recurrence-free survival, respectively *(Kassouf W et al: Eur Urol 52:769–774, 2007).*

TREATMENT

Localized disease

Surgical approaches to superficial bladder cancer

Transurethral resection Most patients with superficial bladder cancer can be treated adequately with transurethral resection (TUR). Such procedures preserve bladder function, entail minimal morbidity, and can be performed repeatedly. Survival rates > 70% at 5 years are expected. Although TUR removes existing tumors, it does not prevent the development of new lesions. Patients should be followed closely.

Laser The neodymium:yttrium-aluminum-garnet (Nd:YAG) laser has achieved good local tumor control when used in the treatment of superficial bladder tumors. However, it has not been adopted for general use because of its limitations in obtaining material for staging and grading of tumors.

Partial cystectomy is an infrequently utilized treatment option for patients whose tumors are not accessible or amenable to TUR but are solitary in location and away from the trigone.

Radical cystectomy is generally not used for the treatment of superficial bladder tumors. The indications for radical cystectomy include:

- Unusually large tumors that are not amenable to complete TUR, even on repeated occasions
- Some high-grade tumors
- Multiple tumors or frequent recurrences that make TUR impractical
- Symptomatic diffuse carcinoma in situ (Tis) that proves unresponsive to intravesical therapy
- Prostatic stromal involvement
- Superficial bacillus Calmette-Guerin (BCG)-refractory high-grade disease.

Intravesical therapy The indications for intravesical therapy include:

- Stage T1 tumors, especially if multiple
- Multifocal papillary Ta lesions, especially grade 2 or 3
- Diffuse Tis
- Rapidly recurring Ta, T1, or Tis disease.

In the United States, four intravesical agents are commonly used: thiotepa, an alkylating agent; BCG, an immune modulator/stimulator; and mitomycin and doxorubicin, both antibiotic chemotherapeutic agents. The dose of BCG varies with the strain (50 mg [Tice] or 60 mg [Connaught]). Mitomycin doses range from 20 to 40 mg.

Although all four agents reduce the tumor recurrence rate, BCG is the most effective particularly for high-grade disease. For the treatment of papillary Ta and T1 lesions, BCG and mitomycin have the greatest efficacy (complete response rate: approximately 50%). For the treatment of Tis, BCG is extremely effective.

In a meta-analysis comparing intravesical BCG and chemotherapy (mitomycin, epirubicin, doxorubicin, or sequential mitomycin/doxorubicin), intravesical BCG was superior in reducing the risk of short- and long-term treatment failure for Tis. Therefore, intravesical BCG appears to be the agent of choice for Tis.

Following radical cystectomy, patients remain at risk of upper tract recurrence, with a previous report estimating the incidence of upper tract recurrence at 2.5%. Only urethral tumor involvement was predictive of upper tract recurrence. Despite routine surveillance of the upper urinary tracts, 78% of these recurrences were detected only upon development of symptoms, with the median survival following recurrence being only 1.7 years. Furthermore, the detection of asymptomatic upper tract recurrences via routine surveillance strategies did not predict lower pathologic stage, absence of nodal metastasis, or the improved survival in patients at time of nephroureterectomy *(Sanderson KM et al: J Urol 177:2088–2094, 2007).*

Surgical approaches to invasive bladder cancer

Radical cystectomy The most standardized treatment for invasive bladder cancer (stage II or higher) is radical cystectomy. Candidates for radical cystectomy include:

- Patients with muscle-invasive tumor
- Patients with high-grade, invasive, lamina propria tumors with evidence of lymphovascular invasion, with or without Tis
- Patients with diffuse Tis or recurrent superficial cancer who do not respond to intravesical therapy.

In men, radical cystectomy with pelvic lymph node dissection and removal of the bladder, seminal vesicles, and prostate. In women, radical cystectomy entails pelvic lymph node dissection and anterior exenteration, including both ovaries, fallopian tubes, uterus, cervix, anterior vaginal wall, bladder, and urethra.

Partial cystectomy is an infrequently utilized treatment option that should only be considered when there is a solitary lesion in the dome of the bladder and when random biopsy results from remote areas of the bladder and prostatic urethra are negative.

Urethrectomy is routinely included in the anterior exenteration performed in female patients. Urethrectomy in male patients is performed if the tumor grossly involves the prostatic urethra or if prior TUR biopsy results of the prostatic stroma are positive. Delayed urethrectomy for positive urethral cytology or biopsy is required in about 10% of male patients.

Urinary reconstruction may involve any one of the following: intestinal conduits (eg, ileal, jejunal, or colonic), continent cutaneous diversion (eg, Indiana or Kock pouch), or orthotopic reconstruction (in both male and female patients).

TABLE 2: Chemotherapy regimens for bladder carcinoma

Drug/combination	Dose and schedule
M-VAC	
Methotrexate	30 mg/m² IV on days 1, 15, and 22
Vinblastine	3 mg/m² IV on days 2, 15, and 22
Adriamycin (doxorubicin)	30 mg/m² IV on day 2
Cisplatin	70 mg/m² IV on day 2

NOTE: Reduce doxorubicin dose to 15 mg/m² in patients who have received prior pelvic irradiation. On days 15 and 22, methotrexate (30 mg/m²) and vinblastine (3 mg/m²) are given only if the white blood cell count is > 2,500 cells/μL and the platelet count is > 100,000 cells/μL.

Repeat cycles every 28–32 days, even if the interim dose is withheld due to myelosuppression or mucositis. Doxorubicin dose is reduced to 15 mg/m² in patients treated with prior pelvic radiation.

von der Maase H, Hansen SW, Roberts JT, et al: J Clin Oncol 18:3068–3077, 2000.

High-dose MVAC + GCSF support	
Methotrexate	30 mg/m² IV on day 1
Vinblastine	3 mg/m² IV on day 2
Adriamycin (doxorubicin)	30 mg/m² IV on day 2
Cisplatin	70 mg/m² IV on day 2
G-CSF	240 μg/m² SC for 7 consecutive days, beginning on day 4 after administration of MVAC chemotherapy (days 4–10 of each 2-week cycle).

NOTE: Treatment with G-CSF can be extended as needed, up to a total of 14 consecutive days.

Repeat cycle every 14 days.

Sternberg CN, de Mulder P, Schornagel JH, et al: Eur J Cancer 42:40–54, 2006; Escudier B, Bellmunt J, Négrier S, et al: J Clin Oncol 28:2144–2150, 2010; Kaufman DS, Shipley WU, Fledman AS: Bladder cancer. Lancet 374:239–249, 2009; Efstathiou JA, Bae K, Shipley WU, et al: Late pelvic toxicity after bladder-sparing therapy in patients with invasive bladder cancer: RTOG 89-03, 95-06, 97-06, 99-06. J Clin Oncol 27:4055–4061, 2009.

Paclitaxel/carboplatin	
Paclitaxel	200 mg/m² IV infused over 3 hours
Carboplatin	Dose calculated by the Calvert formula to an area under the curve of 5 mg/mL/min IV infused over 15 minutes after paclitaxel

Repeat cycle every 21 days.

PREMEDICATIONS: Dexamethasone, 20 mg PO, 12 and 6 hours prior to paclitaxel; as well as ranitidine, 50 mg IV, and diphenhydramine, 50 mg IV, both 30–60 minutes prior to paclitaxel.

Redman B, Smith D, Flaherty L, et al: J Clin Oncol 16:1844–1848, 1998.

Gemcitabine/docetaxel	
Gemcitabine	800 mg/m² IV on days 1, 8, and 15
Docetaxel	60 mg/m² IV on day 1

Repeat cycle every 28 days.

Gitlitz BJ, Baker C, Chapman Y, et al: Cancer 98:1863–1869, 2003.

continued

TABLE 2: Chemotherapy regimens for bladder carcinoma, *continued*

Drug/combination	Dose and schedule
Gemcitabine/cisplatin	
Gemcitabine	1,000 mg/m^2 IV on days 1, 8, and 15
Cisplatin	70 mg/m^2 IV on day 2
Repeat cycle every 28 days.	
von der Maase H, Hansen SW, Roberts JT, et al: J Clin Oncol 18:3068–3077, 2000.	
G-CSF = granulocyte-colony stimulating factor	
Paclitaxel/cisplatin	
Paclitaxel	135 mg/m^2 IV infused over 3 hours
Cisplatin	70 mg/m^2 IV infused over 2 hours
Repeat cycle every 3 weeks until disease progression or for a maximum of 6 cycles.	
PREMEDICATIONS: Dexamethasone, 20 mg PO, 12 and 6 hours prior to paclitaxel; as well as ranitidine, 50 mg IV, or cimetidine, 300 mg IV, prior to paclitaxel, and diphenhydramine, 50 mg IV, 30 minutes prior to paclitaxel.	
Burch PA, Richardson RI, Cha SS, et al: Proc Am Soc Clin Oncol 18:1266a, 1999.	
TCG	
Taxol (paclitaxel)	80 mg/m^2 IV infused over 1 hour on days 1 and 8
Cisplatin	70 mg/m^2 on day 1
Gemcitabine	1,000 mg/m^2 IV on days 1 and 8
Repeat cycle every 21 days.	
PREMEDICATIONS: Dexamethasone, 20 mg PO, 12 and 6 hours prior to paclitaxel; as well as diphenhydramine, 50 mg IV, 30 minutes prior to paclitaxel, and either cimetidine, 300 mg IV, or ranitidine, 50 mg IV, 30 minutes prior to paclitaxel.	
Vaishampayan U, Smith D, Redman B, et al: Proc Am Soc Clin Oncol 18:333a (abstract 1282), 1999.	

Table prepared by Ishmael Jaiyesimi, DO.

Surgical approaches to ureteral and renal pelvic tumors

Optimal surgical management of urothelial malignancies of the ureter and renal pelvis consists of nephroureterectomy with excision of a bladder cuff. Some tumors may respond well to local resection, and tumor specifics may allow for a more conservative intervention particularly in low-grade tumors.

Upper ureteral and renal pelvic tumors (because of similar tumor behavior and anatomic aspects) may be considered as a group, whereas lower ureteral tumors may be considered as a separate group.

Upper ureteral and renal pelvic tumors are best treated with nephroureterectomy. Solitary, low-grade upper tract tumors may be considered for segmental excision or ureteroscopic surgery if close surveillance is feasible. Care should be exercised, however, as multicentricity is more probable, and the risk of recurrence is greater than for lower ureteral lesions.

Lower ureteral lesions may be managed by nephroureterectomy, segmental resection, and neovesical reimplantation or by endoscopic resection. A 15% recurrence rate is seen after segmental resection or endoscopic excision. Careful follow-up is mandatory. Disease progression, the development of a ureteral stricture precluding periodic surveillance, and poor patient compliance are indications to abandon conservative management and perform nephroureterectomy.

Radiation therapy

Radiation therapy for bladder cancer

Primary radiation or chemoradiation therapy Radiation therapy, either alone or, preferably,with chemotherapy, is the modality of choice for patients whose clinical condition precludes surgery, either because of extensive disease or poor overall status. Trials have shown that patients treated with irradiation and cisplatin with or without fluorouracil (5-FU) have improved local control as compared with patients treated with irradiation alone.

The most frequently utilized systemic chemotherapy regimens for urothelial carcinoma are shown in Table 2. Other studies suggest that TUR followed by radiation therapy combined with cisplatin and 5-FU chemotherapy, with cystectomy reserved for salvage, provides a survival equivalent to that achieved with initial radical cystectomy while allowing for bladder preservation in many patients. The extent of TUR and the absence of hydronephrosis are important prognostic factors in studies of bladder-conserving treatment. Updates from institutions in Europe and the United States on over 600 patients with long-term follow-up support the durability of outcomes previously reported.

A randomized phase III study of bladder preservation with or without neoadjuvant chemotherapy following TUR, conducted by the RTOG, revealed no advantage to the use of MCV (methotrexate, cisplatin, and vinblastine) before radiation therapy and concurrent cisplatin. The favorable outcome without neoadjuvant chemotherapy may make bladder preservation a more acceptable option for a wider range of patients.

Radiation dose and technique Initially, a pelvic field is treated to 4,000–4,500 cGy utilizing a three-dimensional conformal technique, with daily or twice-daily fractionation. A cystoscopy is performed with biopsies. If a complete response is confirmed, the bladder tumor site is then boosted to a total dose of 6,480 cGy utilizing multifield techniques.

Radiation therapy for renal pelvic and ureteral cancers

In patients with renal pelvic and ureteral lesions who have undergone nephroureterectomy, postoperative local-field irradiation is offered if there is periureteral, perirenal, or peripelvic extension or lymph node involvement. A dose of approximately 4,500 to 5,580 cGy is delivered utilizing multifield techniques.

Palliative irradiation

Palliative radiation therapy is effective in controlling pain from local and metastatic disease and in providing hemostatic control. A randomized study comparing 3,500 cGy in 10 fractions and 2,100 cGy in three hypofractionated treatments revealed high rates of relief of hematuria, frequency, dysuria, and nocturia with either regimen. In selected cases of bladder cancer, aggressive palliation to approximately

6,000 cGy may be warranted to provide long-term local tumor control. Concurrent chemotherapy should be considered.

Neoadjuvant/adjuvant chemotherapy

Perioperative chemotherapy to improve overall survival and reduce the risk of recurrence before or after cystectomy is a debated topic. Multiple randomized trials of different designs have given various chemotherapy regimens before and/or after cystectomy. Many of these trials had inadequate power or methodologic flaws that limited interpretation. In general, there is likely a small (5%) absolute improvement in survival perioperative chemotherapy given to high-risk patients.

Chemotherapy for advanced disease

Treatment of advanced metastatic urothelial cancer is generally considered to be palliative. Response rates are high with cisplatin-containing regimens (50% to 60%), but the duration of response is short, and median survival is 12 to 14 months. A small subset of patients (5% to 10%; usually with only lymph node metastases) can have a complete response to chemotherapy. This small subset of patients should be considered for post-chemotherapy RPLND. A randomized trial showed an advantage for a regimen of M-VAC (methotrexate, vinblastine, Adriamycin [doxorubicin], and cisplatin) over cisplatin alone with regard to progression-free and overall survival. In another randomized trial, the combination of gemcitabine (Gemzar) and cisplatin exhibited equivalent survival to M-VAC in metastatic bladder cancer but was clinically better tolerated. Thus, cisplatin plus gemcitabine has become a common standard of care in this setting. Similar data do not exist for the perioperative setting. Although carboplatin is an inferior agent to cisplatin in bladder cancer, this agent can be used if a contraindication to cisplatin exists (eg, neuropathy, poor renal function).

KIDNEY CANCER

Approximately 58,240 new cases of renal tumors were diagnosed in the year 2010 in the United States, with an associated 13,040 deaths. There has been a steady increase in the incidence of renal cell carcinoma that is not explained by the increased use of diagnostic imaging procedures. Mortality rates have also shown a steady increase over the past 2 decades.

EPIDEMIOLOGY

Gender and age

This malignancy is twice as common in men as in women. Most cases of renal cell carcinoma are diagnosed in the fourth to sixth decades of life, but the disease has been reported in all age groups.

Ethnicity

Renal cell carcinoma is more common in persons of northern European ancestry than in those of African or Asian descent.

ETIOLOGY AND RISK FACTORS

Renal cell carcinoma occurs most commonly as a sporadic form and rarely (2%) as a familial form. The exact etiology of sporadic renal cell carcinoma has not been determined. However, smoking, obesity, and renal dialysis have been associated with an increased incidence of the disease.

Genetic factors

von Hippel-Lindau disease (VHL)

VHL, an autosomal-dominant disease, is associated with retinal angiomas, CNS hemangioblastomas, and renal cell carcinoma.

Chromosomal abnormalities

Deletions of the short arm of chromosome 3 (3p) occur commonly in renal cell carcinoma associated with VHL disease. In the rare familial forms of renal cell carcinoma, translocations affecting chromosome 3p can be present. Sporadic renal cell carcinoma of the clear cell is also associated with *VHL*-gene silencing.

Associated malignancy

Two studies from large patient databases have reported a higher-than-expected incidence of both renal cell cancer and lymphoma. No explanation for this association has been found.

SIGNS AND SYMPTOMS

Renal cell carcinoma has been associated with a wide array of signs and symptoms. The classic triad of hematuria, flank mass, and flank pain occurs in only 10% of patients and is usually associated with a poor prognosis. With the routine use of CT scanning for various diagnostic reasons, renal cell carcinoma is being diagnosed more frequently as an incidental finding.

Hematuria

More than half of patients with renal cell carcinoma present with hematuria, either gross or microscopic.

Other common signs/symptoms

Other commonly associated signs and symptoms of renal cell carcinoma include normocytic/normochromic anemia, fever, and weight loss.

Less common signs/symptoms

Less frequently occurring, but often described, signs and symptoms include polycythemia, hepatic dysfunction not associated with hepatic metastasis which is termed Stauffer syndrome, and hypercalcemia. Although not a common finding at the time of diagnosis of renal cell carcinoma, hypercalcemia ultimately occurs in up to 25% of patients with metastatic disease.

DIAGNOSIS

Pre- and post-contrast-enhanced CT scanning

This technique has virtually replaced excretory urography and renal ultrasonography in the evaluation of suspected renal cell carcinoma. In most cases, CT imaging can differentiate cystic from solid masses and also supplies information about lymph nodes and renal vein/inferior vena cava (IVC) involvement.

Ultrasonography

Ultrasound is useful in evaluating questionable cystic renal lesions if CT imaging is inconclusive.

Venography and MRI

When IVC involvement by tumor is suspected, either IVC venography or MRI is needed to evaluate its extent. MRI is currently the preferred imaging technique for assessing IVC involvement at most centers. Transesophageal echocardiography is occasionally obtained pre- or intraoperatively to determine the proximal extent of the IVC thrombus particularly in those suspected to be beyond the diaphragm.

Renal arteriography

Renal arteriography is not used as frequently now as it was in the past in the evaluation of suspected renal cell carcinoma. In patients with small, indeterminate lesions, arteriography may be helpful. It is also used by the surgeon as part of the preoperative evaluation and management of a large renal neoplasm.

Evaluation of extra-abdominal disease sites

This includes a chest x-ray or CT imaging of the chest. A bone scan is required if a patient has symptoms suggestive of bone metastasis and/or an elevated alkaline phosphatase level.

Brain CT or MRI

A CT or MRI of the brain is indicated if neurologic signs or symptoms occur or if needed for staging before systemic therapy is given.

PATHOLOGY

Renal cell carcinoma arises from the proximal renal tubular epithelium. Histologically, renal cell carcinoma can be of various cellular types: clear cell (70% to 80%), papillary (10% to 15%), and chromophobe (5%). Oncocytoma is a benign renal tumor. Approximately 10% to 20% of renal cell carcinomas have sarcomatoid features (spindled cells that can occur in any subtype), which is a more aggressive malignancy with a worse prognosis.

TABLE 3: TNM staging of renal cell carcinoma

Primary tumor (T)			
TX	Primary tumor cannot be assessed		
T0	No evidence of primary tumor in the kidneys		
T1	Tumor ≤ 7 cm in greatest dimension, limited to the kidneys		
T1a	Tumor ≤ 4 cm in greatest dimension, limited to the kidneys		
T1b	Tumor > 4 cm but not > 7 cm in greatest dimension, limited to the kidneys		
T2	Tumor > 7 cm in greatest dimension, limited to the kidneys		
T2a	Tumor > 7 cm but not > 10 cm in greatest dimension, limited to the kidneys		
T2b	Tumor > 10 cm in greatest dimension, limited to the kidneys		
T3	Tumor extends into major veins or perinephric issues, but does not invade the adrenal gland or spread beyond Gerota's fascia		
T3a	Tumor spreads into renal vein or its muscles or perirenal and/or renal sinus fat, but not beyond Gerota's fascia		
T3b	Tumor grossly extends into vena cava below the diaphragm		
T3c	Tumor grossly extends into the vena cava above the diaphragm or invades the wall of the vena cava		
T4	Tumor invades beyond Gerota's fascia and extends into the contiguous adrenal gland		
Regional lymph nodes (N)			
NX	Regional lymph nodes cannot be assessed		
N0	No regional lymph node metastasis		
N1	Metastasis to regional nodes		
Distant metastasis (M)			
M0	No distant metastasis		
M1	Distant metastasis		
Stage grouping			
Stage I	T1	N0	M0
Stage II	T2	N0	M0
Stage III	T1	N1	M0
	T2	N1	M0
	T3a	N0–N1	M0
	T3b	N0–N1	M0
	T3c	N0–N1	M0
Stage IV	T4	N0–N1	M0
	Any T	N2	M0
	Any T	Any N	M1

From Edge SB, Byrd DR, Compton CC, et al (eds): AJCC Cancer Staging Manual, 7th ed. New York, Springer 2010.

STAGING AND PROGNOSIS

Staging system

The preferred staging system for renal cell carcinoma is the TNM classification (Table 3).

Prognostic factors

The natural history of renal cell carcinoma is highly variable. However, approximately 30% of patients present with metastatic disease at diagnosis, and one-third of the remainder will develop metastasis during follow-up.

Five-year survival rates after nephrectomy for tumors confined to the renal parenchyma (T1/2) are > 80%. Renal vein involvement without nodal involvement does not affect survival. Lymph node involvement and/or extracapsular spread is associated with a 5-year survival of 10% to 25%. Patients with metastatic disease have a median survival of 2 years.

Several prognostic schemes have been developed for both localized and metastatic renal cell carcinomas. In general, factors such as tumor stage and grade, performance status, hemoglobin value, calcium, and lactate dehydrogenase levels, and time interval to development of metastatic disease are important.

TREATMENT

Surgery

Surgical resection (open and laparoscopic radical or partial nephrectomy) is the established therapy for localized renal cell carcinoma. When performing a radical nephrectomy, the kidneys, adrenal gland, and perirenal fat (structures bound by Gerota's fascia) are removed. Also, limited regional lymph node dissection can be performed for staging purposes. Partial nephrectomy is standard in patients with smaller tumors (eg, < 4 cm) or in whom radical nephrectomy would unacceptably compromise overall renal function.

Because complete resection is the only known cure for renal cell carcinoma, even in locally advanced disease, surgery is considered if the involved adjacent structures can be safely removed. In patients with metastatic renal cell carcinoma, two randomized, controlled trials have shown a survival benefit of 6 months (combined analysis) with a debulking nephrectomy prior to interferon α immunotherapy, as compared with immunotherapy alone. However, patients must be carefully selected prior to the nephrectomy and should have an ECOG performance status of 0 to 1. It is also recommended that patients have a baseline CT or MRI of the brain prior to undergoing surgery. The ECOG performance status of a patient prior to treatment is an important determinant of disease-related outcome and should be considered in making treatment decisions.

TABLE 4: Therapeutic regimens for renal cell carcinoma

Dose and schedule

High-dose IL-2

IL-2: 600,000 or 720,000 IU/kg IV infused over 15 minutes every 8 hours until toxicity develops, or 14 consecutive doses for 5 days

After a 5- to 9-day rest period, an additional 14 doses of IL-2 are administered over a 5-day period. If patients show evidence of tumor regression or stable disease, 1–2 more courses of treatment may be given.

Fyfe G, Fisher RI, Rosenberg SA, et al: J Clin Oncol 13:688–696, 1995.

Low-dose IL-2

IL-2: 72,000 IU/kg by IV bolus every 8 hours to a maximum of 15 doses every 7–10 days for 2 cycles

NOTE: The cycles represent one course of therapy. Patients who are stable or responding after one course of therapy receive a second course. Third and fourth courses are given only if patients demonstrate further tumor regression.

Yang JC, Topalian SL, Parkinson D, et al: J Clin Oncol 12:1572–1576, 1998.

Sunitinib

50 mg PO daily for 4 weeks, followed by 2 weeks off. One cycle of therapy = 6 weeks. Continue therapy until disease progresses or drug intolerance occurs. Repeat every 6 weeks (4 weeks on, 2 weeks off).

Motzer RJ, Hutson TE, Tomczak P, et al: N Engl J Med 356:115–124, 2007; Escudier B, Bellmunt J, Négrier S, et al: J Clin Oncol 28:2144–2150, 2010.

Sorafenib

400 mg PO bid daily continuously until disease progression

Escudier B, Eisen T, Stadler WM, et al: N Engl J Med 356:125–134, 2007.

Bevacizumab/interferon-α

Bevacizumab	10 mg/kg every 2 weeks
Interferon-α	9 million IU SC 3 times weekly

NOTE: Interferon-α dose reductions are acceptable and appear not to compromise the outcome of this combination.

Rini BI, Halabi S, Rosenberg JE, et al: J Clin Oncol 26:5422–5428, 2008; Escudier B, Bellmunt J, Negrier S, et al: J Clin Oncol 28:2144–2150, 2010.

Everolimus

10 mg PO once daily until disease progression

Motzer RJ, Escudier B, Oudard S, et al: Lancet 372:449–456, 2008; Escudier B, Bellmunt J, Négrier S, et al: J Clin Oncol 28:2144–2150, 2010.

Temsirolimus

25 mg IVPB every week

Hudes G, Carducci M, Tomczak P, et al: N Engl J Med 356:2271–2281, 2007.

Pazopanib

800 mg PO daily continuously until disease progression or drug intolerance

Sternberg CN, Szczylik C, Lee E, et al: J Clin Oncol 27(suppl):5021, 2009.

IVPB = intravenous piggyback

Table prepared by Ishmael Jaiyesimi, DO.

Radiation therapy for renal cell carcinoma

Primary radiation therapy

Radiation therapy may be considered for palliation as the primary therapy for renal cell carcinoma in patients whose clinical condition precludes surgery, either because of extensive disease or poor overall condition. A dose of 4,500 cGy is delivered, with consideration of a boost up to 5,580 cGy.

Postoperative radiation therapy

This modality has not been shown to prevent recurrence.

Palliation

Radiation therapy is commonly used for palliation for metastatic, including that affecting the CNS disease.

Systemic therapy for advanced disease

Metastatic renal cell carcinoma is resistant to chemotherapeutic agents. An extensive review of currently available agents concluded that the overall response rate to chemotherapy is 6%.

There is no standard adjuvant therapy for renal cell carcinoma after surgical resection regardless of recurrence risk. Multiple agents, including hormone therapy, radiation, immune therapy, and chemotherapy, have been tried, and none have produced benefit in the adjuvant setting. Thus, observation is the current standard of care. There are ongoing trials testing novel targeted agents in the adjuvant setting.

Interleukin-2 (IL-2, aldesleukin [Proleukin])

The first FDA-approved treatment for metastatic renal cell carcinoma was high-dose IL-2 (Table 4).

High-dose regimen High-dose IL-2 (720,000 IU/kg IV piggyback every 8 hours for 14 doses, repeated once after a 9-day rest) results in a 15% remission rate (7% complete responses, 8% partial responses). The majority of responses to IL-2 are durable, with a median response duration of 54 months.

The major toxicity of high-dose IL-2 is a sepsis-like syndrome, which includes a progressive decrease in systemic vascular resistance and an associated decrease in intravascular volume due to a "capillary leak." Management includes judicious use of fluids and vasopressor support to maintain blood pressure and intravascular volume and at the same time to avoid pulmonary toxicity due to noncardiogenic pulmonary edema from the capillary leak. This syndrome is totally reversible.

Other doses and schedules Because of the toxicity of high-dose IL-2, other doses and schedules have been and are being evaluated. Several trials of low-dose IL-2 (3–18 $\times 10^6$ IU/d), either alone or combined with interferon-α, have reported outcomes similar to those achieved with high-dose IL-2.

Biologic agents

Four oral multikinase inhibitors have been approved by the FDA for the treatment of advanced kidney cancer. In addition, a monoclonal antibody has been tested extensively in treating the disease and, in combination with interferon-α, was FDA-approved to treat metastatic renal cell carcinoma.

Sorafenib (Nexavar) targets several serine/threonine and receptor tyrosine kinases, especially vascular endothelial growth factor, thought to be integral to the biology of renal cell carcinoma. A phase III, placebo-controlled trial was conducted in 769 patients with advanced renal cell carcinoma who had received prior systemic treatment. The recommended oral dose of sorafenib (400 mg twice daily) was used. The median progression-free survival was 5.5 months in the sorafenib group versus 2.8 months in the placebo group. Toxic effects associated with sorafenib included reversible skin rashes in 40% and hand-foot skin reactions in 30% of patients. Notably, the incidence of treatment-emergent cardiac ischemia/infarction events was higher with sorafenib (2.9% vs 0.4%).

Sunitinib (Sutent) targets several receptor tyrosine kinases. Initial phase II trials of sunitinib, given as 50 mg once daily PO for 4 weeks followed by 2 weeks off, to 169 metastatic renal cell cancer patients who had failed prior cytokine-based therapy demonstrated an investigator-assessed objective response rate of 45%, a median duration of response of 11.9 months, and a median progression-free survival of 8.4 months. A phase III trial of sunitinib versus interferon-α in 750 untreated metastatic renal cell cancer patients demonstrated a significant advantage in an independently assessed objective response rate (31%; 95% confidence interval [CI] = 26%–36% vs 6%; $P < .001$) and progression-free survival (11 months vs 5 months). Sunitinib-treated patients had a median overall survival of 26.4 versus 21.8 months for interferon-α-treated patients ($P = .051$).

Temsirolimus (Torisel) and bevacizumab (Avastin) were added to the NCCN Kidney Cancer Guidelines as options for first-line treatment of relapsed or medically unresectable stage IV renal cell carcinoma with predominant clear cell histology and, in the case of temsirolimus, non–clear cell histology. The recommendations were based on the results of large randomized trials. Temsirolimus significantly prolonged median overall survival in a phase III trial of 626 patients ($P = .0078$) and received FDA approval for first-line as well subsequent treatment of advanced renal cell carcinoma.

Bevacizumab Two separate, multicenter, international studies have established bevacizumab-based therapy as robust in the front-line setting. One phase III trial randomized 649 untreated patients with metastatic renal cell carcinoma to treatment with interferon α-2a, recombinant (Roferon) plus placebo infusion or to interferon α-2a plus bevacizumab infusion 10 mg/kg every 2 weeks. A significant advantage for bevacizumab plus interferon α-2a was observed for objective response rate (31% vs 13%, respectively; $P < .0001$) and progression-free survival (10.2 months vs 5.4 months; $P < .0001$). The hazard ratio (HR) for progression in the bevacizumab plus interferon α-2a arm was 0.63 (95% CI = 0.52–0.75; $P = .0001$).

A second multicenter, phase III trial conducted in the United States and Canada through the CALGB was nearly identical in design, except that it lacked a placebo infusion and did not require prior nephrectomy. The median progression-free survival was 8.5 months in patients receiving bevacizumab plus interferon α-2a (95% CI = 7.5–9.7) vs 5.2 months for patients using interferon α-2a monotherapy (95% CI = 3.1–5.6; $P < .0001$). The HR for progression for patients receiving bevacizumab plus interferon α-2a after adjusting for stratification factors was 0.71 ($P < .0001$). Also, among patients with measurable disease, the objective response rate was higher in patients treated with bevacizumab plus interferon α-2a (25.5%) than for those given interferon α-2a monotherapy (13.1%, $P < .0001$).

In the AVOREN trial, bevacizumab significantly increased progression-free survival (10.2 months vs 5.4 months; $P = .0001$) of patients with metastatic renal cell carcinoma when administered in combination with interferon-α 2a.

Pazopanib (Votrient), a multikinase angiogenesis inhibitor, has been used to treat advanced renal cell cancer. In a phase III study, 435 patients with advanced renal cell carcinoma were randomly assigned to treatment with pazopanib (800 mg/d orally) or placebo. Progression-free survival was significantly better in the pazopanib group than in the placebo group (HR, 0.46, $P < .0000001$). This benefit was observed for both treatment-naive patients (HR, 0.40; $P < .0000001$) and for those who had previously received one cytokine-based treatment (HR, 0.54; $P < .001$). The response rate was 30% with pazopanib compared with 3% with placebo, and the median duration of response was 58.7 weeks. Most of the adverse events associated with this therapy were grade 1 or 2. The most common laboratory abnormality was an elevation in alanine aminotransferase The FDA approved pazopanib for advanced renal cell carcinoma in October 2009.

Everolimus (Afinitor) is an oral inhibitor of mTOR kinase that has shown activity in metastatic renal cell carcinoma in phase II studies. Motzer and colleagues presented results of a planned interim analysis of a phase III study assessing the clinical benefit of everolimus in patients who had progressive metastatic renal cell carcinoma after receiving sunitinib, sorafenib, or both. The primary endpoint was progression-free survival. A total of 410 patients were randomized to receive everolimus, 10 mg, or placebo in a 2:1 ratio. Prior bevacizumab and/or cytokine treatment was allowed. The results showed a significant improvement in progression-free survival for everolimus vs placebo (everolimus, 4.0 months; placebo, 1.9 months; $P < .001$)

As always, patients should be encouraged to participate in ongoing clinical trials for metastatic renal cell cancer.

SUGGESTED READING

ON UROTHELIAL CANCER

Barton Grossman H, Natale RB, Tangen CM, et al: Neoadjuvant chemotherapy plus cystectomy compared with cystectomy alone for locally advanced bladder cancer. N Engl J Med 349:859–866, 2003.

Duchesne GM, Bolger JJ, Griffiths GD, et al: A randomized trial of hypofractionated schedules of palliative radiotherapy in the management of bladder carcinoma: Results of Medical Research Council Trial BA09. Int J Radiat Oncol Biol Phys 47:379–388, 2000.

Efstathiou JA, Bae K, Shipley WU, et al: Late pelvic toxicity after bladder-sparing therapy in patients with invasive bladder cancer: RTOG 89-03, 95-06, 97-06, 99-06. J Clin Oncol 27:4055–4061, 2009.

Hudson MA, Herr HW: Carcinoma in situ of the bladder. J Urol 153:564–572, 1995.

Jemal A, Siegel R, Xu J, et al: Cancer statistics, 2010. CA Cancer J Clin 60:277–300, 2010.

Kaufman DS, Shipley WU, Feldman AS: Bladder cancer. Lancet 374:239–249, 2009.

Lotan Y, Gupta A, Shariat SF, et al: Lymphovascular invasion is independently associated with overall survival, cause-specific survival, and local and distant recurrence in patients with negative lymph nodes at radical cystectomy. J Clin Oncol 23:6533–6539, 2005.

Sylvester RJ, van der Meijden AP, Witjes JA, et al: Bacillus calmette-guerin versus chemotherapy for the intravesical treatment of patients with carcinoma in situ of the bladder: A meta-analysis of the published results of randomized clinical trials. J Urol 174:86–92, 2005.

Von der Maase H, Hansen SW, Roberts JT, et al: Gemcitabine and cisplatin versus methotrexate, vinblastine, doxorubicin, and cisplatin in advanced or metastatic bladder cancer: Results of a large, randomized, multinational, multicenter, phase III study. J Clin Oncol 17:3068–3077, 2000.

ON KIDNEY CANCER

Dutcher JP, Szczylik C, Tannir N, et al: Correlation of survival with tumor histology, age, and prognostic risk group for previously untreated patients with advanced renal cell carcinoma receiving temsirolimus or interferon-alpha. J Clin Oncol 25:5033, 2007.

Escudier B, Eisen T, Stadler WM, et al: Sorafenib in advanced clear-cell renal-cell carcinoma. N Engl J Med 356:125–134, 2007.

Escudier B, Koralewski P, Pluzanska A, et al: A randomized, controlled, double-blind phase III study (AVOREN) of bevacizumab/interferon-α 2a vs placebo/interferon-α 2a as first-line therapy in metastatic renal cell carcinoma. J Clin Oncol 25:3, 2007.

Escudier B, Pluzanska A, Koralewski P, et al: Bevacizumab plus interferon alfa-2a for treatment of metastatic renal cell carcinoma: a randomised, double-blind phase III trial. Lancet 370:2103–2111, 2007.

Flanigan RC, Salmon SE, Blumenstein BA, et al: Nephrectomy followed by interferon alfa-2b compared with interferon alfa-2b alone for metastatic renal cell cancer. N Engl J Med 345:1655–1659, 2001.

Hudes G, Carducci M, Tomczak P, et al: Temsirolimus, interferon alfa, or both for advanced renal-cell carcinoma. N Engl J Med 356:2271–2281, 2007.

Mickisch GH, Garin A, van Poppel H, et al: Radical nephrectomy plus interferon-alfa-based immunotherapy compared with interferon alone in metastatic renal-cell carcinoma: A randomized trial. Lancet 358:966–970, 2001.

Motzer RJ, Dror Michaelson MD, Redman BG, et al: Activity of SU11248, a multitargeted inhibitor of vascular endothelial growth factor receptor and platelet-derived growth factor receptor, in patients with metastatic renal cell carcinoma. J Clin Oncol 24:16–24, 2006.

Motzer RJ, Hutson TE, Tomczak P, et al: Sunitinib versus interferon alfa in metastatic renal-cell carcinoma. N Engl J Med 356:115–124, 2007.

Motzer RJ, Rini BI, Bukowski RM, et al: Sunitinib in patients with metastatic renal cell carcinoma. JAMA 295:2516–2524, 2006.

Parkinson DR, Sznol M: High-dose interleukin-2 in the therapy of metastatic renal cell carcinoma. Semin Oncol 22:61–66, 1995.

Rabinovitch RA, Zelefsky MJ, Gaynor JJ, et al: Patterns of failure following surgical resection of renal cell carcinoma: Implications for adjuvant local and systemic therapy. J Clin Oncol 12:206–212, 1994.

Rini BI, Halabi S, Rosenberg JE, et al: Bevacizumab plus interferon alfa compared with interferon alfa monotherapy in patients with metastatic renal cell carcinoma: CALGB 90206. J Clin Oncol 26:5422–5428, 2008.

Stodlen WM, Vogelzang NJ: Low-dose interleukin-2 in the treatment of metastatic renal cell carcinoma. Semin Oncol 22:67–73, 1995.

Zisman A, Pantuck AJ, Dorey F, et al: Improved prognostication of renal cell carcinoma using an integrated staging system. J Clin Oncol 19:1649–1657, 2001.

Abbreviations in this chapter

AJCC = American Joint Committee on Cancer; AVOREN = Avastin for Renal Cell Cancer; CALGB = Cancer and Leukemia Group B; FDA = US Food and Drug Administration; NCCN = National Comprehensive Cancer Network; RTOG = Radiation Treatment Oncology Group; WHO = World Health Organization

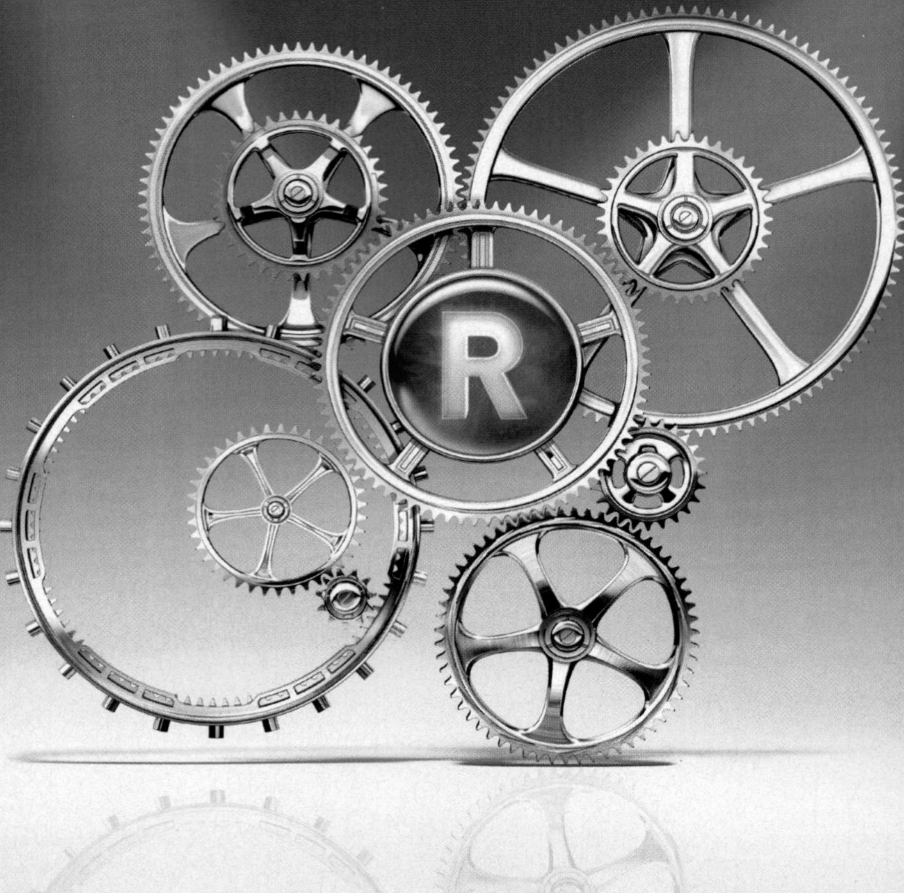

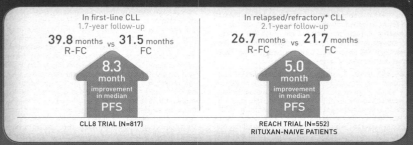

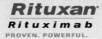

RITUXAN® (Rituximab) Brief summary—Please consult full prescribing information.

WARNING: FATAL INFUSION REACTIONS, TUMOR LYSIS SYNDROME (TLS), SEVERE MUCOCUTANEOUS REACTIONS, and PROGRESSIVE MULTIFOCAL LEUKOENCEPHALOPATHY (PML)

Infusion Reactions: Rituxan administration can result in serious, including fatal infusion reactions. Deaths within 24 hours of Rituxan infusion have occurred. Approximately 80% of fatal infusion reactions occurred in association with the first infusion. Carefully monitor patients during infusions. Discontinue Rituxan infusion and provide medical treatment for Grade 3 or 4 infusion reactions [*see Warnings and Precautions, Adverse Reactions*]. Tumor Lysis Syndrome (TLS): Acute renal failure requiring dialysis with instances of fatal outcome can occur in the setting of TLS following treatment of non-Hodgkin's lymphoma (NHL) patients with Rituxan [*see Warnings and Precautions, Adverse Reactions*]. Severe Mucocutaneous Reactions: Severe, including fatal, mucocutaneous reactions can occur in patients receiving Rituxan [*see Warnings and Precautions, Adverse Reactions*]. Progressive Multifocal Leukoencephalopathy (PML): JC virus infection resulting in PML and death can occur in patients receiving Rituxan [*see Warnings and Precautions, Adverse Reactions*].

INDICATIONS AND USAGE Non-Hodgkin's Lymphoma (NHL) Rituxan® (rituximab) is indicated for the treatment of patients with: Relapsed or refractory, low-grade or follicular, CD20-positive, B-cell NHL as a single agent; Previously untreated follicular, CD20-positive, B-cell NHL in combination with CVP chemotherapy; Non-progressing (including stable disease), low-grade, CD20-positive, B-cell NHL, as a single agent, after first-line CVP chemotherapy; Previously untreated diffuse large B-cell, CD20-positive NHL in combination with CHOP or other anthracycline-based chemotherapy regimens. **Chronic Lymphocytic Leukemia (CLL)** Rituxan® (rituximab) is indicated, in combination with fludarabine and cyclophosphamide (FC), for the treatment of patients with previously untreated and previously treated CD20-positive CLL. **Limitations of use** Rituxan is not recommended for use in patients with severe, active infections.

WARNINGS AND PRECAUTIONS Infusion Reactions Rituxan can cause severe, including fatal, infusion reactions. Severe reactions typically occurred during the first infusion with time to onset of 30–120 minutes. Rituxan-induced infusion reactions and sequelae include urticaria, hypotension, angioedema, hypoxia, bronchospasm, pulmonary infiltrates, acute respiratory distress syndrome, myocardial infarction, ventricular fibrillation, cardiogenic shock, anaphylactoid events, or death. Premedicate patients with an antihistamine and acetaminophen prior to dosing. Institute medical management (e.g. glucocorticoids, epinephrine, bronchodilators, or oxygen) for infusion reactions as needed. Depending on the severity of the infusion reaction and the required interventions, temporarily or permanently discontinue Rituxan. Resume infusion at a minimum 50% reduction in rate after symptoms have resolved. Closely monitor the following patients: those with pre-existing cardiac or pulmonary conditions, those who experienced prior cardiopulmonary adverse reactions, and those with high numbers of circulating malignant cells (≥25,000/mm³). [*See Boxed Warning, Warnings and Precautions, Adverse Reactions.*] **Tumor Lysis Syndrome (TLS)** Acute renal failure, hyperkalemia, hypocalcemia, hyperuricemia, or hyperphosphatemia from tumor lysis, some fatal, can occur within 12–24 hours after the first infusion of Rituxan in patients with NHL. A high number of circulating malignant cells (≥25,000/mm³) or high tumor burden confers a greater risk of TLS. Administer aggressive intravenous hydration and anti-hyperuricemic therapy in patients at high risk for TLS. Correct electrolyte abnormalities, monitor renal function and fluid balance, and administer supportive care, including dialysis as indicated. [*See Boxed Warning.*] **Severe Mucocutaneous Reactions** Mucocutaneous reactions, some with fatal outcome, can occur in patients treated with Rituxan. These reactions include paraneoplastic pemphigus, Stevens-Johnson syndrome, lichenoid dermatitis, vesiculobullous dermatitis, and toxic epidermal necrolysis. The onset of these reactions has varied from 1–13 weeks following Rituxan exposure. Discontinue Rituxan in patients who experience a severe mucocutaneous reaction. The safety of readministration of Rituxan to patients with severe mucocutaneous reactions has not been determined. [*See Boxed Warning, Adverse Reactions.*] **Progressive Multifocal Leukoencephalopathy (PML)** JC virus infection resulting in PML and death can occur in Rituxan-treated patients with hematologic malignancies or with autoimmune diseases. The majority of patients with hematologic malignancies diagnosed with PML received Rituxan in combination with chemotherapy or as part of a hematopoietic stem cell transplant. The patients with autoimmune diseases had prior or concurrent immunosuppressive therapy. Most cases of PML were diagnosed within 12 months of their last infusion of Rituxan. Consider the diagnosis of PML in any patient presenting with new-onset neurologic manifestations. Evaluation of PML includes, but is not limited to, consultation with a neurologist, brain MRI, and lumbar puncture. Discontinue Rituxan and consider discontinuation or reduction of any concomitant chemotherapy or immunosuppressive therapy in patients who develop PML. [*See Boxed Warning, Adverse Reactions.*] **Hepatitis B Virus (HBV) Reactivation** Hepatitis B virus (HBV) reactivation with fulminant hepatitis, hepatic failure, and death can occur in patients with hematologic malignancies treated with Rituxan. The median time to the diagnosis of hepatitis was approximately 4 months after the initiation of Rituxan and approximately one month after the last dose. Screen patients at high risk of HBV infection before initiation of Rituxan. Closely monitor carriers of hepatitis B for clinical and laboratory signs of active HBV infection for several months following Rituxan therapy. Discontinue Rituxan and any concomitant chemotherapy in patients who develop viral hepatitis, and institute appropriate treatment including antiviral therapy. Insufficient data exist regarding the safety of resuming Rituxan in patients who develop hepatitis subsequent to HBV reactivation. [*See Adverse Reactions.*] **Infections** Serious, including fatal, bacterial, fungal, and new or reactivated viral infections can occur during and up to one year following the completion of Rituxan-based therapy. New or reactivated viral infections included cytomegalovirus, herpes simplex virus, parvovirus B19, varicella zoster virus, West Nile virus, and hepatitis B and C. Discontinue Rituxan for serious infections and institute appropriate anti-infective therapy. [*See Adverse Reactions.*] **Cardiovascular** Discontinue infusions for serious or life-threatening cardiac arrhythmias. Perform cardiac monitoring during and after all infusions of Rituxan for patients who develop clinically significant arrhythmias, or who have a history of arrhythmia or angina. [*See Adverse Reactions.*] **Renal** Severe, including fatal, renal toxicity can occur after Rituxan administration in patients with NHL. Renal toxicity has occurred in patients who experience tumor lysis syndrome and in patients with NHL administered concomitant cisplatin therapy during clinical trials. The combination of cisplatin and Rituxan is not an approved treatment regimen. Monitor closely for signs of renal failure and discontinue Rituxan in patients with a rising serum creatinine or oliguria. **Bowel Obstruction and Perforation** Abdominal pain, bowel obstruction and perforation, in some cases leading to death, can occur in patients receiving Rituxan in combination with chemotherapy. In postmarketing reports, the mean time to documented gastrointestinal perforation was 6 (range 1–77) days in patients with NHL. Perform a thorough diagnostic evaluation and institute appropriate treatment for complaints of abdominal pain. [*See Adverse Reactions.*] **Immunization** The safety of immunization with live viral vaccines following Rituxan therapy has not been studied and vaccination with live virus vaccines is not recommended. **Laboratory Monitoring** In patients with lymphoid malignancies, during treatment with Rituxan monotherapy, obtain complete blood counts (CBC) and platelet counts prior to each Rituxan course. During treatment with Rituxan and chemotherapy, obtain CBC and platelet counts at weekly to monthly intervals and more frequently in patients who develop cytopenias. [*See Adverse Reactions*]. The duration of cytopenias caused by Rituxan can extend months beyond the treatment period. **ADVERSE REACTIONS** The most common adverse reactions of Rituxan (incidence ≥25%) observed in clinical trials of patients with NHL were infusion reactions, fever, lymphopenia, chills, infection, and asthenia. The most common adverse reactions of Rituxan (incidence ≥25%) observed in clinical trials of patients with CLL were: infusion reactions and neutropenia. **Clinical Trials Experience in Lymphoid Malignancies** Because clinical trials are conducted under widely varying conditions, adverse reaction rates observed in the clinical trials of a drug cannot be directly compared to rates in the clinical trials of another drug and may not reflect the rates observed in practice. The data described below reflect exposure to Rituxan in 2282 patients, with exposures ranging from a single infusion up to 6–8 months. Rituxan was studied in both single-agent and active-controlled trials (n = 356 and n = 1926). The population included 679 patients with low-grade follicular lymphoma, 927 patients with DLBCL, and 676 patients with CLL. Most NHL patients received Rituxan as infusion of 375 mg/m² per infusion, given as a single agent weekly for up to 8 doses, in combination with chemotherapy for up to 8 doses, or following chemotherapy for up to 16 doses. CLL patients received Rituxan 375 mg/m² as an initial infusion followed by 500 mg/m² for up to 5 doses, in combination with fludarabine and cyclophosphamide. Seventy-one percent of CLL patients received 6 cycles and 90% received at least 3 cycles of Rituxan-based therapy. ***Infusion Reactions*** In the majority of patients with NHL, infusion reactions consisting of fever, chills/rigors, nausea, pruritus, angioedema, hypotension, headache, bronchospasm, urticaria, rash, vomiting, myalgia, dizziness, or hypertension occurred during the first Rituxan infusion. Infusion reactions typically occurred within 30 to 120 minutes of beginning the first infusion and resolved with slowing or interruption of the Rituxan infusion and with supportive care (diphenhydramine, acetaminophen, and intravenous saline). The incidence of infusion reactions was highest during the first infusion (77%) and decreased with each subsequent infusion. [*See Boxed Warning, Warnings and Precautions.*] ***Infections*** Serious infections (NCI CTCAE Grade 3 or 4), including sepsis, occurred in less than 5% of patients with NHL in the single-arm studies. The overall incidence of infections was 31% (bacterial 19%, viral 10%, unknown 6%, and fungal 1%). [*See Warnings and Precautions.*] In randomized, controlled studies where Rituxan was administered following chemotherapy for the treatment of follicular or low-grade NHL, the rate of infection was higher among patients who received Rituxan. In diffuse large B-cell lymphoma patients, viral infections occurred more frequently in those who received Rituxan. ***Cytopenias and hypogammaglobulinemia*** In patients with NHL receiving rituximab monotherapy, NCI-CTC Grade 3 and 4 cytopenias were reported in 48% of patients. These included lymphopenia (40%), neutropenia (6%), leukopenia (4%), anemia (3%), and thrombocytopenia (2%). The median duration of lymphopenia was 14 days (range, 1–588 days) and of neutropenia was 13 days (range, 2–116 days). A single occurrence of transient aplastic anemia (pure red cell aplasia) and two occurrences of hemolytic anemia following Rituxan therapy occurred during the single-arm studies. In studies of monotherapy, Rituxan-induced B-cell depletion occurred in 70% to 80% of patients with NHL. Decreased IgM and IgG serum levels occurred in 14% of these patients. ***Relapsed or Refractory, Low-Grade NHL*** Adverse reactions in Table 1 occurred in 356 patients with relapsed or refractory, low-grade or follicular, CD20-positive, B-cell NHL treated in single-arm studies of Rituxan administered as a single agent. [*See Clinical Studies.*] Most patients received Rituxan 375 mg/m² weekly for 4 doses.

Table 1

Incidence of Adverse Reactions in ≥5% of Patients with Relapsed or Refractory, Low-Grade or Follicular NHL, Receiving Single-agent Rituxan (N = 356)[a,b]

	All Grades (%)	Grade 3 and 4 (%)		All Grades (%)	Grade 3 and 4 (%)
Any Adverse Events	99	57	Respiratory System	38	4
Body as a Whole	86	10	Increased Cough	13	1
Fever	53	1	Rhinitis	12	1
Chills	33	3	Bronchospasm	8	1
Infection	31	4	Dyspnea	7	1
Asthenia	26	1	Sinusitis	6	0
Headache	19	1	Metabolic and Nutritional		
Abdominal Pain	14	1	Disorders	38	3
Pain	12	1	Angioedema	11	1
Back Pain	10	1	Hyperglycemia	9	1
Throat Irritation	9	0	Peripheral Edema	8	0
Flushing	5	0	LDH Increase	7	0
Heme and Lymphatic System	67	48	Digestive System	37	2
Lymphopenia	48	40	Nausea	23	1
Leukopenia	14	4	Diarrhea	10	1
Neutropenia	14	6	Vomiting	10	1
Thrombocytopenia	12	2	Nervous System	32	1
Anemia	8	3	Dizziness	10	1
Skin and Appendages	44	2	Anxiety	5	1
Night Sweats	15	1	Musculoskeletal System	26	3
Rash	15	1	Myalgia	10	1
Pruritus	14	1	Arthralgia	10	1
Urticaria	8	1	Cardiovascular System	25	3
			Hypotension	10	1
			Hypertension	6	1

[a]Adverse reactions observed up to 12 months following Rituxan. [b]Adverse reactions graded for severity by NCI-CTC criteria.

In these single-arm Rituxan studies, bronchiolitis obliterans occurred during and up to 6 months after Rituxan infusion. ***Previously Untreated Low-Grade NHL*** In Study 4, patients in the R-CVP arm experienced a higher incidence of infusional toxicity and neutropenia compared to patients in the CVP arm. The following adverse reactions occurred more frequently (≥5%) in patients receiving R-CVP compared to CVP alone: rash (17% vs. 5%), cough (15% vs. 6%), flushing (14% vs. 3%), rigors (10% vs. 2%), pruritus (10% vs. 1%), neutropenia (8% vs. 3%), and chest tightness (7% vs. 1%). In Study 5, the following adverse reactions were reported more frequently (≥5%) in patients receiving Rituxan following CVP compared to patients who received no further therapy: fatigue (39% vs. 14%), anemia (35% vs. 20%), peripheral sensory neuropathy (30% vs. 18%), infections (19% vs. 9%), pulmonary toxicity (18% vs. 10%), hepato-biliary toxicity (17% vs. 7%), rash and/or pruritus (17% vs. 5%), arthralgia (12% vs. 3%), and weight gain (11% vs. 4%). Neutropenia was the only Grade 3 or 4 adverse reaction that occurred more frequently (≥2%) in the Rituxan arm compared with those who received no further therapy (4% vs. 1%). [*See Clinical Studies*.] ***DLBCL*** In Studies 6 and 7, [*see Clinical Studies*] the following adverse reactions, regardless of severity, were reported more frequently (≥5%) in patients age ≥60 years receiving R-CHOP as compared to CHOP alone: pyrexia (56% vs. 46%), lung disorder (31% vs. 24%), cardiac disorder (29% vs. 21%), and chills (13% vs. 4%). Detailed safety data collection in these studies was primarily limited to Grade 3 and 4 adverse reactions and serious adverse reactions. In Study 7, a review of cardiac toxicity determined that supraventricular arrhythmias or tachycardia accounted for most of the difference in cardiac disorders (4.5% for R-CHOP vs. 1.0% for CHOP). The following Grade 3 or 4 adverse reactions occurred more frequently among patients in the R-CHOP arm compared with those in the CHOP arm: thrombocytopenia (9% vs. 7%) and lung disorder (6% vs. 3%). Other Grade 3 or 4 adverse reactions occurring more frequently among patients receiving R-CHOP were viral infection (Study 7), neutropenia (Studies 7 and 8), and anemia (Study 8). ***CLL*** The data below reflect exposure to Rituxan in combination with fludarabine and cyclophosphamide in 676 patients with CLL in Study 9 or Study 10 [*see Clinical Studies*]. The age range was 30–83 years and 71% were men. Detailed safety data collection in Study 9 was limited to Grade 3 and 4 adverse reactions and serious adverse reactions. Infusion-related adverse reactions were defined by any of the following adverse events occurring during or within 24 hours of the start of infusion: nausea, pyrexia, chills, hypotension, vomiting, and dyspnea. In Study 9, the following Grade 3 and 4 adverse reactions occurred more frequently in R-FC–treated patients compared to FC-treated patients: infusion reactions (9% in R-FC arm), neutropenia (30% vs. 19%), febrile neutropenia (9% vs. 6%), leukopenia (23% vs. 12%), and pancytopenia (3% vs. 1%). In Study 10, the following Grade 3 or 4 adverse reactions occurred more frequently in R-FC–treated patients compared to FC-treated patients: infusion reactions (7% in R-FC arm), neutropenia (49% vs. 44%), febrile neutropenia (15% vs. 12%), thrombocytopenia (11% vs. 9%), hypotension (2% vs. 0%), and hepatitis B (2% vs. <1%). Fifty-nine percent of R-FC–treated patients experienced an infusion reaction of any severity. **Immunogenicity** As with all therapeutic proteins, there is a potential for immunogenicity. The observed incidence of antibody (including neutralizing antibody) positivity in an assay is highly dependent on several factors including assay sensitivity and specificity, assay methodology, sample handling, timing of sample collection, concomitant medications, and underlying disease. For these reasons, comparison of the incidence of antibodies to Rituxan with the incidence of antibodies to other products may be misleading. Using an ELISA assay, anti-human anti-chimeric antibody (HACA) was detected in 4 of 356 (1.1%) patients with low-grade or follicular NHL receiving single-agent Rituxan. Three of the four patients had an objective clinical response. The clinical relevance of HACA formation in Rituxan-treated patients is unclear. **Postmarketing Experience** The following adverse reactions have been identified during post-approval use of Rituxan in hematologic malignancies. Because these reactions are reported voluntarily from a population of uncertain size, it is not always possible to reliably estimate their frequency or establish a causal relationship to drug exposure. Decisions to include these reactions in labeling are typically based on one or more of the following factors: (1) seriousness of the reaction, (2) frequency of reporting, or (3) strength of causal connection to Rituxan.

Hematologic: prolonged pancytopenia, marrow hypoplasia, and late-onset neutropenia, hyperviscosity syndrome in Waldenstrom's macroglobulinemia. *Cardiac:* fatal cardiac failure. *Immune/Autoimmune Events:* uveitis, optic neuritis, systemic vasculitis, pleuritis, lupus-like syndrome, serum sickness, polyarticular arthritis, and vasculitis with rash. *Infection:* viral infections, including progressive multifocal leukoencephalopathy (PML), increase in fatal infections in HIV-associated lymphoma, and a reported increased incidence of Grade 3 and 4 infections in patients with previously treated lymphoma without known HIV infection. *Neoplasia:* disease progression of Kaposi's sarcoma. *Skin:* severe mucocutaneous reactions. *Gastrointestinal:* bowel obstruction and perforation. *Pulmonary:* fatal bronchiolitis obliterans and pneumonitis (including interstitial pneumonitis). **DRUG INTERACTIONS** Formal drug interaction studies have not been performed with Rituxan. In patients with CLL, Rituxan did not alter systemic exposure to fludarabine or cyclophosphamide. **USE IN SPECIFIC POPULATIONS Pregnancy** Category C: There are no adequate and well-controlled studies of rituximab in pregnant women. Postmarketing data indicate that B-cell lymphocytopenia generally lasting less than six months can occur in infants exposed to rituximab in-utero. Rituximab was detected postnatally in the serum of infants exposed in-utero. Non-Hodgkin's lymphoma is a serious condition that requires treatment. Rituximab should be used during pregnancy only if the potential benefit to the mother justifies the potential risk to the fetus. Reproduction studies in cynomolgus monkeys at maternal exposures similar to human therapeutic exposures showed no evidence of teratogenic effects. However, B-cell lymphoid tissue was reduced in the offspring of treated dams. The B-cell counts returned to normal levels, and immunologic function was restored within 6 months of birth. **Nursing Mothers** It is not known whether Rituxan is secreted into human milk. However, Rituxan is secreted in the milk of lactating cynomolgus monkeys, and IgG is excreted in human milk. Published data suggest that antibodies in breast milk do not enter the neonatal and infant circulations in substantial amounts. The unknown risks to the infant from oral ingestion of Rituxan should be weighed against the known benefits of breast-feeding. **Pediatric Use** The safety and effectiveness of Rituxan in pediatric patients have not been established. **Geriatric Use** ***Diffuse Large B-Cell NHL*** Among patients with DLBCL evaluated in three randomized, active-controlled trials, 927 patients received Rituxan in combination with chemotherapy. Of these, 396 (43%) were age 65 or greater and 123 (13%) were age 75 or greater. No overall differences in effectiveness were observed between these patients and younger patients. Cardiac adverse reactions, mostly supraventricular arrhythmias, occurred more frequently among elderly patients. Serious pulmonary adverse reactions were also more common among the elderly, including pneumonia and pneumonitis. ***Low-Grade or Follicular Non-Hodgkin's Lymphoma*** Clinical studies of Rituxan in low-grade or follicular, CD20-positive, B-cell NHL did not include sufficient numbers of patients aged 65 and over to determine whether they respond differently from younger subjects. ***Chronic Lymphocytic Leukemia*** Among patients with CLL evaluated in two randomized active-controlled trials, 243 of 676 Rituxan-treated patients (36%) were 65 years of age or older; of these, 100 Rituxan-treated patients (15%) were 70 years of age or older. In exploratory analyses defined by age, there was no observed benefit from the addition of Rituxan to fludarabine and cyclophosphamide among patients 70 years of age or older in Study 9 or in Study 10; there was also no observed benefit from the addition of Rituxan to fludarabine and cyclophosphamide among patients 65 years of age or older in Study 10 [*see Clinical Studies*]. Patients 70 years or older received lower dose intensity of fludarabine and cyclophosphamide compared to younger patients, regardless of the addition of Rituxan. In Study 9, the dose intensity of Rituxan was similar in older and younger patients, however in Study 10 older patients received a lower dose intensity of Rituxan. The incidence of Grade 3 and 4 adverse reactions was higher among patients receiving R-FC who were 70 years or older compared to younger patients for neutropenia [44% vs. 31% (Study 9); 56% vs. 39% (Study 10)], febrile neutropenia [16% vs. 6% (Study 9)], anemia [5% vs. 2% (Study 9); 21% vs. 10% (Study 10)], thrombocytopenia [19% vs. 8% (Study 10)], pancytopenia [7% vs. 2% (Study 9); 7% vs. 2% (Study 10)] and infections [30% vs. 14% (Study 10)]. **OVERDOSAGE** There has been no experience with overdosage in human clinical trials. Single doses of up to 500 mg/m^2 have been administered in clinical trials. **NONCLINICAL TOXICOLOGY Carcinogenesis, Mutagenesis, Impairment of Fertility** No long-term animal studies have been performed to establish the carcinogenic or mutagenic potential of Rituxan or to determine potential effects on fertility in males or females. **PATIENT COUNSELING INFORMATION** Patients should be provided the Rituxan Medication Guide and provided an opportunity to read prior to each treatment session. It is important that the patient's overall health be assessed at each visit and the risks of Rituxan therapy and any questions resulting from the patient's reading of the Medication Guide be discussed. Rituxan is detectable in serum for up to six months following completion of therapy. Individuals of childbearing potential should use effective contraception during treatment and for 12 months after Rituxan therapy.

Revised 02/2010 (4851501)

Jointly Marketed by:

Biogen Idec Inc. 5200 Research Place San Diego, CA 92122

Genentech USA, Inc. 1 DNA Way South San Francisco, CA 94080-4990

Genentech BIOONCOLOGY | biogen idec

CHAPTER 17

Cervical cancer

Leda Gattoc, MD, Carlos A. Perez, MD, William P. Tew, MD, and Sharmila Makhija, MD

Of the predominant gynecologic cancers, cancer of the uterine cervix is the least common, with only 12,200 new cases anticipated in the United States in 2010. Nevertheless, approximately 4,210 women die of cancer of the uterine cervix annually in the United States.

EPIDEMIOLOGY

Age The peak age of developing cervical cancer is 47 years. Approximately 47% of women with invasive cervical cancer are < 35 years old at diagnosis. Older women (> 65 years) account for another 10% of patients with cervical cancer. Although these older patients represent only 10% of all cases, they are more likely to die of the disease due to their more advanced stage at diagnosis.

Socioeconomic class Carcinoma of the uterine cervix primarily affects women from the lower socioeconomic class and those with poor access to routine medical care.

Geography Although invasive cervical carcinoma is relatively uncommon in the United States compared with the more common cancers in women (breast, endometrial, and ovarian cancers), it remains a significant health problem for women worldwide. In many developing countries, not only is cervical carcinoma the most frequently occurring cancer among middle-aged women, but also it is a leading cause of death. This is due, in part, to poor access to medical care and the unavailability of routine screening in many of these countries.

ETIOLOGY AND RISK FACTORS

Sexual activity Invasive cervical carcinoma can be viewed practically as a sexually transmitted disease.

Human papillomavirus Molecular and epidemiologic evidence clearly indicates that certain types of human papillomavirus (HPV), which is sexually transmitted, are the principal causes of invasive cervical cancer and cervical intraepithelial neoplasia (CIN). More than 100 HPV types have been identified, and about 40 infect the genital tract. HPV-16 and HPV-18 are the types most commonly linked with cancer, present in 70% of cervical cancers and high-grade CINs. Two vaccines to prevent cervical cancer were approved by the FDA and became available in 2006 and 2009, respectively.

Gardasil, a quadrivalent vaccine to prevent cervical cancer, is approved by the FDA to be used in girls and women aged 9 to 26. The vaccine uses virus-like particles to induce immunity to HPV types 16 and 18, which cause approximately 70% of cervical cancers and more than 50% of precancerous lesions of the cervix, vulva, and vagina. It is also reported to be protective against HPV types 6 and 11, which cause more than 90% of genital wart cases. Overall, more than 50,000 women have participated in the phase III trials worldwide. With follow-up ranging from 1 to 4 years, the vaccine has been reported to be 90% to 100% effective in preventing infection and precancerous lesions *(Prescribing information, US FDA. Issued June 2006. No. 9682300)*. Further, Cervarix, a bivalent vaccine, is also approved by the FDA to prevent cervical cancer and precancerous lesions caused by HPV types 16 and 18. It is indicated for use in girls and women ages 10 to 25 years.

Prophylactic vaccination with these HPV virus-like particle (VLP) vaccines against HPV-16 and HPV-18 has transformed the prospects for reducing the incidence of this disease on a global scale, achieving > 98% protection in randomized clinical trials against precursor lesions such as CIN grade 2/3 and adenocarcinoma in situ. However, screening for cervical cancer will have to continue, as only 2 of the 15 oncogenic HPV types are in the vaccines, and for two to three decades at least, unvaccinated sexually active women will remain at risk for the disease. If both vaccination and screening are combined, the virtual elimination of cervical cancer and the other HPV-16– and HPV-18–associated cancers is possible.

Age of onset of sexual activity Population studies of women with invasive cervical carcinoma have demonstrated that early age of onset of sexual activity also plays a role in the later development of the cancer. It is postulated that during the time of menarche in early reproductive life, the transformation zone of the cervix is more susceptible to oncogenic agents, such as HPV. Women who began sexual activity before 16 years of age or who are sexually active within 1 year of beginning menses are at particularly high risk of developing invasive cervical carcinoma.

Other risk factors include multiple sexual partners, a history of genital warts, and multiparity.

Cigarette smoking has been identified as a significant risk factor for cervical carcinoma. It is thought to increase the risk by twofold to fivefold. The mechanism may be related to diminished immune function secondary to a systemic effect of cigarette smoke and its byproducts or a local effect of tobacco-specific carcinogens.

Oral contraceptives may also play a role in the development of invasive cervical carcinoma, although this theory is controversial. Given that most women who use oral contraceptives are more sexually active than women who do not, this may represent a confounding factor rather than a true independent risk factor. The exception may be adenocarcinoma of the cervix; this relatively uncommon histologic subtype may be related to previous oral contraceptive use.

Immune system alterations In recent years, alterations in the immune system have been associated with an increased risk of invasive cervical carcinoma, as exemplified by the fact that patients who are infected with the human immunodeficiency virus

(HIV) have increased rates of both preinvasive and invasive cervical carcinomas. These patients also are at risk for other types of carcinoma, including Kaposi sarcoma, lymphomas, and other squamous cell carcinomas of the head and neck and the anogenital region. (For further discussion of AIDS-related malignancies, see chapter 24.)

Data suggest that patients who are immunocompromised due to immunosuppressive medications also are at risk for both preinvasive and invasive cervical carcinomas. This association is probably due to the suppression of the normal immune response to HPV, which makes patients more susceptible to malignant transformation. An exciting recent development in the prevention of carcinoma of the cervix is the increasing use of HPV vaccines; if used on a timely basis in young women (ideally before they are exposed to the HPV virus), they can decrease this infection and eventually the incidence of cervical cancer.

SIGNS AND SYMPTOMS

A symptom of advanced cervical carcinoma is intermenstrual bleeding in a premenopausal patient. Other commonly reported symptoms include heavier menstrual flow, menorrhagia, and/or postcoital bleeding. With effective screening, cervical cancer is generally asymptomatic.

Less frequently, patients with advanced cancer will present with signs of advanced disease, such as bowel obstruction and renal failure due to urinary tract obstruction. Only rarely are asymptomatic patients with a normal screening Pap smear found to have a lesion on the cervix as their only sign or symptom of cervical cancer. Foul-smelling vaginal discharge, pelvic pain, or both are occasionally observed.

SCREENING AND DIAGNOSIS

Screening

Pap smear The paradigm for a cost-effective, easy-to-use, reliable screening test is the cervical cytology screen, or Pap smear. The introduction of the Pap smear has resulted in a significant reduction in the incidence of invasive cervical carcinoma, as well as a shift toward earlier stages at the time of diagnosis. The success of cervical cytology, as measured by the lowered incidence of cervical cancer, ironically has led to some controversy regarding the most effective application of this screening tool. With the marked reduction in the incidence of cervical carcinoma, more patients are screened and greater costs incurred to detect each additional case of cervical carcinoma.

Current screening recommendations The ACOG recently changed its recommendations to start cervical cancer screening for women at the age of 21 regardless of the age of onset of sexual intercourse. For women between the ages of 21 and 29 years old, cervical cytology screening is recommended every 2 years with either conventional or liquid-based cytology. Women aged 30 and older who have had three consecutive cervical cytology results that are negative for intraepithelial lesions or malignancy may be tested every 3 years.

The current ACS revised guidelines for cervical cancer screening follow: Cervical cancer screening should begin ~3 years after the onset of vaginal intercourse but no later than age 21. Cervical screening should be performed every year with conventional cervical cytology smears, or every 2 years using liquid-based cytology until age 30. After age 30, as an alternative to annual routine cytology, HPV DNA testing may be added to cervical cytology for screening. After this initial dual testing, women whose results are negative by both HPV DNA testing and cytology should not be rescreened before 3 years. Women whose results are negative by cytology but who are high-risk HPV DNA positive (types 16, 18, most commonly) are at a relatively low risk of having high-grade cervical neoplasia, and colposcopy should not be performed routinely in this setting. Instead, HPV DNA testing along with cervical cytology should be repeated in these women at 6 or 12 months. If test results of either modality are positive, colposcopy should then be performed. A randomized study of more than 10,000 women confirmed the evolving role of HPV testing as an accurate screening tool. In this study, women were randomized to undergo either conventional Pap testing or HPV testing as a screening method to identify high-grade CIN. The sensitivity and specificity for CIN 2/3 were 94.6% and 94.1% with HPV testing vs 55.4% and 96.8% for Pap tests. The sensitivity reached 100% when the tests were combined together.

Women who are > 70 years old with an intact cervix and who have had three or more documented, consecutive, technically satisfactory normal cervical cytology tests and no abnormal cytology tests within the 10-year period prior to age 70 may elect to cease cervical cancer screening. Women with a history of cervical cancer, in utero exposure to diethylstilbestrol (DES), and/or who are immunocompromised (including HIV-positive) should continue cervical cancer screening for as long as they are in reasonably good health and do not have a life-limiting chronic condition. Women > 70 years old should discuss their need for cervical cancer screening with a health care professional and make an informed decision about continuing screening based on its potential benefits, harms, and limitations.

Women who have had a supracervical hysterectomy should continue cervical cancer screening as per current guidelines. Cervical cancer screening following total hysterectomy (with removal of the cervix) for benign gynecologic disease is not indicated. Women with a history of CIN 2/3 or for whom it is not possible to document the absence of CIN 2/3 prior to or as the indication for hysterectomy should be screened until three documented, consecutive, technically satisfactory normal cervical cytology tests and no abnormal cytology tests (within a 10-year period) are achieved. Women with a history of in utero DES exposure and a history of cervical carcinoma should continue screening after hysterectomy for as long as they are in reasonably good health and do not have a life-limiting chronic condition.

Techniques designed to improve the sensitivity of the Pap smear have been approved by the FDA. Liquid-based cytologies such as ThinPrep and SurePath are commercially available techniques. Computer-based analysis of these techniques has been developed but is still under evaluation.

Diagnosis

The diagnosis of invasive cervical carcinoma can be suggested by either an abnormal Pap smear or an abnormal physical finding.

Colposcopy In the patient who has an abnormal Pap smear but normal physical findings, colposcopy is indicated. Colposcopic findings consistent with invasive cervical carcinoma include dense white epithelium covering the ectocervix, punctation, mosaicism, and especially, an atypical blood vessel pattern.

Biopsy If the colposcopic findings are suggestive of invasion, biopsies are obtained from the ectocervix and endocervix. If these biopsies demonstrate only precancerous changes but not an invasive carcinoma, the patient should undergo an excisional biopsy of the cervix. In most current clinical settings, the loop electrosurgical excision procedure (LEEP) is the most expedient method for performing an excisional biopsy. This can be easily accomplished in the office with the patient under local anesthesia and provides adequate tissue for diagnosis. Once the diagnosis of either microinvasive or invasive carcinoma has been established, the patient can be triaged accordingly.

Patient with signs/symptoms of advanced disease The patient with signs/symptoms of advanced invasive cervical carcinoma requires a cervical biopsy for diagnosis and treatment planning. In this setting, a Pap smear is superfluous and may be misleading.

PATHOLOGY

Squamous cell carcinoma The most common histology associated with invasive cervical carcinoma is squamous cell carcinoma, which accounts for approximately 80% of all carcinomas of the uterine cervix. For the most part, the decline in the annual incidence of invasive cervical carcinoma has been seen primarily among patients with this subtype.

Adenocarcinoma In the past, adenocarcinoma was relatively uncommon as a primary histology of cervical cancer. As a result of the decrease in the overall incidence of invasive squamous cell cancer and, probably, an increase in the baseline incidence of adenocarcinoma of the uterine cervix, this histology now accounts for approximately 20% of all cervical cancers.

There is controversy over whether patients with adenocarcinoma of the cervix have a worse prognosis than those with the more common squamous cell histology. The poorer prognosis associated with adenocarcinoma may be due to the relatively higher frequency of late stage at the time of diagnosis among patients with this histologic type. In several series in which patients were stratified by stage and tumor size, the outcome of cervical adenocarcinoma appeared to be similar to that of squamous lesions of the cervix.

Among the various subtypes of adenocarcinoma, certain types are particularly aggressive and are associated with a poor prognosis. Among them are the small cell or neuroendocrine tumors, which have a poor prognosis even when diagnosed at an early stage.

TABLE 1: AJCC and FIGO staging for carcinoma of the uterine cervix

AJCC	FIGO	
Primary tumor (T)		
TX		Primary tumor cannot be assessed
T0		No evidence of primary tumor
Tis		Carcinoma in situ
T1	I	Cervical carcinoma confined to the uterus (extension to the corpus should be disregarded)
T1a	1A	Preclinical invasive carcinoma, diagnosed by microscopy only
T1a1	IA1	Minimal microscopic stromal invasion (≤ 3 mm stromal invasion (in depth), ≤ 7 mm in horizontal spread)
T1a2	IA2	Tumor with an invasive component more than 3 mm and not more than 5 mm and 7 mm or less in horizontal spread
T1b	IB	Clinical lesions confined to the cervix or preclinical lesions greater than stage IA
	IB1	Clinical lesions no greater than 4 cm
	IB2	Clinical lesions greater than 4 cm
T2	II	Cervical carcinoma invades beyond the uterus but not to the pelvic wall or to the lower third of the vagina
T2a	IIA	Tumor without parametrial invasion
	IIA1	Tumor less than 4 cm with involvement of less than the upper two-thirds of the vagina
	IIA2	Tumor greater than 4 cm with involvement of less than the upper two-thirds of the vagina
T2b	IIB	Tumor with parametrial invasion
T3	III	Cervical carcinoma extends to the pelvic wall and/or involves the lower third of the vagina and/or causes hydronephrosis or nonfunctioning of the kidneys
T3a	IIIA	Tumor involves the lower third of the vagina, with no extension to the pelvic wall
T3b	IIIB	Tumor extends to the pelvic wall and/or causes hydronephrosis or nonfunctioning of the kidneys
T4a	IVA	Tumor invades the mucosa of the bladder or rectum and/or extends beyond the true pelvis[a]
Regional lymph nodes[b] (N)		
NX		Regional lymph nodes cannot be assessed
N0		No regional lymph node metastasis
N1		Regional lymph node metastasis
Distant metastasis (M)		
MX		Presence of distant metastasis cannot be assessed
M0		No distant metastasis
M1	IVB	Distant metastasis

AJCC = American Joint Committee on Cancer; FIGO = International Federation of Gynecology and Obstetrics

[a] Note: The presence of bullous edema is not sufficient evidence to classify a tumor as T4.

[b] Regional lymph nodes include paracervical, parametrial, hypogastric (obturator), common, internal and external iliac, presacral, and sacral.

Modified from Edge SB, Byrd DR, Compton CC, et al (eds): AJCC Cancer Staging Manual 7th ed. New York, Springer, 2010; Pecorelli S, Zigliani L, Odicino F: Int J Gynaecol Obstet 105:107–108, 2009.

Rare tumor types More rare lesions of the cervix include lymphoma, sarcoma, and melanoma. These histologic subtypes account for < 1% of all cervical cancers.

STAGING AND PROGNOSIS

Clinical staging: Suspected early disease

When a diagnosis of invasive cervical cancer has been established histologically, an evaluation of all pelvic organs should be performed to determine whether the tumor is confined to the cervix or has extended to the adjacent vagina, parametrium, endometrial cavity, bladder, ureters, or rectum. According to the FIGO guidelines for clinical staging (Table 1), diagnostic studies may include intravenous urography (IVU), cystoscopic examination of the bladder and urethra, a proctosigmoidoscopic study, a barium enema (BE), and in the case of early-stage disease, a colposcopic study of the vagina and the vaginal fornices. Colposcopic findings may be used for assigning a stage to the tumor (for instance, FIGO stage IIA), but the results must be confirmed by biopsy.

A pelvic examination must be performed as part of the staging process, and the procedure is best done with the patient completely relaxed by general anesthesia. In up to 20% of patients, the initial clinical classification of the disease has proved to be incorrect at the time of pelvic examination. Such an examination can reveal a more advanced stage of the disease than was originally found; additional biopsies (if indicated) or fractional curettage can be performed as well as colposcopy, cystoscopy, and proctosigmoidoscopy.

Clinical staging: Suspected advanced disease

When studies detect ureteral obstruction, a tumor is classified as a stage IIIB lesion, regardless of the size of the primary lesion. Ureteral obstruction, either hydronephrosis or nonfunction of the kidneys, is well established as an indicator of poor prognosis, as recognized in the FIGO classification.

In women with bulky or advanced-stage tumors, the bladder mucosa also should be inspected cystoscopically for possible bullous edema, which indicates lymphatic obstruction within the bladder wall. Evidence of tumor in the bladder must be confirmed by biopsy before the lesion can be classified as stage IVA. Rectal mucosal lesions also require a biopsy via proctosigmoidoscopy, because they can be related to an inflammatory process rather than to the cervical tumor.

Surgical experience from pelvic lymphadenectomy has confirmed an error rate of 15% to 25% in the clinical staging of patients with stage IB or II lesions. In 10% to 30% of cases with stage II/III tumors, in addition to positive findings of occult pelvic lymph nodes, other metastases may be found in the para-aortic nodes. Unfortunately, pelvic examinations and clinical staging as defined by FIGO cannot detect such metastases.

Consequently, there is a growing body of literature showing the superiority of cross-sectional imaging (CT and MRI) over clinical staging in delineating the extent of disease in patients with cervical cancer. As stated previously, official FIGO guidelines do not incorporate the use of either CT or MRI findings into the staging of cervical

> In a recent study, 129 patients with cervical cancer at stages IB to IV who had pretreatment MRI were randomized to an FDG-PET scan (n = 66) or to no additional study (n = 63). Seven patients (11%) were found to have extrapelvic metastasis on PET scans (six para-aortic nodes and one omental). The 4-year overall survival was 79% and 85%, respectively (P = .65), and the disease-free survival was 75% and 77%, respectively (P = .64; *Tsai C-S et al: Int J Radiat Oncol Biol Phys 76:477–484, 2010*).

cancer. However, as knowledge of prognostic factors and the value of cross-sectional imaging has accumulated, its use in treatment planning has increased without changing the official FIGO clinical staging guidelines. Similarly, although the benefits of laparoscopic extraperitoneal surgical staging have also been reported in this setting, this approach has not been incorporated into the FIGO staging system.

The value of CT scanning in the pretreatment evaluation of patients with cervical cancer is in the assessment of advanced disease (stage IIB and greater) and in the detection and biopsy of suspected lymph node metastasis. The treatment plan for patients with locally advanced disease must be modified if upper abdominal tumor masses and/or distant metastasis is discovered. The soft-tissue contrast resolution of CT scanning does not allow for consistent tumor visualization at the primary cervical site, and, therefore, neither tumor size nor early parametrial invasion can be evaluated reliably. However, T2-weighted MRI allows consistent tumor visualization and has been reported to be over 90% accurate in determining tumor size to within 5 mm of measurements of surgical specimens. Nevertheless, a study by the ACRIN in 208 patients with invasive cervical cancer evaluated with CT scans or MRI before radical hysterectomy showed that MRI was superior to CT and clinical exam in evaluating uterine body involvement and in measuring tumor size, but neither method was accurate in evaluating the cervical stromal depth of tumor invasion.

Recent reports show the value of positron emission tomography (PET) scanning in the pretreatment evaluation, treatment planning, and post-therapy assessment of response in patients with higher-risk invasive carcinoma of the cervix. In a series of 120 newly diagnosed cervical cancer patients with FIGO stage > IB, PET/CT scanning demonstrated a 94% positive predictive value (PPV) and 100% negative predictive value (NPV) in detecting positive para-aortic lymph nodes. There was 100% sensitivity and 99% specificity. When scanning for the presence of distant metastasis, PET/CT scanning had a 63% PPV and 100% NPV, with 100% sensitivity and 94% specificity. In a prospective study of 103 patients who were successfully treated initially with concurrent chemotherapy and radiation therapy, a surveillance FDG-PET (fluorodeoxyglucose-PET) detected asymptomatic recurrent disease earlier, which may be potentially amenable to salvage therapy.

Noteworthy, in 60 patients with stages IA2–IIA cervical cancer up to 4 cm with MRI-negative nodes, preoperative FDG-PET scanning detected 1 para-aortic node metastasis, but only 1 of 10 pelvic node metastases, which led to the conclusion that PET scanning is of little value in evaluating patients with stages IA2–IIA cervical cancer up to 4 cm. A second study showed 3 of 38 patients with no para-aortic uptake on FDG-PET/CT imaging had histologically proven para-aortic node involvement.

Surgical staging

Clinical staging of cervical carcinoma, although widely utilized, is not without controversy. When compared with surgical staging performed by large cooperative groups, clinical staging is frequently inaccurate in predicting locoregional tumor spread. For many cooperative groups, including the GOG, surgical staging may be required for patients who are entering prospective, randomized clinical protocols.

The most common method used to stage patients with advanced disease is extraperitoneal sampling of the pelvic and para-aortic lymph nodes. This approach minimizes the risk of subsequent radiation injury to the small bowel due to surgical adhesions and, in patients with advanced disease, allows for individualized treatment planning. Another approach is sentinel lymph node detection in the pelvis, which is still an active area of research.

Pros and cons of surgical staging The advantage of surgical staging is that patients with microscopic disease in the para-aortic lymph nodes can be treated with extended-field radiation therapy (EFRT) and, possibly, chemotherapy and potentially benefit in terms of long-term survival. The controversy regarding surgical staging stems from the fact that a small number of patients will actually benefit from the procedure; the majority of patients who undergo it will be found not to have metastatic disease and will receive the same treatment as planned prior to surgical staging; if they are found to have metastatic disease, they will be unlikely to benefit from EFRT. Because of this controversy, the GOG considers surgical staging to be *optional* for patients with advanced-stage cervical cancer.

Workup for advanced disease The standard workup of a patient with advanced cervical carcinoma who is not considered a candidate for radical surgery includes an abdominopelvic CT scan with both IV and GI oral contrast. If there is evidence of para-aortic lymph node metastases, the patient should undergo fine-needle aspiration (FNA) of these enlarged lymph nodes. If FNA confirms that there is para-aortic lymph node metastasis, treatment should be individualized, and EFRT should be considered part of the primary treatment regimen.

If the scalene lymph nodes are negative on clinical examination and the patient is known to have positive metastatic disease to the para-aortic lymph nodes, consideration can be given to performing a scalene lymph node biopsy; the incidence of positive scalene nodes when para-aortic lymph nodes are known to be positive ranges from 0% to 17%. The rationale for biopsying the scalene nodes is that if there is disease outside the radiation therapy field, chemotherapy may be appropriate.

If the result of FNA is negative, or if the abdominopelvic CT scan does not demonstrate enlarged para-aortic lymph nodes, the patient can be considered for surgical staging.

Recent data reported the comparison of accuracy between PET and PET/CT for detecting lymph node metastasis in cervical cancer. In a series of 86 patients with stages IB–IVA cervical cancer, a total of 688 lymph node regions were evaluated. PET/CT was more sensitive than PET for detecting small (< 5 mm) lymph node metastases (ASCO 2007). Recent meta-analyses performed by Choi et al showed that PET or PET/CT had an overall higher diagnostic performance (82% sensitivity and 95% specificity) in detecting metastatic lymph nodes in patients with cervical cancer than CT (50% sensitivity and 92% specificity) and MRI (56% sensitivity and 91% specificity).

Laparoscopic surgery The introduction of minimal-access surgery has allowed surgeons to accurately stage patients via the laparoscope prior to initiation of radiation therapy. Laparoscopic para-aortic lymph node dissection has been shown to be feasible in gynecologic malignancies and has been proposed as a diagnostic tool for determining the presence of lymph node metastasis. More recently, robotic surgery has also been used in surgical staging prior to radiation treatment. However, the safety and efficacy of both laparoscopic and robotic surgical staging are areas of ongoing investigation.

Workup for early-stage disease For patients who have early-stage disease for which surgery is contemplated, only a minimal diagnostic workup is indicated prior to surgery. At most institutions, this would include a two-view chest x-ray. Patients who have stage IA cervical carcinoma (microinvasive carcinoma) do not require preoperative CT scanning prior to hysterectomy. For patients with a small stage IB carcinoma of the cervix, a CT scan of the abdomen and pelvis has a low yield and is unlikely to change the treatment plan.

Prognostic factors

Clinical stage The most important determinant of prognosis remains clinical stage, which is defined by tumor volume and extent of disease spread. The overall 5-year survival rate ranges from 95% to 100% for patients with stage IA cancer and from 75% to 90% for those with stage IB disease. Patients with stage IV disease have a ≤ 5% chance of surviving 5 years after diagnosis.

Patients with early disease For patients with early invasive carcinoma (stage IB), the size of the lesion, percentage of cervical stromal invasion, histology, tumor grade, and lymphovascular space involvement are important local factors that predict prognosis. In general, good prognostic signs are lesions that are ≤ 2 cm in diameter, superficially invasive, and well differentiated with no lymphovascular space involvement. In a study of 1,067 patients treated with surgery, HPV-16 was detected in 63.8% and HPV-18, in 16.5% of samples. With a median follow-up of 77 months, HPV was not found to be a significant prognostic factor.

For patients who have undergone radical hysterectomy for early cervical carcinoma, poor prognostic factors, in addition to the local factors previously mentioned, include positive vaginal or parametrial margins and metastasis to the pelvic lymph nodes. For patients with stage IB disease and positive pelvic nodes, the 5-year survival rate drops from approximately 75%–85% to 50%.

Patients with advanced disease For patients with advanced-stage disease (stages IIB–IV), the primary determinants of prognosis are histology and size of the primary lesion. Survival is significantly longer for patients with small stage IIB cervical carcinomas and minimal parametrial involvement than for patients with large bulky tumors and bilateral parametrial involvement. Disease extension beyond the pelvis to the para-aortic nodes is associated with a significant decrease in overall survival rate. With regard to histology, a better prognosis is associated with a large-cell nonkeratinizing squamous cell cancer of the cervix, as opposed to a poorly differentiated adenocarcinoma. In patients with stage IIIB cervical cancer restricted to the pelvis, it was shown that the presence of hydronephrosis at presentation is a significant prognostic factor associated with a poor performance status and a worse survival.

Other prognostic factors Other factors that may predict outcome include the patient's general medical and nutritional status. Patients who are anemic may respond poorly to radiation therapy, as compared with those with normal hemoglobin levels. Patients with significant alterations in their immune system may not respond as well; this result is becoming increasingly apparent with regard to patients who are HIV-seropositive.

A retrospective review of 605 patients from seven institutions in Canada treated with irradiation for cervical cancer described average weekly nadir hemoglobin levels as significant prognostic factors for survival, second only in importance to tumor stage. Interestingly, Winter et al reported that hemoglobin levels during treatment were independent predictors of treatment outcome through a retrospective study of 494 patients from two consecutive prospective GOG trials. The pretreatment level was not a significant predictor of outcome in the multivariate regression model. Hemoglobin levels in the last part of treatment were the most predictive of disease recurrence and survival. However, erythropoietin should not be given outside a clinical trial, as thrombosis is a significant complication and cause/effect has not been proven.

PET scanning is being used to determine response and outcome after therapy. In 152 patients with cervical cancer treated with irradiation alone or in combination with chemotherapy, Grigsby et al reported cause-specific survival of 80% in 114 patients without post-therapy PET abnormalities, 32% in 20 patients with persistent abnormal scans, and no survivors in 18 patients who developed new sites of abnormal uptake.

TREATMENT

SURGICAL TREATMENT OF EARLY-STAGE DISEASE

The standard management of patients with early cervical carcinoma is surgical removal of the cervix. The extent of resection of surrounding tissue depends on the size of the lesion and the depth of tumor invasion.

Stage IA1 disease

Simple hysterectomy Patients who have a microinvasive squamous carcinoma of the cervix with ≤ 3 mm of tumor invasion, ≤ 7 mm of lateral extent, and no lymphovascular space involvement (stage IA1) can be treated with a simple hysterectomy. Vaginal, abdominal, and laparoscopic hysterectomies are equally effective.

Cone biopsy Although simple hysterectomy is considered the standard therapy for patients with microinvasive cervical carcinoma, preservation of future fertility is a strong consideration in some patients. A cone biopsy entails removal of the cervical transformation zone. Provided that the biopsy margins are free of dysplasia and microinvasive carcinoma, cone biopsy is probably a safe treatment for such patients who meet the criteria of having superficial invasion < 3 mm, minimal lateral extension, and no lymphovascular space involvement.

Since there is a small risk of recurrence among this population of patients treated by cone biopsy alone, they should be followed closely. Follow-up includes a Pap smear and pelvic examinations every 3 months for 2 years, every 6 months for 4 years, and then yearly thereafter. An abnormal Pap smear is an indication for a repeat colposcopy. If such patients are successful in achieving pregnancy and have no evidence of recurrent squamous cell carcinoma, there is no need to proceed with hysterectomy at the completion of planned childbearing.

Studies addressing fertility-sparing surgeries such as radical abdominal trachelectomy vs radical vaginal trachelectomy are ongoing. A prospective study included 43 women with stage IB1 cervical cancer; the vaginal approach was performed on 28 patients and the abdominal approach was performed on 15 patients. There was no statistical difference between the two approaches in average blood loss or the number of lymph nodes removed. There was the possibility that the abdominal approach would provide a wider margin of resection of the parametria, but overall, both the radical abdominal and vaginal approaches are potential fertility-sparing options for women with early-stage cervical cancer *(Einstein MH et al: Gynecol Oncol 112:73–77, 2009)*. Another study has compared outcomes associated with radical trachelectomy as a fertility-sparing option vs radical hysterectomy for stage IB1 cervical cancer. Radical trachelectomy was performed in 40 women, and radical hysterectomy was performed in 110 patients. After 5 years, the recurrence-free survival was 96% for those patients undergoing radical trachelectomy and 86% for those undergoing radical hysterectomy. Therefore, there are potential radical surgeries that can be utilized as fertility-sparing options for women with early-stage cervical cancer *(Diaz JP et al: Gynecol Oncol 111:255–260, 2008)*.

Stages IA2, IB1, and nonbulky IIA disease

Radical hysterectomy A standard treatment for patients with small cervical carcinomas (≤ 4 cm) confined to the uterine cervix or with minimal involvement of the vagina (stage IIA) is radical hysterectomy (removal of the uterus, cervix, and parametrial tissue), pelvic lymphadenectomy, and para-aortic lymph node sampling. The overall success of this treatment is similar to that of radiation therapy, and for patients with early lesions, radical hysterectomy may provide an improved quality of life. The benefits of surgical excision include rapid treatment, less time away from normal activities, and preservation of normal ovarian and vaginal function.

A randomized trial for patients with early-stage cervical cancer reported no difference in survival between radical hysterectomy and definitive radiation therapy. Because a significant percentage of patients following radical hysterectomy required postoperative pelvic radiotherapy, the morbidity was increased in the surgery arm. Therefore, patients selected for radical hysterectomy should have small-volume disease so adjuvant pelvic radiation therapy is unnecessary.

Currently, there are no specific contraindications to radical hysterectomy. Several studies have demonstrated that patients ≥ 65 years old tolerate this procedure well, and age alone should not be considered a contraindication. Obesity also is not a contraindication to radical hysterectomy.

Alternatives to radical hysterectomy Reports have described laparoscopically assisted radical vaginal hysterectomy, laparoscopic abdominal radical hysterectomy, laparoscopy-assisted radical vaginal hysterectomy, and robotic-assisted surgery as less invasive alternatives to traditional radical hysterectomy. Robotic-assisted radical hysterectomy has become an area of particular interest. Multiple series have demonstrated the feasibility of performing surgeries on gynecologic malignancies using robotics. The largest case-control series to date by Boggess et al comparing robotic vs open type III radical hysterectomy reported statistically significant differences in operative time, blood loss, and node retrieval in favor of the robotic approach. However, more studies need to be conducted to evaluate intraoperative and postoperative complications with robotic-assisted surgery and to assess data regarding recurrence rates and overall survival in comparison to those with the traditional open and laparoscopic approaches. The use of fertility-preserving surgery by means of pelvic lymphadenectomy combined with radical vaginal trachelectomy (removal of the uterine cervix) has also been evaluated in selected women with early cervical cancer. Successful pregnancies after this procedure have been reported. However, further data are needed to assess the safety and efficacy of fertility-preserving surgery. There is a lack of long-term follow-up data and survival rates between conservative and radical treatments. These techniques should be performed by fully trained surgeons. The role of laparoscopic sentinel lymph node dissection is an area of active investigation. Several studies addressing the utility of intraoperative lymphatic mapping with the use of blue dye and technetium are being conducted in patients with early-stage cervical cancer undergoing radical hysterectomy. Although studies are ongoing, the role of sentinel node detection appears promising.

Complications Due to improved surgical techniques, as well as the use of prophylactic antibiotics and prophylaxis against deep vein thrombosis, the morbidity and mortality associated with radical hysterectomy have declined significantly over the past several decades. The currently accepted complication rate for radical hysterectomy includes approximately a 0.5% to 1.0% incidence of urinary tract injury, a 0.5% to 1.0% incidence of deep vein thrombosis, and an overall mortality of < 1.0%.

The increased awareness of the risks associated with blood transfusion is reflected in the fact that, in many cases, no transfusions are administered. The need for heterologous blood transfusion also can be decreased by encouraging autologous blood donation prior to radical hysterectomy or by using intraoperative hemodilution.

The average hospital stay for patients undergoing radical hysterectomy is between 4 and 7 days. Follow-up should include a vaginal Pap smear with pelvic examination every 3 months for 2 years, twice a year for 3 years, and yearly thereafter.

Stages IB2 and bulky IIA disease

Numerous studies have demonstrated that patients with early-stage "bulky" lesions (> 4 cm) have a worse prognosis than those with nonbulky tumors. Therefore, patients who have undergone radical hysterectomy and pelvic lymphadenectomy for early-stage bulky cervical cancer have traditionally received postoperative adjuvant pelvic radiation therapy. However, a randomized trial from Italy demonstrated that radical hysterectomy plus radiotherapy does not improve overall or disease-free survival in patients with early-stage bulky tumors, as compared with radiation therapy alone, but does significantly increase morbidity. In 92 selected patients with bulky stages IB2, IIA, and IIB disease, without pelvic or para-aortic nodes, preoperative external-beam radiation therapy (EBRT; 40 Gy in 4.5 weeks), low-dose-rate (LDR) brachytherapy (20 Gy), and cisplatin/5-FU (fluorouracil) were administered, followed by class II modified radical hysterectomy. Pathologic residual tumor was observed in 43 patients (47%), and 5-year disease-free survival was 72%. Two severe ureteral complications were noted.

Furthermore, GOG 123 demonstrated the benefit of the addition of cisplatin chemotherapy to pelvic radiation therapy followed by extrafascial hysterectomy in this group of patients (Figure 1). Therefore, many experts believe that patients with stages IB2 and bulky IIA cervical cancer should be treated initially with chemoradiation therapy instead of radical hysterectomy. Others argue that treatment decisions should not be based on tumor size alone, because some studies have demonstrated that significant independent predictors of disease-free survival are lymphovascular space involvement and outer two-thirds depth of invasion. Overall, there are still conflicting data in terms of the efficacy of utilizing chemoradiation therapy alone vs chemoradiation therapy followed by surgery for bulky stage 1B2 cervical disease. The role of curative surgery diminishes once cervical cancer has spread beyond the confines of the cervix and vaginal fornices.

Intracavitary irradiation for central pelvic disease and EBRT for lateral parametrial and pelvic nodal disease are typically combined to encompass the known patterns

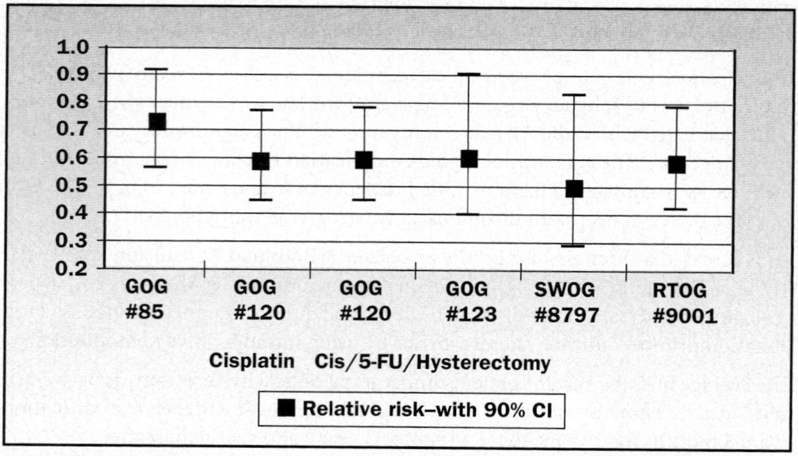

FIGURE 1: Relative risk estimate of survival from five phase III randomized, controlled clinical trials of chemoradiation therapy in women with cervical cancer. A relative risk of 1 indicates no difference in outcome between the treatment arms. A relative risk of < 1 indicates a benefit for the experimental treatment. A relative risk of 0.6, for example, indicates that the treatment has reduced the risk of death by 40%. The relative risks of survival for all five trials, with 90% confidence intervals (CIs) shown, range from 0.70 to 0.50, indicating that the concurrent chemoradiation therapy decreased the risk of death by 30% to 50% (Rose PG, Bundy BN: J Clin Oncol 20:891–893, 2002).

of disease spread with an appropriate radiation dose while sparing the bladder and rectum from receiving full doses. The addition of intracavitary irradiation to EBRT is associated with improved pelvic tumor control and survival over external irradiation alone, as the combination can achieve high central doses of radiation. In some patients, when intracavitary brachytherapy cannot be performed, it is possible to deliver additional irradiation to the central tumor after whole-pelvis radiation therapy. In 44 patients with various clinical stages treated in this fashion, recurrent tumor was noted in 48%. Central recurrence was observed in 16 of 21 patients with recurrent disease. Late grade 3 sequelae were seen in 2% of the patients.

RADIATION THERAPY

Intracavitary brachytherapy Radioactive isotopes, such as cesium-137, can be introduced directly into the uterine cavity and vaginal fornices with special applicators. The most commonly used applicator is the Fletcher-Suit intrauterine tandem and vaginal ovoids.

Calculating dose rates With the advent of computerized dosimetry, the dose rate to a number of points from a particular source arrangement can be calculated. Adjustments in the strength or positioning of the sources can then be made to yield a selected dose rate to one or more points.

Quantification of acceptable implant geometry has been described by Katz and Eifel after review of 808 implants performed in 396 patients with cervical cancer treated with irradiation at M. D. Anderson Cancer Center. These guidelines set the standard for high-quality tandem and ovoid insertions.

Points of interest usually include the maximal rectal and bladder dose, as well as the dose to three standard pelvic points: A, B, and P (see Figure 2). Point A is located 2 cm cephalad from the cervical os and 2 cm lateral to the uterine canal. Anatomically, it represents the medial parametrium/lateral cervix, the approximate point at which the ureter and uterine artery cross. Point B is 5 cm lateral to the center of the pelvis at the same level as point A and approximates the region of the obturator nodes or lateral parametrium. Point P is located along the bony pelvic sidewall at its most lateral point and represents the minimal dose to the external iliac lymph nodes. Publications have advocated the use of imaging (CT or MRI) to delineate tumor/target volumes and to specify more precisely the doses of brachytherapy administered to patients with carcinoma of the cervix (Potter et al).

LDR vs HDR brachytherapy Standard dose rates at point A are typically 50 to 70 cGy/hour; this level is considered LDR brachytherapy. The applicator is placed into the uterus while the patient is under anesthesia in the operating room, and the patient must stay in the hospital for 2 to 3 days during the procedure. One or two implants are usually placed. Despite the fact that two insertions may allow time for regression of disease between placements, there are no data indicating that two insertions improve pelvic tumor control or survival rates over one insertion.

Whereas LDR brachytherapy has been used successfully for decades in the treatment of carcinoma of the cervix, the use of high-dose-rate (HDR) brachytherapy has been increasing in the United States over the past decade. Dose rates are typically 200 to 300 cGy/minute, with short treatment times allowing for stable position of the applicator.

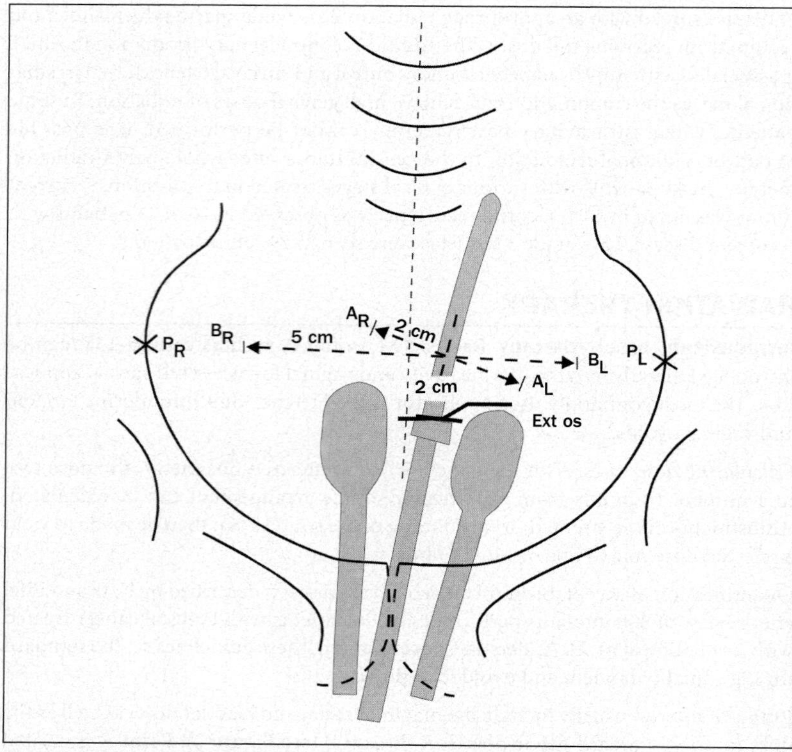

FIGURE 2: GOG definitions of points A, B, and P.

The major benefit of HDR brachytherapy is that the procedure can be performed on an outpatient basis with less radiation exposure to personnel. The major disadvantage is biologic: large single fractions of radiation (5 to 10 Gy) are used with 3 to 10 insertions per patient, which may increase the rate of late complications.

Several series have cited comparable disease control and complication rates with HDR and LDR brachytherapy. A total of 237 patients with previously untreated invasive cervical cancer were enrolled in one randomized study to compare the clinical outcome between HDR and LDR intracavitary brachytherapy. The median follow-up for LDR and HDR groups was 40.2 and 37.2 months, respectively. The 3-year overall and relapse-free survival rates for all patients were 69.6% and 70.0%, respectively. There was no significant difference in the following clinical parameters between LDR and HDR groups: the 3-year overall survival rate was 70.9% and 68.4% (P = .75), the 3-year pelvic control rate was 89.1% and 86.4% (P = .51), and the 3-year relapse-free survival rate in both groups was 69.9% (P = .35). Considering patient convenience, the small number of medical personnel needed, and the decreased radiation exposure to health care workers, HDR intracavitary brachytherapy is an alternative to conventional LDR brachytherapy and is in current GOG and RTOG advanced cervical cancer trials.

Guidelines have been published for HDR brachytherapy for cervical cancer by the ABS (see Suggested Reading).

Pelvic EBRT is used in conjunction with intracavitary radiotherapy for stage IA2 disease and above when the risk of pelvic lymph node involvement is significant. The amount of EBRT delivered and the timing of its administration relative to intracavitary radiation are individualized. For example, the presence of a large exophytic cancer that distorts the cervix would initially preclude successful placement of intracavitary brachytherapy. EBRT would be administered first, and after significant regression of disease, it could be followed by intracavitary radiotherapy.

Various techniques have been developed to optimize EBRT, including CT simulation, conformal blocking, and, more recently, intensity-modulated radiation therapy (IMRT). These techniques reduce the volume of normal tissue having full-dose irradiation while not compromising coverage of the target. MRI has been shown to enhance the accuracy of tumor delineation and design of treatment portals, to avoid geographic misses, particularly in the posterior margin of the lateral pelvic fields.

PET scanning (FDG) has been used to more accurately identify the tumor volume in the cervix and optimize the radiation dose administered with intracavitary brachytherapy (to point A), without increasing the dose delivered to the bladder or the rectum.

Several preliminary reports describing highly conformal dose distributions for patients with carcinoma of the cervix in IMRT have been published. Tumor control has been about 80% for various stages, and no patient has developed > grade 2 GI or genitourinary toxicity.

Advanced tumors require relatively more external irradiation due to the inability of central radioisotope sources to effectively irradiate disease in the lateral parametrium. Typically, external pelvic doses of 4,000 to 5,000 cGy are followed by 4,000 to 5,000 cGy to point A with intracavitary LDR brachytherapy, for a total dose of 8,000 to 9,000 cGy to point A. A parametrial boost completes treatment to the lateral pelvis, for a total dose to point B or P of 6,000 cGy from EBRT and brachytherapy, depending on the extent of disease.

With HDR brachytherapy, equivalent doses are prescribed using the linear quadratic equation.

In a prospective cohort study, 452 patients with cervical cancer were treated with curative intent (135 with IMRT and 317 with non-IMRT external irradiation and brachytherapy); 85% of patients received concurrent chemotherapy. All IMRT patients underwent an FDG-PET/CT simulation. The mean follow-up for all patients alive at the time of the last follow-up was 72 months for non-IMRT and 22 months for IMRT patients. For all patients, the post-therapy FDG-PET response correlated with overall recurrence risk (*P* < .0001) and cause-specific survival (*P* < .0001). Post-treatment FDG-PET findings were not significantly different between the groups. At last follow-up, 178 patients (39 IMRT, 139 non-IMRT) had developed a recurrence (28.9% and 43.8%, respectively). The difference in recurrence-free survival between the two groups did not reach statistical significance, although the IMRT group showed better overall and cause-specific survival. Grade 3 complications were seen in 8 (6%) IMRT patients vs 54 (17%) in the non-IMRT group *(Kidd EA et al: Int J Rad Oncol Bio Phys 77:1085–1091, 2010)*.

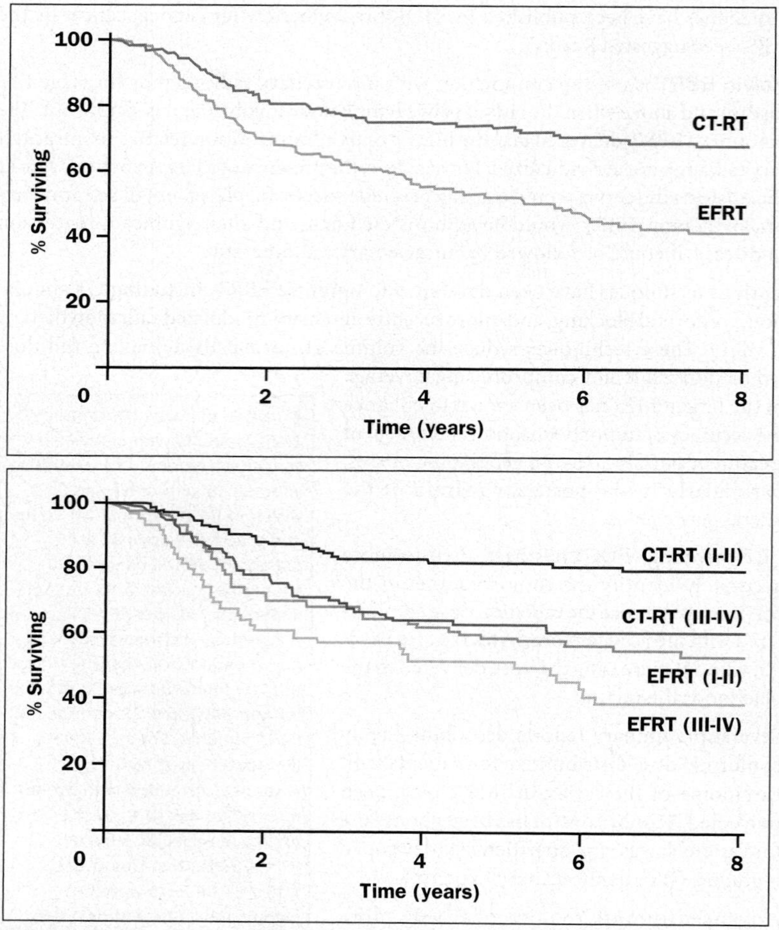

FIGURE 3: Top – Kaplan-Meier estimates of overall survival for patients who received extended-field radiotherapy (EFRT) or concurrent chemotherapy and radiotherapy (CT-RT; $P < .0001$). **Bottom** – Kaplan-Meier estimates of overall survival for patients who received EFRT or CT-RT in subgroups stratified by International Federation of Gynecology and Obstetrics stage ($P < .0001$).

Reprinted with permission from Eifel PJ, Winter K, Morris M, et al: J Clin Oncol 22: 872–880, 2004.

The HDR/LDR dose ratio ranges from .5 to .8 depending on the number of HDR fractions. Deep hyperthermia (administered once weekly) has been combined with pelvic external beam and intracavitary brachytherapy to treat patients with bulky tumors of the cervix.

In 378 patients, overall complete tumor response was 77%; at 5 years, the tumor control rate was 53%, and the disease-free survival was 47%. Late toxicity was observed in 12% of the patients.

Para-aortic EBRT may be used in addition to pelvic EBRT when para-aortic disease is confirmed or suspected. An RTOG trial found that para-aortic EBRT conferred a survival benefit in patients with advanced cervical cancer (stages IB > 4 cm, IIA, and IIB) over pelvic EBRT alone. Although EBRT can successfully sterilize microscopic disease, its value in the treatment of gross para-aortic disease is limited, as the tolerance of surrounding organs (bowel, kidneys, spinal cord) precludes the delivery of sufficiently high doses to the para-aortic region.

In multivariate analysis, treatment factors associated with improved pelvic control for cervical cancer include the use of intracavitary brachytherapy, total point A dose > 8,500 cGy (stage III only), and overall treatment time < 8 weeks.

Definitive radiation therapy

CIS, stage IA disease Carcinoma in situ (CIS) and microinvasive cervical cancer (stage IA) are not associated with lymph node metastases. Therefore, intracavitary LDR brachytherapy alone, delivering approximately 5,500 cGy to point A, can control 100% of CIS and stage IA disease and is an acceptable alternative to surgery for patients who cannot undergo surgery due to their medical condition.

Stage IB disease The most important prognostic factor associated with pelvic tumor control and survival following radiation therapy for stage IB cervical cancer is tumor size. The central tumor pelvic control rate with radiotherapy alone is excellent for tumors < 8 cm (97%), with total pelvic tumor control and survival rates of 93% and 82%, respectively. Therefore, many experts have argued that adjuvant hysterectomy following chemoradiation therapy is unnecessary for cervical cancer < 8 cm. For bulky cervical cancers ≥ 8 cm, pelvic tumor control and survival rates decrease to 57% and 40%, respectively, with irradiation alone, and adjuvant hysterectomy may potentially improve local tumor control and survival rates (Table 2).

Stage III disease Hyperthermia, combined with pelvic irradiation, was introduced into oncology practice several decades ago. A recent meta-analysis showed that 74% of patients treated with this combination had FIGO stage IIIB disease. Outcomes

TABLE 2: Relationship between tumor size and outcome in patients with tumors ≥ 5 cm treated with irradiation alone[a]

Tumor size (cm)	Number of patients	Central pelvic tumor control rate (%)	Total pelvic tumor control rate (%)	DSS (%)
5–5.9	200	93	85	69
6–6.9	99	92	79	69
7–7.9	55	90	81	58
≥ 8	48	69	57	40

[a]Excludes patients who underwent adjuvant hysterectomy DSS = disease-specific survival

were better for patients receiving the combined treatment, with a significantly higher complete response rate (RR = .56; 95% CI = .39–.79; $P < .001$), a significantly reduced local recurrence rate (HR = .48; $P < .001$), and a significantly better overall survival (HR = .67; $P = .05$). No significant difference was observed in treatment-related acute (RR = .99; $P = .99$) or late grade 3 to 4 toxicity (RR = 1.01; $P = .96$) between both treatments. The authors stated that the limited number of patients available for analysis, methodologic flaws, and a significant overrepresentation of patients with FIGO stage IIIB disease prohibited drawing definitive conclusions regarding the impact of adding hyperthermia to standard radiotherapy in cervical cancer. However, the data did suggest that the addition of hyperthermia improves local tumor control and overall survival in patients with locally advanced cervical carcinoma without affecting treatment-related grade 3 to 4 acute or late toxicity.

CHEMORADIATION THERAPY FOR LOCALLY ADVANCED DISEASE

An updated RTOG trial (RTOG 90-01) for advanced cervical cancer (stage IB or IIA with tumor ≥ 5 cm or with biopsy-proven pelvic lymph node involvement and stages IIB–IVA disease) compared pelvic EBRT plus concurrent 5-FU and cisplatin with pelvic and para-aortic EBRT in both arms; these therapies were followed by intracavitary irradiation. The addition of chemotherapy to irradiation improved 5-year survival from 55% to 79% and disease-free survival from 46% to 74% for stage IB/IIA disease by reducing the rates of both local recurrence and distant metastases. For stage III/IVA disease, chemoradiotherapy improved 5-year survival from 45% to 59% and disease-free survival from 37% to 54% (Figures 1 and 3).

GOG 123 randomized patients with stage IB bulky cervical cancer to receive either local treatment alone (external and intracavitary irradiation followed by hysterectomy) or local therapy plus weekly cisplatin. The combination of concurrent weekly cisplatin and irradiation significantly reduced the relapse rate and improved survival by 50%. The 3-year survival rate was significantly improved from 74% to 83% with the use of chemotherapy; this improvement was primarily due to a reduced risk of local recurrence (21% vs 9%).

On the other hand, an Australian gynecologic group randomized study with 76 patients and a Canadian randomized study with 127 patients with stages IB–IIB carcinoma of the cervix treated with chemotherapy and irradiation or irradiation alone showed no significant difference in tumor control or survival. A possible explanation for the discrepancy in the results between the five US trials and the NCIC study has been analyzed by Lehman and Thomas. A review of 4,069 patients with invasive carcinoma of the cervix treated in Ontario, Canada, between 1992 and 2001 documented a significant increase in 3-year survival in patients treated with concurrent chemotherapy-radiotherapy (CT-RT; 75.9%) compared with those treated with irradiation alone (71.1%).

Current treatment recommendations Concurrent CT-RT (usually cisplatin-based) with or without adjuvant hysterectomy is standard treatment for bulky stage IB2 cervical cancer. An alternative approach is radical hysterectomy followed by tailored postoperative CT-RT.

The use of adjuvant hysterectomy is controversial for stage IB2 cervical cancer, since dose-intense external pelvic and intracavitary irradiation plus chemotherapy may obviate the need for adjuvant surgery. The GOG trial suggests that adjuvant hysterectomy reduces the recurrence rate but does not affect survival.

The use of weekly cisplatin for 6 cycles or 5-FU and cisplatin every 3 weeks for 2 cycles concurrently with radiotherapy is the standard treatment approach for bulky stage IB2 cervical cancer.

Stages IIA–IVA disease The most important prognostic factor associated with pelvic tumor control and survival is the bulk of pelvic disease within each stage. For stage IIB, bulky disease is variously defined as bilateral or lateral parametrial infiltration or central bulky disease > 4 cm. For stage IIIB, bulky disease is defined as bilateral sidewall involvement, lower-third vaginal involvement, or hydronephrosis. In the previous GOG experience, in which para-aortic lymph node staging had been mandated, multivariate analysis testing revealed para-aortic lymph node involvement to be the most powerful negative prognostic factor, followed by pelvic lymph node involvement, larger tumor diameter, young age, advanced stage, and lower performance status for patients with negative para-aortic lymph nodes. Five-year survival rates for radiotherapy alone vary from 80% for stage I, 60% for stage II, and 45% for stage III disease, with corresponding pelvic tumor control rates of 90%, 80%, and 50%, respectively.

CT-RT A GOG phase III trial (GOG 120) compared standard pelvic EBRT/intracavitary brachytherapy plus hydroxyurea vs weekly cisplatin vs hydroxyurea, 5-FU, and cisplatin. Both the weekly cisplatin and the 5-FU–cisplatin–hydroxyurea arms produced significantly improved survival and relapse rates compared with hydroxyurea alone. Two-year progression-free survival rates were significantly improved from 47% to 67% and 64% with weekly cisplatin-irradiation and 5-FU–cisplatin–hydroxyurea–irradiation compared with hydroxyurea and radiotherapy (Figure 1). The improved outcome was due to the reduced rates of pelvic failure and lung metastases. Because of an improved therapeutic ratio, weekly cisplatin is the favored regimen. Updated results of this trial confirm the original observations.

GOG 165 compared standard radiation therapy plus concurrent weekly cisplatin vs concurrent protracted venous infusion of 5-FU (225 mg/m^2/day over 5 weeks) as radiation sensitizers. In a randomized trial, 294 patients with advanced cervical cancer were enrolled to compare cisplatin and cisplatin + topotecan (Hycamtin). Patients receiving topotecan had statistically superior outcomes to those receiving cisplatin alone, with median overall survival of 9.4 and 6.5 months ($P = .017$), median progression-free survival of 4.6 and 2.9 months ($P = .014$), and response rates of 27% and 13%, respectively. This study confirms the efficacy of pelvic radiotherapy with weekly cisplatin. The study was closed prematurely when a planned interim analysis indicated that the 5-FU arm had a 35% higher rate of treatment failure. An editorial published with the article highlighted the future difficulties with randomized trials for this population.

A randomized study of patients with stages IIIB–IVA cervical cancer was presented at ASCO 2009. The study had two arms: (1) a standard regimen of weekly cisplatin with pelvic radiation therapy vs (2) concurrent radiation therapy and weekly cisplatin (40 mg/m^2) plus weekly gemcitabine (Gemzar, 125 mg/m^2), followed by 2 additional cycles of higher-dose cisplatin and gemcitabine after radiation therapy was completed. This study enrolled more than 500 patients worldwide, most notably in developing countries. There was a significant survival advantage with the addition of gemcitabine and post-radiation therapy chemotherapy (3-year progression-free survival rate, 65% vs 74%; overall survival HR = .68). Neutropenia and anemia rates were higher in the gemcitabine group. This study did not clarify whether the addition of gemcitabine or the post-radiation chemotherapy, or both, was the reason for the survival improvements.

Current treatment recommendations In view of the multiple randomized trials documenting a survival benefit with concurrent CT-RT, the use of concurrent weekly cisplatin or cisplatin-5-FU every 3 weeks with irradiation is standard therapy for stages IB2–IVA cervical cancer (Figure 1). Further prospective studies should be explored to determine the role of gemcitabine and post-radiation therapy chemotherapy.

Five of six large randomized clinical trials demonstrated a significant survival benefit for patients treated with concurrent CT-RT, using a cisplatin-based regimen, with a 28% to 50% relative reduction in the risk of death. In addition, the results of a meta-analysis of 19 randomized clinical trials of concurrent CT-RT involving 4,580 patients showed that concurrent CT-RT significantly improved overall survival (HR = 0.71; $P < .001$), as well as progression-free survival (HR = .61; $P < .0001$). In line with these results, concurrent CT-RT is currently recommended as standard therapy (Table 3).

A meta-analysis from all randomized trials reaffirms the benefits of concurrent CT-RT. On the basis of 13 trials that compared CT-RT vs the same radiation therapy, there was a 6% improvement in 5-year survival with CT-RT (HR = .81; $P < .001$). A larger survival benefit was seen for the two trials in which CT was administered after CT-RT. There was a significant survival benefit for both the group of trials that used platinum-based (HR = .83; $P < .017$) and non–platinum-based (HR = .77; $P < .009$) CT-RT, but no evidence of a difference in the size of the benefit by radiation therapy or chemotherapy dose or scheduling was seen. CT-RT also reduced local and distant recurrence and disease progression and improved disease-free survival. There was a suggestion of a difference in the size of the survival benefit with tumor stage, but not across other patient subgroups. Acute hematologic and GI toxicities were increased with CT-RT, but data were too sparse for an analysis of late toxicity. This meta-analysis clearly demonstrates the benefit of concurrent CT-RT and suggests further exploration should continue with additional adjuvant chemotherapy and non–platinum-based CT-RT.

Based on the promising responses and acceptable toxicity reported in the phase I/II study, a phase III GOG trial for advanced cervical cancer (stages IB2–IVA) is randomizing patients to undergo pelvic radiotherapy plus cisplatin weekly or pelvic radiotherapy, cisplatin, and tirapazamine (a hypoxic cell sensitizer).

For patients without para-aortic lymph node metastases, pelvic external irradiation (4,000 to 5,000 cGy) should be used, followed by intracavitary LDR brachytherapy (4,000 to 5,000 cGy) to point A, for a total dose of 8,000 to 9,000 cGy to point A. Noteworthy, in a study at the Norwegian Radium Hospital, in 147 patients, the estimates of physician-assessed intestinal, bladder, and vaginal grade 3/4 morbidity

TABLE 3: Large randomized studies of concurrent chemoradiotherapy in cervical cancer

Author	Stage	Design	RT	CT (mg/m², except for HU)	No. of patients	Survival (%) CT/RT vs RT (follow-up)	*P value*
Whitney, GOG 85, 1999	IIB-IVAPAN(-) Washing cytology (-)	WP+PF × 3 vs WP+HU+PAN	IIB: 40 Gy+Ra III, IVA: WP, 51 Gy+Ra III, IV: 61 Gy	P:50/day 1 F:1,000/days 2-5, every 4 weeks HU:80 mg/kg/twice a week	388	55 vs 43 (8.7 years)	.018
Rose, GOG 120, 1999	IIIB-IVA PAN(-)	WP+P weekly vs WP+PF+HU vs WP+HU	IIB: 40 Gy+Ra; III, IVA: WP, 51 Gy +Ra; III, IV: 61 Gy	P:40/week for 4 weeks vs P:50/day 1+F:1,000/days 1-4 HU:2,000/0/week, every 4 weeks vs HU:3,000/2/week of 6 weeks	176	66 vs 67 vs 50 (3 years) 8 vs 71 (4 years)	.0040 .002
Keys GOG 123, 1999	IB ≥ 4 cm	WP+P weekly vs WP Adj TAH	WP:45 Gy + Ra	P:40/week for 6 weeks	369	83 vs 74 (3 years)	.008
Peters SWOG 8797, 2000	IA2-IIA Postsurgical pN1/pT2b/ stump(+)	WP+PF × 4 vs WP + PAN	WP:45 GyWP+PAN	P:70/day 1 + F: 1,000/days 1-4, every 3 weeks	268	81 vs 71 (4 years)	.007
Pearcey NCIC 2002	IB-IVA > 5 cm or pelvic LN (+)	WP+P weekly	WP: 45 Gy + Ra vs WP	P:40 mg/m²	259	62 vs 58 (5 years)	.42
Eifel RTOG 90-01, 2004	IB-IVA > 5 cm PAN(-)	WP+PF × 3 vs WP+PAN	WP: 45 Gy PAN:45 Gy	P:75/day 1 F:1,000/days 2-5, every 3 weeks	403	67 vs 41 (8 years)	.0001

Adj = adjuvant; CT = chemotherapy; F = fluorouracil; HU = hydroxyurea; LN = lymph node; PAN = para-aortic lymph node; P = Platinol (cisplatin); Ra = radium therapy; RT = radiotherapy; TAH = total abdominal hysterectomy; WP = whole pelvis

Adapted with permission from Kuzuya K: Int J Clin Oncol 9:458–470, 2005.

was 15%, 13%, and 23%, respectively, whereas the prevalence of patient-reported severities of the same symptoms was 45%, 23%, and 58%, respectively. The study underscores the importance of incorporating patient assessment in the analysis of treatment morbidity.

Adjuvant radiotherapy following radical hysterectomy

Node-negative disease Local failure rates approach 20% following radical hysterectomy and pelvic lymphadenectomy when pelvic lymph nodes are not involved but the primary tumor has high-risk characteristics (primary tumor > 4 cm, outer-third cervical stromal invasion, and capillary-lymphatic space invasion). A GOG trial randomized these intermediate-risk patients with node-negative disease to receive pelvic EBRT (5,100 cGy/30 fractions) or no further therapy following radical hysterectomy-pelvic lymphadenectomy. Postoperative irradiation produced a significant 44% reduction in recurrence; the recurrence-free rate at 2 years was 88% with irradiation vs 79% without it. Survival analysis awaits further follow-up.

Node-positive disease For patients with positive pelvic lymph nodes following radical hysterectomy-pelvic lymphadenectomy, pelvic radiotherapy reduces the pelvic failure rate from approximately 50% to 25% but does not affect survival, since distant metastases are still seen in 30% of patients. GOG/SWOG 8797 randomized these high-risk patients with node-positive disease (or patients with positive surgical margins) to undergo pelvic EBRT (4,930 cGy/29 fractions) vs pelvic EBRT plus concurrent 5-FU and cisplatin for 4 cycles following radical hysterectomy-pelvic lymphadenectomy. A significant improvement in disease progression-free and overall survival was seen for concurrent 5-FU–cisplatin and radiation therapy compared with radiation therapy alone (4-year survival, 81% vs 71%).

Current treatment recommendations At present, the use of adjuvant pelvic radiotherapy should be considered for patients with negative nodes who are at risk for pelvic failure and remains the standard postoperative treatment for patients with positive lymph nodes. Treatment consists of external pelvic irradiation (45 to 50 Gy), with specific sites boosted with further external-beam or intracavitary irradiation as needed.

Since the combination of radical surgery and irradiation has greater morbidity than either modality alone, complete preoperative assessment is crucial to minimize the need for both.

Since concurrent CT-RT following radical hysterectomy provides a significant benefit in node-positive high-risk cervical cancer, it should be part of the postoperative treatment plan. Postoperative CT-RT following radical hysterectomy should be strongly considered for patients with negative nodes but positive margins or parametria, ≥ middle-third stromal invasion, and lymphovascular space invasion for tumors ≥ 5 cm.

SURGICAL MANAGEMENT OF RECURRENT OR METASTATIC DISEASE

Recurrent advanced disease

Pelvic exenteration For patients whose disease fails to respond to primary radiation therapy or for those with early invasive cervical carcinoma whose disease recurs after surgery or radiation therapy, pelvic exenteration offers the possibility of cure. Patients should be considered for pelvic exenteration only if they have locoregional disease that can be completely removed by this radical surgical procedure. In most cases, patients will require surgical removal of the bladder, uterus, cervix, vagina, and rectum.

Of all patients who are considered candidates for pelvic exenteration, only about half will be found to have resectable disease at the time of exploratory laparotomy. For patients who successfully undergo pelvic exenteration, 5-year survival rates range from 25% to 50%.

When the patient has central recurrence of squamous cell or adenocarcinoma of the cervix, the initial evaluation includes a complete physical examination, as well as a CT, MRI, or PET/CT scan.

Evidence of extrapelvic disease is a contraindication to pelvic exenteration. If no evidence of disease beyond the pelvis is found, the patient can be prepared for pelvic exenteration.

Preparation for exenteration includes complete bowel preparation, a visit with the stomal therapy nurse, and counseling regarding the radical nature of the surgery and the anticipated changes in body image after the operation. In most cases, we counsel the patient that vaginal reconstruction should be performed at the time of pelvic exenteration, both for maintenance of body image and improved healing.

Surgical procedure During surgery, a careful exploration is carried out to confirm that there is no evidence of unresectable disease beyond the pelvis. Explorative laparoscopy prior to pelvic exenteration has been used in this regard to localize the tumor and evaluate the presence of adjacent organ involvement. The pelvic sidewall spaces are opened and resectability is determined. If there is no evidence of adjacent organ involvement, an en bloc resection is usually performed; in some cases, especially when the recurrent tumor involves the lower vagina, a two-team approach can expedite the procedure. The actual exenterative portion of the procedure may take several hours and is usually accompanied by significant blood loss. In cases where surgical margin status may be questionable, the use of intraoperative radiation therapy is considered.

Reconstruction Following the exenterative procedure, the reconstructive portion of the procedure begins. We currently recommend a continent urinary diversion to nearly all patients. Although this step may add approximately 30 to 60 minutes to the surgical procedure, the improvement in quality of life is significant.

In patients who have undergone a supralevator pelvic exenteration, we frequently attempt a stapled reanastomosis of the colon. Unless there is excessive tension on the anastomosis or other problems, a diverting colostomy is not routinely indicated. About one-third of these patients suffer anastomotic breakdown in the postoperative period. At that time, a diverting colostomy can be performed. Unfortunately, Hatch et al found no benefit to the earlier use of colostomy.

Lung metastasis

For the rare patient who presents with a single isolated lung metastasis after treatment of invasive cervical carcinoma, pulmonary resection may offer the possibility of long-term disease-free survival or even cure in selected cases. For patients who have multiple lung metastases or unresectable pelvic disease, surgery offers little or no hope and produces significant morbidity and mortality.

THERAPY FOR RECURRENT OR METASTATIC DISEASE

Local recurrence after radical hysterectomy

Local recurrence confined to the pelvis following radical hysterectomy for cervical cancer can be treated with radiotherapy with curative intent. An experience with 5-FU–based chemotherapy and concurrent pelvic EBRT resulted in a 58% complete response rate and a 45% no-evidence-of-disease rate, at a median follow-up of 57 months. The total pelvic EBRT dose was 5,280 cGy plus a boost to sites of recurrence with twice-daily 160-cGy fractions during the 5-FU infusion. Therefore, radiotherapy, with or without chemotherapy, can provide durable local tumor control, with better results attainable for small, central recurrences, for which brachytherapy is possible.

Local recurrence after definitive radiation therapy

Local recurrence confined to the pelvis following definitive radiation therapy rarely can be cured with exenteration. In a series of patients treated with definitive radiotherapy, 21% of recurrences (80 of 376) were isolated to the pelvis. Only 29% of these localized pelvic recurrences (23 of 80) were explored for curative exenteration, and for the 43% of patients (10 of 23) deemed operable, the 5-year survival rate was 16%. Para-aortic lymph node recurrences are also observed in some of these patients, and some are successfully treated with aggressive irradiation and chemotherapy. Of 758 patients, 42 (6%) had isolated and nonisolated para-aortic lymph node failures. The 5-year survival in the above group was 28%. Careful follow-up, early detection, and aggressive treatment of para-aortic lymph node recurrences may increase the probability of salvage for some of these patients.

Palliation of metastatic disease

Palliative radiation therapy to sites of metastatic cervical cancer is effective. The most common sites of metastasis are distant lymph nodes, bone, and lungs. Reirradiation of the pelvis is possible in selected patients to control local symptoms, such as bleeding, but carries an increased risk of bowel complications. For previously unirradiated sites of metastatic disease, 3,000 cGy in 10 fractions provides palliation of symptoms in the majority of patients.

CHEMOTHERAPY FOR ADVANCED/RECURRENT DISEASE

Chemotherapy has traditionally been used for the palliative management of advanced or recurrent disease that can no longer be managed by surgery or radiation therapy (see Table 3). Various factors complicate the use of chemotherapy in such patients,

TABLE 4: Active agents as defined by a response rate of at least 15%

Drug	No. of patients	Responses	Response rate
Alkylating agents			
CCNU	5	1	20%
Chlorambucil	44	11	25%
Cyclophosphamide	251	38	15%
Dibromodulcitol	120	23	23%
Galactitol	36	7	19%
Ifosfamide	157	35	22%
Melphalan	20	4	20%
Heavy metal complexes			
Carboplatin	175	27	15%
Cisplatin	815	190	23%
Antibiotics			
Doxorubicin	266	45	17%
Mitomycin	18	4	22%
Porfiromycin	78	17	22%
Antimetabolites			
Baker's antifol	32	5	16%
5-Fluorouracil	142	29	20%
Methotrexate	96	17	18%
Plant alkaloids			
Vincristine	55	10	18%
Vindesine	21	5	24%
Vinorelbine	42	6	15%
Other agents			
Irinotecan	55	13	24%
Hexamethylmelamine	64	12	19%
ICRF-159	28	5	18%
Paclitaxel	52	9	17%
Teniposide	32	7	22%
Topotecan	43	8	19%

Adapted with permission from Thigpen T: Cancer J 9:425–432, 2003.

however. Prior radiation treatment can affect the blood supply to the involved field, which may result in decreased drug delivery to the tumor site. Pelvic irradiation also reduces bone marrow reserve, thus limiting the tolerable doses of most chemotherapeutic agents. Moreover, irradiation may produce its cytotoxic effect, in part, through a mechanism similar to that of alkylating agents; thus, it is thought to be cross-resistant with some chemotherapeutic agents. A significant number of patients with advanced disease may also have impaired renal function, further limiting the use of certain chemotherapeutic regimens.

Single agents

Among the chemotherapeutic agents used for cervical cancer, cisplatin and ifosfamide have shown the most consistent activity as single agents (Table 4). The duration of response with any single agent is brief, ranging from 4 to 6 months, with survival ranging from 6 to 9 months.

Cisplatin has been the most extensively evaluated single agent for cervical carcinoma. A dose of 100 mg/m^2 was shown to have a higher response rate than a dose of 50 mg/m^2 (31% vs 21%), but the higher dose was associated with increased toxicity, and overall survival did not differ significantly between the two groups. A 24-hour infusion of cisplatin was tolerated better than a 2-hour infusion, with no difference in therapeutic efficacy.

Ifosfamide produces response rates ranging from 33% to 50% in various dose schedules. A dose of 1.5 g/m^2 over 30 minutes for 5 days (with mesna [Mesnex]) produced an overall response rate of 40% and a complete response rate of 20%.

Lower response rates are generally seen in patients who have had prior chemotherapy. Responses also are decreased in previously irradiated sites.

Taxanes Paclitaxel and docetaxel (Taxotere) have been reported to be active in cervical cancer. A study of paclitaxel (170 mg/m^2 over 24 hours) showed an objective response rate of 17%, and another study of paclitaxel (250 mg/m^2 over 3 hours) demonstrated an objective response rate of 27%. Docetaxel (100 mg/m^2 over 1 hour) has yielded a response rate of 19%.

Camptothecins Irinotecan and topotecan, semisynthetic camptothecins, have shown activity in patients with cervical cancer, even in patients who did not respond to prior chemotherapy and prior radiation therapy. The reported objective response rates were 21% and 19%, respectively.

Targeted therapies Newer biologic agents are being actively studied. Two important receptors in cervical cancer include vascular endothelial growth factor (VEGF) and epidermal growth factor receptor (EGFR). VEGF is a key promoter of tumor progression in cervical cancer. A GOG phase II study of 46 patients with metastatic cervical cancer explored the role of bevacizumab (Avastin), a recombinant humanized anti-VEGF monoclonal antibody. Eleven patients (24%) survived progression free for at least 6 months, and five patients (11%) had objective radiographic responses. This finding compared favorably with results of historic phase II studies in this population. GOG–227E is testing cetuximab (Erbitux), a monoclonocal antibody to the EGFR, in patients with metastatic disease.

TABLE 5: Combination chemotherapy for advanced or recurrent cervical carcinoma

Chemotherapy regimen	Number of patients	Overall response rate
Doublets		
Cisplatin/5-FU	72	48%
	32	47%
	55	22%
Cisplatin/gemcitabine	40	95%
	40	75%
Cisplatin/topotecan	32	28%
Cisplatin/vinorelbine	67	30%
	49	64%
Cisplatin/paclitaxel	41	46%
	34	47%
Cisplatin/ifosfamide	30	50%
	42	38%
Cisplatin/irinotecan	29	59%
	27	37%
Cisplatin/bleomycin	24	54%
Cisplatin/mitomycin	33	42%
Cisplatin/tirapazamine	36	28%
Carboplatin/paclitaxel	25	40%
Carboplatin/ifosfamide	32	59%
Triplets		
Bleomycin/cisplatin/ifosfamide	49	69%
Bleomycin/carboplatin/ifosfamide	35	60%
Paclitaxel/cisplatin/ifosfamide	45	67%
	57	46%
	45	47%
Paclitaxel/cisplatin/5-FU	60	65%
Ifosfamide/cisplatin/5-FU	30	53%
Ifosfamide/cisplatin/mitomycin	44	34%
Ifosfamide/leucovorin/5-FU	30	53%
Vinblastine/bleomycin/cisplatin	33	66%
Quartlets		
Bleomycin/vincristine/cisplatin/mitomycin	20	72%
	90	76%
Methotrexate/vinblastine/doxorubicin/cisplatin	29	66%
	27	52%

5-FU = fluorouracil

Modified from Cadron I, Leunen K, Amant F, et al: Gynecol Oncol 106:354–361, 2007; Long HJ 3rd: J Clin Oncol 25:2966–2974, 2007.

Combination regimens

Various combination chemotherapy regimens have been evaluated in phase II trials, and high response rates (> 50%) were noted, even in patients who had received prior radiation therapy. The results of some of these trials are summarized in Tables 5 and 6. In one study, a subset analysis showed a response rate of 72% with the combination of bleomycin, ifosfamide, and cisplatin as treatment for tumors located in previously irradiated sites. Neoadjuvant regimens of cisplatin combined with gemcitabine in patients with locally advanced cervical cancer demonstrated very high activity, with a clinical response rate of 95%. Neoadjuvant ifosfamide and cisplatin, with or without paclitaxel, produced 87% and 82% response rates, respectively, among 146 evaluable patients in a randomized study.

A randomized trial was reported by Long et al. A total of 146 patients with advanced persistent or recurrent cervical cancer were treated with cisplatin (50 mg/m^2 IV every 21 days), and 147 patients were treated with topotecan (.75 mg/m^2 IV during 30 minutes on days 1, 2, and 3 followed by cisplatin (50 mg/m^2 on day 1) repeated every 21 days. All regimens were administered for a maximum of 6 cycles for nonresponders or until disease progression or unacceptable toxicity prohibited additional chemotherapy. The complete response rate was 3% for cisplatin and 10% for the cisplatin-topotecan combination, and the complete and partial remission rates were 13% and 27%, respectively; the median progression-free survival was 2.9 and 4.6 months, respectively. Chemotherapy remains palliative, with no longevity prolongation of survival in recurrent or metastatic disease.

A randomized phase II GOG study comparing epidermal growth factor (EGF)-based therapy and angiogenesis therapy in women with advanced or recurrent cervical cancer showed favorable results with the use of antiangiogenesis therapy. The study compared lapatinib (Tykerb) vs pazopanib (Votrient). Pazopanib showed improved progression-free survival (HR, 0.66; 90% CI: 0.48–0.91; *P* = .013) and overall survival (HR, 0.67; 90% CI: 0.46–0.99; *P* = .45), with diarrhea as the only grade 3 adverse reaction that occurred in 10% of subjects. Because pazopanib can be administered orally and has a low incidence of serious toxicity, it may prove to be a promising drug in the treatment of advanced and recurrent cervical cancers, especially in developing countries where the treatment is heavily focused on palliation *(Monk B et al: J Clin Oncol 27[15S]: abstract 5520, 2009).*

The most recent phase III GOG randomized trial was presented; it explored four cisplatin-containing doublet combinations in stage IVB, recurrent or persistent cervical carcinoma. A total of 434 evaluable patients received cisplatin (50 mg/m^2 on day 1), combined with either paclitaxel (135 mg/m^2) or vinorelbine (30 mg/m^2 on days 1 and 8) or gemcitabine (1,000 mg/m^2 on days 1 and 8) or topotecan (.75 mg/m^2 on days 1, 2, and 3). Each cycle was repeated every 21 days. In the analysis, the cisplatin and paclitaxel regimen was considered the standard arm, and a 33% death reduction was considered to be a significant endpoint. In the final results, there was no survival difference seen among the four groups. Cisplatin-paclitaxel had the highest radiographic response rate (29.1%) and slightly higher survival rates (2.6 months longer), but still these results were not statistically better than those of the other treatment groups.

TABLE 6: Phase III clinical trials in advanced or recurrent cervical cancer

Protocol	Regimen	N	Response rate	PFS (months)	OS (months)
GOG	Cisplatin (50 mg/m^2/day 1)	150	21%	3.7	7.1
	Cisplatin (20 mg/m^2/days 1–5)	128	25%	3.9	6.1
	Cisplatin (100 mg/m^2/day 1)	166	31%	4.6	7.0
GOG–110	Cisplatin	140	18%	3.2	8.0
	Cisplatin/mitolactol	147	21%	3.3	7.3
	Cisplatin/ifosfamide	151	31%	4.6	8.3
GOG–149	Cisplatin/ifosfamide	146	31%	4.6	8.5
	Bleomycin/ifosfamide/ cisplatin	141	31%	5.1	8.4
GOG–169	Cisplatin	134	19%	2.8	8.8
	Cisplatin/paclitaxel	130	36%	4.8	9.7
GOG–179	Cisplatin	146	13%	2.9	6.5
	Cisplatin/topotecan	147	27%	4.6	9.4

PFS = progression-free survival; OS = overall survival
Modified from Cadron I, Leunen K, Amant F, et al: Gynecol Oncol 106:354–361, 2007; Long HJ 3rd: J Clin Oncol 25:2966–2974, 2007.

Palliative care

Palliation of the dying cervical cancer patient is difficult. Pain due to recurrent pelvic disease can be extreme and requires skillful use of combinations of narcotics, sedatives, and anxiolytics. Fistula from the bladder or rectum demands meticulous local skin care and occasionally surgical diversion procedures in patients with reasonable expected longevity. This patient population often has limited resources, with dependent children requiring careful social service planning. A small percentage has concurrent HIV infection, making the infectious disease specialist part of the palliative care team. The tripod of care in advanced cervical cancer is the judicious use of chemotherapy and radiation therapy, palliation of the symptoms of advancing disease, as well as emotional and social support for the patient and family members.

In the follow-up of patients treated for carcinoma of the cervix, it is important to keep in mind that they are at risk for the development of secondary malignant tumors. In a study of more than 85,000 patients with squamous cell carcinoma and 10,280 with adenocarcinoma, treated in Scandinavian countries and the United States, there were 10,559 second cancers (standardized incidence ratio [SIR], 1.31) in the squamous cell carcinoma and 920 (SIR, 1.29) in the adenocarcinoma patients. Risk of lung cancer was increased in both groups of patients. SIRs for second cancers of the colon, soft tissues, melanoma, and non-Hodgkin lymphoma were significantly higher among the adenocarcinoma survivors than the squamous cell carcinoma survivors.

Carcinoma of the cervix and pregnancy About 1% of patients with cervical cancer are pregnant at diagnosis. Most patients present with an abnormal cytology or vaginal bleeding. Colposcopy during pregnancy is used to rule out invasive carcinoma. This procedure and biopsies of suspicious lesions are safe for these patients. In patients with high-grade dysplasia, a conservative approach is reasonable. Conization during pregnancy was associated with fetal loss of 10% to 20% in some series.

More than 70% of cervical cancer cases diagnosed during pregnancy are stage I disease. Management requires a multidisciplinary approach, involving a gynecologist, radiation oncologist, perinatologist, and psychological counselor. Important elements in the therapeutic decision involve tumor size, tumor stage, gestational status, and the patient's desire to continue the pregnancy.

Invasive cancer in a pregnant woman (< 20 weeks) generally is managed immediately, with loss of the fetus, although there have been reports of delayed treatment in selected patients with small tumors. The majority of patients are treated with a total or radical hysterectomy, which can be performed after a cesarean section and fetal delivery in women with pregnancy in the second or third trimester. An alternative is radiation therapy alone, for stage I/II disease, or combined with chemotherapy, for locally advanced disease. Spontaneous abortion usually occurs at about 4 weeks after initiation of pelvic irradiation (40 Gy). In patients diagnosed during the third trimester, fetal delivery is accomplished with a cesarean section or vaginal delivery, after which definitive treatment with radical surgery or irradiation is instituted. Several reports show comparable results with either therapeutic approach.

SUGGESTED READING

ACOG Committee on Practice Bulletins–Gynecology: ACOG Practice Bulletin no. 109: Cervical cytology screening. Obstet Gynecol 114:1409–1420, 2009.

Barraclough LH, Swindell R, Livsey JE, et al: External beam boost for cancer of the cervix uteri when intracavitary therapy cannot be performed. Int J Radiat Oncol Biol Phys 71:772–778, 2008.

Boggess JF, Gehrig PA, Cantrell L, et al: A case-control study of robot-assisted type III radical hysterectomy with pelvic node dissection compared with open radical hysterectomy. Am J Obstet Gynecol 199:357.e1–7, 2008.

Boughanim M, Leboulleux S, Rey A, et al: Histologic results of para-aortic lymphadenectomy in patients treated for stage IB2/II cervical cancer with negative [18F]fluorodeoxyglucose positron emission tomography scans in the para-aortic area. J Clin Oncol 26:2558–2561, 2008.

Cadron I, Van Gorp T, Amant F, et al: Chemotherapy for recurrent cervical cancer. Gynecol Oncol 107:S113–S118, 2007.

Choi CH, Kim TJ, Lee SJ, et al: Salvage chemotherapy with a combination of paclitaxel, ifosfamide, and cisplatin for the patients with recurrent carcinoma of the uterine cervix. Int J Gynecol Cancer 16:1157–1164, 2006.

Choi HJ, Ju W, Myung SK, Kim Y: Diagnostic performance of computer tomography, magnetic resonance imaging, and positron emission tomography or positron emission tomography/computer tomography for detection of metastatic lymph nodes in patients with cervical cancer: Meta-analysis. Cancer Sci 101:1471–1479, 2010.

Chou HH, Chang TC, Yen TC, et al: Low value of [18F]-fluoro-2-deoxy-D-glucose positron emission tomography in primary staging of early-stage cervical cancer before radical hysterectomy. J Clin Oncol 24:123–128, 2006.

Diaz JP, Sonoda Y, Leitao NM, et al: Oncologic outcome of fertility-sparing radical trachelectomy versus radical hysterectomy for stage IB1 cervical carcinoma. Gynecol Oncol 111:255–260, 2008.

Eifel PJ, Gershenson DM, Kavanagh JJ, et al: M.D. Anderson Cancer Care Series: Gynecologic Cancer. New York: Springer; 2006.

Einstein MH, Park KJ, Sonoda Y, et al: Radical vaginal versus abdominal trachelectomy for stage IB1 cervcal cancer: A comparison of surgical and pathologic outcomes. Gynecol Oncol 112:73–77, 2009.

Franckena M, Lutgens LC, Koper PC, et al: Radiotherapy and hyperthermia for treatment of primary locally advanced cervix cancer: Results in 378 patients. Int J Radiat Oncol Biol Phys 73:242–250, 2009.

FUTURE II Study Group: Quadrivalent vaccine against human papillomavirus to prevent high-grade cervical lesions. N Engl J Med 356:1915–1927, 2007.

Garland SM, Hernandez-Avila M, Wheeler CM, et al: Quadrivalent vaccine against human papillomavirus to prevent anogenital diseases. N Engl J Med 356:1928–1943, 2007.

Huang E-Y, Wang C- J, Chen H- C, et al: Multivariate analysis of para-aortic lymph node recurrence after definitive radiotherapy for stage IB-IVA squamous cell carcinoma of uterine cervix. Int J Radiat Oncol Biol Phys 72:834–842, 2008.

Huguet F, Cojocariu O-M, Levy P, et al: Preoperative concurrent radiation therapy and chemotherapy for bulky stage IB2, IIA, and IIB carcinoma of the uterine cervix with proximal parametrial invasion. Int J Radiat Oncol Biol Phys 72:1508–1515, 2008.

Husain A, Akhurst T, Larson S, et al: A prospective study of the accuracy of 18Fluorodeoxyglucose positron emission tomography (18FDG PET) in identifying sites of metastasis prior to pelvic exenteration. Gynecol Oncol 106:177–180, 2007.

Jemal A, Siegel R, Xu J, et al: Cancer statistics, 2010. CA Cancer J Clin 60:277–300, 2010.

Justino PB, Baroni R, Blasbalg R, et al: Clinical tumor dimensions may be useful to prevent geographic miss in conventional radiotherapy of uterine cervix cancer—A magnetic resonance imaging-based study. Int J Radiat Oncol Biol Phys 74:503–510, 2009.

Kesic V: Management of cervical cancer. Eur J Surg Oncol 32:832–837, 2006.

Keys HM, Bundy BN, Stehman FB, et al: Radiation therapy with and without extrafascial hysterectomy for bulky stage IB cervical carcinoma: A randomized trial of the Gynecologic Oncology Group. Gynecol Oncol 89:343–353, 2003.

Lai CH, Chang CJ, Huang HJ, et al: Role of human papillomavirus genotype in prognosis of early-stage cervical cancer undergoing primary surgery. J Clin Oncol 25:3628–3634, 2007.

Lanciano R, Calkins A, Bundy BN, et al: Randomized comparison of weekly cisplatin or protracted venous infusion of fluorouracil in combination with pelvic radiation in advanced cervix cancer: A Gynecologic Oncology Group Study. J Clin Oncol 23:8289–8294, 2005.

Levenback CF: Status of sentinel lymph node biopsy in gynecological cancers. Ann Surg Oncol 15:18–20, 2008.

Lin LL, Mutic S, Low DA, et al: Adaptive brachytherapy treatment planning for cervical cancer using FDG-PET. Int J Radiat Oncol Biol Phys 67:91–96, 2007.

Loft A, Berthelsen AK, Roed H, et al: The diagnostic value of PET/CT scanning in patients with cervical cancer: A prospective study. Gynecol Oncol 106:29–34, 2007.

Long HJ 3rd: Management of metastatic cervical cancer: Review of the literature. J Clin Oncol 25:2966–2974, 2007.

Long HJ 3rd, Bundy BN, Grendys EC Jr, et al: Randomized phase III trial of cisplatin with or without topotecan in carcinoma of the uterine cervix: A Gynecologic Oncology Group Study. J Clin Oncol 23:4626–4633, 2005.

Lowe MP, Chamberlain DH, Kamelle SA, et al: A multi-institutional experience with robotic-assisted radical hysterectomy for early stage cervical cancer. Gynecol Oncol 113:191–194, 2009.

Lutgens L, van der Zee J, Pijls-Johannesma M, et al: Combined use of hyperthermia and radiation therapy for treating locally advanced cervix carcinoma. Cochrane Database Syst Rev 3:CD006377, 2010.

Maluf FC, Leiser AL, Aghajanian C, et al: Phase II study of tirapazamine plus cisplatin in patients with advanced or recurrent cervical cancer. Int J Gynecol Cancer 16:1165–1171, 2006.

Mayrand MH, Duarte-Franco E, Rodrigues I, et al: Human papillomavirus DNA versus Papanicolaou screening tests for cervical cancer. N Engl J Med 357:1579–1588, 2007.

Mitchell DG, Snyder B, Coakley F, et al: Early invasive cervical cancer: Tumor delineation by magnetic resonance imaging, computed tomography, and clinical examination, verified by pathological results, in the ACRIN 6651/GOG 183 Intergroup Study. J Clin Oncol 24:5687–5694, 2006.

Monk BJ, Huang HQ, Cella D, et al: Quality of life outcomes from a randomized phase III trial of cisplatin with or without topotecan in advanced carcinoma of the cervix: A Gynecologic Oncology Group Study. J Clin Oncol 23:4617–4625, 2005.

Monk BJ, Sill MW, Burger RA, et al: A phase II trial of bevacizumab in the treatment of persistent or recurrent squamous cell carcinoma of the cervix: A GOG study. J Clin Oncol 27:1069–1074, 2009.

Monk BJ, Sill M, McMeekin DS, et al: Phase III trial of four cisplatin-containing doublet combinations in stage IVB, recurrent, or persistent cervical carcinoma: A Gynecologic Oncology Group study. J Clin Oncol 27:4649–4655, 2009.

Odicino F, Pecorelli S, Zigliani L, et al: History of the FIGO cancer staging system. Int J Gynaecol Obstet 101:205–210, 2008.

Pearcey R, Miao Q, Kong W, et al: Impact of adoption of chemoradiotherapy on the outcome of cervical cancer in Ontario: Results of a population-based cohort study. J Clin Oncol 25:2383–2388, 2007.

Pecorelli S, Zigliani L, Odicino F: Revised FIGO staging for carcinoma of the cervix. Int J Gynaecol Obstet 105:107–108, 2009.

Potter R, Haie-Meder C, Van Limbergen E, et al: Recommendations from gynaecological (GYN) GEC ESTRO working group (II): Concepts and terms in 3D image-based treatment planning in cervix brachytherapy-3D dose volume parameters and aspects of 3D image-based anatomy, radiation physics, radiobiology. Radiother Oncol 78:67–77, 2006.

Rose PG, Ali S, Watkins E, et al: Long-term follow-up of a randomized trial comparing concurrent single agent cisplatin, cisplatin-based combination chemotherapy, or hydroxyurea during pelvic irradiation for locally advanced cervical cancer: A Gynecologic Oncology Group Study. J Clin Oncol 25:2804–2810, 2007.

Rose PG, Ali S, Whitney CW, et al: Impact of hydronephrosis on outcome of stage IIIB cervical cancer patients with disease limited to the pelvis, treated with radiation and concurrent chemotherapy: A Gynecologic Oncology Group study. Gynecol Obstet 117:270–275, 2010.

Rotman M, Sedlis A, Piedmonte MR, et al: A phase III randomized trial of postoperative pelvic irradiation in stage IB cervical carcinoma with poor prognostic features: Follow-up of a Gynecologic Oncology Group Study. Int J Radiat Oncol Biol Phys 65:169–176, 2006.

Schneider A, Köhler C, Erdemoglu E: Current developments for pelvic exenteration in gynecologic oncology. Curr Opin Obstet Gynecol 21:4–9, 2009.

Stanley M: Human papillomavirus vaccines versus cervical cancer screening. Clin Oncol (R Coll Radiol) 20:388–394, 2008.

Tierney J: Neoadjuvant chemotherapy for locally advanced cervical cancer: A systematic review and meta-analysis of individual patient data from 21 randomized trials. Eur J Cancer 39:2470–2486, 2003.

Vale C, Meta-Analysis Group: Reducing uncertainties about the effects of chemoradiatiotherapy for cervical cancer: A systematic review and meta-analysis of individual patient data from 18 randomized trials. J Clin Oncol 26:5802–5812, 2008.

Vistad I, Cvancarova M, Fossa SD, et al: Postradiotherapy morbidity in long-term survivors after locally advanced cervical cancer: How well do physicians' assessments agree with those of their patients? Int J Radiat Oncol Biol Phys 71:1335–1342, 2008.

Acknowledgments

The authors would like to thank Dr. Xipeng Wang, Dr. Hye-Sook Chon, Dr. Xi Cheng, and Lora Lothringer for their assistance.

Abbreviations in this chapter

ABS = American Brachytherapy Society; ACOG = American College of Obstetricians and Gynecologists; ACRIN = American College of Radiology Imaging Network; ACS = American Cancer Society; ASCO = American Society of Clinical Oncology; FIGO = International Federation of Gynecology and Obstetrics; NCIC = National Cancer Institute of Canada; RTOG = Radiation Therapy Oncology Group; SWOG = Southwest Oncology Group

CHAPTER 18

Uterine corpus tumors

Kathryn M. Greven, MD, Maurie Markman, MD, and David Scott Miller, MD

ENDOMETRIAL CANCER

Carcinoma of the epithelial lining (endometrium) of the uterine corpus is the most common female pelvic malignancy. Factors influencing its prominence are the declining incidence of cervical cancer, longer life expectancy, and earlier diagnosis. Adenocarcinoma of the endometrium, the most prevalent histologic subtype, is currently the fourth most common cancer in women, with 43,470 new cases, ranking behind breast, lung, and bowel cancers. Endometrial adenocarcinoma is the eighth leading cause of death from malignancy in women, accounting for 7,950 deaths in 2010.

EPIDEMIOLOGY

Age

Endometrial cancer is primarily a disease of postmenopausal women, although 25% of cases occur in premenopausal patients, with 5% of cases developing in patients < 40 years old.

Geography

The incidence of endometrial cancer is higher in Western nations and very low in Eastern countries.

Immigrant populations tend to assume the risks of native populations, highlighting the importance of environmental factors in the genesis of this disease. Endometrial cancers tend to be more common in urban than in rural residents. In the United States, white women have a twofold higher incidence of endometrial cancer than black women.

ETIOLOGY AND RISK FACTORS

Adenocarcinoma of the endometrium may arise in normal, atrophic, or hyperplastic endometrium. Two mechanisms are generally believed to be involved in the development of endometrial cancer. In approximately 75% of women, there is a history of exposure to unopposed estrogen, either endogenous or exogenous (type I). The tumors in these women begin as endometrial hyperplasia and progress to carcinomas, which usually are better differentiated and have a favorable prognosis.

In the other 25% of women, carcinomas appear spontaneously, are not clearly related to a transition from atypical hyperplasia, and rather arise in a background of atrophic or inert endometrium. These neoplasms tend to be associated with a more undifferentiated cell type and a poorer prognosis (type II).

Unopposed Estrogen

It has been hypothesized that long-term estrogenic stimulation of the endometrium unmodified by progesterone has a role in the development of endometrial carcinoma. This hypothesis derives from observations that women who are infertile or obese or who have dysfunctional bleeding due to anovulation are at high risk for this disease, as are women with estrogen-secreting granulosa theca cell ovarian tumors. Also, the recognition that atypical adenomatous (complex) hyperplasia is a precursor of cancer, and that it is associated with unopposed estrogen use in women, underscores the importance of the association among risk factors, estrogens, and cancer. In the late 1970s and early 1980s, several case-control studies demonstrated that the risk of endometrial cancer is increased 4- to 15-fold in long-term estrogen users, as compared with age-matched controls.

It is well established that past use of oral contraceptives (OCs) protects against endometrial cancer. The use of OCs with either high potency progestin or low-potency progestin is associated with a decreased risk of endometrial cancer. The potency of the progestin in most OCs appears adequate to provide a protective effect against endometrial cancer. Higher progestin-potency OCs may be more protective than lower progestin-potency OCs among women with a larger body habitus.

Diet

The high rate of occurrence of endometrial cancer in Western societies and the very low rate in Eastern countries suggest a possible etiologic role for nutrition, especially the high content of animal fat in Western diets. There may be a relationship between high-fat diets and the higher incidence of endometrial carcinoma in women with conditions of unopposed estrogen. Endogenous estrogens rise in postmenopausal women because of increased production of androstenedione or a greater peripheral conversion of this hormone to estrone. In obese women, the extraglandular aromatization of androstenedione to estrone is increased in fatty tissue.

Obesity

Phenotypically, the majority of women who develop endometrial cancer tend to be obese. Women who are 30 pounds over ideal weight have a 3-fold increased risk of developing endometrial cancer, whereas those 50 pounds or more over ideal weight have a 10-fold increased risk.

Parity

Nulliparous women are at 2 times greater risk of developing endometrial cancer, females who undergo menopause after age 52 are at 2.5 times greater risk, and those who experience increased bleeding at the time of menopause are at 4 times greater risk.

Endometrial hyperplasia

It is believed that the majority of endometrioid neoplastic lesions of the endometrium follow a continuum of histologically distinguishable hyperplastic lesions that covers a spectrum ranging from endometrial hyperplasia without atypia (EH) to endometrial hyperplasia with atypia (AEH) to well-differentiated endometrial cancer. Whereas patients found to have simple endometrial hyperplasia have a low risk of disease progression to cancer, 29% of those with complex atypical hyperplasia, if left untreated, will develop adenocarcinoma. However, the reproducibility of these diagnoses has been questioned by many.

As recently reported, GOG0167 estimated the reproducibility of a referring institution's pathologist's diagnosis of AEH and determined the frequency of concomitant adenocarcinoma in the hysterectomy obtained within 12 weeks of the initial diagnosis. The referring institution's pathologist's diagnosis of AEH was supported by the majority of the expert panel in only 38% of cases. The majority diagnosis was adenocarcinoma in 29%, cycling endometrium in 7%, and nonatypical hyperplasia in 18% of cases. Unanimous agreement on any diagnosis was reached among the entire expert panel in only 40% of cases. This study panel found that there was a high incidence (43%) of endometrial cancer in patients who had a biopsy demonstrating AEH.

Other risk factors

Other known risk factors for endometrial cancer include diabetes mellitus; hypertension; endometrial hyperplasia; and a family history of endometrial, breast, and/or colon cancer. Diabetic females have a 3-fold increased risk, and hypertensive patients have a 1.5-fold greater risk of endometrial cancer.

Tamoxifen exerts its primary effect by blocking the binding of estrogen to estrogen receptors. It also exerts mild estrogenic effects on the female genital tract. This weak estrogenic effect presumably accounts for an increased frequency of endometrial carcinoma observed in women receiving prolonged adjuvant tamoxifen therapy for breast carcinoma.

Initially reported in 1985, the increased frequency of endometrial carcinoma in patients treated with tamoxifen was characterized more fully in a study of 1,846 women recorded in the Swedish Cancer Registry. This study reported a 6.4-fold increase in the relative risk of endometrial carcinoma with a daily dose of 40 mg of tamoxifen. The greatest cumulative risk was observed after 5 years of tamoxifen use.

The NSABP subsequently reported on the incidence of other cancers in 2,843 women with node-negative, estrogen receptor-positive breast cancer treated with either tamoxifen or placebo in its B-14 randomized trial and an additional 1,220 patients treated with tamoxifen in another NSABP trial. The relative risk of endometrial carcinoma in the tamoxifen-treated patients was 7.5. The hazard rate was 0.2 per 1,000 cases with placebo and 1.6 per 1,000 cases with tamoxifen therapy. The mean duration of tamoxifen therapy for all patients was 35 months, and 36% of the cancers had developed by 2 years after the initiation of treatment. A more recent review of NSABP treatment and prevention trials revealed that the risk of uterine sarcomas was also increased with tamoxifen. The incidence of sarcomas was very low, however, with a rate of 0.17/1,000 women/year.

These data raise the question of whether tamoxifen should be used as adjuvant therapy for women at relatively low risk for breast cancer recurrence. First, it should be recognized that the endometrial cancers that develop in patients receiving tamoxifen exhibit the same stage, grade, and prognosis distribution as other endometrial cancers. There is some evidence that tamoxifen use is associated with an increased risk of uterine sarcoma; fortunately, this risk is low, and the cure rate should be high. Second, adjuvant tamoxifen reduces the cumulative rate of recurrence of breast cancer from 228 to 124 cases/1,000 women and the cumulative rate of second primary breast cancers from 40.5 to 23.5 cases/1,000 women.

When all of these facts are taken into account, there is an overall 38% reduction in the cumulative hazard rate for recurrence of breast cancer in tamoxifen-treated patients. Thus, the benefits of tamoxifen may outweigh the risks of endometrial cancer.

The current recommendations for screening women on tamoxifen are to educate patients about the significance of abnormal spotting, bleeding, or discharge and to investigate promptly any of these abnormalities.

Some experts have proposed that tamoxifen-treated women be screened with transvaginal ultrasonography. However, recent data suggest a high false-positive rate and a low frequency of significant findings, leading to the conclusion that endometrial screening is not warranted.

SIGNS AND SYMPTOMS

Postmenopausal women

Symptoms of early endometrial carcinoma are few but common. However, 90% of patients complain of abnormal vaginal discharge, and 80% of these women experience abnormal bleeding, usually after menopause. In the general population, 15% of postmenopausal women presenting with abnormal bleeding will be found to have endometrial carcinoma. Signs and symptoms of more advanced disease include pelvic pressure and other symptoms indicative of uterine enlargement or extrauterine tumor spread.

Premenopausal women

The diagnosis of endometrial cancer may be difficult to make in premenopausal patients. The physician must maintain a high index of suspicion in this group of patients and perform endometrial sampling in any women who complain of prolonged, heavy menstrual periods or intermenstrual spotting.

SCREENING AND DIAGNOSIS

Screening

There is no role for screening of asymptomatic patients for endometrial cancer.

Outpatient endometrial sampling

These procedures, such as endometrial biopsy or aspiration curettage coupled with endocervical sampling, are definitive if results are positive for cancer. The results of endometrial biopsies correlate well with endometrial curettings, and these biopsy procedures have the advantage of avoiding general anesthesia. However, if sampling techniques fail to provide sufficient diagnostic information or if abnormal bleeding persists, formal dilation and curettage is required.

Dilation and curettage

This is the gold standard for assessing uterine bleeding and diagnosing endometrial carcinoma. Before dilating the cervix, the endocervix should be curetted. Next, careful sounding of the uterus is accomplished. Dilation of the cervix is then performed, followed by systematic curetting of the entire endometrial cavity. Cervical and endometrial specimens should be kept separate and forwarded for pathologic interpretation.

The American Cancer Society has concluded that there is insufficient evidence to recommend routine screening for endometrial cancer for average-risk women. However, the ACS recommends that at the time of menopause, all women should be informed about the risks and symptoms of endometrial cancer and strongly encouraged to report any unexpected bleeding or spotting to their physicians. Women at elevated risk for endometrial cancer from tamoxifen therapy should be informed about the risk and symptoms of endometrial cancer and strongly encouraged to report any unexpected bleeding or spotting to their physicians.

In addition, results from three HNPCC (hereditary nonpolyposis colorectal cancer) registries have shown a 10-fold increased risk of endometrial cancer for women who carry the HNPCC genetic abnormality, with a cumulative risk for endometrial cancer of 43% by age 70. Women with or at risk for HNPCC can be offered endometrial screening annually beginning at age 35, but informed decision-making after a discussion of options, including benefits, risks, and limitations of testing, is appropriate. Additional investigation is needed to determine the appropriate monitoring for endometrial cancer in HNPCC carriers.

PATHOLOGY

Adenocarcinoma

Endometrioid adenocarcinoma is the most common form of endometrial carcinoma, comprising 75% to 80% of cases. It varies from well differentiated to undifferentiated. The former demonstrates well-preserved glands in at least 95% of the tumor, whereas in the latter, less than half of the neoplasm shows glandular differentiation. Squamous differentiation can be seen in 30% to 50% of cases.

Adenocarcinoma with benign squamous differentiation has been termed adenoacanthoma and generally has a good prognosis.

If the squamous component resembles squamous carcinoma, the tumor is designated an adenosquamous carcinoma. These lesions tend to have a worse prognosis due to their association with a poorly differentiated glandular component.

Serous carcinoma

This is an aggressive form of endometrial cancer that accounts for < 10% of these tumors. Serous cancer of the endometrium closely resembles serous carcinoma of the ovaries and fallopian tubes and is usually found in an advanced stage in older women.

Clear-cell carcinomas

Clear-cell carcinomas of the endometrium closely resemble their counterparts in the cervix, vagina, and ovaries. As with serous cancers, these tumors generally occur in older women and have a poor prognosis due to their propensity for early intraperitoneal spread.

Table 1: 2009 FIGO staging system for carcinoma of the endometrium

Stage I[a]	Tumor contained to the corpus uteri		
	IA	No or less than half myometrial invasion	
	IB	Invasion equal to or more than half of the myometrium	
Stage II		Tumor invades the cervical stroma but does not extend beyond the uterus[b]	
Stage III[a]		Local and/or regional spread of tumor[c]	
	IIIA	Tumor invades the serosa of the corpus uteri and/or adnexas	
	IIIB	Vaginal and/or parametrial involvement	
	IIIC	Metastases to pelvis and/or para-aortic lymph nodes	
		IIIC1	Positive pelvic nodes
		IIIC2	Positive para-aortic lymph nodes with or without positive pelvic lymph nodes
Stage IV[a]			Tumor invades bladder and/or bowel mucosa and/or distant metastases
	IVA		Tumor invasion of bladder and/or bowel mucosa
	IVB		Disant metastases, including intra-abdominal metastases and or inguinal lymph nodes

FIGO = International Federation of Gynecology and Obstetrics

[a] Includes grades 1, 2, or 3

[b] Endocervical glandular involvement only should be considered as stage I and no longer as stage II.

[c] Positive cytology has to be reported separately without changing the stage.

Secretory adenocarcinoma

This is an uncommon endometrial cancer that resembles secretory endometrium with its associated progestational changes. These cancers tend to be of low grade and have a good prognosis.

STAGING AND PROGNOSIS

Two large prospective GOG surgical staging trials reported in 1984 and 1987 helped define the prognostic factors for endometrial carcinoma and the current treatment approach. In addition to evaluating the predictive value of such factors as age, race, and endocrine status, the studies confirmed that prognosis is directly related to the presence or absence of easily determined uterine and extrauterine risk factors. Uterine prognostic factors include histologic cell type, tumor grade, depth of myometrial invasion, occult extension of disease to the cervix, and vascular space invasion. Extrauterine prognostic factors include adnexal metastases, intraperitoneal spread of disease to other extrauterine structures, positive peritoneal cytology, pelvic lymph node metastases, and aortic node involvement.

The revised staging system takes into account the nearly equivalent survival rates among low to intermediate grade IA and IB tumors, the lack of prognostic significance of endocervical gland involvement, and the marked survival differences of pelvic node or para-arotic node involvement. A revised staging system can be seen in Table 1.

Peritoneal cytology

Peritoneal cytology is no longer included in the staging system. It is to be reported separately without changing the stage. Several reports of patients with positive peritoneal cytology have failed to demonstrate that peritoneal cytology is a poor prognostic factor.

Uterine size

The size of the uterus was previously believed to be a risk factor and was part of the older clinical staging system. However, recent information indicates that uterine size is *not* an independent risk factor but rather relates to cell type, grade, and myometrial invasion.

Surgical staging

Cell type and grade can be determined before hysterectomy, although in some series, grade, as determined by dilation and curettage, has an overall inaccuracy rate of 31% compared with grade in the hysterectomy specimen, and grade 3 tumors have an inaccuracy rate of 50%. Recognition of all of the other factors requires an exploratory laparotomy, peritoneal fluid sampling, and hysterectomy with careful pathologic interpretation of all removed tissue. This primary surgical approach led the FIGO to define endometrial cancer as a surgically staged disease in 1988, incorporating many of the prognostic factors into the staging process (Table 2).

TABLE 2: 1988 FIGO surgical staging for endometrial cancer

Stage	Grade	Characteristic
IA	G1,2,3	Tumor limited to the endometrium
IB	G1,2,3	Tumor invasion to less than half of the myometrium
IC	G1,2,3	Tumor invasion to more than half of the myometrium
IIA	G1,2,3	Endocervical glandular involvement only
IIB	G1,2,3	Cervical stromal invasion
IIIA	G1,2,3	Tumor invades serosa or adnexa or positive peritoneal cytology
IIIB	G1,2,3	Vaginal metastases
IIIC	G1,2,3	Metastases to pelvic or para-aortic lymph nodes
IVA	G1,2,3	Tumor invades the bladder and/or bowel mucosa
IVB		Distant metastases, including intra-abdominal and/or inguinal lymph nodes

Histopathology—Degree of differentiation[a]

G1	≤ 5% of a nonsquamous or nonmorular solid growth pattern
G2	6%–50% of a nonsquamous or nonmorular solid growth pattern
G3	> 50% of a nonsquamous or nonmorular solid growth pattern

FIGO = International Federation of Gynecology and Obstetrics
[a] Cases should be grouped by the degree of differentiation of the adenocarcinoma.

TREATMENT

Surgery

Approximately 90% of patients with a diagnosis of endometrial cancer are medically able to undergo surgery. Preparation for this surgery should include evaluation of such concurrent medical problems as hypertension and diabetes, which are frequently found in patients with endometrial cancer.

Open surgical procedure

The operative procedure is performed through an adequate abdominal incision that allows for thorough intra-abdominal exploration and retroperitoneal lymph node removal if necessary. On entry into the peritoneal cavity, fluid samples are obtained for subsequent cytologic determination (intraperitoneal cell washings). Next, thorough intra-abdominal and pelvic exploration is undertaken, with biopsy or excision of any suspicious lesions. In particular, the uterus should be observed for tumor breakthrough of the serosal surface. The distal ends of the fallopian tubes are clipped or ligated to prevent possible tumor spillage during uterine manipulation.

These procedures should be followed by total extrafascial hysterectomy and bilateral salpingo-oophorectomy. The excised uterus is opened away from the operating table, and the depth of myometrial penetration is determined by clinical observation or microscopic frozen section. The depth of myometrial invasion can be accurately assessed in over 90% of cases.

Laparoscopic surgery

An alternative method of surgically staging patients with clinical stage I endometrial cancer is gaining in popularity. This approach combines laparoscopically assisted vaginal hysterectomy with laparoscopic lymphadenectomy.

Laparoscopy-assisted surgical staging (LASS) is feasible in a select group of patients. However, it is not yet known whether this approach is applicable to all patients with clinical stage I disease. In particular, patients who are overweight or have intra-abdominal adhesions may not be ideal candidates. Para-aortic lymphadenectomy is technically more difficult through the laparoscope. To obtain adequate exposure, it is necessary to elevate the small bowel mesentery into the upper abdomen, which becomes increasingly difficult as the patient's weight increases, especially when weight exceeds 180 pounds.

Walker et al recently reported the results of GOGLAP2, which randomized patients between laparoscopic vs open laparotomy surgical staging. Laparoscopy was initiated in 1,682 and completed without conversion in 1,248 cases (74%). Conversion from laparoscopy to laparotomy was secondary to poor visibility in 246 patients (15%), metastatic cancer in 69 patients (4%), and bleeding in 49 patients (3%). Patients randomized to undergo laparoscopy had significantly fewer moderate to severe (> Common Toxicology Criteria grade 2) postoperative (14% vs 21%; $P < .0001$) complications and similar rates of intraoperative complications. Length of hospital stay was significantly shorter for those randomized to undergo laparoscopy (median 3 days vs 4 days; $P < .001$), but operative time was significantly longer (median 204 minutes vs 130 minutes; $P < .001$). Pelvic and para-aortic nodes were removed in 92% of laparoscopy patients and 96% of laparotomy patients ($P < .0001$), and cytology was performed in 96% vs 98% ($P = .052$). Neither treatment arm demonstrated an improved ability to detect metastatic disease ($P = .841$). Laparoscopic surgical staging is feasible and safe for patients with uterine cancer and results in fewer complications and a shorter hospital stay. Quality of life evaluation found a better body image and return to normal activities for the laparoscopy patients. A reduction in para-aortic node evaluation is a potential risk of laparoscopic staging. Follow-up of these patients will determine whether surgical technique affects recurrence-free survival.

Lymph node evaluation

Any suspicious pelvic or para-aortic lymph nodes should be removed for pathologic evaluation. If there is no gross residual intraperitoneal tumor, pelvic and para-aortic lymph nodes should be removed for the following indications:

- invasion of more than one-half of the outer myometrium
- presence of tumor in the isthmus-cervix
- adnexal or other extrauterine metastases
- presence of serous, clear-cell, undifferentiated, or squamous types
- palpably enlarged lymph nodes.

Lymph nodes need not be removed in patients whose tumor is limited to the endometrium, regardless of grade, because < 1% of these patients have disease spread to pelvic or para-aortic lymph nodes. The decision of whether to perform lymph node sampling is less clear-cut for patients whose only risk factor is invasion of the inner half of the myometrium, particularly if the tumor grade is 1 or 2. This group has a ≤ 5% chance of node positivity.

Lymphadenectomy

The extent of lymph node removal has been the subject of debate. Recently, GOG defined the extent of lymphadenectomy required for entry into its studies:

Pelvic lymphadenectomy

- The skin incision may be of the surgeon's choosing, including midline vertical, transverse, and lateral vertical. The procedure may be performed via laparoscopy or a retroperitoneal approach.
- Identify the bifurcation of the common iliac, external iliac, and hypogastric arteries; veins; and the ureters bilaterally.
- Any enlarged or suspicious nodes will be excised or biopsied if unresectable.
- Remove bilaterally all nodal tissue and skeletonization of all vessels from the mid portion of the common iliac artery superiorly, to the circumflex iliac vein inferiorly.
- Remove bilaterally all nodal tissue from the mid portion of the psoas muscle laterally to the ureters medially, including the hypogastric arteries and veins and from the obturator fossas anterior to the obturator nerves.
- An adequate dissection requires that a minimum of four lymph nodes be demonstrated pathologically from each side (right and left) of the pelvis, preferably from multiple sites.

Para-aortic lymphadenectomy

- The bifurcation of the aorta, the inferior vena cava, the ovarian vessels, the inferior mesenteric artery, the ureters, and duodenum should be identified.
- The nodal tissue over the distal vena cava from the level of the inferior mesenteric artery to the mid right common iliac artery is removed.
- The nodal tissue between the aorta and the left ureter from the inferior mesenteric artery to the left mid common iliac artery is removed.
- An adequate dissection requires that lymphatic tissue be demonstrated pathologically from each side (right and left).

Surgical staging

After these procedures, the patient should be surgically staged according to the 2009 FIGO criteria. The overall surgical complication rate after this type of staging is approximately 20%. The rate of serious complications is 6%, and they include vascular, ureteral, and bowel injuries.

Whether lymph node dissections are therapeutic or merely prognostic has been debated. A recent phase III trial comparing endometrial cancer patients who received systematic lymphadenectomy with those without lymphadenectomy demonstrated improved staging but with an increased complication rate with lymphadenectomy. There was no improvement in disease-free or overall survival. In another study known as the ASTEC trial, 1,408 women were randomized to undergo a lymphadenectomy or no lymphadenectomy at the time of total abdominal hysterectomy/bilateral salpingo-oophorectomy. There was no benefit in terms of survival or recurrence-free survival for women treated with lymphadenectomy.

Grossly involved lymph nodes

These can often be completely resected. A retrospective study revealed 5-year disease-specific survival rates of 50% in the patients with grossly positive lymph nodes who underwent complete resection, compared with 63% in those with microscopic metastatic disease and 43% in the women with residual macroscopic lymph node metastasis.

Adjuvant radiation therapy

Following surgical staging, adjuvant radiation therapy is offered to patients based on prognostic factors found at the time of surgery. A pelvic recurrence rate of 7% to 14% is predictable for all stage I patients after surgery alone, although certain subgroups with more risk factors may have a higher incidence of recurrence of endometrial carcinoma. Well-described prognostic factors include disease extent (cervical involvement, extrauterine involvement of the serosa, adnexa, lymph nodes or intra-abdominal spread), as well as histologic grade of the tumor, depth of myometrial penetration, pathologic subtype, and presence of lymphovascular space invasion.

Teletherapy

Adjuvant irradiation has been delivered primarily using external-beam radiotherapy (EBRT) directed to the pelvis, which allows for treatment of the pelvic nodes. There have now been three large randomized trials demonstrating that radiation can decrease local recurrence but has no demonstrable effect on overall survival.

One trial, GOG0099, compared the results of pelvic irradiation with those of observation following hysterectomy and lymphadenectomy. The estimated 2-year cumulative incidence of recurrence was 12% in the observation arm and 3% in those irradiated ($P = .007$). The treatment difference was particularly evident among a "high-intermediate risk" subgroup defined as those (1) with moderate to poorly differentiated tumor, presence of lymphovascular invasion, and outer-third myometrial invasion; (2) age 50 or older with any two risk factors previously listed; or (3) age of at least 70 with any risk factor previously listed, where the cumulative incidence of recurrence in the observed patients was 26% vs 6% in the treated patients. Overall survival rates at 3 years did not differ significantly between the two groups.

However, one-third of patients were found to be in a high-risk group that included patients who were older, had lymph-vascular space invasion, deep myometrial penetration, and high-grade disease. When outcomes were stratified by these factors, the addition of pelvic irradiation was found to reduce the recurrence and death rate from 36% to 17%, the cancer death rate from 17% to 10%, and the distant metastatic rate from 19% to 10%. This finding suggests that pelvic irradiation may not only influence pelvic recurrence in these patients but that there is a subgroup of patients who may benefit in terms of distant metastasis and death. A larger trial with high-risk patients is needed to validate this assumption.

Of the 18 pelvic recurrences in the no adjuvant treatment arm, 13 were in the vagina. Thirteen other sites of recurrence were outside the pelvis. It has been speculated that vaginal irradiation alone could have controlled these vaginal recurrences, leading to interest in treatment with vaginal irradiation instead of pelvic irradiation.

The findings of a multicenter trial with 754 patients from the Netherlands, called the PORTEC study, have been reported. Eligible patients had stage IC grade 1 tumors (21%), stage IB or IC grade 2 tumors (69%), or stage IB grade 3 tumors (10%). After total abdominal hysterectomy without lymphadenectomy, patients were randomized to receive pelvic radiotherapy (46 Gy) or no further treatment.

Pelvic irradiation decreased the incidence of locoregional tumor recurrence but did not affect survival. Patients with grade 3 histology demonstrated the highest risk of distant metastases and death caused by endometrial cancer. Most of the locoregional relapses were located in the vagina (30 of 40 cases). It is possible that vaginal brachytherapy could have prevented the majority of these cases. When patients were subdivided into a high-risk subgroup with two or three risk factors, including age ≥ 60, grade 3 histology, and myometrial depth ≥ 50%, the 10-year locoregional relapse rate was 4.6% in the radiotherapy group vs 23% in the control group.

PORTEC also registered patients on a prospective trial who had deep myometrial invasion and grade 3 histology. All patients were treated with pelvic irradiation following hysterectomy. Notably, these patients had a distant recurrence rate at 5 years of 31%, and a pelvic recurrence rate at 5 years of 14%. The information from this report as well as from the subgroup of patients in the GOG 99 trial suggests that there may be a role for systemic therapy as well as pelvic irradiation in this high-risk subgroup.

A third randomized trial was recently published. More than 900 patients with stage I or IIa endometrial cancer from the NCIC and the MRC were randomized to receive pelvic radiation therapy or no pelvic radiation therapy. Notably, vaginal radiation therapy was optional, and 52% of patients in each arm received it. There was no difference in survival and only a minimal difference in local or regional tumor recurrence rates.

Brachytherapy

Several reports have demonstrated excellent local tumor control with vaginal irradiation alone. A review of the world literature included 1,800 patients with low- to intermediate-risk disease. Overall, the vaginal control rate was 99.3% following adjuvant high-dose-rate (HDR) vaginal brachytherapy.

In a randomized study from the Norwegian Radium Hospital, pelvic irradiation significantly decreased the incidence of locoregional tumor recurrences compared with vaginal irradiation alone. Patients with deeply invasive, grade 3 tumors had lower death and recurrence rates when treated with pelvic plus vaginal irradiation than patients treated with vaginal irradiation alone.

Many women with endometrial cancer are being treated with lymphadenectomy at the time of hysterectomy. There has been some interest in using vaginal irradiation alone to treat women who have negative nodes but deep myometrial penetration or high-grade histology. Several small retrospective reports have demonstrated excellent outcomes for such patients. However, more experience is needed to determine whether vaginal irradiation alone is adequate.

The results of a phase III randomized trial from PORTEC were recently published. This trial included patients who had a high-intermediate risk endometrial cancer: age > 60 and stage IC grade 1/2 or stage IB grade 3; any age and stage IIA grade 1/2 or grade 3 with < 50% invasion. They were randomized to receive pelvic radiation or vaginal brachytherapy. A total of 427 patients were randomized between 2002 and 2006. At a median follow-up of 34 months, 3-year actuarial rates of vaginal relapse were 0.9% in the vaginal brachytherapy arm and 2.0% after EBRT (P = .97), with standard error of the difference 1.4%. Three-year rates of pelvic recurrence were 3.6% and 0.7% (P = .03). There were no significant differences in 3-year overall survival (90.4% vs 90.8%; P = .55) and RFS (89.5% vs 89.1%; P = .38). As patient-reported quality of life after vaginal brachytherapy was shown to be better than after EBRT, vaginal brachytherapy should be the treatment of choice for patients with high- or intermediate-risk endometrial carcinoma.

Vaginal irradiation alone is appropriate for patients at low risk for pelvic node metastasis. Because of increased rectal and vaginal sequelae, treatment of the entire length of the vagina is usually not recommended.

Irradiation of the pelvis and vagina has been combined for the adjuvant treatment of some patients. Patients with cervical involvement or extrauterine disease, who may have an increased incidence of local failure, may benefit from the two treatments combined, although there are no data to suggest that the addition of brachytherapy improves outcome over EBRT alone. Patients with uterine-confined disease have excellent local tumor control following treatment with either type of irradiation. Combining the two treatments has not been shown to benefit these patients.

TABLE 3: Recommendations for adjuvant irradiation

	Stage		
Histologic grade	**IA**	**IB**	**IC**
G1	–	–	–
G2	–	–	VB
G3	VB	VB	+[a]
Vascular space invasion[b]	+	+	+

[a] After full lymphadenectomy, consider brachytherapy alone because of excess complications.
[b] Any grade
\+ = irradiation recommended
– = irradiation not recommended
VB = vaginal brachytherapy

Vaginal irradiation

Vaginal irradiation can be delivered with HDR or low-dose-rate (LDR) equipment. Both techniques have resulted in excellent local tumor control rates and low morbidity when administered by experienced practitioners. Each technique has its advantages. HDR treatments require multiple insertions, generally with one or two insertions performed every week for 3 to 6 weeks. However, hospitalization is not required, and each insertion takes only a brief amount of time. LDR treatments are delivered once but require hospitalization for 2 to 3 days.

Stage I disease

Current recommendations for the treatment of patients with pathologic stage I disease include adjuvant pelvic irradiation for women with deep myometrial penetration, and grade 3 histology, or evidence of vascular space invasion (Table 3). Data support the use of vaginal irradiation alone for women with more superficial tumors and low-grade histology.

Radiation doses are generally 45 to 50 Gy with standard fractionation. The technique should include multiple fields treated daily, with attempts to protect the small bowel. Complications from adjuvant pelvic irradiation are related to technique and the extent of lymphadenectomy.

If full lymphadenectomy has been performed, the incidence of complications increases significantly with pelvic irradiation. For these patients, consideration should be given to adjuvant brachytherapy rather than pelvic irradiation.

Papillary serous histology

The high rate of upper abdominal, pelvic, and vaginal recurrences in patients with uterine papillary serous cancers has led some clinicians to recommend that these patients receive whole abdominal irradiation (WAI, with doses up to 30 Gy) and additional treatments to bring the pelvic dose to 50 Gy. A vaginal cylinder or colpostats may be used to boost the surface dose with 40 Gy. This treatment has resulted in a 5-year survival rate of 50%.

The most common treatment for this rare cancer is combination chemotherapy and radiation therapy (either vaginal brachytherapy or EBRT). Surgical staging is usually similar to that for ovarian cancer, as these patients have a high propensity of distant and abdominal tumor spread.

Stage II disease

Patients whose endometrial cancer extends to the cervix usually represent a heterogeneous group, with differing histologic grades and varying degrees of cervical involvement, myometrial penetration, and nodal involvement. Similar outcomes with preoperative and postoperative irradiation suggest that initial surgical treatment with tailored postoperative irradiation is a reasonable approach.

Current treatment recommendations frequently include adjuvant pelvic irradiation to a dose of 45 to 50 Gy, in addition to insertion of a vaginal cylinder or colpostats to raise the total dose to the vaginal surface to 80 to 90 Gy. This treatment should result in a 5-year disease-free survival rate of 80%, with a locoregional tumor control rate of 90%. Of course, outcome varies with the extent of myometrial penetration, degree of cervical involvement, and histologic grade of tumor.

Patients who have a large amount of cervical involvement that precludes initial hysterectomy are candidates for preoperative irradiation. A multiple-field technique is used to deliver a dose of 40 to 45 Gy with standard fractionation. A midline block may be inserted for the last 20 Gy to protect the rectum.

Intracavitary insertion with a standard Fletcher applicator, consisting of a uterine tandem and vaginal colpostats, delivers 20 to 25 Gy to point A (defined as 2 cm caudally and 2 cm laterally to the cervical os). Hysterectomy should follow in approximately 4 to 6 weeks. The expected 5-year disease-free survival rate for patients with extensive disease is 70% to 80%.

Stage III disease

More favorable patients have an isolated extrauterine site (eg, adnexa alone), low-grade histology, and/or disease confined to the pelvis. Greven et al reported that 17 patients with an isolated extrauterine site who had low-grade histology and received postoperative pelvic radiation therapy had a 100% disease-free survival rate. However, patients with grade 2 or 3 disease or more than one extrauterine site had progressively worse outcomes.

One subgroup found to have a relatively favorable prognosis includes women with isolated ovarian metastasis. Five-year disease-free survival rates ranging from 60% to 82% have been reported in these women after hysterectomy and pelvic irradiation, depending on the histologic grade of the tumor and the depth of myometrial penetration. Pelvic irradiation usually includes a dose of 45 to 50 Gy using standard fractionation. A vaginal boost with a cylinder or colpostats may add 30 to 35 Gy to the vaginal surface.

Patients with pelvic node involvement alone have much better outcomes than patients with extension to periaortic nodes, despite the fact that they are both considered stage IIIC patients. Morrow et al demonstrated 5-year recurrence-free survival rates of 70% and 35% for patients with pelvic nodes compared with patients with para-aortic nodes, respectively. Patients with pelvic nodes and negative para-aortic nodes are generally treated with adjuvant pelvic radiation therapy. Those with para-aortic nodes are treated with extended-field irradiation, which includes 45 to 50 Gy to a volume encompassing the pelvic and periaortic regions.

Because upper abdominal failures have been reported previously in patients with stage III disease, attention has focused on the role of WAI. Although subsets of patients have done well with WAI, it is unclear whether this more aggressive therapy has any benefit over pelvic irradiation. A GOG phase II trial of WAI demonstrated a 3-year progression-free survival rate of 35%. The GOG completed a trial of WAI compared with chemotherapy, GOG0122. (The outcomes from this trial are discussed in the "Chemotherapy" section.) Unfortunately, because most studies have combined patients who have favorable stage III disease with patients who have unfavorable stage IV disease, it is impossible to determine whether there are some subgroups of patients who might best be managed with a particular therapy.

Because many of these patients are at increased risk of pelvic recurrence as well as distant recurrence, there is interest in combining pelvic radiation therapy with systemic therapy. RTOG 9708 combined pelvic radiation therapy with cisplatin and followed it with cisplatin and paclitaxel. Toxicity was predominantly hematologic. For stage III patients, 4-year survival and disease-free survival rates were 77% and 72%, respectively. There were no recurrences for patients with stage IC, IIA or IIB disease.

GOG0184 was instituted following the completion of GOG0122, based on the assumption that combined-modality therapy with radiation therapy and chemotherapy in advanced but optimally cytoreduced endometrial carcinoma may lead to a better result than either modality used alone. Patients with stages III and IV adenocarcinoma of the endometrium with less than 2 cm of residual disease were treated with radiation therapy tailored to include the volume at risk followed by randomization to cisplatin plus doxorubicin or to cisplatin, doxorubicin and paclitaxel. As reported by Homesley et al, the addition of paclitaxel to cisplatin and doxorubicin did not improve progression-free survival.

Definitive radiation treatment

For patients who are poor operative risks, definitive treatment with irradiation has produced excellent local tumor control and survival rates. Such treatment is considered to be justified when the operative risk exceeds the 10% to 15% uterine recurrence rate expected with irradiation alone.

A more favorable outcome with definitive irradiation is related to low clinical tumor stage, less aggressive histologic variant, and use of brachytherapy for at least part of the treatment. Five-year disease-specific survival rates as high as 87%, 88%, and 49% have been reported in patients with stages I, II, and III or IV disease, respectively. Ten-year local tumor control rates in patients with stages I/II, III, and IV disease were 84%, 87%, and 68%, respectively.

For patients with early-stage disease and low-grade histology, treatment techniques with irradiation alone consist of uterine intracavitary insertions with Heyman or Simon capsules or an afterloading intrauterine tandem. Doses for intracavitary treatment range from 40 to 45 Gy prescribed to point A. One report used an HDR endometrial applicator and prescribed twice-daily fractions of 700 Gy given for five treatments to 2 cm. Patients with more advanced disease, a large uterus, or aggressive histology generally receive both an intrauterine intracavitary insertion and external pelvic irradiation. External irradiation typically delivers 40 to 45 Gy to the pelvis, followed by intracavitary treatment that delivers 30 to 35 Gy to point A.

Rates of serious complications attributable to irradiation range from 4% to 5% with intracavitary treatment alone to 10% to 15% with combined external and intracavitary irradiation.

Adjuvant systemic therapy

Only a few trials of adjuvant systemic therapy have been conducted in patients with early-stage endometrial cancer. At present, we believe that such therapy should not be recommended outside the clinical trial setting.

Endocrine therapy

Early uncontrolled trials suggested that progestin therapy might prolong the disease progression-free interval and time to recurrence in patients with stages I and II lesions treated with initial surgery and irradiation. However, at least three subsequent randomized trials failed to show any survival benefit for progestins, and a meta-analysis has demonstrated no advantage of adjuvant progestin therapy.

Chemotherapy

Three studies have evaluated the role of chemotherapy in early-stage endometrial carcinoma. The EORTC compared pelvic radiation plus brachytherapy versus pelvic radiation and chemotherapy. The Japanese gynecologic oncology group compared pelvic radiation versus cisplatin-based chemotherapy, and the consistent finding was a lower incidence of distant metastasis with minimal impact on survival. The EORTC trial had an overall survival benefit at 5 years of 8%; however, the trial as well as the Japanese trial included some patients with positive pelvic nodes. These trials do lead to enthusiasm for the addition of chemotherapy as adjuvant treatment for high-risk patients with early-stage disease.

The current GOG trial is randomizing patients with high-risk stage I and II disease between pelvic radiation and no chemotherapy or vaginal brachytherapy with three cycles of carboplatin and paclitaxel.

Results from a GOG trial , GOG0122, compared adjuvant chemotherapy (doxorubicin plus cisplatin) with WAI. The patient population included patients with stages III and IV disease (75% and 25%, respectively) with 50% endometrioid histologies. Patients treated with chemotherapy had significantly improved progression-free (38% vs 50%) and overall (42% vs 55%) survival at 5 years. However, serious adverse effects were also more common in the chemotherapy group than in the radiotherapy group, with treatment-related deaths twice as high in the former group, at 4% vs 2%. Pelvic and abdominal recurrences were the predominant pattern of recurrence for both treatment arms. Distant recurrences were slightly less frequent for patients treated with chemotherapy. This finding leads to the support of the concept of combining chemotherapy with involved-field irradiation for patients with more advanced disease.

The next GOG trial (184) randomized patients to receive involved field external beam radiation with either doxorubicin and cisplatin or paclitaxel, docetaxel, and cisplatin. There was a 10% locoregional recurrence at 3 years with no difference in survival. Subset analysis suggested that paclitaxel benefited patients with gross residual disease, papillary serous histology, and grade 3 histology. The current GOG study (258) is randomizing patients to concurrent cisplatin and external beam radiation followed by adjuvant carboplatin with paclitaxel or carboplatin and paclitaxel alone. The ongoing PORTEC 3 trial randomizes such patients to either pelvic radiation and concurrent cisplatin or radiation therapy with adjuvant carboplatin and paclitaxel.

Hormone replacement therapy (HRT)

Whether HRT increases the likelihood of recurrence has been studied, with several retrospective reports showing no adverse outcomes. Thus, GOG undertook a large randomized placebo-controlled trial of HRT after treatment for earlier stage endometrial cancer. However, there were too few events, and it was closed after the findings of the Women's Health Initiative were released. HRT was not associated with a significant incidence of recurrent disease, mortality, or new malignancy.

TREATMENT OF RECURRENT OR METASTATIC DISEASE

Patterns of recurrence

Recurrent endometrial cancer is initially confined to the pelvis in 50% of patients. The major sites of distant metastasis are the abdominal cavity, liver, and lungs.

Following diagnosis and initial treatment, periodic evaluation, including history, physical examination, and pelvic examination, is recommended at 3- to 6-month intervals for the first 5 years and yearly thereafter. More extensive and more costly procedures, such as chest x-ray, CT imaging, and marker studies, used in asymptomatic patients are of questionable value and are unlikely to have a major impact on survival. Symptomatic patients should be evaluated as appropriate.

Radiation therapy

After hysterectomy alone for endometrial cancer, approximately 50% of recurrences are pelvic and 50% are extrapelvic. It is clear that locoregional recurrences can develop in isolation, without distant metastasis, and salvage can be accomplished with high-dose irradiation.

Pelvic recurrences

Five-year disease-specific survival rates as high as 51% have been reported in patients with isolated locoregional recurrences treated with radiation therapy. Factors that have an adverse impact on outcome are increased size of tumor at recurrence, young age, pelvic vs vaginal involvement, and treatment of recurrence with EBRT only vs the addition of vaginal brachytherapy.

The PORTEC group has published its experience with salvage of vaginal recurrence in patients who did not receive adjuvant irradiation. At 5 years, the survival rate after vaginal relapse was 65% in the control group, compared with 43% in the irradiated group.

TABLE 4: Results of a phase III, dose-response trial of progestins in advanced or recurrent endometrial carcinoma

Parameter	Oral medroxyprogesterone 200 mg/day (n = 145)	Oral medroxyprogesterone 1,000 mg/day (n = 154)
Response rate (%)	25	15
Complete response rate (%)	17	9
Median disease progression–free survival (mo)	3.2	2.5
Median survival (mo)	11.1	7.0

Radiation treatment for pelvic recurrence usually consists of EBRT with the addition of a brachytherapy boost that may include colpostats, a cylinder, interstitial needles, or seeds. Treatment must be individualized based on the location and size of the recurrence and the boost method selected. The tolerance of normal tissues must be respected, but combined doses > 60 Gy have been associated with improved local tumor control.

Extrapelvic recurrences

For patients with recurrences outside the pelvis, irradiation is effective in producing responses in localized symptomatic lesions. Therefore, irradiation may be effective for palliation of such lesions in the lymph nodes, brain, or bones. Doses and protocols vary, depending on the site of recurrence.

Pelvic exenteration for pelvic recurrences after irradiation

Isolated pelvic central recurrence after irradiation is rare. Selected patients in whom it does occur may benefit from pelvic exenterative surgery. No large series have been published, but some long-term survivors have been reported.

Although the long-term survival rate after this procedure is only 20%, it remains the only potentially curative option for the few patients with central recurrence of endometrial cancer who have not responded to standard surgery and radiation therapy.

Endocrine therapy

Progestins

These produce complete and partial response rates of 15% to 25% in patients with locoregional recurrence or distant metastases. The route, type, and dose of progestins do not appear to be related to response; hence, oral therapy is preferred.

In clinical practice, oral administration of 200 mg of medroxyprogesterone or 160 mg of megestrol produces blood levels similar to those achieved with parenteral therapy (400 to 1,000 mg of medroxyprogesterone IM weekly). A phase III trial conducted by GOG comparing 200 mg and 1,000 mg of medroxyprogesterone given orally daily found no differences between the two regimens, although it is noteworthy that the trends all favored the low-dose regimen (Table 4). Doses higher than 200 mg/d of medroxyprogesterone, therefore, are clearly not warranted.

Several factors are predictive of a favorable response to progestin therapy. Patients with well-differentiated lesions are more likely to respond than those with poorly differentiated tumors. A related observation is that a much higher percentage of grade 1 tumors have significant levels of estrogen and progesterone receptors; data show that lesions with higher receptor levels respond much more frequently to progestins than those with lower receptor levels. Response is almost always associated with better progression-free and overall survival.

The median time to disease progression for all patients treated with progestins is 3 to 4 months, and the median survival is 10 months.

Tamoxifen

Tamoxifen has a 0% to 13% response rate, is not as active as progestins, and is of little value as second-line therapy in patients who do not respond to progestins.

GOG has evaluated combined therapy with tamoxifen plus a progestin given sequentially in the hope that tamoxifen may increase progesterone receptor expression and, thus, increase the likelihood of response to progestins. Continuous tamoxifen and medroxyprogesterone given every other week was an active treatment, with a 33% response rate. A subsequent study found a 27% response rate for alternating megestrol, with several prolonged responses. As with prior hormonal studies, patients with well-differentiated cancers were more likely to respond. Nevertheless, this trial was relatively unique in that 22% of patients with poorly differentiated tumors responded.

Other hormonal agents

Drugs such as gonadotropin-releasing hormone analogs and aminoglutethimide (Cytadren) have been studied to some extent in endometrial carcinoma. These agents do not appear to have sufficient activity to warrant further study.

Chemotherapy

Single agents

Chemotherapy for advanced endometrial cancer focuses on three groups of agents with demonstrated activity: anthracyclines, platinum compounds, and taxanes.

The anthracyclines studied include doxorubicin and epirubicin. In a total of 298 patients, doxorubicin produced a 27% response rate. Epirubicin, primarily in European studies including 27 patients, yielded a 26% response rate. Two platinum compounds have activity. Cisplatin, in 86 patients, elicited responses in 29%. Carboplatin produced a 31% response rate in 52 patients. Paclitaxel, in two GOG studies, yielded responses in 36% of chemotherapy-naive and 27% of previously treated patients.

For all of these studies, the progression-free interval ranged from 4 to 7 months, with an overall survival range of 8 to 12 months. Approximately one-third of the responses were clinical complete responses, with a substantially longer duration and better survival than partial responders.

Other single agents with modest activity in endometrial cancer include ifosfamide and topotecan (Hycamtin).

Combination regimens

A number of phase II trials of combination regimens have been conducted. The combination of carboplatin and paclitaxel has been demonstrated to be active in advanced endometrial cancer (50%–60% response rate). Ultimately, the relative merits of combination chemotherapy with carboplatin and paclitaxel must be judged in the context of a randomized trial that is being performed by GOG (GOG0209). A randomized trial of cisplatin and doxorubicin with or without paclitaxel following surgery and radiation therapy did not show any improvement in recurrence-free survival but did have more toxicity.

Following encouraging phase II results, a phase III trial of circadian timed administration of cisplatin and doxorubicin found no significant benefit. GOG then compared this two-drug (cisplatin [50 mg/m^2]/doxorubicin [60 mg/m^2]) regimen with a three-drug combination of cisplatin (50 mg/m^2), doxorubicin (45 mg/m^2), and paclitaxel (160 mg/m^2 as a 3-hour infusion), with G-CSF (granulocyte colony-stimulating factor, filgrastim [Neupogen]) support (GOG 177). The three-drug combination of the paclitaxel-containing program produced a higher response rate (57% vs 35%) and an improved progression-free survival (8.3 months vs 5.3 months). Overall survival was also modestly improved (15.3 months vs 12.3 months; $P = .037$) with the three-drug program but with considerably greater toxicity, particularly peripheral neuropathy (grade 3, 12% vs 1%).

There has been concern about the potential effect of "high-risk" endometrial histologies on response to chemotherapy. It has been suggested that papillary serous and clear cell tumor adenocarcinomas should be treated differently. McMeekin et al correlated histology with chemotherapy outcomes in several of the above-mentioned trials and found no significant difference in response or survival based on the histologic type of endometrial cancer.

Chemotherapy plus progestins

Combinations of chemotherapy plus progestins have been studied in a number of phase II trials. The only large, randomized trial evaluating this approach (GOG29) allocated patients with advanced or recurrent disease to receive either cyclophosphamide, doxorubicin, cisplatin, and megestrol or melphalan (Alkeran), fluorouracil (5-FU), and megestrol. In pilot studies, these two regimens had been reported to yield response rates of 75% and 94%, respectively. The randomized trial produced response rates of 36% and 38%, respectively, with no evident advantage of either combination over single-agent doxorubicin (from prior studies) with regard to response rate, progression-free interval, or overall survival. These results do not suggest any advantage for the combined use of chemotherapy and progestins.

Treatment recommendations

Patients who have advanced or recurrent endometrial carcinoma should be considered for systemic therapy. Patients should first be offered the opportunity to participate in a clinical trial. Those who are ineligible or who choose not to participate should be treated according to current evidence.

Patients who have a grade 1 tumor and/or known progesterone receptor-positive disease clearly benefit from treatment with progestins (response rate, 40%; median progression-free interval, 9 months; overall median survival, 14 months) and should be so treated. Those with a grade 2 to 3 tumor and/or known progesterone receptor-negative disease do not do well with progestin therapy (response rate, 12%; median progression-free interval, 3 months; overall median survival, 10 months) and should be considered for initial treatment with single-agent chemotherapy (eg, paclitaxel, doxorubicin, carboplatin) or a combination regimen. Options include cisplatin/doxorubicin, cisplatin/doxorubicin/paclitaxel, and carboplatin/paclitaxel. Chemotherapy should also be considered for patients who do not respond to initial hormonal therapy.

Regimens that include both chemotherapy and hormonal therapy should not be considered outside a clinical trial because of the lack of data supporting any advantage of these combinations.

UTERINE SARCOMAS

Carcinosarcomas and other uterine sarcomas are uncommon tumors, accounting for less than 4% of all cancers of the uterine corpus. Carcinosarcomas, the most common histologic subtype, demonstrate both epithelial and stromal differentiation. Endometrial stromal sarcomas and leiomyosarcomas are characterized by differentiation toward one or more stromal tissues. Leiomyosarcomas occur at an earlier age than do carcinosarcomas, with a plateau observed in middle age. There is strong epidemiologic evidence that prior exposure to pelvic irradiation may increase the risk for the development of uterine sarcomas. Generally, these tumors are characterized by aggressive growth, with early lymphatic or hematogeneous spread. The overall survival rate is poor, with the majority of deaths occurring within 2 years of diagnosis.

PATTERNS OF SPREAD

Lymphatic metastases are a significant route of spread for carcinosarcoma, with a reported incidence of 40% to 60% occurring with stage I disease. Leiomyosarcoma has a propensity for extra-abdominal spread, often involving the lungs. For carcinosarcoma, the initial site for recurrence after surgical resection is likely to be the pelvis or abdomen, whereas leiomyosarcomas tend to fail to recur distantly. In a prospective surgical staging trial by GOG, the recurrence rate for early-stage carcinosarcoma was 53% and for leiomyosarcoma was 71%.

TREATMENT

Surgery

Surgery is the mainstay of treatment for uterine sarcomas. For carcinosarcoma, this usually consists of total abdominal hysterectomy and bilateral salpingo-oophorectomy, with washings to be obtained for peritoneal cytology. The GOG prospective staging study reported a 17% incidence of nodal metastasis for this histologic subtype, so retroperitoneal nodes should be sampled as for poorly differentiated endometrial cancers. For patients with advanced/recurrent disease, aggressive surgical debulking does not appear to improve outcome.

Hysterectomy with oophorectomy is also standard therapy for uterine leiomyosarcoma. Retroperitoneal nodal sampling is not usually performed, because lymph node involvement is unusual. For late recurrences of leiomyosarcoma, surgery must be individualized. Five-year survival rates of 30% to 50% have been reported following pulmonary resection for lung metastases. Patients with unilateral metastases have a significantly better prognosis than those with bilateral disease. Local and regional recurrences may also be amenable to surgical resection of disease.

Hysterectomy with oophorectomy is the standard of care for patients with low-grade endometrial stromal sarcomas. Removal of the ovaries was thought to be critical, as these tumors tend to have very high concentrations of estrogen and progesterone receptors and often respond to hormonal therapy. However, Li et al reviewed a multi-institutional experience and reported that bilateral salpingo-oophorectomy did not appear to affect time to recurrence or overall survival. Retention of ovarian function may be an option for premenopausal women with low-grade endometrial stromal sarcomas. Because these tumors have a tendency to spread via the lymphatics, resection of all disease, especially extension into the parametrium, should be attempted. This approach may require radical hysterectomy.

Adjuvant irradiation

Pelvic recurrence is a pattern of failure for most uterine sarcomas; isolated pelvic recurrences are uncommon. Adjuvant irradiation can decrease local recurrence, but there is no evidence that it improves survival. Patients will often experience recurrence distantly and treatment failure. Pelvic irradiation may be indicated for improvement of quality of life, however, because pelvic recurrence can be associated with pain, bleeding, and intestinal obstruction.

Radiotherapy

Uterine sarcomas represent only 2% to 5% of all uterine malignancies. These patients have a high incidence of distant, as well as pelvic, recurrences. In a nonrandomized prospective GOG study, patients with stages I and II mixed mesodermal sarcomas and leiomyosarcomas had fewer pelvic recurrences following irradiation than did those patients who did not undergo pelvic irradiation. No difference in overall or disease-free survival was noted.

Several retrospective reports have suggested improved pelvic control rates following pelvic irradiation for stages I and II uterine sarcomas. A randomized trial from the EORTC demonstrated that patients with carcinosarcoma randomized to receive pelvic radiation compared with no adjuvant treatment benefitted from pelvic radiation, with decreased local failures but no survival improvement. Patients with leiomyosarcoma did not demonstrate any benefit with the addition of pelvic radiation.

As reported by Wolfson et al, GOG 0150 was a randomized study of patients with stages I–IV carcinosarcoma of the uterus with less than 1 cm of residual disease and no extra-abdominal spread. Patients were treated with either cisplatin (20 mg/m^2/day for 4 days) plus ifosfamide (1.5 g/m^2/day for 4 days every 3 weeks for 3 cycles) or WAI to a total dose of 3,000 cGy and the pelvis treated to a total dose of 4,980 cGy. The abdomen received 150 cGy per fraction, with 5 fractions per week. The pelvis was boosted an additional 11 fractions at 180 cGy per fraction. The study tested whether patients treated with systemic treatment or locoregional treatment differ in progression-free interval, survival, and failure patterns. There were 105 patients in the WAI and 101 in the chemotherapy cohorts, respectively.

Of 206 study patients, there were 112 total recurrences (54%), with 60 (57%) in the radiotherapy and 52 (51%) in the chemotherapy treatment arms. Although patients may have had several different sites of failure, there were more vaginal failures in the chemotherapy group (10%) than in the WAI group (4%). However, there were more abdominal relapses in the WAI arm (28%) than in the chemotherapy cohort (19%). Pelvic and distant failures were essentially the same. Although acute toxicities of anemia and neuropathy were more frequent in the chemotherapy arm, there were more severe grade 3/4 gastrointestinal late effects in the WAI group, and two patients died as a direct result of radiation hepatitis. The estimated probability of surviving 5 years was 35% vs 45% for WAI vs chemotherapy. After adjusting for stage and age, there was no definite survival advantage but rather a trend favoring chemotherapy (the estimated death rate was 29% lower for chemotherapy patients than for WAI patients [HR = 0.712; 95% CI: 0.484–1.048; $P = .085$, two-tail test]).

GOG0150 has shown that adjunctive chemotherapy has less toxic long-term side effects and is more likely than radiotherapy to improve survival for these patients. Because chemotherapy did not reduce the risk of vaginal relapses, less toxic vaginal brachytherapy with chemotherapy would be an appropriate experimental arm for future adjuvant therapeutic trials in this group of patients.

Chemotherapy

There is no proven role for adjuvant chemotherapy in stage I disease following complete surgical resection. A GOG study looking at adjuvant doxorubicin vs no further therapy showed no differences in recurrence rate, progression-free survival, or overall survival. As reported by Sutton et al, GOG0117 showed that adjuvant ifosfamide and cisplatin after primary surgery for stage I or II carcinosarcoma of the uterus was tolerable. That combination was then compared with WAI in GOG 0150 (described in detail above), which showed a trend in survival favoring those treated with that chemotherapy combination.

For patients with advanced/recurrent disease, single-agent chemotherapy or combination chemotherapy can be used with a palliative intent. For carcinosarcomas, ifosfamide or paclitaxel appears to be the agent of choice. Because GOG 0108 showed that ifosfamide plus cisplatin had no greater progression-free interval or survival than ifosfamide alone, GOG 0161 randomized patients to receive ifosfamide (2.0 g/m^2 for 3 days every 3 weeks for 8 cycles) vs ifosfamide (1.6 g/m^2 for 3 days) plus paclitaxel (135 mg/m^2 by 3-hour infusion on day 1 repeated every 3 weeks for eight cycles). Homesley et al reported that there was a survival advantage for combination chemotherapy (13.5 months vs 5.8 months).

Doxorubicin has traditionally been used for leiomyosarcomas. Hensley et al reported that the combination of gemcitabine (Gemzar) plus docetaxel (Taxotere) produced a 36% response rate in LMS. Hormonal agents, specifically progestins, are the treatment of choice for advanced/recurrent endometrial stromal sarcomas.

GESTATIONAL TROPHOBLASTIC DISEASES

Gestational trophoblastic diseases (GTDs) encompass a spectrum of neoplastic disorders that arise from placental trophoblastic tissue after abnormal fertilization. In the United States, GTDs account for less than 1% of gynecologic malignancies.

Forty years ago, women with choriocarcinoma had a 95% mortality rate. Today, with the advent of effective chemotherapy and the development of a reliable tumor marker (β-subunit human chorionic gonadotropin [β-hCG]), the cure rate for choriocarcinoma is 90% to 95%.

CLINICAL PRESENTATION

Complete mole

The classic signs of a molar pregnancy include the absence of fetal heart sounds, physical evidence of a uterus that is larger than expected for gestational age, and vaginal bleeding. Although an intact fetus may coexist with a partial mole, this occurs in fewer than 1 in 100,000 pregnancies.

The most common presenting symptom of molar pregnancy is vaginal bleeding, reported in up to 97% of patients. Intrauterine clots may undergo oxidation and liquefaction, producing pathognomonic prune juice–like fluid. Prolonged or recurrent bleeding may result in iron-deficiency anemia. Symptoms of anemia occur in approximately 50% of patients at the time of diagnosis. Early toxemia (hypertension, proteinuria, and edema) presenting during the first or second trimester is common (20%–30%) in molar pregnancy.

Hyperthyroidism is seen clinically in approximately 7% of molar pregnancies. An elevation of triiodothyronine (T_3) and thyroxine (T_4) levels is observed more commonly than are the clinical manifestations of tachycardia, sweating, weight loss, and tremor. These hormonal elevations are presumed to be secondary to the structural similarity of hCG to thyroid-stimulating hormone (TSH).

Partial mole

Patients with partial mole have different clinical features than those with complete mole. Fewer than 10% of patients with partial mole have uterine enlargement. Patients with partial mole do not have prominent theca-lutein cysts, hyperthyroidism, or respiratory insufficiency. They experience toxemia only rarely. The diagnosis of partial mole is usually made after histologic review of curettage specimens.

Gestational trophoblastic neoplasia (GTN)

GTN develops in 6% to 19% of patients after molar evacuation. Metastases sometimes have an identical histology to that of molar disease, but the vast majority are choriocarcinomas. Metastatic spread is hematogeneous. Because of its extensive vascular network, metastatic GTN often produces local, spontaneous bleeding. The New England Trophoblastic Disease Center reported that the common metastatic sites of GTD are the lungs (80%); vagina (30%); pelvis (20%); liver (10%); brain (10%); and bowel, kidneys, and spleen (5% each).

Pulmonary metastases are common (80% of patients with metastatic disease) and occur when trophoblastic tissue enters the circulation via uterine venous sinuses. The radiologic features may be protean or subtle and include alveolar, nodular, and miliary patterns. Pleural effusions may also be present. Pulmonary metastases can be extensive and can cause respiratory failure and death.

Right upper-quadrant pain has been observed when hepatic metastases stretch Glisson's capsule. GI lesions may result in severe hemorrhage or in perforation with peritonitis, both of which require emergency intervention. Vaginal examination may reveal bluish metastatic deposits; these and other metastatic sites should not undergo biopsy because severe uncontrolled bleeding may occur.

CNS involvement from metastatic GTN suggests widespread disease and has a poor prognosis. CNS metastases are clinically evident in 7% to 28% of patients with metastatic choriocarcinoma. Cerebral metastases tend to respond favorably to both radiotherapy and chemotherapy.

Diagnostic studies

Although the clinical presentation may suggest a diagnosis of GTN, certain laboratory studies, particularly a determination of the patient's β-hCG level, and radiographic studies are needed to confirm this diagnosis.

Laboratory studies

Thyroid function studies should be performed in all patients with a clinical history or physical examination suggestive of hyperthyroidism. Abnormal thyroid function, manifested as an elevated T_4 level, is common in GTD. Metastatic deposits in the kidneys or GI tract may reveal themselves by hematuria or hematochezia.

Tumor markers

A well-characterized glycoprotein hormone secreted by the syncytiotrophoblast, hCG is essential to maintaining normal function of the corpus luteum during pregnancy. Because all trophoblastic tumors secrete β-hCG, this hormone serves as an excellent marker for tumor activity in the nonpregnant patient. Serial β-hCG levels should be monitored during therapy to ensure adequate treatment. The level of β-hCG is roughly proportional to the tumor burden and inversely proportional to the therapeutic outcome.

Radiologic studies

A chest x-ray should always be performed because 70% to 80% of patients with metastatic GTN have lung involvement. Although this x-ray usually demonstrates nodular metastases, the patterns of metastatic disease can range from atelectatic areas to subtle pleural abnormalities. A CT scan is often helpful in evaluating these nonspecific findings.

Since it has been demonstrated that 97% to 100% of patients with CNS disease from choriocarcinoma have concomitant pulmonary metastases, a CNS workup in asymptomatic patients with normal chest x-rays is not routinely warranted. If the chest x-ray is abnormal, or if β-hCG levels plateau or rise during treatment, a more thorough evaluation for metastatic disease is indicated. MRI of the brain, brain stem, and cerebellum as well as CT scans of the abdomen and pelvis should be performed to evaluate other likely sites of metastatic spread. The presence of intrauterine or ovarian disease also may be detected by MRI of the pelvis. Ultrasonography is a reliable, safe, economical, and relatively simple method for confirming the diagnosis of intrauterine GTD. It is also useful in identifying embryonic remnants.

The proposed FIGO 2000 anatomic staging system is a straightforward system based on anatomic criteria. In GTD, stage I disease is confined to the uterus; stage II disease

GOG0174 was the first randomized prospective frontline chemotherapy trial in 240 patients with GTN. The primary endpoint was normalization of the β-human chorionic gonadotropin (hCG) levels. Eligible patients were those with untreated, histologically confirmed low-risk GTN (WHO risk score, 0–6) defined as one of the following: < 10% decrease in hCG level over 3 consecutive weeks, persistently elevated hCG level for more than 4 months following initial curettage, or histologically proven nonmetastatic choriocarcinoma. Among eligible patients, complete response was observed in 53% of those given methotrexate and 69% of those given dactinomycin (Cosmegen; *P* = .015). Both regimens were well tolerated; only two patients experienced grade 4 toxicity, and no patient experienced grade 5 toxicity. This study demonstrates that biweekly dactinomycin (at 1.25 mg/m²) is statistically superior to weekly parenteral methotrexate (at 30 mg/m²) as initial management for low-risk GTN *(Osborne R et al: Gynecol Oncol 108: abstract SGO #2, 2008)*.

is outside the uterus but limited to the genital structures; stage III disease extends to the lungs with or without known genital tract involvement; and stage IV disease includes all other metastatic sites. The FIGO 2000 scoring system is based on a method (adapted from WHO) to identify patients at high risk for treatment failure. With the FIGO 2000 scoring system, patients are classified as being in a low-, middle-, or high-risk category. A total score of up to 4 is considered low risk; 5 to 7, middle risk; and 8 or greater, high risk. (Some centers recommend a low-risk score of 6 or less, a high-risk score of 7 or greater, and no middle-risk score.)

TREATMENT

The treatment strategy for GTD must be individualized for each patient. The stratification of risk groups enables physicians to direct an appropriate treatment strategy. Low-risk disease responds readily to single-agent chemotherapy and is virtually 100% curable. High-risk disease is not likely to be cured with single-agent therapy and therefore requires multidrug regimens.

Molar pregnancy

For patients with complete or partial hydatidiform mole, evacuation of the mole by suction and sharp curettage should be performed. Oxytocics also are given to produce uterine involution and to control bleeding. However, these agents should be used judiciously, as they may cause hyponatremia and fluid overload. A baseline chest x-ray and β-hCG measurement should be obtained prior to surgery. After molar evacuation, 80% of patients will need no further intervention.

Follow-up

As mentioned previously, all patients with molar disease should obtain a baseline chest x-ray. Serial β-hCG levels should be obtained every 1 to 2 weeks until the level is normal for three consecutive assays. Complete remission is defined by three consecutive normal β-hCG levels. Once this has occurred, β-hCG levels should be checked monthly for 12 months, every 4 months for the following year, and then yearly for 2 years. However, a single undetectable human chorionic gonadotropin level after evacuation is sufficient follow-up to ensure remission in patients with partial hydatidiform moles.

Although the use of OCs during the surveillance period remains controversial, strict contraception is required, because pregnancy would obviate the usefulness of β-hCG as a tumor marker. In general, once 12-month surveillance establishes a disease-free status, conception is acceptable. These women are always at high risk for future molar disease and will require close observation during future pregnancies. A pelvic ultrasonographic examination should be performed during the first trimester of all subsequent pregnancies to confirm that gestation is normal.

Chemotherapy is indicated when there is a plateau or increase in β-hCG levels on consecutive measurements, failure to reach normal levels by 16 weeks, or metastatic disease. Such patients are usually at low risk and will respond to single-agent chemotherapy. Methotrexate is the most commonly initiated single agent. Therapy is continued for one to two courses after a normal β-hCG level is achieved.

Low-risk metastatic disease

In more than 30 years of experience, single-agent chemotherapy with methotrexate has produced a high cure rate in patients with low-risk GTN. Likewise, methotrexate plus leucovorin induces remission in 90% of patients with low-risk metastatic disease with low toxicity. GOG conducted two phase II trials; both showed that a single dose of dactinomycin (Cosmegen) every other week (GOG0069) or weekly IM methotrexate (GOG0079) had good compliance, comparable activity, and tolerable toxicity. The use of dactinomycin in methotrexate-resistant patients increased the cure rate to more than 95%. The first prospective multicenter phase II trial of salvage therapy for failed low-risk GTN, GOG0176, found that pulse actinomycin D (1.24 mg/m^2 IV every 2 weeks) is an active regimen.

High-risk metastatic disease

The discovery that etoposide is an effective agent against trophoblastic disease led to the development of the EMA-CO regimen (etoposide, methotrexate, actinomycin D [dactinomycin], cyclophosphamide, Oncovin [vincristine]), with a reported survival rate of 83% in patients with high-risk choriocarcinoma.

EMA-CO is the preferred regimen for high-risk GTN. This regimen is also used for patients with middle-risk GTN, as defined by the FIGO 2000 criteria. EMA-CO is generally well tolerated, with no life-threatening toxic effects. Alopecia occurs universally, and anemia, neutropenia, and stomatitis are mild. Reproductive function is preserved in approximately 75% of patients.

Within hours of receiving chemotherapy, patients with a significant tumor burden are at risk of hemorrhage into tumors and surrounding tissues. Thus, any acute organ toxicity that begins shortly after the induction of chemotherapy should be considered as possibly related to this phenomenon. Some researchers have advocated a reduction in dosage at the beginning of therapy in patients with large-volume disease to minimize these sequelae.

Salvage therapy

Unfortunately, about 25% of women with high-risk metastatic disease become refractory to EMA-CO and fail to achieve a complete remission. Currently, there is no standard salvage chemotherapy regimen for patients not responding to EMA-CO. However, salvage regimens that combine cisplatin, etoposide, vinca alkaloids, and bleomycin have been administered.

Early studies show cisplatin-based regimens to be an effective salvage therapy in GTD. A recent dose-intensive regimen, EMA-CE, utilizes cisplatin (100 mg/m²) and etoposide (200 mg/m²) combined with EMA, with favorable results.

Another alternative is to give cisplatin in the EMA-POMB regimen (Platinol [cisplatin], Oncovin [vincristine], methotrexate, bleomycin). POMB is administered as vincristine, 1 mg/m² IV, and methotrexate, 300 mg/m² IV (day 1); bleomycin, 15 mg IV over 24 hours by continuous infusion (CI), and folinic acid, 15 mg twice daily for four doses (day 2); bleomycin, 15 mg IV over a 24-hour CI (day 3); and cisplatin, 120 mg/m² IV (day 4).

A new PEBA regimen (Platinol [cisplatin], etoposide, bleomycin, Adriamycin [doxorubicin]) was reported from China and was found to be effective in EMA-CO–resistant disease. A complete remission was achieved in 96% of the women, and 73% had a sustained complete remission that lasted at least 1 year. In a small study, ifosfamide alone and combined in the VIP regimen (VePesid [etoposide], ifosfamide, and Platinol [cisplatin]) showed promise as being an effective salvage drug in GTD. The experience of the Brewer Trophoblastic Disease Center in patients with persistent or recurrent high-risk GTN showed that those who develop resistance to methotrexate-containing treatment protocols should be treated with drug combinations employing a platinum agent and etoposide with or without bleomycin or ifosfamide.

Another consideration in the treatment of refractory GTN is the use of high-dose chemotherapy with autologous bone marrow transplantation.

SUGGESTED READING

ON ENDOMETRIAL CANCER

ASTEC/EN.5 Study Group, Blake P, Swart AM, et al: Adjuvant external beam radiotherapy in the treatment of endometrial cancer (MRC ASTEC and NCIC CTG EN.5 randomised trials): Pooled trial results, systematic review, and meta-analysis. Lancet 373:137-146, 2009.

Blake P, Swart AM, Orton J, et al: Adjuvant external beam radiotherapy in the treatment of endometrial cancer (MRC ASTEC and NCIC CTG EN.5 randomised trials): Pooled trial results, systematic review, and meta-analysis. Lancet 373:137–146, 2009.

Benedetti Panici P, Basile S, Maneschi F, et al: Systematic pelvic lymphadenectomy vs no lymphadenectomy in early-stage endometrial carcinoma: Randomized clinical trial. J Natl Cancer Inst 100:1707–1716, 2008.

Homesley HD, Filiaci V, Gibbons SK, et al: A randomized phase III trial in advanced endometrial carcinoma of surgery and volume directed radiation followed by cisplatin and doxorubicin with or without paclitaxel: A Gynecologic Oncology Group study. Gynecol Oncol 112:543–552, 2009.

Jemal A, Siegel R, Xu J, et al: Cancer statistics, 2010. CA Cancer J Clin 60:277–300, 2010.

Kitchener H, Swart AM, Qian Q, et al, on behalf of the ASTEC Study Group: Efficacy of systematic pelvic lymphadenectomy in endometrial cancer (MRC ASTEC trial): A randomised study. Lancet 373:125–136, 2009.

Kornblith AB, Huang HQ, Walker JL, et al: Quality of life of patients with endometrial cancer undergoing laparoscopic international federation of gynecology and obstetrics staging compared with laparotomy: A Gynecologic Oncology Group study. J Clin Oncol 27:5337–5342, 2009.

Maxwell GL, Tian C, Risinger JI, et al: Racial disparities in recurrence among patients with early-stage endometrial cancer: Is recurrence increased in black patients who receive estrogen replacement therapy? Cancer 113:1431–1437, 2008.

Miller DS, Fleming G, Randall ME, et al: Chemo- and radiotherapy in adjuvant management of optimally debulked endometrial cancer. J Natl Compr Canc Netw 7:535–541, 2009.

Nout RA, Putter H, Jurgenliemk-Schulz IM, et al: Quality of life after pelvic radiotherapy or vaginal brachytherapy for endometrial cancer: First results of the randomized PORTEC-2 trial. J Clin Oncol 27:3547–3556, 2009.

Nout RA, Smit VT, Putter H, et al: Vaginal brachytherapy versus pelvic external beam radiotherapy for patients with endometrial cancer of high-intermediate risk (PORTEC-2): An open-label, non-inferiority, randomised trial. Lancet 375:816-823, 2010.

Pecorelli S: Revised FIGO staging for carcinoma of the vulva, cervix, and endometrium. Int J Gynaecol Obstet 105:103–104, 2009.

Pectasides D, Xiros N, Papaxoinis G, et al: Carboplatin and paclitaxel in advanced or metastatic endometrial cancer. Gynecol Oncol 109:250–254, 2008.

Susumu N, Sagae S, Udagawa Y, et al: Randomized phase III trial of pelvic radiotherapy versus cisplatin-based combined chemotherapy in patients with intermediate- and high-risk endometrial cancer: A Japanese Gynecologic Oncology Group study. Gynecol Oncol 108:226–233, 2008.

Walker JL, Piedmonte MR, Spirtos NM, et al: Laparoscopy compared with laparotomy for comprehensive surgical staging of uterine cancer: Gynecologic Oncology Group Study. J Clin Oncol Oct 5, 2009 [Epub ahead of print].

ON GESTATIONAL TROPHOBLASTIC DISEASES

Hoekstra AV, Lurain JR, Rademaker AW, et al: Gestational trophoblastic neoplasia: Treatment outcomes. Obstet Gynecol 112:251–258, 2008.

Lurain JR, Hoekstra AV, Schink JC: Results of treatment of patients with gestational trophoblastic neoplasia referred to the Brewer Trophoblastic Disease Center after failure of treatment elsewhere (1979-2006). J Reprod Med 53:535–540, 2008.

ON UTERINE SARCOMAS

Hensley ML, Blessing JA, Mannel R, et al: Fixed-dose rate gemcitabine plus docetaxel as first-line therapy for metastatic uterine leiomyosarcoma: A Gynecologic Oncology Group phase II trial. Gynecol Oncol 109:329–334, 2008.

Homesley HD, Filiaci V, Markman M, et al: Phase III trial of ifosfamide with or without paclitaxel in advanced uterine carcinosarcoma: A Gyncologic Oncology Group Study. J Clin Oncol 25:526–531, 2007.

Kapp DS, Shin JY, Chan JK: Prognostic factors and survival in 1396 patients with uterine leiomyosarcomas: Emphasis on impact of lymphadenectomy and oophorectomy. Cancer 112:820–830, 2008.

Makker V, Abu-Rustum NR, Alektiar KM, et al: A retrospective assessment of outcomes of chemotherapy-based versus radiation-only adjuvant treatment for completely resected stage I-IV uterine carcinosarcoma. Gynecol Oncol 111:249–254, 2008.

Reed NS, Mangioni C, Malmstrom H, et al: Phase III randomised study to evaluate the role of adjuvant pelvic radiotherapy in the treatment of uterine sarcomas stages I and II: An European Organisation for Research and Treatment of Cancer Gynaecological Cancer Group Study (protocol 55874). Eur J Cancer 44:808–818, 2008.

Abbreviations in this chapter

ACS = American Cancer Society; ASTEC = Adjuvant External-Beam Radiotherapy in the Treatment of Endometrial Cancer; FIGO = International Federation of Gynecologists and Obstetricians; GOG = Gynecologic Oncology Group; JGOG = Japanese Gynecologic Oncology Group; MRC = Medical Research Council; NCIC = National Cancer Institute of Cancer; NSABP = National Surgical Adjuvant Breast and Bowel Project; PORTEC = Postoperative Radiation Therapy in Endometrial Carcinoma; RTOG = Radiation Therapy Oncology Group; WAI = whole abdominal irradiation

CHAPTER 19

Ovarian cancer

Stephen C. Rubin, MD, Paul Sabbatini, MD,
and Akila N. Viswanathan, MD, MPH

Despite the fact that it is highly curable if diagnosed early, ovarian cancer causes more mortality in American women each year than all other gynecologic malignancies combined. An estimated 21,880 new cases of this cancer will be diagnosed in the United States in 2010, and about 13,850 women will succumb to the disease.

Notable advances in chemotherapy and surgery over the past several decades have begun to translate into improved survival. According to American Cancer Society data, the overall 5-year survival rate from ovarian cancer has increased significantly, from 37% in the mid-1970s to 46% in the mid-2000s ($P < .05$). Recent data from the National Cancer Institute show a similar increase in stage-specific survival. It is expected that data from the current decade, reflecting continued improvements in chemotherapy and surgery, will continue this trend.

This chapter will focus on epithelial cancers of the ovaries, which account for about 90% of ovarian malignancies.

EPIDEMIOLOGY

Age Ovarian cancer is primarily a disease of postmenopausal women, with the large majority of cases occurring in women between 50 and 75 years old. The incidence of ovarian cancer increases with age and peaks at a rate of 61.5 per 100,000 women in the 75–79-year-old age group.

Race The incidence of ovarian cancer appears to vary by race, although the effects of race are difficult to separate from those of environment related to culture, geography, and socioeconomic status. In the United States, the age-adjusted rate of ovarian cancer for Caucasians is estimated to be 17.9 per 100,000 population, which is significantly higher than 11.9 per 100,000 for the African-American population.

Geography There are distinct geographic variations in the incidence of ovarian cancer, with the highest rates found in industrialized countries and the lowest rates seen in underdeveloped nations. Japan, with an incidence of only about 3.0 per 100,000 population, is a notable exception to this observation. It has been postulated that geographic variations in the incidence of ovarian cancer are related, in part, to differences in family size.

Some of the highest rates are seen in women of Eastern European Jewish ancestry, who have an estimated incidence of 17.2 per 100,000 population, a probable result of the relatively high frequency of *BRCA1* and *BRCA2* mutations in this population.

ETIOLOGY AND RISK FACTORS

The cause of epithelial ovarian cancer remains unknown. Although it now appears certain that, at the cellular level, ovarian cancer results from the accumulation of multiple discrete genetic defects, the mechanism(s) by which these defects develop have yet to be determined. Epidemiologic studies have identified a number of factors that may increase or decrease the risk of the disease. In addition, a small proportion of ovarian cancers in the United States, approximately 5% to 10%, result from inherited defects in the *BRCA1* gene or other genes, including *BRCA2* and the hereditary nonpolyposis colorectal cancer *(HNPCC)* genes.

Diet It has been suggested that numerous dietary factors increase the risk of ovarian cancer, although the magnitude of the reported increase is relatively modest.

A low-fat diet may reduce the incidence of ovarian cancer among postmenopausal women.

Populations with a high dietary intake of lactose who lack the enzyme galactose-1-phosphate uridyltransferase have been reported to be at increased risk.

Conflicting reports have been published regarding the role of coffee consumption and the risk of ovarian cancer.

Environmental factors Various environmental risk factors also have been suggested.

Exposure to talc (hydrous magnesium trisilicate) used as dusting powder on diaphragms and sanitary napkins has been reported in some studies to increase the risk of ovarian cancer, although other studies have failed to find an association.

No association between exposure to ionizing radiation and the risk of ovarian cancer has been documented.

Several studies have examined the effect of viral agents, including mumps, rubella, and influenza viruses, on the risk of ovarian cancer. No clear relationship has been demonstrated.

Physical activity may decrease the risk of ovarian cancer.

Hormonal and reproductive factors In contrast to the conflicting data on dietary and environmental factors, some clear associations have been drawn between certain hormonal and reproductive factors and the risk of developing ovarian cancer.

Several analyses have documented that women with a history of low parity or involuntary infertility are at increased risk of ovarian cancer.

Tubal ligation significantly decreases the risk of ovarian cancer, as demonstrated by several epidemiologic studies.

Evidence suggests that treatment with ovulation-inducing drugs, particularly for prolonged periods, may be a risk factor, although it is difficult to separate the increased risk related to the infertility itself from the risk carried by use of ovulation-inducing agents.

Breastfeeding for long durations may decrease ovarian cancer risk.

Although the data are not consistent, some studies have shown an association between the use of postmenopausal hormone replacement and the development of ovarian cancer. Data from the Women's Health Initiative randomized trial of estrogen plus progestin showed a slight increase in the risk of ovarian cancer in users of hormone replacement therapy, although it was not statistically significant.

Several large case-controlled studies have documented a marked protective effect of oral contraceptives against ovarian cancer. Women who have used oral contraceptives for at least several years have approximately half the risk of ovarian cancer as do nonusers, and the protective effect of oral contraceptives appears to persist for years after their discontinuation. It is estimated that the routine use of oral contraceptives may prevent nearly 2,000 cases of ovarian cancer yearly in the United States. Evidence suggests that the protective effect of oral contraceptives also applies to women carrying *BRCA* mutations.

Hereditary cancer syndromes There has been a fascinating evolution in our understanding of the role of hereditary factors in the development of ovarian cancer. It has been recognized for many years that women with a family history of cancer, particularly cancer of the ovaries or breasts, are themselves at increased risk of ovarian cancer. In the 1980s, Lynch and colleagues refined these observations by delineating several apparently distinct syndromes of hereditary cancer involving the ovaries, including breast-ovarian cancer syndrome, site-specific ovarian cancer syndrome, and Lynch II syndrome (HNPCC).

Epidemiologically, these syndromes appear to be inherited as an autosomal-dominant trait with variable penetrance. During the past decade, the specific genes responsible for HNPCC (*MSH1* and *MLH2*) and for most cases of hereditary ovarian cancer have been identified, allowing fundamental observations to be made regarding their molecular pathophysiology.

The *BRCA1* gene is classified as a tumor suppressor, since mutations in this gene increase the risk of breast and ovarian cancers. Definitive identification of the function of the protein translated from this gene remains to be elucidated, although evidence suggests that it plays a role in the repair of oxidative damage to DNA. Part of the protein appears to contain a DNA-binding domain, suggesting that it also functions as a transcriptional regulator.

The frequency of *BRCA1* mutations in the general population is estimated at approximately 1 in 800, and in Jewish women of Eastern European descent, 1 in 100.

Women carrying a germline mutation of *BRCA1* have a significantly elevated risk of both breast and ovarian cancers compared with the general population. The average population risk of developing breast cancer is about 12.5% (one in eight) and of developing ovarian cancer, 1.5%. However, in the presence of a germline *BRCA1* mutation and a strong family history of cancer, these risks rise to about 90% and 40% for breast and ovarian cancers, respectively.

It is important to recognize that these risk estimates are derived from families identified with multiple cases of breast and/or ovarian cancer. The risk for women with *BRCA1* mutations from families with less impressive family histories is probably lower for ovarian cancer, perhaps in the range of 15% to 20%.

Although the presence of germline mutations in *BRCA1* is not limited to women with a strong family history of breast cancer, data from several laboratories suggest that

BRCA1 mutations usually are not a feature of sporadic ovarian cancer. Mutations in this gene appear to play a role in the development of approximately 50% of familial breast cancer cases and may account for the majority of hereditary ovarian cancers. Evidence from multiple studies suggests that *BRCA1*-related ovarian cancers may have a less aggressive clinical course than do sporadic ovarian cancers.

Hereditary ovarian cancers not related to *BRCA1* are most often related to mutations in the *BRCA2* gene.

For patients having a *BRCA1* or *BRCA2* mutation, laparoscopic prophylactic risk-reducing salpingo-oophorectomy after childbearing can reduce the risk of both breast and ovarian carcinomas.

SIGNS AND SYMPTOMS

Early-stage disease In the early stages, ovarian cancer may be an insidious disease, but nonspecific symptoms that may be clues to the diagnosis are present more often than previously thought. A case-controlled series by Goff et al proposed that a symptom index could be devised which might suggest a diagnosis of ovarian cancer. It was based on the presence of any of the following symptoms more than 12 times in a given month, but with overall duration less than 1 year. When these criteria were met, the specificity for a diagnosis of ovarian cancers was 90% for women > 50 years of age.The symptoms were pelvic/abdominal pain, urinary frequency, increased abdominal size, and difficulty eating (feeling full). This illustrates the diffuse nature of ovarian cancer symptoms, and taken alone will not yield early diagnosis in most patients. Thus, more than 70% of patients with ovarian cancer will present with disease beyond the confines of the ovaries at initial diagnosis.

The impact of screening patients with serum CA-125 levels and transvaginal ultrasonography on mortality is being addressed in the PLCO Trial. In this study, 39,115 women were randomized to undergo screening. To date, screening has identified both early- and late-stage cancers, and the predictive value is low (3.7% for abnormal CA-125 levels, 1.0% for abnormal transvaginal ultrasonography, and 23.5% for both). Follow-up is ongoing to determine whether there is an effect on mortality.

Early ovarian cancer also may be detected as a pelvic mass noted fortuitously at the time of a routine pelvic examination. Imaging with sonography, CT, or MRI will confirm the presence of a mass. The size, internal architecture, and blood flow of the mass can be used to make an educated guess as to whether it is benign or malignant, but imaging findings are not diagnostic in this regard. Approximately 50% of patients with early ovarian cancers have an elevated serum CA-125 level.

Advanced-stage disease Patients may complain of abdominal bloating or swelling if ascites is present, and large pelvic masses may produce bladder or rectal symptoms. Occasional patients may have respiratory distress as a result of a large pleural effusion, which is more common on the right side. Infrequently, there may be a history of abnormal vaginal bleeding.

Most patients with advanced disease have ascites detectable by physical examination or imaging. Complex pelvic masses and an omental tumor cake may be present, and nodules can frequently be palpated in the pelvic cul-de-sac on rectovaginal examination. It should be noted that some patients with advanced ovarian cancer have essentially normal-sized ovaries. Approximately 80% of patients with advanced ovarian cancer will have an elevated serum CA-125 level.

SCREENING AND DIAGNOSIS

Screening Unfortunately, no effective strategy exists for screening of the general population for ovarian cancer. Imaging techniques, including abdominal and transvaginal sonography, have been studied extensively, as has the serum marker CA-125. None of these techniques, alone or in combination, is specific enough to serve as an appropriate screening test, even in populations targeted by age.

Both the National Institutes of Health Consensus Conference (see full page of NIH guidelines) and the American College of Obstetricians and Gynecologists have issued statements advising against routine screening for ovarian cancer, which, due to its high false-positive rate, leads to an unacceptable amount of invasive interventions in women without significant disease.

The NIH PLCO Screening Trial accrued its full complement of 152,000 patients in 2001. For the ovarian cancer segment of the trial, half of the women are being screened via physical examination, CA-125 level, and vaginal ultrasonography, and the other half, via standard medical care. Since patients will be followed for 13 years or more, final results are not yet available. It is not expected that these screening modalities will have a significant impact on the general population.

Recent studies using serum proteomics to screen for early ovarian cancer have yielded disappointing results. Work in this area is ongoing and may result in a clinically useful assay.

Management of women from families with hereditary ovarian cancer is controversial. Evidence suggests that surveillance of such women with serum markers and sonography is of limited benefit in early detection of ovarian cancer. Most experts recommend prophylactic laparoscopic excision of the ovaries and fallopian tubes after age 35 if the woman has completed childbearing, as several studies have shown that it will dramatically reduce the risk of ovarian cancer. Evidence also suggests that prophylactic oophorectomy substantially lowers the risk of breast cancer in women from high-risk families.

In September 2009, the FDA approved a test called OVA1 as an adjunct to other clinical and radiographic tests to help detect ovarian cancer. OVA1 uses a blood sample to test for levels of five proteins that change due to ovarian cancer. The test combines the five separate results into a single numerical score between 0 and 10 to indicate the likelihood that a pelvic mass known to require surgery is benign or malignant. Approval of OVA1 was based on the FDA's review of a study of 516 patients that compared OVA1 results with biopsy results. A total of 269 of these patients were evaluated by non-gynecologic oncologists. Results of the study also indicated that OVA1 may help identify patients who might benefit from referral to a gynecologic oncologist. The study was presented earlier in 2009 at a meeting of the Society of Gynecologic Oncologists *(Ueland F et al: Gynecol Oncol 116[suppl 1]:S23, 2010)*.

Patients with suspected ovarian cancer should undergo a thorough evaluation prior to surgery. This assessment should include a complete history and physical examination and serum CA-125 level determination. In women younger than age 30, determinations of β-human chorionic gonadotropin (β-hCG) and α-fetoprotein (AFP) levels are useful, as germ-cell tumors are more common in this age group.

Abdominal CT and MRI In apparent early-stage cases, abdominal scanning by CT or MRI adds little to the diagnostic evaluation, and, thus, these studies are not routinely necessary. CT and MRI may be useful in providing a preoperative assessment of disease extent in probable advanced-stage cases.

Exploratory laparotomy The diagnosis of ovarian cancer is generally made by histopathologic study following exploratory laparotomy. The stage of the disease can only be determined by surgery, as discussed later.

Preoperative endometrial sampling Women with abnormal vaginal bleeding should undergo preoperative endometrial sampling.

Preoperative cytologic or histologic evaluation of effusions or tumor masses is neither necessary nor desirable. Often, patients with ascites and large pelvic masses, for whom exploration is necessary, are subjected to paracentesis or needle biopsy. These procedures only delay definitive management and may lead to seeding of tumor cells along needle tracks.

PATHOLOGY

The ovaries are notable for their ability to give rise to a large variety of neoplasms with distinct embryologic origins and differing histologic appearances.

Epithelial adenocarcinoma Approximately 90% of all ovarian malignancies are of epithelial origin, arising from the cells on the surface of the ovaries. These cells give rise to a variety of adenocarcinomas, including serous, mucinous, endometrioid, and clear-cell types. These tumors have benign counterparts of similar histologic appearance and can also exist as "borderline" cancers, also known as "tumors of low malignant potential." There is some prognostic significance to the cell type of the tumor, with clear-cell and mucinous varieties tending to be especially virulent.

Pathologists also classify adenocarcinomas according to the degree of histologic differentiation. Those tumors retaining clear-cut glandular features are considered grade 1, or well differentiated, whereas those that are largely composed of solid sheets of tumor are considered grade 3, or poorly differentiated. Tumors showing both glandular and solid areas are assigned to grade 2. The histologic grade seems to correlate roughly with biologic aggressiveness.

Stromal and germ-cell tumors Malignancies can also arise from the ovarian stroma or the primordial germ cells contained within the ovaries. Stromal tumors are often hormone-producing and include such types as the granulosa tumor, Sertoli-Leydig tumor, and several variants. Germ-cell tumors, which tend to be highly aggressive, include the dysgerminoma, endodermal sinus tumor, malignant teratoma, embryonal carcinoma, and rare primary choriocarcinoma of the ovaries. Malignant germ-cell tumors occur primarily in younger patients, with an average age at diagnosis of about 19 years.

NIH GUIDELINES ON SCREENING FOR OVARIAN CANCER

Until clinical trials gather enough information, no evidence supports routine screening for ovarian cancer in women without first-degree relatives affected by the disease, according to a consensus development panel convened by the NIH.

The panel did recommend that physicians take a comprehensive family history of their female patients. The panel also advised women to undergo routine annual rectovaginal pelvic examinations.

There are no conclusive data that screening is beneficial, even for women with two or more first-degree relatives with ovarian cancer, the panel stated. However, these women have a significant chance of having a hereditary ovarian cancer syndrome and should be counseled by a gynecologic oncologist or other qualified specialist regarding their individual risk.

Patients with hereditary ovarian cancer syndrome

Patients with hereditary ovarian cancer syndrome (assuming autosomal-dominant inheritance with 80% penetrance) have a 40% lifetime risk of developing ovarian cancer. Recent data suggest that screening these women reduces their mortality from ovarian cancer.

High-risk women

The three known hereditary syndromes that place a woman at exceedingly high risk are familial site-specific ovarian cancer syndrome, breast-ovarian cancer syndrome, and breast-ovarian-endometrial-colorectal cancer syndrome. Annual rectovaginal pelvic examinations, CA-125 level determinations, and transvaginal ultrasonography are recommended for these women until their childbearing is completed or until age 35, at which time prophylactic bilateral oophorectomy is recommended.

Prophylactic oophorectomy performed in women undergoing abdominal surgery for other indications, such as benign uterine disease, is also associated with a significant reduction in the risk of ovarian cancer. The appropriateness of hormonal replacement therapy is not straightforward, given that many of these women are at higher risk for breast cancer. In addition, the report from the study by the Women's Health Initiative in postmenopausal women raised questions regarding the role of long-term hormonal replacement, particularly showing no benefit in terms of cardiovascular risk reduction. Women should discuss the potential for estrogen replacement vs other agents for the prevention of osteoporosis, for example, with their healthcare provider.

Other panel recommendations

Women with ovarian masses who have been identified preoperatively as having a significant risk of ovarian cancer should be advised to have their surgery performed by a gynecologic oncologist.

Aggressive attempts at cytoreductive surgery as the primary management of ovarian cancer will improve the chances for long-term survival.

Women with stages IA and IB, grade 1 ovarian cancer do not require postoperative adjuvant therapy, although many remaining patients with stage I disease do require chemotherapy. Subsets of stage I must be fully defined and ideal treatment determined.

Second-look laparotomy should not be employed as routine care for all patients but should be performed for patients enrolled in clinical trials or for patients in whom the surgery will affect clinical decision-making and the clinical course.

From Ovarian cancer: Screening, treatment and follow-up. NIH Consensus Statement. 12:1–30, 1994 ; US Preventive Services Task Force. Screening for ovarian cancer: Recommendation statement. May 2004. Agency for Healthcare Research and Quality, Rockville, MD. http://www.ahrq.gov/clinic/3rduspstf/ovariancan/ovcanrs.htm

TABLE 1: FIGO staging system for ovarian cancer

Stage	Characteristics
I	Growth limited to the ovaries
IA	Growth limited to one ovary; no ascites; no tumor on the external surfaces, capsule intact
IB	Growth limited to both ovaries; no ascites; no tumor on the external surfaces, capsule intact
IC	Tumor either stage IA or IB but on the surface of one or both ovaries; capsule ruptured; ascites-containing malignant cells present; or positive peritoneal washings
II	Growth involving one or both ovaries with pelvic extension of disease
IIA	Extension of disease and/or metastases to the uterus and/or fallopian tubes
IIB	Extension of disease to other pelvic tissues
IIC	Tumor either stage IIA or IIB but on the surface of one or both ovaries; capsule(s) ruptured; ascites-containing malignant cells present; or positive peritoneal washings
III	Tumor involving one or both ovaries with peritoneal implants outside the pelvis and/or positive retroperitoneal or inguinal nodes; superficial liver metastasis equals stage III; tumor is limited to the true pelvis but with histologically verified malignant extension to the small bowel or omentum
IIIA	Tumor grossly limited to the true pelvis with negative nodes but with histologically confirmed microscopic seeding of abdominal peritoneal surfaces
IIIB	Tumor of one or both ovaries; histologically confirmed implants on abdominal peritoneal surfaces, none > 2 cm in diameter; nodes negative
IIIC	Abdominal implants > 2 cm in diameter and/or positive retroperitoneal or inguinal nodes
IV	Growth involving one or both ovaries with distant metastases; if pleural effusion is present, there must be positive cytologic test results to allot a case to stage IV; parenchymal liver metastasis equals stage IV

FIGO = International Federation of Gynecology and Obstetrics

STAGING AND PROGNOSIS

Staging system

The staging system for ovarian cancer shown in Table 1, developed by the International Federation of Gynecology and Obstetrics (FIGO), is used uniformly in all developed countries. It is based on the results of a properly performed exploratory laparotomy, a fact that bears emphasis, since inadequate surgical staging has been and continues to be a significant problem.

Surgical staging The surgical staging of ovarian cancer is based on an understanding of the patterns of disease spread and must be conducted in a systematic and thorough manner. It should include a complete evaluation of all visceral and parietal surfaces within the peritoneal cavity, omentectomy, and biopsy of aortic and pelvic

TABLE 2: Procedures for surgical staging for apparent early ovarian cancer

Appropriate incision
Multiple cytologic washings
Intact tumor removal
Complete abdominal exploration
Removal of remaining ovaries, uterus, fallopian tubes[a]
Omentectomy
Lymph node sampling
Random peritoneal biopsies, including the diaphragm

[a] May be preserved in selected patients who wish to preserve fertility

lymph nodes. It generally includes removal of the internal reproductive organs as well, although exceptions to this rule can be made for younger women with limited disease who may wish to retain fertility.

The issue of adequate surgical staging becomes particularly acute in just the patient population likely to be operated upon by individuals with no specialized training in gynecologic oncology: patients with adnexal masses that are not obvious cancers on preoperative evaluation. At the time of exploration, if the mass is shown to be malignant on frozen section and there is no obvious metastatic disease, a complete staging operation is essential to search for occult metastatic spread, which may be present in 20% to 30% of such cases. Also, if the tumor is documented to be stage IA by thorough staging and the patient wishes to preserve the potential for future fertility, it may be appropriate to conserve the uterus and uninvolved ovaries and fallopian tubes.

The elements of surgical staging for apparent early ovarian cancer are listed in Table 2.

Prognostic factors

The prognosis of epithelial ovarian cancer depends on a number of factors.

Disease stage Of primary importance is the disease stage, which, when properly determined, is of strong prognostic significance. The distribution of ovarian cancer cases by stage follows: stage I, 26%; stage II, 15%; stage III, 42%; stage IV, 17%. For patients with advanced ovarian cancer, the amount of residual tumor at the conclusion of the initial operation is of major importance. Patients with stage III disease who have minimal or no residual tumor may have a 30% to 50% chance of 5-year survival, whereas those patients with stage III disease left with bulky tumor masses have a 5-year survival rate of only about 10%.

Histologic grade and type Most studies have found the histologic grade of the tumor to have prognostic significance; the histologic cell type of the tumor is of less importance, although patients with clear-cell and possibly mucinous tumors may have a worse prognosis.

Molecular markers In recent years, a great deal of effort has been devoted to the identification of molecular markers of prognosis in ovarian cancer. Studies of HER2, *p53, ras*, and other oncogenes and tumor-suppressor genes have had varying results relative to prognostic significance. Currently, the assessment of molecular markers is ongoing in numerous studies in the hope of identifying clinically relevant targets that are susceptible to available agents. The continued progress in developing high-throughput techniques for determining gene and protein expression increases the likelihood that good candidates will be found.

Predictors of chemosensitivity Despite a continued effort to assess in vitro methods to predict the sensitivity or resistance of ovarian cancers to various chemotherapeutic drugs, the clinical usefulness of such an approach remains under investigation. The American Society of Clinical Oncology (ASCO) recently reviewed the relevant literature on the subject and reached the same conclusion for cancers in general.

TREATMENT

Surgery plays a crucial role in all phases of the management of ovarian cancer and, when applied as part of a multidisciplinary approach, affords patients the highest likelihood of a favorable outcome. For most patients with ovarian carcinoma, surgery is not curative due to dissemination of tumor cells throughout the abdominal cavity. Therefore, successful management generally requires additional treatment.

The use of postoperative chemotherapy is standard for all patients with advanced-stage disease and for many patients with early-stage disease. Adjunctive chemotherapy significantly prolongs survival, with most current data supporting the use of platinum- and taxane-based regimens.

Despite a long history of the use of radiation therapy in ovarian carcinoma, due to the relatively high sensitivity of ovarian cancer to radiation in general, opinions on indications for its use differ widely. Presumably, this controversy is due to the limited amount and adequacy of data comparing radiotherapy with modern chemotherapy regimens, as well as concerns regarding potential toxicities. Studies using radiation in both radical and palliative settings have been published, but standardization of the use of radiation varies significantly worldwide.

MANAGEMENT OF EARLY-STAGE DISEASE

Clearly, comprehensive surgical staging is necessary to properly identify patients with stages I and II ovarian carcinoma. Beyond surgery, the need for adjuvant treatment with chemotherapy has been recently supported, with the exception of patients with stage I disease and well-differentiated histology.

Surgery

Suspicious adnexal masses should be excised intact and submitted for frozen section. If a malignancy is confirmed and there is no obvious metastatic spread, complete surgical staging should be undertaken. As discussed previously (see section on "Staging and prognosis"), it is of critical importance that surgical staging be performed systematically and completely. Inadequate staging may result in inappropriate postoperative treatment, which can severely compromise the chances for cure.

Data from the American College of Surgeons community hospital-based tumor registry show that almost 75% of the primary surgeries for ovarian cancer performed in this country are done so without the involvement of a gynecologic oncologist. This finding is unfortunate given the fact that, with physical examination, measurement of CA-125 levels, and appropriate imaging tests, the majority of cases of ovarian cancer can be identified preoperatively. Results from other studies suggest that when a gynecologic oncologist is not present at the initial operation, staging is more often inadequate, cytoreduction is more often suboptimal, and long-term survival is poorer.

Conservation of reproductive organs In a woman of reproductive age with cancer limited to one ovary, it may be possible to conserve the uterus and opposite fallopian tube and ovary if she wishes to maintain the option of future fertility. To facilitate such intraoperative decision-making, it is essential that the surgeon's preoperative discussion with the patient and her family address the possibility of malignancy and review the surgical options for both benign and malignant diseases.

Operative laparoscopy Recent advances in the instrumentation for operative laparoscopy have led to an increase in the proportion of adnexal masses being managed with this technique. Physicians should exercise caution in selecting patients with adnexal masses for operative laparoscopic approaches. Unless the surgeon's laparoscopic skills are extraordinary, suspicious masses are best managed by laparotomy. For masses that are approached laparoscopically, the same surgical principles of removal without spill and complete surgical staging apply.

Systemic chemotherapy for early-stage disease

The current management of patients with early-stage disease focuses on comprehensive surgical staging and the identification of high-risk features. Patients with stage IA or IB tumors with well-differentiated histology have excellent 5-year survival rates, and adjuvant chemotherapy is generally not used in such patients. High-risk features include moderately to poorly differentiated tumors, stage IC or II disease, and clear-cell histology.

The reported survival rates of 60% to 80% in patients who have early-stage tumors with high-risk features suggested a potential role for adjuvant therapy. The IICG conducted two randomized trials to evaluate the role of adjuvant therapy in patients with stage I disease. The first trial compared cisplatin, 50 mg/m^2 q28d × 6, with observation in 85 patients with stage IA or IB, grade 2–3 disease. The 5-year disease-free survival rate was higher in patients treated with cisplatin than in those who were observed (83% vs 63%), but the 5-year overall survival rate was similar in the two groups (88% vs 82%).

The second trial compared cisplatin (same dose) to phosphorus-32 (P-32) administration in 161 patients with stages IA–IB, grade 2, or stage IC disease. The 5-year disease-free survival rate again favored the platinum arm (85% vs 65%), but the 5-year overall survival rate was unchanged and similar to that reported in the previous trial. P-32 administration was associated with more long-term toxicity.

More recent data have provided support for a survival benefit to the immediate use of adjuvant chemotherapy in patients with early-stage disease. The results of the EORTC–ACTION trial and the ICON1 trial were combined and reported. A 5-year survival rate improvement of 8% was reported for those receiving immediate chemotherapy compared with reserving chemotherapy for those who relapsed (74% vs 82%; 95% CI: 2%–12%).

Improvements in systemic chemotherapy for advanced ovarian cancer with associated improvements in survival are relevant to the design of regimens for early-stage disease. GOG 157 evaluated 3 vs 6 cycles of paclitaxel and carboplatin in patients with stage IA or IB, grade 2–3; stage IC; or stage II disease. The trial completed accrual in 1995, and final results showed no significant benefit to the longer regimen. The GOG replacement trial evaluated 3 cycles of paclitaxel plus carboplatin with or without additional weekly paclitaxel (40 mg/m^2) in patients with early-stage disease. These data are reported in abstract form, but no benefit to extended-schedule paclitaxel was seen.

In the absence of additional data, taxane- and platinum-based systemic chemotherapy should be considered the standard approach for patients who have early-stage disease with the exception of well-staged IA or IB, grade 1 disease. The optimal number of cycles is currently unclear, but 3 cycles were considered the standard arm in the GOG 157 trial, although many clinicians offer 6 cycles of therapy in the absence of prohibitive toxicity.

Past GOG trials have established that patients with stages IA–IB, well-differentiated or moderately differentiated tumors have a 5-year survival rate of 90% to 98%, which does not seem to improve with adjuvant chemotherapy. However, patients with less favorable neoplasms by virtue of higher grade or stage have poorer outcomes (80% 5-year survival rate among treated patients).

Radiation therapy

Whole-abdominal irradiation A study by Hepp et al found whole-abdominal irradiation (WAI) to be an effective adjuvant therapy in patients with optimally debulked tumors. In a series of 60 patients, the 5-year survival rate was 55%, with a median follow-up of 96.5 months. Patients who received chemotherapy (n = 41) fared slightly worse than those who received radiation therapy only. The abdominal control rate was 83%, and the grade 3 and 4 late toxicity rates were 7% and 3%, respectively.

The findings indicate that 5- and 10-year survival rates obtained with WAI are at least equivalent to results obtained using modern systemic agents. However, in view of the recognized limitations of these trials, more rigorously gathered data will be required to establish the role of WAI in these patients.

MANAGEMENT OF ADVANCED DISEASE

Surgery

In the majority of cases, surgeons operating on patients with ovarian cancer find obvious evidence of widespread metastatic disease. Ascites is often present, with diffuse peritoneal tumor studding and extensive omental involvement. In such cases, it is still important to document the surgical stage (usually a substage of stage III) and carefully evaluate and describe the extent and location of tumor identified at both the beginning and conclusion of surgery.

Optimal cytoreduction The primary function of surgery in patients with advanced ovarian cancer is cytoreduction or debulking. When surgery is performed by experienced gynecologic cancer surgeons, at least 50% of patients with stage III ovarian cancer can be left with "optimal" residual tumor (ie, ≤ 1 cm). The morbidity associated with such surgery is low, and operative mortality is rare.

Patients with optimally debulked disease have an increased likelihood of achieving a complete clinical response to chemotherapy. Disease progression-free interval, median survival, and long-term survival are all improved in patients who have optimal cytoreduction.

Even among patients with suboptimal residual disease (> 1 cm) after primary surgery, those left with smaller tumor volumes (1 to 2 cm) have a survival advantage over those with a larger residuum. It is thus clear that aggressive surgical cytoreduction, if successful in reducing tumor to small volumes, improves several measures of outcome.

Interval cytoreduction In an EORTC trial, 299 patients with suboptimal advanced ovarian cancer were randomized to receive 6 cycles of cisplatin plus cyclophosphamide with or without interval surgical cytoreduction after the third cycle. Median survival for patients who underwent interval debulking surgery was 27 months, vs 19 months for patients who did not have interval debulking ($P = .01$). The GOG then completed a randomized trial of interval cytoreduction using a cisplatin-paclitaxel chemotherapy regimen. These results show no benefit for interval cytoreduction (median overall survival, 32 vs 33 months). Taxane-based chemotherapy and more standardized aggressive initial debulking by experienced gynecologic oncologists in the GOG trial have been offered as possible explanations for the discordant outcomes. If an aggressive initial surgical attempt is provided by a gynecologic oncologist, interval surgical cytoreduction cannot be routinely recommended.

Chemotherapy

Primary treatment The results of two randomized trials support a survival advantage for patients treated with combinations of IV platinum and paclitaxel, as compared with those given a platinum plus cyclophosphamide. McGuire et al found a 37- vs 24-month median survival advantage for the platinum-paclitaxel arm. Similarly, an analysis of the intergroup trial by Piccart et al showed an improvement in median survival from 25 to 35 months ($P = .001$) in favor of the paclitaxel arm. In contrast, the initial analysis of the ICON 3 trial evaluating a control arm (carboplatin or CAP [cyclophosphamide, Adriamycin (doxorubicin), Platinol (carboplatin)] chemotherapy) vs paclitaxel and carboplatin has failed to show a survival advantage for the taxane-containing arm. Many factors in the study have been proposed to explain this difference, and for the present, taxane- and platinum-based therapy remains the standard.

A randomized trial (GOG 158) comparing paclitaxel (175 mg/m^2 via a 3-hour infusion) plus carboplatin (dosed to achieve an area under the concentration-time curve [AUC] of 7.5) vs the standard regimen of paclitaxel (135 mg/m^2 via a 24-hour infusion) plus cisplatin (75 mg/m^2) in patients with optimally debulked disease showed the shorter schedule with carboplatin to be as effective as the older regimen. Due to its decreased toxicity and ease of administration, the shorter schedule with carboplatin is the preferred treatment.

Two GOG studies have indicated that the major survival benefit of cytoreductive surgery was in those patients who were optimally cytoreduced to no macroscopic residual disease.
In the first series, 1,895 patients with stage III disease received cisplatin and paclitaxel in standard IV regimens. Optimal cytoreduction to no macroscopic disease was achieved in 23%. This resulted in significantly better ($P < .001$) progression-free and overall survival rates (PFS = 33.0 months; OS = 71.9 months) vs patients with residual disease of 0.1 to 1 cm residual disease (PFS = 16.8 months; OS = 42.4 months) or residual disease greater than 1 cm (PFS = 14.1 months; OS = 35.0 months).
In a subsequent GOG report on 360 patients with stage IV disease who received cisplatin and paclitaxel in standard IV regimens, 8% were optimally cytoreduced to no macroscopic residual tumor, yielding a PFS of 20.1 months and an OS of 64.1 months. For those patients with residual disease less than or equal to 1 cm, or between 1.1 and 5 cm, PFS and OS rates were similar (PFS = 13.0 months in both groups; OS = 28.7 and 31 months, respectively; *Winter WE III et al: J Clin Oncol 25:3621–3627, 2007; Winter WE III et al: J Clin Oncol 26:83–89, 2008*).

In addition, the SCOTROC trial suggested that, as primary treatment, docetaxel (Taxotere) and paclitaxel have similar efficacy when combined with carboplatin and that docetaxel produces less neuropathy.

A five-arm international randomized study of primary therapy for patients with stage III or IV disease evaluated carboplatin and paclitaxel as the control arm and studied two triplets (carboplatin + paclitaxel with either gemcitabine [Gemzar] or liposomal doxorubicin [Doxil]) and two sequential doublets (topotecan [Hycamtin]/carboplatin + carboplatin/paclitaxel or carboplatin/gemcitabine + carboplatin/paclitaxel). No difference in progression-free or overall survival rates was seen among the arms, and therefore paclitaxel and carboplatin remains the standard. Based on the variety of phase III trials employing IV paclitaxel and carboplatin therapy following maximal surgical cytoreduction, the expected progression-free and overall survival rates of stage III patients follow: stage III optimal (progression-free survival, 21 to 28 months; overall survival, 52 to 57 months) and stage III suboptimal (progression-free survival, 18 months; overall survival, 38 months).

Neoadjuvant chemotherapy In patients with an inadequate performance status to undergo aggressive primary debulking, a "neoadjuvant" approach with paclitaxel and carboplatin is often considered for several cycles prior to a maximal cytoreductive effort. A large randomized trial reported by Vergote et al evaluated the use of neoadjuvant chemotherapy in 718 patients with stages IIIC–IV ovarian cancer. Patients were randomized to undergo primary debulking followed by 6 courses of paclitaxel and carboplatin chemotherapy (arm A) vs 3 courses of neoadjuvant chemotherapy, interval debulking, and then 3 additional courses (arm B). In the reported data in abstract form, median overall survival was 29 and 30 months for arms A and B, respectively (HR, 0.098; CI: 0.85–1.14); the median progression-free survival was 11 months in both arms (HR, 0.99; CI: 0.87–1.13). The overall survival in both arms was lower than expected, but there was no difference between them. The approach is still controversial, and most gynecologic oncologists still consider primary surgical debulking the standard of care, reserving neoadjuvant therapy only for those patients in whom primary optimal debulking will not be achieved. Further developments in this area will be forthcoming.

The role of bevacizumab in primary treatment Bevacizumab (Avastin) has shown activity in patients with recurrent ovarian cancer. Response rates of 16% and 21% have been reported when it is used as a single agent and of 24% when it is used in conjunction with oral cyclophosphamide. The progression-free intervals across trials range from 4.4 months to 7.2 months, and the median overall survival ranges from 10.7 months to 17 months. An important and large first-line chemotherapy trial was reported at ASCO 2010. This trial randomized patients with stages III and IV ovarian cancer following surgical debulking to receive paclitaxel and carboplatin + placebo followed by placebo maintenance (total therapy, 15 months), paclitaxel and carboplatin + bevacizumab followed by placebo maintenance, or paclitaxel and carboplatin + bevacizumab with bevacizumab maintenance. This trial evaluated toxicity, progression-free, and overall survival. A total of 1,873 patients were enrolled in the study. The baseline clinical characteristics were well balanced. Adverse events were typical of those seen in other bevacizumab-containing studies. Hypertension was seen in 16%–22% of the bevacizumab-containing arms, and bowel perforations occurred in < 3%. The median PFS was 10.3 months for patients treated with chemotherapy alone vs 14.1 months for those receiving extended-schedule bevacizumab (HR, 0.717; CI: 0.625–0.824, $P < .0001$). No difference in overall survival was seen, although it is early for this assessment.

As a result of these preliminary data, there are many questions to consider. They will be answered in time with additional studies or clarified once details are available. Will there be an overall survival benefit? If not, is a strategy that prolongs only progression-free survival sufficient? How long should bevacizumab be given? Should it be continued longer than 15 months, until disease progression, or for life? What happens when bevacizumab is discontinued? Is the phenotype of relapsed disease on bevacizumab more aggressive? Is there rebound at its discontinuation? Finally, is the "cure" proportion improved with prolonged bevacizumab use?

Intraperitoneal chemotherapy

The randomized study by Armstrong et al employed intraperitoneal (IP) therapy as part of primary treatment. They showed a median overall survival of 65.6 months for the IP arm vs 49 months in the IV group. This finding represents the largest difference to date between two treatment arms in any study evaluating primary therapy. The study is the third in a series of studies supporting the IP administration of primary chemotherapy to optimally debulked stage III patients.

The first study by Alberts et al predated paclitaxel and carboplatin use and simply asked the question of whether the IV or IP administration of cisplatin was better, showing an advantage for the latter (median overall survival, 49 vs 41 months; $P = .02$) This first IP study has been criticized because it does not contain paclitaxel and thus does not reflect contemporary treatment.

The second study by Markman et al included paclitaxel, but the experimental arm not only included IP delivery of cisplatin but also added high-dose IV carboplatin in an attempt to "chemically debulk" the tumor prior to IP administration. The Markman study, while also showing an advantage for the IP-containing experimental arm (overall survival, 52 vs 63 months; $P = .05$), was criticized because more than one variable was changed and the benefit could not be directly attributed to IP therapy.

Early treatment of relapse immediately after testing positive for elevated CA-125 levels in women with ovarian cancer in clinical complete remission does not improve survival over delaying treatment until the occurrence of clinical symptoms of relapse such as pelvic pain or bloating. This was according to data presented at ASCO 2009. In this study, investigators compared overall survival between 265 women with ovarian cancer in remission after initial chemotherapy who began second-line chemotherapy after experiencing a rise in CA-125 level, and 264 women with rising CA-125 level whose treatment was delayed until symptoms of relapse appeared. Second-line chemotherapy was started in the early treatment group a median 5 months before the delayed treatment group. At the time the study was presented, overall survival was the same between both groups (HR, 1.01, 95% CI: 0.82–1.25: $P = .91$). Researchers concluded that there was no survival benefit from early treatment based on a raised serum marker level alone. They added that consequently, there was no value in the routine measurement of CA-125 levels in the follow-up of ovarian cancer patients *(Rustin GJ et al: J Clin Oncol 27[18S]: abstract P1, 2009).*

As previously discussed, the third and well-designed trial by Armstrong et al showed a median overall survival of 65.6 months for the IP arm vs 49 months for the IV group. This study used IV paclitaxel (135 mg/m^2) over 24 hours on day 1, IP cisplatin (100 mg/m^2) on day 2, and IP paclitaxel (60 mg/m^2) on day 8 for 6 total cycles. Due to increased toxicity in the IP arm (metabolic, neuropathy), only 42% of patients completed all 6 cycles. However, a quality-of-life analysis at 12 months showed no difference between the IP and IV groups, suggesting the toxicity was reversible.

The general consensus opinion is that patients with stage III optimally debulked disease should be offered IP primary therapy. Studies are under way to modulate the regimen in an attempt to preserve the benefit and lessen toxicity. Initial modifications have included changing the IV paclitaxel to 135 mg/m^2 over 3 hours on day 1 and lowering the IP cisplatin dose to 75 mg/m^2 on day 2. If toxicity becomes prohibitive for a given patient, therapy is completed using IV paclitaxel and carboplatin. For patients not suited for IP treatment or for suboptimally debulked stage III patients or those with stage IV disease, IV paclitaxel with carboplatin also remains the standard. The next logical step to be addressed in upcoming cooperative groups is how to combine IP therapy with bevacizumab-containing treatment while also reducing the toxicity of IP therapy.

Radiation therapy as a single modality

In ovarian cancer, no prospective randomized trial has compared WAI, performed with modern techniques and equipment, with a paclitaxel-containing chemotherapy regimen. It has been demonstrated that the ability of WAI to sterilize macroscopic deposits of ovarian carcinoma is limited. Patients with any site of residual disease > 1 cm have compromised outcomes. The limited radiation tolerance of the abdominal organs also limits the radiation dose. Chemotherapy remains the standard of care for the adjuvant treatment of ovarian cancer.

Chemotherapy plus radiation therapy

Sequential combined-modality therapy (CMT) employing chemotherapy and irradiation has been shown in randomized trials to significantly increase survival over patients treated with chemotherapy alone. A phase III prospective randomized trial in patients with stage III ovarian cancer from the SNG showed a significant 20% improvement in 5-year progression-free survival for patients treated with chemotherapy and WAI vs chemotherapy alone.

In another European study, 64 of 94 patients with stages IC–IV disease who had undergone "radical" surgery and had no evidence of gross residual disease after 6 courses of chemotherapy (carboplatin, epirubicin, and prednimustine) were randomized to receive either consolidation WAI (30 Gy), followed by a boost to the para-aortic region and pelvis (12.0 and 21.6 Gy, respectively), or no further therapy. Relapse-free survival rates were significantly higher in patients who received adjuvant chemoradiation therapy than in those who received adjuvant chemotherapy only (2- and 5-year relapse-free survival rates, 68% vs 56% and 49% vs 26%, respectively); the same was true of overall survival rates (2- and 5-year overall survival rates, 87% vs 61% and 59% vs 33%, respectively). The differences between the two treatment groups were more pronounced in patients with stage III disease (2- and 5-year relapse-free survival rates, 77% vs 54% and 45% vs 19%, respectively; 2- and 5-year overall survival rates, 88% vs 58% and 59% vs 26%, respectively).

Einhorn et al, from the Karolinska Hospital in Stockholm, treated 75 patients with stages IIB–IV ovarian carcinoma with combined surgery, chemotherapy, and WAI to 40 Gy, utilizing a "six-field" approach. Outcomes were compared with those of 98 patients treated in subsequent years with only surgery and chemotherapy. After different prognostic factors were controlled statistically, it was found that patients who received WAI had a significantly better survival rate than those who did not. The authors suggest that, given the results of this and other studies combined with the limited success of modern combination chemotherapy regimens, the role of abdominal radiation therapy should be further investigated in a prospective fashion.

Despite these successful European trials, the regimen of chemotherapy and radiation in the up-front management of stage III ovarian cancer has not been implemented in the United States due to many factors. Paclitaxel-based chemotherapy provides a significant benefit for patients, as does IP chemotherapy. The use of radiation may increase potential bowel toxicity, particularly IP chemotherapy, and in some patients may cause bone marrow suppression, which theoretically may hinder future administration of chemotherapy.

Recurrent disease

Patients who respond to primary chemotherapy with paclitaxel and platinum agents and who relapse ≥ 6 months after the completion of treatment often have additional responses when retreated with the same agents. Response rates to repeat treatment with carboplatin are ~30% in those patients who relapse 12 months after primary therapy and 57% if the relapses occur > 24 months after primary therapy. In addition, a plethora of new agents have demonstrated modest phase II activity in patients with refractory disease.

TABLE 3: Chemotherapy regimens for ovarian carcinoma

Drug/combination	Dose and schedule
Paclitaxel/carboplatin	
Paclitaxel	175 mg/m² IV infused over 3 hours on day 1
Carboplatin	Dose calculated by the Calvert formula to an AUC of between 5.0 and 7.5 mg/mL/min IV infused over 30 minutes
	Carboplatin is given after paclitaxel
Repeat cycle every 21 days for 6 courses.	
PREMEDICATIONS: Dexamethasone, 20 mg PO 12 and 6 hours prior to paclitaxel; as well as diphenhydramine, 50 mg IV, and ranitidine, 50 mg IV, both 30 to 60 minutes prior to paclitaxel.	
Coleman RL, Bagnell KG, Townley PM: Cancer J Sci Am 3:246–253, 1997.	
Paclitaxel/cisplatin IP regimen[a]	
Paclitaxel	135 mg/m² IV over 24 hours on day 1 60 mg/m² IP on day 8 for 6 total cycles
Cisplatin	100 mg/m² IP on day 2
Armstrong DK, Bundy B, Wenzel L, et al: N Engl J Med 354:34–43, 2006.	
Single-agent topotecan[b] **(refractory or recurrent disease)**	
Topotecan	1.5 mg/m² IV over 30 minutes daily for 5 days
Repeat cycle every 21 days.	
Iva B, Ondrej B, Milan B, et al: Proc Am Soc Clin Oncol 19:1570a, 2000.	
Single-agent liposomal doxorubicin[a] **(refractory or recurrent disease)**	
Liposomal doxorubicin	50 mg/m² IV on day 1 at an initial rate of 1 mg/min; if tolerated, complete administration over 1 hour
Repeat cycle every 4 weeks.	
Muggia FM, Hainsworth JD, Jeffers S, et al: J Clin Oncol 15:987–993, 1997.	

[a] For the IP regimen, some are considering administering the IV paclitaxel at 135 mg/m² over day 1 as an outpatient, and lowering the IP cisplatin dose on day 2 to 75 mg/m² to reduce toxicity.
[b] NOTE: Clinical experience is accumulating to suggest that liposomal doxorubicin (at doses of 40 mg/m² every 4 weeks) and topotecan (at 1.0 mg/m²/d × 5 days or 4 mg/m²/wk) are equally efficacious and better tolerated than these agents at initial phase II doses. Definitive trials are ongoing.
AUC = area under the concentration-time curve
Table prepared by Ishmael Jaiyesimi, DO.

Topotecan has received FDA approval for the treatment of patients with refractory disease (Table 3). An oral preparation is in phase III trials.

An open, randomized study compared topotecan (1.5 mg/m²/d for 5 days) with paclitaxel (175 mg/m² q21d) in 226 women whose ovarian cancer had recurred after first-line platinum therapy. There were no statistically significant differences between the treatment groups with respect to response rate (20.5% vs 14.0%), response duration (25.9 vs 21.6 weeks), or median survival (63 vs 53 weeks).

Topotecan has efficacy comparable to that of paclitaxel in this setting and is being evaluated in combination with platinum and other agents.

Liposomal doxorubicin also has received FDA approval for the treatment of patients with metastatic platinum- and paclitaxel-refractory disease. A randomized trial by Gordon et al compared liposomal doxorubicin with topotecan in this setting; similar response rates, time to disease progression, and overall survival (60.0 vs 56.7 weeks) were seen with these two agents.

Other agents Phase II trials have demonstrated the activity of other agents in patients with recurrent ovarian cancer. They include gemcitabine, vinorelbine, oral altretamine (Hexalen), oral etoposide, irinotecan, and bevacizumab. In general, these agents have similar response rates, ranging from 10% to 15% in patients with platinum-resistant disease and 30% in patients with platinum-sensitive disease, with a median duration of response ranging from 4 to 8+ months. With the judicious selection and dosing of available agents to keep symptoms from disease and treatment to a minimum, a good quality of life can be maintained throughout much of the disease course.

A randomized ICON 4/AGO-OVAR 2.2 study addressed the issue of using single-agent carboplatin vs paclitaxel with carboplatin for patients with platinum-sensitive recurrent disease (defined generally as patients relapsing more than 6 months from prior platinum therapy). Both progression-free (HR, 0.76; 95% CI: 0.66–0.80; *P* = .0004) and 1-year overall survival rates (50% vs 40%) favored combination therapy. An AGO study evaluating carboplatin vs carboplatin with gemcitabine in a similar population was reported. This study likewise showed an improved response rate (47.2% vs 30.9%; *P* = .0016) and disease progression-free survival (8.6 vs 5.8 months; *P* = .0031) favoring the combination.

Preliminary results of the CALYPSO study have been reported in abstract form in the platinum-sensitive population. This study compared paclitaxel and carboplatin with liposomal doxorubicin and carboplatin. It showed an extended progression-free survival favoring the liposomal doxorubicin and carboplatin combination, from 9.4 months to 11.3 months (HR, 0.82; 95% CI: 0.72–0.94). Taken together, these data at a minimum suggest a benefit for platinum-based combination therapy over single-agent carboplatin in patients with platinum-sensitive recurrence. Survival data from the CALYPSO study are not yet mature.

The role of antivascular agents in recurrent disease

The single-agent and combination chemotherapy response rates for bevacizumab in patients with recurrent disease are reviewed in the section justifying the clinical trials and evaluating its potential use in the first-line setting. Several large important phase III studies are also ongoing in patients with platinum-sensitive recurrent disease (defined as > 6 months from prior platinum treatment). The GOG trial (NCT0056551) is randomizing recurrent patients to a secondary debulking or not and then to paclitaxel and carboplatin with or without bevacizumab. Primary objectives are to determine whether secondary surgical cytoreduction followed by adjuvant chemotherapy with or without bevacizumab prolongs overall survival. Bevacizumab continues in responders to evaluate the potential benefit of maintenance. Secondary objectives are to evaluate progression-free survival and quality of life, with a planned enrollment of 660 patients.

TABLE 4: Possible prognostic factors for salvage radiation therapy following chemotherapy

Residual tumor before WAI	Lymph node status
Location of residual disease	Chemotherapy duration
Initial FIGO stage	Type of prior chemotherapy
Histologic grade	Completion of WAI
Disease bulk at diagnosis	Response to chemotherapy
Patient age	Histologic type
Disease-free interval from initial treatment to relapse	CA-125 level CA-125 level trend
Performance status	Parameters of WAI
Number of sites of residual disease	Interval debulking/second-look surgery

FIGO = International Federation of Gynecology and Obstetrics; WAI = whole-abdominal irradiation

The ICON 6 study (NCT00544973) is evaluating patients with paclitaxel and carboplatin with or without AZ2171 (cediranib) and includes both a concurrent arm as well as a concurrent approach followed by maintenance therapy. Primary endpoints are safety, progression-free survival, and overall survival, with a planned enrollment estimate of 2,000 patients. Finally, the OCEANS study (NCT00434642) is evaluating the use of gemcitabine and carboplatin with or without bevacizumab in patients with platinum-sensitive disease. The primary endpoint is progression-free survival, with secondary endpoints to include overall survival and safety, particularly characterizing the incidence of gastrointestinal perforation. Planned enrollment is 440 patients.

Salvage and palliative radiotherapy after chemotherapy

In the setting of small-volume residual disease detected after chemotherapy, external-beam irradiation has been used with some success. Favorable experiences with salvage radiation therapy in chemotherapy-refractory ovarian carcinomas continue to be reported. Table 4 lists possible prognostic variables in these patients.

In a report of 20 patients who received multiple chemotherapy regimens for recurrent disease located in the pelvis, surgical debulking of the recurrent mass was followed by postoperative radiation therapy to 50.4 Gy. Patients who were able to have complete debulking and radiation had a 3-year overall survival of 50%, a disease-free survival of 72%, and local relapse-free survival of 89%; those with residual disease had corresponding values of 19%, 22%, and 42%, respectively. Radiation therapy should be considered for patients with localized recurrence of ovarian cancer who have failed to respond to multiple chemotherapy regimens, given the general sensitivity of ovarian cancer to radiation therapy.

Sedlacek et al described 27 patients who had not responded to aggressive cytoreductive surgery followed by multiple-drug platinum-based chemotherapy and who received WAI (30 to 35 Gy at 100 to 50 cGy/fraction, with a pelvic boost to a total dose of 45 Gy). The 5-year survival rate was 15%. The extent of residual disease at the initiation of radiation therapy strongly correlated with the length of survival.

Baker et al analyzed the efficacy of salvage WAI in 47 patients with ovarian cancer who had not responded to one or more chemotherapy regimens. Actuarial 4-year survival and disease-free survival rates were 48% and 37%, respectively, in patients with microscopic residual disease, vs 11% and 5%, respectively, in patients with macroscopic residual disease. In addition, patients with disease limited to the pelvis after laparotomy (including gross disease) had a 4-year actuarial survival rate of 60% and a disease-free survival rate of 54%, as compared with 16% and 4%, respectively, in patients with upper abdominal involvement.

This finding was confirmed by Firat and Erickson, who described their experience with selective radiotherapy in 28 patients with recurrent or persistent disease involving the vagina and/or rectum. Pelvic radiotherapy was uniformly successful in palliating vaginal bleeding. Furthermore, there were eight long-term survivors (five with no evidence of disease), implying that pelvic radiotherapy alone can be effective salvage therapy, particularly when there is no extrapelvic disease.

Fujiwara and colleagues reported high rates of objective and symptomatic responses using local radiotherapy in 20 patients (42 evaluable lesions) with recurrent ovarian cancer following chemotherapy. Lymph node metastases appeared to be particularly responsive.

Tinger et al reported an overall response rate of 73% in 80 patients with advanced and recurrent disease treated with palliative intent. Responses were maintained until death in all but 10 patients. Toxicity was limited, and there was no grade 4 toxicity. It was suggested that response rate, survival, and toxicity with palliative radiotherapy compared favorably with those of second- and third-line chemotherapies.

Based on these and other studies, certain treatment guidelines can be suggested:

- Palliation of vaginal bleeding, pelvic pain, or bowel or bladder blockage due to tumor compression may be feasible.
- Salvage radiation therapy may also be considered in selected patients after a localized pelvic recurrence following maximal debulking.

Novel approaches

The randomized trials evaluating the role of antivascular strategies in patients with ovarian cancer are all nearing completion, and results will be available soon to guide their use in both the primary and recurrent settings. Other clinical trials evaluating PARP (poly [ADP-ribose] polymerase) inhibitors and other targeted agents are ongoing, and clinical trial participation should be supported whenever possible.

High-dose chemotherapy In a trial conducted largely in patients with platinum-resistant (66%) and bulky disease (61%), the median progression-free and overall survival intervals were short (7 and 13 months, respectively) in those treated with high-dose chemotherapy and stem cell support, suggesting no benefit. There is no role for high-dose chemotherapy in the standard management of patients with epithelial ovarian cancer.

Treatment recommendations and unresolved issues

For advanced ovarian cancer, current front-line management should incorporate a taxane with platinum-based therapy, utilizing an IV and/or IP route. Results also support the use of a taxane and platinum-based therapy in patients with high-risk early-stage disease.

Issues that are evolving include (1) considering a variety of IP doses and schedules to reduce the toxicity of this approach, which has been shown to prolong overall survival; (2) the role of maintenance or consolidation treatment with standard chemotherapy or with novel agents following primary therapy; (3) the optimal use of platinum vs nonplatinum agents, and whether they should be used as single agents or in combination, for patients with recurrent disease; and (4) the role of novel drugs, notably bevacizumab and other antivascular agents, in both the adjuvant and recurrent-disease settings.

SUGGESTED READING

Albuquerque KV, Singla R, Potkul RK, et al: Impact of tumor volume-directed involved field radiation therapy integrated in the management of recurrent ovarian cancer. Gynecol Oncol 96:701–704, 2005.

Anderson GL, Judd HL, Kaunitz AM, et al: Effects of estrogen plus progestin on gynecologic cancers and associated diagnostic procedures: The Women's Health Initiative randomized trial. JAMA 290:1739–1748, 2003.

Armstrong DK, Bundy B, Wenzel L, et al: Intraperitoneal cisplatin and paclitaxel in ovarian cancer. N Engl J Med 354:34-43, 2006.

Burger RA, Brady MF, Bookman MA, et al: Phase III trial of bevacizumab (BEV) in the primary treatment of advanced epithelial ovarian cancer (EOC), primary peritoneal cancer (PPC), or fallopian tube cancer (FTC): A Gynecologic Oncology Group study. J Clin Oncol 28(18S):abstract 1, 2010.

Buys SS, Partridge E, Greene MH, et al: Ovarian cancer screening in the Prostate, Lung, Colorectal and Ovarian (PLCO) cancer screening trial: Findings from the initial screen of a randomized trial. Am J Obstet Gynecol 193:1630–1639, 2005.

Cannistra SA, Matulonis UA, Penson RT, et al: Phase II study of bevacizumab in patients with platinum resistant ovarian cancer or peritoneal serous cancer. J Clin Oncol 25:5180–5186, 2007.

Garcia AA, Hirte H, Fleming G, et al: Phase II clinical trial of bevacizumab and low-dose metronomic oral cyclophosphamide in recurrent ovarian cancer: A trial of the California, Chicago, and Princess Margaret Hospital phase II consortia. J Clin Oncol 26:76–82, 2008.

Goff BA, Mandel LS, Drescher CW, et al: Development of an ovarian cancer symptom index: Possibilities for earlier detection. Cancer 109:221–227, 2007.

ICON and AGO collaborators: Paclitaxel plus platinum based chemotherapy versus conventional platinum based chemotherapy in women with relapsed ovarian cancer: The ICON 4/AGO-OVAR 2.2 trial. Lancet 361:2099–2106, 2003.

ICON and EORTC-ACTION investigators: International Collaborative on Ovarian Neoplasm Trial 1 and Adjuvant Treatment in Ovarian Neoplasm Trial: Two parallel randomized phase III trials of adjuvant chemotherapy in patients with early stage ovarian cancer. J Natl Cancer Inst 95:105–112, 2003.

Jemal A, Siegel R, Xu J, et al: Cancer statistics, 2010. CA Cancer J Clin 60:277–300, 2010.

Kauff ND, Domchek SM, Friebel TM, et al: Risk-reducing salpingo-oophorectomy for the prevention of BRCA1- and BRCA2-associated breast and gynecologic cancer: A multicenter, prospective study. J Clin Oncol 26:1331–1337, 2008.

Kauff ND, Satagopan JM, Robson ME, et al: Risk-reducing salpingo-oophorectomy in women with a BRCA1 or BRCA2 mutation. N Engl J Med 346:1609–1615, 2002.

Markman M, Liu PY, Wilczynski S, et al: Phase III randomized trial of 12 versus 3 months of maintenance paclitaxel in patients with advanced ovarian cancer after complete response to platinum and paclitaxel based chemotherapy: A Southwest Oncology Group and Gynecologic Oncology Group Trial. J Clin Oncol 21:2460–2465, 2003.

Ozols RF, Bundy BN, Greer E, et al: Phase III trials of carboplatin and paclitaxel compared with cisplatin and paclitaxel in patients with optimally resected stage III ovarian cancer: A Gynecologic Oncology Group Study. J Clin Oncol 21:3194–3200, 2003.

Pfisterer J, Plante M, Vergote I, et al: Gemcitabine/carboplatin (GC) vs carboplatin (C) in platinum-sensitive recurrent ovarian cancer (OVCA): Results of a Gynecologic Cancer Intergroup randomized phase III trial of the AGO OVAR, the NCIC CTG, and the EORTC GCG (abstract 5005). J Clin Oncol 22:14S, 2004.

Pujade-Lauraine E, Mahner S, Kaern J, et al: A randomized phase III study of carboplatin and pegylated doxorubicin versus carboplatin and paclitaxel in relapsed platinum-sensitive ovarian cancer. CALYPSO Study of the Gynecologic Cancer Intergroup (GCIG) (abstract LBA5509). J Clin Oncol 27:18S, 2009.

Rose PG, Nerenstone S, Brady MF, et al: Secondary surgical cytoreduction for advanced ovarian carcinoma. N Engl J Med 351:2489–2497, 2004.

Sorbe B, for the Swedish-Norwegian Ovarian Cancer Study Group: Consolidation treatment of advanced (FIGO stage III) ovarian carcinoma in complete surgical remission after induction chemotherapy: A randomized, controlled clinical trial comparing whole abdominal radiotherapy, chemotherapy, and no further treatment. Int J Gynecol Cancer 13:278–286, 2003.

Vasey PA, Jayson GC, Gordon A, et al; Scottish Gynaecological Cancer Trials Group: Phase III randomized trial of docetaxel-carboplatin versus paclitaxel-carboplatin as first-line chemotherapy for ovarian cancer. J Natl Cancer Inst 96:1682–1691, 2004.

Vergote I, Trope CG, Amant F, et al: EORTC-GCG/NCIC-CTG randomised trial comparing primary debulking surgery with neoadjuvant chemotherapy in stage IIIc–IV ovarian, fallopian tube and peritoneal cancer (OvCa) (abstract 1767). Presented at the 12th Biennial Meeting of the International Gynecologic Cancer Society, Bangkok, October 25–28, 2008.

Abbreviations in this chapter

ACTION = Adjuvant Treatment in Ovarian Neoplasms; AGO-OVAR = Arbeitsgemeinschaft Gynaekologische Onkologie Studiengrappe Ovarialkarzinom; CTG = Clinical Trials Group; EORTC = European Organisation for Research and Treatment of Cancer; GCG = Gynecologic Cancer Group; GOG = Gynecologic Oncology Group; ICON = International Collaborative on Ovarian Neoplasms; IICG = Italian Interregional Cooperative Group; NCIC = National Cancer Institute of Canada; PLCO = Prostate, Lung, Colorectal, and Ovarian Trial; SCOTROC = Scottish Randomized Trial in Ovarian Cancer; SNG = Swedish-Norwegian Group

MELANOMA

CHAPTER 20

Melanoma and other skin cancers

Mary S. Brady, MD, Aradhana Kaushal, MD, Christine Ko, MD, and Keith Flaherty, MD

Skin cancer is the single most common form of cancer, accounting for more than 75% of all cancer diagnoses. More than 1 million cases of squamous cell and basal cell carcinomas are diagnosed annually, with a lifetime risk of more than one in five. The vast majority of skin cancers can be cured with surgery alone. Resection is the mainstay of therapy, even for skin cancer involving regional lymph nodes or, in some cases, more distant metastatic sites.

Sun exposure is the predominant risk factor for squamous cell and basal cell skin cancer, and is the only known environmental risk factor for melanoma. Genetic susceptibility to melanoma clearly varies across the population and correlates to a large degree with light skin, hair, and eye color. Melanoma contributes to 75% of deaths from skin cancer. Melanoma was diagnosed in 68,130 Americans in 2010 and accounted for 8,700 deaths (12.8% of patients diagnosed). Melanoma accounted for 4% of new cancer cases in women and 5% in men in 2010. Death from melanoma increased by 5.8% in the United States between 1990 and 2005 due to an increase in melanoma deaths in men, although there was a slight decrease in mortality from melanoma in women. The lifetime risk of melanoma for Caucasians is 1 in 39 for men and 1 in 58 for women in the United States. The 5-year survival was 92% of patients diagnosed with melanoma in the United States between 1996 and 2004, an increase of 10% compared with the years 1975 through 1977. This is almost certainly due to an increase in early detection.

The superficial nature of melanoma and other skin cancers supports campaigns to raise public awareness and healthcare provider expertise in detecting skin cancers at the earliest possible stage. High-risk groups, for whom screening efforts might make the largest impact, are families with numerous cases of melanoma and older men. Screening initiatives would be less likely to benefit the 10% of melanomas that are nonpigmented or arise from the choroid of the eyes or mucosal surfaces.

SKIN CANCERS

EPIDEMIOLOGY

Age

The relationship between the incidence of melanoma and age is somewhat unique in comparison to other common cancers. There is not an exponential increase in risk with age but rather a more even distribution across age groups. The median age of diagnosis of melanoma is 53 years, almost 10 years younger than the median age of diagnosis of most common cancers. Forty-two percent of cases present in people younger than age 55, contributing to the third highest number of years of life lost across all cancers. In contrast, the incidence of squamous cell and basal cell carcinomas increases exponentially with age.

Gender

Men are more likely than women to develop melanoma (67% higher incidence), and their prognosis is worse (136% higher risk of death from melanoma). The risk of recurrence in the setting of resected primary melanoma is higher, and their expected survival in the setting of regionally advanced disease is significantly shorter.

Location

Basal cell cancers arise exclusively from cutaneous sites and are closely related to sites of skin that receive the most sun exposure, such as the scalp, face, neck, and arms. Squamous cell cancers can arise from numerous sites in the body, but the term squamous cell skin cancer is reserved for cutaneous sites. The vast majority of melanomas arise from cutaneous sites, but most cases of melanoma arise from intermittently sun-exposed skin. A small percentage of melanomas arise on acral surfaces of the hands and feet, which tend to be diagnosed at a later stage. Melanoma can arise from melanocytes adjacent to the retina or within mucosal surfaces in the oropharynx, sinuses, rectum, or vulva. These lesions typically present with greater local invasion and risk of distant spread than cutaneous melanoma.

Geography

The rates of melanoma and other skin cancers are highest where fair-skinned Caucasians migrated to lower latitudes, with annual sun exposure that is substantially higher than their historically native climates. Australia, New Zealand, South Africa, and Israel bear a disproportionate burden of skin cancer. In Australia, melanoma is the third most common cancer. In the United States, Hawaii and the desert Southwest have the highest rates of skin cancer of all kinds and melanoma.

Race

Caucasians are by far the most susceptible race for melanomas, as well as squamous cell and basal cell cancers. Hispanics have a lower incidence but represent the group at next highest risk. Asians and African-Americans have the lowest rates of skin cancer. For those populations, cutaneous melanomas arising from sun-exposed sites are uncommon but not unseen. All racial groups are equally likely to develop melanoma on the acral surfaces of the hands and feet or mucosal surfaces. Therefore, melanomas arising from these sites represent nearly all cases of melanoma in these more darkly pigmented racial groups.

Survival

Skin cancers that are confined to the skin at presentation and with adequate staging evaluation have a high rate of cure. The 10-year survival for patients with invasive melanomas that are 1 mm or less in thickness and that lack ulceration is 97%. Melanoma that is microscopically present in regional lymph nodes is associated with a 10-year survival of 50% to 60%; when macroscopic or clinically apparent lymph nodes are detected, the 10-year survival is only 30% to 40%. The presence of more distant metastatic disease is associated with only a 5% possibility of survival 10 years from initial recognition.

ETIOLOGY AND RISK FACTORS

Genetic predisposition

Although there are families in which melanoma can occur with high likelihood, an underlying genetic predisposition can only be found in 3% all cases. The pedigrees have been identified because of their high likelihood of a mutation carrier developing melanoma. Lower penetrance genotypes remain to be elucidated. Nonetheless, the identification of the genes responsible for familial melanoma has contributed greatly to the understanding of the molecular pathophysiology of melanoma.

The clinical observations that patients with multiple dysplastic nevi were at greater risk of developing melanoma and that many such patients came from families with multiple affected individuals provided the first insight into a melanoma progression model that might be accelerated based on inborn genetic abnormalities. Two highly related genes were discovered to harbor germline mutations in roughly 50% of melanoma pedigrees: *CDKN2A* and *CDK4*. *CDKN2A* enocodes two products via alternate splicing of messenger RNA: p16INK4A and p14ARF. Each of these tumor suppressor genes exerts an inhibitory effect on cell cycle progression.

Xeroderma pigmentosum is a rare inherited disorder in which DNA repair mechanisms are compromised, particularly in response to ultraviolet (UV) light. Mutations in *XP* genes *A* through *G* have been identified as the underlying molecular event. Squamous cell and basal cell carcinomas and melanoma are prevalent in this population and at a young age. The near-complete penetrance of melanoma in these patients emphasizes the critical balance between UV-induced DNA damage and repair in risk for skin cancer. As DNA damage repair is mediated by a complex network of sensor and effector proteins, variability in the function of this system almost certainly underlies the variability in risk among the fair-skinned population.

Genetic variability in the melanocortin-1 receptor (*MC1R*) has been clearly implicated in pigmentation of skin and hair and, more recently, in melanoma predisposition. It has been known for decades that melanoma is more prevalent among fair-skinned individuals with red or blond hair. Furthermore, blond-haired individuals with an inability to tan are at substantially greater risk of developing melanoma than blond-haired individuals who tan readily. Polymorphisms, distinct from mutations, in

MC1R appear to account for skin and hair color differences among Caucasians. It appears that individuals with melanocortin receptors that have a muted response to increased melanocortin expression following sun exposure suffer the greatest UV-induced genetic damage, leading to a greater risk of melanoma.

Exposure

Even the inheritance of *CDKN2A* and *CDK4* mutations is insufficient to lead to melanoma in all carriers. It is clear that multiple genetic changes are required to give rise to invasive disease. UV damage is the best-described modifiable risk factor for melanoma, as well as squamous cell and basal cell skin cancers. It is believed that the acquired or somatic genetic changes that give rise to melanoma occur as a consequence of UV-induced genetic damage.

Epidemiologic data relate the risk of melanoma most closely to a connection between cumulative sun exposure, severe sun burns, or sun exposure during childhood, depending on the study. The disagreement between studies likely stems from methodologic differences in obtaining a sun exposure history, a heterogeneous effect of sun exposure and risk depending on the underlying genetic composition of the study population, or both. It has been clarified that melanoma arising on intermittently sun-exposed skin (such as the trunk) has its peak incidence among younger individuals and declines severely with increasing age. On the other hand, melanoma arising from chronically sun-damaged skin (such as the face, neck, and upper extremities) has the highest incidence in older individuals. With the rise in popularity of indoor tanning salons, data indicate that those who use them are at higher risk of melanoma than those who are sun-exposed. There is little dispute regarding the causal link between sun exposure or tanning salon use and risk of melanoma; however, there is disagreement regarding the constituents of light (UV-A or UV-B) that contribute most to genetic damage. Laboratory studies support a connection for both and suggest that prevention strategies must take the entire UV light spectrum into account.

Prevention

With the incidence of melanoma still rising, it is clear that primary prevention efforts have not yet taken hold. The only approach firmly rooted in evidence is to minimize sun exposure. The use of sun-protective clothing appears to be the next best strategy. There are conflicting data regarding the protective effect of suncreens for melanoma, although there is no controversy regarding their ability to prevent squamous cell and basal cell carcinomas. Protection against UV-A has been a long-standing feature of widely available suncreens, whereas UV-B protection has more recently been engineered into all mainstream products. It is possible that the more widespread of these wide-spectrum sunscreens will provide more meaningful protective effects over the coming decades.

Immunosuppression

There is incontrovertible evidence linking immunosuppression and squamous cell skin cancer. This increased risk applies to patients with acquired immunodeficiency syndrome as well as transplant recipients on chronic immunosuppressive medications. The risk of developing primary melanoma in the setting of immunosuppression is less well established, but there is some evidence that patients who have a history of melanoma are more likely to develop disease recurrence in the setting of immunosuppression.

Nevi

Patients with numerous benign nevi (small, regularly shaped, and uniformly pigmented moles) are at increased risk of melanoma, as are patients with relatively few dysplastic nevi (large, irregularly shaped, and heterogeneously pigmented moles). Patients in either group may have a fivefold increased risk of developing melanoma compared with those with few benign nevi or without dysplastic nevi. However, it is critical to recognize that these preexisting moles represent a risk factor for melanoma, rather than precursor lesions, in most cases. The vast majority of dysplastic nevi do not give rise to melanoma. There seems to be little value in resecting every nevus that appears dysplastic on clinical grounds. Surveying the skin regularly for new or changing moles has been most widely adopted strategy for educating patients and healthcare providers. Beyond the age of 25 to 30, new mole formation warrants examination by a provider who is comfortable making the diagnosis of melanoma.

Congenital nevi

These are relatively rare compared with acquired nevi. In general, they do not suggest a predisposition to melanoma. A small number of children are born with so-called giant congenital nevi, also referred to as bathing trunk nevi. Melanoma arising from within a giant congenital nevus is a well described phenomenon and is one reason that staged resection of such lesions is recommended for many children and adolescents.

History of melanoma

Perhaps the single greatest clinical risk factor for melanoma is a personal history of melanoma. In addition to having surveillance for local and distant recurrence related to their prior melanoma, these individuals require lifelong observation for the emergence of a new primary melanoma; their risk is 10 times greater than that of the general population.

Actinic keratoses

These lesions represent the precursor lesion for the vast majority of squamous cell skin cancers. They manifest as raised, nonpigmented lesions with a plaque-like surface. Typically, they have an erythematous base and arise on heavily sun-exposed skin. These lesions are typically treated with either excision, cryotherapy, topical chemotherapy (5-fluorouracil [5-FU]), or immunotherapy (imiquimod). It is unclear what effect nonsurgical therapy has on the long-term risk of progression to squamous cell carcinoma, but the relatively indolent nature of most actinic keratoses suggests that nonsurgical therapy followed by close observation is reasonable, particularly for lesions arising on cosmetically sensitive areas such as the face.

Burns

Burns (unrelated to sun exposure) predispose to the formation of squamous cell carcinoma on permanently scarred areas. Although not particularly prevalent among those with a burn history, a high clinical suspicion for malignancy must be taken for the patient with a new nonpigmented lesion or an area of ulceration on a preexisting healed burn.

Signs and symptoms

The diagnosis of melanoma is based on complete pathologic evaluation of a clinically suspicious lesion. A growing or changing skin lesion is the easiest description that a patient can provide a physician to assist in determining which skin lesions should be biopsied. The "ABCDs" is a simple method for identifying lesions that should be brought to medical attention and referral for consideration of biopsy. This system, which is based on asymmetry of the skin lesion, irregular edges, color appearance, and diameter, can be helpful to patients, but it does not describe all lesions that are ultimately diagnosed as melanoma upon pathologic review.

DIAGNOSIS

Early diagnosis of melanoma

Beyond prevention, early detection is the next priority in limiting the life-threatening potential of melanoma. Although tumor invasion into the dermis (the definition of invasive melanoma) cannot be assessed clinically, there are hallmarks of melanoma that can be appreciated by visual inspection. The "ABCD" algorithm, promoted by the ACS, has not proved to be a particularly effective method of educating the general population, but healthcare providers may be better suited to implementing this system in clinical practice. (See the color atlas following this chapter.) 'A' indicates gross asymmetry of a pigmented lesion. 'B' refers to irregular or indistinct borders. 'C' regards color, which, in the case of melanoma, refers to black, dark brown, or blue color for newly formed lesions. In the case of preexisting moles, the loss of pigmentation in a portion of the lesion can indicate regression, which is worrisome for melanoma. Additionally, a focus of darker pigmentation within a preexisting mole is grounds for concern. 'D', or diameter of 6 mm or greater, raises concern for melanoma, whereas smaller lesions are rarely indicative of invasive lesions. None of these single criteria can be considered as grounds for performing a biopsy, rather lesions that satisfy multiple criteria warrant either close observation or biopsy of the most abnormal portion. Not included in the ABCD system is the papular or nodular characteristic of most melanomas. If melanoma arises within a preexisting mole, the raised element of an otherwise flat or macular lesion should be considered suspicious for melanoma. Some primary melanomas do not produce melanin and therefore lack the classic appearance.

Atypical nevi

These lesions represent a risk factor for melanoma in that individual lesions can occasionally progress to invasive melanoma. More commonly, the presence of dysplastic nevi suggests an individual at risk for melanoma formation at other sites. The clinical definition of atypical nevi has never been formally established but generally refers to the presence of one or two of the ABCD features. Cutaneous photography has been routinely incorporated in the follow-up of patients with multiple clinically dysplastic nevi in specialized pigmented lesion clinics. Full-body cutaneous photography is increasingly available to patients and provides an objective baseline from which to judge change of preexisting lesions or the appearance of new lesions. In general, excision of all atypical nevi is impractical and does not adequately address the risk that patients face of developing melanoma in sites where no precursor lesion is found.

Nodular melanoma

This represents the most difficult subset of melanomas to diagnose at an early stage. These lesions are more rapidly proliferative than typical melanomas and are generally not pigmented. Furthermore, they are generally raised early in their development and have symmetric and well-demarcated boundaries. Thus, they do not meet the ABCD criteria. Nodular melanomas account for approximately 10% of melanoma cases but account for a disproportionate percentage of fatalities. The most useful clinical rule to apply in the assessment of lesions that have these features is that the de novo appearance of such lesions over a short time (months) warrants consideration of biopsy. As the features of nodular melanoma are common to some benign skin lesions, as well as basal cell carcinoma, the yield of biopsies for such lesions may be relatively low. Nonetheless, heightened awareness of this small but lethal subset of melanoma is needed.

Nonmelanoma skin cancers

Classically, basal cell skin cancers are nodular and have a pearly, nonpigmented surface. Squamous cell carcinomas typically have a scaly, nonpigmented surface and can occasionally be ulcerated. Both types are generally slow to evolve. In most cases, squamous cell carcinomas are believed to arise from actinic keratoses. The differentiation between the two is based largely on size, with actinic keratoses being less than 1 cm in diameter. The appearance of nodularity or induration in preexisting keratinized lesions raises concern for tumor invasion into the dermis and warrants biopsy.

Skin examination

Examination of the entire body should be performed for any patient who presents with numerous benign-appearing nevi, any dysplastic nevi, or a history of even a single melanoma. The entire skin is at risk in these individuals and must be investigated for the appearance of new or changing lesions. Patients who fit into any of these risk groups should be instructed to perform monthly skin self-examination. Two mirrors are required to adequately examine the back if a partner is not available to assist in examining the back longitudinally.

Skin examination should be performed in a well-lit room with the patient completely disrobed. For patients with numerous moles, full-body cutaneous photography is extremely helpful to provide an objective baseline from which to judge change. For patients with only a few atypical moles, close-up photographs of those lesions may facilitate careful evaluation of those lesions while the remainder of the skin is surveyed for new lesions. A focused method for examining individual lesions, dermoscopy employs low-level magnification of the epidermis with tangential light applied to a liquid-skin interface. Examination of pigmented lesions with dermoscopy allows more precise visualization of patterns of pigmentation than is possible with the unaided eye. This method requires some degree of training and the availability of appropriate equipment. When regression of part or all of a preexisting mole is suspected, a Wood's lamp can be helpful in bringing out the contrast in pigmentation between normally pigmented surrounding skin and an area where immunologic destruction of melanocytes has occurred.

Lymph node examination

This should be performed in all patients who are suspected of having invasive melanoma or large squamous cell or basal cell carcinomas. The closest lymph node basin is the most essential area to examine. The presence of a palpable lymph node mandates biopsy of the suspicious node, generally with fine needle aspiration (FNA). If the result of FNA is negative, a formal lymph node biopsy should be pursued for a clinically suspicious node. Whereas sentinel lymph node biopsy (SLNB) is performed routinely for patients with primary melanomas 1 mm or greater in depth, palpable lymphadenopathy with histologic evidence of melanoma or nonmelanoma skin cancer warrants proceeding directly to a regional lymph node dissection.

Biopsy techniques

Excisional biopsy is recommended for any lesion that is suspected of being melanoma, squamous cell cancer, or basal cell carcinoma. This is especially true for lesions that can be entirely excised without concern for causing an unacceptable cosmetic result. Local anesthesia is generally all that is required. Narrow margins of 1 to 2 mm are sufficient when making an initial diagnosis of skin cancer. The biopsy should extend to the subcutaneous tissue to provide an adequate estimate of the depth of invasion, particularly for melanoma. Biopsy specimens should be placed in formalin and submitted for expert pathologic preparation including embedding in paraffin.

Incisional biopsy is an acceptable alterative for large lesions, especially when located on the face, neck, or distal extremities. In the case of possible melanoma, the most abnormal-appearing area should be biopsied. As with excisional biopsies, the biopsy should include subcutaneous tissue to allow an estimation of thickness. A punch biopsy, of sufficient diameter to encompass the most abnormal-appearing area, is the preferred method. Should the biopsy identify a melanocytic lesion with dysplasia or atypia, the entire lesion should be removed, when possible, with radial margins to 1 to 2 mm.

Techniques to avoid For lesions that are suspicious for melanoma, every attempt should be made to preserve the ability to assess involvement of margins and to perform immunohistochemistry of the primary tumor. The latter is critically important in borderline cases, where the diagnosis of melanoma is uncertain. Thus, shave biopsies and serial thin section techniques (such as Mohs surgery) are strictly contraindicated. Frozen biopsy assessment is inadequate for the diagnosis of melanoma and does not allow adequate material for review in difficult pathologic cases.

Pathology

Nonmelanoma skin cancers

The two most common skin cancers are basal and squamous cell carcinomas. Both of these skin cancers arise predominately on sun-exposed areas and may be considered

TABLE 1: TNM staging for cutaneous melanoma

Primary Tumor (T)		
Classification	**Thickness (mm)**	**Ulceration status/mitoses**
Tis	NA	NA
T1	≤ 1.00	a: Without ulceration and mitosis < 1/mm^2 b: With ulceration and mitosis ≥ 1/mm^2
T2	1.01–2.00	a: Without ulceration b: With ulceration
T3	2.01–4.00	a: Without ulceration b: With ulceration
T4	> 4.00	a: Without ulceration b: With ulceration
Regional nodes (N)		
Classification	**No. of metastatic nodes**	**Nodal metastatic burden**
N0	0	NA
N1	1	a: Micrometastasis[a] b: Macrometastasis[b]
N2	2–3	a: Micrometastasis[a] b: Macrometastasis[b] c: In-transit metastases/satellites without metastatic nodes
N3	4+ metastatic nodes, or matted nodes, or in-transit metastases/ satellites with metastatic nodes	
Distant metastases (M)		
	Site	**Serum LDH**
M0	No distant metastases	NA
M1a	Distant skin, subcutaneous, or nodal metastases	Normal
M1b	Lung metastases	Normal
M1c	All other visceral metastases Any distant metastasis	Normal Elevated

NA = not applicable; LDH = lactate dehydrogenase

[a] Micrometastases are diagnosed after sentinel lymph node biopsy.

[b] Macrometastases are defined as clinically detectable nodal metastases confirmed pathologically.

From Balch CM, Gershenwald JE, Soong SW, et al: Final version of 2009 AJCC melanoma staging and classification. J Clin Oncol 27:6199–6206, 2009.

in the differential diagnosis with melanoma. The diagnosis of these skin cancers should be made after pathologic analysis of the skin specimen.

STAGING AND PROGNOSIS OF MELANOMA

A great deal of information is available regarding factors that correlate with clinical outcome in patients with melanoma. In patients with clinically localized disease, the most important prognostic factors are Breslow's thickness, ulceration, and SLN

TABLE 2: Anatomic stage groupings for cutaneous melanoma

Clinical staging[a]				Pathologic staging[b]			
Stage	**T**	**N**	**M**	**Stage**	**T**	**N**	**M**
0	Tis	N0	M0	0	Tis	N0	M0
IA	T1a	N0	M0	IA	T1a	N0	M0
IB	T1b	N0	M0	IB	T1b	N0	M0
	T2a	N0	M0		T2a	N0	M0
IIA	T2b	N0	M0	IIA	T2b	N0	M0
	T3a	N0	M0		T3a	N0	M0
IIB	T3b	N0	M0	IIB	T3b	N0	M0
	T4a	N0	M0		T4a	N0	M0
IIC	T4b	N0	M0	IIC	T4b	N0	M0
III	Any T	N > N0	M0	IIIA	T1–4a	N1a	M0
					T1–4a	N2a	M0
				IIIB	T1–4b	N1a	M0
					T1–4b	N2a	M0
					T1–4a	N1b	M0
					T1–4a	N2b	M0
					T1–4a	N2c	M0
				IIIC	T1–4b	N1b	M0
					T1–4b	N2b	M0
					T1–4b	N2c	M0
					Any T	N3	M0
IV	Any T	Any N	M1	IV	Any T	Any N	M1

[a] Clinical staging includes microstaging of the primary melanoma and clinical/radiologic evaluation for metastases. By convention, it should be used after complete excision of the primary melanoma with clinical assessment for regional and distant metastases.

[b] Pathologic staging includes microstaging of the primary melanoma and pathologic information about the regional lymph nodes after partial (ie, sentinel node biopsy) or complete lymphadenectomy. Pathologic stage 0 or stage IA patients are the exception; they do not require pathologic evaluation of their lymph nodes.

From Balch CM, Gershenwald JE, Soong SW, et al: Final version of 2009 AJCC melanoma staging and classification. J Clin Oncol 27:6199–6206, 2009.

status. Overall, however, 85% of melanoma patients present with clinically normal lymph nodes. In clinically node-negative patients, most investigators have found the microscopic degree of invasion of the melanoma, or microstaging, to be of critical importance in predicting outcome (Tables 1 and 2; Figure 1).

Microstaging

Primary melanoma

Three microscopic characteristics of primary melanoma are now incorporated into the AJCC staging system for melanoma, as each has a significant contribution in predicting risk of regional lymph node involvement and long-term risk of metastatic disease and death.

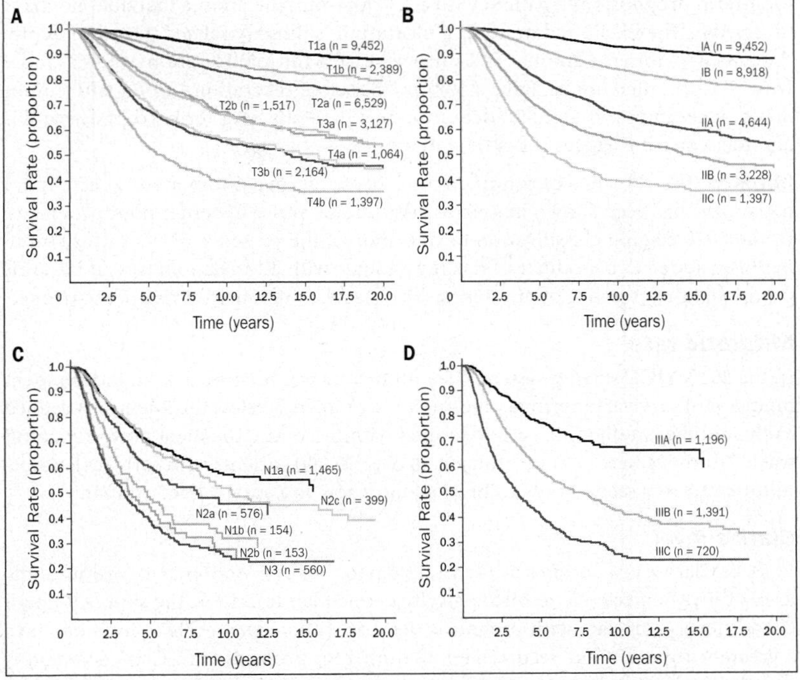

FIGURE 1: Survival curves from the American Joint Committee on Cancer Melanoma Staging Database comparing (A) the different T categories and (B) the stage groupings for stages I and II melanoma. For patients with stage III disease, survival curves are shown comparing (C) the different N categories and (D) the stage groupings.

From Balch CM, Gershenwald JE, Soong SW, et al: Final version of 2009 AJCC melanoma staging and classification. J Clin Oncol 27:6199–6206, 2009.

Breslow's thickness First described by Alexander Breslow, this method of describing tumor thickness measures from the top of the granular layer of the epidermis to the deepest contiguous tumor cell at the base of the lesion using a micrometer in the microscope eyepiece. It is the primary determinant of T staging and has the highest prognostic value of any primary tumor characteristic. In the 2010 AJCC 7th Edition Cancer Staging Manual, Clark's level was removed from stage groupings, as it is not predictive of outcome when the three cardinal features are considered.

Ulceration The presence of ulceration in a primary melanoma is one of the strongest negative predictive factors for long-term survival. Ulceration is defined as the lack of a complete epidermal layer overlying the melanocytic lesion. The presence of ulceration essentially upstages affected patients to the next highest T level. In other words, a patient with a 1.1- to 2-mm melanoma that is ulcerated will carry the same long-term prognosis as a patient with a 2.1- to 4-mm melanoma that does not have ulceration. The likelihood of finding ulceration is directly related to tumor depth: Patients with thin melanomas (≤ 1 mm) have a 6% rate of ulceration, whereas those with > 4-mm melanomas have a 63% incidence of ulceration. Along with tumor depth, ulceration is integral in determining a patient's long-term prognosis and is an independent predictor of patient outcome.

Mitoses The presence of mitotic figures in the dermal component of a primary melanoma has been shown in several institutional series to confer poor prognosis. In the 2010 staging classification for melanoma, the presence of ≥ 1 mitosis/mm^2 has been added as a modifier of risk for patients with T1 melanomas, as it is in this group that the presence of mitoses has the greatest influence on risk of recurrence.

Mitototic rate

In the 2010 AJCC staging system, the mitotic rate was identified as an independent predictor of survival for primary melanoma < 1 mm in Breslow thickness. It is defined as the number of dividing cells identified within 1 mm^2. The most powerful cutoff was < 1/mm^2 versus > 1/mm^2. Indeed, in over 10,000 patients with early melanoma, mitotic rate was second only to Breslow thickness as a survival determinant.

Clark's level

Wallace Clark and associates devised a system to classify melanomas according to the level of invasion relative to histologically defined landmarks in the skin. Although Clark's levels correlate with prognosis (lesions with deeper levels of invasion have a greater propensity for recurrence), the inherent problem with Clark's system is that the thickness of the skin and hence the distance between the various landmark dermal layers varies greatly in different parts of the body. When initially described, the Clark's level was a standard way to stage patients with melanoma and predict outcome. Over the years, it has proven much less reliable than Breslow thickness, and the 2002 AJCC staging system was used only for lesions < 1 mm. In the 2010 AJCC staging system, the mitotic index has replaced the Clark's level in staging lesions < 1 mm. The Clark's level is only used when mitotic index is unavailable for lesions < 1 mm.

Regional lymph node involvement

In patients with intermediate-risk melanoma (1 to 4 mm in thickness), lymph node involvement is the strongest prognostic indicator in the staging of melanoma. Patients with nodal involvement at the time of their diagnosis have significantly decreased survival compared with those who do not, independent of the prognostic factors associated with the primary lesion. There is a direct relationship between the depth of invasion of the primary lesion and the potential for lymph node involvement. Among node-positive patients, the prognosis is more favorable in those with microscopic as opposed to macroscopic or clinically apparent disease. In addition, the increased number of nodes involved is associated with decreased survival in both microscopically detected and clinically apparent regional nodal metastasis. The worst prognosis occurs in patients with large, matted regional lymph nodes, whose outcome is similar to that of patients with stage IV disease.

TABLE 3: Differences between the 6th edition (2002) and the 7th edition (2010) of the AJCC melanoma staging system

Factor	6th edition criteria	7th edition criteria	Comments
Thickness	Primary determinant of T staging	Same	Thresholds of 1.0, 2.0, and 4.00 mm
Level of invasion	Used only for defining T1 melanomas	Same	Used as a default criterion only if mitotic rate cannot be determined
Ulceration	Included as a secondary determinant of T and N staging	Same	Signifies a locally advanced lesion; dominant prognostic factor for grouping stages I, II, and III
Mitotic rate/mm^2	Not used	Used for categorizing T1 melanoma	Mitosis $\geq 1/mm^2$ used as a primary criterion for defining T1b melanoma
Satellite metastases	In N category	Same	Merged with transit lesions
Immunochemical detection of nodal metastases	Not included	Included	Must include at least one melanoma-associated marker (eg, HMB-45, Melan-A [MART-1]) unless diagnostic cellular morphology is present
0.2-mm threshold of defined N+	Implied	No lower threshold of staging N+ disease	Isolated tumor cells or tumor deposits < 0.1 mm meeting the criteria for histologic or immunohistochemical detection of melanoma should be scored as N+
Number of nodal metastases	Primary determinant of N staging	Same	Thresholds of 1 vs 2–3 vs 4+ nodes
Metastatic volume	Included as a second determinant of N staging	Same	Clinically occult (microscopic) nodes are diagnosed as sentinel node biopsy vs clinically apparent (macroscopic) nodes diagnosed by palpation or imaging studies, or by the finding of gross (not microscopic) extracapsular extension in a clinically occult node
Lung metastases	Separate category as M1b	Same	Has a somewhat better prognosis than other visceral metastases
Elevated serum LDH	Included as a second determinant of M staging	Same	Recommend a second confirmatory LDH level if elevated
Clinical vs pathologic staging	Sentinel node results incorporated into definition of pathologic staging	Same	Large variability in outcome between clinical and pathologic staging; sentinel node staging is encouraged for standard patient care and should be required prior to entry into clinical trials

HMB-45 = human melanoma black-45; LDH = lactate dehydrogenase; MART-1 = melanoma antigen recognized by T-cells

From Balch CM, Gershenwald JE, Soong SW, et al: Final version of 2009 AJCC melanoma staging and classification. J Clin Oncol 27:6199–6206, 2009.

In the 2010 version of the AJCC staging system, there was no change in nodal basin staging. Importantly, despite reports from some centers that a low burden of disease in the regional node predicts no additional nodal metastasis, the current staging system does not identify a minimal nodal tumor burden that would be considered essentially negative.

Melanoma of unknown primary

Melanoma of unknown primary (MUP) occurs in up to 5% of patients who present to tertiary cancer referral centers. Lymphadenopathy is the most common clinical presentation followed by identification of visceral metastases and cutaneous nodules. Patients should be evaluated by a dermatologist and should undergo a complete physical examination, including an anorectal and genital evaluation. A CT scan of the chest, abdomen, and pelvis and/or a whole-body PET scan are useful for staging patients with MUP. In the absence of other sites of disease, surgical resection of the metastatic lesion (or complete regional lymphadenectomy) is appropriate. In the absence of symptoms, an ophthalmologic consultation is probably not warranted unless liver metastases are the only site of disease, given the propensity for ocular melanoma to metastasize to this site.

Single dermal nodules with no identifiable primary lesion are typically treated in similar fashion to primary melanomas, with wide local excision and regional nodal evaluation SLNB if appropriate. The prognosis for patients who present with MUP is similar to that for somewhat more favorable patients with metastatic disease from a known primary (AJCC M1a).

Clinical and pathologic staging

TNM staging system

The melanoma staging committee of the AJCC revised the TNM staging system to reflect more accurately the impact of statistically significant prognostic factors that were validated on a multi-institution sample of 38,918 melanoma patients. The AJCC 2010 Staging System is shown in Tables 1, 2, and 3. Survival curves from the AJCC Melanoma Staging Database comparing different T categories and stage groupings for stages I and II melanoma are shown in Figure 1; in addition, for patients with stage III disease, survival curves in this figure compare the different N categories and the stage groupings.

Changes in the staging system are summarized in Table 3. The most significant change to the 2010 AJCC staging classification is the replacement of Clark's level by presence of mitoses in the stage I group. This involves the use of mitotic rate in the staging of patients with clinically localized melanoma $\leq$ 1 mm. Patients without ulceration and a mitosis $< 1/mm^2$ are categorized as T1a, whereas those with more than mitosis are T1b.

For patients with stage IV disease (distant metastases), there are few long-term survivors, but significant differences in prognosis for disease limited to the skin, for subcutaneous and nodal sites vs visceral sites, and for patients with levels of LDH in the serum.

Other prognostic factors

Age

Overall, patients who are ≥ 65 years old have a survival rate that is decreased by 10% to 15% compared with their younger counterparts. This trend has been demonstrated in numerous studies. A different relationship between age and risk of lymph node involvement, however, is emerging. Data from the prospective Sunbelt Melanoma Trial and retrospective studies reveal that younger patients are significantly more likely to harbor nodal disease than older patients with similar lesions.

Gender

Many studies have identified improved survival in women compared with men with melanoma when stratified by stage. The reasons for this are unclear.

Anatomic location

There is a correlation between anatomic location and prognosis of primary melanoma. Those with lesions on the back, upper arms, neck, and scalp (BANS area) have a worse prognosis than those with lesions on the extremities. This may be due to the simple fact that these lesions cannot be evaluated easily by the patient because of their inopportune location rather than a manifestation of true differences in tumor biology. Men are more likely to develop truncal melanomas, whereas women are most likely to develop melanoma on their extremities.

Desmoplastic melanoma

Desmoplastic melanomas represent a less common but clinically distinct spindle cell variant of melanoma with dense fibrosis and frequent neurotropism. Clinically, they are raised, firm nodules that are amelanotic in up to 40% of patients, commonly leading to a delay in diagnosis.They are usually deep lesions but have a more favorable prognosis than do conventional melanomas of a similar depth. The association of desmoplastic melanoma with local recurrence may be due to the fact that many of these lesions are misdiagnosed and undertreated, with regard to an appropriate radial margin of excision.

Additionally, although many of these lesions are deeply invasive at the time of diagnosis, desmoplastic melanomas are less likely to involve regional lymph node basins. Patients with "pure" desmoplastic melanoma are extremely unlikely to harbor regional nodal metastasis, and SLN biopsy is unlikely to provide useful information. Patients with "mixed" desmoplastic melanoma, containing a component of conventional melanoma, have a risk of regional nodal metastasis that is approximately half that of patients with purely conventional melanoma, and SLN mapping should be considered in these patients.

Despite the fact that these lesions are often relatively thick at presentation, patients with desmoplastic melanomas tend to have survival rates that are favorable compared with patients with conventional melanomas of a similar depth.

Angiolymphatic invasion

Defined as invasion of tumor cells into the wall and/or lumen of vessels or lymphatics of the dermis or deeper structures, angiolymphatic invasion is uncommon in malignant melanoma. However, this finding is clearly associated with more aggressive tumors. Multiple large studies have shown worsened long-term survival and more frequent lymph node involvement in patients with angioinvasive melanomas. In fact, risk of lymphatic involvement increases as much as threefold, whereas 5-year survival is reduced by as much as 50%, in patients with vascular invasion compared with matched patients without vascular invasion.

Regression

The finding of regression represents host immune response to invasive melanoma. Areas where invasive cells may have once existed are replaced by inflammatory reaction and fibrosis, which may make it impossible to determine the precise depth of the initial lesion histologically. There is continuing debate regarding the prognostic importance of regression; however, many clinicians believe that thin lesions that show signs of regression should be given higher consideration for surgical nodal staging, given the fact that the initial lesion may have originally been more deeply invasive. Although some studies have shown that regressed lesions have a higher propensity for lymph node metastases than nonregressed primary tumors of the same thickness, this finding has not been universally observed. Indeed, a recent retrospective single-institution study demonstrated no increased risk of SLN metastasis in patients with regressed melanoma, suggesting that SLNB should not be performed for lesions that would otherwise not be considered based on the presence of regression.

Tumor-infiltrating lymphocytes (TILs)

Variable numbers of TILs are observed in melanoma. Tumors with a high number of TILs should carry an improved prognosis because of the active host response to tumor. In fact, many studies have shown this tendency. The absence of TILs in the primary melanoma has been associated with a higher risk of positive SLNs in a recent, large, single-institution study.

TREATMENT

Surgical treatment of cutaneous melanoma

Excision of primary lesion

It was recognized over a century ago that tumor cells could extend within the skin for several centimeters beyond the visible borders of a melanoma, so that the risk of local recurrence relates to the width of normal skin excised around the primary tumor. Only much more recently was it realized that the thickness of the primary tumor influenced the likelihood of contiguous spread and that not all melanomas require the same excision margin. This realization prompted a number of randomized trials to determine the optimal excision margins for melanomas of different Breslow's thicknesses.

Initially, a "one-size-fits-all" approach of taking a 5-cm margin around all cutaneous melanomas was adopted. With such wide margins, skin grafts were required after removal of melanomas on most parts of the body. Modern melanoma surgical care is based on level I medical evidence, and many large, prospective randomized trials have been conducted to determine the appropriate radial margin for cutaneous melanoma based on Breslow thickness.

A randomized trial conducted by the WHO found that when a 1-cm margin of normal skin was taken around a melanoma < 1 mm thick, the local recurrence rate was exceedingly low (< 1%), and patient survival was just as good as if 3-cm margins were taken. For melanomas 1 to 2 mm in thickness, patient survival was the same for both margins of excision, but the local recurrence rate was higher with the 1-cm margin (3.3% after 10-year follow-up).

The Intergroup Melanoma Trial compared 2- vs 4-cm margins for all cutaneous melanomas of the trunk or proximal extremity between 1 and 4 mm in thickness. Most patients in this trial had melanomas less than or equal to 2 mm in thickness. In the Intergroup trial, both local recurrence and survival were the same regardless of whether 2- or 4-cm margins were obtained. Skin grafts were less frequent and hospital stays shorter with the narrower margin.

A recent trial conducted in the United Kingdom addressed patients with primary melanoma greater than or equal to 2 mm in depth. Patients who underwent a 1-cm radial margin of excision had a higher risk of local/regional recurrence than those who underwent excision with 3-cm margins.

Current recommendations

Based on these important studies, it is possible to make rational recommendations for excision margins for melanoma patients.

- Patients with melanoma less than or equal to 1 mm should undergo excision of skin and subcutaneous tissue for a radial margin of 1 cm.
- Patients with melanoma between 1 and 2 mm should undergo excision of skin and subcutaneous tissue for a radial margin of 1 to 2 cm.
- Patients with melanoma greater than 2 mm in depth should undergo a wide excision of skin and subcutaneous tissue of 2 to 3 cm.
- When the anatomic location of the primary tumor precludes excision of the margin (eg, on the face), at least 1 cm should be taken when feasible.

TNM staging system

Clinically apparent lymphadenopathy

Melanoma patients with clinically enlarged nodes and no evidence of distant disease (AJCC stage IIIB) should undergo complete regional lymphadenectomy. The first step in evaluating palpable nodes is generally FNA. A negative or inadequate sample FNA may be repeated, with image guidance if necessary, or may lead directly to an open node biopsy, followed by complete lymphadenectomy in the event of a positive frozen section or touch-prep cytologic determination of metastasis.

Clinically normal nodes

The surgical management of clinically normal nodes is determined by the characteristics of the primary lesion. A direct relationship between thickness of the primary lesion and nodal involvement has long been recognized. When the depth of the primary is unknown because of the biopsy technique or other factors, consideration should be given to SLN mapping.

SLNB is the primary method for regional nodal staging. All potentially involved basins should initially be examined as part of a thorough history and physical examination.

Thin melanomas Patients with thin melanomas (< 1 mm Breslow depth) have a low risk of occult nodal involvement (< 5%). Some patients with melanomas 0.76 to 1 mm have a high enough risk of lymph node involvement to justify consideration of SLNB in addition to wide excision.

When ulceration is present, consideration should be given to SLNB. In addition, a high mitotic count should prompt consideration of regional nodal basin staging.

Intermediate-thickness melanomas Risk of nodal metastasis rises significantly with increasing depth of invasion. Patients with a 1-mm thick melanoma have approximately a 10% chance of nodal involvement, whereas those with a 4-mm melanoma have a 35% to 40% risk of nodal metastases. For these reasons, wide excision of the primary tumor is generally accompanied by SLNB for staging of the nodal basin. Patients who have evidence of metastasis in the SLN are offered completion lymphadenectomy as a standard approach. An alternative approach of wide excision alone with observation and serial physical examination of nodal basins has been advocated by some clinicians and has not been shown to reduce long-term survival if complete lymph node dissection is performed at the identification of clinically positive nodes. This approach is justified in a recently completed prospective randomized clinical trial of wide excision and SLN mapping compared with wide excision and nodal basin observation. There was no evidence that SLN mapping contributed to an overall survival benefit, but it was a powerful predictor of outcome. The use of SLNB vs observation continues to be an area of intense debate.

Regional lymphadenectomy

The identification and management of nodal disease have evolved significantly over the past 20 years. Historically, complete lymph node dissections were performed on all patients with intermediate and thick melanomas with the belief that this would lead to a survival benefit. This was based on the observation that there was an approximately 20% survival advantage to patients found to have microscopic involvement of lymph nodes at "elective" lymph node dissection when compared with those patients who had clinically apparent nodal metastasis and underwent a "therapeutic" lymph node dissection. With elective node dissection, however, a significant percentage (80% to 85%) of patients underwent complete lymphadenectomy only to find that their nodal basin was free of disease. More importantly, a series of prospective randomized clinical trials failed to demonstrate a survival advantage for patients undergoing elective lymphadenectomy over wide excision only. For this reason, the standard approach prior to the use of SLN mapping was wide excision alone and clinical observation of the nodal basin.

SLN mapping is performed by injecting radiolabeled colloid into the dermis surrounding the primary melanoma. The radiotracer migrates via the lymphatics to the regional nodal basin(s), which is visualized with a gamma camera. The patient is then taken to the operating room, where a hand-held gamma probe is used to identify the sentinel node(s). This technique, in combination with the use of vital blue dye, has led to a success rate exceeding 99% in most large current trials.

The intuitive hope that SLN mapping and biopsy followed by completion lymphadenectomy would result in improved survival was not borne out in a recently reported prospective randomized clinical trial. Even in the absence of a proven survival benefit, however, the staging advantages of SLNB are sufficiently compelling to justify its routine use in healthy patients with melanomas and a significant risk of nodal involvement. A large, prospective clinical trial is currently being conducted to determine the role of completion lymphadenectomy compared with close surveillance in SLN-positive patients.

Thick melanomas Deep melanomas harbor nodal metastases in up to 60% of patients; surgical evaluation of the nodal basin may be appropriate, as most studies suggest that SLN status retains prognostic status in patients with deep primary melanoma. Unless the information will direct further management, however, it is unlikely to be of benefit for these patients. In addition, a completion lymphadenectomy for those at high risk for local and regional recurrence may subject the patients to undue morbidity. The lymphedema associated with complete node dissection may complicate treatment of subsequent recurrences in patients with deep melanoma of the extremity. Although elective or completion lymph node dissection (LND) has not proven beneficial in these patients, SLNB has been used extensively to guide diagnostic, prognostic, and therapeutic decision-making.

Surgical treatment of noncutaneous melanoma

Ocular melanomas

These lesions generally do not have access to lymphatic channels, so the surgical principles outlined previously do not apply here. However, the unique propensity to metastasize hematogeneously, often to the liver after a long relapse-free interval, warrants further study of the biology associated with this primary site. Advances in understanding the biology of ocular melanomas may lead to adjuvant approaches different from therapies now under investigation for cutaneous primaries.

A diagnosis of ocular melanoma with no evidence of distant disease signifies that a decision must be made as to whether or not the eye can be spared. Some small melanomas situated peripherally in the retina can be excised with minimal loss of vision, but most cannot. For larger lesions, treatment options are enucleation (total removal of the eye) or implanted radiotherapy with a radioactive gold plaque fitted to the back of the eyeball immediately behind the tumor. A multi-institution, randomized trial comparing implanted radiotherapy with enucleation for local disease control and overall survival was completed by the COMSG; it appears that both techniques provide similar outcomes for all sizes of tumors.

Melanomas of the anus and vulva

These pose challenges in the treatment of both the primary lesion and regional nodes. These "mucosal" melanomas are notoriously difficult to cure and are almost always associated with a poor outcome. The surgical management of anal melanoma is controversial, but most surgeons prefer a wide excision, when possible, over an abdominoperineal resection (APR). In the past, an APR was more commonly used for patients with less-advanced disease who were viewed as potentially curable. This almost certainly explains the reported association of APR with long-term survivors.

More recently, APR is reserved for patients with bulky disease or recurrent disease that is not amenable to wide excision, which is favored for patients with more localized/potentially curable disease. Not surprisingly, more recent studies demonstrate no survival advantage to APR, which appears to be equivalent to wide excision.

Radical resection is also less commonly performed for patients with vulvar melanoma, who also have a high risk for relapse and death. Function-preserving resection and nodal basin staging in the setting of relatively early disease are appropriate, but, as in patients with anal primaries, preemptive nodal staging in patients with advanced primary tumors is unlikely to impart a benefit to those whose nodal basin can be followed clinically.

Nasal sinuses or nasopharyngeal melanomas

Melanomas arising in the nasal or nasopharyngeal mucosa should be widely excised to include adjacent bony structures, if needed. As in patients with anal or vulvar melanoma, node dissection is reserved for patients who have proven nodal involvement. Radiotherapy should be considered for those patients whose primary tumor cannot be fully removed from this site with adequate margins or as adjuvant therapy in patients unlikely to be controlled with surgical resection alone.

Adjuvant therapy for melanoma

Interferon α-2b (IFN-α; Intron A) was approved as a standard therapy on the basis of an adjuvant therapy trial conducted in patients with deep primary or N1 disease (ECOG). Interferon α-2b was administered by IV, 20 mU/m^2 for 5 consecutive days every 7 days for 4 weeks, during the "induction" phase. For a subsequent 48 weeks, 10 mU/m^2 was administered by subcutaneous injection on alternate days for a total of three doses every 7 days in the "maintenance" phase.

This "high-dose" regimen was compared with observation. A statistically significant improvement in overall survival was demonstrated with interferon, compared with the observation arm; relapse-free survival was also improved. Three-quarters of the interferon patients experienced severe toxicities, most commonly fatigue, asthenia, fever, depression, and elevated liver transaminase levels. A quality-of-life analysis found that the toxicity associated with this regimen was largely compensated for by the prevention of disease relapse.

Due to uncertainty regarding the optimal dose and schedule of interferon, a second trial was initiated comparing the high-dose regimen and a low-dose regimen (3 mU by subcutaneous injection 3 times weekly for 24 months) as well as observation. No significant improvement in overall survival for either the high-dose or low-dose arm was observed compared with observation; relapse-free survival was improved by 22% in the high-dose arm compared with observation. A pooled analysis of E1684 and E1690, with longer follow-up for both trials, revealed a continued, statistically significant impact on relapse-free survival but not on overall survival.

High-dose interferon has been consistently shown to improve relapse-free survival compared with either observation or ganglioside GM2/keyhole limpet hemocyanin (GM2-KLH) vaccination but does not clearly confer an overall survival advantage. A recent prospective randomized trial conducted by the HCOG compared outcome in patients treated with high-dose interferon as an adjuvant for 1 month vs 1 year and found no difference in overall survival or disease-free survival; however, this trial was of insufficient size to firmly conclude that 1 month of interferon therapy is truly equivalent to the full-year regimen with regard to relapse-free survival. Due to the significant toxicity associated with 1 year of high-dose interferon and the lack of an overall survival advantage, consensus is lacking regarding the use of interferon in the adjuvant setting.

Intermediate-dose regimens with interferon have been evaluated in several trials; they have less consistently demonstrated a relapse-free survival advantage compared with observation and have never resulted in a survival advantage. A recent trial conducted by the EORTC demonstrated no survival advantage for patients undergoing 13 months or 25 months of intermediate-dose adjuvant interferon after resection of stage IIB (deep primary melanoma) or stage III nodal disease when compared with observation.

The EORTC reported the results of a prospective randomized trial of observation vs pegylated interferon-α for 5 years. Again, there was an advantage to treatment in terms of relapse-free survival but no overall survival advantage for patients with high-risk resected melanoma. Nearly one-third of the patients in the treated arm discontinued therapy due to toxicity.

Adjuvant chemotherapy

Single-agent chemotherapy or combination chemotherapy regimens have not been systematically evaluated for the adjuvant treatment of melanoma because of the low response rates seen in patients with advanced disease. The largest randomized trial compared an IV administered regimen of carmustine (BiCNU; 80 mg/m^2) every 4 weeks, dactinomycin (Cosmegen, 10 μg/kg), and vincristine (1.0 mg/m^2) every 2 weeks for 6 months with observation among patients with resected stage III or IV melanoma. A significant improvement in relapse-free survival, but not overall survival, was observed in this small study. A randomized trial comparing dacarbazine and observation failed to demonstrate an improvement in either relapse-free or overall survival.

There is currently no widely accepted adjuvant therapy following resection of metastatic melanoma. Therefore, observation remains a standard of care for patients in this setting, and some investigational therapies are currently being evaluated in comparison to placebo in light of the significant percentage of patients who choose not to pursue interferon therapy.

Neoadjuvant therapy for resectable stage IIIC or IV melanoma remains an investigational approach. Neoadjuvant biochemotherapy (cisplatin, dacarbazine, vinblastine, interleukin-2 [IL-2], and interferon) was evaluated in a small study of patients with stage III melanoma. In the 50 patients with measurable disease, the response rate was 26%. High-dose interferon, however, produced a 55% clinical response and 15% pathologic response when used in a neoadjuvant setting in a small group of patients with clinically apparent nodal metastasis. Currently available chemotherapy regimens for melanoma are not sufficiently active to support use in neoadjuvant therapy.

Radiation therapy

In vitro data from the 1970s demonstrated radiation resistance among melanoma cell lines and thus have led to the reluctance to use radiation therapy in the treatment of melanoma. More modern data have shown that many melanomas are sensitive to radiation, but the disinclination toward the use of radiation therapy for melanoma continues.

Another unanswered question is the proper fraction size to use in melanoma. In a large series of patients studied by Overgaard and colleagues, they found that the response rate of metastatic melanoma lesions was dependent on the fraction size. The complete response rate was 57% when fractions greater than 4 Gy were used, compared with 24% for those of less than 4 Gy. RTOG 83-05 is the only randomized trial that compared hypofractionated (8 Gy for 4 fractions) and conventional (2.5 Gy for 20 fractions) schedules of radiation therapy. In this study, they noted no difference in the complete and partial responses. Though a wide spectrum of fraction sizes have been used, this does not preclude the use of radiation but emphasizes the need for more research to better understand and create an effective fractionation schedule.

Adjuvant radiation treatment

Radiation treatment has been increasingly employed in the postoperative setting to improve locoregional tumor control in a select group of patients. In the past decade, there have been multiple reports regarding patient outcomes with the use of adjuvant radiation treatment. The 5-year regional control has ranged from 87% to 94%, and the 5-year overall survival has ranged from 36% to 46% with the addition of radia-

TABLE 4: Selected chemotherapy agents – Results from phase II and phase III trials in melanoma

Chemotherapy	Patients (N)	Objective response rate
Alkylating agents		
Dacarbazine	2,470	18%
Temozolomide	350	15%
Nitrosoureas		
Lomustine	270	13%
Fotemustine	153	24%
Platinum analog		
Cisplatin	188	23%
Carboplatin	43	16%
Microtubule stabilizing/destabilizing		
Paclitaxel	85	13%
Docetaxel	105	11%
Vincristine	52	12%
Vinblastine	62	13%
Vindesine	273	14%

tion to surgery. Single institutions have reported that local recurrence is reduced to 6% to 11% when postoperative radiotherapy is used for high-risk lesions, relative to 19% seen in the O'Brien study and 30% in previous studies. High risk is defined as having a thick primary, desmoplasia or neurotropism, a head and neck site, close or positive (unresectable) margins, and multiple previous recurrences. In these reports, they found that serious complication rates after radiation therapy were low, which is likely secondary to the superficial nature of the treated volumes.

At the Royal Prince Alfred Hospital, 143 patients with melanoma metastases to the parotid and/or cervical lymph nodes were treated with surgery alone or surgery and postoperative radiation therapy. The patients who received radiation therapy had more aggressive features such as at least two lymph nodes, and extracapsular extension; there was a trend toward higher regional control in the group that received surgery and postoperative radiation therapy (94%) than with surgery alone (91%, $P = .065$).

In a retrospective study of 615 patients at Roswell Park and M. D. Anderson who had advanced regional nodal metastasis, adjuvant radiotherapy was associated with improved regional control when compared with surgery alone. The results of a prospective randomized trial of adjuvant radiotherapy in melanoma patients with high-risk nodal metastasis confirmed this observation. In this trial, there was no impact of radiation on survival. The risk of long-term lymphedema is known to be high in patients with inguinal lymph node metastases; thus, it would be prudent to consider a higher threshold for treatment of these patients. Indeed, in a recent large, retrospective review, there was no improvement in regional control in patients at high risk for nodal basin failure undergoing adjuvant radiotherapy to the inguinal nodes as compared with patients having surgery alone. In a review on the use of radiation therapy in malignant melanoma, Stevens and McKay offered the following recommendations for postoperative radiation therapy after regional lymph node dissection:

- Multiple involved nodes (greater than one for parotid, three to four in other regions)
- Any involved node greater than 3 to 4 cm in maximum diameter
- Extranodal spread
- Incomplete dissection
- Recurrence after previous lymph node dissection (no previous radiation therapy)

Radiation therapy can provide some benefit and should be considered in the palliative treatment of melanoma metastatic to bone or other symptomatic sites.

In November 2009, results of the ANZMTG/TROG 02.01 trial were reported at the annual ASTRO meeting. Patients were eligible for the trial if they had involvement of at least one parotid node, at least two cervical or axillary nodes, or at least three groin nodes; extranodal extension; or a minimum metastatic node diameter of 3 cm in the neck or axilla or of 4 cm in the groin. Patients were randomized to observation after surgery or to adjuvant radiation (48 Gy in 20 fractions). At a median follow-up of 38 months, the rate of lymph node recurrence was 68% in the group having surgery and external-beam radiotherapy and 80% in the group having surgery alone.

The radiation treatment compliance rate was 79%. There was a higher rate of acute toxicity (dermatitis and pain) with radiotherapy, but no grade 4 toxicity was seen.

Vaccines and other immunotherapy

These remain an investigational approach and are currently being tested among patients with resected stages II, III, and IV melanoma. The goal of this immunotherapy is to reverse immune tolerance of microscopic residual melanoma following surgery through the amplification of melanoma-specific cytolytic T cells. This approach is distinct from conventional immunization against pathogens to which the host is naive, where long-lasting, antibody-mediated immunity is sought by induction of memory B cells.

Melanoma peptide vaccines are currently being intensely evaluated in clinical trials. Peptides have been selected from two classes for clinical development: melanocyte-specific proteins and so-called cancer-testis antigens. The latter are proteins that have a restricted spatiotemporal expression and are not detectable in adult tissues outside the immunologic sanctuary site of the testes. The most widely studied peptides are derived from gp-100, tyrosinase, melan-A (all melanocyte-specific), and *NY-ESO-1* and melanoma antigen-encoding gene (*MAGE*) proteins (cancer-testis antigens). Preliminary evidence suggests that this approach may successfully engender specific and potent immunologic responses to the protein fragments being administered. Protection against disease recurrence in patients at high risk following surgery has not yet been demonstrated. Notably, no randomized data suggesting a detrimental effect from peptide vaccination in melanoma have been presented. Indeed, a recent prospective randomized trial reported a survival advantage for patients treated with a peptide vaccine (gp100:209-217). Patients with metastatic melanoma were randomized to receive a multivalent peptide vaccine and high-dose IL-2 vs high-dose IL-2 alone. This approach may prove promising in the adjuvant setting.

CTLA-4 blockade

Ipilimumab (MDX-010) is a promising new agent for the treatment of patients with metastatic melanoma. Ipilimumab is a monoclonal antibody against CTLA-4 (cytotoxic T-lymphocyte–associated molecule-4). It has been used in patients with metastatic melanoma and renal cell carcinoma refractory to other immunotherapies. The overall response rate is 10%, with a significant percentage of patients having a durable complete response.

The efficacy of ipilimumab is due to its ability to block the normal activity of CTLA-4, a molecule that tempers the immune system's response to antigen. Although the exact antitumor activity of anti–CTLA-4 is unclear, it is thought that by inhibiting the activity of CTLA-4, the threshold for a full immune response to antigen may be lowered, and an immune response against tumor antigens is facilitated.

In 2010, the results of the first phase III trial comparing ipilimumab combined with GP-100 peptide vaccine to vaccine alone or ipilimumab alone were reported. This trial demonstrated overall survival benefit for both of the ipilimumab-containing arms, compared with peptide vaccine alone. The rates of overall survival at 12 months for ipilimumab plus GP-100 and ipilimumab alone were 44% and 46%, compared with 25% for peptide vaccine alone. The rates of overall survival at 24 months for the ipilimumab-containing arms were 22% and 24%, compared with 14% for peptide vaccine alone. These data confirm a durable benefit associated with this novel immunotherapy in metastatic melanoma patients who had failed one prior therapy. Ongoing trials of ipilimumab as a therapeutic agent and as an adjuvant therapy will provide further guidance regarding the role this new drug will play in the treatment of patients with melanoma.

B-raf inhibition is an appealing target in patients with cutaneous melanoma, as 50% to 65% of patients have tumors with an activating mutation. Despite this, sorafenib (Nexavar), a first-generation *B-raf* targeting drug, was disappointing and ineffective. PLX4032 is a more specific *B-raf* target, and in the extension cohort (fixed dose, all melanoma patients) of a recently completed phase II trial, Flaherty et al reported a remarkable 81% response rate with a median progression-free survival time of 7 months. Of the patients, 78% had been treated with at least one prior chemotherapy regimen, and 38% of the patients had been treated with three or more. A phase III trial is in progress in which patients with melanoma and *B-raf* mutation are randomized to DTIC vs PLX4032. The trial is rapidly accruing owing to the exciting phase II results.

Treatment of advanced melanoma

Surgery

The surgical treatment of patients with isolated or limited distant metastasis is controversial, as there are only a few systemic agents with demonstrated tumor responses, and only a few patients may be eligible for surgery. A number of retrospective studies have shown the validity of resecting pulmonary metastases in patients with melanoma, and more recent studies have shown similar survival rates for patients undergoing resection of limited number and sites of disease (usually up to four) for metastases to distant lymph nodes, skin and subcutaneous tissue, and lungs. Patients with isolated metastases in the liver, adrenal, brain, and gastrointestinal tract may undergo resection, but the survival of these patients may be less favorable.

Surgical resection may also be an important component of palliation. Bleeding or obstruction from small intestine metastases may be managed by resection. Although palliative resection can provide short-term effective relief of patient symptoms, numerous studies have shown that incomplete resection does nothing to enhance the length of survival.

Single-agent chemotherapy

Melanoma is regarded as a relatively chemotherapy-refractory tumor. Durable objective responses have been observed in a small minority of patients with metastatic melanoma treated with single-agent chemotherapy, providing perhaps the most compelling reason to offer these agents routinely.

In a phase III trial comparing temozolomide (Temodar) and dacarbazine as first-line therapy, 3% of patients on either arm experienced complete responses. The highest response rates have been observed with alkylating agents, platinum-analog, and mictrotubule-interactive drugs (Table 4). The reference standard to which novel agents and regimens are compared is dacarbazine. In the majority of trials, dacarbazine was administered IV at daily doses of 200 mg/m^2 for 5 days every 3 or 4 weeks; however, 1,000 mg/m^2 once every 3 or 4 weeks has been given in recent trials. The most common toxicities are myelosuppression and nausea. The severity of myelosuppression rarely requires the use of growth factor support, and the advent of potent antiemetics in recent years has significantly improved the tolerability of this agent. In the largest phase III trial that included a single-agent dacarbazine arm, the objective response rate was 3.5%, and the median progression-free survival was 1.5 months. Overall survival for dacarbazine-treated patients is 6 to 9 months and does not clearly differ from the natural history of metastatic melanoma. Fotemustine, a nitrosourea with modestly superior activity compared with dacarbazine, is available for clinical use in Europe but not in the United States.

Combination chemotherapy regimens

As with other types of cancer, combinations of agents with some measurable single-agent activity in melanoma have been empirically developed. Clinical trials combining chemotherapy have produced promising response rates in single-arm, single-institution studies but have never demonstrated an improvement in overall survival compared with single-agent chemotherapy in multicenter, randomized trials. Given the increased toxicity associated with such regimens, the absence of a survival advantage limits their consideration as standard therapies. These treatments include cisplatin, vinblastine, and dacarbazine (CVD) and the Dartmouth regimen (cisplatin, carmustine, dacarbazine, and tamoxifen). Inpatient treatment is standard for these regimens, and the severity of myelosuppression often requires growth factor support not needed for single-agent chemotherapies. Given that longevity is not impacted for these patients who have such a short life expectancy, the quality-of-life detriment associated with combination therapy cannot be justified.

Tamoxifen

Based on anecdotes of tumor regression associated with single-agent tamoxifen and laboratory evidence suggesting synergy with chemotherapy, clinical trials were undertaken combining tamoxifen with individual chemotherapy agents or combination regimens. As with other combination chemotherapy trials, single-arm trials of regimens containing tamoxifen appeared promising. However, in randomized trials where the same chemotherapy regimen was administered to all patients, and tamoxifen given only to the experimental arm, no evidence of clinical benefit was observed with the addition of tamoxifen.

Biologic therapies

IL-2 was approved by the FDA as a treatment for metastatic melanoma on the basis of durable complete and partial remissions associated with the "high-dose" regimen. This regimen requires patients to be in excellent overall health to tolerate the physiologic stress of 5 days of inpatient therapy. The standard dose is 200,000 U/m^2 repeated every 8 hours, for a maximum of 14 doses. This treatment is followed by a treatment break of 10 to 14 days and readmission for another course of therapy. Patients who demonstrate some degree of tumor regression are offered additional courses of therapy. Typical toxicities include fever, malaise, hypotension complicated by renal dysfunction, elevated levels of liver transaminases, and mood alterations. Clinical expertise among physicians and nurses is required to safely and effectively administer this therapy. As a consequence, the use of high-dose IL-2 has largely been restricted to high-volume referral centers.

Interferon-α has demonstrated single-agent activity in metastatic melanoma that is comparable to chemotherapy, including occasional durable responses. A randomized trial comparing interferon-α with dacarbazine in metastatic disease has never been conducted. Given the significant toxicity associated with chronic administration of interferon, its use in the metastatic setting is limited.

Biochemotherapy regimens

The distinct mechanism of action of biologic agents and evidence of single-agent activity have led investigators to combine these agents with chemotherapy for the treatment of metastatic melanoma. Given the toxicity associated with high-dose IL-2, it is not possible to safely administer chemotherapy concurrently. However, lower-dose IL-2 regimens can be safely coadministered with combination chemotherapy. Likewise, the high-dose interferon regimen that is the current standard therapy for adjuvant treatment of stages II and III melanoma cannot be easily combined with chemotherapy, whereas modified schedules of interferon can.

The first biochemotherapy regimens tested in phase II trials and then subsequently in large, randomized phase III trials combined interferon-α with dacarbazine. Despite early evidence suggesting a substantially higher response rate associated with the combination, definitive phase III trials failed to identify a survival advantage to this regimen over with dacarbazine alone.

More intensive regimens combining chemotherapy with biologic agents, requiring inpatient administration, have more recently been evaluated. A regimen containing cisplatin, vinblastine, dacarbazine, with concurrent interferon and IL-2, was evaluated in several phase II trials, a small, single-institution phase III trial, and a multicenter phase III trial in comparison to multiagent chemotherapy without the biologic agents. Although progression-free survival appeared modestly superior to that of the chemotherapy backbone alone, no improvement in overall survival could be demonstrated. Likewise, a trial in which the contribution of IL-2 to a regimen of cisplatin, dacarbazine, and interferon-α was isolated failed to demonstrate a significant improvement in outcome.

Targeted therapy

The discovery of somatic genetic mutations in melanoma, underlying aberrant signal transduction in melanoma cells, has provided leads for the development of molecularly targeted therapy. The MAP kinase pathway, which is activated in the vast majority of melanomas due to mutations in *B-raf*, *NRAS*, and *c-kit*, has been the focus of most clinical investigations of signal transduction (kinase) inhibitors. Angiogenesis, necessary for the progression of all solid tumors, has proved to be a valuable therapeutic target in the treatment of other metastatic cancers and is currently being investigated in randomized trials in melanoma.

Promising early results have been generated in clinical trials with potent and selective inhibitors of *B-raf* among patients whose tumors harbor activating mutations in this gene. The orally available therapies have been associated with very high objective response rates (70%–80%) but highly variable duration of response. Confirmatory clinical trials are under way attempting to establish these agents as standard therapies for the treatment of metastatic melanoma. This represents a particularly exciting development given the presence of *B-raf* mutations in 50% of the metastatic melanoma population.

Activating mutations in the c-kit receptor were recently identified in patients with acral, mucosal, and lentigo maligna melanoma. The successful development of c-kit–targeted therapies in gastrointestinal carcinoma, where mutations in the same gene are found, has provided the opportunity for immediate investigation of these oral agents in patients with metastatic melanoma harboring *c-kit* mutations. Early reports suggests that a subset of *c-kit* mutant melanomas respond to inhibitors of the signaling portion of this receptor.

Palliative radiation therapy

Unfortunately, many patients with malignant melanoma will present with CNS metastases. These patients can be symptomatic, with complaints of headache, seizures, motor loss, or impaired mentation; these symptoms can be relieved with the use of whole-brain radiation therapy (WBRT). WBRT has been used with multiple different fractionation schemes, although none has been found to be superior to standard fractionation (300 cGy × 10). These patients have a median survival of 2.2 to 4.9 months with the addition of WBRT, with local tumor control rates in the brain in the 70% to 80% range.

Stereotactic radiosurgery (SRS) involves the use of a large, single fraction of radiation to a limited target volume and rapid dose falloff outside the target. A standard linear accelerator is used to deliver one dose, usually between 15 and 24 Gy. Most centers that perform SRS have an upper size limit for the metastatic lesion (approximately 4 cm). Proponents of this treatment have shown less cognitive decline due to the limited area of radiation. There has been a small prospective series of patients with one to three brain metastases from melanoma, renal cell carcinoma, and sarcoma treated with SRS alone; they were found to have a 32% intracranial recurrence rate outside the SRS volume, suggesting there is a need for WBRT.

RTOG 95-08 was a randomized trial that looked at the addition of SRS to WBRT in patients with one to three brain metastases (including those with metastatic melanoma). Both treatment modalities produced an improvement in Karnofsky Performance Status (KPS) at 6-month follow-up, with no difference in mental status or neurologic death. Patients with only one brain metastasis who underwent WBRT and SRS had a survival advantage (median survival time, 6.5 vs 4.9 months; $P = .0393$).

Patients with recurrent disease or metastasis at multiple sites may require palliative radiation therapy. Common examples include skin metastases that have bleeding and fungation, painful bony metastases or lymph nodes metastases that push against soft tissue, bony metastases, neurologic compromise, and spinal cord compression from vertebral metastases. These patients may experience improvement in quality of life with a short course of radiation treatment.

Future directions

In addition to the previously mentioned trials in active research, there are multiple studies being performed at different institutions around the United States, some of which are assessing the use of radiosensitizers. The University of Utah is performing a phase II study looking at the response rate of measurable melanoma lesions with the use of cisplatin, a known radiomodifier, with radiation treatment. The M. D. Anderson Cancer Center is performing a phase I trial looking at the toxicity of using docetaxel (Taxotere)/temozolomide/cisplatin in patients with melanoma. There is still much to be understood about radiation treatment for patients with melanoma and how best to use it to its maximal efficacy in this subset of patients.

INITIAL TREATMENT OF NONMELANOMA SKIN CANCER

Surgery

Most nonmelanoma skin cancers can be conservatively excised with much narrower margins than are required for cutaneous melanomas. Excision margins of 0.5 to 1.0 cm are adequate for most nonrecurrent basal cell and squamous cell cancers and yield local recurrence rates under 5%, provided that histologically negative margins are achieved. For most tumors in most anatomic sites, these excision margins can be achieved using standard surgical techniques with local anesthesia and primary closure.

Radiation therapy

Radiation therapy is effective for the treatment of squamous cell and basal cell skin cancers, and is associated with a similar likelihood of cure as surgery. However, this practice is only considered standard in areas of the body where surgery would be disfiguring or debilitating. In instances where negative margins cannot be obtained without an unacceptable cosmetic result, adjuvant radiation therapy to treat microscopic residual disease appears effective. This practice is also typically extended to Merkel cell skin cancers and sarcomas of the skin. The use of radiation therapy to the surgical bed when negative margins have been obtained is more controversial and is not well supported by data.

Topical and intralesional therapy

Topical therapy is a consideration for patients with large areas of skin affected by numerous or recurrent squamous cell or basal skin cancers. Immunocompromised patients and occasional patients with extremes of cumulative lifetime sun exposure are candidates for topical 5-FU or imiquimod. These therapies are generally not offered to patients who are otherwise good candidates for surgical resection. 5-FU is an antimetabolite chemotherapy that is effective in eradicating both actinic keratoses and squamous cell skin cancers. Following treatment, patients typically develop significant erythema in treated skin lasting for several weeks until the treated skin has adequately regenerated its epithelium. Imiquimod stimulates the activity of antigen-presenting cells in the skin when applied topically, which engenders an immune response in treated tumors. Complete regression of treated tumors is typically achieved. However, patients who are offered this therapy are typically at high risk for local recurrence and appearance of new lesions elsewhere and thus require lifelong surveillance and, potentially, repeated treatment.

Intralesional therapy for unresectable or recurrent basal cell skin cancers has been investigated. The only readily available agent that has been employed for this purpose is interferon-α. Comparative trials have not been conducted with intralesional vs topical therapies.

Management of recurrent nonmelanoma skin cancer

Local recurrence complicates approximately 5% of cases of nonmelanoma skin cancer; if possible, surgical resection should be performed. In areas of skin where surgery would result in an unacceptable cosmetic result, radiation therapy can be offered. The vast majority of recurrent nonmelanoma skin cancers can be cured with re-excision or radiation therapy.

Regional lymph node involvement Among nonmelanoma skin cancers, Merkel cell carcinoma is the most likely to be associated with regional lymph node involvement. The prognosis of patients with lymph node involvement appears to be significantly worse than that of patients with localized disease. Thus, SLNB is justified as a staging procedure in patients with primary Merkel cell carcinoma. Squamous cell skin cancer is less likely to involve regional lymph nodes (5% of all cases), and SLNB is generally reserved for patients with primary tumors that are large, deeply invasive, or poorly differentiated. Lymph nodes should be evaluated with FNA to determine the need for lymph node dissection. Basal cell carcinoma infrequently spreads to regional lymph nodes.

Distant metastases occur infrequently in squamous cell carcinoma (2% of all cases) and generally are limited to patients who are immunocompromised. Fewer than 1 in 1,000 cases of basal cell carcinoma develop metastatic disease. Therefore, clinical trials in these patients have not been conducted. Combination chemotherapy regimens employed for squamous cell carcinoma from other sites are typically employed for patients with metastatic squamous cell carcinoma of the skin, although responses appear to be infrequent and usually short-lived.

SUGGESTED READING

ON SKIN CANCERS

Balch CM, Gershenwald JE, Soong SW, et al: Final version of 2009 AJCC melanoma staging and classification. J Clin Oncol 27:6199–6206, 2009.

Swetter SM, Geller AC, Kirkwood JM: Melanoma in the older person. Oncology 18:1187–1196, 2004.

Tsao H, Atkins MB, Sober AJ: Management of cutaneous melanoma. N Engl J Med 351:998–1012, 2004.

ON BIOLOGY AND EPIDEMIOLOGY OF MELANOMA

Chao C, McMasters KM: Relationship between age and other prognostic factors in melanoma. Am J Oncol Rev 3:446–454, 2004.

Curtin JA, Fridlyand J, Kgeshita T, et al: Distinct sets of genetic alterations in melanoma. N Engl J Med 353:2135–2147, 2005.

Demierre MF, Merlino G: Chemoprevention of melanoma. Curr Oncol Rep 6:406–413, 2004.

Kashani-Sabet M: Melanoma genomics. Curr Oncol Rep 6:401–405, 2004.

Tucker MA, Fraser MC, Goldstein AM, et al: A natural history of melanomas and dysplastic nevi: An atlas of lesions in melanoma-prone families. Cancer 94:3192–3209, 2002.

ON SURGICAL TREATMENT AND IMAGING

Agrawal S, Kane JM, Guadagnolo A, et al: The benefits of adjuvant radiation therapy after therapeutic lymphadenectomy for clinically advanced, high risk, lymph node-metastatic melanoma. Cancer 115:5836–5844, 2009.

DuBay D, Cimmino V, Lowe L, et al: Low recurrence rate after surgery for dermatofibrosarcoma protuberans: A multidisciplinary approach from a single institution. Cancer 100:1008–1016, 2004.

Hawkins WG, Busam KJ, Ben-Porat L, et al: Desmoplastic melanoma: A pathologically and clinically distinct form of cutaneous melanoma. Ann Surg Oncol 12:207–213, 2005.

Kammula US, Ghossein R, Bhattacharya S, et al: Serial follow-up and the prognostic significance of reverse transcriptase-polymerase chain reaction—Staged sentinel lymph nodes from melanoma patients. J Clin Oncol 22:3989–3996, 2004.

McMasters KM, Reintgen DS, Ross MI, et al: Sentinel lymph node biopsy for melanoma: Controversy despite widespread agreement. J Clin Oncol 19:2851–2855, 2001.

Mijnhout GS, Hoekstra OS, van Lingen A, et al: How morphometric analysis of metastatic load predicts the (un)usefulness of PET scanning: The case of lymph node staging in melanoma. J Clin Pathol 56:283–286, 2003.

Morton DL, Thompson JF, Cochran AJ, et al: Sentinel-node biopsy or nodal observation in melanoma. N Engl J Med 355:1307–1317, 2006.

Pawlik TM, Sondak VK: Malignant melanoma: Current state of primary and adjuvant treatment. Crit Rev Oncol Hematol 45:245–264, 2003.

Statius Muller MG, van Leeuwen PA, de Lange-de Klerk ES, et al: The sentinel lymph node status is an important factor for predicting clinical outcome in patients with stage I or II cutaneous melanoma. Cancer 91:2401–2408, 2001.

Thomas JM, Newton-Bishop J, A'Hern R, et al: Excision margins in high-risk malignant melanoma. N Engl J Med 350:757–766, 2004.

ON ADJUVANT THERAPY

Ang KK, Byers RM, Peters LJ, et al: Regional radiotherapy as adjuvant treatment for head and neck malignant melanoma: Preliminary results. Arch Otolaryngol Head Neck Surg 116:169–172, 1990.

Ang KK, Peters LJ, Weber RS, et al: Postoperative radiotherapy for cutaneous melanoma of the head and neck region. Int J Radiat Oncol Biol Phys 30:795–798, 1994.

Ballo MT, Ang KK: Radiotherapy for cutaneous malignant melanoma: Rationale and indications. Oncology 18:99–108, 2004.

Ballo MT, Garden AS, Myers JN, et al: Melanoma metastatic to cervical lymph nodes: Can radiotherapy replace formal dissection after local excision of nodal disease? Head Neck 27:718–721, 2005.

Ballo MT, Zagars GK, Gershenwald JE, et al: A critical assessment of adjuvant radiotherapy for inguinal lymph node metastases from melanoma. Ann Surg Oncol 11:1079–1084, 2004.

Bonnen MD, Ballo MT, Myers JN, et al: Elective radiotherapy provides regional control for patients with cutaneous melanoma of the head and neck. Cancer 100:383–389, 2004.

Buchsbaum JC, Suh JH, Lee SY, et al: Survival by radiation therapy oncology group recursive partitioning analysis class and treatment modality in patients with brain metastases from malignant melanoma: A retrospective study. Cancer 94:2265–2272, 2002.

Kirkwood JM, Manola J, Ibrahim J, et al: A pooled analysis of Eastern Cooperative Oncology Group and Intergroup trials of adjuvant high-dose interferon for melanoma. Clin Cancer Res 10:1670–1677, 2004.

Stevens G, McKay MJ: Dispelling the myths surrounding radiotherapy for treatment of cutaneous melanoma. Lancet Oncol 7:575–583, 2006.

ON SYSTEMIC THERAPY

Eichler AF, Loeffler JS: Multidisciplinary management of brain metastases. Oncologist 12:884–898, 2007.

Flaherty KT, Hodi FS, Bastian BC: Mutation-driven drug development in melanoma. Curr Opin Oncol 22:178–183, 2010.

Flaherty KT, Puzanov I, Kim KB, et al: Inhibition of mutated, activated BRAF in metastatic melanoma. N Engl J Med 363:809–819, 2010.

Panelli MC, Wang E, Monsurro V, et al: Overview of melanoma vaccines and promising approaches. Curr Oncol Rep 6:414–420, 2004.

Ribas A, Butterfield LH, Glaspy JA, et al: Current developments in cancer vaccines and cellular immunotherapy. J Clin Oncol 21:2415–2432, 2003.

Rosenberg SA: Shedding light on immunotherapy for cancer. N Engl J Med 350:1461–1463, 2004.

Rosenberg SA, Dudley ME: Cancer regression in patients with metastatic melanoma after the transfer of autologous antitumor lymphocytes. Proc Natl Acad Sci 101(suppl 2):14639–14645, 2004. Cancer Res 10:1670–1677, 2004.

Weber JS, O'Day S, Urba W, et al: Phase I/II study of ipilimumab for patients with metastatic melanoma. J Clin Oncol 26:5950–5956, 2008.

ON METASTATIC DISEASE TREATMENT

Andrews DW, Scott CB, Sperduto PW, et al: Whole brain radiation therapy with or without stereotactic radiosurgery boost for patients with one to three brain metastases: Phase III results of the RTOG 9508 randomised trial. Lancet 363:1665–1672, 2004.

Abbreviations in this chapter

ACS = American Cancer Society, AJCC = American Joint Committee on Cancer; ANZMTG = Australia and New Zealand Melanoma Trials Group; COMSG = Collaborative Ocular Melanoma Study Group; DCOG = Dermatologic Cooperative Oncology Group; ECOG = Eastern Cooperative Oncology Group; EORTC = European Organization for Research and Treatment of Cancer; HCOG = Hellenic Cooperative Oncology Group; RTOG = Radiation Therapy Oncology Group; TROG = Trans-Tasman Radiation Oncology Group; WHO = World Health Organization

The ABCDEs of moles and melanomas

Concept and photographs:
The Skin Cancer Foundation, www.skincancer.org

MOLES/MELANOMAS

People at high risk of developing melanoma are those who have:

- A family history of melanoma, or who have had a melanoma in the past
- Unusual moles on the skin, or changing moles
- Fair skin, light hair and eye color, and who sunburn easily or tan with difficulty
- A record of painful or blistering sunburns as children or in their teenage years
- Indoor occupations and outdoor recreational habits.

When you inspect moles, pay special attention to their sizes, shapes, edges, and color. A handy way to remember these features is to think of the A, B, C, D, and E of skin cancer—asymmetry, border, color, diameter, and evolving.

Asymmetry: If you draw a line through an asymmetrical mole, the two halves will not match.

Border: The borders of an early melanoma tend to be uneven. The edges may be scalloped or notched.

Color: Having a variety of colors is another warning signal. A number of different shades of brown, tan, or black could appear. A melanoma may also become red, blue, or some other color.

Diameter: Melanomas usually are larger in diameter than the size of the eraser on your pencil (1/4 inch or 6 mm), but they may sometimes be smaller when first detected.

Evolving: Any change in a mole—in size, shape, color, elevation, or another trait, or any new symptom such as bleeding, itching, or crusting—points to suspicion and possible danger.

A
Asymmetry

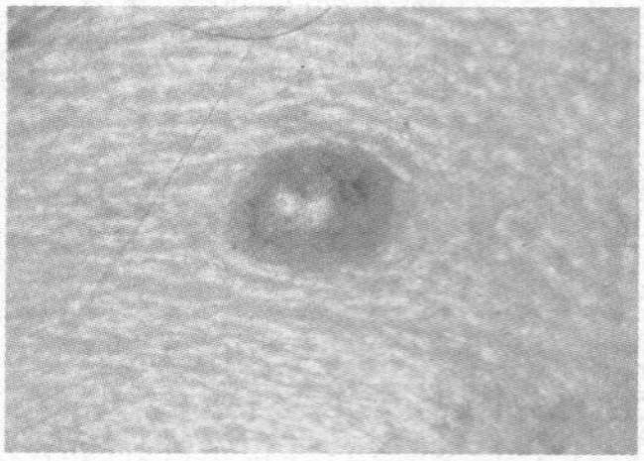

Benign **Symmetrical**

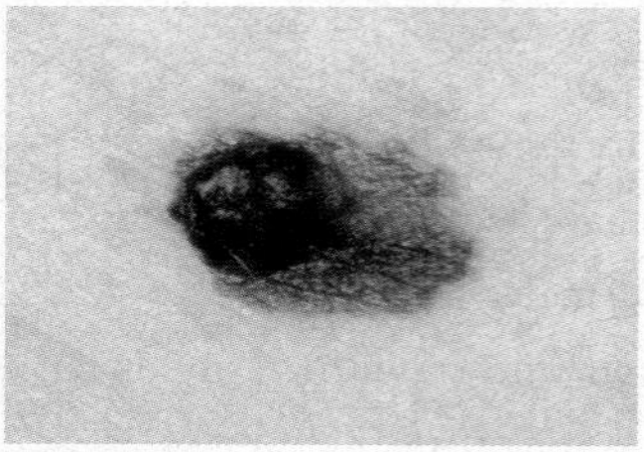

Malignant **Asymmetrical**

B
Border

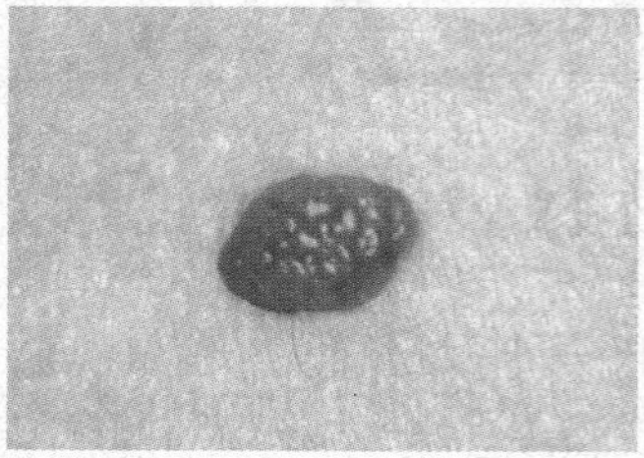

Benign **Even edges**

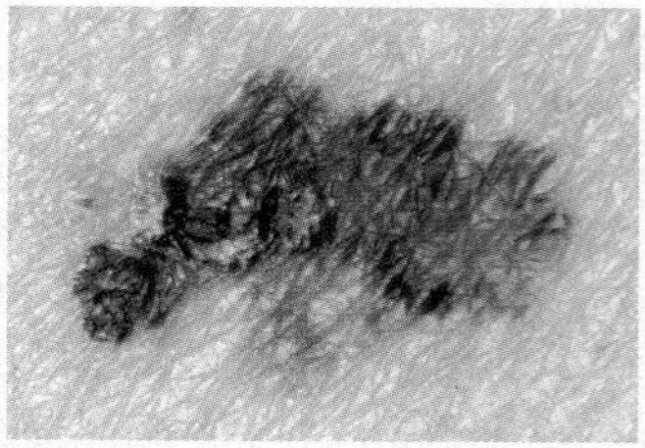

Malignant **Uneven edges**

C
Color

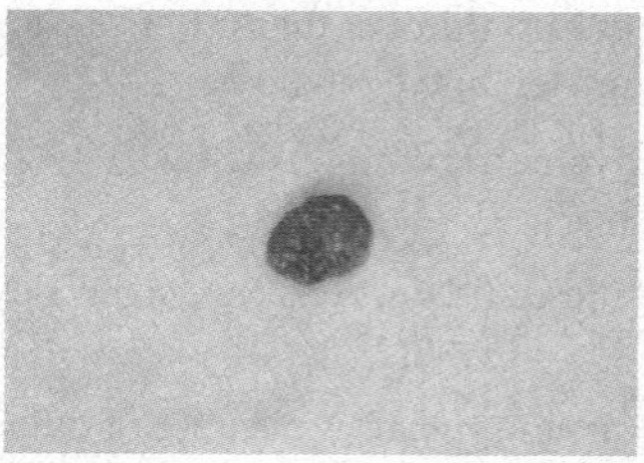

Benign **One shade**

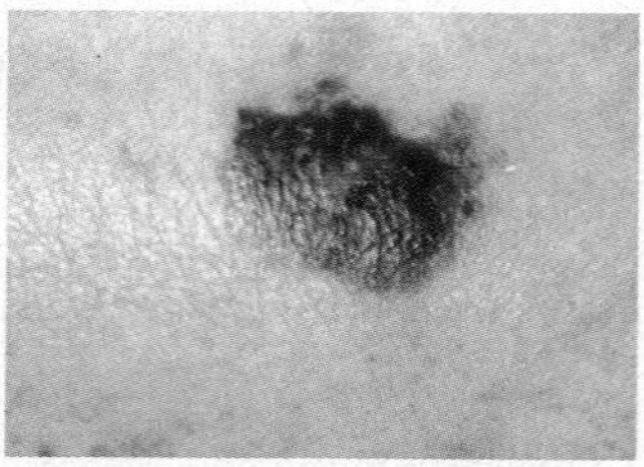

Malignant **Two or more shades**

D
Diameter

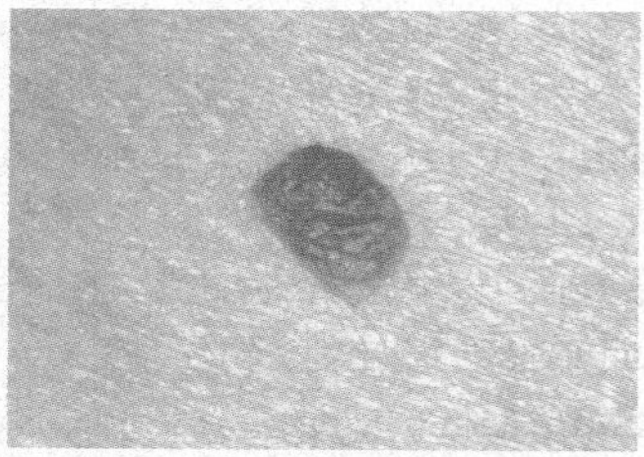

Benign **Smaller than 6 mm**

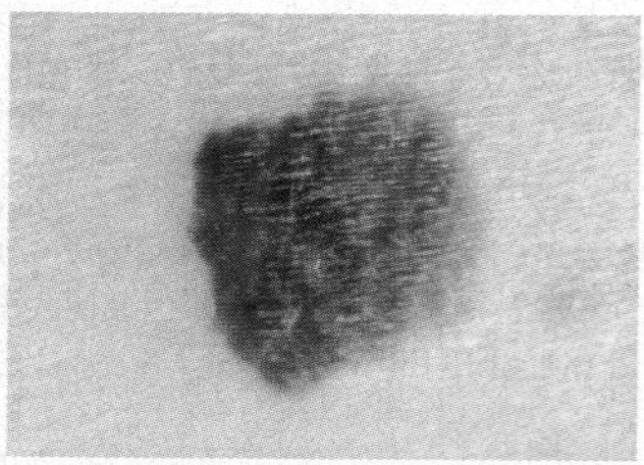

Malignant **Larger than 6 mm**

E
Evolving

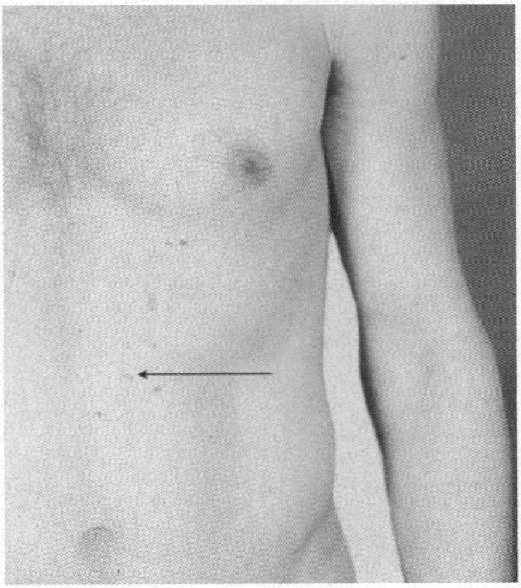

Benign

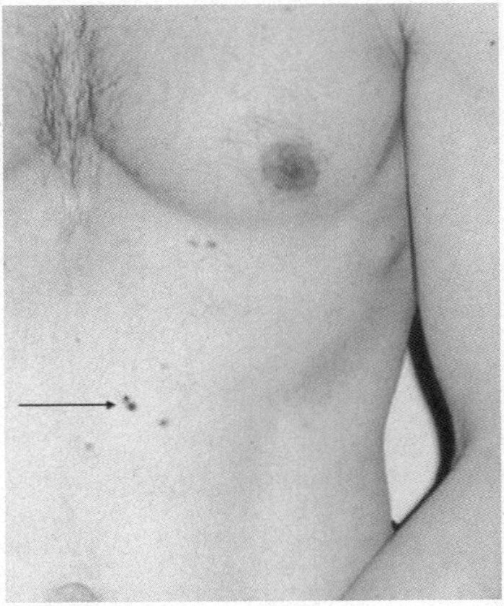

Malignant

A color atlas of skin lesions

Prepared by The Skin Cancer Foundation, www.skincancer.org, and the American Academy of Dermatology

SKIN LESIONS

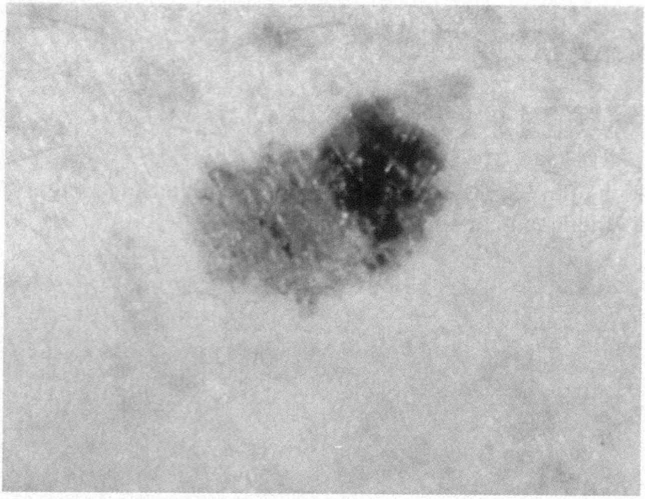

FIGURE 1: Malignant melanoma
The heterogeneous color and asymmetry of the lesion point to the diagnosis of melanoma. Particularly note the black color of the right side of the lesion. (Figures 1 and 2 courtesy of the American Academy of Dermatology)

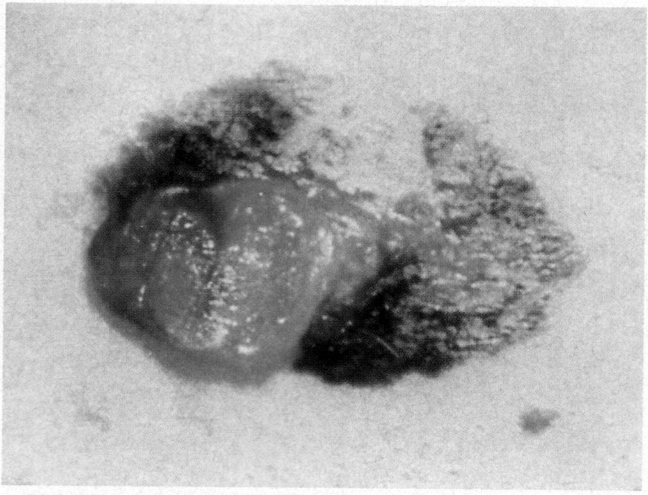

FIGURE 2: Malignant melanoma
There are several colors clearly visible in this lesion, consistent with melanoma. There are mottled black areas of the lesion, with central tumor growth that is eroded and less pigmented.

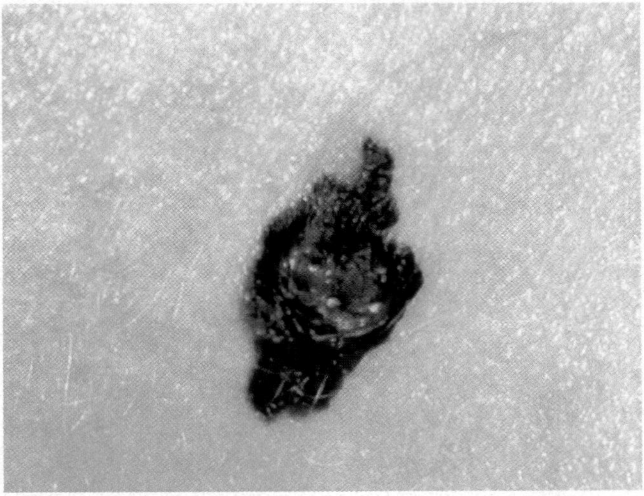

FIGURE 3: Thick melanoma
Thick melanomas (> 4 mm in thickness) tend to have a nodular shape. While this lesion is dark, some thick melanomas may be pale. (Figures 3 through 11 courtesy of The Skin Cancer Foundation)

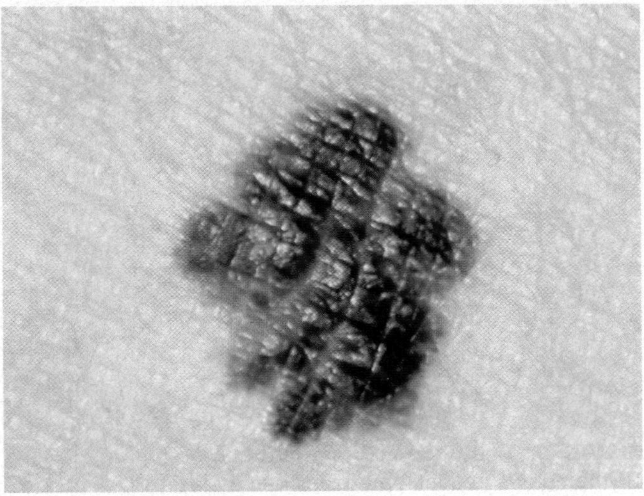

FIGURE 4: Thin melanoma
Thin melanomas (1 mm or less in thickness) are frequently diagnosed and are considered highly curable.

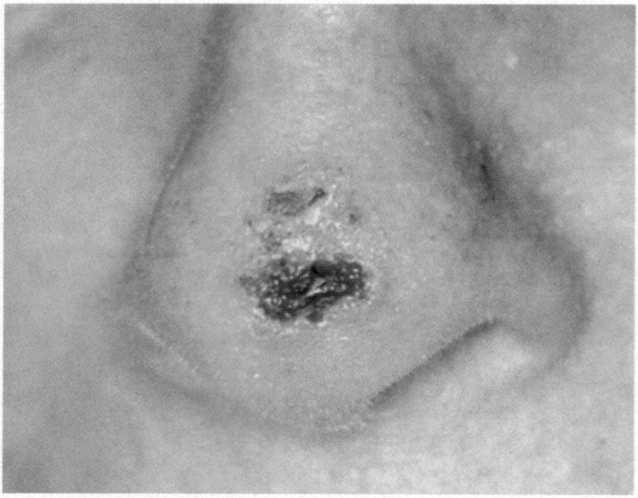

FIGURE 5: Squamous cell carcinoma
This infiltrated red plaque has central erosion and crust.

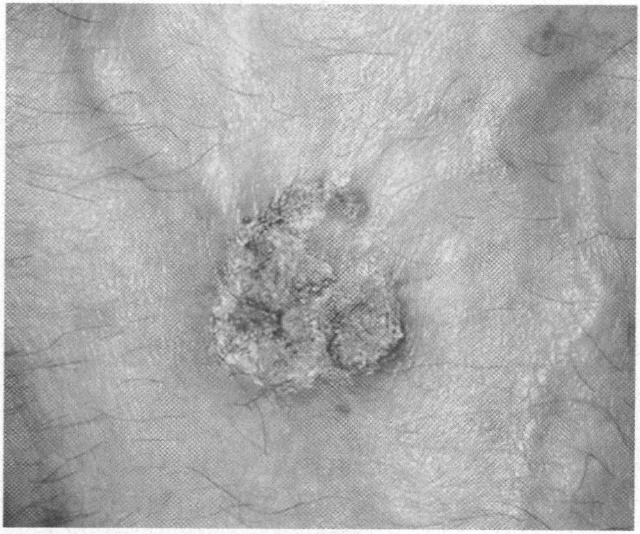

FIGURE 6: Squamous cell carcinoma
Erythematous and infiltrated lesion in a maximally sun-exposed area, with an erosive center.

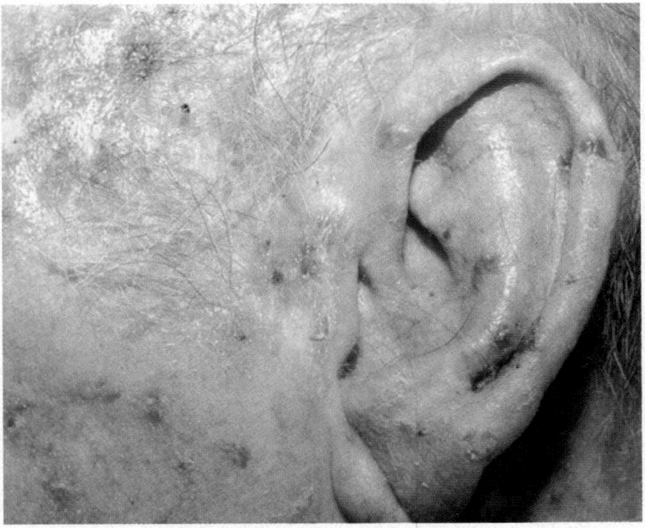

FIGURE 7: Actinic keratosis
Actinic keratosis is considered the earliest stage in skin cancer development.

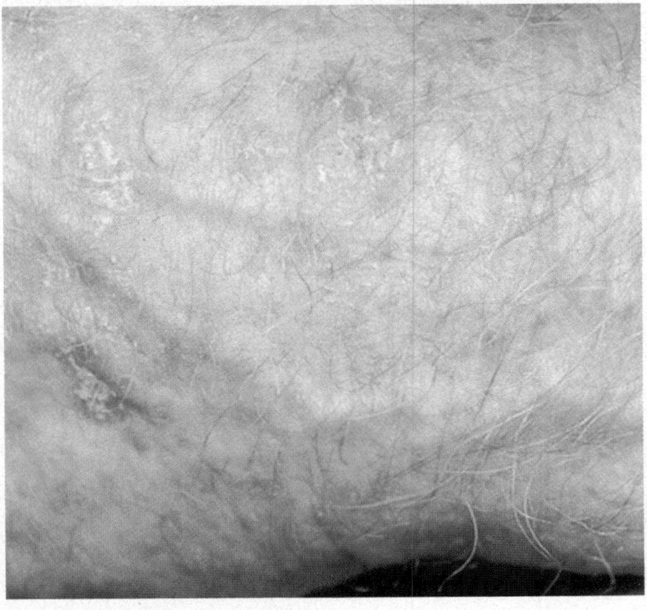

FIGURE 8: Actinic keratosis
Actinic keratosis may present as a dry, rough-textured patch on the skin.

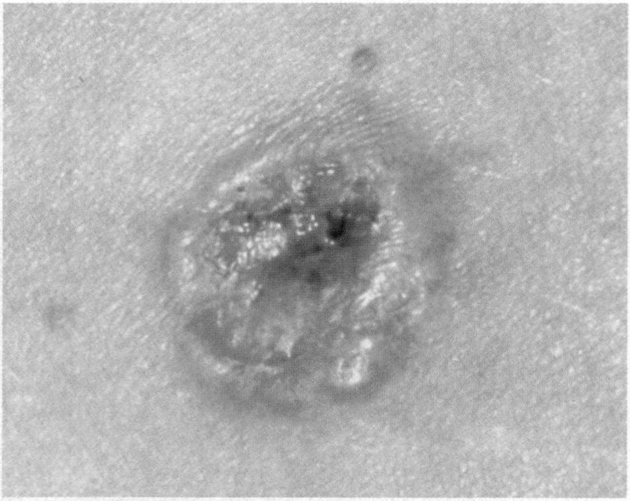

FIGURE 9: Basal cell carcinoma
Basal cell carcinoma is a type of non-melanoma. It begins as a papule and enlarges into a crater.

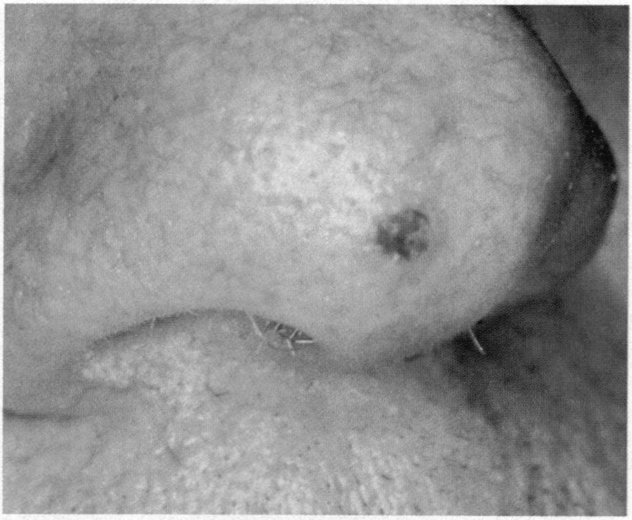

FIGURE 10: Basal cell carcinoma
Basal cell carcinoma is the most common type of skin cancer and often presents on the face and head.

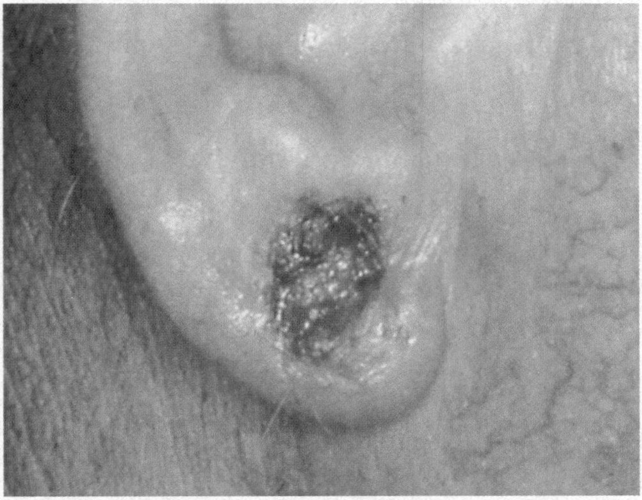

FIGURE 11: Basal cell carcinoma
Basal cell carcinoma may crust and bleed. Metastasis is rare.

CHAPTER 21

Bone sarcomas

Alan W. Yasko, MD,* Warren Chow, MD, and Karl Haglund, MD, PhD

Bone sarcomas are extremely rare neoplasms, which precludes determination of their true incidence. In 2010, approximately 2,650 new cases of cancer of the bones and joints were diagnosed in the United States, and some 1,460 patients will have died from the disease. Population-based tumor registries seldom separate bone sarcomas into various histologic types.

Osteosarcoma is the most common malignant primary bone tumor (excluding multiple myeloma), comprising 30% of all such malignancies. The annual incidence of osteosarcoma is approximately 800 cases per year in the United States. Chondrosarcoma is the second most common malignant primary tumor of bone; its annual incidence is approximately half that of osteosarcoma. Ewing's sarcoma represents approximately 6% of all primary malignant bone tumors, with an annual incidence of 200 cases. Malignant fibrous histiocytoma (MFH) comprises < 1% of primary bone sarcomas.

EPIDEMIOLOGY

Gender

The incidence of primary bone sarcomas is higher in males than in females, regardless of histologic type. A low-grade variant of osteosarcoma (parosteal osteosarcoma) is observed more frequently in females.

Age

Osteosarcoma and Ewing's sarcoma develop primarily in children and adolescents. A biphasic pattern of incidence of osteosarcoma has been observed; peaks have been noted among adolescents (rapid growth of long bones) and in the elderly (secondary tumors arising in association with Paget's disease or within previously irradiated tissue). Chondrosarcomas are rarely seen in skeletally immature patients. They usually develop in middle-aged and older adults. MFH is observed in adults.

Race

No predilection has been noted in any particular race. However, Ewing's sarcoma is extremely rare in American and African blacks.

*Dr. Alan W. Yasko, 1958–2010. The editors of *Cancer Management: A Multidisciplinary Approach*, would like to acknowledge the significant contributions that Dr. Yasko has made to the book and express our sadness at his passing.

Disease site

Any bone and any site within a given bone may be affected. Most osteosarcomas occur in the metaphyseal region of skeletally immature long bones (ie, distal femur, proximal tibia, and proximal humerus), which have the greatest growth potential. Ewing's sarcoma is classically described as a diaphyseal lesion, but it may arise in any region within an involved long bone. It commonly arises in the flat bones of the pelvis and scapula. Primary bone tumors of any histologic type are extremely rare in the spine and sacrum.

Survival

Low-grade sarcomas are associated with the most favorable survival, which approaches 90% in patients with adequately treated tumors. With regard to high-grade sarcomas, survival has improved dramatically in patients with osteosarcoma or Ewing's sarcoma due to the advent of effective multiagent chemotherapy regimens. Survival has improved with multimodality therapy from historic rates of < 20% to current rates of 50% to 75%.

ETIOLOGY AND RISK FACTORS

For the majority of bone sarcomas, no specific etiology has been established. A few predisposing factors have been identified.

Genetic factors

Children with familial retinoblastoma have a 13q chromosome deletion and an increased incidence of osteosarcoma. Li-Fraumeni syndrome is also associated with an increased risk of bone sarcomas, as well as such other cancers such as breast, leukemia, soft-tissue sarcoma, brain, and adrenal cortical tumors. Li-Fraumeni syndrome results from a genetic loss of *TP53*.

Radiation therapy

Bone sarcomas constitute a rare, but devastating, consequence of therapeutic irradiation. Radiation-associated sarcomas develop within the radiation field, usually after a latent period of at least 3 years. The majority of these tumors are osteosarcomas. MFH and other histologies also can arise within a radiation field.

Chemotherapy

Alkylating agents and anthracyclines administered for unrelated cancers have been implicated as etiologic factors in the development of second malignant neoplasms, particularly osteosarcoma.

Preexisting benign tumors/conditions

Osteosarcomas can arise in association with Paget's disease and rarely in association with benign bone tumors (ie, fibrous dysplasia). Chondrosarcomas can develop in the cartilaginous component of osteochondromas (solitary and multiple hereditary exostosis) and in patients with enchondromatosis (Ollier's disease and Maffucci's syndrome). MFH can arise in association with bone infarcts.

Trauma

A traumatic event often prompts medical intervention, at which time the bone sarcoma is detected. The short temporal relationship between the traumatic event and the diagnosis of the tumor usually rules out a causal relationship.

Orthopedic implants

Case reports of bone sarcomas arising in the region in which a metallic prosthetic device has been implanted have been published. The rarity of these clinical situations relative to the vast number of devices implanted makes a causal relationship unlikely.

SIGNS AND SYMPTOMS

Local symptoms

Localized pain and swelling are the hallmark clinical features of bone sarcomas. The pain, which initially is insidious and transient, becomes progressively more severe and unremitting. Localized soft-tissue swelling, with or without associated warmth and erythema, may be present. A joint effusion may be observed, and range of motion of the adjacent joint may be limited and painful. Movement or weight-bearing of the involved extremity may exacerbate local symptoms.

Patients with tumors arising in the lower extremities can present with a painful limp. The neurovascular examination of the affected extremity is usually normal. Regional lymph nodes are rarely involved.

Pathologic fracture may also be a presenting sign, although a history of pain prior to fracture usually can be elicited.

Constitutional symptoms

These are rare in patients with bone sarcoma, but such symptoms as fever, malaise, and weight loss can be observed in those with Ewing's sarcoma.

SCREENING AND DIAGNOSIS

Currently, there is no screening test for primary bone sarcomas. The diagnosis must be made by clinical and radiographic evaluations and confirmed by histopathologic analysis of biopsy-obtained tissue.

Physical examination

Physical examination should include an assessment of the local extent of the soft-tissue mass, if present, and its relationship to the adjacent joint.

Laboratory studies

A CBC may demonstrate anemia and/or leukocytosis associated with Ewing's sarcoma, but, in general, results of these studies fall within the normal range. Alkaline phosphatase and lactic dehydrogenase (LDH) levels may be elevated in patients with osteosarcoma or Ewing's sarcoma. An abnormal glucose tolerance test may be observed in patients with chondrosarcomas.

X-rays

Biplanar (anteroposterior and lateral) plain radiographs of the affected extremity provide critical information on the nature of the bone lesion. The specific site of involvement within the bone, the pattern and extent of bone destruction, type of periosteal changes, and the presence of matrix mineralization within the tumor, and of soft-tissue extension may be gleaned from plain films.

CT

Standard CT scans provide further delineation of many of these changes.

MRI

MRI is the imaging study of choice for evaluating the extent of an associated soft-tissue mass and the relationship of the tumor to the neurovascular structures, surrounding soft tissues, and the adjacent joint. The intramedullary extent of the tumor and presence of skip metastases within the bone are best demonstrated by MRI.

Bone scan

A bone scan is performed to screen for distant osseous metastases.

Chest radiographic studies

A plain film of the chest is required in any patient suspected of having a bone sarcoma. Once the diagnosis of malignancy has been established, a CT scan of the chest is a critical part of initial staging.

Biopsy

With few exceptions, a biopsy must be obtained to confirm the diagnosis. Tissue may be obtained by percutaneous (closed) or surgical (open) techniques. The biopsy should be performed by personnel expert in percutaneous biopsy techniques who are familiar with bone tumors and their treatment.

Biopsies performed at referring institutions have been reported to be associated with a higher incidence of misdiagnosis and complications, which may affect patient outcome. Optimally, the biopsy should be performed at the institution where definitive treatment will be given.

PATHOLOGY

Histologic subtypes

Current histopathologic classification of bone neoplasms is based on the putative cell of origin. Malignant tumors may arise from any cellular constituent present in bone, including osteogenic (osteosarcoma), chondrogenic (chondrosarcoma), hematopoietic (multiple myeloma, lymphoma), vascular (angiosarcoma, hemangioendothelioma, leiomyosarcoma), lipogenic (liposarcoma), neurogenic (neurofibrosarcoma, chordoma), and histiocytic and fibrohistiocytic (MFH, Ewing's sarcoma) elements. Histologic subtyping is based on the predominant cellular pattern present within the tumor, the degree of anaplasia, and the relationship of the tumor to the bone (intramedullary vs surface).

A monoclonal antibody (CD99) that recognizes a cell-surface glycoprotein (p30/32MIC2) in human Ewing's sarcoma and primitive neuroectodermal tumor (PNET) has been developed. There is strong immunoreactivity of CD99 in Ewing's sarcoma and PNET that aids in distinguishing these tumors from other small, round-cell tumors of childhood and adolescence. Additional experience with CD99, however, demonstrates that it is not exclusively specific for Ewing's sarcoma and PNET.

Dedifferentiation

Primary bone sarcomas can exhibit the phenomenon of "dedifferentiation." These neoplasms demonstrate a dimorphic histologic pattern, which is characterized by the presence of a borderline malignant or low-grade malignant tumor juxtaposed against a high-grade, histologically different sarcoma. Enchondromas, low-grade chondrosarcomas, low-grade variants of osteosarcoma (surface and intramedullary), and chordomas may all develop an area of high-grade spindle-cell tumor, usually MFH.

Metastatic spread

Approximately 10% to 20% of patients with osteosarcoma and 15% to 35% of patients with Ewing's sarcoma have evidence of metastatic disease at initial presentation. In approximately 90% of patients with bone sarcomas, the initial site of distant metastasis is the lungs. Distant osseous sites, bone marrow, and viscera may also be involved as a manifestation of advanced disease, but involvement of these sites is less common and usually occurs after the development of pulmonary metastases. Regional lymph node involvement is rare.

STAGING AND PROGNOSIS

Staging system

The staging system of the MTS is currently used (Table 1). This system is based on tumor grade (I = low or II = high), tumor extent (A = intraosseous involvement

TABLE 1: Surgical staging of bone sarcomas

Stage	Grade	Site
IA	Low	Intracompartmental
IB	Low	Extracompartmental
IIA	High	Intracompartmental
IIB	High	Extracompartmental
III	Any regional or distant metastasis	Any

Enneking WF, Spanier SS, Goodman MA: A system for the surgical staging of musculoskeletal sarcoma. Clin Orthop 153:106–120, 1980.

only or B = extraosseous extension), and presence of distant metastases, regardless of the extent of local disease (III). Patients with a localized tumor may have stage IA, IB, IIA, or IIB disease.

Prognostic factors

Many studies have demonstrated that tumor response to preoperative chemotherapy, as determined by histologic analysis of the resected specimen, is the most powerful predictor of survival for patients with osteosarcoma. Adverse prognostic indicators, such as an axial primary tumor or elevated LDH and alkaline phosphatase levels, signal an even worse outcome.

Tumor size (low volume) and anatomic site (peripheral), absence of metastases at initial presentation, and good histologic response to chemotherapy are prognostic variables associated with better outcome in patients with osteosarcomas and Ewing's sarcoma. The translocation t(11;22), which results in the type 1 EWS-FLI1 fusion, is also a significant positive predictor of overall survival in Ewing's sarcoma.

For low-grade malignant tumors, adequacy of surgery is the most significant predictor of outcome.

TREATMENT

Primary treatment of bone sarcomas

Surgical excision is the mainstay of treatment for patients with low-grade sarcomas. For high-grade tumors, multimodality therapy is indicated. For most high-grade bone sarcomas, excluding chondrosarcoma, preoperative multiagent chemotherapy (3 to 4 cycles) is followed by surgical extirpation of the primary tumor. Chemotherapy is reinitiated postoperatively after wound healing has occurred (usually 2–3 weeks after surgery).

For patients with Ewing's sarcoma, the optimal therapy for local tumor control is less well defined. Historically, radiotherapy has been a mainstay of local treatment. However, there has been a recent trend toward surgery, with or without radiotherapy, to achieve local tumor control. No prospective, randomized studies have been performed to define the relative role of each of these treatment modalities, but several retrospective studies suggest improvements in local tumor control and patient survival when surgery is satisfactorily performed. Patients with unresectable tumors or microscopic or macroscopic residual disease following tumor excision clearly require adjuvant radiotherapy to consolidate their local treatment.

Surgical treatment strategy

The MTS recognizes wide excision, either by amputation or a limb-salvage procedure, as the recommended surgical approach for high-grade sarcomas. A wide excision removes the primary tumor en bloc along with its reactive zone and a cuff of normal tissue in all planes. Conceptually, this strategy is applicable to all high-grade sarcomas. Wide excision successfully controls local disease in ≥ 90% of patients.

The timing of surgery must be coordinated with the patient's chemotherapy schedule and with bone marrow recovery to minimize the period of systemic therapy. Generally, surgical intervention is postponed until the patient's absolute neutrophil count has recovered to a level of ≥ 1,500/μL and the platelet count ≥ 70,000/μL.

Limb-salvage procedures

Wide tumor excision with limb preservation has supplanted amputation as the principal surgical method for eradicating local disease in patients with primary sarcomas of bone, regardless of histology or grade. Local tumor control and patient survival have not been compromised by this more conservative operative strategy. Refinements in surgical techniques and advances in bioengineering have increased the number of patients eligible for limb-salvage surgery. Currently, 75% to 80% of patients may be treated with conservative surgery.

Successful limb-salvage surgery for the patient with a high-grade bone sarcoma is predicated on complete extirpation of the tumor, effective skeletal reconstruction, and adequate soft-tissue coverage. Planning for the operative procedure must begin far in advance to permit adequate time to procure the implant for reconstruction.

Types of resection Limb-sparing tumor resection falls into one of three types based on the anatomic site and extent of involved bone to be excised. Resection can involve (1) tumor-bearing bone and the adjacent joint (osteoarticular), (2) tumor-bearing bone only (intercalary), or (3) whole bone and adjacent joints (whole bone).

Since most bone sarcomas arise in the metaphysis of the long bone near the joint, the majority of procedures performed for these tumors involve resection of both the segment of tumor-bearing bone and the adjacent joint (osteoarticular resection). Most of these resections are performed through the adjacent joint (intra-articular). When the tumor extends along the joint capsule or ligamentous structures and/or invades the joint, the entire joint should be resected (extra-articular) to avoid violating areas that have tumor involvement.

Reconstruction Prosthetic arthroplasty is the most common method by which the skeletal defect and adjacent joint are reconstructed. Osteoarticular allografts, intercalary allografts, and vascularized and nonvascularized autografts are also used, depending on the extent of resection and requirements for successful reconstruction.

Soft-tissue coverage Adequate soft-tissue coverage is critical to the success of any limb-salvage procedure. Local transposition muscle flaps and free tissue transfers are extremely useful for providing a healthy, well-vascularized soft-tissue envelope to cover the reconstruction and reduce the risk of deep infection.

Tumors in the immature skeleton Tumors arising in the immature skeleton pose a unique problem for the orthopedic oncologist, particularly in patients with substantial projected growth of the involved extremity. The surgical management of bone sarcomas in young patients, with few exceptions, has entailed amputation or rotationplasty.

Custom-manufactured expandable metallic joint prostheses can be implanted to allow for skeletal growth in those children deemed candidates for limb-salvage surgery. The long-term outcome of this technique has been promising. However, multiple operative procedures should be anticipated to maintain a functional extremity.

Preoperative chemotherapy

MTX	CDP ADM	MTX	IFO CDP	IFO ADM	Surgery
0	1	4	5	8	10 .... 11 wk

MTX: Methotrexate (MTX) 12 g/m^2 as 6-h intravenous (IV) infusion. The dose of MTX was escalated by 2 g/m^2 if after 6 h the serum measurement of the drug in the previous course was < 1,000 µmol/L (top dose 24 g).

CDP/ADM: 120 mg/m^2 cisplatin CDP intra-arterially (IA) or IV as a 72-h continuous infusion and 60 mg/m^2 doxorubicin (ADM) as an 8-h infusion starting 48 h after the beginning of the CDP infusion.

IFO/CDP: 3 g/m^2/d ifosfamide (IFO) as a 1-hr infusion for 2 consecutive days followed by 120 mg/m^2 CDP IA or IV as a 72-h continuous infusion.

IFO/ADM: 3 g/m^2/d IFO as a 1-h infusion for 2 days followed by 30 mg/m^2/d ADM in a 4-h infusion for 2 days.

Postoperative chemotherapy

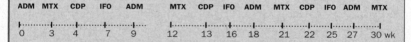

ADM	MTX	CDP	IFO	ADM	MTX	CDP	IFO	ADM	MTX	CDP	IFO	ADM	MTX
0	3	4	7	9	12	13	16	18	21	22	25	27	30 wk

ADM: 45 mg/m^2/d as an 8-h infusion for 2 consecutive days

MTX: as in preoperative treatment

CDP: 150 mg/m^2 as a 72-h continuous infusion

IFO: 2 g/m^2/d as a 1-h infusion for 5 consecutive days.

In patients with localized disease and total necrosis, the last 3 cycles of chemotherapy were omitted.

Figure 1: The IOR/OS-4 protocol for neoadjuvant/adjuvant chemotherapy for osteosarcoma of the extremities, from the Rizzoli Institute, Bologna, Italy.
Bacci G, Briccoli A, Ferrari S, et al: Eur J Cancer 37:2030–2039, 2001.

Surgical treatment of metastatic disease

The most common site of metastatic involvement for bone sarcoma is the lungs. Patients who present with pulmonary metastases (10%–20% of patients with osteosarcoma) have a poor prognosis (5-year survival rate < 15%). Approximately 30% to 40% of patients who present with localized disease and who subsequently develop resectable pulmonary metastases can undergo salvage treatment with reinduction chemotherapy and metastasectomy (see section on "Treatment of advanced osteosarcoma"). Patients with extrapulmonary metastases or unresectable pulmonary metastases have a uniformly poor prognosis. The objective of any surgical intervention in these patients, therefore, would be palliative.

Osteosarcoma

Chemotherapy

The probability of 5-year disease-free survival for patients with osteosarcoma of the extremities treated with either amputation or limb-salvage surgery alone is < 20%. Although the incidence of local recurrence is low, microscopic dissemination is likely to be present in 80% of patients at the time of diagnosis, leading to distant metastases, mostly in the lungs and bones, within the first 6 to 12 months. The incorporation of chemotherapy as part of the standard therapeutic plan for osteosarcoma (Figure 1) has improved both relapse-free and overall survival.

Neoadjuvant/adjuvant chemotherapy To achieve better systemic control and decrease the degree of functional defect following surgery, neoadjuvant (presurgical) treatment programs have been developed by several centers. Early trials incorporated high doses of methotrexate given weekly for 4 weeks with leucovorin rescue prior to surgery. Subsequent modifications included the incorporation of bleomycin, dactinomycin (Cosmegen), and cyclophosphamide into the regimen, with the further addition of doxorubicin.

The next generation of trials adjusted the adjuvant (postoperative) chemotherapeutic regimen, depending on the degree of tumor necrosis found at the time of surgery. Patients who had a good tumor response (> 90% necrosis) were treated with additional cycles of the neoadjuvant regimen; those who had a poor response received cisplatin and doxorubicin. It remains controversial whether altering the adjuvant chemotherapeutic regimen for patients with poor histologic response truly changes their event-free survival.

The addition of ifosfamide did not improve survival in pediatric patients with osteosarcoma in one study. A COG study reported no difference in outcome between a three-drug combination of cisplatin, doxorubicin, and high-dose methotrexate and a four-drug regimen of the same drugs plus ifosfamide. The EOI reported no difference in histopathologic response to preoperative chemotherapy and overall survival in patients randomized to receive a two-drug regimen with doxorubicin and cisplatin or a complex multidrug protocol containing doxorubicin, cisplatin, and high-dose methotrexate, among other agents.

The EOI also investigated standard-dose versus increased-dose intensity (dose-dense) cisplatin and doxorubicin for patients with operable osteosarcoma of the extremity. The overall dose intensity was increased by 24% for cisplatin and 25% for doxorubicin. Good histologic response (≤ 10% viable tumor) was significantly higher in the intensified arm (51% vs 36%). Unfortunately, overall survival at 4 years was not significantly different (61% for standard and 64% for intensified).

The actuarial 5-year event-free survival rate in patients presenting with localized, primarily extremity osteosarcoma is > 70%. Regardless of the multidrug therapy used, event-free survival correlates with histologic response. Patients with > 90% tumor necrosis have a > 80% probability of 5-year event-free survival. Complete responses are more likely to occur in patients with the nonchondroblastic subtype and in those whose peak serum methotrexate levels are > 700 µmol/L. Chemosensitivity also seems to be diminished in patients with metastatic disease at presentation.

A joint protocol of four of the world's leading multi-institutional osteosarcoma groups (COG, EOI, COSG, and Scandinavian Sarcoma Group) is currently accruing patients with localized osteosarcoma (EURAMOS). All patients will receive induction chemotherapy with two cycles of cisplatin and doxorubicin along with four cycles of high-dose methotrexate (MAP). Patients will then proceed to surgical resection. Postoperative therapy will be determined by histologic response. Good responders will be randomized to continue with MAP or receive MAP with pegylated interferon alfa-2b as maintenance therapy after MAP. Poor responders will be randomized to continue with MAP or receive the same regimen with the addition of ifosfamide and etoposide.

Treatment of advanced osteosarcoma

Axial primary tumor For the 10% to 15% of patients who present with axial primary osteosarcoma, neoadjuvant chemotherapy should be considered to reduce the tumor burden prior to surgery or radiation therapy. The COSG reported that 11.4% of its patients treated before 1999 had proven metastases at diagnosis. Actuarial survival at 5 and 10 years was 29% and 24%, respectively, when treated with preoperative and postoperative multiagent chemotherapy as well as aggressive surgery for all resectable lesions. Multivariate Cox regression analysis demonstrated that multiple metastases at diagnosis and macroscopically incomplete surgical resection are significantly associated with inferior outcomes in patients with primary metastatic osteosarcoma.

Pulmonary metastasis Patients with metastatic disease to the lungs should be evaluated for resection. Following aggressive pulmonary metastasectomy, < 25% of patients will achieve prolonged relapse-free survival. Hence, these patients may also benefit from aggressive "secondary" adjuvant chemotherapy.

Chemotherapy should also be considered for patients whose pulmonary metastases are unresectable, with the intention of performing surgery in those who have a sufficient response; approximately 10% of such patients may become long-term survivors.

Poor-risk patients or patients with recurrent disease are candidates for clinical trials that evaluate newer therapeutic agents. The COG demonstrated stabilization of disease in patients with recurrent or refractory osteosarcoma employing the combination of cyclophosphamide and topotecan (Hycamtin), although objective responses were rare. A team from the University of Michigan reported that the combination of gemcitabine (Gemzar) and docetaxel (Taxotere) is moderately active in recurrent osteosarcoma, Ewing's sarcoma, and other soft-tissue sarcomas.

The prognosis for patients who develop metachronous skeletal osteosarcoma has been considered grave compared with that for patients with relapse limited to the lungs. Investigators at MSKCC reported that in a small subset of patients who developed metachronous osteosarcoma at 24 months or more from the initial diagnosis (11 of 23 patients with osteosarcoma), combined-modality therapy with surgery and aggressive chemotherapy resulted in a 5-year postmetachronous survival rate of 83%, versus 40% for patients receiving monotherapy (usually surgery) only. These results refute an earlier pessimistic sentiment.

Radiotherapy

Although the routine use of adjuvant radiotherapy for osteosarcoma is unnecessary, certain patients may benefit from treatment. Patients with positive margins and poor response to chemotherapy are particularly at risk for local recurrence. Primary lesions in the axial skeleton are more likely to be difficult to resect with wide margins. DeLaney et al have reported a local control rate of 78% in patients with subtotal resections followed by radiotherapy. Doses in the range of 60 Gy or more are recommended. Patients who have unresectable disease should be considered for high-dose radiotherapy following chemotherapy. Local tumor control may be achieved in 40% to 55% of patients. Sophisticated planning with intensity-modulated radiotherapy and/or proton therapy may be required for unresectable lesions in the pelvis, or those located adjacent to radiosensitive structures such as the spinal cord. The use of radiosensitizing chemotherapy has been studied by investigators at MDACC; it may improve the chances of controlling locally advanced disease.

Investigators at the Mayo Clinic reported significant palliation of pain in patients with osteosarcoma and symptomatic bone metastases who were treated with high doses of samarium 153 ethylene diamine tetramethylene phosphonate (^{153}Sm EDTMP), a bone-seeking radiopharmaceutical, in conjunction with stem-cell rescue. Escalating doses up to 30 mCi/kg were studied. Nonhematologic side effects were minimal. ^{153}Sm at a dose of 1 mCi/kg has been used for palliation of bone pain from skeletal metastases without the need for stem-cell support. Investigators at the Johns Hopkins Hospital have determined that a 1.21-mCi/kg dose can be administered to heavily pretreated patients without significant toxicity.

Long-term follow-up is necessary for patients treated for osteosarcoma. Late side effects of neoadjuvant chemotherapy for osteosarcoma were assessed in a retrospective review performed by investigators at the Rizzoli Institute in Italy. Of the 755 patients with localized osteosarcoma treated with six subsequent protocols, the following side effects were noted: symptomatic cardiomyopathy (1.7%), second malignant neoplasms (2.1% after a median of 7 years), permanent azoospermia (100% in men who received 60–75 g/m^2 of ifosfamide), subclinical renal impairment (48% in those who received > 60 g/m^2 of ifosfamide), and hearing impairment (40% of those who received cisplatin.

Ewing's sarcoma

Chemotherapy

Prior to the availability of effective chemotherapeutic agents, < 10% of patients with Ewing's sarcoma survived beyond 5 years. The first intergroup Ewing's sarcoma study demonstrated an improved survival rate for patients receiving systemic therapy with the VAC regimen (vincristine, Actinomycin D [dactinomycin], cyclophosphamide, for those receiving the VACA regimen (the VAC regimen plus Adriamycin [doxorubicin]), and for patients receiving VAC plus bilateral pulmonary irradiation. In the future, selection of a specific therapeutic regimen may be influenced by the presence of molecular markers in addition to standard clinical criteria.

In the second intergroup study, the addition of doxorubicin to VAC, when given on an intermittent schedule and at a higher dose, improved the 5-year relapse-free survival

Dose intensification is defined as the amount of drug given over unit time. Therapy may be intensified by keeping the interval stable while escalating chemotherapeutic doses or shortening the interval between cycles. Dose-intensification of alkylating agents with similar cumulative doses between the two arms did not demonstrate a significant difference in 5-year event-free survival between a standard or intensified regimen in a phase II trial conducted by the COG *(Granowetter L et al: J Clin Oncol 27:2536–2541, 2009)*. In contrast, a trial of dose-intensification via interval compression in patients with localized Ewing's sarcoma demonstrated a significant improvement in 3-year event-free survival (P = .028) between the experimental arm of VAC alternating with IE every 2 weeks (75%) versus the standard arm of the same regimen every 3 weeks *(65%; Womer RB et al: J Clin Oncol 26: abstract 10504, 2008)*.

rate to 73%; this rate was almost double that of the cohort of patients not receiving doxorubicin as part of their treatment. The worst results were observed in patients with pelvic, proximal extremity, and lumbar vertebral lesions.

In a phase III study, the addition of ifosfamide and etoposide to standard VACA chemotherapy for patients with Ewing's sarcoma and PNET of the bone significantly improved overall survival for patients with localized disease (72% vs 61%), but it did not affect the outcome for patients with metastatic disease (overall survival = 34% vs 35%). In addition to biologic adverse features at presentation (male sex, age, high LDH levels, anemia, fever, axial locations, non-type 1 fusion transcripts, and lack of feasibility of surgical resection), independent prognostic factors also include the type of chemotherapy and degree of tumor necrosis.

Advanced disease Aggressive combination chemotherapy and irradiation can lead to prolonged progression-free survival, even in patients with metastatic disease. The combination of ifosfamide (1.6 g/m^2) and etoposide (100 mg/m^2 given on days 1–5; IE) results in high response rates of > 80%. Unfortunately, late recurrences are not uncommon.

Autologous stem cell rescue has not been definitively shown to significantly improve survival of patients with poor-risk, metastatic, and recurrent Ewing's sarcoma and PNET. Newer therapeutic agents should continue to be tested in this population of patients.

In patients with recurrent or refractory Ewing's sarcoma, the combination of cyclophosphamide and topotecan was shown to possess significant antitumor activity by COG.

Radiotherapy

Local control Definitive radiotherapy is recommended for patients with unresectable primary tumors or in those for whom morbidity from resection is judged to be excessive. Patients treated with radiotherapy alone tend to have larger, less favorable tumors. In modern series of patients treated without surgery, local failure rates are on the order of 20%, compared with 4% to 10% with surgery or surgery plus radiotherapy. Patients treated definitively with chemotherapy and radiation therapy alone generally receive 45 Gy to the initial prechemotherapy volume plus a 2-cm margin, followed by a 10.8-Gy boost to a smaller volume, including the site of the original lesion plus any residual soft-tissue disease after chemotherapy.

Postoperative radiotherapy is indicated for microscopic or gross positive margins after resection or when > 10% of tumor is viable in the pathologic specimen. A dose of 45 Gy is recommended for microscopic positive margins. Lower doses appeared to be associated with higher recurrence rates, based on data from two Cooperative Ewing's Sarcoma Study trials. If gross disease is left, total doses on the order of 55.8 Gy similar to those used for definitive radiotherapy are utilized.

Metastatic disease Patients with lung metastases at presentation should be considered for "consolidative," low-dose, whole-lung irradiation following completion of chemotherapy. Doses in the range of 15 to 18 Gy are typically utilized in 1.5-Gy fractions. Radiotherapy may also be used to treat isolated bone metastases following chemotherapy. Patients with painful bone metastases can benefit from palliative radiotherapy for pain control, with up to 55% achieving complete pain relief and an additional 30% achieving partial relief.

SUGGESTED READING

Anderson P, Aguilera D, Pearson M, et al: Outpatient chemotherapy plus radiotherapy in sarcomas: Improving cancer control with radiosensitizing agents. Cancer Control 15:38–46, 2008.

Bacci G, Ferrari C, Longhi A, et al: Second malignant neoplasm in patients with osteosarcoma of the extremities treated with adjuvant and neoadjuvant chemotherapy. J Pediatr Hematol Oncol 28:774–780, 2006.

Bölling T, Schuck A, Paulussen M, et al: Whole lung irradiation in patients with exclusively pulmonary metastases of Ewing tumors. Toxicity analysis and treatment results of the EICESS-92 trial. Strahlenther Onkol 184:193–197, 2008.

Chow WA: Update on chondrosarcomas. Curr Opin Oncol 19:371–376, 2007.

Ferrari S, Smeland S, Mercuri M, et al: Neoadjuvant chemotherapy with high-dose ifosfamide, high-dose methotrexate, cisplatin, and doxorubicin for patients with localized osteosarcoma of the extremity: A joint study by the Italian and Scandinavian Sarcoma Groups. J Clin Oncol 23:8845–8852, 2005.

Frink SJ, Rutledge J, Lewis VO, et al: Favorable long-term results of prosthetic arthroplasty of the knee for distal femur neoplasms. Clin Orthop Relat Res 438:65–70, 2005.

Granowetter L, Womer R, Devidas M, et al: Dose-intensified compared with standard chemotherapy for nonmetastatic Ewing sarcoma family of tumors: A Children's Oncology Group Study. J Clin Oncol 27:2536-2541, 2009.

Grier HE, Krailo MD, Tarbell NJ, et al: Addition of ifosfamide and etoposide to standard chemotherapy in Ewing's sarcoma/primitive neuroectodermal tumor of bone. N Engl J Med 384:694–701, 2003.

Grimer RJ, Carter SR, Tillman RM, et al: Chondrosarcoma of bone: An assessment of outcome. J Bone Joint Surg Am 82:1203–1204, 2000.

Indelicato DJ, Keole SR, Shahlaee AH, et al: Long-term clinical and functional outcomes after treatment for localized Ewing's tumor of the lower extremity. Int J Radiat Oncol Biol Phys 70:501–509, 2008.

Jeys LM, Kulkarni A, Grimer RJ, et al: Endoprosthetic reconstruction for the treatment of musculoskeletal tumors of the appendicular skeleton and pelvis. J Bone Joint Surg Am 90:1265–1271, 2008.

Kager L, Zoubek A, Pötschger U, et al: Primary metastatic osteosarcoma: Presentation and outcome of patients treated on neoadjuvant Cooperative Osteosarcoma Study Group protocols. J Clin Oncol 21:2011–2018, 2003.

Koontz BF, Clough RW, Halperin EC: Palliative radiation therapy for metastatic Ewing sarcoma. Cancer 106:1790–1793, 2006.

La TH, Meyers PA, Wexler LH, et al: Radiation therapy for Ewing's sarcoma: Results from Memorial Sloan-Kettering in the modern era. Int J Radiat Oncol Biol Phys 64:544–550, 2006.

Ladanyi M: EWS-FLI1 and Ewing's sarcoma: Recent molecular data and new insights. Cancer Biol Ther 1:330–336, 2002.

Lewis IJ, Nooij MA, Whelan J, et al: Improvement in histologic response but not survival in osteosarcoma patients treated with intensified chemotherapy: A randomized phase III trial of the European Osteosarcoma Intergroup. J Natl Cancer Inst 99:112–128, 2007.

Loeb D, Garret-Mayer E, Hobbs R, et al: Dose-finding study of 153Sm-EDTMP in patients with poor-prognosis osteosarcoma. Cancer 115:2514–2522, 2009.

Longhi A, Ferrari S, Bacci G, et al: Long-term follow-up of patients with doxorubicin-induced cardiac toxicity after chemotherapy for osteosarcoma. Anticancer Drugs 18:737–744, 2007.

Machak GN, Tkachev SI, Solovyev YN, et al: Neoadjuvant chemotherapy and local radiotherapy for high-grade osteosarcoma of the extremities. Mayo Clin Proc 78:147–155, 2003.

Meyers PA, Schwartz CL, Krailo M, et al: Osteosarcoma: A randomized, prospective trial of the addition of ifosfamide and/or muramyl tripeptide to cisplatin, doxorubicin, and high-dose methotrexate. J Clin Oncol 23:2004–2011, 2005.

Miser JS, Goldsby RE, Chen Z, et al: Treatment of metastatic Ewing sarcoma/primitive neuroectodermal tumor of bone: Evaluation of increasing the dose intensity of chemotherapy—a report from the Children's Oncology Group. Pediatr Blood Cancer 49:894–900, 2007.

Rodriguez-Galindo C, Navid F, Liu T, et al: Prognostic factors for local and distant control in Ewing sarcoma family of tumors. Ann Oncol 19:814–820, 2008.

Schuck A, Ahrens S, Paulussen M, et al: Local therapy in localized Ewing tumors: Results of 1058 patients treated in the CESS 81, CESS 86, and EICESS 92 trials. Int J Radiat Oncol Biol Phys 55:168–177, 2003.

Womer RB, West DC, Krailo MD, et al: Randomized comparison of every-two-week v. every-three-week chemotherapy in Ewing sarcoma family tumors. J Clin Oncol 26: abstract 10504, 2008.

Yock TI, Krailo M, Fryer CJ, et al: Local control in pelvic Ewing sarcoma: Analysis from INT-0091—a report from the Children's Oncology Group. J Clin Oncol 24:3838–3843, 2006.

Abbreviations in this chapter

COG = Children's Oncology Group; COSG = Cooperative Osteosarcoma Study Group; EOI = European Osteosarcoma Intergroup; EURAMOS = European and American Osteosarcoma Study Group ; IOR/OS-4 = Istituto Ortopedico Rizzoli/Osteosarcoma-4; MDACC = The University of Texas MD Anderson Cancer Center; MSKCC = Memorial Sloan-Kettering Cancer Center; MTS = Musculoskeletal Tumor Society

CHAPTER 22

Soft-tissue sarcomas

Peter W. T. Pisters, MD, Mitchell Weiss, MD, and Robert Maki, MD, PhD

The soft-tissue sarcomas are a group of rare but anatomically and histologically diverse neoplasms. This is due to the ubiquitous location of the soft tissues and the nearly three dozen recognized histologic subtypes of soft-tissue sarcomas. In the United States, approximately 10,500 new cases of soft-tissue sarcoma are identified annually, and about 3,800 patients die of the disease each year. The age-adjusted incidence is 2 cases per 100,000 persons.

EPIDEMIOLOGY

Unlike the more common malignancies, such as colon cancer, little is known about the epidemiology of soft-tissue sarcomas. This, again, reflects the uncommon nature of these lesions.

Gender There is a slight male predominance, with a male-to-female ratio of 1.1:1.0.

Age The age distribution in adult soft-tissue sarcoma studies is < 40 years, 20.7% of patients; 40 to 60 years, 27.6% of patients; and > 60 years, 51.7% of patients.

Race Studies in large cohorts of patients demonstrate that the race distribution of soft-tissue sarcomas mirrors that of the American population (86% Caucasian, 10% African American, 1% Asian American, and 3% other).

Geography Studies have suggested that the incidence and mortality of soft-tissue sarcomas may be increasing in New Zealand. There are no currently available data addressing this possibility in the United States.

ETIOLOGY AND RISK FACTORS

In the majority of cases of patients with soft-tissue sarcoma, no specific etiologic agent is identifiable. However, a number of predisposing factors have been recognized.

Radiation therapy Soft-tissue sarcomas are recognized to originate in radiation fields following therapeutic irradiation for a variety of malignancies. Frequently, they are seen in the lower-dose regions at the edge of the radiation target volume. By definition, radiation-induced sarcomas arise no sooner than 3 years after radiation therapy and often develop decades later. The majority of these sarcomas are high-grade lesions (90%), and high-grade undifferentiated pleomorphic sarcoma (formerly termed MFH, malignant fibrous histiocytoma) is a predominant histology. Osteosarcoma, angiosarcoma, and other histologic subtypes have also been reported.

Chemical exposure Exposure to various chemicals in specific occupations or situations has been linked with the development of soft-tissue sarcoma. These chemicals include the phenoxy acetic acids (forestry and agriculture workers), chlorophenols (sawmill workers), vinyl chloride (individuals working with this gas, used in making plastics and as a refrigerant), and arsenic (vineyard workers).

Chemotherapy Soft-tissue sarcomas have been reported after previous exposure to alkylating chemotherapeutic agents, most commonly after treatment of pediatric acute lymphocytic leukemia. The drugs implicated include cyclophosphamide, melphalan (Alkeran), procarbazine (Matulane), nitrosoureas, and chlorambucil (Leukeran). The relative risk of sarcoma appears to increase with cumulative drug exposure.

Chronic lymphedema Soft-tissue sarcomas have been noted to arise in the chronically lymphedematous arms of women treated with radical mastectomy for breast cancer (Stewart-Treves syndrome). Lower-extremity lymphangiosarcomas have also been observed in patients with congenital lymphedema or filariasis complicated by chronic lymphedema.

Trauma and foreign bodies Although a recent history of trauma is often elicited from patients presenting with soft-tissue sarcoma, the interval between the traumatic event and diagnosis is often short; thus, a causal relationship is highly unlikely. Chronic inflammatory processes, however, may be a risk factor for sarcoma. Foreign bodies, such as shrapnel, bullets, and implants, have also been implicated.

SIGNS AND SYMPTOMS

Signs and symptoms of soft-tissue sarcoma depend, in large part, on the anatomic site of origin. Due to the ubiquitous location of the soft tissues, these malignancies may arise at any site in the body where soft tissues are located. Since 50% of soft-tissue sarcomas arise in an extremity, the majority of patients present with a palpable soft-tissue mass. Pain at presentation is noted in only one-third of cases.

Extremity and superficial trunk Extremity and superficial trunk sarcomas account for 60% of all soft-tissue sarcomas. The majority of patients present with a painless primary soft-tissue mass. Lipomas are at least 100 times more common than soft-tissue sarcomas; however, any growing lesion or even a deep-seated fatty lesion should be biopsied to rule out a sarcoma.

Retroperitoneum Retroperitoneal sarcomas account for 15% of all soft-tissue sarcomas. Most patients (80%) present with an abdominal mass, with 50% of patients reporting pain at presentation. Due to the considerable size of the retroperitoneum and the relative mobility of the anterior intra-abdominal organs, these tumors often grow to substantial size before the patient's nonspecific complaints are evaluated or even before an abdominal mass is noted on physical examination.

Viscera Visceral soft-tissue sarcomas, which comprise 15% of all soft-tissue sarcomas, present with signs and symptoms unique to their viscus of origin. For example, gastrointestinal stromal tumors (GISTs) present with GI symptoms that are usually indistinguishable from those of the more common adenocarcinomas, such as anemia, melena, abdominal pain, or weight loss. Similarly, uterine leiomyosarcomas frequently present with painless vaginal bleeding, such as that often noted in patients with more common uterine malignancies.

Head and neck Head and neck sarcomas comprise 10% of all soft-tissue sarcomas. Although generally smaller than sarcomas in other sites, they may present with important mechanical problems related to compression or invasion of adjacent anatomy (eg, orbital contents, airway, or pharynx). In addition, their proximity to critical anatomy can pose management difficulties due to compromise in the delivery of both surgery and radiotherapy.

PATHOLOGY

Histopathologic classification As a consequence of the wide spectrum of soft tissues, a variety of histologically distinct neoplasms have been characterized. The current histopathologic classification is based on the putative cell of origin of each lesion. Such classification based on histogenesis is reproducible for the more differentiated tumors. However, as the degree of histologic differentiation declines, it becomes increasingly difficult to determine a potential cellular origin.

In addition, many of these tumors appear to have the ability to dedifferentiate. This process results in a variety of overlapping patterns, making uniform classification difficult. Experienced soft-tissue pathologists frequently disagree as to the cell of origin of an individual tumor. Comparative studies have demonstrated concordance in histopathologic diagnosis in only two-thirds of cases. MFH used to be the most common histologic subtype of soft-tissue sarcoma. However, in one study, reanalysis histologically, immunohistochemically, and ultrastructurally allowed reclassification of most of tumors to a specific line of differentiation. As a result, the term "malignant fibrous histiocytoma" is increasingly being replaced by the term "high-grade undifferentiated pleomorphic sarcoma" (UPS). GIST is now recognized as the most common form of sarcoma.

STAGING AND PROGNOSIS

AJCC/UICC staging system

The relative rarity of soft-tissue sarcomas, the anatomic heterogeneity of these lesions, and the presence of more than 30 recognized histologic subtypes of variable grade have made it difficult to establish a functional system that can accurately stage all forms of this disease. The staging system of the AJCC and the UICC, now in its 7th edition (2010), is the most widely employed staging classification for soft-tissue sarcomas (Table 1). In the 7th edition, the staging for GIST has been separated from other sarcomas for the first time (Table 2). All soft-tissue sarcoma subtypes are included, except desmoid tumors (deep fibromatosis), Kaposi sarcoma, and infantile fibrosarcoma. In keeping with the FNCLCC (Fédération Nationale des Centres de Lutte Contre la Cancer) sarcoma grading system, three distinct histologic grades are recognized, based on the degree of differentiation, mitotic activity, and necrosis.

Histologic grade and tumor size are the primary determinants of clinical stage. In the 6th version of the AJCC staging system, tumor size was further substaged as "a" (a superficial tumor that arises outside the investing fascia) or "b" (a deep tumor

TABLE 1: AJCC version 7 staging for soft tissue sarcomas

Primary Tumor (T)

TX	Primary tumor cannot be assessed
T0	No evidence of primary tumor
T1	Tumor 5 cm or less in greatest dimension
T1a	Superficial tumor
T1b	Deep tumor
T2	Tumor more than 5 cm in greatest dimension
T2a	Superficial tumor
T2b	Deep tumor

Note: Superficial tumor is located exclusively above the superficial fascia without invasion of the fascia; deep tumor is located either exclusively beneath the superficial fascia, superficial to the fascia with invasion of or through the fascia, or both superficial yet beneath the fascia.

Regional Lymph Nodes (N)

NX	Regional lymph nodes cannot be assessed
N0	No regional lymph node metastasis
N1	Regional lymph node metastasis

Note: Presence of positive nodes (N1) in M0 tumors is considered Stage III.

Distant Metastasis (M)

M0	No distant metastasis
M1	Distant metastasis

ANATOMIC STAGE/PROGNOSTIC GROUPS

Stage IA	T1a	N0	M0	G1, GX
	T1b	N0	M0	G1, GX
Stage IB	T2a	N0	M0	G1, GX
	T2b	N0	M0	G1, GX
Stage IIA	T1a	N0	M0	G2, G3
	T1b	N0	M0	G2, G3
Stage IIB	T2a	N0	M0	G2
	T2b	N0	M0	G2
Stage III	T2a	N0	M0	G3
	T2b	N0	M0	G3
	Any T	N1	M0	Any G
Stage IV	Any T	Any N	M1	Any G

From Edge SB, Byrd DR, Compton CC, et al (eds): AJCC Cancer Staging Manual, 7th ed. New York, Springer, 2010.

TABLE 2: AJCC version 7 staging for GIST

Primary Tumor (T)				
TX	Primary tumor cannot be assessed			
T0	No evidence for primary tumor			
T1	Tumor 2 cm or less			
T2	Tumor more than 2 cm but not more than 5 cm			
T3	Tumor more than 5 cm but not more than 10 cm			
T4	Tumor more than 10 cm in greatest dimension			
Regional Lymph Nodes (N)				
NX	Regional lymph nodes cannot be assessed			
N0	No regional lymph node metastasis			
N1	Regional lymph node metastasis			
Distant Metastasis (M)				
M0	No distant metastasis			
M1	Distant metastasis			
Low mitotic rate: five or fewer per 50 high-power field (HPF); High mitotic rate: more than five per 50 HPF				
ANATOMIC STAGE/PROGNOSTIC GROUPS				
Gastric (GIST)[a]				
Group	**T**	**N**	**M**	**Mitotic rate**
Stage IA	T1–T2	N0	M0	Low
Stage IB	T3	N0	M0	Low
Stage II	T1	N0	M0	High
	T2	N0	M0	High
	T4	N0	M0	Low
Stage IIIA	T3	N0	M0	High
Stage IIIB	T4	N0	M0	High
Stage IV	Any T	N1	M0	Any rate
	Any T	Any N	M1	Any rate
Small Intestinal Gastric (GIST)[b]				
Group	**T**	**N**	**M**	**Mitotic rate**
Stage I	T1–T2	N0	M0	Low
Stage II	T3	N0	M0	Low
Stage IIIA	T1	N0	M0	High
	T4	N0	M0	Low
Stage IIIB	T2	N0	M0	High
	T3	N0	M0	High
	T4	N0	M0	High
Stage IV	Any T	N1	M0	Any rate
	Any T	Any N	M1	Any rate

[a]Also to be used for omentum; [b]Also to be used for esophagus, colorectal, mesentery and peritoneum.
GIST = gastrointestinal stromal tumor
From Edge SB, Byrd DR, Compton CC, et al (eds): AJCC Cancer Staging Manual, 7th ed. New York, Springer, 2010.

that arises beneath the fascia or invades the fascia). While these data are collected in AJCC/UICC version 7, these data are not used to stage the tumor.

The AJCC/UICC system is designed to optimally stage extremity tumors but is also applicable to the trunk and head and neck. It is more difficult to employ for retroperitoneal or visceral (GI or other viscera) tumors, since the designation of superficial or deep is meaningless here, as all are deeply seated tumors in these anatomic sites.

Anatomic site is itself an important determinant of outcome. Patients with retroperitoneal, head and neck, and visceral sarcomas have an inferior overall prognosis compared with patients with extremity tumors. Although the anatomic site is not incorporated as a specific component of any current staging system, outcome data should be reported on a site-specific basis.

At Memorial Sloan-Kettering Cancer Center, a retrospective review of 369 patients with high-grade soft-tissue sarcoma of the extremity treated with postoperative radiation therapy was conducted to evaluate the influence of tumor site on local control and complications. The tumor site was upper extremity in 103 patients (28%) and lower extremity in 266 patients (72%). With a median follow-up of 50 months, the 5-year actuarial rates of local control, distant relapse–free, and overall survival for the entire population were 82%, 61%, and 71%, respectively. The 5-year local control rates in patients with upper extremity lesions vs lower extremity lesions were 70% and 86%, respectively ($P = .0004$). On multivariate analysis, upper extremity site ($P = .001$) and positive resection margin ($P = .02$) were significant predictors of poor local control.

Prognostic factors

Understanding relevant clinicopathologic prognostic factors is important in treatment planning for patients with soft-tissue sarcoma. Several reports document the adverse prognostic significance of tumor grade, anatomic site, tumor size, and depth relative to the investing fascia (for extremity and body wall tumors). Patients with high-grade lesions, large (T2) sarcomas, a nonextremity subsite, or deep tumor location are at increased risk for disease relapse and sarcoma-specific death.

Sarcoma-specific nomogram Kattan and colleagues from Memorial Sloan-Kettering Cancer Center developed a sarcoma-specific nomogram for estimation of sarcoma-specific 12-year survival. The nomogram takes into account pretreatment clinicopathologic factors, including anatomic site, histologic subtype, tumor size, histologic grade, tumor depth, and patient age. The nomogram is based on prospectively collected data and has been validated in a population of 2,136 patients with sarcoma. The nomogram can be found at www.nomograms.org. The sarcoma nomogram may be useful for patient stratification for clinical trials and for risk assessment and treatment planning for individual patients. Similar nomograms have been generated for specific sarcoma subtypes, such as synovial sarcoma or the family of liposarcomas, and are validated for both 4-grade and 3-grade staging systems.

Risk assessment in GIST Beyond the cumbersome AJCC/UICC staging system for GIST, there are other ways to assess tumor risk. Perhaps the most useful of these is the risk-stratification strategy from the Armed Forces Institute of Pathology (AFIP). Tumors are classified by anatomic site, size, and mitotic rate, and risk of recurrence (Table 3). This simple method allows one to discuss with a patient the risk of a particular GIST with respect to mortality or potential benefit of adjuvant imatinib (Gleevec). What is notable from this table is that even large gastric GISTs with a low mitotic rate, one of the most common scenarios for diagnosis, have a low recurrence rate (≤ 12%); thus, for the average patient adjuvant imatinib can be avoided.

Prognostic factors for local vs distant recurrence Unlike other solid tumors, the adverse prognostic factors for local recurrence of a soft-tissue sarcoma differ from those that predict distant metastasis and tumor-related mortality. In other words, patients with a constellation of adverse prognostic factors for local recurrence are not necessarily at increased risk for distant metastasis or tumor-related death.

This concept has been validated by an analysis of the SSG prospective database. In 559 patients with soft-tissue sarcomas of the extremities and trunk treated with surgery alone, inadequate surgical margin was found to be a risk factor for local recurrence but not for distant metastasis. Therefore, staging systems that are designed

TABLE 3: AFIP risk stratification strategy

Tumor parameters

Group	Size	Mitotic Rate
Stage 1	≤ 2 cm	≤ 5 per 50 HPFs
Stage 2	> 2 ≤ 5 cm	≤ 5 per 50 HPFs
Stage 3a	> 5 ≤ 10 cm	≤ 5 per 50 HPFs
Stage 3b	> 10 cm	≤ 5 per 50 HPFs
Stage 4	≤ 2 cm	> 5 per 50 HPFs
Stage 5	> 2 ≤ 5 cm	> 5 per 50 HPFs
Stage 6a	> 5 ≤ 10 cm	> 5 per 50 HPFs
Stage 6b	> 10 cm	> 5 per 50 HPFs

Patients with progressive disease during long-term follow-up and characterization of the risk for metastasis (%)

Group	Gastric GISTs	Jejunal and ileal GISTs	Duodenal GISTs	Rectal GISTs
Stage 1	0 none	0 none	0 none	0 none
Stage 2	1.9 very low	4.3 low	8.3 low	8.5 low
Stage 3a	3.6 low	24 moderate		
Stage 3b	12 moderate	52 high	34 high[b]	57[a] high[b]
Stage 4	0[a]	50[a]	See note[c]	54 high
Stage 5	16 moderate	73 high	50 high	52 high
Stage 6a	55 high	85 high		
Stage 6b	86 high	90 high	86 high[b]	71 high[b]

Based on previously published long-term follow-up studies on 1,055 gastric, 629 small intestinal, and 111 rectal GISTs.

[a] Denotes tumor categories with very small numbers of cases.

[b] Groups 3a and 3b or 6a and 6b combined in duodenal and rectal GISTs because of small numbers of cases.

[c] No tumors of such category were included in the study. Note that small intestinal and other intestinal GISTs show a markedly worse prognosis in many mitosis and size categories than gastric GISTs.

From Miettinen M, Lasota J. Gastrointestinal stromal tumors: Pathology and prognosis at different sites. Semin Diagn Pathol 23:70-83, 2006.

to stratify patients for risk of distant metastasis and tumor-related mortality using these prognostic factors (such as the AJCC/UICC system) do not stratify patients for risk of local recurrence.

SCREENING AND DIAGNOSIS

Currently, there are no screening tests for soft-tissue sarcomas. Since the majority of patients with soft-tissue sarcoma have lesions arising in the extremities or superficial trunk, most of the comments here apply to soft-tissue lesions in those sites. A separate algorithm is usually employed for the evaluation of a primary retroperitoneal mass or visceral sarcoma.

Physical examination should include an assessment of the size of the mass and its mobility relative to the underlying soft tissues. The relationship of the mass to the investing fascia of the extremity (superficial vs deep) and nearby neurovascular and bony structures should be noted. Site-specific neurovascular examination and assessment of regional lymph nodes should also be performed.

Biopsy Any soft-tissue mass in an adult extremity should be biopsied if it is symptomatic or enlarging, is > 5 cm, or has persisted beyond 4 to 6 weeks.

Percutaneous approaches Percutaneous tissue diagnosis can usually be obtained with fine-needle aspiration (FNA) for cytology or by percutaneous core biopsy for histology. The needle track should be placed in an area to be excised or that can be encompassed in adjuvant radiotherapy fields if they are to be used. In most instances, when an experienced cytopathologist and/or histopathologist examines the specimen, a diagnosis of malignant soft-tissue sarcoma can be made. FNA is often viewed as a suboptimal method of establishing an initial diagnosis of soft-tissue sarcoma. Histology is usually preferred to cytology because more tissue is obtained, which allows for a more accurate delineation of tumor type and grade. Percutaneous tissue diagnosis is preferred to facilitate subsequent treatment planning and to permit surgical resection to be performed as a one-stage procedure.

Open biopsy In some cases, an adequate histologic diagnosis cannot be secured by percutaneous means. Open biopsy is indicated in these instances, with the exception of relatively small superficial masses, which can be easily removed by excisional biopsy with clear margins.

Biopsies should be incisional and performed with a longitudinal incision parallel to the long axis of the extremity. This approach facilitates subsequent wide local excision of the tumor, and the incisional scar results in minimal difficulties in wound closure. It also facilitates inclusion of any scars within the area of the tumor in adjuvant radiation fields without the excessive morbidity of large-field radiotherapy planning. The incision should be centered over the mass at its most superficial location. Care should be taken not to raise tissue flaps. Meticulous hemostasis should be ensured after the biopsy to prevent dissemination of tumor cells into adjacent tissue planes by hematoma.

Retroperitoneal or intra-abdominal mass Biopsy of primary retroperitoneal soft-tissue masses is generally not required for radiographically resectable masses, nor is biopsy recommended for suspected GISTs. The circumstances under which percutaneous or preoperative biopsy of retroperitoneal masses should be strongly considered include:

- tissue diagnosis for radiographically unresectable disease
- clinical suspicion of lymphoma or germ-cell tumor
- tissue diagnosis for neoadjuvant treatment, including radiotherapy and/or chemotherapy
- suspected metastases from another primary tumor.

Primary tumor imaging Optimal imaging of the primary tumor depends on the anatomic site. For soft-tissue masses of the extremities, MRI has been regarded as the imaging modality of choice because it enhances the contrast between tumor and muscle and between tumor and adjacent blood vessels and also provides multiplanar definition of the lesion. However, a study by the RDOG that compared MRI and CT in 183 patients with malignant bone and 133 patients with soft-tissue tumors showed no specific advantage of MRI over CT from a diagnostic standpoint.

For pelvic lesions, the multiplanar capability of MRI may provide superior single-modality imaging. In the retroperitoneum and abdomen, CT usually provides satisfactory anatomic definition of the lesion. Occasionally, MRI with gradient sequence imaging can better delineate the relationship of the tumor to midline vascular structures, particularly the inferior vena cava and aorta. In the future, MRI–CT fusion techniques may facilitate treatment planning using conformal radiotherapy techniques.

More invasive studies, such as angiography and cavography, are almost never required for the evaluation of soft-tissue sarcomas. The role of PET scan in sarcoma management is not well defined, although it correlates well with contrast-enhanced CT scans in patients with GIST. In particular, if the lack of IV contrast uptake as a sign of a responding tumor is taken into account, contrast-enhanced CT scans appear to yield results similar to PET scans in patients with GIST.

Imaging for metastatic disease Cost-effective imaging to exclude the possibility of distant metastatic disease depends on the size, grade, and anatomic location of the primary tumor. In general, patients with low-grade soft-tissue sarcomas < 10 cm or intermediate-/high-grade tumors < 5 cm in diameter require only a chest x-ray for satisfactory staging of the chest. This reflects the fact that these patients are at comparatively low risk of presenting with pulmonary metastases. In contrast, patients with very large (≥ 10 cm) low-grade tumors or high-grade tumors ≥ 5 cm should undergo more thorough staging of the chest by CT.

Patients with retroperitoneal and intra-abdominal visceral sarcomas should undergo single-modality imaging of the liver to exclude the possibility of synchronous hepatic metastases. The liver is a common site for a first metastasis from these lesions.

TREATMENT

TREATMENT OF LOCALIZED DISEASE

Surgical resection is the cornerstone of therapy for patients with localized disease. Over the past 20 years, there has been a gradual shift in the surgical management of soft-tissue sarcoma of the extremities away from radical ablative surgery, such as amputation or compartment resection, and toward limb-sparing approaches combining wide local resection with preoperative or postoperative radiotherapy. The development of advanced surgical techniques (eg, microvascular tissue transfer, bone and joint replacement, and vascular reconstruction) and the application of multimodality approaches have allowed most patients to retain a functional extremity without any compromise in survival.

Surgery

The surgical approach to soft-tissue sarcomas depends on careful preoperative staging with MRI or CT for lesions of the extremities and a percutaneous histologic diagnosis and assessment of tumor grade. In most instances, preoperative imaging studies allow for accurate prediction of resectability.

The surgical approach to soft-tissue sarcomas is based on an awareness that these lesions tend to expand and compress tissue planes, producing a pseudocapsule comprising normal host tissue interlaced with tumor fimbriae. Conservative surgical approaches in which the plane of dissection is immediately adjacent to this pseudocapsule, such as intracapsular or marginal excision, are associated with prohibitive local recurrence rates of 33% to 63%.

Wide local resection encompassing a rim of normal tissue around the lesion has led to improvements in local tumor control, with local recurrence rates of approximately 30% in the absence of adjuvant therapies. However, studies indicate that carefully selected patients with localized, small (T1), low-grade soft-tissue sarcomas of the extremity can be treated by wide resection alone, with local recurrence rates of < 10%.

A prospective trial examining local recurrence rates for T1 primary soft-tissue sarcomas of the trunk and extremities has been conducted. Patients underwent function-preserving surgery. Postoperative radiation was delivered for microscopically positive margins (R1 resection). No radiation was delivered if margins were negative (R0 resection). A total of 88 patients were evaluated in this trial. A total of 16% had R1 resection and received adjuvant radiation therapy, whereas 84% had R0 resection and did not receive radiation therapy. With a median follow-up of 75 months, isolated local recurrence was observed in six patients in the R1 arm (43%) and six patients in the R0 arm (8%). The 5- and 10-year local recurrence rates in the R0 arm were 7.9% and 10.6%, respectively, and the sarcoma-specific death rates were 3.2% at both 5 and 10 years in the R0 arm.

The need for adjuvant irradiation in small (< 5 cm), high-grade lesions has been studied. A retrospective review of 204 patients with stage IIB soft-tissue sarcoma of the extremity treated at Memorial Sloan-Kettering Cancer Center has been completed. A total of 57% of patients did not receive adjuvant radiation therapy, whereas 43% received either brachytherapy or external-beam radiation therapy. With a median follow-up of 67 months, there was no significant difference in 5-year local tumor control, distant relapse–free survival, or disease-specific survival when adjuvant irradiation was delivered.

Further studies will be required to define which subsets of patients with primary extremity sarcoma can be treated by wide excision surgery alone. Preoperative or postoperative radiotherapy should be employed for patients with primary T1 sarcomas in whom a satisfactory gross surgical margin cannot be attained without compromise of functionally important neurovascular structures.

Limb-sparing surgery plus irradiation Limb-sparing surgery employing adjuvant irradiation to facilitate maximal tumor local control has become the standard approach for large (T2) soft-tissue sarcomas of the extremities. In most centers, upward of 90% of patients are treated with limb-sparing approaches. Amputation is reserved as a last-resort option for local tumor control and is used with the knowledge that it does not affect survival. This approach was validated in a prospective National Cancer Institute (NCI) study, in which patients with a limb-sparing surgical option were randomized to receive limb-sparing surgery with postoperative radiation therapy or amputation. Both arms of the study included postoperative therapy with doxorubicin, cyclophosphamide, and methotrexate.

Surgical procedure The planned resection should encompass the skin, subcutaneous tissues, and soft tissues adjacent to the tumor, including the previous biopsy site and any associated drain sites. The tumor should be excised with a 2- to 3-cm margin of normal surrounding tissue whenever possible. Since good adjuvant approaches are available to facilitate local tumor control, this ideal margin is sometimes compromised rather than attempting resection of adjacent, possibly involved bone or neurovascular structures that would result in significant functional loss. In the rare circumstance of gross involvement of neurovascular structures or bone, they can be resected en bloc and reconstructed.

Metal clips should be placed at the margins of resection to facilitate radiation field planning, when and if external irradiation is indicated. Drain sites should be positioned close to the wound to allow inclusion in radiation therapy fields. As noted earlier, avoidance of transverse incisions greatly facilitates the ability to include the tissues at risk in radiation target volume without unduly large fields.

Regional lymphadenectomy Given the low, 2% to 3%, prevalence of lymph node metastasis in adult sarcomas, there is no role for routine regional lymphadenectomy. Patients with angiosarcoma, embryonal rhabdomyosarcoma, synovial sarcoma, and epithelioid histologies have an increased incidence of lymph node metastasis and should be carefully examined and radiographically imaged for lymphadenopathy. Clinically apparent lymphadenopathy should be treated with therapeutic lymphadenectomy. A recent analysis suggested that select patients undergoing lymphadenectomy, particularly in the absence of systemic metastases, may have a 5-year survival rate of 57%, far superior to the survival expected for patients with AJCC stage IV disease, as this is presently defined. As a result, the AJCC staging system (version 7) for sarcomas treats patients with lymph node metastasis as a different category from those patients with overt blood-borne metastases.

Radiotherapy

Radiation therapy is usually combined with surgical resection in managing soft-tissue sarcomas of the extremities. The decision of whether to use preoperative (neoadjuvant) or postoperative (adjuvant) irradiation remains somewhat controversial, but has been addressed in a phase III randomized trial.

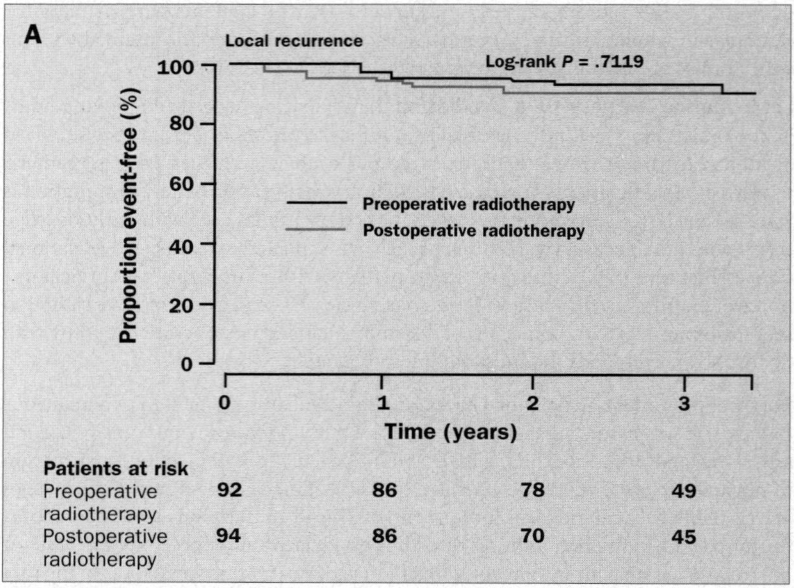

FIGURE 1A: Kaplan-Meier plots for probability of local recurrence in the National Cancer Institute of Canada Clinical Trials Group phase III trial.

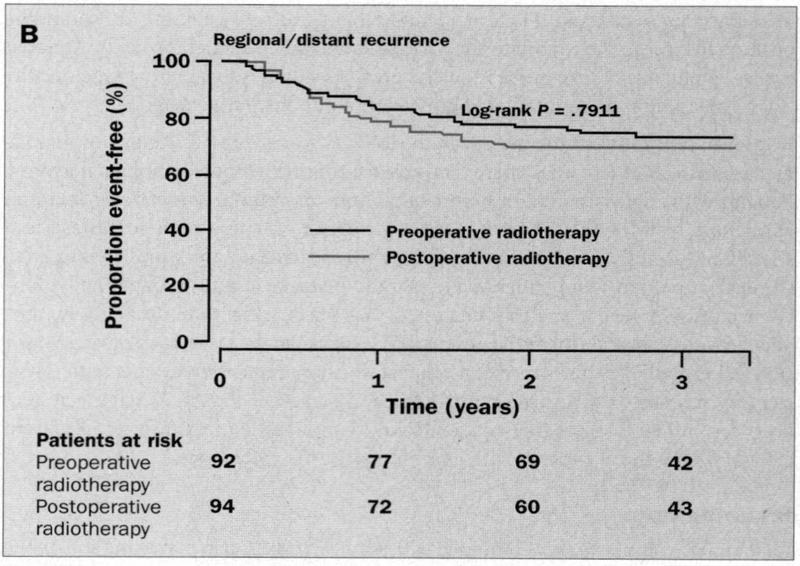

FIGURE 1B: Kaplan-Meier plots for probability of metastatic (regional and distant) recurrence in the National Cancer Institute of Canada Clinical Trials Group phase III trial.

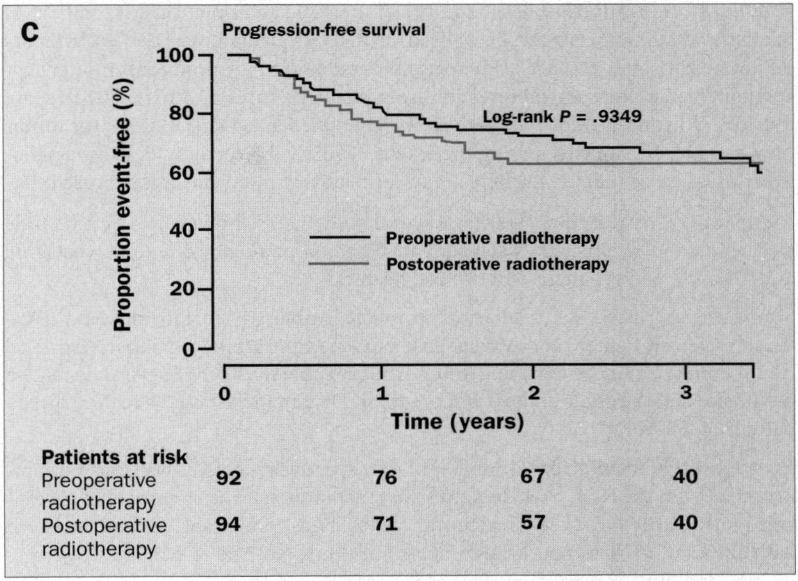

FIGURE 1C: Kaplan-Meier plots for probability of progression-free survival in the National Cancer Institute of Canada Clinical Trials Group phase III trial.

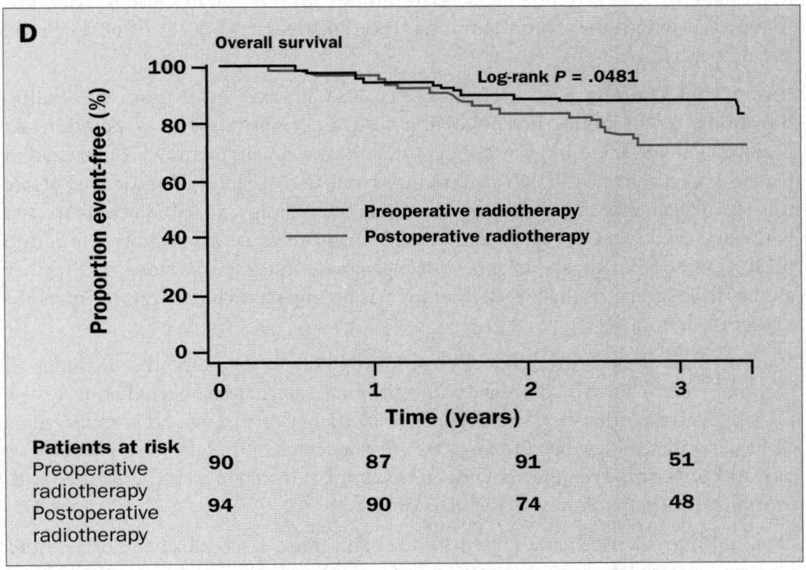

FIGURE 1D: Kaplan-Meier plots for probability of overall survival in the National Cancer Institute of Canada Clinical Trials Group phase III trial.

From O'Sullivan R, Davis AM, Turcotte R, et al: Lancet 359:2235–2241, 2002.

Preoperative irradiation has a number of theoretic and practical advantages: (1) Smaller radiation portals can be utilized, as the scar, hematomas, and ecchymoses do not need to be covered. (2) Preoperative irradiation may produce tumor encapsulation, facilitating surgical resection from vital structures. (3) It is easier to spare a strip of skin and thereby reduce the risk of lymphedema. (4) The size of the tumor may be reduced, thus decreasing the extent of surgical resection. (5) Lower radiation doses can be utilized, as there are fewer relatively radioresistant hypoxic cells.

Preoperative irradiation also has several drawbacks, however. They include (1) the inability to precisely stage patients based on pathology due to downstaging and (2) increased problems with wound healing.

Studies of preoperative irradiation from the University of Florida, M. D. Anderson Cancer Center, and Massachusetts General Hospital demonstrated local tumor control rates of 90% using doses of approximately 50 Gy. Survival depended on the size and the grade of the primary tumor. Distant metastases were the primary pattern of failure.

Postoperative irradiation A number of retrospective reports, as well as a randomized trial from the NCI, have demonstrated that limb-sparing surgery plus postoperative irradiation produces local tumor control rates comparable to those achieved with amputation. Five-year local tumor control rates of 70% to 90%, survival rates of 70%, and limb-preservation rates of 85% can be expected.

Equivocal or positive histologic margins are associated with higher local recurrence rates, and, therefore, adjuvant external-beam irradiation should be considered in all patients with sarcoma of the extremities with positive or close microscopic margins in whom reexcision is impractical. Postoperative doses of 60 to 65 Gy should be used.

Interstitial therapy with iridium-192 is used at some institutions as a radiation boost to the tumor bed following adjuvant external-beam irradiation. At Memorial Sloan-Kettering Cancer Center, adjuvant brachytherapy is often used in place of external irradiation. In a randomized trial, the 5-year local tumor control rate was 82% in patients who received adjuvant brachytherapy, vs 69% in those treated with surgery alone. On subset analysis, the local tumor control rate was found to be 89%, vs 66% for those patients with high-grade lesions. This study and further studies have indicated that brachytherapy has no impact on local tumor control for low-grade lesions.

If an implant alone is used, the dose is 40 to 45 Gy to a volume that includes all margins; when a boost is combined with additional external-beam irradiation, a dose of 20 to 25 Gy is utilized. Some data suggest a higher rate of wound complications and a delay in healing when implants are afterloaded prior to the third postoperative day. Although some centers load implants sooner, this step must be performed with caution and strict attention to the incision site.

Over a 15-year period, 202 patients with high-grade sarcoma of the extremities underwent complete gross resection and adjuvant brachytherapy to a median dose of 45 Gy, delivered over 5 days. With a median follow-up of 61 months, the 5-year local tumor control, distant relapse-free survival, and overall survival rates were 84%, 63%, and 70%, respectively. These rates compared favorably with data on external-beam irradiation. Morbidity of brachytherapy was considered acceptable, with reoperation rates of 12%, bone fractures in 3%, and nerve damage in 5%.

Comparison of irradiation techniques Comparable local tumor control results (90%) are obtained with preoperative, postoperative, and interstitial techniques, although rates of wound complications are higher with preoperative techniques. Brachytherapy can offer a number of advantages. When brachytherapy is employed as the sole adjuvant, the entire treatment (surgery and irradiation) is completed in a 10- to 12-day period, compared with the 10 to 12 weeks required for typical external-beam irradiation (6 to 7 weeks) and surgery (4- to 6-week break before or after irradiation). Generally, smaller volumes can be irradiated with brachytherapy, which could improve functional results. However, smaller volumes may not be appropriate, depending on the tumor size, grade, and margin status.

The NCI of Canada Clinical Trials Group published 3-year median follow-up results of a randomized phase III trial comparing preoperative and postoperative radiotherapy for limb soft-tissue sarcoma (Figures 1A–1D). Wound complications were observed in 31 of 88 patients (35%) in the preoperative group and 16 of 94 patients (17%) in the postoperative group (difference, 18% [95% CI: 5–30]; $P = .01$). Tumor size and anatomic site were also significant risk factors in multivariate analysis. Local tumor control was identical in both arms of the trial. Five-year outcomes have been reported, and no difference in metastases, cause-specific survival, or overall survival was noted. Because preoperative radiotherapy is associated with a greater risk of wound complications than postoperative radiotherapy, but less late fibrosis and edema, the choice of regimen for patients with soft-tissue sarcoma should take into account the timing of surgery and radiotherapy and the size and anatomic site of the tumor.

Regardless of the technique employed, local control is a highly achievable and worthwhile endpoint, as demonstrated in a study of 911 patients treated by various techniques at Memorial Sloan-Kettering Cancer Center. Of the 116 patients who developed local recurrence, 38 patients subsequently developed metastases and 34 patients died. Metastases after local recurrence were predicted in patients with high-grade or large (> 5 cm) tumors.

Treatment recommendations Adjuvant radiotherapy should be employed for virtually all high-grade sarcomas of the extremities and larger (≥ 5 cm) low-grade lesions. If small (T1) lesions can be resected with clear margins, radiotherapy can be omitted. Postoperative therapy with either external-beam irradiation (with or without an interstitial implant boost) or an implant alone will achieve a high likelihood of local tumor control and, therefore, limb preservation. Preoperative irradiation, although equally efficacious, does carry a higher wound complication rate than the postoperative approach.

Primary radiation therapy

Several studies on radiation therapy alone in the treatment of unresectable or medically inoperable soft-tissue sarcomas have reported 5-year survival rates of 25% to 40% and local tumor control rates of 30%. Local tumor control depends largely on the size of the primary tumor. Radiation doses should be at least 65 to 70 Gy, if delivery of such doses is feasible. The tumor's location may be particularly important in determining this dose because of the potential for damage to critical structures (eg, the spinal cord) with the higher doses normally used.

Radiation therapy in retroperitoneal sarcomas

Only 50% of patients with retroperitoneal sarcomas are able to undergo complete surgical resection. Of patients undergoing complete resection, one-half develop local recurrence. This significant local failure rate suggests a potentially important role for adjuvant treatment in all patients with retroperitoneal sarcomas. However, the role of radiation therapy for retroperitoneal sarcomas remains controversial due to the rarity of the tumor, the paucity of data, the retrospective nature of available studies, the low doses of radiation used in many studies, and the lack of consistent policies in determining the indications for radiation therapy.

Preoperative irradiation The advantages of preoperative radiotherapy have already been discussed for soft-tissue sarcomas of the extremities. In the retroperitoneum, an additional advantage is that bowel is frequently displaced significantly by the tumor. In contrast to the postoperative setting, the bowel being treated is also unlikely to be tethered by adhesions from prior surgery. These features significantly offset acute toxicity of large-field intra-abdominal radiotherapy (eg, nausea, vomiting, and diarrhea) as well as the potential for late-onset bowel toxicity. Conformal techniques capable of sparing normal tissues are also more easily applied in the preoperative setting, when the tumor can be visualized and the target area more readily defined.

Intraoperative irradiation In a prospective trial from the NCI, 35 patients with completely resected retroperitoneal sarcomas were randomized to receive either intraoperative electron-beam irradiation (IORT) followed by low-dose (30 to 40 Gy) postoperative external-beam irradiation or high-dose postoperative external-beam irradiation (35 to 40 Gy plus a 20-Gy boost). Absolute local recurrence rates were significantly lower in the IORT group ($P < .05$), but disease-specific and overall survival rates did not differ between the two groups.

Similarly, a nonrandomized series from the Massachusetts General Hospital has suggested improved local tumor control with IORT for patients with retroperitoneal sarcoma. In 16 patients who underwent irradiation, complete gross resection, and IORT, overall survival and local tumor control rates were 74% and 83%, respectively. These numbers diminished to 30% and 61%, respectively, in the 13 patients treated with irradiation and complete gross resection without IORT. Although these local tumor control results are encouraging, IORT remains investigational and cannot be advocated on a routine basis at this time.

Postoperative irradiation Two-year local tumor control rates of 70% have been reported with the addition of postoperative irradiation. However, irradiation of the retroperitoneum/abdomen in doses that have effected local tumor control in soft-tissue sarcoma of the extremities (50 to 65 Gy) is usually associated with significant GI toxicity. Obviously, the incidence of GI toxicity depends on the exact fields and technique used. However, as most retroperitoneal sarcomas are > 10 to 15 cm, the radiation fields employed are generally also quite large, and bowel is often located and/or tethered in the high-risk area. Three-dimensional treatment planning and conformal techniques can now be utilized to maximize the radiation dose to the tumor bed while minimizing the dose to the surrounding normal tissues.

Isolated limb perfusion

Recent studies have evaluated the role of isolated limb perfusion (ILP) in the management of sarcomas of the extremities. These studies have generally been extrapolations from protocols initially designed to treat locally advanced melanoma.

The agents most commonly employed for ILP have been melphalan and tumor necrosis factor-alpha (TNF-α), with or without interferon-gamma (IFN-γ-1b [Actimmune]). The results of the largest series of ILP in patients with locally advanced soft-tissue sarcoma of the extremities were reported by Eggermont and colleagues. TNF-α has now been approved in Europe for ILP in patients with locally advanced, grade 2/3 soft-tissue sarcomas of the extremities.

The Netherlands Cancer Institute published its results in patients with unresectable soft-tissue sarcoma of the extremities who were perfused with melphalan and TNF-α. A total of 49 patients were treated and followed for a median of 26 months. One patient died shortly after perfusion, but 31 patients (63%) were able to undergo resection of the tumor. Based on clinical and pathologic grounds, an overall response was seen in 31 patients (63%), and a complete response was seen in 4 patients (8%). A total of 28 patients (57%) had local tumor control with limb preservation. Toxicity was frequent but usually mild.

ROLE OF ADJUVANT CHEMOTHERAPY

The striking success of combined-modality therapy in children with osteogenic sarcoma, rhabdomyosarcoma, and the Ewing sarcoma family of tumors has provided the stimulus for the use of aggressive combined-modality approaches in adults. The literature is replete with reports of the apparent benefit of combined-modality therapy in patients with resectable soft-tissue sarcoma. Yet most series are either retrospective or small nonrandomized trials.

Preoperative chemotherapy

Preoperative chemotherapy has been adopted at many centers for patients with large high-grade sarcoma. The specific regimens employed have evolved over the years but generally contain both an anthracycline and ifosfamide.

Aside from theoretic considerations, there are several pragmatic reasons to favor preoperative over postoperative treatment. First, a reduction in the size of a large lesion may permit surgical resection with less morbidity. Second, compliance may be better with preoperative therapy. One observation that supports the neoadjuvant approach is that response to preoperative chemotherapy, whether pathologic or radiographic, predicts improved tumor control and survival.

Neoadjuvant chemotherapy has been explored in a prospective randomized trial initiated by the EORTC. The trial was open to patients who had a sarcoma measuring at least 8 cm (of any grade), a primary or recurrent intermediate- to high-grade (grade 2/3) sarcoma of any size, or a locally recurrent or inadequately excised grade 2/3 sarcoma. In spite of these broad eligibility criteria, accrual was slow, and the trial was closed after only 150 patients entered.

Patients were randomized to receive either immediate surgery, followed by radiation therapy for close or positive margins, or 3 cycles of chemotherapy with doxorubicin (50 mg/m^2 by IV bolus) plus ifosfamide (5 g/m^2 by 24-hour continuous infusion) with mesna (Mesnex). Among the 134 eligible patients, over 80% had primary tumors of the extremities, but only 4% had grade 2/3 lesions > 8 cm. Among 49 patients evaluable for response, 29% had major objective responses, including four complete responses. Only 18% had progression of disease before surgery. Chemotherapy was generally well tolerated and never prevented surgery. With a median follow-up of 7.3 years, the estimated 5-year survival rate was similar for both groups.

Trials have explored the role of neoadjuvant chemotherapy and radiation therapy to decrease the rate of distant failure and possibly impact survival. A study reported from Massachusetts General Hospital enrolled patients with high-grade soft-tissue sarcomas (8 cm or larger). Patients were treated with 3 cycles of preoperative chemotherapy consisting of MAID (mesna, doxorubicin [Adriamycin], ifosfamide, dacarbazine) interdigitated with 44 Gy of radiation therapy. This regimen was followed by surgical resection and 3 cycles of postoperative MAID chemotherapy. In cases with positive surgical margins, an additional 16 Gy of radiation therapy was delivered.

This regimen resulted in a significant improvement in 5-year freedom from distant metastasis (75% vs 44%; $P = .0016$) when compared with historic control patients. Additionally, 5-year disease-free and overall survival rates were 70% vs 42% ($P = .0002$) and 87% vs 58% ($P = .0003$) for the MAID and control groups, respectively. There was a 29% rate of wound healing complications in the MAID group.

These data have been extended in a follow-up study of similar interdigitated chemotherapy/radiation therapy in a phase II study from the RTOG. In this study, 66 patients with primary high-grade soft-tissue sarcoma ≥ 8 cm in diameter received a modified MAID regimen plus granulocyte colony-stimulating factor (G-CSF, filgrastim [Neupogen]) and radiation therapy, followed by resection and postoperative chemotherapy. Preoperative radiotherapy and chemotherapy were successfully completed by 89% and 79% of patients, respectively. Grade 4 hematologic and nonhematologic toxicities affected 80% and 23% of patients, respectively. Two patients developed acute myelogenous leukemia (AML) following therapy. Delayed wound healing was noted in 31%. The estimated 3-year survival, disease-free survival, and local tumor control rates were 75%, 55%, and 79%, respectively.

The M. D. Anderson Cancer Center conducted a phase I trial to define the maximum tolerated dose of continuous infusion doxorubicin administered with preoperative radiation therapy to a dose of 50 Gy. In total, 27 patients with intermediate- or high-grade sarcomas were enrolled in the trial. The maximum tolerated dose of doxorubicin was 17.5 mg/m^2/week. Twenty-six patients underwent surgery, and all had a macroscopic complete resection (R0 or R1). Two patients had a pathologic complete response. These studies suggest that further investigation of a preoperative approach combining chemotherapy and radiation therapy is warranted. The lack of randomized data regarding the addition of chemotherapy to radiation therapy for extremity sarcomas limits the ability to apply these treatment regimens outside the setting of a study.

Postoperative chemotherapy

A number of published trials have compared postoperative chemotherapy with observation alone in adults who had undergone resection of a primary or recurrent soft-tissue sarcoma. Most of these trials included fewer than 100 patients, and even the largest trial had inadequate statistical power to detect a 15% difference in survival. Other flaws confound the interpretation of many of the studies. Some trials included low-risk patients with small and/or low-grade sarcomas. In some trials, patient ineligibility rates were as high as 20%, and in none of the trials published before 2000 was ifosfamide part of the combination evaluated.

In five of the six trials in which doxorubicin monotherapy was studied, including one study limited to patients with uterine sarcoma, a significant improvement in survival could not be demonstrated. Among the trials of combination chemotherapy, most used the combination known as CyVADIC (cyclophosphamide, vincristine, doxorubicin [Adriamycin], dacarbazine). A significant survival advantage was seen in only one combination chemotherapy trial.

Nonetheless, some of the trials showed a trend or a statistically significant improvement in disease-free survival among patients who were administered adjuvant chemotherapy, especially among those with high-grade sarcomas of the extremities. Analyses of the pooled results of the published literature are consistent with this observation.

Ifosfamide-containing trials Only one trial included in a meta-analysis by SMAC used an ifosfamide-containing regimen; that trial involved only 29 patients. An attempt to conduct a large prospective trial of postoperative chemotherapy with the MAID regimen in the United States failed because of insufficient patient accrual.

An Italian cooperative group conducted a trial in which patients 18 to 65 years old with high-grade (> 5 cm) or any recurrent sarcoma of the extremities were randomized to receive postoperative chemotherapy or observation alone. The treatment consisted of 5 cycles of epirubicin, 60 mg/m^2 on days 1 and 2, plus ifosfamide, 1.8 g/m^2 on days 1 to 5. G-CSF was used to support the granulocyte counts during therapy.

The trial had been planned for 200 patients but was interrupted after accrual of 104 patients, when an interim analysis showed a significant survival advantage for the chemotherapy-treated group. At 36 months after the last randomization, with a median follow-up of 59 months, median overall survival among the patients who received adjuvant chemotherapy was 75 months, vs 46 months for control patients (P = .03). In a longer-term follow-up analysis, survival was not improved on an intention-to-treat analysis, although 5-year overall survival rates still favored the patients receiving chemotherapy.

An analysis of adjuvant chemotherapy using doxorubicin and ifosfamide was conducted by the EORTC. This study examined surgery and adjuvant radiation therapy vs the same local therapy and adjuvant chemotherapy with 5 cycles of doxorubicin (75 mg/m^2) and ifosfamide (5 g/m^2) every 21 days. The data indicated no benefit in overall survival for the chemotherapy arm and tempered some of the enthusiasm regarding adjuvant chemotherapy as demonstrated in a positive Italian study of epirubicin and ifosfamide.

Since the time of the original Italian study, two other randomized studies have been performed. They do not indicate a benefit for chemotherapy but were underpowered to detect small differences in outcome.

SMAC and newer meta-analyses A formal meta-analysis of individual data from 1,568 patients who participated in randomized trials of postoperative adjuvant chemotherapy vs no chemotherapy control patients was performed by the SMAC and published in 1997. Although not all data were available for all patients, the analysis demonstrated a significant reduction in the risk of local or distant recurrence in patients who received adjuvant chemotherapy.

The overall hazard ratio (HR) for distant relapse-free survival was 0.70; ie, the risk of distant relapse (metastasis) was reduced by 30% in treated patients. The absolute benefit at 10 years was 10%, so the recurrence-free survival rate at 10 years was improved from 60% to 70%. Also, the HR for local recurrence-free survival was 0.73 (27% reduction in the risk of local recurrence), and the absolute benefit was 6%.

The HR for overall survival, however, was 0.89, which did not meet the criteria for statistical significance. The observed survival at 10 years was 54% for patients who received chemotherapy and 50% for those who did not. Subset analysis failed to show that the effects of chemotherapy differed by primary site, although the best evidence for an effect of adjuvant chemotherapy was seen in patients with sarcoma of the extremities.

A newer meta-analysis, including more ifosfamide-based studies, although excluding the large randomized EORTC 62931 study, confirms the trend seen in the SMAC meta-analysis, with a modest overall survival benefit of chemotherapy in the adjuvant setting. In this updated meta-analysis, 18 trials, representing 1,953 patients, were examined. The odds ratio (OR) for local recurrence was 0.73 in favor of chemotherapy ($P = .02$). In terms of overall survival, use of doxorubicin-based therapy without ifosfamide had an OR of 0.84, which was not statistically significant ($P = .09$). However, the OR for doxorubicin/ifosfamide-based therapy was 0.56 ($P = .01$) in favor of chemotherapy. The updated meta-analysis confirmed the SMAC meta-analysis in that there was modest efficacy of adjuvant chemotherapy for resected soft-tissue sarcoma with respect to local recurrence, distant recurrence, overall recurrence, and overall survival. The authors concluded that benefits were further improved with the addition of ifosfamide to doxorubicin-based regimens but must be weighed against the toxicity of the addition of ifosfamide.

Analyses of other collected prospective data regarding adjuvant chemotherapy from large referral centers have yielded conflicting data. In two analyses of patients with synovial sarcoma and one involving myxoid/round cell liposarcoma, chemotherapy appeared to improve overall survival. In a large analysis of two prospective databases, patients receiving chemotherapy initially had superior survival but then suffered inferior survival compared with those who received no adjuvant chemotherapy. Notably, patients were not randomized as part of their treatment. Given the fact that this was a registry instead of a randomized study, there was by definition a bias to treat patients who had higher-risk tumors with chemotherapy, although this did not appear to correlate with a specific single variable in the analysis. The data from the most recent meta-analysis appear to be consistent with data from prior studies when taken as a whole. If there is a benefit in terms of overall survival with the use of adjuvant chemotherapy, it is a small one, and the risks and benefits should be discussed with patients on an individual basis.

Treatment recommendations

- Multidisciplinary treatment planning should precede the initiation of any therapy. An experienced multidisciplinary team should evaluate pathologic material and imaging studies and coordinate the integration of surgical resection, irradiation, and systemic therapy.
- Ideally, patients should be offered participation in clinical trials. Unfortunately, there are no active trials in the United States that will definitively answer the most important questions. Thus, a decision to treat must be made on an individual basis.
- Preoperative chemotherapy should be considered for fit, high-risk patients after a discussion of the risks and potential benefits. Older patients, especially those with cardiac or renal disease, are not optimal candidates for such treatment.
- Patients who do not receive preoperative chemotherapy may still be offered postopertive treatment. Adjuvant anthracycline/ifosfamide combinations improves relapse-free survival in selected patients and can be considered for the treatment of those with tumor size > 5 cm, deep tumor location, and high histologic grade. Overall survival was superior in the most recent meta-analysis for patients receiving doxorubicin-ifosfamide based therapy, and this should be the standard combination to consider if adjuvant therapy is to be administered.
- For patients who opt for preoperative or postoperative chemotherapy, a regimen that includes doxorubicin (60 to 75 mg/m^2) or epirubicin (120 mg/m^2) plus ifosfamide (9 to 10 g/m^2), given for a total of four to six cycles, is a reasonable choice for patients younger than age 60.
- Outside the context of a clinical trial, it is difficult to recommend concurrent doxorubicin and radiation therapy, or closely spaced doxorubicin-based chemotherapy with radiation therapy, owing to the observed risk of second malignancies such as AML in clinical trials to date.

TREATMENT OF LOCAL RECURRENCE

Despite optimal multimodality therapy, local recurrence develops in 10% to 50% of patients, with a median local recurrence-free interval of ~24 months. Local recurrence rates are a function of the primary site and are highest for patients with retroperitoneal and head and neck sarcomas, for which adequate surgical margins are difficult to attain. In addition, high-dose adjuvant irradiation of these sites is often limited by the relative radiosensitivity of surrounding structures. These factors result in local recurrence rates of 40% for retroperitoneal sarcomas and up to 50% for head and neck sarcomas, which are substantially higher than the 10% proximity typically seen for extremity sarcomas.

A large retrospective analysis of patients with high-grade sarcoma of the extremities was reported from UCLA. Local recurrence required amputation in 38% of cases and was associated with a threefold decrement in survival. This finding accentuates the necessity for adequate local therapy for sarcomas presenting primarily as well as for multidisciplinary management of local recurrence.

Reoperation Following staging evaluation, patients with isolated local recurrence should undergo reoperation. The results of reoperation in this setting are good, with two-thirds of patients experiencing long-term survival.

Adjuvant radiation therapy If no prior radiation therapy had been employed, adjuvant irradiation (50 to 65 Gy) should be used before or after surgery for locally recurrent disease. Radiation therapy (external-beam irradiation or brachytherapy) should be considered in patients for whom previous radiation doses were subtherapeutic or the previous radiation field design permitted additional treatment.

Reports from Memorial Sloan-Kettering Cancer Center, M. D. Anderson Cancer Center, and Princess Margaret Hospital suggest that patients who develop local recurrence following previous full-dose irradiation represent a difficult local tumor control challenge. A report from Memorial Sloan-Kettering Cancer Center suggests that limb-sparing surgery combined with adjuvant brachytherapy may produce excellent local tumor control and function in this group.

ILP Ongoing clinical investigations are defining the role of ILP in the management of patients with locally recurrent sarcoma. ILP is approved in Europe for treatment of otherwise unresectable extremity sarcomas.

TREATMENT OF LIMITED PULMONARY METASTASIS

Thoracotomy and metastasectomy The most common site of metastatic disease involvement of soft-tissue sarcoma is the lungs. Rates of 3-year survival following thoracotomy for pulmonary metastasectomy range from 23% to 42%. This fact, combined with the limited efficacy of systemic therapy, is the basis for the recommendation that patients with limited pulmonary metastases and no extrapulmonary disease should undergo thoracotomy and metastasectomy.

Appropriate patient selection for this aggressive therapeutic approach to metastatic disease is essential. The following are generally agreed upon criteria: (1) the primary tumor is controlled or controllable; (2) there is no extrathoracic metastatic disease; (3) the patient is a medical candidate for thoracotomy; and (4) complete resection of all disease appears to be possible.

Preresection chemotherapy Chemotherapy is sometimes recommended before resection of pulmonary metastases. Although occasional patients may have tumor shrinkage to a degree that an unresectable tumor becomes resectable, there are no convincing data that chemotherapy impacts favorably on patient survival. It is also worth remarking that there are no randomized data on which to base this judgment.

CHEMOTHERAPY FOR UNRESECTABLE LOCALLY ADVANCED OR METASTATIC DISEASE

Single agents

Doxorubicin Early trials of doxorubicin reported major responses in approximately 30% of patients with advanced soft-tissue sarcoma. In more recent randomized series, however, the rate of response has been closer to 17%.

Subset analysis of patients with soft-tissue sarcoma from a broad phase II trial in which patients were randomized to receive various doses of doxorubicin demonstrated a steep dose-response relationship; patients treated with doses below 60 mg/m^2 rarely responded. Whether dose intensification of doxorubicin is associated with improved survival remains an open question (see section on "Intensifying chemotherapy").

Pegylated liposomal doxorubicin (Doxil in the United States, Caelyx in Europe) has demonstrated limited activity in phase II trials, especially in patients whose disease is refractory to standard doxorubicin. In a randomized comparison among 95 previously untreated patients, however, the response rates to pegylated liposomal doxorubicin (50 mg/m^2 every 4 weeks; 10%) and to standard doxorubicin (75 mg/m^2 every 3 weeks; 9%) were similar, with no significant difference in time to disease progression or survival. Response rates improved to 14% and 12%, respectively, when GIST cases were excluded.

Ifosfamide In a randomized phase II trial conducted by EORTC, 18% of patients treated with ifosfamide (5 g/m^2) experienced major responses, in contrast to 12% of patients treated with cyclophosphamide (1.5 g/m^2), despite the greater myelosuppression with the latter agent. In a large American phase II trial, 17 of 99 patients with soft-tissue sarcoma responded to ifosfamide (8 g/m^2). All of the patients had been treated previously with doxorubicin-based therapy, suggesting a degree of non–cross-resistance.

Increasing ifosfamide dose Responses to ifosfamide ($\geq$ 12 g/m^2) have been observed in patients whose disease progressed while receiving lower doses, supporting the concept of a dose-response relationship.

In a randomized trial, the response to 9 g/m^2 of ifosfamide (17.5%) was superior to the 3% response observed among patients treated with 5 g/m^2. The reason for the low response to the lower dose was unclear. In a subsequent trial by the same investigators, the response to 12 g/m^2 was only 14%, however.

Among 45 evaluable patients enrolled in a Spanish phase II trial of ifosfamide (14 g/m^2 given by continuous infusion over 6 days), the response rate was 38%, but 47% of patients developed febrile neutropenia and 32%, grade 3 neurotoxicity.

At M. D. Anderson Cancer Center, ifosfamide (14 g/m^2 given by continuous infusion over 3 days) yielded responses in 29% of 37 patients with soft-tissue sarcoma and 40% of patients with bone sarcoma. Also within that report was a small cohort of patients in whom the response to the same total dose of ifosfamide was higher when the drug was given by an intermittent bolus rather than a continuous infusion; this finding led the authors to suggest that bolus therapy is more efficacious than continuous infusion. Pharmacokinetic studies, however, have shown no difference between a 1-hour infusion and bolus injection of ifosfamide with respect to the area under the concentration-time curve (AUC) for serum ifosfamide or its metabolites or the levels of ifosfamide metabolites in urine.

In an EORTC phase II trial, ifosfamide (12 g/m^2 given as a 3-day continuous infusion every 4 weeks) yielded a response rate of 17% among 89 chemotherapy-naive patients and 16% among 25 previously treated patients.

Ifosfamide doses as high as 14 to 20 g/m^2 have been given with hematopoietic growth factor support; reported response rates are high, but neurologic and renal toxicities often are dose-limiting. The available data suggest that synovial sarcoma is particularly sensitive to ifosfamide.

Dacarbazine The activity of dacarbazine in soft-tissue sarcoma has been recognized since the 1970s and was confirmed in a formal phase II trial. This marginally active agent has been used mostly in doxorubicin-based combinations. In particular, patients with leiomyosarcoma respond better to dacarbazine than do patients with other sarcoma subtypes.

Ecteinascidin (ET-743, trabectedin), a novel compound derived from a marine organism, has demonstrated promising activity as well. In phase I trials, trabectedin demonstrated activity in heavily pretreated patients with advanced sarcoma. Three phase II trials of trabectedin (1,500 mg/m^2 over 24 hours every 3 weeks) in refractory non-GIST soft-tissue sarcoma have been reported.

In one trial, two partial responses and four minor responses were seen among 52 patients; 9 additional patients had stable disease for at least 6 months. Twenty-four percent of patients were free of disease progression at 6 months. The median survival was 12.8 months, with 30% of patients alive at 2 years.

In a second trial, responses were observed in 3 of 36 patients, with one complete response and two partial responses, for an overall response rate of 8% (95% CI: 2–23). Responses, however, were durable, lasting up to 20 months.

Finally, a phase II study of patients treated in first line with the 24-hour infusion schedule of trabectedin demonstrated a 17% response rate. These data confirm that trabectedin is an active compound in the treatment of soft-tissue sarcomas, with a response rate similar to the 10% to 30% range seen for either doxorubicin or ifosfamide. The predominant toxicities were neutropenia and elevation of transaminase levels. Two phase II trials of trabectedin in patients with GIST showed no therapeutic activity. Trabectedin was approved for use in chemotherapy-refractory sarcomas in Europe in 2007.

Other agents Gemcitabine (Gemzar) has demonstrated modest activity in several phase II trials, although results of a recent SWOG trial were disappointing. Taxanes, vinca alkaloids, and platinum compounds have demonstrated only marginal activity, however. It should be noted that the taxanes, gemcitabine, and vinorelbine (Navelbine) have been observed to be active in angiosarcoma, especially involving the scalp and face.

TABLE 4: Chemotherapy regimens for soft-tissue sarcoma

Drug/combination	Dose and schedule
AIM	
Adriamycin (doxorubicin)	30 mg/m^2 IV on days 1 and 2 by rapid IV infusion
Ifosfamide	3,750 mg/m^2 on days 1 and 2 by IV infusion over 4 hours
Mesna	750 mg/m^2 IV infused immediately preceding and 4 and 8 hours after ifosfamide administration on days 1 and 2
Repeat cycle every 21 days.	
NOTE: IV hydration at 300 mL/h beginning 3 hours before each treatment cycle and for 3 days at 100 mL/h after each day-1 ifosfamide infusion. Granulocyte colony-stimulating factor, 5 μg/kg subcutaneously, may be given, starting at 24 to 48 hours, daily for 10 days or until a granulocyte count of 1,500/μL is reached. Appropriate supportive measures should be given.	
Edmonson JH, Ryan LM, Blum RH, et al: J Clin Oncol 11:1269–1275, 1993.	
EIM	
Epirubicin	60 mg/m^2 IV infused on days 1 and 2, total dose of 120 mg/m^2 per cycle
Ifosfamide	1.8 $g/m^2/d$ on days 1–5, total dose of 9 g/m^2 per cycle
Mesna	360 mg/m^2 IV infused immediately before and 4 and 8 hours after ifosfamide infusion
Repeat cycle every 3 weeks for a total of five cycles.	
Granulocyte colony-stimulating factor, 300 μg subcutaneously given on days 8–15.	
Hydration (1,500–2,000 mL) of fluids IV given after ifosfamide.	
Frustaci S, Gherlinzoni F, De Paoli A, et al: J Clin Oncol 19:1238–1247, 2001.	
Gemcitabine and docetaxel	
Gemcitabine	900 mg/m^2 IV on days 1 and 8
Docetaxel	100 mg/m^2 on day 8
Repeat cycle every 21 days.	
NOTE: Lower docetaxel doses are typically used off study. Granulocyte colony-stimulating factor is given subcutaneously on days 9 and 15. Patients who have undergone prior pelvic radiation therapy receive 25% dose reduction of both agents. Gemcitabine is delivered over 30 to 90 minutes in cycles 1 and 2 and by 90-minute infusion in all subsequent cycles.	
Hensley ML, Maki R, Venkatraman E, et al: J Clin Oncol 20:2824–2831, 2002.	

Table prepared by Ishmael Jaiyesimi, DO.

Combination chemotherapy

Combination chemotherapy regimens have been used widely in the management of patients with soft-tissue sarcoma (Table 4). High response rates have been reported in a number of single-arm phase II trials. Most combination regimens include an anthracycline (either doxorubicin or epirubicin) plus an alkylating agent, dacarbazine, or both agents. Overall response rates are higher in these single-arm trials than when the same regimens are tested in larger, randomized studies.

CyVADIC and doxorubicin/dacarbazine regimens Combinations of doxorubicin with other agents have not proved to be superior to doxorubicin alone in terms of overall survival. Also, for over a decade, the CyVADIC regimen was widely accepted as the standard of care. In a prospective, randomized trial, however, CyVADIC did not prove to be superior to doxorubicin alone.

Doxorubicin (or epirubicin) plus ifosfamide Combinations of doxorubicin (or epirubicin) plus ifosfamide have consistently yielded responses in over 25% of patients in single-arm trials. In sequential trials conducted by the EORTC, doxorubicin at 75 mg/m^2 plus ifosfamide (5 g/m^2) was superior to doxorubicin at 50 mg/m^2 plus ifosfamide (5 g/m^2). A prospective randomized EORTC trial with 314 patients compared the two regimens. There was no difference in response rate or overall survival, but disease progression-free survival favored the more intensive regimen.

The strategy of intensifying the dosing of ifosfamide within the context of combination chemotherapy was explored in a randomized phase II trial. This study included both patients with localized disease treated with four cycles of preoperative chemotherapy as well as patients with metastatic disease. Overall, there was no survival benefit for patients treated with doxorubicin (60 mg/m^2) plus 12 g/m^2 of ifosfamide over those treated with doxorubicin (60 mg/m^2) plus 6 g/m^2 of ifosfamide. Also, there was no advantage to the patients with localized disease in terms of disease-free survival.

MAID regimen The MAID regimen yielded an overall response rate of 47% in patients in a large phase II trial. In a randomized comparison of AD (Adriamycin [doxorubicin]/dacarbazine) vs MAID regimens, the response to MAID was 32%, vs 17% with the two-drug regimen ($P < .002$). However, the price paid for the higher response was toxicity; of eight toxic deaths reported in this trial, seven occurred among the 170 patients treated with MAID. All treatment-related deaths occurred in patients > 50 years old. During the study, the doses of MAID were reduced to lessen toxicity. The median survival did not differ significantly between the two regimens, although a trend favoring the AD regimen was noted.

Combination chemotherapy vs single-agent doxorubicin Combination chemotherapy has been compared with single-agent doxorubicin in eight randomized phase III trials. Two trials were limited to patients with uterine sarcoma. Some of these studies showed superior response rates with combination chemotherapy, but none of the trials found a significant survival advantage. Kaplan-Meier plots of survival are virtually superimposable within each trial and from trial to trial. A meta-analysis confirmed the higher response rate when ifosfamide is added to other agents and showed no benefit at 1 year of combination therapy over single agents, likely due to the lack of synergy between anthracyclines and ifosfamide. Patients can achieve equal benefit by sequential use of such agents rather than by combinations.

It should be emphasized that approximately 20% to 25% of patients entered into such trials are alive 2 years after therapy was initiated. Complete responses are uncommon and do not appear to translate into prolonged survival.

Gemcitabine plus docetaxel In a phase II study of 34 patients with unresectable leiomyosarcoma, mostly uterine in origin, 53% responded to a combination of gemcitabine (given by 90-minute infusion) plus docetaxel (Taxotere), with G-CSF support. An additional 20% had stable disease. Almost half of the patients had disease progression after anthracycline-based therapy. The median time to disease progression was 5.6 months, and grade 3/4 toxicity was uncommon. The activity of the gemcitabine-docetaxel combination was confirmed in a variety of other sarcoma subtypes in another study, which also confirmed the rationale for the sequence used in the study in vitro.

A prospective, randomized trial comparing gemcitabine-docetaxel with gemcitabine alone in a spectrum of histologic types of sarcoma has been completed. The response rates were 8% for gemcitabine alone and 16% for gemcitabine-docetaxel. Time to disease progression and overall survival were superior with gemcitabine-docetaxel (17.9 months vs 11 months). Although this is one of the few studies in metastatic sarcoma to show a survival advantage, enthusiasm is tempered by toxicity, causing treatment discontinuation in up to 50% of patients after 6 months of gemcitabine-docetaxel chemotherapy. These data suggest that a dose reduction is needed in the off-study use of the therapy.

In the authors' experience, weekly administration of lower doses of each agent is more tolerable than the large day-8 dose of docetaxel and remains an active regimen. The randomized study previously noted that the response rate was higher in patients with high-grade undifferentiated pleomorphic sarcoma (UPS, formerly termed MFH [malignant fibrous histiocytoma]) than in patients with leiomyosarcoma.

Gemcitabine plus vinorelbine These agents given together were also active in one phase II study. It is not clear whether either vinorelbine or docetaxel is synergistic for all histologies tested or synergy is only observed for specific subtypes.

Kinase-targeted agents in non-GIST sarcomas Several of the commercially available tyrosine kinase inhibitors have been examined for activity in the setting of metastatic disease. In general, response rates have been low, and use of the agents is not recommended outside a clinical trial.

Exceptions to this statement may include a 15% response rate of patients with synovial sarcoma to pazopanib (Votrient), a 14% response rate of patients with angiosarcoma to sorafenib (Nexavar) (particularly those induced by therapeutic radiation) and similar activity of bevacizumab (Avastin) in angiosarcomas, and reports of the utility of imatinib in patients with the rare sarcoma subtype dermatofibrosarcoma protuberans. There appears to be at least modest activity of sunitinib (Sutent) in alvelolar soft part sarcoma, clear cell sarcoma, and solitary fibrous tumor/hemangiopericytoma, and of cediranib (Recentin) in patients with metastatic alveolar soft-part sarcoma.

Intensifying chemotherapy Hematopoietic growth factors have facilitated the evaluation of dose-intensive chemotherapy in patients with sarcoma. The nonhematologic toxicities (cardiac, neurologic, and renal) of the agents most active in soft-tissue sarcoma prevent dramatic dose escalation.

Phase I/II trials of dose-intense anthracycline/ifosfamide regimens with hematopoietic growth factor support have shown that doxorubicin (70 to 90 mg/m^2) can be used in combination with ifosfamide (10 to 12 g/m^2) in selected patients. Response rates as high as 69% have been reported. Although toxicity increases, often dramatically, with these relatively modest dose escalations, the clinical benefit in terms of survival or palliation in patients with metastatic disease remains uncertain.

No randomized trial has demonstrated a survival advantage for patients treated with these more aggressive regimens. In one randomized trial, however, the FFCCSG demonstrated that, in comparison with standard doses, a 25% escalation in doses of MAID with G-CSF support did not improve outcome.

High-dose therapy with autologous stem-cell transplantation Most trials are small and presumably involve highly selected patients. In one trial involving 30 patients with metastatic or locally advanced sarcoma accrued over 6 years, more than 20% were free of disease progression at 5 years after high-dose therapy with stem-cell rescue. Complete response to standard induction chemotherapy predicted superior 5-year survival. Based on these favorable results, the investigators suggested a prospective randomized trial examining this approach. Although some groups are still exploring this approach, the appropriateness of generalizing these results to most patients with soft-tissue sarcoma remains speculative.

Prognostic factors for response to therapy Over the past 20 years, the EORTC has collected data on more than 2,000 patients with metastatic disease who participated in first-line anthracycline-based chemotherapy trials. Multivariate analysis of these data indicated that the patients most likely to respond to chemotherapy are those without liver metastases ($P < .0001$), younger patients, individuals with high histologic grade, and those with liposarcoma. In this Cox model, the factors associated with superior survival were good performance status, absence of liver metastases, low histologic grade, a long time to metastasis after treatment of the primary tumor, and young age.

More recently, these same investigators have reported that the observed response rate is superior in patients who have pulmonary metastases only, as compared with those who have metastases to the lungs and other sites or to other sites only. These findings highlight the danger of reaching broad conclusions based on extrapolations from small trials that include highly selected patients. The EORTC data are also consistent with the observation that patients with metastatic GI sarcoma rarely respond to standard chemotherapy regimens. This increasingly recognized observation has been used to explain the low response rates seen in some trials.

Targeted therapy for GISTs

Advances in our understanding of the biology of GIST, and the availability of an effective therapy for patients with advanced disease, have resulted in intense interest in this entity and rapid expansion of diagnosis of this disease. Because this entity had not been recognized, the incidence of GIST was underappreciated. GIST is the most common nonepithelial tumor of the GI tract, with an estimated annual incidence of 3,000 to 3,500 cases in the United States. Approximately 50% to 60% of GISTs arise in the stomach, and 25% in the small bowel. Other sites include the rest of the GI tract, the omentum, mesentery, and retroperitoneum. These tumors may range in size from millimeters to huge masses. It is not clear how many of these GISTs become clinically relevant and how many are noted anecdotally at the time of endoscopic ultrasonography or other abdominal procedures.

The demonstration of the efficacy of imatinib in GIST has been among the most dramatic and exciting observations in solid-tumor oncology. A randomized multicenter trial evaluated two doses of oral imatinib (400 vs 600 mg) in 147 patients with advanced GISTs. With a median follow-up of 288 days, 54% had a partial response, and 28% had stable disease, but there were no complete responses. Response was sustained, with a median duration exceeding 6 months. Most patients had mild grade 1 or 2 toxicity, but only 21% had severe grade 3 or 4 toxicity. GI or intra-abdominal hemorrhage occurred in 5% of patients. There was no difference in response or toxicity between the two doses.

These observations were expanded in two parallel, multi-institution trials in which patients with GISTs were randomized to receive imatinib (400 or 800 mg daily). The results were remarkably similar. In the American trial, among 746 registered patients, the overall response rate was 43% for patients treated with 400 mg and 41% for those treated with 800 mg. There were no differences in survival between the two arms. At 2 years, progression-free and overall survival rates in the 400-mg arm were 50% and 78%, respectively. In the 800-mg arm, the rate of progression-free survival at 2 years was 53%, and the rate of overall survival was 73%.

In a large European trial, 946 patients were randomized to receive imatinib (400 mg daily or twice a day). Among the 615 patients whose response could be evaluated, there was no difference in response frequency (43%) or survival between the two arms. Complete responses were seen in 3% and 2% of the lower-dose and higher-dose patients, respectively. Sixty-nine percent of patients whose disease was progressing on 400 mg of imatinib were allowed to cross over to the higher dose (800 mg). Further therapeutic activity was seen, with 26% of these patients free of disease progression at 1 year.

Based on these results, the EORTC, in conjunction with the ISG and the AGG, has reported its results to further identify factors predicting early and late resistance to imatinib in patients with GIST. Initial resistance was defined as disease progression within 3 months of randomization, and late resistance was disease progression beyond 3 months. Initial resistance was noted in 116 of 934 patients (12%). Low hemoglobin level, high granulocyte count, and the presence of lung and the absence of liver metastases were independent predictors of initial resistance. Late resistance occurred in 347 of 818 patients. Independent predictors were high baseline granulocyte count, primary tumor outside the stomach, large tumor size, and low initial imatinib dose. The impact of the dose on late resistance was significant in patients with high baseline granulocyte counts and in patients with GI tumors originating outside the stomach and small intestine.

Among a group of 127 patients with advanced GISTs, activating mutations of *KIT* or *PDGFRA* were identified in 87.4% and 3.9% of patients, respectively. In patients harboring an exon 11 mutation of *KIT*, the partial remission rate was 83.5%, whereas in patients without a discernible mutation in *KIT* or *PDGFRA*, the partial remission rate was 9.1%. The presence of an exon 11 mutation in *KIT* correlated with clinical response, decreased risk of treatment failure, and improved overall survival.

The National Comprehensive Cancer Network (NCCN) has established a GIST Task Force to develop guidelines for the evaluation and treatment of patients with GIST. This group recommended 400 mg daily as the initial starting dose of imatinib. Dose escalation should be considered in patients who do not respond initially or who demonstrate unequivocal disease progression. Surgery remains the primary modality for treatment of primary GIST, but adjuvant and neoadjuvant trials are ongoing.

The efficacy, dose, and duration of imatinib therapy in these settings have not been established, so participation of patients in such trials should be encouraged.

Recent data indicate that sunitinib is an active agent in imatinib-refractory GIST. In both phase I/II and III studies, the response rate is on the order of 10%, with a greater than 60% chance of these patients remaining on treatment for 6 months or longer. Notably, the patients that showed the most benefit were those with the converse *KIT* genetic phenotype (exon 9 mutation or wild type *KIT*) to those who were sensitive to imatinib (exon 11 mutation). Nonetheless, imatinib remains the first line of therapy regardless of mutation type, because there is still a response rate seen for imatinib in patients with wild-type or exon 9 *KIT* mutations and because imatinib is less toxic than sunitinib in its present schedule (4 weeks on at 50 mg oral daily, 2 weeks off). Some studies are examining new schedules of sunitinib (eg, 37.5 mg oral daily continuously), whereas other studies are evaluating the benefit of other small-molecule inhibitors of *KIT*. Newer tyrosine kinase inhibitors such as sorafenib may have some activity in the imatinib- and sunitinib-refractory settings. A phase III study of Hsp90 (heat shock protein 90) inhibitor vs placebo for kinase inhibitor-resistant GIST was closed due to deaths observed on study.

The FSG has initiated a phase III randomized trial looking at intermittent vs continuous imatinib therapy after completion of 1 year of continuous imatinib therapy. A total of 159 patients have enrolled in the trial. A partial or complete response was achieved in 52% of patients. Twenty-three patients were randomized to join the intermittent arm, and 23 the continuous arm. After 3 months, five patients (21%) in the intermittent arm had evidence of disease progression, vs no patients in the continuous arm. Reintroduction of imatinib resulted in tumor control in all patients.

Assessment of response and treatment after disease progression on imatinib

The use of standard (RECIST) response criteria in patients with GIST may be misleading. On CT or MR imaging, large tumor masses may become completely necrotic without a reduction in size for months in spite of dramatic clinical improvement. Indeed, such masses may actually increase. ^{18}F-FDG (^{18}F-fluorodeoxyglucose)–PET imaging may be extremely useful in selected patients, because response may be seen as early as 24 hours after a dose of imatinib. It should be noted that the survival of patients with stable disease parallels that of patients with major objective responses using RECIST criteria.

Surgery does not cure GIST that recurs after resection of primary disease and should be managed as metastatic disease. However, multimodality therapy should be considered in patients with limited sites of disease. It has also been recognized that patients with disease progression in limited sites of disease, occasionally with a growing nodule within a previously necrotic metastasis, may experience rapid disease progression of previously controlled areas. Thus, imatinib should be continued indefinitely in such patients, who should be referred for investigational therapy.

FDA-approved therapy for metastatic disease includes imatinib in first-line and sunitinib in second-line. If there is disease progression on second-line sunitinib, patients may be able to receive another kinase inhibitor such as sorafenib or nilotinib (Tasigna), but neither drug is FDA approved for GIST. The results of the ACOSOG phase III study of adjuvant imatinib for 48 weeks vs placebo have been reported. The study examined patients with any GIST of at least 3 cm in maximum dimension. Dematteo et al indicated that there was only a 3% chance of disease progression after the 48 weeks of therapy, in comparison to 17% in those who underwent surgery alone. However, there was a decay in the progression-free survival curve after approximately 2 to 2.5 years of therapy back toward that of the untreated patients. Furthermore, overall survival was no different between the two study arms, although median survival was only 15 months at the time of the report. These data indicate that although imatinib is a good salvage strategy for patients with recurrent GIST, it cannot be considered a new standard of care, given the lack of overall survival benefit noted with evidence of disease progression after therapy is complete. Thus, longer exposure to imatinib may be necessary; this is the subject of two studies in Europe (0 vs 2 years of imatinib, 1 vs 3 years of imatinib) and future studies by ACOSOG. Greater follow up in the potential use of adjuvant imatinib based on mutation status has been reported in preliminary form at ASCO 2010. In the presentation by Corless et al (Proc ASCO 2010, 28: abstract 10006), there was no improvement in overall survival with adjuvant imatinib, since relapsing patients so frequently responded to imatinib in the metastatic setting. Furthermore, there were certain mutational subtypes in which it was clear that 400 mg oral daily for 48 weeks did not improve progression-free survival over placebo, including patients with exon 9 mutations in *KIT*, so-called wild type GIST, and those patients with *PDGFRA* mutation D842V.

Thus, if adjuvant therapy is to be given, patients with the more common exon 11 *KIT* mutations (or the rare *PDGFRA* mutant non-D842V) could be considered for therapy. It is not clear if longer exposure (eg, the 2 or 3 years' experimental arm of two European clinical trials) will demonstrate improved overall survival, the ultimate proof of the utility of adjuvant therapy.

If relapse-free survival is improved several years after the completion of therapy, one could deduce that this reflects a higher cure rate for patients, even without a presently demonstrable overall survival advantage. The cost of saving even one life with adjuvant remains unknown, however, given the ability to salvage nearly all recurring patients with imatinib in the metastatic setting—understanding that systemic therapy for recurrent metastatic disease is lifelong. Greater follow-up is needed to make definitive conclusions about this important topic.

Recommendations for the treatment of metastatic sarcoma

- For patients with rapidly progressive disease or with symptoms, combination chemotherapy with an anthracycline/ifosfamide combination is indicated. For most patients, however, sequential single-agent therapy is less toxic and not inferior in terms of survival.
- The management of metastatic GIST involves imatinib as first-line therapy, and increasing doses of imatinib, when feasible, before changing to sunitinib. Some patients can be maintained with good responses to imatinib for more than 5 years.
- Schedules other than the 50 mg oral daily dose of sunitinib (4 weeks on, 2 off) can be considered in an attempt to minimize the drug's toxicity (eg, 25 to 37.5 mg oral daily without interruption).

- Surgery is increasingly being performed at the time of best response (typically 6 to 9 months) and at the time of limited disease progression. There are no data that indicate that early surgery (at the time of best response) leads to superior survival than later surgery (at the time of limited disease progression). Surgery should generally be avoided in patients with multifocal progressive disease; a change in medical therapy is appropriate in this setting.
- The importance of histology relevant to selection of therapy is increasingly being appreciated. It is especially significant to distinguish GISTs from GI leiomyosarcomas. Patients with GIST that is progressive on standard therapy should be referred to subspecialty centers experienced in the multimodality management of this disease. Data regarding kinase-targeted agents will likely lead to the use of such agents for a limited number of rare sarcoma subtypes.
- Periods of watchful waiting may be appropriate for many patients with metastatic sarcoma who have no or only minimal symptoms.

SUGGESTED READING

Blay JY, Le Cesne A, Ray-Coquard I, et al: Prospective multicentric randomized phase III study of imatinib in patients with advanced gastrointestinal stromal tumors comparing interruption versus continuation of treatment beyond 1 year: The French Sarcoma Group. J Clin Oncol 25:1107–1113, 2007.

Cherix S, Speiser M, Matter M, et al: Isolated limb perfusion with tumor necrosis factor and melphalan for non-resectable soft tissue sarcomas: Long-term results on efficacy and limb salvage in a selected group of patients. J Surg Oncol 98:148–155, 2008.

Choi H, Charnsangavej C, Faria SC, et al: Correlation of computed tomography and positron emission tomography in patients with metastatic gastrointestinal stromal tumor treated at a single institution with imatinib mesylate: Proposal of new computed tomography response criteria. J Clin Oncol 25:1753–1759, 2007.

Chugh R, Wathen JK, Maki RG, et al: Phase II multicenter trial of imatinib in 10 histologic subtypes of sarcoma using a bayesian hierarchical statistical model. J Clin Oncol 27:3148–3153, 2009.

Corless CL, Fletcher JA, Heinrich MC, et al: Biology of gastrointestinal stromal tumors. J Clin Oncol 22:3813–3825, 2004.

Cormier JN, Huang X, Xing Y, et al: Cohort analysis of patients with localized, high-risk, extremity soft tissue sarcoma treated at two cancer centers: Chemotherapy-associated outcomes. J Clin Oncol 22:4567–4574, 2004.

Davis A, O'Sullivan B, Turcotte R, et al: Late radiation morbidity following randomization to preoperative versus postoperative radiotherapy in extremity soft tissue sarcoma. Radiother Oncol 75:48-53, 2005.

DeLaney TF, Spiro IJ, Suit HD, et al: Neoadjuvant chemotherapy and radiotherapy for large extremity soft-tissue sarcomas. Int J Radiat Oncol Biol Phys 56:1117–1127, 2003.

Demetri GD, van Oosterom AT, Garrett CR, et al: Efficacy and safety of sunitinib in patients with advanced gastrointestinal stromal tumour after failure of imatinib: A randomised controlled trial. Lancet 368:1329–1338, 2006.

Dileo P, Morgan JA, Zahrieh D, et al: Gemcitabine and vinorelbine combination chemotherapy for patients with advanced soft tissue sarcomas: Results of a phase II trial. Cancer 109:1863–1869, 2007.

Eggermont AM, Schraffordt Koops H, Klausner JM, et al: Isolated limb perfusion with tumor necrosis factor and melphalan for limb salvage in 186 patients with locally advanced soft tissue extremity sarcomas: The cumulative multicenter European experience. Ann Surg 224:756–764, 1996.

Eilber FC, Eilber FR, Eckardt J, et al: The impact of chemotherapy on the survival of patients with high-grade primary extremity liposarcoma. Ann Surg 240:686–695, 2004.

Eilber FC, Rosen G, Nelson SD, et al: High-grade extremity soft-tissue sarcomas: Factors predictive of local recurrence and its effect on morbidity and mortality. Ann Surg 237:218–226, 2003.

Feng M, Murphy J, Griffith KA, et al: Long-term outcomes after radiotherapy for retroperitoneal and deep truncal sarcoma. Int J Radiat Oncol Biol Phys 69:103–110, 2007.

Ferrari A, Gronchi A, Casanova M, et al: Synovial sarcoma: A retrospective analysis of 271 patients of all ages treated at a single institution. Cancer 101:627–634, 2004.

Frustaci S, De Paoli A, Bidoli E, et al: Ifosfamide in the adjuvant therapy of soft tissue sarcomas. Oncology 65(suppl 2):80–84, 2003.

Heinrich MC, Corless CL, Blanke CD, et al: Molecular correlates of imatinib resistance in gastrointestinal stromal tumors. J Clin Oncol 24:4764–4774, 2006.

Heinrich MC, Maki RG, Corless CL, et al: Primary and secondary kinase genotypes correlate with the biological and clinical activity of sunitinib in imatinib-resistant gastrointestinal stromal tumor. J Clin Oncol 26:5352–5359, 2008.

Kraybill WG, Harris J, Spiro IJ, et al: Phase II study of neoadjuvant chemotherapy and radiation therapy in the management of high-risk, high-grade, soft tissue sarcomas of the extremities and body wall: Radiation Therapy Oncology Group Trial 9514.J Clin Oncol 24:619–625, 2006.

Le Cesne A, Blay JY, Judson I, et al: Phase II study of ET-743 in advanced soft tissue sarcomas: A European Organisation for the Research and Treatment of Cancer (EORTC) soft tissue and bone sarcoma group trial. J Clin Oncol 23:576–584, 2005.

Maki RG, D'Adamo DR, Keohan ML, et al: Phase II study of sorafenib in patients with metastatic or recurrent sarcomas. J Clin Oncol 27:3133–3140, 2009.

O'Sullivan B, Bell RS, Bramwell VHC: Sarcomas of the soft tissues, in Souhami RL, Tannock I, Hohenberger P, et al (eds): Oxford Textbook of Oncology, 2nd ed, pp 2495–2523. Oxford, Oxford University Press, 2002.

O'Sullivan B, Davis AM, Turcotte R, et al: Preoperative versus postoperative radiotherapy in soft-tissue sarcoma of the limbs: A randomized trial. Lancet 359:2235–2241, 2002.

Pervaiz N, Colterjohn N, Farrokhyar F, et al: A systematic meta-analysis of randomized controlled trials of adjuvant chemotherapy for localized resectable soft-tissue sarcoma. Cancer 113:573–581, 2008.

Pisters PW, Patel SR, Prieto VG, et al: Phase I trial of preoperative doxorubicin-based concurrent chemoradiation and surgical resection for localized extremity and body wall soft tissue sarcomas. J Clin Oncol 22:3375–3380, 2004.

Pisters PW, Pollock RE, Lewis VO, et al: Long-term results of prospective trial of selective use of radiation for patients with T1 extremity and trunk soft tissue sarcomas. Ann Surg 246:675–682, 2007.

Riad S, Griffin AM, Liberman B, et al: Lymph node metastasis in soft tissue sarcoma in an extremity. Clin Orthop Sep:129–134, 2004.

Van den Abbeele AD, Badawi RD: Use of positron emission tomography in oncology and its potential role to assess response to imatinib mesylate therapy in gastrointestinal stromal tumors (GISTs). Eur J Cancer 38(suppl 5):S60–S65, 2002.

Verma S, Younus J, Stys-Norman D, et al: Meta-analysis of ifosfamide-based combination chemotherapy in advanced soft tissue sarcoma. Cancer Treat Rev 34:339–347, 2008.

Wendtner C-M, Abdel-Rahman S, Krych M, et al: Response to neoadjuvant chemotherapy combined with regional hyperthermia predicts long-term survival for adult patients with retroperitoneal and visceral high-risk soft-tissue sarcomas. J Clin Oncol 20:3156–3164, 2002.

Zalcberg JR, Verweij J, Casali PG, et al: Outcome of patients with advanced gastro-intestinal stromal tumours crossing over to a daily imatinib dose of 800 mg after progression on 400 mg. Eur J Cancer 41:1751–1757, 2005.

Abbreviations in this chapter

ACOSOG = American College of Surgeons Oncology Group; AGG = Australasian Gastrointestinal Group; AJCC = American Joint Committee on Cancer; EORTC = European Organization for Research on the Treatment of Cancer; FFCCSG = French Federation of Cancer Centers Sarcoma Group; FSG = French Sarcoma Group; ISG = Italian Sarcoma Group; RDOG = Radiation Diagnostic Oncology Group; RTOG = Radiation Therapy Oncology Group; SMAC = Sarcoma Meta-Analysis Collaboration; SSG = Scandinavian Sarcoma Group; SWOG = Southwest Oncology Group; UICC = International Union Against Cancer

CHAPTER 23

Primary and metastatic brain tumors

Lisa M. DeAngelis, MD, Jay S. Loeffler, MD, John de Groot, MD, and Nicole Shonka, MD

Intracranial neoplasms can arise from any of the structures or cell types present in the cranial vault, including the brain, meninges, pituitary gland, skull, and even residual embryonic tissue. The overall annual incidence of primary brain tumors in the United States is 18.7 cases per 100,000 population.

The most common primary brain tumors are meningiomas, representing 30% of all primary brain tumors, and gliomas, representing 40% of all primary brain tumors; many of these tumors are clinically aggressive and high grade. Primary brain tumors are the most common of the solid tumors in children and the second most frequent cause of cancer death after leukemia in children.

Brain metastases occur in approximately 15% of cancer patients as a result of hematogeneous dissemination of systemic cancer, and the incidence may be rising due to better control of systemic disease. Lung and breast cancers are the most common solid tumors that metastasize to the central nervous system (CNS). Melanoma and testicular and renal carcinomas have the greatest propensity to metastasize to the brain, but their relative rarity explains the low incidence of these neoplasms in large series of patients with brain metastases. Patients with brain metastases from nonpulmonary primaries have a 70% incidence of lung metastases. Although many physicians presume that all brain metastases are multiple, in fact, half are single and many are potentially amenable to focal therapies.

EPIDEMIOLOGY

Gender There is a slight predominance of primary brain tumors in men.

Age Primary brain tumors have a bimodal distribution, with a small peak in the pediatric population and a steady increase in incidence with age, beginning at age 20 years and reaching a maximum of 20 cases per 100,000 population between the ages of 75 and 84 years.

ETIOLOGY AND RISK FACTORS

The cause of primary brain tumors is unknown, although genetic and environmental factors may contribute to their development.

Genetic factors Clear heritable factors play a minor role in the genesis of primary brain tumors; less than 5% of patients with glioma have a family history of brain tumor. Several inherited diseases, such as tuberous sclerosis, neurofibromatosis type I, Turcot syndrome, and Li-Fraumeni cancer syndrome, predispose patients to the development of gliomas. However, these tumors tend to occur in children or young adults and do not account for the majority of gliomas that appear in later life. A large genomic study identified five risk loci for glioma susceptibility: 5p15.33 (TERT), 8q24.21 (CCDC26), 9p21.3 (CDKN2A-CDKN2B), 20q13.33 (RTEL1), and 11q23.3 (PHLDB1).

Loss of heterozygosity (LOH) on chromosomes 9p and 10q and p16 deletions are frequently observed in high-grade gliomas, with low-grade gliomas having the fewest molecular abnormalities. In oligodendrogliomas, 1p and 19q LOH and IDH1 mutations are associated with significantly improved survival.

Molecular markers One of the most useful markers, the epigenetic silencing of the *MGMT* (O6-methylguanine-DNA methyltransferase) DNA-repair gene by promoter methylation, is an independent prognostic factor in patients with glioblastoma and has been associated with longer survival in patients who received the alkylating agent temozolomide (Temodar). Epidermal growth factor receptor (EGFR) amplification and overexpression are present in about 60% of glioblastomas. Molecular markers of brain tumors can predict survival and will become increasingly important in the diagnosis and treatment of glioma.

Environmental factors Prior cranial irradiation is the only well-established risk factor for intracranial neoplasms.

Lifestyle characteristics Brain tumors are not associated with lifestyle characteristics such as cigarette smoking, alcohol intake, or cellular phone use.

SIGNS AND SYMPTOMS

Brain tumors produce both nonspecific and specific signs and symptoms.

Nonspecific symptoms include headaches, which occur in about half of patients but are rarely an isolated finding of intracranial tumors, and nausea and vomiting, which are caused by an increase in intracranial pressure. Because of the widespread availability of CT and MRI, papilledema is now seen in < 10% of patients, even when symptoms of raised intracranial pressure are present.

Specific signs and symptoms are usually referable to the particular intracranial location of the tumor and are similar to the signs and symptoms of other intracranial space–occupying masses.

Mutations of the isocitrate dehydrogenase genes (*IDH1* and *IDH2*) are early glioma-initiating events and are seen in the majority of low-grade gliomas *(Yan H et al: N Engl J Med 360:765–773, 2009).*

Lateralizing signs, including hemiparesis, aphasia, and visual-field deficits, are present in ~50% of patients with primary and metastatic brain tumors.

Seizures are a common presenting symptom, occurring in ~25% of patients with high-grade gliomas, at least 50% of patients with low-grade tumors, and 50% of patients with metastases from melanoma, perhaps due to their hemorrhagic nature. Otherwise, seizures are the presenting symptom in 15% to 20% of patients with brain metastases. Seizures may be generalized, partial, or focal.

Stroke-like presentation Hemorrhage into a tumor may present like a stroke, although the accompanying headache and alteration of consciousness usually suggest an intracranial hemorrhage rather than an infarct. Hemorrhage is usually associated with high-grade gliomas, occurring in 5% to 8% of patients with glioblastoma. However, oligodendrogliomas have a propensity to bleed, and hemorrhage occurs in 7% to 14% of these low-grade neoplasms. Sudden visual loss and fatigue may be seen with bleeding into or infarction of pituitary tumors, termed *pituitary apoplexy*.

Several studies have identified glioblastoma subtypes based on gene expression profiles. Proneural, neural, classic, and mesenchymal subtypes were described. Proneural tumors were more likely to carry mutations of *IDH1* and *p53* and were associated with improved overall survival. Classic tumors frequently (95%) showed amplification of *EGFR*. Mesenchymal tumors were most likely to have mutations or deletions of *NF1*, several of which were comutated with *PTEN*. They also had higher activity of mesenchymal and astrocytic markers CD44 and MERTK, as well as high expression of *CHI3L* and *MET*, and had the shortest overall survival *(Verhaak RG et al: Cancer Cell 17:98–110, 2010)*.

Altered mental status Approximately 75% of patients with brain metastases, and as many as half of patients with malignant gliomas, have impairment of consciousness or cognitive function. Some patients with multiple bilateral brain metastases may present with an altered sensorium as the only manifestation of metastatic disease; this finding can be easily confused with metabolic encephalopathy.

SCREENING FOR METASTATIC BRAIN TUMORS

Screening for brain metastases is performed in only a few clinical situations.

Lung cancer Approximately 10% of patients with small-cell lung cancer (SCLC) have brain metastases at diagnosis, and an additional 20% to 25% develop such metastases during their illness. Therefore, cranial CT or MRI is performed as part of the initial evaluation for extent of disease.

Occasionally, patients with non–small-cell lung cancer (NSCLC) undergo routine cranial CT or MRI prior to definitive thoracotomy, because the presence of brain metastases may influence the choice of thoracic surgical procedure. This approach is particularly valuable in patients with suspected stage IIB or III disease for whom thoracotomy is considered following neoadjuvant therapy.

DIAGNOSIS

Radiographic appearance of primary lesions

MRI The diagnosis of a brain tumor is best made by cranial MRI. This should be the first test obtained in a patient with signs or symptoms suggestive of an intracranial mass. MRI is superior to CT and should always be obtained with and without contrast material such as gadolinium.

High-grade or malignant primary brain tumors appear as contrast-enhancing mass lesions that arise in white matter and are surrounded by edema (Figure 1). Multifocal malignant gliomas are seen in ~5% of patients.

Low-grade gliomas typically are nonenhancing lesions that diffusely infiltrate and tend to involve a large region of the brain. Low-grade gliomas are usually best appreciated on T2-weighted or fluid-attenuated inversion recovery (FLAIR) MRI scans (Figure 2). As many as 40% of nonenhancing tumors may harbor foci of high-grade glioma.

CT A contrast-enhanced CT scan may be used if MRI is unavailable or the patient cannot undergo MRI (eg, because of a pacemaker). CT is adequate to exclude brain metastases in most patients, but it can miss low-grade tumors or small lesions located in the posterior fossa. Tumor calcification is often better appreciated on CT than on MRI.

PET Body positron emission tomography (PET) scans performed for staging of systemic malignancies have a sensitivity of only 75% and a specificity of 83% for

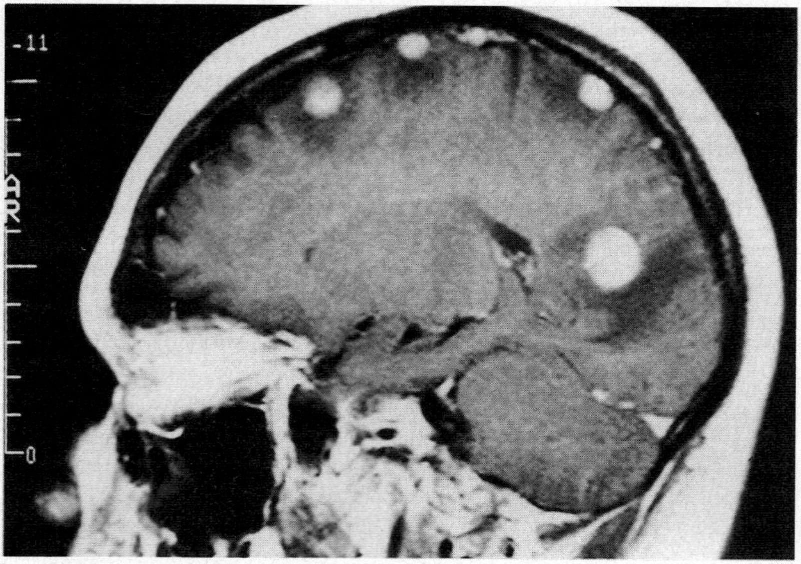

FIGURE 1: T1-weighted MRI with gadolinium contrast showing a typical appearance of a glioblastoma. Non–contrast-enhanced images of this lesion (not shown) revealed the presence of some hemorrhage.

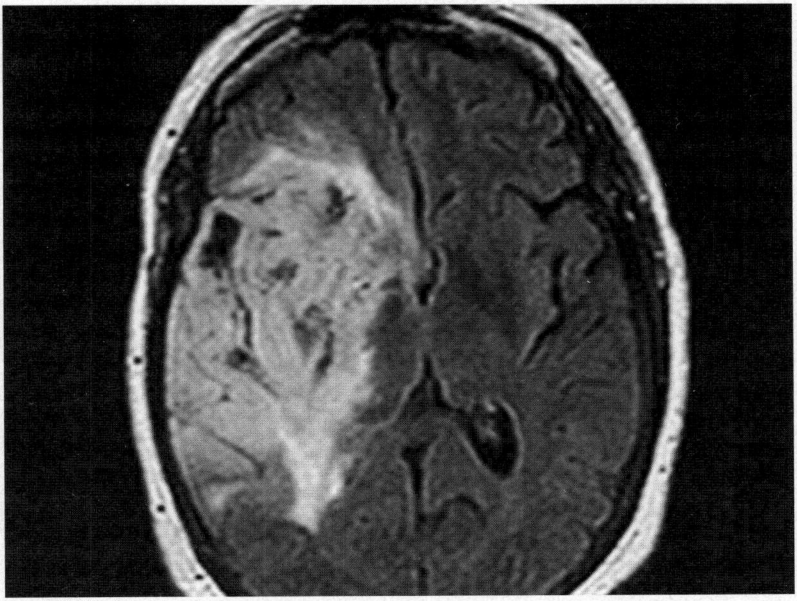

FIGURE 2: FLAIR MRI demonstrating a diffusely infiltrating, low-grade oligodendroglioma involving the right frontal and temporal lobes. This lesion did not enhance with gadolinium.

identification of cerebral metastases. Therefore, they are less accurate than MRI, which remains the gold standard.

Radiographic appearance of metastatic lesions On CT or MRI, most brain metastases are enhancing lesions surrounded by edema, which extends into the white matter (Figure 3). Unlike primary brain tumors, metastatic lesions rarely involve the corpus callosum or cross the midline.

The radiographic appearance of brain metastases is nonspecific and may mimic other processes, such as infection. Therefore, the CT or MRI scan must always be interpreted within the context of the clinical picture of the individual patient, particularly as cancer patients are vulnerable to opportunistic CNS infections or may develop second primaries, which can include primary brain tumors.

Other imaging tools Magnetic resonance spectroscopy (MRS) and perfusion imaging can help differentiate low-grade from high-grade brain tumors but cannot distinguish different tumor types of the same grade.

PATHOLOGY

Glial tumors arise from astrocytes, oligodendrocytes, or their precursors and exist along a spectrum of malignancy. The astrocytic tumors are graded, using the four-tier World Health Organization (WHO) system. Grade I tumors are localized

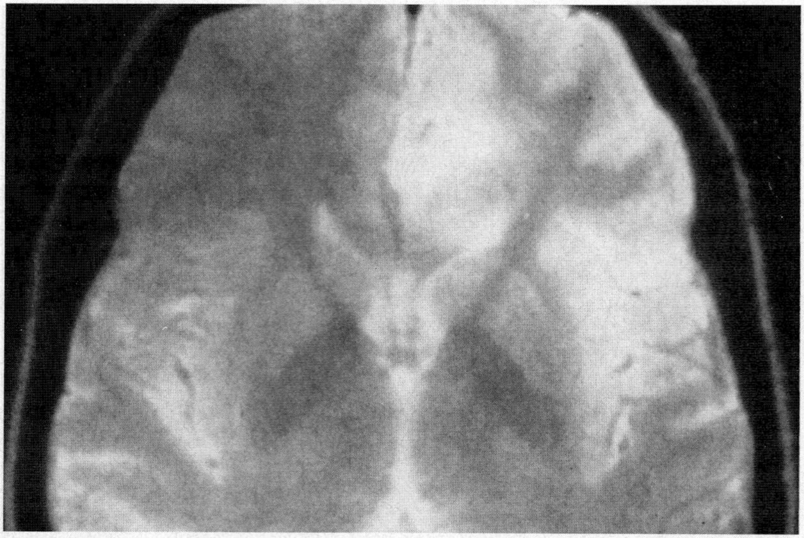

FIGURE 3: Gadolinium-enhanced MRI scan demonstrating multiple brain metastases. Note the edema surrounding each lesion.

tumors called pilocytic astrocytomas, which are usually found in children and may be associated with neurofibromatosis type I. Grade II tumors are low-grade diffuse fibrillary astrocytomas. Grade III (anaplastic astrocytoma) and IV (gliobastoma) tumors are high-grade malignant neoplasms. Grading is based on pathologic features, such as endothelial proliferation, cellular pleomorphism, mitoses, and necrosis. The oligodendroglial neoplasms are classified as either the low-grade oligodendroglioma (grade II) or the anaplastic oligodendroglioma (grade III).

Low-grade glial tumors (such as astrocytoma and oligodendroglioma) and mixed neuronal-glial tumors (such as ganglioglioma) grow slowly but have a propensity to transform into malignant neoplasms over time. Transformation is usually associated with progressive neurologic symptoms and the appearance of enhancement on MRI.

The high-grade gliomas include glioblastoma, gliosarcoma, anaplastic astrocytoma, and anaplastic oligodendroglioma. These tumors are extremely invasive, with tumor cells often found up to 4 cm away from the primary tumor.

Ependymomas Intracranial ependymomas are relatively rare, accounting for < 2% of all brain tumors. They are most frequently seen in the posterior fossa or spinal cord, although they may also arise in the supratentorial compartment. Ependymomas are typically low grade histologically, but their high rate of recurrence indicates malignant behavior.

Medulloblastomas are uncommon in adults but are one of the two most common primary brain tumors in children (the other being cerebellar astrocytomas). Medulloblastomas arise in the cerebellum and are always high-grade neoplasms.

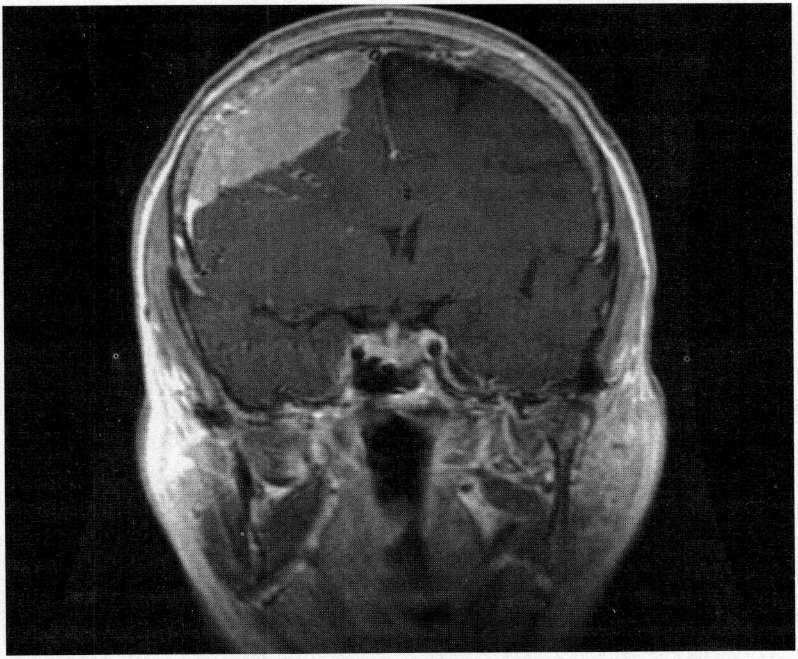

FIGURE 4: T1-weighted MRI with gadolinium contrast showing the typical appearance of a meningioma. Note the dural-based 'tail.'

Primitive neuroectodermal tumors (PNETs) are high-grade, aggressive tumors that usually occur in children. They include pineoblastoma and neuroblastoma. Histologically, they are identical to medulloblastomas, but their prognosis is usually worse than that for medulloblastomas. Thus, their biology is different, even though they may be similar pathologically.

Extra-axial tumors The most common extra-axial tumor is the meningioma. Meningiomas are usually benign tumors that arise from residual mesenchymal cells in the meninges. They produce neurologic symptoms by compressing the underlying brain. Meningiomas rarely are malignant or invade brain tissue (Figure 4).

Other common extra-axial tumors include pituitary adenoma, epidermoid or dermoid tumors, and acoustic neuroma (vestibular schwannoma). Most extra-axial tumors have a benign histology but can be locally invasive. Many extra-axial benign tumors are incidentally identified on MRI imaging performed for nonspecific symptoms such as headache. Most of these tumors do not require therapy and do not enlarge. Many benign extra-axial tumors identified in this way can be observed with serial imaging studies alone.

Metastatic brain tumors The pathology of metastatic brain lesions recapitulates the pathology of the underlying primary neoplasm. This feature often enables the pathologist to suggest the primary source in patients whose systemic cancer presents as brain metastasis. However, even after a complete systemic evaluation, the site of the primary tumor remains unknown in 5% to 13% of patients with brain metastases.

STAGING AND PROGNOSIS

Staging is not applicable to most primary brain tumors because they are locally invasive and do not spread to regional lymph nodes or distant organs. Staging with an enhanced complete spinal MRI and cerebrospinal fluid (CSF) evaluation is important for a few primary tumor types, such as medulloblastoma, ependymoma, and PNET, because they can disseminate via the CSF. All systemic cancers are stage IV when they present with brain metastasis.

Prognostic factors For patients with primary brain tumors, prognosis is inversely related to several important factors, including pathologic grade and patient age, and is directly related to the overall clinical condition at diagnosis. Several molecular markers that correlate well with prognosis have been identified recently, such as *IDH1* mutations and LOH on chromosomes 1p and 19q in anaplastic oligodendroglioma.

With conventional treatment, including surgical resection, radiotherapy, and chemotherapy, median survival is 3 years for patients with an anaplastic astrocytoma and 15 to 18 months for those with glioblastoma. In a population of patients with low-grade tumors, including astrocytoma and oligodendroglioma, median survival is 5 to 10 years; most of these individuals die of malignant transformation of their original tumor. Patients with low-grade oligodendroglioma can survive a median of 16 years in some series. Patients ≥ 40 years old with low-grade glioma generally have a more aggressive disease; their median survival is usually < 5 years.

For a large proportion of patients with brain metastases, median survival is only 4 to 6 months after whole-brain radiotherapy. However, some patients (ie, those who are < 60 years old, have a single lesion, or have controlled or controllable systemic disease) can achieve prolonged survival, and these individuals warrant a more aggressive therapeutic approach. Furthermore, most of these patients qualify for vigorous local therapy for their brain metastases, such as surgical resection or, stereotactic radiosurgery. These approaches can achieve a median survival of 40 weeks or longer, and rarely some patients are cured.

TREATMENT

Treatment of primary brain tumors and brain metastases consists of both supportive and definitive therapies.

SUPPORTIVE THERAPY

Supportive treatment focuses on relieving symptoms and improving the patient's neurologic function. The primary supportive agents are anticonvulsants and corticosteroids.

Anticonvulsants

Anticonvulsants are administered to the 25% of patients who have a seizure at presentation. Traditionally, phenytoin was the most commonly used medication, but carbamazepine and valproic acid are equally efficacious. Doses of all these anticonvulsants can be titrated to the appropriate serum levels to provide maximal protection.

Newer anticonvulsants, such as levetiracetam (Keppra), gabapentin, lamotrigine (Lamictal), and topiramate (Topamax), are preferred and have become the first choice in many patients. Most of these agents have the advantages of causing fewer cognitive side effects, and because they do not induce the hepatic microsomal system, they do not alter the metabolism of chemotherapeutic agents. Serum levels of these agents are less reliable than those of older drugs. These agents should replace the older drugs as first-line antiepileptic therapy in most patients.

Prophylaxis Prospective studies have failed to show the efficacy of prophylactic anticonvulsants for patients with brain tumors who have not had a seizure. Consequently, prophylactic anticonvulsants should not be administered, except during the perioperative period, when their use may reduce the incidence of postoperative seizures; the drugs can be tapered off within 2 weeks of surgery. Increasingly, the new agents are being used for prophylaxis.

Corticosteroids

Corticosteroids reduce peritumoral edema, diminishing mass effect and lowering intracranial pressure. This effect produces prompt relief of headache and improvement of lateralizing signs. Dexamethasone is the corticosteroid of choice because of its minimal mineralocorticoid activity. The starting dose is ~16 mg/d, but this dose is adjusted upward or downward to reach the minimum dose necessary to control neurologic symptoms. In patients whose MRI is suggestive of CNS lymphoma, urgent biopsy should precede the initiation of steroids.

Long-term corticosteroid use is associated with hypertension, diabetes mellitus, a nonketotic hyperosmolar state, myopathy, weight gain, insomnia, and osteoporosis. Thus, the steroid dose in patients with a brain tumor should be tapered as rapidly as possible once definitive treatment has begun. Most patients can stop taking steroids by the time they have completed cranial irradiation. All patients taking corticosteroids for more than 6 weeks should be on antibiotic prophylaxis for *Pneumocystis jiroveci* (formerly *carinii*) pneumonia. Prophylaxis should continue for 1 month after the steroids have been discontinued. This practice is without supporting evidence (as shown in a large Cochrane review), although it is routinely used.

DEFINITIVE THERAPY: PRIMARY BRAIN TUMORS

Definitive treatment of brain tumors includes surgery, radiation therapy, and chemotherapy. The first step is to devise an overall therapeutic plan that should outline the sequence and elements of multidisciplinary therapy.

Surgery

Various surgical options are available, and the surgical approach should be carefully chosen to maximize tumor resection while preserving vital brain structures and minimizing the risk of postoperative neurologic deficits. The goals of surgery include (1) obtaining an accurate histologic diagnosis; (2) reducing tumor burden and associated mass effect caused by the tumor and/or peritumoral edema; (3) maintaining or re-establishing pathways for CSF flow; (4) achieving a potential "cure" by gross total removal; and (5) reducing tumor burden prior to adjuvant irradiation or chemotherapy. Surgery for a primary brain tumor rarely achieves cure but can reduce tumor burden so that the tumor becomes more amenable to adjuvant irradiation or chemotherapy. In glioblastomas, resection of greater than 98% of tumor, as measured by postoperative MRI, is associated with improved survival. Similarly, improved survival has also been demonstrated for low-grade gliomas when gross total resection is achieved.

Surgical tools A variety of tools are available to help the neurosurgeon achieve these goals, including stereotactic and image-based guidance systems and electrophysiologic brain mapping.

Stereotactic frames provide a rigid, three-dimensional (3D) coordinate system for accurate targeting of brain lesions identified on CT or MRI scans and are particularly well suited for obtaining tissue for biopsy from tumors located in sites where aggressive tissue removal would produce unacceptable neurologic deficits. Limitations of stereotactic biopsy are that small volumes of tissue are obtained and that tissue sampling errors may result in a failure to reach a correct diagnosis. Stereotactic biopsy may be nondiagnostic in 3% to 8% of cases and has a surgical morbidity of approximately 5%.

Image-based guidance system "Frameless" or "image-guided" stereotactic systems use computer technology to coregister preoperative imaging studies with intraoperative head position, thereby establishing stereotactic accuracy without the need for a frame. These systems are useful for stereotactic biopsy or achieving maximal resections of predefined tumor volumes and minimizing surgical morbidity. Intraoperative MRI accomplishes similar goals but is limited by a requirement for specialized operating suites.

Intraoperative brain mapping, also termed cortical mapping, uses electrical stimulation of the cortical surface to define the primary motor, sensory, or speech cortex. By identifying the exact location of these areas prior to tumor resection, the surgeon can avoid these structures, thereby preserving neurologic function. These tools enable the neurosurgeon to perform more complete removal of tumors with less morbidity. Intraoperative MRI is being used in a number of centers to facilitate the complete removal of a tumor. Images are obtained before the operation is completed to assure removal of all visible tumor.

Pathology-based surgical approach for primary brain tumors The surgical approach to an intracranial lesion is strongly influenced by the suspected or previously confirmed pathology. Guidelines for the management of the most common tumors are discussed.

Meningiomas and other extra-axial tumors Benign extra-axial tumors, such as meningiomas, usually have a well-defined plane separating them from the surrounding brain parenchyma. In general, total extirpation can be achieved by open craniotomy, particularly when the tumor is located over the convexity. Firm attachment of the tumor to the dura, cranial nerves, vascular structures, or skull base may make this impossible. Subtotal resections that preserve neural or vascular structures while reducing mass effect are often favored for extensive skull base tumors.

The surgical management of other benign extra-axial tumors, such as acoustic neuroma, pineocytoma, choroid plexus papilloma, and pituitary adenoma, closely parallels that of meningiomas. Gross total resection is generally curative and should be attempted whenever safe.

Low-grade gliomas Gross total resection, whenever possible, is the goal of surgery for low-grade gliomas and mixed neuronal-glial tumors (eg, astrocytoma, oligodendroglioma, pilocytic astrocytoma, and ganglioglioma). Long-term survival is better in patients who have undergone gross total resection than in those who have had subtotal resection (5-year survival rates > 80% for gross total resection vs ~50% for subtotal resection).

If radiographically proven gross total resection is attained, postoperative irradiation or chemotherapy can often be withheld until there is evidence of tumor progression (see section on "Radiation therapy"). If a postoperative scan reveals a small but surgically accessible residual lesion, immediate reoperation should be considered, particularly in children or in those with pilocytic astrocytomas (WHO grade I).

When low-grade tumors are found in patients with medically refractory chronic epilepsy, surgical management should be oriented toward curing the epilepsy, as well as achieving total tumor removal.

Ependymomas Gross total resection is the goal of surgery whenever possible for ependymomas. Because ependymomas arise in the ventricular system, they can disseminate in the CSF. Therefore, all patients should be assessed for subarachnoid metastases with complete cranial and spinal MRI performed with gadolinium.

High-grade gliomas More extensive resections improve the quality of life and neurologic function of patients with high-grade gliomas (glioblastoma, anaplastic astrocytoma, and anaplastic oligodendroglioma) by reducing mass effect, edema, and steroid dependence. Resection of > 98% of the tumor volume prolongs survival relative to subtotal or partial resections, but extensive subtotal resections do not appear to confer any survival advantage over biopsy. For this reason, most neurosurgeons attempt to achieve maximal resection while minimizing the risk to critical areas of the brain.

Recurrent or progressive tumors When a brain tumor recurs or enlarges, reoperation is often necessary to reduce mass effect. Although rarely curative, these procedures can improve quality of life and modestly extend survival. In general, reoperation is not considered in patients with a Karnofsky performance status (KPS) score ≤ 60 or in those patients who are not candidates for additional therapy following surgery.

Pseudoprogression describes an increase in contrast enhancement independent of tumor growth in patients who have recently received radiation therapy. It occurs most frequently (58%) within the first 3 months following radiation therapy and is more commonly seen after concurrent chemoradiation therapy. It is estimated that up to 50% of patients with an increase in enhancement have true tumor progression. However, in practice, current treatment is usually continued for at least 3 months to avoid discontinuing an effective therapy. Pseudoprogression may represent a more robust response to therapy and may correlate with *MGMT* promoter methylation and a better therapeutic outcome. A recurrent tumor cannot be distinguished from radiation necrosis on routine MRI. Both disorders may cause severe mass effect and edema, and resection is the optimal treatment for both if the patient is symptomatic.

Occasionally, PET or MRS can distinguish tumor from treatment effect, but these imaging modalities are unreliable.

Initial resection or reoperation followed by intracavitary or intraparenchymal administration of chemotherapy, immunotherapy, or liquid I-125 radiotherapy (GliaSite) is being explored but is still investigational. Carmustine (BiCNU)-impregnated wafers (Gliadel) are the only form of intracavitary chemotherapy currently approved by the FDA for glioblastoma.

Radiation therapy

Radiation therapy plays a central role in the treatment of brain tumors in adults. It is the most effective nonsurgical therapy for patients with malignant gliomas and also has an important role in the treatment of patients with low-grade gliomas and metastatic brain tumors.

Whole-brain vs partial-brain irradiation Whole-brain irradiation is reserved for multifocal lesions, lesions with significant subependymal or leptomeningeal involvement, and metastatic brain tumors. For the majority of patients with unifocal disease, limited-field treatment results in less morbidity and appears to produce equal, albeit poor, overall survival.

Intensity-modulated radiotherapy (IMRT) is an advanced technique to deliver high-precision radiotherapy to a tumor. Treatment is planned using 3D CT images to design a dose that will conform to the 3D shape of the tumor. Using multiple beams, a uniform dose of RT is delivered to the whole tumor while sparing normal tissues.

Radiation therapy for low-grade gliomas Retrospective studies suggest a limited radiation dose response in low-grade gliomas. However, selection bias may play a role in these studies.

Several randomized studies addressed the question of optimal timing and dose of radiotherapy in patients with low-grade gliomas. An American intergroup randomized trial compared 50.4 vs 64.8 Gy of radiation in patients with low-grade glioma. An EORTC trial compared 45.0 vs 59.4 Gy of radiation in patients with low-grade astrocytoma. Both studies confirmed the superiority or equivalent efficacy of the lower radiation dose and less toxicity.

A second EORTC trial tested immediate vs delayed radiotherapy in individuals with low-grade glioma. Although immediate radiotherapy significantly improved 5-year progression-free survival, overall survival was identical in the two treatment arms. Furthermore, quality of life was better in patients whose radiotherapy was deferred until clinical or radiographic disease progression was evident.

Recommended treatment approach for low-grade astrocytomas The role of postoperative radiotherapy in the management of incompletely resected low-grade astrocytomas has not been firmly established. However, based on the available data, the following principles appear reasonable:

- Complete surgical resection of hemispheric astrocytomas should be attempted.
- If complete surgical resection has been attained, radiation therapy can be withheld until MRI or CT studies clearly indicate a recurrence that cannot be approached surgically.

- When complete surgical resection is not performed, postoperative irradiation may be recommended, depending upon the patients' clinical condition. Patients with controlled seizures and no neurologic deficit can be followed and radiation therapy deferred until clinical or radiographic disease progression occurs. Patients with progressive neurologic dysfunction, such as language or cognitive difficulties, require immediate therapy. Astrocytomas must be treated with radiotherapy, but oligodendrogliomas or mixed gliomas may benefit from chemotherapy as initial treatment (see later in this chapter).
- Radiation therapy should be delivered, using a megavoltage machine, in 1.7- to 2.0-Gy daily fractions, to a total dose of about 50 Gy. The treatment fields should include the primary tumor volume only, as defined by MRI, and should not encompass the whole brain.
- In low-grade astrocytomas, radiation therapy can be expected to produce a 5-year survival rate of 50% and a 10-year survival rate of 20%. Patients with low-grade oligodendrogliomas survive even longer.
- Cognitive impairment may develop in long-term survivors of low-grade gliomas. This may be due to the disease itself, surgical resection, antiepileptic drug use, and radiotherapy if used.

Radiation therapy for high-grade gliomas An analysis of three studies of high-grade gliomas performed by the BTSG showed that postoperative radiotherapy doses > 50 Gy were significantly better in improving survival than no postoperative treatment and that 60 Gy resulted in significantly prolonged survival compared with 50 Gy. Doses greater than 60 Gy used in the American intergroup protocol resulted in competing morbidity.

Based on these data, involved-field radiotherapy to 60 Gy in 30 to 33 fractions is standard treatment for high-grade histologies; this amount corresponds to a dose just above the threshold for radionecrosis. About half of patients with anaplastic astrocytomas exhibit radiographic evidence of response following 60 Gy of radiation, compared with 25% of patients with glioblastoma. Complete radiographic response is rare in either case. Elderly patients with glioblastoma have a particularly poor prognosis, with a median survival of 4 to 6 months in most series. Some of these patients are not treated at all, but a randomized controlled study demonstrated that 50 Gy yields a significantly longer survival than supportive care alone (median of 29.1 weeks vs 16.9 weeks; $P = .002$) without compromising quality of life. Such an abbreviated course of radiotherapy should be considered in patients older than 70 years of age.

Alternatives to conventional radiotherapy

The results of standard radiation treatment in patients with malignant gliomas are poor. Patients with glioblastoma have a median survival of 12 to 15 months, whereas patients with anaplastic astrocytomas survive a median of 3 years. To improve these poor results, a number of new approaches have been tried, including hyperfractionated radiotherapy (HFRT), focal dose escalation with interstitial brachytherapy, and radiosurgery, but none improved survival. Brachytherapy and HFRT have been abandoned.

Antiangiogenic therapy was found to be a highly effective treatment for radiation necrosis. All 5 of the 14 patients with radionecrosis initially randomized to receive bevacizumab (Avastin) and the 7 patients who crossed over from the placebo arm had significant radiographic response and clinical improvement *(Levin VA et al: Int J Radiat Oncol Biol Phys Apr 15, 2010 [E-pub ahead of print]).*

Radionecrosis Both brachytherapy and stereotactic radiosurgery can induce focal radionecrosis. This complication produces symptoms of mass effect in about 50% of patients with malignant glioma, requiring resection to remove the necrotic debris. Occasionally, treatment with corticosteroids can control the edema around the radionecrotic area, but often the patient becomes steroid-dependent, with all of the attendant complications of chronic steroid use. Radionecrosis can be a significant limitation of the focal radiotherapy techniques.

Recommended approach for extra-axial tumors Surgery alone is curative in the vast majority of patients with benign tumors. However, in certain subsets of patients, postoperative radiotherapy may control further growth of these lesions.

Pituitary adenomas For hormonally inactive pituitary adenomas that persist or recur after surgery, 45 to 50 Gy is delivered in 25 to 28 fractions to the radiographic boundaries of the tumor. For Cushing disease and acromegaly, higher doses are required for biochemical remission. Coronal-enhanced MRI is critical for treatment planning, because CT often does not visualize the skull base and the entire extent of disease.

The most common indications for radiotherapy are invasion of the cavernous sinus or the suprasellar space and incomplete resection of macroadenomas (> 1.5 cm). Most pituitary lesions do not grow following radiotherapy, and hormonally active tumors usually demonstrate a hormonal response, with a reduction in hormone hypersecretion in 1 to 3 years. Following radiation therapy, 20% to 50% of patients develop panhypopituitarism, requiring hormone replacement therapy. Other significant complications (ie, damage to the visual apparatus) are rare today.

Meningiomas are readily curable with complete surgical resection. However, base of skull lesions and lesions involving a patent venous sinus often cannot be resected completely. For some patients with these lesions, a course of postoperative radiotherapy is indicated. In general, 54 Gy is delivered in 30 fractions to the radiographic tumor region utilizing 3D treatment planning. Malignant meningiomas always require postoperative radiotherapy, even after gross total resection. Radiosurgery may also be useful in treating meningiomas, and doses of 13 to 18 Gy are associated with a high rate of control 10 years following therapy.

Acoustic neuroma has classically been considered a surgical disease. Following total resection, recurrence rates are < 5%. When only subtotal resection is possible, disease recurs in at least 60% of patients.

The benefit of adding temozolomide (Temodar) to radiotherapy in newly diagnosed glioblastoma persists throughout 5 years of follow-up *(Stupp R et al: Lancet Oncol 10:459–466, 2009).*

Radiosurgery has been used as an alternative to surgery for acoustic neuroma. Tumor control rates of > 80% at 20 years have been reported. For patients with useful hearing prior to radiosurgery, that function is preserved in < 50%. After radiosurgery, 10% of patients experience facial weakness, and 25% have trigeminal neuropathy. The risk of cranial neuropathies is related to the size of the lesion treated.

> The NOA-04 trial randomized patients with newly diagnosed anaplastic gliomas to receive either radiation (RT) followed by chemotherapy (randomized to either temozolomide [Temodar] or PCV) or chemotherapy followed by RT at the time of disease progression. Neither initial treatment selection nor chemotherapy type adversely affected progression-free survival, although time to disease progression after RT may be longer than after chemotherapy. In this study, *IDH1* mutations more strongly influenced survival than codeletion of 1p/19q or *MGMT* methylation *(Wick W et al: J Clin Oncol 27:5874–5880, 2009).*

Chemotherapy

Malignant gliomas Chemotherapy has a limited but measurable benefit in the treatment of patients with malignant gliomas, and temozolomide is the most active agent.

In a large phase III trial, patients with newly diagnosed glioblastoma were randomized to receive radiotherapy alone or radiotherapy with concurrently administered temozolomide followed by adjuvant temozolomide. A total of 573 patients were studied, and median survival was significantly prolonged from 12.1 months to 14.6 months with the addition of temozolomide to radiotherapy. The 2-year survival rate was only 10% in those treated with radiotherapy alone compared with 27% in those who received radiotherapy plus temozolomide. The combined-modality regimen was well tolerated and associated with minimal additional toxicity. This regimen has now become the standard for all newly diagnosed patients with glioblastoma and combines the potential radiosensitizing effect of concurrent temozolomide with the benefit of adjuvant chemotherapy.

This study demonstrates clear benefit in patients with glioblastoma, and many investigators have extrapolated this regimen for use in patients with gliomas of all grades. Current practice varies from treating anaplastic astrocytoma with radiation therapy alone, to sequential radiotherapy and chemotherapy, to concurrent chemoradiation therapy. Two ongoing phase III trials are addressing this question.

Studies designed to improve upon the standard of care for newly diagnosed glioblastoma add another agent to chemoradiation therapy with temozolomide. Based on data that the glutaminergic system plays a role in glioblastoma cell proliferation and migration, talampanel, an alpha-amino-3-hydroxy-5-methyl-4-isoxazolepropionic acid (AMPA) receptor blocker, was given in addition to standard radiation and temozolomide. Median survival was 18.3 months, and those younger than 71 years had a median survival of 20.3 months. This finding compares favorably with a median survival in the EORTC study of radiation therapy and temozolomide of 14.6 months, despite having fewer patients on study with methylated *MGMT*.

Despite initial treatment, all malignant gliomas eventually recur. At relapse, patients may benefit from re-resection or different chemotherapeutic agents such as procarbazine or lomustine (CeeNU). However, re-challenging with temozolomide at higher doses and using an alternate schedule may improve outcome. Patients with progressive grade III or IV glioma after standard temozolomide (150 to 200 mg/m² days 1–5) were given metronomic temozolomide at 50 mg/m² daily for up to 1 year or until disease progression. Six-month progression-free survival was 24%,

Patients with newly diagnosed glioblastoma were given standard chemoradiation with temozolomide (Temodar) and were then randomized to receive 6 cycles of dose-dense (150 mg/m² on days 1–7 and 15–21) or metronomic (50 mg/m² daily) temozolomide. This regimen was followed by maintenance cis-retinoic acid. Median overall survival was 17.1 months, with an 80% 1-year survival in the dose-dense group, compared with 15.1 months and 69%, respectively, in the metronomic arm *(Clarke JL et al: J Clin Oncol 27:3861–3867, 2009).*

and 1-year survival was 27% for glioblastoma and 36% and 61%, respectively, for anaplastic glioma. Those deriving the greatest benefit from temozolomide re-challenge were patients whose disease progressed in the first 6 months of therapy and those whose disease progressed after initial treatment discontinuation.

Molecularly targeted agents have been a major focus of glioblastoma treatment in recent years. Randomized phase II trials have generated attention for their ability to expedite clinical testing of new agents. Unfortunately, targeted therapy has not been shown to be effective as single-agent therapy.

Cilengitide, an integrin receptor inhibitor, was given in a randomized phase II trial to patients with recurrent glioblastoma. Those receiving a dose of 2,000 mg twice weekly had an overall survival of 9.9 months. In another randomized phase II trial, patients with progressive glioblastoma were given either erlotinib (Tarceva) or cytotoxic chemotherapy with temozolomide or carmustine. Erlotinib compared unfavorably, with progression-free survival at 6 months of only 11% vs 24% in the control group. EGFRvIII mutation did not correlate with efficacy.

Recently, a phase III trial randomized patients to receive enzastaurin, a PKC-beta inhibitor, or lomustine for progressive glioblastoma. The 6-month progression-free survival rate was 11% for enzastaurin and 19% for lomustine.

Targeting anigogenesis has proven to be an effective approach to prolong progression-free survival at recurrence. Bevacizumab (Avastin), a monoclonal antibody that targets vascular endothelial growth factor (VEGF), recently received accelerated FDA approval for recurrent glioblastoma based on two studies. In the one study, patients with recurrent glioblastoma were given either bevacizumab alone or with irinotecan. Six-month progression-free and overall survival rates were 43% and 9.2 months, respectively, in the bevacizumab-alone group and 50% and 8.7 months in the combination group. Although bevacizumab frequently is combined with irinotecan, it is not clear how much benefit chemotherapy adds to bevacizumab alone. AZD2171 (cediranib), a VEGF receptor inhibitor, demonstrated a high radiographic response rate and was shown to normalize tumor vessels in recurrent glioblastoma patients and is undergoing further study.

Disease progression after vascular targeted agents may occur at the primary tumor site or a distant site in the brain. It may have an atypical imaging pattern with diffuse infiltration that is nonenhancing and seen only on MRI FLAIR sequences or more recently described on diffusion-weighted sequences. There has been no increase in intratumoral hemorrhage with the antiangiogenic agents, which makes them safe for use in patients with malignant gliomas. Hydroxyurea and imatinib (Gleevec) may also provide antitumor activity in some patients at recurrence. Current studies are using multitargeted approaches to enhance efficacy.

Astrocytomas Chemotherapy has no role in the initial treatment of low-grade astrocytomas, and often they have progressed to malignant tumors at the time of recurrence.

Oligodendroglioma In contrast, the oligodendroglioma is now recognized as a particularly chemosensitive primary brain tumor. This finding was first observed with the anaplastic oligodendroglioma but has recently been seen with the more common low-grade oligodendroglioma. Chemosensitivity of anaplastic and low-grade tumors is associated with loss of chromosomes 1p and 19q.

Several alkylating agents are active, but the best studied regimen is procarbazine (Matulane), lomustine, and vincristine (PCV), which produces response rates of 75% and 90% in malignant and low-grade oligodendrogliomas, respectively. However, two randomized controlled studies of newly diagnosed patients with anaplastic oligodendroglioma showed a significant delay in progression-free survival with the addition of PCV to radiotherapy but no prolongation of overall survival. PCV is an active regimen but has largely been supplanted by temozolomide because of the significant myelosuppression, neuropathy, and asthenia associated with PCV. Consequently, chemotherapy is an important therapeutic modality and may be used as initial treatment in patients with low-grade tumors who require therapeutic intervention. This approach defers or eliminates the late cognitive toxicity associated with cranial irradiation in patients with low-grade tumors who can have relatively prolonged survival. Patients with malignant oligodendrogliomas require radiotherapy with or without chemotherapy for initial treatment.

DEFINITIVE THERAPY: BRAIN METASTASES

Surgery

Surgical approach for metastatic tumors Most patients with brain metastases have a life expectancy of < 6 months, but the majority who undergo resection of a metastatic lesion followed by irradiation will die of systemic rather than intracranial disease.

Excision of metastatic brain tumors is rarely curative, however, as microscopic cells may be left behind. Nevertheless, the reduced tumor burden becomes more amenable to adjuvant irradiation and/or chemotherapy.

Criteria The decision whether to recommend surgery for metastatic brain tumors should be based on the following factors:

Extracranial oncologic status A comprehensive workup of the patient's extracranial oncologic status is necessary. Extensive critical organ metastases preclude surgery in favor of palliative irradiation as the sole therapy. Brain surgery should not be performed in patients with limited expected survival (3 to 6 weeks) based on extracranial disease.

Number of metastases In general, only patients harboring a single metastasis are considered for resection. Occasionally, a large tumor will be removed in the presence of multiple smaller nodules if the edema and mass effect of this lesion are causing a substantial neurologic deficit that could be improved by tumor removal.

If brain metastasis is the presenting sign of systemic cancer and no clear primary source can be identified with routine staging, surgery may be required to establish a tissue diagnosis and plan further therapy.

In addition, surgical removal of a brain metastasis often reverses the neurologic deficits caused by compression of local structures by the tumor and reduces intracranial hypertension. After complete excision of a single brain metastasis, postoperative whole-brain radiotherapy improves control of neurologic disease but does not prolong survival.

Three studies have concluded that when multiple (up to three distinct locations) metastases are resected, either with or without radiotherapy, survival times are identical to those in patients with a surgically resected single metastasis and almost twice as long as those in patients treated by radiation therapy or radiosurgery alone. These studies suggest that a more aggressive surgical approach may be justified in patients with multiple brain metastases who have stable systemic disease.

Recurrence of solitary metastases Up to 20% of single metastases may recur in long-term survivors. In these cases, a second operation may be warranted to remove the recurrent lesion and confirm the histologic diagnosis (ie, exclude radionecrosis).

Radiotherapy

Radiation therapy for metastatic brain tumors For symptomatic patients with brain metastases, median survival is about 1 month if untreated and 3 to 6 months if whole-brain radiation therapy is delivered, with no significant differences among various conventional radiotherapy fractionation schemes (20 Gy in 5 fractions, 30 Gy in 10 fractions, 40 Gy in 20 fractions). A more protracted schedule is used for patients who have limited or no evidence of systemic disease or for those who have undergone resection of a single brain metastasis, as these patients have the potential for long-term survival or even cure. The use of hypofractionated regimens is associated with an increased risk of neurologic toxicity.

The addition of the radiosensitizer motexafin gadolinium to whole-brain radiotherapy did not improve survival or time to neurologic disease progression in a randomized phase III trial. Subgroup analysis suggested a prolonged time to neurocognitive disease progression in patients with brain metastases from lung cancer. A new study has confirmed these findings.

Relief of neurologic symptoms The major result of whole-brain radiation therapy is an improvement in neurologic symptoms, such as headache, motor loss, and impaired mentation. The overall response rate ranges from 70% to 90%. Unfortunately, symptomatic relief is not permanent, and symptoms recur with intracranial tumor progression.

Multiple lesions Patients with multiple lesions are generally treated with whole-brain radiation therapy alone. Retreatment with a second course of whole-brain radiation therapy can provide further palliation for patients with progressive brain metastases (who have at least a 6-month or longer remission of symptoms after the initial course of cranial irradiation).

Concomitant steroid therapy Because the radiographic and clinical responses to whole-brain irradiation take several weeks, patients with significant mass effect should be treated with steroids during whole-brain radiation therapy. Dexamethasone (16 mg/d) is started prior to therapy, and the dose may be tapered as tolerated during treatment. Occasionally, higher doses are necessary to ameliorate neurologic symptoms. However, most patients can be safely tapered off corticosteroids at the completion of whole-brain radiotherapy.

Radiosurgery for metastatic brain tumors

In patients with one to three brain metastases, aggressive local therapy (surgical resection or radiosurgery) produces superior survival and quality of life compared with whole-brain radiation therapy alone. Radiosurgery may be the optimal choice for elderly patients at greater risk for surgical morbidity. Radiosurgery has been used as sole therapy, as a boost to whole-brain radiation therapy, or for recurrent lesions in patients with brain metastases. Radiosurgery has the advantage of delivering effective focal treatment, usually in a single dose, without irradiating the normal brain. Radiosurgery of brain metastases < 1 cm achieves 1- and 2-year local tumor control rates of 86% and 78%, respectively, significantly better than 56% and 24% for lesions > 1 cm. It is particularly useful for patients who have one to three lesions, each < 4 cm in diameter. Patients with numerous lesions are not good candidates for radiosurgery because some of the ports may overlap, and, more importantly, these patients likely harbor other microscopic lesions in the brain that are not being treated effectively with such focal therapy.

Brain metastases are particularly amenable to treatment with radiosurgery. Metastatic tumors do not infiltrate the brain and tend to have well-circumscribed borders; therefore, they can be targeted effectively with highly focused irradiation techniques that maintain a sharp delineation between the enhancing tumor seen on neuroimaging and normal brain. Furthermore, radiosurgery does not have the operative morbidity that may be associated with resection of a brain metastasis. Consequently, it can be used safely in many patients who are not surgical candidates, and it can even treat lesions in surgically unapproachable locations such as the brainstem.

Radiosurgery can achieve crude local tumor control rates of 73% to 98% over a median follow-up of 5 to 26 months. Radiosurgery was initially used as a boost after treatment with whole-brain radiotherapy. Three randomized trials have reported on the value of radiosurgery in addition to whole-brain radiotherapy for patients with multiple brain metastases. Although all three studies show a local tumor control advantage and an improvement in quality-of-life endpoints with the addition of a radiosurgical boost, none shows a statistical advantage in survival. For patients with multiple brain metastases, adding radiosurgery to whole-brain radiotherapy only offers an improved neurologic quality of life with no impact on survival.

Motexafin gadolinium combined with prompt whole-brain radiotherapy (WBRT) prolonged neurologic disease progression and neurocognitive decline compared with WBRT alone in patients with brain metastases from non–small-cell lung cancer ***(Mehta MP et al: Int J Radiat Oncol Biol Phys 73:1069–1076, 2009)*****.**

A prospective, randomized RTOG trial compared whole-brain radiotherapy alone vs whole-brain radiotherapy plus radiosurgery in patients with one to three metastases. Although there was no statistical improvement in overall survival in the two arms of the trial, a subset analysis showed improved survival for those patients with a single lesion. Local tumor control, neurologic function, and steroid doses were improved in patients with a single lesion treated with radiosurgery.

Radiosurgery is often considered an alternative to standard surgical resection, but it is unclear whether they are equivalent. Most retrospective studies suggest that the two techniques produce similar results; however, some reports indicate that surgery offers improved local tumor control, whereas others suggest that radiosurgery is superior.

Increasingly, radiosurgery is being used as the sole therapy for one to three brain metastases. A prospective randomized trial compared radiosurgery with or without whole-brain radiotherapy in patients with one to four brain metastases. Results were similar to those of the phase III trial of surgical resection of a single brain metastasis with or without radiotherapy: improved local tumor control but no survival benefit. Therefore, whole-brain radiotherapy reduced CNS relapse but had no impact on survival.

Median survival from the time of radiosurgery is 6 to 15 months, and some patients can live for years without recurrence. Most patients exhibit clinical improvement and decreased steroid requirement after radiosurgery, and only 11% to 25% of patients eventually die of neurologic causes.

Chemotherapy

Metastatic brain tumors Chemotherapy usually has a limited role in the treatment of brain metastases and has not proven to be effective as adjuvant therapy after irradiation or surgery. However, it may have some efficacy in patients with recurrent brain metastases who are not eligible for further whole-brain radiation therapy or stereotactic radiosurgery. In addition, chemotherapy has proven active in patients with asymptomatic brain metastases (discovered on screening neuroimaging) who are scheduled to receive chemotherapy for their systemic disease. We have seen patients with brain metastases from a variety of primary tumors respond in this situation. A recent phase III trial of chemotherapy with early vs delayed whole-brain radiotherapy in NSCLC patients with brain metastases showed an identical intracranial response rate and survival. Thus, systemic chemotherapy had some efficacy against brain metastases.

A recently completed phase II trial of temozolomide (75 $mg/m^2/d$) and concurrent whole-brain radiotherapy (40 Gy in 20 fractions) vs whole-brain radiotherapy alone demonstrated improved response rates and neurologic improvement in the combined-modality arm. In addition, there is growing recognition that systemic chemotherapy, including targeted agents, can be effective against brain metastases when the drugs are selected based on the primary tumor. Capecitabine (Xeloda) is effective against brain metastases from breast cancer. High-dose methotrexate has activity against a number of primaries. Temozolomide has activity against recurrent brain metastases, particularly from NSCLC and melanoma.

Erlotinib has efficacy against brain metastases from lung cancer with the appropriate EGFR mutations.

SUGGESTED READING

ON PRIMARY INTRACRANIAL TUMORS

Bauman G, Fisher B, Watling C, et al: Adult supratentorial low-grade glioma: Long-term experience at a single institution. Int J Radiat Oncol Biol Phys 75:1401–1407, 2009.

Brandes AA, Franceschi E, Tosoni A, et al: MGMT promoter methylation status can predict the incidence and outcome of pseudoprogression after concomitant radiochemotherapy in newly diagnosed glioblastoma patients. J Clin Oncol 26:2192–2197, 2008.

Correa DD, Shi W, Thaler HT, et al: Longitudinal cognitive follow-up in low grade gliomas. J Neurooncol 86:321–327, 2008.

Friedman HS, Prados MD, Wen PY, et al: Bevacizumab alone and in combination with irinotecan in recurrent glioblastoma. J Clin Oncol 27:4733–4740, 2009.

Grossman SA, Ye X, Chamberlain M, et al: Talampanel with standard radiation and temozolomide in patients with newly diagnosed glioblastoma: A multicenter phase II trial. J Clin Oncol 27:4155–4161, 2009.

Grossman SA, Ye X, Piantadosi S, et al: Survival of patients with newly diagnosed glioblastoma treated with radiation and temozolomide in research studies in the United States. Clin Cancer Res 16:2443–2449, 2010.

Iwamoto FM, Abrey LE, Beal K, et al: Patterns of relapse and prognosis after bevacizumab failure in recurrent glioblastoma. Neurology 73:1200–1206, 2009.

Keime-Guibert F, Chinot O, Taillandier L, et al: Radiotherapy for glioblastoma in the elderly. N Engl J Med 356:1527–1535, 2007.

Kreisl TN, Kim L, Moore K, et al: Phase II trial of single-agent bevacizumab followed by bevacizumab plus irinotecan at tumor progression in recurrent glioblastoma. J Clin Oncol 27:740–745, 2009.

Perry JR, Bélanger K, Mason WP, et al: Phase II trial of continuous dose-intense temozolomide in recurrent malignant glioma: RESCUE study. J Clin Oncol 28:2051–2057, 2010.

Prados MD, Chang SM, Butowski N, et al: Phase II study of erlotinib plus temozolomide during and after radiation therapy in patients with newly diagnosed glioblastoma multiforme or gliosarcoma. J Clin Oncol 27:579–584, 2009.

Quant EC, Norden AD, Drappatz J, et al: Role of a second chemotherapy in recurrent malignant glioma patients who progress on bevacizumab. Neuro Oncol 11:550–555, 2009.

Reardon DA, Fink KL, Mikkelsen T, et al: Randomized phase II study of cilengitide, an integrin-targeting arginine-glycine-aspartic acid peptide, in recurrent glioblastoma multiforme. J Clin Oncol 26:5610–5617, 2008.

Scott BJ, Quant EC, McNamara MB, et al: Bevacizumab salvage therapy following progression in high-grade glioma patients treated with VEGF receptor tyrosine kinase inhibitors. Neuro Oncol 12:603–607, 2010.

van den Bent MJ, Brandes AA, Rampling R, et al: Randomized phase II trial of erlotinib versus temozolomide or carmustine in recurrent glioblastoma: EORTC brain tumor group study 26034. J Clin Oncol 27:1268–1274, 2009.

Wick W, Hartmann C, Engel C, et al: NOA-04 randomized phase III trial of sequential radiochemotherapy of anaplastic glioma with procarbazine, lomustine, and vincristine or temozolomide. J Clin Oncol 27:5874–5880, 2009.

ON PRIMARY EXTRA-AXIAL TUMORS

Korah MP, Nowlan AW, Johnstone PA, et al: Radiation therapy alone for imaging-defined meningiomas. Int J Radiat Oncol Biol Phys 76:181–186, 2010.

Yang SY, Park CK, Park SH, et al: Atypical and anaplastic meningiomas: Prognostic implication of clinicopathological features. J Neurol Neurosurg Psychiatry 79:574–580, 2008.

ON METASTATIC BRAIN TUMORS

Aoyama H, Tago M, Kato N, et al: Neurocognitive function of patients with brain metastasis who received either whole brain radiotherapy plus stereotactic radiosurgery or radiosurgery alone. Int J Radiat Oncol Biol Phys 68:1388–1395, 2007.

Chang EL, Wefel JS, Hess KR, et al: Neurocognition in patients with brain metastases treated with radiosurgery or radiosurgery plus whole-brain irradiation: A randomised controlled trial. Lancet Oncol 10:1037–1044, 2009.

Ekenel M, Hormigo AM, Peak S, et al: Capecitabine therapy of central nervous system metastases from breast cancer. J Neurooncol 85:223–227, 2007.

Kim JE, Lee DH, Choi Y, et al: Epidermal growth factor receptor tyrosine kinase inhibitors as a first-line therapy for never-smokers with adenocarcinoma of the lung having asymptomatic synchronous brain metastasis. Lung Cancer 65:351–354, 2009.

Lin NU, Dieras V, Paul D, et al: Multicenter phase II study of lapatinib in patients with brain metastases from HER2-positive breast cancer. Clin Cancer Res 15:1452–1459, 2009.

Omlin A, D'Addario G, Gillessen S, et al: Activity of pemetrexed against brain metastases in a patient with adenocarcinoma of the lung. Lung Cancer 65:383–384, 2009.

Abbreviations in this chapter

BTSG = Brain Tumor Study Group; EORTC = European Organisation for Research and Treatment of Cancer; RTOG = Radiation Therapy Oncology Group

CHAPTER 24

AIDS-related malignancies

Ronald T. Mitsuyasu, MD, Deepa Reddy, MD, and Jay S. Cooper, MD

AIDS MALIGNANCIES

Malignancies have been detected in approximately 40% of all patients with acquired immunodeficiency syndrome (AIDS) sometime during the course of their illness. These cancers have been both a primary cause of death in some patients and also a source of considerable morbidity. In the current era of highly active antiretroviral therapy (HAART), patients infected with the human immunodeficiency virus (HIV) are surviving longer than ever. HAART appears to have substantially reduced the incidence of, and mortality from, Kaposi's sarcoma (KS) and non-Hodgkin lymphoma (NHL) and may enhance the efficacy of treatment for those patients who do develop these tumors. Unfortunately, HAART has not shown a similar effect on the development of other types of neoplasms, and caring for patients who develop malignancies in the setting of HIV remains a challenge. Furthermore, HAART is not available universally, with many patients in resource-poor developing countries not having access to antiretroviral drugs.

KAPOSI SARCOMA

Kaposi sarcoma (KS) has been the most common tumor associated with HIV infection, but it currently develops in < 10% of homosexual men with AIDS in the United States and in 1% to 2% of other HIV-infected persons. The incidence of KS has declined substantially, from 4.8 per 100 person-years in 1990 to 1.5 per 100 person-years in 1997. In 2003, a European study found that the incidence of KS among HIV-infected individuals was less than 10% of the incidence seen a decade earlier in 1994.

In a multicenter national study of changes in cancer mortality among HIV-infected adults in France in 2005, there was an increasing proportion of lethal non-AIDS/non-hepatitis cancers (38% in 2000 vs 50% in 2005) and a stable proportion of AIDS-related cancers *(Bonnet F et al: Clin Infect Dis 48:633–639, 2009)*.

EPIDEMIOLOGY

Gender

Among AIDS patients in the United States, the incidence of KS is higher in males than in females. There is also a higher incidence of KS in men than in women in Africa (male-female ratio, 2:1), despite the equal prevalence of HIV infection among men and women.

Age

The age distribution of AIDS-related KS follows the distribution of HIV infection. As such, AIDS-related KS can occur in all age groups. In American adult males, the most common age of onset of AIDS-related KS is 30 to 40 years old. No peak age has been reported.

Race

No racial or ethnic differences in the incidence of AIDS-related KS have been observed.

Geography

In the United States, KS is seen in < 10% of homosexual men with AIDS. The proportion of KS among AIDS-defining diagnoses is lower in parts of Europe, where there are proportionately fewer male homosexual AIDS cases (eg, 6.8% of Italian AIDS patients), and higher in parts of Africa, where KS is endemic in the non–HIV-infected population. Among AIDS cases in the United States, the proportion of patients with KS has declined from the beginning of the AIDS epidemic, possibly as a result of changes in high-risk sexual behavior among homosexual men and the wider use of more effective antiretroviral combination regimens.

ETIOLOGY AND RISK FACTORS

Viruses

In 1994, unique viral DNA sequences were identified in tumor tissues from patients with AIDS-related KS, which led to the identification of a new virus called KS-associated herpesvirus or human herpesvirus type 8 (HHV-8). HHV-8 has been found in > 90% of AIDS-KS tumors, as well as in classic KS, endemic African KS, and post–organ transplant-related KS. It has also been identified in body cavity–based lymphoma/primary effusion lymphoma, multicentric Castleman's disease, and angioimmunoblastic lymphadenopathy with dysproteinemia in HIV-infected patients.

HHV-8 may be transmitted through sexual contact, blood products, or organ transplantation. The seroprevalence of HHV-8 in AIDS-related KS is nearly 100%. HHV-8 has been found in high concentration in the saliva of patients with KS.

HHV-8 is critical in the pathogenesis of AIDS-related KS. The mechanism by which HHV-8 induces KS in susceptible individuals is the subject of intense current investigations.

> In black South Africans in Kwazulu Natal, there has been an increased incidence of KS from < 1:100,000 in 1990 to at least 15:100,000 in 2006. This increase has been observed in both men and women *(Mosam A et al: Int J STD AIDS 30:553–556, 2009)*.

Environmental and host factors

Various environmental and host factors, including HIV- and HHV-8–induced cytokines, AIDS-associated infections, the host's hormonal milieu, immunosuppression, and antiretroviral therapy, may induce or suppress the development of KS and alter its growth.

SIGNS AND SYMPTOMS

The manifestations of KS in patients with AIDS are variable and range from small, innocuous-looking cutaneous lesions to symptom-producing visceral or oral lesions, which may be troublesome and even life-threatening. Although KS occasionally may involve just about every internal organ, it is rarely seen in the bone marrow or CNS.

Skin lesions

KS tumors typically begin as flat or raised lesions that may progress to plaque-like or nodular tumors. Lesions vary in size and shape but are generally nonpruritic and painless. They range in color from light pink to red to deep purple. KS lesions may be cosmetically disfiguring and may result in social stigmatization that far exceeds any actual physical impairment.

Dermal and lymphatic infiltration

Involvement of the skin and lymph glands with tumor can result in edema of the extremities, periorbital areas, and genitals and may be complicated by skin breakdown and bacterial cellulitis. Edema can be marked and may prevent patients from wearing shoes and/or walking.

Podiatric involvement

Lesions on the feet can cause pain and hamper walking.

Oral lesions

These are often asymptomatic but can produce pain and swallowing difficulties.

GI tract involvement

KS involves the GI tract in up to 50% of patients. Most lesions are asymptomatic; however, obstruction, bleeding, or enteropathy can occur occasionally.

Pulmonary KS

Lung involvement usually presents as dyspnea without fever and may become severely debilitating and rapidly fatal if untreated.

SCREENING AND DIAGNOSIS

Currently, there are no screening tests for KS. Although most KS lesions are readily recognized, early lesions may be difficult to diagnose, and the lesions of other diseases (eg, bacillary angiomatosis) may mimic those of KS. Once clinically suspected, the diagnosis of KS is made by biopsy and histologic examination of skin lesions, an excised lymph node, or other tissue or by presumptive diagnosis based on the bronchoscopic or endoscopic appearance of a visceral lesion. Staining for HHV-8 antigen in a biopsy specimen can confirm diagnosis of KS.

GI KS

These lesions have a typical red, raised appearance and are difficult to diagnose by biopsy because many of them have a submucosal location.

Pulmonary KS

In patients with pulmonary KS, chest radiographs typically demonstrate diffuse, reticular-nodular infiltrates, mediastinal enlargement, and, sometimes, pleural effusion. Bronchoscopy may reveal extensive endobronchial involvement with tumor. Definitive diagnosis requires transbronchial or open-lung biopsy. Transbronchial biopsies, however, often yield negative results. A presumptive diagnosis of pulmonary KS may be made, in the absence of fever, based on typical radiographic and endobronchial findings of KS-appearing lesions and after the exclusion of infections.

Thallium and technetium-99m scanning may help differentiate KS from other pulmonary diseases. Patients with KS have been found to have thallium- and technetium-avid scans, whereas pulmonary lymphomas and infections are more typically gallium-avid.

PATHOLOGY

Skin

Cutaneous KS is a lesion of the dermis composed of a proliferation of aberrant vascular structures lined by abnormal-appearing, spindle-shaped endothelial cells and with extravasated erythrocytes and leukocytes within the structures. These spindle cells are generally sparse in early stages but become more numerous and "stack up" between the vascular structures as the tumor advances. Infiltration of mononuclear leukocytes, including plasma cells, T cells, and monocytes, is more prominent in earlier lesions. The histologic appearance of KS in AIDS patients is similar to that seen in non–HIV-infected patients.

Cell of origin

The KS tumor cell is believed to be of mesenchymal, endothelial origin. Several endothelial cell markers are positive in KS, including stains for CD31, CD34, and EN-4. In addition, the tumor stains with factor VIIIa, CD68, and alpha-actin but not with pathologische anatomie leiden endothelium (PAL-E).

STAGING AND PROGNOSIS

Prognostic factors

Although it is difficult to predict from the initial presentation which patients are most likely to have rapidly progressive tumors, several retrospective studies have shown a correlation of survival with the degree of T-cell immunodeficiency, as reflected in the absolute number of T-helper cells in blood. Prior opportunistic infections or the presence of such symptoms as fevers, night sweats, and weight loss (B symptoms) also portends a poor prognosis. Patients who develop KS or whose tumor growth accelerates after an opportunistic infection often have a more aggressive clinical course. Patients with pulmonary involvement generally have a poor prognosis.

Staging system

A tumor classification system has been proposed for AIDS-related KS by the oncology committee of the ACTG. This system segregates patients into good or poor prognostic groups based on tumor characteristics, immune system function, and systemic illness (the tumor-immune system-systemic illness [TIS] system; see Table 1). A retrospective analysis of 294 patients with AIDS-related KS has shown that the TIS system is a valid predictor for survival.

TREATMENT

The treatment of AIDS-related KS requires an individualized approach, based on the extent and location of the lesions, the wishes and treatment needs of the patient, the presence of tumor-associated symptoms (eg, pain, bleeding, edema), the presence of other AIDS-associated illnesses, and the patient's tolerance of medications. Nevertheless, the following general statements can be made:

- Patients with widespread symptomatic disease or life-threatening visceral involvement require prompt, cytoreductive treatment with one or more chemotherapeutic drugs.
- Even in the absence of symptomatic visceral disease, the disfigurement and emotional distress of having these visible reminders of AIDS may mandate treatment for psychological reasons.
- For patients with asymptomatic indolent lesions, aggressive treatment is not mandatory, but these patients may derive substantial benefits from local treatment or investigational therapies that are directed against HIV or HHV-8 or that may interrupt the pathogenesis of KS and/or restore immune competence.
- Given the heterogeneity and unpredictable growth of this tumor, it is often difficult to gauge objective responses. The peculiarities of this multicentric tumor make some subjectivity almost inevitable in gauging treatment responses.

TABLE 1: Staging classification for AIDS-related KS[a]

	Risk status	
Characteristic	**Good risk (0)**	**Poor risk (1)**
	All of the following:	Any of the following:
Tumor (T)	Tumor confined to skin and/or lymph nodes and/or minimal oral disease[b]	Tumor-associated edema or ulceration; extensive oral KS; GI KS; KS in other non-nodal viscera
Immune system (I)	CD4 cells ≥ 150/μL	CD4 cells < 150/μL
Systemic illness (S)	No history of opportunistic infection or thrush; no B symptoms[c]; performance status ≥ 70 (KPS)	History of opportunistic infection and/or thrush; B symptoms; performance status < 70 (KPS); other HIV-related illness (eg, neurologic disease, lymphoma)

AIDS = acquired immunodeficiency syndrome; GI = gastrointestinal; KPS = Karnofsky Performance Status scale; KS = Kaposi sarcoma

[a] Patients are assigned a disease state TxIxSx, where X corresponds to the risk designation (0 or 1) for each risk category.

[b] Minimal oral disease is non-nodular KS confined to the palate.

[c] B symptoms: unexplained fever, night sweats, > 10% involuntary weight loss, or diarrhea persisting for more than 2 weeks.

Treatment options

With the introduction of protease inhibitors and non-nucleoside reverse transcriptase inhibitors for HIV, cases of KS regression with combination antiretroviral therapy have been reported. Because KS seems to be influenced by the state of HIV infection, it is particularly important for patients with AIDS-related KS to have their HIV infection under optimal control. There is no one best anti-HIV regimen, and oncologists should consult with infectious disease specialists familiar with the treatment of HIV infection. Occasionally, a flare in KS tumor progression may be seen when antiretroviral therapy is initiated. Eventually, even with good anti-HIV therapy, some patients with AIDS-related KS will require some form of treatment for their tumor.

Local treatments, including cryotherapy, topical retinoic acid, intralesional chemotherapy and other sclerosing agents, and local irradiation, can produce good local control of tumors. Interferon-alfa (Intron A, Roferon-A) and cytotoxic chemotherapy are effective systemic treatments for patients with more extensive or symptomatic disease. Single-agent or combination chemotherapy is effective in controlling tumors, even in patients with extensive disease and severe immune deficiencies (Table 2). The use of hematopoietic growth factors has facilitated the administration of myelosuppressive treatments, such as interferon-alfa and chemotherapy.

Interferon-alfa

The first treatment licensed for AIDS-related KS was recombinant interferon-alfa. Tumor responses have been seen in approximately 30% of patients treated with subcutaneous (SC) interferon given daily or three times weekly. Current practice is to administer interferon-alfa SC three times weekly. Unmaintained response durations in trials of interferon-alfa monotherapy have ranged from 12 to 24 months in complete responders and from 8 to 12 months in partial responders.

Duration of therapy The optimal duration of interferon-alfa treatment is unknown; however, many patients relapse within a few months after discontinuation of therapy. Reinduction of second responses with interferon-alfa after relapse may be unreliable and often is of short duration. It is therefore generally recommended that treatment with interferon-alfa be continued for as long as drug tolerance and tumor responses continue.

In a prospective cohort study performed from 1996 to 2008, 63 patients with T0 category KS were treated with HAART alone. Only one died of KS, and only 37 required chemotherapy, giving a 5-year systemic treatment-free survival of 74% and a 5-year overall survival of 91% *(Bower M et al: AIDS 23:1701–1706, 2009).*

Dose The optimal dose of interferon-alfa also has not been clearly established. Interferon-alfa is generally administered at either 3 or 5 million units SC three times weekly together with antiretroviral therapy.

Major dose-limiting toxicities of interferon-alfa include fever, chills, rigor, and other flu-like symptoms. They are dose-related and often observed at the initiation of treatment but lessen somewhat with continued use. Neutropenia, elevation of transaminase levels, depression, peripheral neuropathy, and other neuropsychiatric abnormalities may also occur.

Other side effects include headaches, cognitive impairments, paresthesias, and mild thrombocytopenia. As the subjective side effects of interferon-alfa are also common in HIV-related or other conditions, care must be taken to avoid ascribing all of these symptoms to drug toxicity and overlooking treatable infections and other conditions.

Retinoids

Alitretinoin gel 0.1% (9-*cis*-retinoic acid [Panretin]) has received approval of the US FDA for the topical treatment of localized cutaneous KS. This compound inhibits the growth of KS and induces apoptosis of KS cells by binding to retinoic acid receptors on the cell surface.

Phase III clinical trials comparing application of alitretinoin three to four times daily versus placebo gel demonstrated a 35% rate of complete and partial responses in the alitretinoin-treated patients, vs a rate of 18% in controls. The median time to response to alitretinoin was 29 to 34 days, with a median duration of response of 12 to 16 weeks. Responses were seen in both previously untreated and previously treated KS patients and were not dependent on patients' CD4 cell count.

Local cutaneous adverse reactions to alitretinoin include erythema, skin irritation, skin cracking, flaking, peeling, and desquamation. The severity of these reactions can be mitigated by less frequent dosing, thinner application, or use of topical vitamin E.

TABLE 2: Chemotherapy for AIDS–related KS

Regimen	Dose	Response rate[a] (%)
Vincristine	2 mg/wk IV	20–60
Vinblastine	0.05–0.1 mg/kg/wk IV	25–30
Doxorubicin	20 mg/m^2 IV every other wk	50–60
Etoposide	150 mg/m^2 IV every d × 3 q3–4wk	75
Vinorelbine	30 mg/m^2 IV q2wk	47
Liposomal daunorubicin	40 mg/m^2 IV q2–4wk	25–70
Liposomal doxorubicin	20 mg/m^2 IV q2–4wk	58–63
Paclitaxel	100–135 mg/m^2 IV over 3 h q2–4 wk	60–72
Irinotecan	150 mg/m^2 IV days 1–10	75
Vincristine/ vinblastine	2 mg IV vincristine alternating with 0.1 mg/kg IV vinblastine every other wk	45
Vincristine/ bleomycin	2 mg IV vincristine + 10 mg/m^2 IV bleomycin q2wk	23–70
Doxorubicin/ bleomycin/ vincristine	10 mg/m^2 IV doxorubicin + 10 mg/m^2 IV bleomycin + 1–2 mg IV vincristine q2wk	87

AIDS = acquired immunodeficiency syndrome; IV = intravenous; KS = Kaposi sarcoma
[a] Complete responses plus partial responses

Alitretinoin should be reserved for patients who do not require systemic treatment for visceral disease. However, it may be used in conjunction with other treatments for cutaneous disease.

Oral alitretinoin has been investigated in patients with AIDS-related KS, and it was found to have a 37% response rate.

Bexarotene (Targretin), an oral retinoid X receptor (RXR)-selective agonist, has been studied in patients with AIDS-related KS, with an overall response rate of 33% in one study.

Chemotherapy

For patients with more widely disseminated, rapidly progressive, or symptomatic disease, systemic chemotherapy is generally warranted. Chemotherapy drugs are included in Table 2.

Antiretroviral drugs A total of 25 anti-HIV drugs have received FDA approval, and more are in various stages of clinical development. When evaluated by an oncologist, the majority of HIV-infected individuals will be taking some anti-HIV drugs. The interactions between cytotoxic chemotherapy and the various anti-HIV drugs have not been fully studied. Thus, oncologists treating patients with AIDS-related KS should continue to monitor them frequently for side effects. Withholding antiretroviral therapy during chemotherapy and then immediately restarting it after giving the chemotherapy drugs may avoid some toxic effects of drug interactions, especially with high-dose therapy.

Combination regimens The two most frequently utilized combination chemotherapy regimens are doxorubicin, bleomycin, and vincristine (ABV) and bleomycin and vincristine (BV). These regimens were initially reported to yield tumor response rates in excess of 70% to 90%, with good palliation of symptoms, including decreased edema, decreased pain, and, in patients with pulmonary KS, respiratory improvement and alleviation of obstructive symptoms. A beneficial effect of these combinations on survival has not been clearly demonstrated, however.

Early reports of a high response rate with these combination regimens have not been reproduced by later multicenter trials. A conservative response rate of 50% to 60% has been reported in more contemporary phase III trials. The discrepancy in response rates most likely stems from differences in the response criteria used.

Liposomal anthracyclines (eg, liposomal doxorubicin [Doxil] and liposomal daunorubicin [DaunoXome]) are also effective in inducing tumor regression in KS. Clinical trials have shown that liposomal anthracyclines as single agents can achieve a response rate equal to or better than that obtained with the ABV combination regimen. As such, the liposomal anthracyclines have become first-line chemotherapy for AIDS-related KS.

The dose-limiting toxicity is neutropenia, and many patients will require the use of granulocyte colony-stimulating factor (filgrastim [Neupogen]) after several cycles of treatment. Other common side effects include nausea, fatigue, anemia, and thrombocytopenia. A palmar-plantar syndrome, characterized by acute painful erythematous swelling of the hands and feet, has been reported with the use of liposomal doxorubicin. Once the symptoms resolved, readministration of liposomal doxorubicin did not necessarily reproduce the syndrome. Neither of the liposomal anthracyclines has been reported to depress left ventricular function.

Paclitaxel has been shown to produce responses in both chemotherapy-naive KS patients and patients with refractory tumors, including those refractory to liposomal anthracyclines. The dosage is typically 100 to 135 mg/m^2 IV given over 3 hours every 2 to 4 weeks. This agent is widely considered the primary second-line chemotherapy for KS.

The dose-limiting toxicity is neutropenia. Other reported toxicities include anemia, stomatitis, alopecia, and fatigue. Neuropathy has not been a major problem with this low-dose approach.

Investigational agents Other drugs under investigation for the treatment of KS include a number of other antiangiogenesis compounds. Compounds that may affect HHV-8 gene expression (eg, valproic acid) or signal transduction pathways in KS-infected cells (eg, imatinib [Gleevec] and sunitinib [Sutent]) and a mammalian target of rapamycin inhibitor (eg, sirolimus [rapamycin]) are also in development or in early clinical testing in KS patients. Cidofovir (Vistide) does not appear to be clinically active.

Radiation therapy

Although radiation therapy can easily produce sufficient regression of KS to be useful for palliation of symptomatic disease or cosmetic improvement of disfiguring lesions, this practice has become less common as HAART has changed the natural history of AIDS. More than 90% of lesions will respond (complete responses [CRs] and partial responses [PRs]). Local radiation therapy commonly alleviates pain and bleeding, lessens edema, and shrinks obstructing lesions.

Treatment technique For most superficial lesions, a single, shaped, en face beam of relatively limited penetration (approximately 100 kV) works well. A relatively low-energy electron beam (eg, 6 MeV) often can be used with shielding as an alternative to superficial x-rays.

Large lesions For large lesions, electron beams are used more often, due to the limited penetration of kilovoltage x-ray beams and the limited width of the treatment cones attached to most superficial x-ray units. For patients with more widespread tumors of the legs with edema, parallel opposed megavoltage x-ray beams and overlying bolus material are often used to provide homogeneous irradiation to the entire area.

Dose fractionation regimens Several dose fractionation regimens have proved effective in AIDS-related KS. As this tumor is radiosensitive, almost any dose of radiation therapy can produce some response. Interestingly, in vitro irradiation of KS cell cultures induces the cells to produce interleukin-6 (IL-6) and oncostatin M, which, in turn, make the cells more sensitive to radiation therapy.

A recent review of the possible radiosensitizing effects of HIV concluded that the available data are universally weak and often insufficient to warrant a recommendation. When the data were deemed insufficient, the authors recommended that "standard" radiation therapy be used to treat the various cancers that occur in HIV-infected patients, with the caveat that KS patients should be monitored closely for toxicity *(Housri N et al: Cancer 116:273–283, 2010)*.

For most cutaneous lesions, a single treatment of 800 cGy will produce a short-term response. For lesions on sensitive structures (eg, penis, hands, conjunctivae), some radiation oncologists attenuate treatment to a total dose of 2,000 cGy administered in 300 cGy increments (accepting a 50% decrease in CR rate), whereas 3,000 cGy delivered over 2 weeks is more typically used for lesions in general.

Prospectively acquired data clearly demonstrate a dose-response relationship for radiation therapy in AIDS-related KS. When compared with 2,000 cGy given in 10 fractions or 800 cGy given in 1 fraction, a dose of 4,000 cGy delivered in 20 fractions over 4 weeks was significantly more effective, as measured by a higher response rate, longer duration of tumor control, and the absence of residual hyperpigmentation. However, the short- and medium-term effects of moderately intense but briefer regimens, such as 3,000 cGy in 10 fractions over 2 weeks, probably are equivalent to those of higher total dose and more protracted regimens, and the moderately intense regimens require only half the time to deliver.

For patients with an anticipated survival of < 3 months, in whom the response duration may be of less overall importance, a single fraction of 800 cGy is likely to provide the same benefit as the more intensive regimens. In contrast, small lesions in patients who are expected to survive for at least 1 year should be treated with fractionated radiation therapy, such as 3,000 cGy in 10 fractions over 2 weeks.

NON-HODGKIN LYMPHOMA (NHL)

The incidence of NHL is 60 times higher in individuals with HIV infection than in the general population. The overall occurrence of lymphoma as a manifestation of AIDS has declined somewhat as treatment of HIV has improved.

Although NHL currently comprises < 5% of all initial AIDS-defining conditions, it accounts for as many as 28% of all AIDS-related deaths. The majority of patients present with advanced-stage, high- or intermediate-grade, B-cell lymphoma and have a high frequency of extranodal involvement. Primary CNS lymphoma occurs in approximately 0.5% of patients with AIDS.

The majority of patients with AIDS-related lymphoma have advanced HIV disease. Median CD4 cell counts in patients with systemic lymphoma range from 100 to 200 cells/μL, although NHL can occur at any CD4 count.

EPIDEMIOLOGY

At-risk groups

NHL occurs with approximately equal frequency in all population groups infected by HIV, including IV drug users, homosexual-bisexual men, transfusion recipients, and patients with hemophilia.

Gender and race

AIDS-related NHL is seen more frequently in men than in women and occurs more often in whites than in blacks.

Age

The age distribution of AIDS-related NHL follows the distribution of HIV infection. Primary CNS lymphoma occurs with the same frequency in all age groups.

Geography

Current data do not indicate any geographic differences in the incidence of AIDS-related NHL.

ETIOLOGY AND RISK FACTORS

AIDS-related NHL is believed to arise as a consequence of continued stimulation of B-cell proliferation as a result of HIV, Epstein-Barr virus (EBV), and other infections, all of which occur in the setting of profound T-cell immunodeficiency. An association between the polyomavirus, simian virus 40 (SV40), and diffuse large B-cell and follicle-type lymphoma has been detected. HIV also induces the expression of a number of cytokines (eg, IL-6 and IL-10) that can further increase B-cell activation.

Small noncleaved lymphomas

Genetic errors are increased in the setting of chronic B-cell proliferation, and a variety of chromosomal translocations resulting in oncogene activation can lead to polyclonal and monoclonal B-cell expression. Other molecular biological abnormalities associated with small noncleaved lymphomas include expression of an abnormal *TP53* (alias *p53*) tumor-suppressor gene and the c-*myc* or *ras* oncogene.

Immunoblastic lymphoma

The pathogenesis of AIDS-related immunoblastic lymphoma appears to be distinct from that of small noncleaved lymphoma and is more likely related to EBV infection without c-*myc* dysregulation. Clonal integration of EBV within tumor cells, with expression of various latent EBV proteins, has been demonstrated in essentially all cases of AIDS-related primary CNS lymphoma and in as many as two-thirds of systemic lymphomas.

Diffuse large cell lymphoma

The specific molecular aberrations described in patients with AIDS-related diffuse large cell lymphoma appear distinct as well, with recent descriptions of abnormal *BCL6* expression in approximately 40% of cases.

Body cavity–based lymphoma/primary effusion lymphoma

This appears to be highly associated with HHV-8 and EBV. The tumor cells stain positive for CD45. The disease appears to occur predominantly in males and may coexist with KS in patients with AIDS.

SIGNS AND SYMPTOMS

B symptoms

These events (ie, fever, weight loss, and night sweats) are seen in approximately 80% of patients with systemic AIDS-related NHL. In these patients, it is mandatory to exclude the presence of occult opportunistic infections before ascribing B symptoms to the lymphoma itself.

Extranodal involvement

Advanced-stage disease is expected in the majority of patients, with extranodal involvement reported in 60% to 90% of patients in most series. Common sites of extranodal involvement include the CNS (occurring in approximately 30% of patients), GI tract (25%), and bone marrow (25%). Essentially any other site in the body can also be involved, including the rectum, soft tissue, oral cavity, lungs, and heart.

CNS lymphoma

Patients with primary CNS lymphoma often present with focal neurologic deficits, seizures, and/or altered mental status. Any site in the brain may be involved, and one to four space-occupying lesions are usually seen on MRI or CT scan.

Other sites

Changes in bowel habits, GI bleeding, weight loss, pain, and hepatomegaly are common presenting symptoms in patients with GI involvement. Pancytopenia may indicate bone marrow involvement.

Primary effusion lymphoma

Patients usually present with pleural or pericardial effusion without an identifiable mass. Pain, shortness of breath, and B symptoms are the main initial complaints.

SCREENING AND DIAGNOSIS

Diagnosis of NHL in patients with AIDS requires histologic confirmation by biopsy with immunophenotypic and/or molecular gene-rearrangement studies.

Evaluation

A complete staging evaluation should be done. This should include:

- CT or MRI of the head
- positron-emission tomography/CT scan of whole body
- bone marrow aspiration and biopsy
- liver function studies
- spinal fluid analysis.

Assessing spinal fluid for EBV

The presence of EBV DNA in cerebrospinal fluid, as determined by polymerase chain reaction, appears to have a high specificity and sensitivity for the diagnosis of primary CNS lymphoma.

PATHOLOGY

Common tumor types

Over 95% of AIDS-related NHL cases are of B-lymphocyte origin. Most AIDS-related NHL tumors are high-grade types, including the immunoblastic and small noncleaved lymphomas. Diffuse large cell lymphoma constitutes up to 30% of AIDS lymphomas.

Less common tumor types

Although not considered part of the AIDS epidemic, several cases of T-cell lymphoma occurring in HIV-infected patients have been described. In addition, cases of Ki-1–positive, large cell anaplastic lymphoma and plasmablastic lymphoma have been reported in HIV-infected patients. The clinical and pathologic characteristics of these forms of lymphoma are similar to those seen in non–HIV-infected individuals.

CNS lymphomas

These are typically of the immunoblastic or large cell type.

GI and oral cavity lymphomas

Large cell or immunoblastic lymphomas are also more likely to involve the GI tract and oral cavity than are small noncleaved lymphomas.

Primary effusion lymphomas

The cells are large and pleomorphic with prominent nucleoli and immunoblastic morphology. Clonal immunoglobulin DNA rearrangement demonstrates clonality of the tumor cells but not surface immunoglobulin expression.

STAGING AND PROGNOSIS

Staging system

Staging of AIDS-related NHL is the same as that for non–AIDS-related NHL. The Ann Arbor classification system for staging of NHL is utilized (see chapter 27), and the staging workup includes imaging studies, as well as bone marrow and CNS evaluation for lymphomas.

Prognostic factors

Five factors have been shown to correlate most closely with a shorter survival in patients with systemic AIDS-related NHL:

- a history of opportunistic infection prior to the lymphoma
- CD4 cell count < 100 cells/μL
- International Prognostic Index score
- Karnofsky Performance Status (KPS) score < 70
- stage IV disease, especially if due to bone marrow or meningeal involvement.

TABLE 3: Chemotherapy for AIDS-related NHL

Regimen	Drugs and dosage	Cycle length	CR rate (%)	Median survival
m-BACOD	Methotrexate, 500 mg/m² IV on day 15, with leucovorin, 25 mg PO q6h × 4, after completion of methotrexate	q28d	41	35 wk
	Bleomycin, 4 U/m² IV on day 1			
	Doxorubicin, 25 mg/m² IV on day 1			
	Cyclophosphamide, 300 mg/m² IV on day 1			
	Vincristine, 1.4 mg/m² IV on day 1 (maximum, 2 mg)			
	Dexamethasone, 3 mg/m² PO on days 1–5			
CDE	Cyclophosphamide, 800 mg/m²/96 h IV	q28d	46	8.2 mo
	Doxorubicin, 50 mg/m²/96 h IV			
	Etoposide, 240 mg/m²/96 h IV			
R-EPOCH	Rituximab, 375 mg/m² IV day 1	q3–4wk	79	53 mo+
	Etoposide, 200 mg/m²/96 h IV			
	Prednisone, 60 mg/m² PO on days 1-6			
	Vincristine, 1.6 mg/m²/96 h IV			
	Cyclophosphamide, 187 mg/m² IV on day 5 (if CD4 cell count < 100 cells/μL) or 375 mg/m² IV on day 5 (if CD4 cell count ≥ 100 cells/μL)[a]			
	Doxorubicin, 40 mg/m²/96 h IV			
CEOP	Cyclophosphamide, 750 mg/m² IV on day 1	q3–4wk	47	10 mo
	Epirubicin, 50 mg/m² IV on day 1			
	Vincristine, 2 mg IV on day 1			
	Prednisone, 100 mg PO on days 1–5			
R-CHOP	Rituximab, 375 mg/m² IV day 1	q21d	63	9 mo
	Cyclophosphamide, 750 mg/m² IV on day 1			
	Doxorubicin, 50 mg/m² IV on day 1			
	Vincristine, 1.4 mg/m² IV on day 1 (maximum, 2 mg)			
	Prednisone, 60 mg PO on days 1–5			

AIDS = acquired immunodeficiency syndrome; CR = complete response; IV = intravenous; NHL = non-Hodgkin lymphoma; PO = orally

[a] With dose escalation as tolerated with each subsequent cycle, to a maximum of 750 mg/m²

In patients without these findings, the median survival is typically 11 to 12 months, as compared with a median survival of approximately 4 to 5 months in those with one or more of these adverse prognostic features.

Three factors correlate with *better* survival in patients with primary CNS lymphoma:

- KPS score > 70
- age < 35 years
- adequate dose of radiation therapy.

Type of lymphoma

To date, no major differences have been seen in response or survival among the various pathologic types of systemic AIDS-related NHL. Patients with polyclonal lymphomas appear to have better tumor responses to chemotherapy and better survival. Patients with primary CNS lymphoma have an extremely poor prognosis, with a median survival of only 2 to 3 months despite therapy; treatment with potent antiretroviral therapy does seem to improve survival. The prognosis for patients with primary effusion lymphoma is also poor, with a median survival of only 5 months.

TREATMENT

Systemic NHL

Chemotherapy

The mainstay of treatment for patients with systemic AIDS-related NHL is chemotherapy. As the likelihood of tumor dissemination is great, AIDS patients who develop NHL must be assumed to have widespread disease at presentation and should be treated with systemic chemotherapy, even if tumor dissemination is not confirmed on routine staging evaluation.

Some of the commonly used regimens designed for AIDS-related NHL are listed in Table 3. No regimen appears to be superior to any other, although early findings show that the EPOCH regimen (etoposide, prednisone, vincristine [Oncovin], cyclophosphamide, doxorubicin) gives the best results to date.

CNS prophylaxis with either intrathecal cytarabine (Ara-C; 50 mg) or intrathecal methotrexate (10–12 mg) every week for four treatments has been shown to be effective in reducing the incidence of CNS relapse.

The role of rituximab in AIDS-related lymphoma is not clearly defined, given that it induces greater remissions but can cause more cellular and humoral immunodeficiency and may predispose to life-threatening infections. Prospective trials evaluating the use of rituximab in AIDS lymphoma have had mixed results. Given

> Whereas earlier studies initially suggested that rituximab may cause more infectious complications and greater mortality in the treatment of AIDS-NHL with chemotherapy, the recent AMC 034 phase II study of rituximab given either concomitantly or sequentially with EPOCH chemotherapy, HAART, and prophylactic antibiotics, demonstrated complete response in 35 of 40 patients given concurrent rituximab (*Sparano J et al: Blood 225:3008–3016, 2010*).

these data, clinicians should consider using rituximab in patients with CD20-positive NHL who have CD4 counts > 50/mm^3 or using it in combination with multiple prophylactic antibiotics.

Dose intensity Standard-dose chemotherapy (eg, cyclophosphamide, doxorubicin, vincristine, and prednisone [CHOP]) is generally recommended for most patients with AIDS-related NHL. Results from trials using continuous infusion therapy (eg, EPOCH or CDE) have shown better CR (complete response) rates and long disease progression-free and overall survival.

Certain subsets of patients with high CD4 cell counts (> 100 cells/μL), no B symptoms, lower disease stage at presentation (stage I or II), and good performance status (0 or 1) may enjoy prolonged survival (> 2 years) when treated with either a standard-dose or intensive, high-dose regimen.

Growth factor and other support The major dose-limiting toxic effect of multiagent chemotherapy regimens is myelosuppression. Studies of methotrexate with leucovorin, bleomycin, doxorubicin, cyclophosphamide, vincristine, and dexamethasone (m-BACOD) or CHOP chemotherapy demonstrated that coadministration of myeloid hematopoietic growth factors enhanced patient tolerance of these regimens. In addition, prophylaxis with trimethoprim/sulfamethoxazole, azithromycin, fluconazole, valganciclovir (Valcyte), and ciprofloxacin can also reduce the risk of infection during intensive chemotherapy and rituximab.

Salvage chemotherapy Patients in whom initial treatment fails or relapse occurs after initial remission rarely achieve a prolonged second remission. Studies of various salvage regimens with or without autologous stem-cell support have demonstrated some early promising results.

Second-line chemotherapy (eg, etoposide, methylprednisolone, high-dose cytarabine, cisplatin [ESHAP]) has been shown to produce a CR of up to 31% and a PR of 23%, with a median survival of 7.1 months, in patients with refractory or relapsed AIDS-related NHL.

A multicenter collaboration of 33 European cohorts showed that the incidence rates of both NHL and primary CNS lymphoma are substantially reduced in patients on HAART and that, in the era of HAART, two-thirds of patients diagnosed with systemic HIV-associated lymphoma survive longer than 1 year from diagnosis. Survival was poorer (54%) for those with primary CNS lymphoma (*Bohlius J et al: Antiviral Ther 14:1065–1074, 2009; The COHERE Study Group: AIDS 23:2029–2037, 2009*).

Radiation therapy

The role of radiotherapy in systemic lymphoma is limited to consolidation of the effects of chemotherapy. Treatment principles are similar to those used for aggressive NHL in the non-HIV setting and typically involve the use of involved or extended fields only.

Lymphomatous meningitis For patients with lymphomatous meningitis and/or radiographically detectable cerebral deposits, "step-brain" irradiation (including the covering meninges) is administered along with intrathecal chemotherapy to control microscopic spinal disease. Focal radiation therapy may be required for known tumor deposits in the spine. Unfortunately, many such patients develop multiple deposits anywhere along the spinal axis, either synchronously or metachronously.

Fractionated doses of 3,000 to 4,500 cGy may be used to control local lymphoma deposits in nodal areas. Patients who have lymphomatous meningitis typically have a poor prognosis and are best treated with regimens that do not unduly occupy their time (eg, 3,000 cGy in 10 fractions over 2 weeks).

Treatment of Primary CNS Lymphoma

An effective therapy for patients with AIDS-related CNS lymphoma has not yet been found, although many AIDS oncologists find high-dose methotrexate with leucovorin rescue more effective than radiation therapy.

Radiation therapy

The conventional standard of treatment is step-brain irradiation, which can result in response rates of 50% and improve survival, as compared with untreated patients, even when adjusted for antiretroviral therapy, CD4 cell count, and time to diagnosis. Treatment is directed to the entire cranial contents, including the meninges down to C2.

Doses equivalent to 3,900 cGy (or more) delivered at 200 cGy/fraction appear to be associated with increased survival. KPS scores and younger age at the time of treatment are also associated with longer survival. Mean survival ranges from 2 to 6 months, with death often due to complicating opportunistic infections.

CERVICAL CARCINOMA

Cervical carcinoma in the setting of HIV infection has been recognized as an AIDS-defining malignancy since 1993. Unfortunately, in some women, cervical carcinoma may be the first indication that they have HIV infection.

Cervical intraepithelial neoplasia (CIN) is also seen in association with HIV infection. These premalignant lesions, also known as squamous intraepithelial lesions (SILs), may foretell a higher incidence of cervical carcinoma among HIV-infected women. SILs have been associated with human papillomavirus (HPV), particularly those subtypes with greater oncogenic potential, such as serotypes 16, 18, 31, 33, and 35.

EPIDEMIOLOGY

Prevalence of HIV infection and cervical abnormalities

The risk of HIV infection in women with an abnormal Pap smear varies with the prevalence of HIV infection in the given population. Screening in clinics in high-prevalence areas has yielded HIV-positivity rates of between 6% and 7% (and up to 10% in parts of Africa). In such high-prevalence areas, among women younger than age 50 with cervical carcinoma, up to 19% of women were found to be HIV positive. HIV-positive women have up to a 10-fold increased risk of abnormal cervical cytology. Several centers have reported abnormal cytology rates of 30% to 60% in HIV-positive women and Pap smears consistent with cervical dysplasia in 15% to 40%. The prevalence of cervical dysplasia increases with declining CD4 cell counts in HIV-infected women.

Nationwide, invasive cervical carcinoma was found in 1.3% of women with AIDS. In New York, invasive cervical carcinoma constitutes 4% of AIDS-defining illnesses in women. Recent findings from linkage studies in the US and Italy clearly have shown increased rates of cervical cancer in women with HIV.

Race and geography

The prevalence of invasive cervical carcinoma among American Hispanic and black women is lower than that in white women. However, this difference may stem from a difference in access to health care. The southern and northeastern sections of the United States have a higher reported number of cases of HIV-associated invasive cervical carcinoma.

ETIOLOGY AND RISK FACTORS

The severe cellular immunodeficiency associated with advanced HIV infection may allow oncogenic viruses to flourish and may also compromise the body's immunologic defenses that control the development of these tumors.

HPV

There is abundant evidence that HPV infection is related to malignant and premalignant neoplasia in the lower genital tract. HPV serotypes 16, 18, 31, 33, and 35 are the most oncogenic strains and have been associated with invasive cervical carcinoma and progressive dysplasia. The prevalence of cervical SILs among HIV-infected women may be as high as 20% to 30%, with many having higher cytologic and histologic grade lesions.

SIGNS AND SYMPTOMS

The majority of cervical SILs are detected on routine cytologic evaluation of Pap smears in women with HIV infection.

Advanced invasive disease

Postcoital bleeding with serosanguineous and/or foul-smelling vaginal discharge is usually the first symptom of more advanced invasive disease. Lumbosacral pain or urinary obstructive symptoms may indicate advanced disease.

SCREENING AND DIAGNOSIS

Because the majority of patients with cervical dysplasia or early invasive cancer are asymptomatic, frequent cytologic screening of women at risk for HIV infection must be undertaken. The role of newly developed HPV vaccines in preventing HPV infection or disease progression in HIV-infected women has yet to be determined.

Screening of HIV-positive women

Current screening recommendations call for women with HIV infection to have pelvic examinations and cytologic screening every 6 months during the first year after HIV diagnosis and then annually if the test results are normal. Pap smears indicating cervical SILs must be taken seriously, and abnormalities justify immediate colposcopy. Although abnormalities are sometimes missed by relying solely on cytologic screening, recommendations for routine colposcopy have not yet been established.

Screening of women with a history of cervical SILs

For women who have a history of cervical SILs, more frequent reevaluation and cytologic screening should be undertaken. Since these women are at high risk for recurrence or development of lesions in other areas of the lower genital tract, post-therapy surveillance with repeat colposcopy also is warranted.

Workup of women with invasive carcinoma

For women with invasive carcinoma, complete staging should be undertaken; this should include pelvic examination, CT of the pelvis and abdomen, chest x-ray, and screening laboratory tests for hepatic and bone disease. In addition, full evaluation and treatment for HIV and related complications should be initiated.

PATHOLOGY

Squamous cell carcinoma

Most cases of cervical carcinoma are of the squamous cell type.

STAGING AND PROGNOSIS

The staging classification for cervical carcinoma (see chapter 17), as adopted by the FIGO, also applies to AIDS patients.

Cervical dysplasia in HIV-infected women is often of higher cytologic and histologic grade. These women are more likely to have CIN II–III lesions with extensive cervical involvement, multisite (vagina, vulva, and anus) involvement, and endocervical lesions.

HIV-infected women with cervical carcinoma typically present with more advanced disease and appear to have a more aggressive clinical course. Tumors are typically high grade with a higher proportion of lymph node and visceral involvement at presentation. Mean time to recurrence after primary treatment is short, and many patients have persistent disease after primary therapy. The median time to death in one series was 10 months in HIV-infected women, as compared with 23 months in HIV-negative patients.

TREATMENT

Treatment of preinvasive disease

Cryotherapy, laser therapy, cone biopsy, and loop electrosurgical excision procedure have all been used to treat preinvasive disease in HIV-infected patients. Short-term recurrence rates of 40% to 60% have been reported.

Determinants of recurrence

Immune status of the patient seems to be the most important determining factor for recurrence. Close surveillance after initial therapy is critical, and repetitive treatment may be necessary to prevent progression to more invasive disease.

Treatment of cervical carcinoma

The same principles that guide oncologic management of the immunocompetent patient with cervical carcinoma (see chapter 17) are utilized in AIDS patients with this cancer.

Resection

Resection can be undertaken for the usual indications, and surgical decisions should be based on oncologic appropriateness and not on HIV status.

Radiation therapy

As most AIDS patients with cervical cancer present with advanced disease, radiation therapy is indicated more often than surgery. If the patient's overall physical condition permits, treatment regimens are identical to those used for the same stage disease in uninfected individuals (see chapter 17). It is important to note that the standard of care for advanced carcinoma of the cervix (stages III–IV, without hematogeneous dissemination) now includes a combination of irradiation and concurrent cisplatin-based chemotherapy. At present, there is insufficient evidence to suggest that irradiation or other treatments for cervical carcinoma in AIDS patients is any less effective than in similar non–HIV-infected individuals.

Chemotherapy

Antineoplastic regimens, such as cisplatin (50 mg/m^2) or carboplatin (200 mg/m^2), bleomycin (20 U/m^2; maximum, 30 U), and vincristine (1 mg/m^2), have been used in patients with metastatic or recurrent disease. Vigorous management of side effects and complications of these treatments and of AIDS itself must be provided.

ANAL CARCINOMA

Although anal carcinoma is not currently an AIDS-defining illness, the incidence of this tumor is increasing in the population at risk for HIV infection. The incidence of anal carcinoma in homosexual men in a San Francisco study was estimated at between 25 and 87 cases per 100,000, compared with 0.7 case per 100,000 in the entire male population.

ETIOLOGY AND RISK FACTORS

HPV

Precursor lesions of anal intraepithelial neoplasia (AIN), also known as anal SILs, have been found to be associated with HPV infection, typically with oncogenic serotypes, eg, types 16 and 18. Cytologic abnormalities occur in nearly 40% of patients, especially those with CD4 cell counts < 200 cells/μL. Abnormal cytology may predict the later development of invasive carcinoma.

SIGNS AND SYMPTOMS

Rectal pain, bleeding, discharge, and symptoms of obstruction or a mass lesion are the most frequent presenting symptoms.

SCREENING AND DIAGNOSIS

Studies to evaluate the usefulness of anoscopy with frequent anal cytology have been undertaken to determine whether early detection of AIN may result in interventions that would prevent the development of invasive tumors.

Workup of patients with anal carcinoma

For patients with anal carcinoma, determination of the extent of local disease, as well as full staging for dissemination, should be undertaken (see chapter 13).

PATHOLOGY

Squamous cell carcinoma

The majority of anal carcinomas are of the squamous cell type.

Histologic grading

The grading for AIN is similar to that for CIN, with AIN-1 denoting low-grade dysplasia and AIN-2 and AIN-3 referring to higher grade dysplastic lesions. The gross appearance of lesions on anoscopy does not predict histologic grade. Higher grade dysplastic lesions are seen in patients with lower CD4 cell counts.

STAGING AND PROGNOSIS

The staging of squamous cell carcinoma of the anus in HIV-infected individuals is the same as that in non–HIV-infected patients (see chapter 13). Patients with severe immunosuppression (ie, CD4 cell counts < 50 cells/μL) may present with more advanced, more aggressive disease. The true natural history of this tumor in the AIDS population has yet to be defined, however.

TREATMENT

AIN and carcinoma in situ

Treatment of patients with local AIN is similar to that of women with CIN. Ablative therapy may be used.

Invasive anal squamous cell carcinoma

Anal cancer can be controlled with chemotherapy and radiation therapy despite HIV infection. However, patients who have low CD4 cell counts appear to be more likely to experience severe toxicity and to require colostomy for salvage therapy than those with higher CD4 cell counts. For patients with squamous cell carcinoma of the anus, chemotherapy with mitomycin (10 mg/m^2 on day 1) and fluorouracil (5-FU; 1,000 mg/m^2 by continuous infusion on days 1–4) combined with radiation therapy can produce high rates of complete remission.

Concomitant radiation therapy, 5-FU, and mitomycin have been reported to produce a CR in 9 of 11 patients with AIDS-associated invasive anal carcinoma (median CD4 cell count at diagnosis of 209 cells/μL) and a 60% 2-year actuarial survival rate. Two patients remain alive more than 8 years following treatment, but severe toxicity (three grade 3 hematologic, one grade 3 dermatologic, one grade 4, and one grade 5 GI toxicity) and one death resulted from treatment.

Evidence appears to suggest that 5-FU plus cisplatin may be better tolerated than 5-FU plus mitomycin in HIV patients. Tolerance to treatment seen in patients who have relatively intact immune systems is similar to that seen in HIV-infected patients. The role of cetuximab (Erbitux) and other target therapies in this disease population also has not yet been determined. However, the appropriate dose of radiation therapy for patients with anal carcinoma in the context of HIV infection remains unsettled. Patients who are unable to tolerate chemoradiation therapy and those in whom treatment fails (defined as a positive biopsy after a CR) should be considered for abdominoperineal resection.

OTHER NON–AIDS-DEFINING MALIGNANCIES

As more effective control of HIV has become possible, patients are living longer and are being affected by types of cancers that are not directly induced by HIV. A growing number of reports from around the world now indicate that other malignant tumors, including Hodgkin lymphoma (HL), nonmelanomatous skin cancers, lung cancer, germ-cell tumors, myeloid or lymphoid leukemias, multiple myeloma, renal cell carcinoma, head and neck cancer, brain tumors, squamous tumor of the conjunctiva, and leiomyosarcoma in pediatric patients, are occurring in HIV-infected individuals.

Rates of other non–AIDS-defining cancers appear to be increasing among HIV-infected individuals. In an Australian cancer data base, 196 cases of non–AIDS-defining cancers were noted in 13,067 individuals (1.5%) including 8,351 notified with HIV infection and 8,118 registered with AIDS. As HIV-infected individuals are surviving longer with currently available combination anti-HIV drugs, clinicians should anticipate seeing the development of more tumors in these patients. Greater vigilance for these tumors is warranted.

These non-AIDS defining cancers are generally treated with the same stage-adjusted strategies as would be used in individuals not infected with HIV.

HODGKIN LYMPHOMA (HL)

Studies showing a possible increased incidence of HL in HIV-infected individuals have been reported from Europe, Australia, and the United States. The most common histology is mixed cellularity and lymphocyte-depleted. Male predominance, a higher prevalence of B symptoms, and more extranodal disease on presentation are the main characteristics of HL in HIV-infected patients.

Chemotherapy is recommended for this group of patients, due to the high proportion of stage III or IV disease. Standard treatments include doxorubicin, bleomycin, vinblastine, and dacarbazine (ABVD) or ABVD alternating with vincristine mechlorethamine (Mustargen), vincristine, procarbazine (Matulane), and prednisone (MOPP). More recently, early results with bleomycin, etoposide, doxorubicin, cyclophosphamide, vincristine, procarbazine, and prednisone (BEACOPP) and the Stanford V regimen (mechlorethamine, doxorubicin, vinblastine, vincristine, bleomycin, etoposide, and prednisone) look promising.

NONMELANOMATOUS SKIN CANCERS

As in the general population, basal cell carcinoma is more common than squamous cell carcinoma in the setting of HIV infection. The risk factors for the development of these tumors are the same as in the general population: namely, fair skin, history of sun exposure, and family history.

LUNG CANCER

Patients with HIV appear to have a higher relative risk of developing lung cancer than do age-matched controls (relative risk = 4.5; 95% confidence interval, 4.2–4.8). These tumors tend to present at later stages than do tumors with a similar histologic distribution in the general population.

PEDIATRIC LEIOMYOSARCOMA

Cases of aggressive leiomyosarcoma developing in HIV-positive children have been reported. Leiomyosarcoma is a rare tumor, occurring in < 2 cases per 10 million non–HIV-infected children. However, a much higher than expected frequency of leiomyosarcoma has been reported in HIV-infected children. Visceral sites (eg, the lungs, spleen, and GI tract) are commonly involved.

SUGGESTED READING

ON KS

Franceschi S, Maso LD, Rickenbach M, et al: Kaposi sarcoma incidence in the Swiss HIV Cohort Study before and after highly active antiretroviral therapy. Br J Cancer 99:800–804, 2008.

Housri N, Yarchoan R, Kaushal A: Radiotherapy for patients with the human immunodeficiency virus: Are special precautions necessary? Cancer 116:273–283, 2010.

Spano JP, Costagliola D, Katlama C, et al: AIDS-related malignancies: State of the art and therapeutic challenges. J Clin Oncol 26:4834–4842, 2008.

Sullivan RJ, Pantanowitz L, Casper C, et al: HIV/AIDS: Epidemiology, pathophysiology and treatment of Kaposi sarcoma-associated herpes virus disease: Kaposi sarcoma, primary effusion lymphoma, and multicentric Castleman disease. Clin Infect Dis 47:1209–1215, 2008.

Sullivan RJ, Pantanowitz L, Dezube BJ: Targeted therapy for Kaposi's sarcoma. BioDrugs 23:69–75, 2009.

ON NHL

Lewden C, May T, Rosenthal E, et al: Changes in causes of death among adults infected by HIV between 2000 and 2005: The "Mortalite 2000 and 2005" surveys (ANRS EN19 and Mortavic). J Acquir Immune Defic Synd 48:590–598, 2008.

Lin L, Lee JY, Kaplan LD, et al: Effects of chemotherapy in AIDS-associated non-Hodgkin's lymphoma on Kaposi's sarcoma herpes virus DNA in blood. J Clin Onc 27:2496–2502, 2009.

Marti-Carvajal AJ, Cardona AF, Lawrence A: Interventions for previously untreated patients with AIDS-associated non-Hodgkin's lymphoma. Cochrane Database Syst Rev 8: CD005419, 2009.

Mwanda WO, Orem J, Fu P, et al: Dose-modified oral chemotherapy in the treatment of AIDS-related non-Hodgkin's lymphoma in East Africa. J Clin Onc 27:3480–3488, 2009.

Re A, Michieli M, Casari S, et al: High-dose therapy and autologous peripheral blood stem cell transplantation as salvage treatment for AIDS-related lymphoma: Long-term results of the Italian Cooperative Group on AIDS and Tumors (GICAT) study with analysis of prognostic factors. Blood 114:1306–1313, 2009

Sparano JA, Lee JY, Kaplan LD, et al: Rituximab plus concurrent infusional EPOCH chemotherapy is highly effective in HIV-associated B-cell non-Hodgkin's lymphoma. Blood 115:3008–3016, 2010.

ON CERVICAL AND ANAL CARCINOMAS

Chaturvedi AK, Madeleine MM, Biggar RJ, et al: Risk of human papillomavirus-associated cancers among persons with AIDS. J Natl Cancer Inst 101:1120–1130, 2009.

Cranston RD, Hirschowitz SL, Cortina G, et al: A retrospective clinical study of the treatment of high-grade anal dysplasia by infrared coagulation in a population of HIV-positive men who have sex with men. Int J STD AIDS 19:118–120, 2008.

De Vuyst H, Clifford GM, Nascimento MC, et al: Prevalence and type distribution of human papillomavirus in carcinoma and intraepithelial neoplasia of the vulva, vagina and anus: A meta-analysis. Int J Cancer 124:1626–1636, 2009.

Seo Y, Kinsella MT, Reynolds HL, et al: Outcomes of chemoradiotherapy with 5-Fluorouricil and mitomycin C for anal cancer in immunocompetent versus immunodeficient patients. nt J Radiat Oncol Biol Phys 75:143–149, 2009.

Stier EA, Goldstone SE, Berry JM, et al: Infrared coagulator treatment of high-grade anal dysplasia in HIV-infected individuals: An AIDS malignancy consortium pilot study. J Acquir Immune Defic Syndr 47:56–61, 2008.

ON NON–AIDS-DEFINING MALIGNANCIES

Bedimo RJ, McGinnis KA, Dunlap MM, et al: Incidence of non-AIDS-defining malignancies in HIV-infected versus non-infected patients in the HAART era: Impact of immunosuppression. J Acquir Immune Def Syndr 52:203–208, 2009.

Crum-Cianflone N, Hullsiek KH, Marconi V, et al: Trends in the incidence of cancers among HIV-infected persons and the impact of antiretroviral therapy: A 20-year cohort study. AIDS 23:41–50, 2009.

Deeken JF, Pantanowitz L, Dezube BJ: Targeted therapies to treat non-AIDS defining cancers in patients with HIV on HAART therapy: Treatment considerations and research outlook. Curr Opin Oncol 21:445–454, 2009.

Patel P, Hanson DL, Sullivan PS, et al: Incidence of types of cancer among HIV-infected persons compared with the general population in the United States, 1992–2003. Ann Intern Med 148:728–736, 2008.

Powles T, Robinson D, Stebbing J, et al: Highly active antiretroviral therapy and the incidence of non-AIDS-defining cancers in people with HIV infection. J Clin Oncol 27:884–890, 2009.

Abbreviations in this chapter

ACTG = AIDS Clinical Trials Group; AMC = AIDS Malignancy Consortium; ANRS = Agence Nationale de Recherche sur le Sida et les Hépatites Virales; FDA = US Food and Drug Administration; FIGO = International Federation of Gynecology and Obstetrics; SEER = Surveillance, Epidemiology and End Results

Acknowledgment: Supported, in part, by grants from the California HIV/AIDS Research Program, the UCLA Network for AIDS Research in Los Angeles (MC08-LA-710) and USPHS, NIH grants AI-69424, AI28697, CA-121947, and RR00865.

CHAPTER 25

Carcinoma of an unknown primary site

John D. Hainsworth, MD, and Lawrence M. Weiss, MD

UNKNOWN PRIMARY

Carcinoma of an unknown primary site is a common clinical syndrome, accounting for approximately 3% of all oncologic diagnoses. Patients in this group are heterogeneous, having a wide variety of clinical presentations and pathologic findings. A patient should be considered to have carcinoma of an unknown primary site when a tumor is detected at one or more metastatic sites, and routine evaluation (see below) fails to define a primary tumor site.

Although all patients with cancer of an unknown primary site have advanced, metastatic disease, universal pessimism and nihilism regarding treatment are inappropriate. Subsets of patients with specific treatment implications can be defined using clinical and pathologic features. In addition, trials of empiric chemotherapeutic regimens incorporating new antineoplastic agents have suggested improved response rates and survival in unselected groups of patients with carcinoma of an unknown primary site.

Epidemiology

Gender

Unknown primary cancer occurs with approximately equal frequency in men and women and has the same prognosis in the two genders.

Age

As with most epithelial cancers, the incidence of unknown primary cancer increases with advancing age, although a wide age range exists. Some evidence suggests that younger patients are more likely to have poorly differentiated histologies.

Disease sites

Autopsy series performed prior to the availability of CT resulted in the identification of a primary site in 70% to 80% of patients. Above the diaphragm, the lungs were the most common primary site, whereas various gastrointestinal (GI) sites (pancreas, colon, stomach, liver) were most common below the diaphragm. Several frequently occurring cancers, particularly those of the breast and prostate, were rarely identified in autopsy series.

With improved radiologic diagnosis, the spectrum of unknown primary cancer has probably changed. Limited recent autopsy data suggest a lower percentage of primary sites identified, particularly in patients with poorly differentiated histology.

Signs and symptoms

Patients with unknown primary cancer usually present with symptoms related to the areas of metastatic tumor involvement.

Sites of metastatic involvement

Sites of metastatic involvement include the lungs, liver, and skeletal system; therefore, symptoms referable to these areas are common.

Symptoms and physical findings

Constitutional symptoms, such as anorexia, weight loss, weakness, and fatigue are common.

Pathologic evaluation

Optimal pathologic evaluation is critical in the evaluation of patients with carcinoma of an unknown primary site and can aid with the following:

- distinguishing carcinoma from other cancer types,
- determining histologic type,
- identifying the primary site,
- identifying specific characteristics that may direct specific treatments.

Initial approach

Although cytologic evaluation, including fine-needle aspiration biopsy, can often determine whether a lesion is malignant, a tissue biopsy will probably be needed to further evaluate the neoplasm. Tissue is required for paraffin-section immunohistochemistry, which is currently the usual methodology of choice in the workup. Immunohistochemical methods can reliably distinguish carcinoma from other neoplasms, and can sometimes suggest a specific primary site when interpreted in conjunction with clinical features. Gene expression profile studies are now available as an additional tool in determining the tissue of origin, although more experience in the clinical setting is needed to determine how valuable this technology will be in practice. Electron microscopy, which optimally requires glutaraldehyde fixation, is usually no longer required.

Carcinoma versus other neoplasms

It is important to rule out the possibility of malignant lymphoma, malignant melanoma, and sarcoma. A battery of antibodies is utilized in an attempt to distinguish carcinoma from other types of neoplasms, as summarized in Table 1. The staining

TABLE 1: Immunohistochemical studies useful in the differential diagnosis of carcinoma vs another neoplasm

	Immunoperoxidase stains			
Tumor type	Pan-keratin	CD45 and other markers	S-100 protein	Vimentin
Carcinoma	+	–	–	–/+
Malignant lymphoma	–	+	–	–/+
Malignant melanoma	–	–	+	+
Sarcoma	–	–	–	+

result obtained with any single marker is unreliable, as exceptions may occur for each antibody. For example, although keratin is a relatively reliable marker of carcinoma, some carcinomas (eg, adrenal cortical carcinoma or undifferentiated carcinoma of the thyroid) may be keratin-negative, whereas some types of sarcoma are characteristically keratin-positive (eg, epithelioid sarcoma).

Determination of histologic type

There may be clues on initial histologic examination. For example, the presence of gland formation or mucin production would indicate an adenocarcinoma, whereas the presence of keratinization would indicate a squamous cell carcinoma. Evidence of neuroendocrine differentiation may be suggested by the presence of a characteristic, relatively fine chromatin pattern. Immunohistochemistry can also be of use, as expression of keratin subtypes 7 and 20 would favor adenocarcinoma, and expression of *p63* or keratin subtypes 5/6 and 14 would favor squamous cell carcinoma. Reliable neuroendocrine markers include chromogranin A and synaptophysin.

Determination of primary site in metastatic adenocarcinoma

Immunohistochemical staining can suggest the primary site in patients with adenocarcinoma of unknown primary site in about two-thirds of cases. Useful stains are listed in Table 2, however most of these stains must be interpreted in conjunction with tumor histology and clinical features. An exception is the prostate-specific antigen (PSA) stain, which is highly sensitive and specific for prostate adenocarcinoma.

Identification of specific treatment target characteristics

Even if the primary site is not determined, characteristics of the carcinoma may suggest specific treatment options or impart prognostic information. Examples of the former may include determination of estrogen or progesterone receptors or expression of members of the epidermal growth factor receptor family (eg, HER2/*neu*). Examples of the latter may include Ki-67, which is a surrogate marker of the proliferation rate of a neoplasm.

TABLE 2: Most useful organ-specific markers

Organ or type of cancer	Antibody
Breast	GCDFP-15, estrogen receptor
Lung	TTF-1
Gastrointestinal carcinoma	CDX-2
Stomach	CDX-2 + Hep-Par
Colon	CDX-2 + CK20
Liver	Hep-Par
Kidney	CD10 + PAX-2
Prostate	Prostate-specific antigen
Urinary bladder	CK7, CK20, CK5/6
Seminoma/embryonal carcinoma	OCT-4
Ovarian, serous	WT-1
Mesothelioma	Calretinin, CK5/6, WT1
Thyroid	TTF-1 + thyroglobulin
Neuroendocrine	Chromogranin + synaptophysin

Molecular genetic tumor profiling

Specific gene expression profiles based on the tissue of origin have been identified for many tumor types. Several assays using either quantitative reverse transcriptase polymerase chain reaction or gene microarray techniques are now available; they can be performed on tumor tissue from formalin-fixed, paraffin-embedded biopsy specimens. In tumors of a known primary, these assays can correctly identify the tissue of origin in over 85% of metastases; in unknown primary cancers, they yield diagnoses that are usually compatible with clinical features and response to empiric treatment. Clinical identification of a primary site is unusual in patients with the initial diagnosis of unknown primary cancer; however, this group provides an ideal subset for evaluating the accuracy of molecular profiling predictions. In a recent study, molecular profiling of the original biopsy yielded the "correct" diagnosis in 15 of 20 such patients.

The value of the molecular profiling diagnosis in directing therapy and improving treatment outcome is unknown, but it is being evaluated in ongoing prospective trials.

Although information is still incomplete, it is likely that gene expression profiling will be a valuable addition to the diagnosis and management of patients with these malignancies.

Clinical evaluation

After a biopsy has established metastatic carcinoma, a relatively limited clinical evaluation is indicated to search for a primary site. Recommended evaluation includes a complete history, physical examination, chemistry profile, CBC, chest radiograph, and CT scan of the abdomen.

Symptomatic areas

Specific radiologic and/or endoscopic evaluation of symptomatic areas should be pursued. In addition, mammography, ultrasonography, and breast MRI should be performed in women with clinical features suggestive of metastatic breast cancer (eg, estrogen receptor-positive tumor and/or specific metastatic involvement including axillary nodes, bones, or pleura), and serum PSA level should be measured in men with features suggestive of prostate cancer (eg, blastic bone metastasis). In young men with poorly differentiated carcinoma, serum human chorionic gonadotropin (hCG) and alpha-fetoprotein (AFP) levels should always be measured.

Asymptomatic areas

In general, radiologic or endoscopic evaluation of asymptomatic areas is not productive and should be avoided. An exception is positron emission tomography (PET) scanning, which detects a primary site in almost 40% of cases and frequently changes the approach to treatment. The PET scan is now considered a standard part of the initial evaluation of patients with carcinoma of an unknown primary site.

Cervical lymphadenopathy

Metastatic squamous carcinoma in cervical lymph nodes usually involves upper or mid-cervical locations. All patients should undergo a thorough search for a primary site in the head and neck region, including direct endoscopic examination of the oropharynx, hypopharynx, nasopharynx, larynx, and upper esophagus. Any suspicious areas should be biopsied. Fiberoptic bronchoscopy should be considered in patients with involvement of low cervical or supraclavicular nodes. This type of evaluation will identify a primary site, usually in the head and neck, in 85% to 90% of these patients. Further evaluation with PET scanning can identify a primary site in 15% to 30% of the remaining patients and should be considered. Low cervical adenopathy (level IV, supraclavicular) may also represent an upper GI primary.

Inguinal lymphadenopathy

Patients with metastatic squamous cell cancer presenting in inguinal lymph nodes almost always have an identifiable primary site in the perineal area. Women should undergo careful examination of the vulva, vagina, and cervix; men should have careful inspection of the penis. Anoscopy should be performed to exclude lesions in the anorectal area.

Treatment

Table 3 summarizes the recommended treatment for various recognized clinicopathologic subsets.

TABLE 3: Recommended treatment for recognized clinicopathologic subsets

Histopathology	Clinical subset	Treatment
Adenocarcinoma	Women with isolated axillary adenopathy	Treat as stage II breast cancer
	Women with peritoneal carcinomatosis	Treat as stage III ovarian cancer
	Men with blastic bone metastases or elevated serum PSA level	Treat as metastatic prostate cancer
	Colon cancer "profile"	Treat as metastatic colon cancer
	Single metastatic site	Local excision and/or radiation therapy
Squamous cell carcinoma	Cervical adenopathy	Treat as head/neck primary (combined-modality therapy)
	Inguinal adenopathy	Node dissection ± radiation therapy
Poorly differentiated carcinoma	Young men with a mediastinal/retroperitoneal mass	Treat as extragonadal germ-cell tumor
	Neuroendocrine features by immunoperoxidase staining or electron microscopy	Treat with platinum/etoposide-based regimen
	All others with good performance status	Treat with taxane/platinum or platinum/etoposide-based regimen
Neuroendocrine carcinoma	Well differentiated (low grade)	Treat as advanced carcinoid tumor
	Poorly differentiated or small cell	Treat with platinum/etoposide-based regimen

PSA = prostate-specific antigen

Adenocarcinoma

When evaluating patients with adenocarcinoma of an unknown primary site, several clinical subsets should be identified and treated specifically. Empiric therapy for patients not included in any of these subsets is outlined in the final section of this chapter.

Women with isolated axillary adenopathy Treatment appropriate for stage II breast cancer should be administered. Mastectomy reveals an occult primary cancer in 50% to 60% of these patients, even when physical examination and mammography are normal. Axillary dissection with breast irradiation is also a reasonable treatment, although there are no definitive comparisons of this approach versus mastectomy. Adjuvant systemic therapy, following standard guidelines for stage II breast cancer, is also indicated.

Women with peritoneal carcinomatosis Often, the histopathology in these patients suggests ovarian cancer (ie, serous cystadenocarcinoma or papillary adenocarcinoma). However, all women with this syndrome should be treated as if they had stage III ovarian cancer. Initial cytoreductive surgery should be followed by chemotherapy with a taxane/platinum combination, as recommended for advanced ovarian cancer. In these patients, serum CA-125 can often be used as a tumor marker.

Men with bone metastasis Metastatic prostate cancer should be suspected and usually can be diagnosed with either an elevated serum PSA level or positive tumor staining for PSA. In such patients, androgen deprivation therapy, as recommended for advanced prostate cancer, is often of palliative benefit.

Patients with a colon cancer "profile" Treatment with modern regimens for advanced colon cancer (eg, fluorouracil/leucovorin/oxaliplatin [Eloxatin]; FOLFOX/bevacizumab [Avastin]) should be considered for patients with a metastatic pattern (liver with or without peritoneal involvement) and pathologic findings (adenocarcinoma, CK20-positive/CK7-negative) strongly suggestive of metastatic colorectal cancer. Although clinical data to support this recommendation are still developing, the improved efficacy of advanced colon cancer regimens (versus the taxane/platinum regimens used empirically for carcinoma of an unknown primary site) provides a strong rationale.

Patients with a single metastatic site Surgical resection or radiation therapy should be administered to patients who present with clinical evidence of a single metastasis. Prior to proceeding with local therapy in these patients, PET scanning should be considered to rule out additional metastatic sites. Some of these patients have prolonged survival after local therapy, particularly those who present with a sole metastasis in an isolated peripheral lymph node group. The role of "adjuvant" systemic therapy is undetermined in these patients.

Squamous cell carcinoma

Squamous cell cancer accounts for only 10% of light microscopic diagnoses in patients with unknown primary cancer. Isolated cervical adenopathy is the most common presentation for squamous cell carcinoma of an unknown primary site; other patients have isolated inguinal adenopathy at presentation. Specific management is essential for both of these subgroups, since both have the potential for long-term survival following treatment.

Patients with cervical lymphadenopathy in whom no primary site is identified should be treated as if they had a primary site in the head and neck. Concurrent treatment with chemotherapy and radiation therapy has recently proved superior to local treatment alone and to these treatment modalities used sequentially. Radiation therapy doses and techniques should be identical to those used in treating patients with known head and neck primaries. In addition to the involved neck, the nasopharynx, oropharynx, and hypopharynx should be included in the radiation field. Radical neck dissection should be considered in patients who have any evidence of residual cancer following combined-modality therapy.

Five-year survival rates with combined-modality therapy are 60% to 70% and appear superior to results with local modalities alone (30% to 50%). The extent of cervical lymph node involvement is the most important prognostic factor. (For additional discussion, see "Unknown head and neck primary site" in chapter 1 on "Head and Neck Tumors.")

Patients with inguinal lymphadenopathy Identification of a primary site in the perineal area is important in patients with inguinal lymphadenopathy, as curative therapy is available for some patients, even after metastasis to inguinal lymph nodes. In the uncommon patient for whom no primary site is identified, inguinal node dissection, with or without radiation therapy, can result in long-term survival. Although limited data exist on this uncommon subgroup, the demonstrated superiority of combined-modality therapy versus local treatment alone for primary squamous cell cancers in the perineal area (eg, cervix, anus) has led to a suggestion that the addition of platinum-based chemotherapy may improve treatment results.

Poorly differentiated carcinoma

This heterogeneous group includes a minority of patients with highly responsive neoplasms and therefore requires special attention in initial clinical and pathologic evaluations. Specialized pathologic techniques can identify some patients with tumor types known to be treatable; these patients should be treated using standard guidelines for the appropriate tumor type.

In the remaining patients, several investigators have documented an increased responsiveness to platinum-based chemotherapy when compared with patients with adenocarcinoma of an unknown primary site. In addition, several series have described a small cohort of long-term survivors following platinum-based treatment. Patients with poorly differentiated adenocarcinoma have usually been included in this group when making treatment decisions. Although most patients in this group should receive an empiric trial of treatment, several specific subsets can be recognized.

Men with extragonadal germ-cell cancer syndrome Young men with a predominant tumor location in the mediastinum and retroperitoneum and/or high levels of serum hCG or AFP should be treated as if they had a poor prognosis germ-cell tumor (ie, four courses of chemotherapy with cisplatin/etoposide/bleomycin, followed by surgical resection of residual radiographic abnormalities).

Molecular genetic analysis can identify an i(12p) chromosomal abnormality diagnostic of a germ-cell tumor in some of these patients, even when the diagnosis cannot be made by any other pathologic evaluation. Patients with germ-cell tumors diagnosed in this manner have been shown to be as responsive to treatment as patients with extragonadal germ-cell tumors of typical histology.

Patients with poorly differentiated neuroendocrine carcinoma With the improved immunoperoxidase stains now available, neuroendocrine features are recognized more frequently in patients with poorly differentiated carcinoma. These tumors are distinct in biology and therapeutic implications from well-differentiated neuroendocrine tumors (eg, carcinoid tumors, islet-cell tumors) of an unknown primary site, which almost always present with multiple liver metastases. In contrast to typical carcinoid tumors, poorly differentiated neuroendocrine tumors are difficult to recognize by light microscopic examination alone, although some of the latter tumors have neuroendocrine or “small-cell” features.

Patients with poorly differentiated neuroendocrine carcinoma of an unknown primary site should receive a trial of chemotherapy with a regimen containing a platinum and etoposide. In a group of 51 such patients, the complete response rate was 28% following treatment with cisplatin and etoposide, with or without bleomycin; the overall response rate was 71%. Eight patients (16%) had durable complete remissions.

The combination of paclitaxel, carboplatin (Paraplatin), and etoposide is also highly active in the treatment of poorly differentiated neuroendocrine tumors (response rate, 53%; 2-year survival, 33%). However, the addition of paclitaxel increases myelosuppression and is not clearly superior to platinum/etoposide therapy.

Although the identity of most poorly differentiated neuroendocrine tumors remains unknown, this group of chemotherapy-responsive patients can be reliably identified using specialized, but widely available, pathologic evaluation.

Other patients with poorly differentiated carcinoma Most patients with poorly differentiated carcinoma do not have neuroendocrine features or clinical features of germ-cell tumor. Patients in this group should receive an empiric trial of chemotherapy, unless an extremely poor performance status precludes this possibility. In a group of 220 such patients treated with cisplatin-based regimens effective for germ-cell tumor at a single institution, the overall response rate was 64%, with 27% complete responses. Median survival of this group was 20 months, and 13% of patients have been disease-free for more than 8 years and are considered cured. Although the young median age of 39 years indicates that this was a select patient group, the extreme chemosensitivity of some patients in this large, heterogeneous group is clearly demonstrated.

Empiric chemotherapy - adenocarcinoma - nonspecific subgroup

Systemic therapy for patients not included in any specific treatable subgroup has been difficult. Unfortunately, this group includes the majority of patients with adenocarcinoma of an unknown primary site; some patients with poorly differentiated carcinoma and no “favorable” clinical features also respond poorly to current therapy.

‘Old’ regimens Table 4 summarizes results compiled from phase II trials of empiric chemotherapy. Most patients in these trials had adenocarcinoma, but 5% to 10% had poorly differentiated carcinoma. Regimens initially evaluated included historic regimens for GI malignancy and breast cancer, as well as various cisplatin-based

TABLE 4: Results of empiric chemotherapy for carcinoma of an unknown primary site[a]

Regimen	Number of patients	Response rate (%)	Median survival (mo)
Old regimens			
FAM	120	20	8
AM	197	29	5
CAF/CMeF	72	17	5
Cisplatin/5-FU–based	186	24	6
Other cisplatin-based	90	30	5
New regimens			
Paclitaxel/carboplatin/etoposide	71	46	11
Paclitaxel/carboplatin	72	41	12
Docetaxel/platinum	76	24	8
Paclitaxel/carboplatin/gemcitabine	120	25	9
Gemcitabine/cisplatin	40	42	8
Gemcitabine/docetaxel	35	40	10

A = Adriamycin (doxorubicin); C = cyclophosphamide; F = 5-FU (fluorouracil); M = mitomycin; Me = methotrexate
[a]Reported series using similar regimens have been compiled; response rates and median survivals are averages.

regimens. Most of these regimens have produced response rates of 20% to 35% and median survival durations of 5 to 8 months. There is little evidence of prolongation of median survival or long-term complete remission with any of these regimens, and none is considered "standard treatment" in this group of patients.

Regimens incorporating newer cytotoxic agents The taxanes, gemcitabine (Gemzar), and the topoisomerase I inhibitors are all broad-spectrum cytotoxic agents with potential efficacy in the treatment of an unknown primary cancer. Most experience to date has been with taxane/platinum-based regimens. Results of phase II trials suggest higher response rates and longer median survivals along with a moderate decrease in toxicity with these regimens versus previous cisplatin-based regimens (Table 4). Long-term follow-up of patients treated with paclitaxel/carboplatin/etoposide shows actual 2-year and 3-year survival rates of 20% and 14%, respectively. Recently, other combinations (eg, gemcitabine/cisplatin and gemcitabine/docetaxel

[Taxotere]) have also shown substantial activity, but further experience is required before comparisons are possible.

Targeted agents have undergone limited evaluation in patients with carcinoma of an unknown primary site. In a phase II trial, the combination of bevacizumab/erlotinib (Tarceva) showed activity in a group of previously treated patients (objective response or stable, 71%; 1-year survival, 33%). Recently, a phase II trial of first-line paclitaxel/carboplatin/bevacizumab/erlotinib produced a 53% response rate, and median progression-free and overall survivals of 8 and 13 months, respectively. Further evaluation of targeted agents is ongoing.

At present, paclitaxel/carboplatin, with or without etoposide, should be considered for empiric therapy for patients with adenocarcinoma of an unknown primary site and a good performance status.

SUGGESTED READING

Anderson, GG, Weiss L: Determining tissue of origin for metastatic cancers. Appl Immunohistochem Mol Morphol 18:3–8, 2010.

Hainsworth JD, Spigel DR, Clark BL, et al: Paclitaxel/carboplatin/etoposide versus gemcitabine/irinotecan in the first-line treatment of patients with carcinoma of unknown primary site. Cancer 16:70–75, 2010.

Hainsworth JD, Spigel DR, Thompson DS, et al: Paclitaxel/carboplatin plus bevacizumab/erlotinib in the first-line treatment of patients with carcinoma of unknown primary site. Oncologist 14:1189–1197, 2009.

Hainsworth JD, Spigel DR, Litchy S, et al: Phase II trial of paclitaxel, carboplatin, and etoposide in advanced poorly differentiated neuroendocrine carcinoma: A Minnie Pearl Cancer Research Network study. J Clin Oncol 24:3548–3554, 2006.

Horlings HM, van Laar RK, Kerst JM, et al: Gene expression profiling to identify the histogenetic origin of metastatic adenocarcinomas of unknown primary. J Clin Oncol 26:4435–4441, 2008.

Monzon FA, Lyons-Weiler M, Buturovic LJ, et al: Multicenter validation of a 1,550-gene expression profile for identification of tumor tissue of origin. J Clin Oncol 27:2503–2508, 2009.

Park SY, Yim BH, Kim JH, et al: Panels of immunohistochemical markers help determine primary sites of metastatic adenocarcinoma. Arch Pathol Lab Med 131:1561–1567, 2007.

Varadhachary GR, Raber MN, Matamoros A, et al: Carcinoma of unknown primary with a colon-cancer profile—Changing paradigm and emerging definitions. Lancet Oncol 9:561–601, 2008.

Varadhachary GR, Talantov D, Raber MN, et al: Molecular profiling of carcinoma of unknown primary and correlation with clinical evaluation. J Clin Oncol 26:4442–4448, 2008.

CHAPTER 26

Hodgkin lymphoma

Joachim Yahalom, MD, and David Straus, MD

In 2010 approximately 8,490 new cases of Hodgkin lymphoma (HL) will be diagnosed in the United States. Over the past 4 decades, advances in radiation therapy and the advent of combination chemotherapy have tripled the cure rate of patients with HL. In 2010, more than 80% of all newly diagnosed patients can expect a normal, disease-free life span.

EPIDEMIOLOGY

Gender

The male-to-female ratio of HL is 1.3:1.

Age

The age-specific incidence of the disease is bimodal, with the greatest peak in the third decade of life and a second, smaller peak after the age of 50 years.

Race

HL occurs less commonly in African-Americans (2.3 cases per 100,000 persons) than in Caucasians (3.0 per 100,000 persons).

Geography

The age-specific incidence of HL differs markedly in various countries. In Japan, the overall incidence is low, and the early peak is absent. In some developing countries, there is a downward shift of the first peak into childhood.

ETIOLOGY AND RISK FACTORS

The cause of HL remains unknown, and there are no well-defined risk factors for its development. However, certain associations have been noted that provide clues to possible etiologic factors.

Studies of young adult HL developing in one of a pair of monozygotic twins suggest a common T helper (Th) cell type 2 (Th2) cytokine profile in each twin with elevated interleukin (IL)-6 levels and decreased IL-12 levels when compared with controls. This inherited cytokine phenotype may increase the likelihood of HL development *(Cozen W et al: Blood 103:3216–3221, 2004; Cozen W et al: Blood 111:3377–3382, 2008)*. Environmental factors also may play a role. The hygiene hypothesis explains a propensity for atopy with an associated lack of a healthy Th cell type 1 response to antigenic challenge noted among patients having decreased fecal-oral exposure during early childhood. Monozygotic twins developing HL showed less fecal-oral exposure and more atopy than did unaffected twins of the same pairs *(Cozen W et al: Blood 112(11): abstract 1457, 2008)*. Thus, genetic and environmental factors may contribute to a Th2 milieu that favors HL development.

HODGKIN

Familial factors

Same-sex siblings of patients with HL have a 10 times higher risk for developing the disease. Patient-child combinations are more common than spouse pairings. Higher risk for HL is associated with few siblings, single-family houses, early birth order, and fewer playmates—all of which decrease exposure to infectious agents at an early age. The monozygotic twin sibling of a patient with HL has a 99 times higher risk of developing HL than a dizygotic twin sibling of a patient with HL. These associations suggest a genetic predisposition and/or a role for an infectious or environmental agent during childhood or early adolescence in the etiology of the disease.

Viruses

Familial aggregation may imply genetic factors, but other epidemiologic findings mentioned previously suggest an abnormal response to an infective agent. Both factors may play a role in the pathogenesis of the disease. The Epstein-Barr virus (EBV) has been implicated in the etiology of HL by both epidemiologic and serologic studies, as well as by the detection of the EBV genome in 20% to 80% of tumor specimens.

There have been no conclusive studies regarding the possible increased frequency of HL in patients with human immunodeficiency virus (HIV) infection. However, HL in HIV-positive patients is associated with an advanced stage and poor therapeutic outcome. (For further discussion of HL in patients with HIV infection, see chapter 24.)

Smoking

The incidence of HL is increased by approximately two-fold in smokers.

SIGNS AND SYMPTOMS

HL is a lymph node-based malignancy and commonly presents as an asymptomatic lymphadenopathy that may progress to predictable clinical sites.

Location of lymphadenopathy

More than 80% of patients with HL present with lymphadenopathy above the diaphragm, often involving the anterior mediastinum; the spleen may be involved in about 30% of patients. Less than 10% to 20% of patients present with lymphadenopathy limited to regions below the diaphragm. The commonly involved peripheral lymph nodes are located in the cervical, supraclavicular, and axillary areas; para-aortic pelvic and inguinal areas are involved less frequently. Disseminated lymphadenopathy is rare in patients with HL, as is involvement of Waldeyer's ring and occipital, epitrochlear, posterior mediastinal, and mesenteric sites.

Systemic symptoms

About 30% of patients experience systemic symptoms. They include fever, night sweats, or weight loss (so-called B symptoms) and chronic pruritus. These symptoms occur more frequently in older patients and have a negative impact on prognosis (see section on "Staging and prognosis").

Extranodal involvement

HL may affect extranodal tissues by direct invasion (contiguity; the so-called E lesion) or by hematogenous dissemination (stage IV disease). The most commonly involved extranodal site is the lungs. Liver, bone marrow, and bone may also be involved.

DIAGNOSIS

The initial diagnosis of HL can only be made by biopsy. Because reactive hyperplastic nodes may be present, multiple biopsies of a suspicious site may be necessary. Needle aspiration is inadequate because the architecture of the lymph node is important for diagnosis and histologic subclassification.

PATHOLOGY

Reed-Sternberg cell

In a biopsied lymph node, the R-S cell is the diagnostic tumor cell that must be identified within the appropriate cellular milieu of lymphocytes, eosinophils, and histiocytes. HL is a unique malignancy pathologically in that the tumor cells constitute a minority of the cell population, whereas normal inflammatory cells are the major cell component. As a result, it may be difficult to identify R-S cells in some specimens. Also, other lymphoproliferations may have cells resembling R-S cells.

The R-S cell is characterized by its large size and classic binucleated structure with large eosinophilic nucleoli. Two antigenic markers are thought to provide diagnostic information: CD30 (Ber-H2) and CD15 (Leu-M1). These markers are present on R-S cells and their variants but not on background inflammatory cells. It is also important to obtain a stain for CD20, since it may be positive in the minority of patients with classic HL (nodular sclerosis or mixed cellularity). The prognostic significance of CD20-positive R-S cells in classic HL is controversial.

Studies have confirmed the B-cell origin of the R-S cell. Single-cell polymerase chain reaction (PCR) analysis of classic R-S cells shows a follicular center B-cell origin for these cells with clonally rearranged but crippled V heavy-chain genes, presumably leading to inhibition of apoptosis. Also, high levels of the nuclear transcription factor-kappa-B (NF-kB) have been found in R-S cells; these high NF-kB levels may play a role in pathogenesis by interfering with apoptosis. A molecular link between R-S cells and tumor cells of mediastinal diffuse large B-cell lymphoma has been recently found in gene-profiling studies.

Histologic subtypes

According to the Rye classification (based on the number and appearance of R-S cells, as well as the background cellular milieu), there are four histologic subtypes of HL.

Nodular sclerosis

As the most common subtype, nodular sclerosis is typically seen in young adults (more commonly in females) who have early-stage supradiaphragmatic presentations. Its distinct features are the presence of (1) broad birefringent bands of collagen that divide the lymphoid tissue into macroscopic nodules and (2) an R-S cell variant, the lacunar cell.

Mixed cellularity

This is the second most common histology. It is more often diagnosed in males, who usually present with generalized lymphadenopathy or extranodal disease and with associated systemic symptoms. R-S cells are frequently identified; bands of collagen are absent, although fine reticular fibrosis may be present; and the cellular background includes lymphocytes, eosinophils, neutrophils, and histiocytes.

Lymphocyte-predominant HL

This is an infrequent form of HL in which few R-S cells or their variants may be identified. The cellular background consists primarily of lymphocytes in a nodular or sometimes diffuse pattern. The R-S variants express a B-cell phenotype (CD20-positive, CD15-negative). B-cell clonality has also been demonstrated by PCR of the immunoglobulin heavy-chain genes in single R-S variant cells in biopsy material from patients with lymphocyte-predominant HL.

This finding has led investigators to propose that lymphocyte-predominant HL is a B-cell malignancy with a mature B-cell phenotype, distinct from the other three histologic types of HL. Lymphocyte-predominant HL is often clinically localized, is usually treated effectively with irradiation alone, and may relapse late (a clinical feature reminiscent of low-grade lymphoma). The 15-year disease-specific survival is excellent (> 90%).

The WHO classification recognizes a new subtype of lymphocyte-rich classic HL that has morphologic similarity to nodular lymphocyte-predominant HL. However, the R-S cells have a classic morphology and phenotype (CD30-positive, CD15-positive, CD20-negative), and the surrounding lymphocytes are reactive T cells. This disease subtype does not show a tendency toward late relapse and should be managed like other classic HL histologies.

A recent analysis of long-term outcome in a cohort of 164 French patients with nodular lymphocyte–predominant Hodgkin lymphoma confirmed an excellent outcome regardless of treatment strategy, with a 15-year overall survival of 89%. Studies have shown that treatment, such as radiation or combined-modality therapy, compared with "watch and wait" reduces relapses (10-year progression-free survival rate of 66% vs 41%, respectively; *P* = .002), but does not yield improved overall survival; 15-year overall survival was 89% in both groups *(Biasoli I et al: Cancer 116:631–639, 2010)*. Some investigators argue that radiation-based treatment increases the chances of cure. A recent retrospective analysis of radiation treatment in 93 patients with stages I and II NLPHL showed a 10-year PFS of 85% and 61%, respectively, for patients with stage I disease. However, due to late relapses and the long indolent natural history of NLPHL, one must not overinterpret these results as definitive for the curative potential of radiation therapy *(Chen RC et al: J Clin Oncol 28:136–141, 2010)*. Histologic transformation to T-cell/histiocyte-rich diffuse large B-cell lymphoma (TCRLBCL) can also occur; it was reported in 12% of patients from one series and was associated with a lower survival rate (76%) at 10 years. This supports aggressive early diagnosis by biopsy of patients with new rapidly growing disease. These results reflect the variable albeit usually indolent behavior of NLPHL and indicate that the treatment strategy should be tailored to the clinical situation.

Lymphocyte depletion

This is a rare diagnosis, particularly since the advent of antigen marker studies, which led to the recognition that many such cases represented T-cell non-HLs (NHLs). R-S cells are numerous, the cellular background is sparse, and there may be diffuse fibrosis and necrosis. Patients usually have advanced-stage disease, extranodal involvement, an aggressive clinical course, and a poor prognosis.

Because of the limited treatment outcome predictability of current models based on pretreatment clinical factors, new predictive models have been developed using molecular and other biological markers. A model using gene expression of 10 genes determined from paraffin-embedded biopsies integrating four gene signatures (cell cycle, apoptosis, NF-kB, and monocyte-macrophage) has been found to predict 5-year freedom from progression *(Sánchez-Espiridión B et al: Blood 114 [abstract]: 3660, 2009)*. Gene-expression profiling identified a gene signature of tumor-associated macrophages in Hodgkin lymphoma biopsy specimens that was associated with primary treatment failure. An increased number of these macrophages that were CD68-positive in pretreatment biopsy samples was associated with a decreased disease-specific survival and outperformed the International Prognostic Score in multivariate analysis *(Steidl C et al: N Engl J Med 362:875–885, 2010)*.

STAGING AND PROGNOSIS

Precise definition of the extent of nodal and extranodal involvement with HL according to a standard staging classification system is critical for selection of the proper treatment strategy.

Staging system

The staging system is detailed in Table 1, and the anatomic regions that provide the basis for the staging classification are illustrated in Figure 1. The assignment of stage is based on:

- the number of involved sites
- whether lymph nodes are involved on both sides of the diaphragm and whether this involvement is bulky (particularly in the mediastinum)
- whether there is contiguous extranodal involvement (E sites) or disseminated extranodal disease
- whether typical systemic symptoms (B symptoms) are present.

In defining the disease stage, it is important to note how the information was obtained, since this fact reflects on remaining uncertainties in the evaluation for extent of disease. Clinical staging refers to information that has been obtained by initial biopsy, history, physical examination, and laboratory and radiographic studies only. A pathologic stage is determined by more extensive surgical assessment of potentially involved sites, eg, by surgical staging laparotomy and splenectomy.

Also, various designations relating to the presence or absence of B symptoms or bulky disease (see Table 1) can be applied to any disease stage. For example, a patient with no B symptoms but with a bulky mediastinal mass and involvement of the cervical lymph nodes would be defined as having CS IIAX disease. A patient with axillary disease and fever who underwent a staging laparotomy that revealed involvement of the para-aortic lymph nodes and spleen would be staged as PS III2B.

TABLE 1: The Cotswald's staging classification for Hodgkin lymphoma

Stage	Description
I	Involvement of a single lymph node region or lymphoid structure (eg, spleen, thymus, Waldeyer's ring)
II	Involvement of two or more lymph node regions on the same side of the diaphragm (ie, the mediastinum is a single site, hilar lymph nodes are lateralized). The number of anatomic sites should be indicated by a subscript (eg, II_2).
III	Involvement of lymph node regions or structures on both sides of the diaphragm: III_1: With or without involvement of splenic, hilar, celiac, or portal nodes III_2: With involvement of para-aortic, iliac, or mesenteric nodes
IV	Involvement of extranodal site(s) beyond that designated E
Designations applicable to any disease stage[a]	
A	No symptoms
B	Fever, drenching sweats, weight loss
X	Bulky disease: > 1/3 the width of the mediastinum > 10 cm maximal dimension of nodal mass
E	Involvement of a single extranodal site, contiguous or proximal to a known nodal site
CS	Clinical stage
PS	Pathologic stage

[a] For examples of how these designations are applied to disease stage, see text discussion.

Most recent studies in stage I/II disease distinguish between favorable and unfavorable early-stage disease, according to the EORTC definitions outlined in Table 2.

Clinical staging evaluation

Disease-associated symptoms

As mentioned previously, disease-associated symptoms may occur in up to one-third of patients. They may include B symptoms, pruritus, and, less commonly, pain in involved regions after ingestion of alcohol. In each anatomic stage, the presence of B symptoms is an adverse prognostic indicator and may strongly affect treatment choices. B symptoms are carefully defined in the staging system. Unexplained fever should be > 38°C and recurrent during the previous month, night sweats should be drenching and recurrent, and unexplained weight loss should be significant only if > 10% of body weight has been lost within the preceding 6 months. Although pruritus is no longer considered to be a B symptom, the presence of generalized itching may be considered to be an adverse prognostic symptom.

Certain combinations of B symptoms are more prognostically significant than others. For example, the combination of fever and weight loss has a worse prognosis than do night sweats alone.

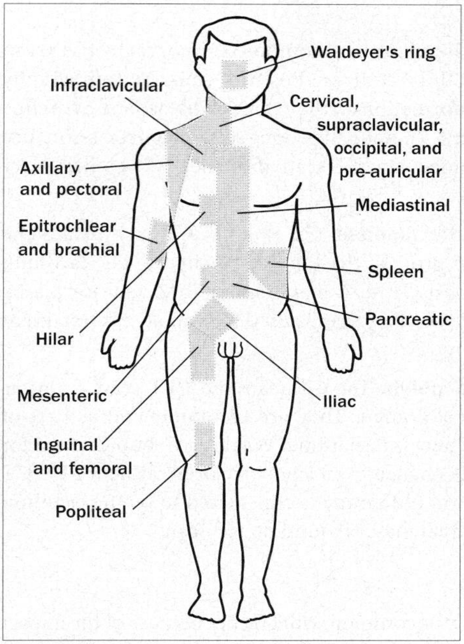

FIGURE 1: Anatomic regions for staging of Hodgkin lymphoma.

Physical examination

The physician should carefully determine the location and size of all palpable lymph nodes. Inspection of Waldeyer's ring, detection of splenomegaly or hepatomegaly, and evaluation of cardiac and respiratory status are important.

Laboratory studies

These should include a complete blood cell count with white blood cell (WBC) differential and platelet count, the erythrocyte sedimentation rate (ESR), tests for liver and renal function, and assays for serum alkaline phosphatase and lactate dehydrogenase (LDH). A moderate to marked leukemoid reaction and thrombocytosis are common, particularly in symptomatic patients, and usually disappear with treatment.

ESR studies may provide helpful prognostic information. At some centers, treatment programs for patients with early-stage disease are influenced by the degree of ESR elevation. In addition, changes in the ESR following therapy may correlate with response and relapse.

Abnormalities of liver function studies should prompt further evaluation of that organ, with imaging and possible biopsy.

Alkaline phosphatase An elevated alkaline phosphatase level may be a nonspecific marker, but it may also indicate bone involvement that should be appropriately evaluated by a radionuclide bone scan and directed skeletal radiographs.

TABLE 2: EORTC prognostic definition of early-stage disease

Favorable	CS I and II (maximum 3 involved areas) and < 50 years and ESR < 50 mm/h (no B symptoms) or ESR < 30 mm/h (B symptoms present) and MT ratio < 0.33
Unfavorable	CS II ≥ 4 nodal areas involved or age ≥ 50 years or ESR ≥ 50 mm/h (no B symptoms) or ESR ≥ 30 mm/h (B symptoms present) or MT ratio ≥ 0.33

CS = Cotswald's staging; EORTC = European Organization for Research and Treatment of Cancer; ESR = erythrocyte sedimentation rate; MT = mediastinal/thoracic

Imaging studies

Radiologic studies should include a chest x-ray and computed tomography (CT) scan of the chest, abdomen, and pelvis with IV contrast. Positron emission tomography (PET) scan will provide important information on the extent of disease and a baseline for evaluation of response to treatment. Radionuclide bone scan, magnetic resonance imaging (MRI) of the chest or abdomen, and CT scan of the neck are contributory only under special circumstances.

Evaluation for supradiaphragmatic disease The thoracic CT scan details the status of intrathoracic lymph node groups, the lung parenchyma, pericardium, pleura, and chest wall. Since the chest CT scan may remain abnormal for a long time after the completion of therapy, the PET scan is used to evaluate pretreatment involvement and response to therapy.

Evaluation of the abdomen and pelvis The CT scan and PET scan are basic imaging studies for evaluating the abdomen. They are recommended as part of initial staging and are critical in the new International Working Group Criteria for assessing response after treatment. A change from a positive pretreatment PET/CT scan to negative following completion of therapy is considered to be the criterion for complete response even if a residual mass is found on CT scan.

Bone marrow biopsy

Bone marrow involvement is relatively uncommon with HL, but because of the impact of a positive biopsy on further staging and treatment, unilateral bone marrow biopsy should be part of the staging process of patients with stage IIB disease or higher.

Lymphangiography and staging laparotomy

These two old methods of staging have been replaced by modern imaging techniques using high-resolution CT scanning and ^{18}F-fluorodeoxyglucose (FDG)-PET.

TREATMENT

HL is sensitive to radiation and many chemotherapeutic drugs, and, in most stages, there is more than one effective treatment option. Disease stage is the most important determinant of treatment options and outcome. All patients, regardless of stage, can and should be treated with curative intent.

Treatment of stage I/II disease

A common treatment choice for favorable and unfavorable early-stage HL is brief chemotherapy followed by involved-field radiotherapy (IFRT). Most of the experience that yielded excellent treatment results with low toxicity was with ABVD (Adriamycin [doxorubicin], bleomycin, vinblastine, and dacarbazine) for 4 cycles and IFRT of 30 to 36 Gy. Table 3 summarizes data from randomized studies that reported on the combination of short chemotherapy (4 or even only 2 cycles) followed by IFRT. The three top randomized studies have also indicated that adding extended-field radiotherapy (EFRT) to chemotherapy is not necessary and the small involved field is adequate.

Table 3: Results of prospective randomized studies with short chemotherapy followed by IFRT for early-stage HL

Study (# of patients)	Prognostic group	Treatment	RFS or FFTF	OS (median follow-up)
Milan (133)	Favorable and unfavorable	ABVD (4) + IFRT (36 Gy)	94%	94% (12 years)
GHSG HD8 (1,064)	Unfavorable	COPP/ABVD (4) + IFRT (30 Gy + 10 Gy to bulk)	84%	92% (5 years)
EORTC H8U (995)	Unfavorable	MOPP/ABV (4) + IFRT (36 Gy)	96%	93% (4 years)
GHSG HD10 (1,131)	Favorable	ABVD (2 or 4) + IFRT (20 or 30 Gy)	97%	99% (2 years)
GHSG HD11 (1,363)	Unfavorable	ABVD (4) or BEACOPP (4) + IFRT (20 or 30 Gy)	90%	97% (2 years)

Abbreviations: For chemotherapy, see Table 4
COPP = cyclophosphamide, Oncovin (vincristine), procarbazine, and prednisone; EORTC = European Organisation for Research and Treatment of Cancer; FFTF = freedom from treatment failure; GHSG = German Hodgkin's Study Group; HL = Hodgkin lymphoma; IFRT = involved-field radiation therapy; OS = overall survival; RFS = relapse-free survival

The most recent (and, as yet, not fully mature) excellent results are with shortening the duration of chemotherapy to only 2 cycles of ABVD in favorable patients and reducing the IFRT dose to 20 Gy (Table 3). The addition of consolidative IFRT to chemotherapy for patients with bulky disease, which usually appears in the mediastinum, remains standard treatment. However, the role of PET scans in assessing response during or after chemotherapy and the possibility of omitting radiotherapy in patients with negative PET scans are both controversial and the subject of ongoing and planned clinical trials.

Subtotal lymphoid irradiation

This therapeutic modality (ie, treatment of the mantle and para-aortic fields only) remains an adequate alternative treatment of clinically or pathologically staged favorable (nonbulky and without B symptoms) early-stage HL (stage I/II). Yet this option is no longer the treatment of choice due to the risk of second tumors and (to a lesser degree) coronary artery disease in long-term survivors of extensive radiotherapy alone as practiced in the past. In classic (non–lymphocyte-predominant) HL, subtotal lymphoid irradiation is adequate for patients who are not candidates for a chemotherapy-containing strategy.

In patients who underwent pathologic staging (laparotomy) and were treated with primary irradiation alone, several large series reported a 15- to 20-year survival rate of nearly 90% and a relapse-free survival rate of 75% to 80%. Most relapses (75%) occurred within 3 years after the completion of therapy; late relapses were uncom-

The mature data from two large randomized trials in early-stage patients with HL were recently presented by the German Hodgkin Study Group (GHSG). The HD 10 trial studied the efficacy of reducing both the number of chemotherapy cycles and the involved field radiation dose in a combined modality program *(Engert A et al: N Engl J Med 363:640–652, 2010)*. A total of 1,370 favorable patients were randomized into four arms: ABVDX4 + radiotherapy at 30 Gy; ABVDX4 + 20Gy; ABVDX2 + 30 Gy; ABVDX2 + 20 Gy. With a median follow-up of > 7 years, there were no differences in progression-free survival (PFS), freedom-from treatment failure (FFTF), and overall survival between the arms. These rates were excellent at 93% and 98%, respectively. The arm with the least treatment was almost identical to the one with the most treatment. However, toxicity from chemotherapy was significantly higher for patients randomized to ABVDX4 compared with ABVDX2, and it was slightly higher for IFRT 30 Gy than for 20 Gy. This study demonstrated the efficacy of safety of reducing treatment in favorable patients. The twin GHSG trial HD 11 *(Eich HT et al: J Clin Oncol 28:4199–4206, 2010)* randomized 1,395 patients with unfavorable early-stage HL into four arms: ABVDX4 + 30 Gy; ABVDX4 + 20 Gy; baseline BEACOPPX4 + IFRT 30 Gy. The CR rate was same for all arms: 94%. The 5-year FTTF was 85%, PFS was 86%, and OS was 94.5%. More acute side effects were recorded with baseline BEACOPP than with ABVD and with 30 Gy vs 20 Gy. When IFRT of 30 Gy was used, there was no difference in FTTF between ABVD and BEACOPP. Yet with only 20 Gy IFRT, FTTF with BEACOPP was better than with ABVD by 5.7%. The study thus suggests that in unfavorable patients, ABVDX4 should be supplemented by IFRT of 30 Gy, while if baseline BEACOPP is used, the RT dose can safely be reduced to 20 Gy.

mon. More than half of the patients who relapsed after radiotherapy alone were still curable with standard chemotherapy.

Two recently published, large, randomized trials, the EORTC H7-F trial and the GHSG HD7 trial, further established significant decreases in relapse rates at 7 and 10 years, respectively, for combined modality chemotherapy and IFRT as compared with EFRT alone. However, neither study showed a difference in survival between the two arms.

Canadian and European studies have reported excellent overall survival results in patients selected for radiotherapy on the basis of clinical prognostic factors alone. Thus, irradiation alone can be safely offered to clinically staged patients with favorable prognostic factors who are not candidates for combined-modality treatment.

Chemotherapy alone

Early results of two prospective randomized trials found extended field radiation therapy to be as effective as or superior to MOPP (mechlorethamine, [Mustargen], vincristine [Oncovin], procarbazine and prednisone) chemotherapy in improving the survival of patients with early-stage Hodgkin lymphoma. However long-term follow-up of one of the studies demonstrated significantly higher disease-free and overall survival rates at 25 years for MOPP as compared with extended-field radiation therapy.

More recently, five prospective randomized studies compared chemotherapy alone with chemotherapy followed by IFRT or regional radiotherapy in patients with early-stage HL. The Children's Cancer Group tested the role of radiation therapy in young patients (< 21 years old) who attained a complete response with risk-adapted chemotherapy (mostly COPP [cyclophosphamide, Oncovin (vincristine), procarbazine, and prednisone)/ABV [Adriamycin (doxorubicin), bleomycin, and vinblastine], 4 to 6 cycles). They enrolled 829 patients into the study (68% had early-stage disease); 501 patients who achieved a complete response were then randomized to receive either low-dose (21 Gy) IFRT or no further treatment. The accrual was stopped earlier than planned because of a significantly higher number of relapses on the no-radiotherapy arm. The 3-year event-free survival rate with an intent-to-treat analysis was 92% for patients randomized to receive radiotherapy and 87% for those randomized to receive no further treatment ($P = .057$).

The EORTC/Group d'Etude des Lymphomes de l'Adulte (GELA) conducted a large randomized trial in patients with favorable early-stage classic HL. All patients received 6 cycles of EBVP (epirubicin, bleomycin, vinblastine, and prednisone). Only patients who achieved a complete response were randomized to receive either IFRT of 36 Gy, IFRT of 20 Gy, or no irradiation. After an interim analysis, the EORTC/GELA groups closed the entry to the no-radiotherapy arm because of the excessive number of relapses. It should be noted that in previous EORTC studies, EBVP with IFRT was found to be inferior to MOPP/ABV with IFRT hybrid in patients with unfavorable disease but provided excellent results when combined with radiotherapy and was compared with radiotherapy alone in patients with favorable disease.

The NCIC and ECOG included 405 patients with nonbulky stage I/II disease. They were randomized to receive either "standard therapy," namely, subtotal nodal irradiation (STNI) for favorable patients, and ABVD (2 cycles) followed by STNI for unfavorable (B symptoms, elevated ESR, ≥ 3 sites, age ≥ 40, mixed cellularity histology) patients or experimental therapy consisting of 6 cycles or 4 cycles (if complete response was attained after 2 cycles) of ABVD and no radiotherapy. At a median follow-up of 4.2 years, progression-free survival with ABVD alone was significantly inferior ($P = .006$; hazard ratio [HR] = 2.6; 5-year estimates of disease progression-free survival, 87% vs 93%). At 5 years, no event-free or overall survival difference has been detected. The study was planned for 12 years' analysis of survival.

The MSKCC trial included 152 patients with nonbulky, early-stage HL. Patients were randomized up front to receive either ABVD for 6 cycles alone or ABVD for 6 cycles followed by radiotherapy. At 60 months, the duration of complete response and freedom from disease progression for ABVD and radiotherapy versus ABVD alone were 91% versus 87% ($P = .61$) and 86% versus 81% ($P = .61$), respectively. Overall survival was 97% with ABVD and radiotherapy vs 90% with ABVD alone ($P = .08$). Although the differences between the outcome of the two treatment groups were not statistically significant, the study was not powered to detect differences between the treatment strategies that were smaller than 20%, due to the small number of patients and events.

In a prospective, randomized study reported from India, patients with HL who achieved a complete response after ABVD were randomized to receive either IFRT or no further therapy. The 8-year event-free and overall survival rates were significantly better for the patients who received consolidation with IFRT than for those who received ABVD alone. Subset analysis indicated that the benefit from added IFRT was more prominent in advanced-stage than in early-stage disease.

A systematic review and meta-analysis of randomized controlled trials comparing chemotherapy alone versus the same chemotherapy plus radiotherapy (combined modality therapy, or CMT) in early-stage HL was performed by the Cochrane Hematological Malignancies Group. Five randomized studies involving 1,245 patients were identified. The meta-analysis showed that the patients receiving CMT had significantly better tumor control and overall survival compared with those receiving same chemotherapy alone. The hazard ratio (HR) for tumor control in CMT patients was 0.41 (CI 0.25–0.66) compared with chemotherapy alone and for overall survival HR was 0.40 (CI 0.27–0.59) in favor of CMT *(Herbst C et al: Haematologica 95:494–500, 2010).*

The NCCN guidelines recommend combined-modality therapy or ABVD or Stanford V alone as treatment options for favorable or unfavorable classic HL. For patients with bulky mediastinal involvement, combined-modality therapy remains the standard of care. The standard treatment by NCCN category 1 is ABVD + RT and by category 2B is chemotherapy alone.

However, because of concern about the late morbidity and mortality related to radiotherapy, including second malignancies and cardiovascular complications, some medical oncologists favor the use of chemotherapy only for patients with nonbulky stages I and II HL. The treatment regimen employed is usually 6 cycles of ABVD or 4–6 cycles of ABVD (complete response + 2 additional cycles).

Technical aspects of radiation therapy

IFRT and involved-node radiotherapy (INRT)

In a combined-modality setting, irradiation of the involved lymph node chain, with or without adjacent sites, and tailoring of the field borders to the postchemotherapy tumor volume (in critical areas such as the mediastinum) are recommended. IFRT is the most appropriate irradiation approach after chemotherapy. IFRT or regional radiotherapy alone is used for lymphocyte-predominant HL. Recommendations for IFRT for HL are detailed in an article by Yahalom and Mauch. Recently, further reduction in IFRT has been introduced and implemented in EORTC/GELA studies. The INRT field is limited to the prechemotherapy lymph node(s) volume, and, in the mediastinum, it also accounts for the reduction of mass after chemotherapy.

The transition into INRT fields or reduced IFRT markedly reduces the exposure of normal structures in most cases; the safety of field reduction has recently been reported.

Extended radiation fields

Successful therapy with irradiation alone in classic HL requires treatment of all clinically involved lymph nodes and all nodal and extranodal regions at risk for subclinical involvement (Figure 2). The HL radiation fields were designed to conform to the philosophy of treating regions beyond the immediately involved area while accounting for normal tissue tolerance and the technical constraints of field size. The extended radiation fields are inappropriate when radiation is administered as consolidation following chemotherapy and, thus, they are rarely used today.

Dose considerations

When irradiation alone is used to treat HL, the standard total dose to each field is 3,600 cGy, delivered in daily fractions of 180 cGy over 4 weeks. In addition, clinically involved areas are given a boost of 360 to 540 cGy in 2 to 3 fractions to bring the total dose to these areas up to 3,960 to 4,140 cGy. Patients who receive irradiation as consolidation after chemotherapy receive a total dose of 2,000 to 3,600 cGy in 150- to 180-cGy fractions. We normally use opposed anterior and posterior fields that are evenly weighted and treat both fields daily. Three-dimensional conformal radiotherapy and intensity-modulated radiation therapy (IMRT) are employed for selected cases.

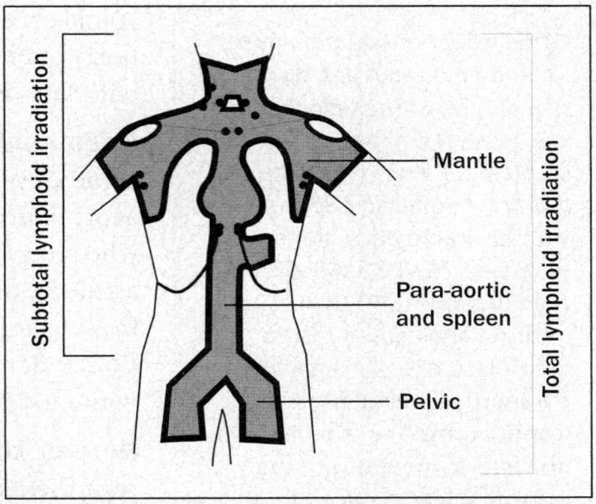

FIGURE 2: Extended radiation fields used for treatment of classic Hodgkin lymphoma with irradiation alone.

Recent studies suggest that a reduction in the size of radiation fields and doses delivered may decrease the risk of breast cancer.

Side effects and complications of radiotherapy

Side effects of radiotherapy depend on the irradiated volume, dose administered, and technique employed. They are also influenced by the extent and type of prior chemotherapy, if any, and by the patient's age.

Acute effects

The potential acute side effects of involved fields in the upper body include mouth dryness, change in taste, pharyngitis, nausea, dry cough, dermatitis, and fatigue. These side effects are usually mild and transient.

The main potential side effects of subdiaphragmatic irradiation are loss of appetite, nausea, and increased bowel movements. These reactions are usually mild and can be minimized with standard antiemetic medications.

Irradiation of more than one field, particularly after chemotherapy, can cause myelosuppression, which may necessitate treatment delays.

Delayed effects

Delayed side effects may develop anywhere from several weeks to several years after the completion of radiotherapy.

Lhermitte's sign Approximately 15% of patients who receive the full dose of radiation to the neck may note an electric shock sensation radiating down the backs of both legs when the head is flexed (Lhermitte's sign) 6 weeks to 3 months after mantle-field radiotherapy. Possibly secondary to transient demyelinization of the

The effect of radiation dose and field reduction on the risk of long-term complications was analyzed in two recent studies. A French collaborative group randomized 188 patients with favorable early-stage HL to receive ABVDX3 followed by radiotherapy at 40 Gy to the involved sites and 30 Gy to uninvolved sites, including the paraaortic and splenic areas (control arm). The experimental arm was same but with the radiation dose reduced to 30 Gy to involved areas and 24 Gy to uninvolved sites. While FFTF and OS were the same in both arms, long-term severe adverse events, either cardiac or second tumors, at a median follow-up of 10 years were observed only in the control arm with the higher radiation doses. Rates of complications in the control group were similar to those of patients in an older study who were treated with the higher doses of RT (and ABVDX3) *(Arakelyan N et al: Cancer 116:4054–4062, 2010)*. In a recent study, researchers from the Netherlands Cancer Institute analyzed 1,122 female 5-year survivors treated for HL between 1965 and 1995; 806 were irradiated (36–44 Gy) to a mantle field that includes the bilateral axillae or axillae alone, while in 126 patients who received radiation only to the mediastinum, the axillae (and thus most of the breast tissue) were spared from radiation. Sparing the axillae markedly reduced the risk of breast cancer (by 2.7-fold) compared with patients who received a full mantle field. Nowadays, in most patients treated with involved field RT, the axillae are not included *(De Bruin ML et al: J Clin Oncol 27:4239–4246, 2009)*.

spinal cord, Lhermitte's sign resolves spontaneously after a few months and is not associated with late or permanent spinal cord damage.

Pneumonitis and pericarditis During the same period, radiation pneumonitis and/or acute pericarditis may occur in < 5% of patients who receive large fields of radiation to the mediastinum; these side effects occur more often in those who have extensive mediastinal disease. Both inflammatory processes have become rare with modern radiation techniques.

Herpes zoster infection Patients with HL, regardless of treatment type, have a propensity to develop herpes zoster infection within 2 years after therapy. Usually, the infection is confined to a single dermatome and is self-limited. If the cutaneous eruption is identified promptly, treatment with systemic acyclovir will limit its duration and intensity.

Subclinical hypothyroidism

Radiotherapy of the neck can induce subclinical hypothyroidism in about one-third of patients. This condition is detected by elevation of thyroid-stimulating hormone. Thyroid replacement with levothyroxine is recommended, even in asymptomatic patients, to prevent overt hypothyroidism and decrease the risk of benign thyroid nodules.

Infertility

Irradiation of the pelvis may have deleterious effects on fertility. In most patients, this problem can be avoided by appropriate gonadal shielding. In females, the ovaries can be moved into a shielded area laterally or inferomedially near the uterine cervix. Irradiation fields that spare the pelvis do not increase the risk of sterility.

Secondary malignancies

The rate of second malignancies following radiation therapy with or without chemotherapy for HL is approximately 1% per year. The most common second malignancies were breast cancer, gastrointestinal cancers, lung cancer, thyroid cancer, soft tissue and bone sarcomas, and acute leukemias, which are associated with chemotherapy as mentioned earlier in this chapter. The risk of developing breast cancer following radiation therapy increases with length of follow-up. Addition of alkylating agent–containing chemotherapy of the MOPP type seems to reduce this risk, probably because of effects on the ovaries that reduce estrogen production. The risk is increased with larger fields and higher doses of RT. Among solid tumors, only alkylating agent–based regimens of the MOPP type are associated with an increased risk of lung cancer. Second malignancies are the leading cause of late morbidity and mortality in early-stage patients cured of HL.

Lung cancer Patients who are smokers should be strongly encouraged to quit the habit because the increase in lung cancer that occurs after irradiation or chemotherapy with alkylating agents has been detected mostly in smokers. Alkylating agents (such as in the MOPP regimen) and radiation therapy were associated with an increased risk of lung cancer in an additive and dose-dependent fashion. These effects were multiplied by tobacco use (see "Suggested Reading").

Breast cancer The increase in breast cancer risk is inversely related to the patient's age at HL treatment; no increased risk has been found in women irradiated after 30 years of age. The risk of breast cancer is increased with higher radiation breast dose and is reduced in patients who received chemotherapy or ovarian irradiation that induced early menopause.

In most situations, modern IFRT should spare the breast. Breast cancer is curable in its early stages, and early detection has a significant impact on survival. Breast examination should be part of the routine follow-up for women cured of HL, and routine mammography should begin about 8 years after treatment.

Cardiovascular disease

An increased risk of cardiovascular morbidity has been reported among patients who have received mediastinal irradiation. In a retrospective study evaluating the cardiac risks of 450 patients cured of HL with radiotherapy alone or in combination, 42 patients (10%) developed coronary artery disease (CAD) at a median of 9 years after treatment, 30 patients (7%) developed carotid and/or subclavian artery disease at a median of 17 years after treatment, and 25 patients (6%) developed clinically significant valvular dysfunction at a median of 22 years after treatment. The most common valve lesion was aortic stenosis, which occurred in 14 valves. The only treatment-related factor associated with the development of CAD was use of a radiation technique that resulted in a higher total dose to a portion of the heart (relative risk [RR] = 7.8; 95% CI = 1.1–53.2; *P*=.04). No specific treatment-related factor was associated with carotid or subclavian artery disease or valvular dysfunction. Freedom from cardiovascular morbidity was 88% at 15 years and 84% at 20 years.

To reduce this hazard, radiation fields should conform to the involved postchemotherapy volume, and the dose should be reduced to 20 to 30 Gy, if possible. Patients who have received radiation to the mediastinum should be monitored and advised about other established CAD risk factors, such as smoking, hyperlipidemia, hypertension, and poor dietary and exercise habits. Cholesterol levels should be monitored and treated if elevated.

> **In a cohort of 2,201 people who were 5-year survivors of Hodgkin lymphoma treated between 1965 and 1995, irradiation of the neck and mediastinum was associated with a 2.55 increased risk of ischemic cerebrovascular disease** *(De Bruin ML et al: J Natl Cancer Inst 101:928–937, 2009).*

The risk of late mortality from MI is increased with use of supradiaphramatic radiotherapy, especially total nodal radiation therapy. The risk also was higher in patients given various chemotherapy regimens (particularly ABVD) with, and even without, supradiaphragmatic radiotherapy.

Effects on bone and muscle growth

In children, high-dose irradiation will affect bone and muscle growth and may result in deformities. Current treatment programs for pediatric HL are chemotherapy-based; radiotherapy is limited to low doses.

Treatment of stage III/IV disease

Chemotherapy has become curative for many patients with advanced stages of HL. MOPP has been the primary effective combination chemotherapy regimen for advanced-stage disease since the 1960s. Over the past several years, ABVD has been shown to be more effective and less toxic than MOPP, particularly with respect to sterility and secondary leukemia.

Combination chemotherapy regimens

Doxorubicin-containing regimens A doxorubicin-containing regimen, such as ABVD (Table 4), is the treatment of choice for patients presenting with stage III or IV disease, as demonstrated by a randomized phase III trial undertaken by the CALGB. This trial showed higher complete response rates with ABVD and ABVD/MOPP (82% and 83%, respectively) than with MOPP alone (65%).

One reason for the improved response rate in the groups treated with doxorubicin-containing regimens was the higher percentage of patients who were able to receive ≥ 85% of the expected chemotherapy dose, particularly in the ABVD group. In addition, rates of significant and life-threatening neutropenia were higher in patients treated with the MOPP-containing regimens than in those treated with other regimens.

Subsequent trials compared ABVD, alternating MOPP/ABVD, and a MOPP/ABV hybrid. Alternating MOPP/ABVD and the MOPP/ABV hybrid was found to be equally effective in treating advanced-stage HL. However, an intergroup study that compared ABVD with MOPP/ABV hybrid (without irradiation) was closed early because of concerns of excess treatment-related deaths and second malignancies (mostly acute myelogenous leukemia and lung cancer) in the MOPP/ABV hybrid arm. ABVD and MOPP/ABV hybrid yielded similar 5-year failure and overall survival rates.

Shortened dose-intense regimens Shortened dose-intense regimens have shown promise. For example, the 12-week Stanford V regimen (see Table 4) combined with IFRT produced a 5-year overall survival rate of 96% and a freedom-from-disease-progression rate of 89%. The freedom-from-disease-progression rate was significantly superior among patients with a prognostic score of 0–2, compared with those with a score of 3 and higher (94% vs 75%; $P = .0001$). Of interest, in 142 patients from Stanford, no secondary leukemia was observed, and 42 pregnancies were reported.

TABLE 4: Chemotherapeutic regimens used for the treatment of Hodgkin lymphoma

Regimen	Dosage and schedule	Frequency
MOPP		
Mechlorethamine	6 mg/m^2 IV on day 1	
Vincristine (Oncovin)	1.4 mg/m^2 IV on day 1 (maximum dose, 2.0 mg)	
Procarbazine	100 mg/m^2 PO on days 1–7	Repeat cycle
Prednisone[a]	40 mg/m^2 PO on days 1–14	every 28 days.
ABVD		
Doxorubicin (Adriamycin)	25 mg/m^2 IV on days 1 and 15	
Bleomycin	10 mg/m^2 IV on days 1 and 15	
Vinblastine	6 mg/m^2 IV on days 1 and 15	Repeat cycle
Dacarbazine	375 mg/m^2 IV on days 1 and 15	every 28 days.
BEACOPP		
Bleomycin	10 mg/m^2 IV on day 8	
Etoposide	100 mg/m^2 (200 mg/m^2)[b] IV on days 1–3	
Doxorubicin (Adriamycin)	25 mg/m^2 (35 mg/m^2)[b] IV on day 1	
Cyclophosphamide	650 mg/m^2 (1,200 mg/m^2)[b] IV on day 1	
Vincristine (Oncovin)	1.4 mg/m^2 IV on day 8[c]	
Procarbazine	100 mg/m^2 PO on days 1–7	
Prednisone	40 mg/m^2 PO on days 1–14	Repeat cycle
G-CSF from day 8		every 21 days.
Stanford V		
Doxorubicin	25 mg/m^2 IV on days 1 and 15	Repeat cycle
Vinblastine	6 mg/m^2 IV on days 1 and 15	every 28 days for
Mechlorethamine	6 mg/m^2 IV on day 1	a total of 3 cycles.
Vincristine[d]	1.4 mg/m^2 IV on days 8 and 22	Radiotherapy to
Bleomycin	5 U/m^2 IV on days 8 and 22	initial sites ≥ 5 cm
Etoposide	60 mg/m^2 IV on days 15 and 16	(dose: 36 cGy).
Prednisone[e]	40 mg/m^2 PO every other day	

[a] In the original report, prednisone was given only in cycles 1 and 4.
[b] Increased dose for BEACOPP
[c] Maximal dose of 2 mg
[d] Vinblastine dose was decreased to 4 mg/m^2 and vincristine dose to 1 mg/m^2 during cycle 3 for patients ≥ 50 years of age.
[e] Tapered by 10 mg every other day starting at week 10
G-CSF = granulocyte colony-stimulating factor

An escalated dose version of BEACOPP (bleomycin, etoposide, Adriamycin [doxorubicin], cyclophosphamide, Oncovin [vincristine], procarbazine, and prednisone) was found to have a statistically significant superior freedom from treatment failure at 5 years compared with standard-dose BEACOPP and alternating monthly COPP and ABVD for patients with advanced stages of HL. Short-term hematologic toxicity was greatest for escalated BEACOPP, and a significant increased risk for secondary acute leukemias was also seen as compared with standard-dose BEACOPP and COPP/ABVD.

In advanced-stage disease, PET scanning during or after chemotherapy is emerging as a powerful predictor of outcome. Patients with advanced-stage disease who have positive PET scans after 2 cycles of ABVD are at a higher risk of relapse following treatment than are patients who have negative PET scans. Risk-adapted clinical trials based on this finding, which also holds true in early-stage HL, currently are ongoing and opening in the United States and Europe. At present, a change in therapy due to PET scan results during treatment cannot be recommended outside of the setting of a clinical trial. The PET scan currently is standard for assessing response after the completion of therapy.

Combined-modality therapy

Although the role of consolidation radiotherapy after induction chemotherapy remains controversial, irradiation is routinely added in patients with advanced-stage disease who present with bulky disease or who remain in uncertain complete remission after chemotherapy. Retrospective studies have demonstrated that adding low-dose radiotherapy to all initial disease sites after chemotherapy-induced complete response decreases the relapse rate by ~25% and significantly improves overall survival.

Interpretation of the impact of irradiation in prospective studies has been controversial. However, a SWOG randomized study of 278 patients with stage III or IV HL suggested that the addition of low-dose irradiation to all sites of initial disease after a complete response to MOP-BAP (mechlorethamine, Oncovin [vincristine], prednisone, bleomycin, Adriamycin [doxorubicin], and procarbazine) chemotherapy improves the duration of remission in patients with advanced-stage disease. An intention-to-treat analysis showed that the advantage of combined-modality therapy was limited to patients with nodular sclerosis. No survival differences were observed.

A meta-analysis demonstrated that the addition of radiotherapy to chemotherapy reduced the rate of relapse but did not show a survival benefit for the combined-modality approach.

The EORTC conducted a randomized trial in patients with stages III and IV HL in which those achieving a complete remission with MOPP/ABV hybrid were randomized to receive either low-dose IFRT or no radiotherapy. Of the 739 patients enrolled, 421 achieved a complete remission. The median follow-up was 79 months. There was no statistically significant difference in 5-year event-free or overall survival. Partial responders received low-dose IFRT, and their event-free and overall survival rates were similar to those patients who achieved a complete remission.

More recently, an analysis of data collected prospectively within a randomized controlled trial of induction chemotherapy that included ABVD showed that patients who received consolidation radiotherapy had significantly better 5-year PFS and OS compared with those who had not received radiation (see sidebar).

The Medical Research Council (MRC) clinical trial unit (London, UK) reported on the effect of consolidation radiotherapy in patients with advanced-stage Hodgkin lymphoma treated in the UKLG LY09 randomized controlled trial. A total of 807 patients with advanced-stage HL were randomized to receive either six to eight cycles of ABVD or two prespecified multidrug regimens. A total of 706 patients achieved an objective response, and at a median follow-up of 7 years there were no outcome differences between the chemotherapy regimens. Post-chemotherapy radiotherapy (RT) consolidation was given to 300 patients on a physician's-choice basis. (The protocol provided only guidance for considering RT for patients with residual masses or to sites of original bulk.) Thus when comparing RT patients vs no-RT patients, in the RT group there were significantly more patients with partial response or with bulky disease, while other baseline characteristics were similar. The 5-year progression-free survival (PFS) and overall survival (OS) rates were significantly superior in patients who received RT, compared with those who received only chemotherapy, 86% vs 71%; *P* < .0001 (for PFS), and 93% vs 87%; *P* = .0014 (for OS), respectively. There was no evidence of heterogeneity of radiation treatment effect across subgroups *(Johnson PW et al: J Clin Oncol 28:3352–3359, 2010)*.

Long-term toxicities of combination chemotherapy

The CALGB trial and the intergroup trials mentioned previously (see section on "Combination chemotherapy regimens") noted differences in the long-term toxicities of various combination chemotherapeutic regimens.

Myelodysplasia and acute leukemia

MOPP therapy is known to be related to the development of myelodysplastic syndromes and acute leukemia. These secondary hematologic malignancies begin 2 years following therapy and decline by 10 years, with the maximum risk between 5 and 9 years. Patients with these malignancies have a poor prognosis.

The incidence of secondary leukemia appears to increase with cumulative doses of chemotherapy, age > 40 years when receiving chemotherapy for HL, and splenectomy. It is controversial whether combined-modality therapy increases the risk of leukemia compared with chemotherapy alone.

Cytogenetic studies of secondary leukemias reveal a loss of the long arm of chromosome 5 and/or 7. Less frequently, there is a loss of chromosome 18 or rearrangement of the short arm of chromosome 17. A balanced rearrangement of 11q23 and 2lq22 also has been described with etoposide therapy.

Other malignancies

Other types of cancer also are being observed with increasing frequency after chemotherapy (most regimens included alkylating agents), particularly for lung cancer and NHL. These malignancies have a longer latency period and usually are not observed until 15 years after therapy.

Infertility

The inability to conceive a child after trying for 1 year is another long-term complication seen with combination chemotherapy. At least 80% of males have permanent azoospermia or oligospermia following more than 3 cycles of MOPP chemotherapy; < 10% of men will have recovery of spermatogenesis within 1–7 years following the end of chemotherapy. The risk of infertility with ABVD chemotherapy is significantly lower (~ 15%–25%) than that with MOPP. All men who desire childbearing potential following therapy should be counseled regarding sperm banking.

In females, there is a 50% rate of primary ovarian failure overall. The risk is 25% to 30% in patients treated at age 25 or younger but increases to 80% to 100% in women older than age 25. Many women who maintain ovarian function during chemotherapy will have premature menopause following therapy.

Female fertility appears to be well preserved following administration of ABVD, which does not contain alkylating agents of the nitrogen mustard type or procarbazine. Male fertility also probably is better preserved with such treatment, although this finding is not as well documented.

Pulmonary complications

Lung problems have been reported with ABVD chemotherapy and are related to bleomycin-induced lung toxicity. In a MSKCC study of 60 patients with early-stage HL receiving ABVD chemotherapy with or without mediastinal irradiation, bleomycin was discontinued in 23% of patients. Following ABVD therapy, there was a significant decline in median forced vital capacity (FVC) and diffusing capacity of the lungs for carbon monoxide. Radiotherapy following ABVD chemotherapy resulted in a further decrease in FVC but did not significantly affect functional status. In a study from the Mayo Clinic, bleomycin pulmonary toxicity (BPT) was observed in 18% of patients. Increasing age and use of ABVD and granulocyte colony-stimulating factor were associated with development of BPT. Patients with BPT had a 5-year overall survival of only 63% as compared with 90% (P = .001) in patients without BPT. Mortality from BPT was 4.2% in all patients and 24% in those who developed BPT. The omission of bleomycin had no effect on obtaining complete remission or on progression-free or overall survival.

In the CALGB trial, there were 3 fatal pulmonary complications in 238 patients; all 3 patients were older than age 40.

Pulmonary fibrosis has also been described after combined-modality therapy. Pulmonary function testing usually reveals a decreased diffusion capacity and restrictive changes prior to the onset of symptoms.

Cardiomyopathy

Deteriorated myocardial function is a recognized complication of doxorubicin therapy but is not commonly seen in patients receiving ABVD chemotherapy. Patients who are treated with 6 cycles of ABVD chemotherapy receive a total doxorubicin dose of 300 mg/m^2; cardiac toxicity is rarely seen in patients who receive a total dose ≤ 400 mg/m^2.

Management of relapsed disease

Relapse after radiation therapy

Patients with early-stage HL who relapse after initial therapy with irradiation alone have excellent complete remission rates and 50% to 80% long-term survival rates when treated with MOPP or ABVD. The dose regimens used for salvage therapy are the same as those outlined in Table 4.

An increase in acute myeloid leukemias, possibly partly related to etoposide, has been reported at 10 years with the BEACOPP regimen (bleomycin, etoposide, doxorubicin [Adriamycin], cyclophosphamide, vincristine [Oncovin], procarbazine, and prednisone), in both the standard-dose (1.5%) and escalated (3.0%) versions, as compared with cyclophosphamide, vincristine, procarbazine, prednisone (COPP)/ABVD (0.4%) *(Engert A et al: J Clin Oncol 27:4548–4554, 2009).*

Relapse after combination chemotherapy

Among patients with advanced-stage HL, 70% to 90% will have a complete response to treatment; however, up to one-third of patients with stage III or IV disease will relapse, usually within the first 3 years after therapy.

Various studies have identified the following poor prognostic factors for response to first-line chemotherapy: B symptoms, age > 45 years, bulky mediastinal disease, extranodal involvement, low hematocrit, high ESR, high levels of CD30, and high levels of serum interleukin-10 (IL-10) and soluble IL-2 receptor.

An International Prognostic Index (IPI) has been devised for advanced HL based on a retrospective analysis of 1,618 patients from 25 centers. In the final model, seven factors were used: albumin < 4 g/dL, hemoglobin < 10.5 g/dL, male gender, stage IV disease, age ≥ 45 years, WBC ≥ 15,000/µL, and lymphocytes < 600/µL (or 8% of the WBC count). The worst prognostic group (7%) had a 5-year overall survival rate of 56% and a failure-free survival rate of 42%.

In a comparison of seven well-known prognostic models for HL applied retrospectively to a population of patients with advanced-stage disease, three were found to be the most predictive of outcome. One was the IPI, and the other two were the MSKCC model (employing age, LDH, hematocrit, inguinal nodal involvement, and mediastinal mass bulk) and the Database on Hodgkin Lymphoma model (employing stage, age, B symptoms, albumin level, and gender). Integration of the three models in a linear model improved their predictive power.

High-dose therapy with autologous stem-cell transplantation The preferred salvage method for patients who relapsed after combined-modality therapy or chemotherapy alone or remained refractory to those programs is high-dose chemoradiotherapy with autologous stem-cell transplantation (ASCT).

Two randomized studies (from Great Britain and Germany) demonstrated an event-free survival advantage with the high-dose therapy approach. Although a significant survival advantage was not observed due to the crossover design of the studies, most patients with refractory disease or postchemotherapy relapse are currently managed with high-dose chemoradiation therapy and ASCT.

> **S**everal new and novel agents have recently shown promise for treatment of relapsed and refractory Hodgkin lymphoma. These include an immunotoxin SGN-35 (anti-CD30 antibody conjugated with anti-tubulin agent monomethyl auristatin E)*(Bartlett N et al: J Clin Oncol 27[15s]:8500, 2009)*, panobinostat (LBH589; pan-deacetylase inhibitor; *Younes A et al: Blood 114 [abstract]:923, 2009)*, lenalidomide (Revlimid; immune-modulatory inhibitor; *Fehniger TA et al: Blood 114 [abstract]:3693, 2009)* and bendamustine (Treanda; novel alkylating agent; *Moskowitz AJ et al: Blood 114 [abstract]:720, 2009)*. A phase II trial of everolimus (Afinitor; m-TOR inhibitor) in relapsed and refractory Hodgkin lymphoma has also been opened recently (http://clinicaltrials.gov/show/NCT01022996).

No standard conditioning regimen has been used in this setting, as patients have had prior treatment with a variety of combinations of chemotherapy and radiation therapy. Most patients who have received bone marrow have been treated with several regimens or have had poorly responsive disease from initial diagnosis, but the complete response rate has ranged from 50% to 80%, with approximately 40% to 80% of responding patients achieving durable remission.

Analysis of prognostic factors in patients receiving high-dose salvage therapy indicated that B symptoms at relapse, extranodal disease, and short (< 1 year) remission or no remission are associated with a poor outcome.

A study from MSKCC reported the results of high-dose chemotherapy with ASCT in 65 patients with relapsed or refractory HL. At a median follow-up of 43 months, overall survival was estimated to be 73%, and event-free survival was estimated to be 58% by intent-to-treat analysis. In a multivariate logistic regression model, there were three adverse prognostic factors: extranodal sites of relapse or refractory disease, complete remission duration of < 1 year or refractory disease, and B symptoms. Patients with no or one adverse factor had an overall survival of 90% and an event-free survival of 83%, those with two adverse factors had an overall survival of 57% and an event-free survival of 27%, and those with three adverse factors had an overall survival of 25% and an event-free survival of 10%. A follow-up study of a risk-adapted approach based on the study previously described suggested that patients with adverse prognostic factors may benefit from further augmentation of high-dose programs, including a "double-transplant" for selected patients.

SUGGESTED READING

Aleman BM, Raemaekers JM, Tomisic R, et al: Involved-field radiotherapy for patients in partial remission after chemotherapy for advanced Hodgkin's lymphoma. Int J Radiat Oncol Biol Phys 67:19–30, 2007.

Aleman BM, van den Belt-Dusebout AW, De Bruin ML, et al: Late cardiotoxicity after treatment for Hodgkin lymphoma. Blood 109:1878–1886, 2007.

Bartlett NL: Modern treatment of Hodgkin lymphoma. Curr Opin Hematol 15:408–414, 2008.

Brice P: Managing relapsed and refractory Hodgkin lymphoma. Br J Haematol 141:3–13, 2008.

Cheson BD, Pfistner B, Juweid ME, et al: Revised response criteria for malignant lymphoma. J Clin Oncol 25:579–586, 2007.

Chetaille B, Bertucci F, Finetti P, et al: Molecular profiling of classical Hodgkin lymphoma tissues uncovers variations in the tumor microenvironment and correlations with EBV infection and outcome. Blood 113:2765–3775, 2009.

Eichenauer DA, Bredenfeld H, Haverkamp H, et al: Hodgkin's lymphoma in adolescents treated with adult protocols: A report from the German Hodgkin study group. J Clin Oncol 27:6079–6085, 2009.

Engert A, Diehl V, Franklin J, et al: Escalated-dose BEACOPP in the treatment of patients with advanced-stage Hodgkin's lymphoma: 10 years of follow-up of the GHSG HD9 study. J Clin Oncol 27:4548–4554, 2009.

Engert A, Franklin J, Eich HT, et al: Two cycles of doxorubicin, bleomycin, vinblastine, and dacarbazine plus extended-field radiotherapy is superior to radiotherapy alone in early favorable Hodgkin's lymphoma: Final results of the GHSG HD7 trial. J Clin Oncol 25:3495–3502, 2007.

Gallamini A, Hutching M, Rigacci L, et al: Early interim 2-[18F]fluoro-2-deoxy-D-glucose positron emission tomography is prognostically superior to international prognostic score in advanced-stage Hodgkin's lymphoma: A report from a joint Italian-Danish study. J Clin Oncol 25:3746–3752, 2007.

Girinsky T, Specht L, Ghalibafian M, et al: The conundrum of Hodgkin lymphoma nodes: To be or not to be included in the involved node radiation fields. The EORTC-GELA lymphoma group guidelines. Radiother Oncol 88:202–210, 2008.

Goodman KA, Riedel E, Serrano V, et al: Long-term effects of high-dose chemotherapy and radiation for relapsed and refractory Hodgkin's lymphoma. J Clin Oncol 26:5240–5247, 2008.

Hodgson DC: Hodgkin lymphoma: The follow-up of long-term survivors. Hematol Oncol Clin North Am 22:233–244, vi, 2008.

Hodgson DC, Pintille M, Gitterman L, et al: Fertility among female Hodgkin lymphoma survivors attempting pregnancy following ABVD chemotherapy. Hematol Oncol 25:11–15, 2007.

Hoppe RT, Hira Advani R, Ambinder RF, et al: NCCN physician guidelines: Hodgkin Lymphoma 2010. Available at: www.nccn.org.

Kobe C, Dietlein M, Franklin J, et al: Positron emission tomography has a high negative predictive value for progression or early relapse for patients with residual disease after first-line chemotherapy in advanced-stage Hodgkin lymphoma. Blood 112:3989–3994, 2008.

Ma Y, Visser L, Roelofsen H, et al: Proteomics analysis of Hodgkin lymphoma: Identification of new players involved in the cross-talk between HRS cells and infiltrating lymphocytes. Blood 111:2339–2346, 2008.

Moskowitz C, Sweetenham J: The role of hematopoietic stem cell transplantation in hodgkin lymphoma. Cancer Treat Res 144:1–16, 2009.

Moskowitz CH, Yahalom J, Zelenetz AD, et al: High-dose chemo-radiotherapy for relapsed or refractory hodgkin lymphoma and the significance of pre-transplant functional imaging. Br J Haematol, 148:890–897, 2010.

Noordijk EM, Carde P, Dupouy N, et al: Combined-modality therapy for clinical stage I or II Hodgkin's lymphoma: Long-term results of the European Organisation for Research and Treatment of Cancer H7 randomized controlled trials. J Clin Oncol 24:3128–3135, 2006.

Sarina B, Castagna L, Farina L, et al: Allogeneic transplantation improves the overall and progression-free survival of Hodgkin lymphoma patients relapsing after autologous transplantation: A retrospective study based on the time of HLA typing and donor availability. Blood 115:3671–3677.

Tsai HK, Mauch PM: Nodular lymphocyte-predominant hodgkin lymphoma. Semin Radiat Oncol 17:184–189, 2007.

van der Kaajj MAE, Heutte N, Le Stange N, et al: Gonadal function in males after chemotherapy for early-stage Hodgkin's lymphoma treated in four subsequent trials by the European Organisation for Research and Treatment of Cancer: EORTC Lymphoma Group and the Groupe d'Etude des Lymphomes de l'Adulte. J Clin Oncol 25:2825–2832, 2007.

Yahalom J: Role of radiation therapy in Hodgkin's lymphoma. Cancer J 15:155–160, 2009.

Abbreviations in this chapter

CALGB = Cancer and Leukemia Group B; ECOG = Eastern Cooperative Oncology Group; EORTC = European Organisation for Research and Treatment of Cancer; GELA = Groupe d'Etudes des Lymphomes de l'Adulte; GHSG = German Hodgkin's Study Group; MSKCC = Memorial Sloan-Kettering Cancer Center; NCCN = National Comprehensive Cancer Network; NCIC = National Cancer Institute of Canada; SEER = Surveillance, Epidemiology and End Results; SWOG = Southwest Oncology Group; WHO = World Health Organization

CHAPTER 27

Non-Hodgkin lymphoma

Andrew M. Evens, DO, MS, Jane N. Winter, MD, Leo I. Gordon, MD, Brian C.-H. Chiu, PhD, Richard Tsang, MD, and Steven T. Rosen, MD

The incidence rates of non-Hodgkin lymphoma (NHL) in the United States have almost doubled between 1970 and 1990, representing one of the largest increases of any cancer. Although the overall incidence rates of NHL began to stabilize in the late 1990s, the temporal trends varied by histologic subtype. Some of this increase may be artifactual, resulting from improved diagnostic techniques and access to medical care, or directly related to the development of NHL in 25- to 54-year-old men with human immunodeficiency virus (HIV) infection. However, additional factors must be responsible for this unexpected increase in frequency of NHL that has been observed throughout the United States.

The incidence of NHL overall per 100,000 persons rose from 8.8 in 1972–1974 to 19.6 in 2003–2007 in the United States. The increases have been more pronounced in whites, males, the elderly, and those with NHL diagnosed at extranodal sites. Similar findings have been reported in other developed countries. In the United States, incidence rates of B-cell lymphomas increased significantly during 1992–2001 for marginal zone lymphoma (21% per year), mantle cell lymphoma (8% per year), and Burkitt lymphoma (8% per year) and decreased significantly for diffuse large B-cell lymphoma (–0.5% per year) and chronic lymphocytic leukemia/small lymphocytic lymphoma (–2.7% per year). During the same period, the incidence of T/NK-cell lymphomas rose about 4% per year, due especially to the increase in peripheral T-cell lymphomas (6.6% per year).

Currently, NHL represents approximately 4.6% of all cancer diagnoses (4.8% in males and 4.4% in females), being the fifth most common cancer in women and the sixth in men. Estimates from the ACS indicate that in 2010, some 65,540 new cases of NHL will be diagnosed in the United States and approximately 20,210 people will die of this disease.

EPIDEMIOLOGY

Gender The overall incidence of lymphoma is higher in men than in women. The incidence rate (per 100,000 population) between 2002 and 2006 was 40% higher in males than in females. Only thyroid NHL is more common in women than in men. Overall, NHL incidence rates remained unchanged during 1992–2001 among women but decreased at the rate of 1% per year among men, in part due to improved HIV treatment.

The 6p21 chromosomal region, which contains the major histocompatibility complex, has been shown to be important in the etiology of NHL. Wang et al showed that HLA class II alleles *HLA-DRB1*0101* predicted for risk of follicular lymphoma (OR = 2.14; *P* = .0004), whereas *HLA-DRB1*0401* and *HLA-DRB1*13* were associated with DLBCL (OR = 0.45; *P* = .006) and follicular lymphoma (OR = 0.48; *P* = .008), respectively *(Wang SS et al: Blood 115:4820–4823, 2010).*

Age The incidence of NHL overall and of most histologic subtypes rises exponentially with increasing age. In persons older than age 65, the incidence is 87.2 per 100,000 population. Except for high-grade lymphoblastic and Burkitt lymphomas (the most common types of NHL seen in children and young adults), the median age at presentation for all subtypes of NHL exceeds 50+ years. Low-grade lymphomas account for 37% of NHLs in patients between the ages of 35 and 64 years at diagnosis but for only 16% of cases in those younger than age 35. Substantially higher rates were observed for diffuse large B cell lymphoma (DLBCL) and Burkitt lymphoma among white and black men aged 25 to 54 years.

Race The incidence of NHL varies by race, with whites at higher risk than blacks and Asian-Americans (incidence rates increased 40% to 70% in whites compared with blacks). Most histologies, particularly low-grade small lymphocytic and follicular lymphomas, are more common in whites than in blacks. Only peripheral T-cell lymphoma (PTCL), mycosis fungoides, and Sézary syndrome are more common in blacks than in whites.

Geography NHL is most common in developed countries, with the United States having the highest rate worldwide. The lowest NHL rates are found in Eastern and south central Asia (2 to 3 per 100,000 population). Certain endemic geographic factors appear to influence the development of NHL in specific areas.

Human T-cell lymphotrophic virus-1 (HTLV-1)-associated adult T-cell lymphoma/leukemia (ATLL) occurs more frequently where HTLV-1 is endemic, in southern Japan and the Caribbean, and occurs sporadically in Brazil, sub-Saharan Africa, the Middle East, and the southeastern United States. The seroprevalence in southwest Japan is 16%, although the lifetime risk of ATLL for these persons is 2% to 6%.

The incidence (per 100,000 population) of Burkitt NHL in Africa (Nigeria and Tanzania) is 6 to 8, as compared with 0.1 in the United States. The clinical features of Burkitt lymphoma in Africa differ from those of cases reported to the American Burkitt Lymphoma Registry. Etiologic endemic factors include malaria as a source of chronic B-cell antigenic stimulation and Epstein-Barr virus (EBV)-induced immortalization of B lymphocytes.

Heavy-chain disease is a disorder of B-lymphoid cells characterized by diffuse thickening of the small intestine due to a lymphoplasmacytic infiltrate with secretion of incomplete IgA heavy chains. Pathologically, it is a mucosa-associated lymphoid tissue (MALT) lymphoma of the small bowel. This clinicopathologic entity is rarely encountered in individuals other than those of Mediterranean ethnic origin.

Follicular lymphomas are more common in North America and Europe but are rare in the Caribbean, Africa, China, Japan, the Middle East, and Latin America.

PTCLs are more common in Europe and China than in North America. They represent 7% to 12% of lymphomas in Western countries.

Disease site The NHLs are a heterogeneous group of neoplasms that usually arise or present in lymphoid tissues, such as lymph nodes, spleen, and bone marrow, but they may arise in almost any tissue. The most frequent sites for extranodal lymphomas, which constitute about 20% to 30% of all lymphomas (peripheral T-cell NHL, 70% to 80%; follicular, 8% to 10%), are the stomach, skin, oral cavity and pharynx, small intestine, and CNS. Although primary CNS lymphomas are rare, there has been a threefold increase in incidence, even if patients with HIV infection and other types of immunosuppression are excluded. Each of these sites may be involved singularly (ie, primary extranodal lymphoma) or as secondary extranodal sites concomitantly with other systemic disease.

Survival The 5-year relative survival rate of patients with NHL increased from 28% between 1950 and 1954 to 63% between 1990 and 2003. These improvements in survival occurred mainly in patients with intermediate-to-high–grade histologies. The potential for cure varies among the different histologic subtypes and is related in part to stage at presentation and response to initial therapy. The natural history (survival rates) for indolent lymphomas was unchanged from the 1950s to the early 1990s, but recent data, including an analysis from Iowa of SEER data (1979–1999), show improving overall survival rates for patients with follicular lymphoma.

ETIOLOGY AND RISK FACTORS

Chromosomal translocations and molecular rearrangements Nonrandom chromosomal and molecular rearrangements play an important role in the pathogenesis of many lymphomas and correlate with histology and immunophenotype (Table 1). The most commonly associated chromosomal abnormality in NHL is the t(14;18)(q32;q21) translocation, which is found in 85% of follicular lymphomas and 25% to 30% of higher-grade NHLs. This translocation results in the juxtaposition of the *bcl-2* apoptotic inhibitor "oncogene" at chromosome band 18q21 to the heavy-chain region of the immunoglobulin locus within chromosome band 14q32.

The t(11;14)(q13;q32) translocation results in overexpression of *bcl-1* (cyclin D1/PRAD 1), a cell-cycle–control gene on chromosome 11q13, and is characteristically associated with mantle cell lymphoma (MCL). The t(3;16)(q27;p11) translocation makes the gene for the interleukin-2 (IL-2) receptor a partner of *bcl-6*, which is expressed in DLBCL.

Chromosomal translocations involving 8q24 lead to c-*myc* deregulation, which is seen in nearly all cases of Burkitt lymphoma including those associated with HIV infection.

Environmental factors also may play a role in the development of NHL. Chemicals that have been linked to the development of NHL include a variety of pesticides and herbicides (2,4-D-organophosphates, chlorophenols), solvents and organic chemicals (benzene, carbon tetra-chloride), and wood preservatives. There is some evidence that the association between pesticides and NHL risk was limited to t(14;18)-positive NHL cases.

Viruses Several viruses have been implicated in the pathogenesis of NHL, including EBV; HTLV-1; Kaposi sarcoma–associated herpesvirus (KSHV, also known as human

TABLE 1: Correlation of chromosomal abnormalities in NHL with histology, antigen rearrangement, and oncogene expression

Cytogenetic abnormality	Histology	Antigen rearrangement	Oncogene expression	% of cases
B-cell lymphoma				
t(14;18)(q32;q21)	FL	IgH	*bcl-2*	≈ 90%
	DLBCL	IgH	*bcl-2*	15%–30%
t(11;14)(q13;q32)	Mantle cell	IgH	*bcl-1*	> 95%
t(1;14)(p22;q32)	MALT lymphoma	IgH	*bcl-10*	≈ 5%
t(11;18)(q21;q21)	MALT lymphoma		*API2* on chromosome II *MALT-1* on chromosome 18	≈ 30%
t(9;14)(p13;q32)	Lymphoplasmacytic lymphoma	IgH	*PAX-5*	
8q24 translocations	Burkitt lymphoma and variants		*c-myc*	≈ 99%
t(8;14)(q24;q32)		IgH		
t(2;8)(p11-12;q24)		Ig-κ		
t(8;22)(q24;q11)		Ig-λ		
(3;22)(q27;q11)	Diffuse (large cell, small cleaved cell)	Ig-κ	*bcl-6* (*LAZ3*)	
(3;14)/(q27;q32)	DLBCL	IgH	*bcl-6*	≈ 35%
T-cell lymphoma				
14q11 abnormalities				
inv 14(q11;q32)	Variable	TCR-α	*tcl-1*	
t(10;14)(q24;q11)	Variable	TCR-α	*hox-11* (*tcl-3*)	
i(7q)(q10)	Hepatosplenic	TCR-α	*ALK*	
2p23 translocations				
t(2;5)(p23;q35)	ALCL	TCR-α	*Npm*	
t(1;2)(p21;p23)	ALCL	TCR-α	*TPM3*	
t(2;3)(p23;p20)	ALCL	TCR-α	*TFG*	
t(2;22)(p23;q11)	ALCL	TCR-α	*CLTCL*	
inv(2)(p23;q35)	ALCL	TCR-α	*ATIC*	

ALCL = anaplastic large cell lymphoma; ATIC = 5-aminoimidazole-4-carboxamide-1-beta-D-ribonucleotide transformylase/inosine monophosphate cyclohydrolase; CLTCL = clathrin heavy polypeptide-like gene; inv = inversion; MALT = mucosa-associated lymphoid tissue; TFG = tropomyosin receptor kinase-fused gene; TPM3 = nonmuscle tropomyosin

herpesvirus 8, or HHV-8); and hepatitis C virus (HCV). Meta-analyses have shown a 13% to 15% HCV seroprevalence in certain geographic regions among persons with B-cell NHL, especially marginal zone NHL.

EBV is a DNA virus that has been associated with Burkitt lymphoma, particularly in endemic areas of Africa; Hodgkin lymphoma; lymphomas in immunocompromised patients (ie, organ transplantation and HIV infection); sinonasal lymphoma (Asia and South America); and sporadically in other B- and T-cell lymphomas. In contrast to studies performed in European patients, Mexican patients with intestinal lymphomas show a high frequency of EBV positivity; this finding is not limited to T-cell NHLs but rather includes a significant portion of B-cell NHLs. EBV can transform lymphocytes in culture. B lymphocytes from normal EBV-positive subjects have been shown to grow as tumors in mice with severe combined immunodeficiency.

HTLV-1 is a human retrovirus that establishes a latent infection via reverse transcription in activated T-helper cells. A minority (3% to 5%) of carriers develop ATLL. An HTLV-1–like provirus has been detected in some patients with mycosis fungoides, although conflicting findings have been reported.

KSHV-like DNA sequences are frequently detected in primary effusion lymphomas, in patients with Kaposi sarcoma, and in those with multicentric (plasma cell variant) Castleman disease.

HCV infection is associated with the development of clonal B-cell expansions and certain subtypes of NHL, particularly in the setting of essential (type II) mixed cryoglobulinemia. HCV may predispose B cells to malignant transformation by enhancing signal transduction upon binding to the CD81 (TAPA-1) molecule.

Bacterial infections Infection with *Borrelia burgdorferi*, the etiologic agent in Lyme disease, has been detected in about 35% of patients with peripheral cutaneous B-cell lymphoma (PCBCL) in Scotland. A near-complete clinical and histologic remission of a primary marginal zone B-cell lymphoma was observed after eradication of *B burgdorferi* with antibiotic treatment. Gastric MALT lymphoma is seen most frequently, but not exclusively, in association with *Helicobacter pylori* infection. Recent studies indicate that *Campylobacter jejuni* and immunoproliferative small intestinal disease (α-heavy chain disease) are related.

Some reports noted an association between infection with *Chlamydia psittaci* and ocular adnexal lymphoma. The infection was found to be highly specific and does not reflect a subclinical infection widespread among the general population. Responses to antibiotics have been reported. Attempts to confirm this association in the Western hemisphere have been unsuccessful.

Immune modulation Congenital and acquired states of immunosuppression that are at increased risk include ataxia-telangiectasia, Wiskott-Aldrich syndrome, common variable hypogamma-globulinemia, X-linked lymphoproliferative syndrome, and severe combined immunodeficiency.

Acquired immunodeficiency states such as HIV infection are associated with relative increased risk of NHL of 75 to 100 compared with the general population, although recent data in the post-HAART (highly active antiretroviral therapy) era suggest it has decreased. These NHLs are usually high grade and extranodal. Furthermore, iatrogenic immunosuppression (ie, solid organ transplantation [SOT] or hematopoietic stem cell transplantation recipients) have a significantly increased risk of NHL. The risk of NHL after SOT is 1% to 3% after liver or kidney transplant versus >10% for intestinal

Two recent analyses showed the prognostic importance of *MYC* oncogene rearrangement in DLBCL. Savage et al reported that *MYC*+ DLBCL treated with R-CHOP was associated with an inferior 5-year progression-free survival (66% vs 31%) and overall survival (72% vs 33%). Further, *MYC*+ DLBCL was associated with a significantly increased risk of secondary CNS disease *(Savage KJ et al: Blood 114:3533–3537, 2009)*. A subsequent report confirmed the presence of *MYC* as a significant adverse prognostic factor in DLBCL *(Barrans S et al: J Clin Oncol 28:3360–3365, 2010)*.

or multiorgan transplants, the latter of which warrant much higher immunosuppressive therapy.

An increased incidence of GI lymphomas is seen in patients with celiac (nontropical) sprue and inflammatory bowel disease, particularly Crohn's disease. An aberrant clonal intraepithelial T-cell population can be found in up to 75% of patients with refractory celiac sprue prior to the development of overt T-cell lymphoma using immunophenotyping and T-cell receptor gamma gene rearrangement PCR (polymerase chain reaction) techniques. Systemic lupus erythematosus and rheumatoid arthritis have been associated with B-cell lymphoma. Sjögren syndrome has been associated with NHL overall, DLBCL, and marginal zone lymphoma.

Patients who receive chemotherapy and/or radiation therapy are also at increased risk of developing NHL.

Lifestyle factors Several studies have reported an excess risk of NHL in association with diets high in fat and meat products. Some studies have suggested that ultraviolet radiation exposure and alcohol intake may be linked inversely with NHL risk.

Genetic susceptibility Several reports have implicated a role for genetic variants in the risk of NHL, including genes that influence DNA integrity and methylation; genes that alter B-cell survival and growth; and genes that involve innate immunity, oxidative stress, and xenobiotic metabolism. Of note, replication studies are needed to rule out false-positive associations.

SIGNS AND SYMPTOMS

Fever, weight loss, and night sweats, referred to as systemic B symptoms, as well as fatigue and weakness, are more common in advanced or aggressive NHL but may be present in all stages and histologic subtypes.

Low-grade lymphomas Painless, slowly progressive peripheral adenopathy is the most common clinical presentation in patients with low-grade lymphomas. Patients sometimes report a history of waxing and waning adenopathy before seeking medical attention. Spontaneous regression of enlarged lymph nodes can occur and can cause a low-grade lymphoma to be confused with an infectious condition.

Primary extranodal involvement and B symptoms are uncommon at presentation; however, both are more common in advanced or end-stage disease. Bone marrow is frequently involved, sometimes in association with cytopenias. Splenomegaly is seen in about 40% of patients, but the spleen is rarely the only involved site at presentation.

Aggressive-histology lymphomas The clinical presentation of aggressive-histology lymphomas is more varied. Although the majority of patients present with adenopathy, more than one-third present with extranodal involvement, the most common sites being the GI tract (including Waldeyer's ring), skin, bone marrow, sinuses, genitourinary (GU) tract, thyroid, and CNS. B symptoms are more common, occurring in about 30% to 40% of patients.

Lymphoblastic lymphoma often typically presents with an anterior superior mediastinal mass with possible superior vena cava syndrome, and leptomeningeal disease with possible cranial nerve palsies.

American patients with Burkitt lymphoma often present with a large abdominal mass and symptoms of bowel obstruction.

SCREENING AND DIAGNOSIS

No effective methods are available for screening or identifying populations at high risk of developing NHL. A definitive diagnosis can be made only by biopsy of pathologic lymph nodes or tumor tissue. It is critical to perform an excisional lymph node biopsy (fine-needle aspiration [FNA] is insufficient for diagnostic purposes) to avoid false-negative results and inaccurate histologic classification. One study showed that when FNAs and biopsy results for the diagnosis of NHL and Hodgkin lymphoma were compared, only 12% of FNAs correlated with subsequent excisional biopsy results. When clinical circumstances make surgical biopsy of involved lymph nodes or extranodal sites prohibitive, a core biopsy obtained under CT or ultrasonographic guidance may suffice but often requires the integration of histologic examination for diagnosis. A formal review by an expert hematopathologist is mandatory. Additional studies, such as immunophenotyping and genotyping, are often necessary.

Initial diagnostic evaluation of patients with lymphoproliferative malignancy should include the following:

- Careful history (night sweats, weight loss, fever; neurologic, musculoskeletal, or GI symptoms)
- Physical examination (lymph nodes, including submental, infraclavicular, epitrochlear, iliac, femoral, and popliteal nodes; pericardial rub, pleural effusion, distended neck and/or upper extremity veins in superior vena cava syndrome; breast masses; hepatosplenomegaly, bowel obstruction, renal mass, and testicular or ovarian mass; focal neurologic signs, such as plexopathy, spinal cord compression, nerve root infiltration, and meningeal involvement; skin lesions)
- Biopsy of peripheral lymphadenopathy (excisional biopsy)
- CT scan of the neck (cervical lymph nodes, Waldeyer's ring) and chest (mediastinal, hilar, or parenchymal pulmonary disease)
- CT scan of the abdomen and pelvis (enlarged lymph nodes, splenomegaly, filling defects in the liver and spleen)
- Bilateral bone marrow biopsy and aspirate
- FDG-PET scans (selected cases: aggressive histologies) for staging at diagnosis, response, assessment, and relapse; off of a clinical trial, "early" repeat PET scans (eg, following 2 cycles) are not advocated, in part due to the frequent disparate interpretation of PET scans.
- CBC with differential and platelet count (peripheral blood lymphocytosis with circulating malignant cells is common in low-grade lymphoma and MCL). Bone marrow and peripheral blood involvement may be present, and the distinction between leukemia and lymphoma is difficult to make in some cases.

TABLE 2: Immunophenotypic and histochemical markers of B-cell lymphomas/leukemias

	sIg	cIg	CD5	CD10	CD20	CD23	CD43	CD103	Cyclin D1
Follicular	+	–	–	+	+	–(+)	–	–	–
CLL/SLL	dim+	–(+)	+	–	dim+	+	+	–	–
Mantle	+	–	+	–	+	–(+)^	+	–	+
MZL/ MALT	+/+	–(+)/(+)	–/–	–/–	+/+	–/–	–(+)/–(+)	+	–/–
B-cell-PLL*	+	–	–(+)	–	+	+(–)	+	+	–
DLBCL#	+(–)	–(+)	–(+)	–(+)	+	–	–	–	–
HCL	+	–	–	–	+	–	+	–	+(–)
BL/BLL	+	–	–	+	+	–	+	NA	–
LPL	+	+	–	–	+	–	–(+)	–	–

+ = > 90% positive; +(–) = > 50% positive; –(+) = < 50% positive; – = < 10% positive; BL/BLL = Burkitt lymphoma/Burkitt-like lymphoma; cIg = cytoplasmic immunoglobulin; CLL = chronic lymphocytic leukemia; B-cell PLL = B-cell prolymphocytic leukemia; DLBCL = diffuse large B-cell lymphoma; HCL = hairy cell leukemia; LPL = lymphoplasmacytic lymphoma; MZL/MALT = splenic marginal zone/mucosa-associated lymphoid tissue; sIg = surface immunoglobulin; SLL = small lymphocytic leukemia

* = A T-cell variant is present in approximately 20% to 30% of PLL cases.

= A T-cell histiocyte-rich B-cell lymphoma variant is present in approximately 1% to 3% of DLBCL cases.

^ = 20% to 25% of cases are CD23+ by flow cytometric immunophenotyping; testing for *bcl-1* is essential.

- General chemistry panel (including lactate dehydrogenase [LDH] level determination) is mandatory.
- Hepatitis B virus (HBV) and HCV panels should be considered, especially in patients anticipated to receive monoclonal antibody therapy and/or chemotherapy (HBV:HBV surface antigen and HBV core antibody; HCV:HCV antibody).
- HIV serology in at-risk patients with DLBCL and other aggressive and Burkitt histologies; HTLV-1 serology in select patients with cutaneous T-cell lymphoma, especially if they have hypercalcemia.
- Cytogenetic and molecular analyses of lymph node, bone marrow, and peripheral blood (selected cases).
- Immunophenotyping can be of particular benefit in distinguishing B-cell chronic lymphocytic leukemia/small lymphocytic lymphoma (CLL/SLL) from other lymphomas (Table 2). Immunophenotyping and histochemical markers may also be of benefit in distinguishing T-cell lymphomas/leukemias (Table 3).
- Examination of CSF and consideration of intrathecal chemotherapy prophylaxis in patients with (1) diffuse aggressive NHL with bone marrow, epidural, testicular, paranasal sinus, breast, or multiple extranodal sites; (2) high-grade lymphoblastic lymphoma and Burkitt lymphoma and its variants; (3) primary CNS lymphoma if no evidence of increased intracranial pressure.

- Upper GI endoscopy and/or GI series with small bowel follow-through in patients with head and neck involvement (tonsil, base of tongue, nasopharynx) and those with a GI primary; MCL is associated with a high incidence of occult GI involvement.
- Ultrasonography of opposite testis in patients with a testicular primary.
- Spinal MRI scan for epidural disease when clinically indicated (useful in the evaluation of suspected spinal cord involvement).

PATHOLOGY

The Working Formulation was proposed in 1982 as a modification of the Rappaport classification of NHL based on morphology and biologic aggressiveness. Although many subtypes were not recognized, including T-cell lineage lymphomas, a revised European-American classification of lymphoid neoplasms (REAL classification) was introduced in 1994 incorporating T-cell malignancies, subtypes of Hodgkin lymphoma, and newer defined lymphoma-proliferative disorders. The WHO (World Health Organization) classification for lymphomas (introduced in 1999 and updated in 2008) uses the principles of the REAL classification defining each entity according to morphologic features, immunophenotype, genetic features, postulated normal counterpart, and clinical features.

WHO CLASSIFICATION

The modifications in the 2008 WHO classification included incorporation of further site-specific lymphoma subtypes, recognition of age as a defining feature of some diseases, and inclusion of several borderline and provisional categories (Table 4). The most frequently occurring clinical entities recognized within the WHO classification are DLBCL (31%), follicular lymphoma (22%), marginal zone/MALT lymphoma (8%), SLL (7%), and MCL (6%), whereas all noncutaneous T-cell lymphomas represent approximately 10% of NHL diagnoses in the United States.

The WHO classification includes three types of follicular lymphoma (grades 1/2, 3a, and 3b). Grading of follicular lymphoma is based in part on the number of centroblasts or large cells per high-powered field. Notably, the presence of any diffuse areas (ie, nonfollicular pattern) with large B cells should be designated as DLBCL. Further, some cases may include a composite of different histologic subtypes within the same lymph node excision (eg, follicular lymphoma and DLBCL). Grade 3b follicular lymphoma indicates sheets of large cells within a follicle (ie, maintained follicular architecture). Grade 3b follicular lymphoma more closely resembles DLBCL at the molecular level. The WHO classification considers B-cell SLL to be synonymous with CLL.

In the updated WHO classification, further clinicopathologic subtypes were added, namely DLBCL associated with inflammation and EBV and DLBCL in the elderly. In terms of T-cell lymphomas (TCLs), anaplastic large cell lymphoma (ALCL), ALK-positive, is considered a distinct disease, which is distinguished from the provisional entity of ALCL, ALK-negative. In addition, three new variants of primary cutaneous TCL were introduced (Table 4).

TABLE 3: Immunophenotypic and histochemical markers of T-cell lymphomas/leukemias

Histology	CD3	CD5	CD7	CD4	CD8	CD30	NK16/56	Cytotoxic granules	TCR
T-PLL	+	–	+	+(–)	–(+)	–	–	–	α/β
T-LGL disease*	+	–	+	–	+	–	+/–	+	α/β >> γ/δ
Mycosis fungoides	+	+	+	+	–(+)	–(+)	–	–	α/β
Cutaneous ALCL	+	+(–)	+(–)	+(–)	(–)	++	–(+)/–(+)	+/–	α/β
Primary systemic ALCL^	+(–)	+(–)	+(–)	–(+)	–(+)	++	–	–	α/β
Peripheral T-cell lymphoma, unspecified	+(–)	+(–)	–(+)	+(–)	–(+)	–(+)	–(+)/–(+)	–(+)	α/β > γ/δ
Subcutaneous panniculitis-like T-cell	+	+	+	–(+)	+(–)	–(+)	–/–(+)	+	γ/δ >> α/β
Hepatosplenic T-cell lymphoma	+	–	+	–	–	–	+/+(–)	+	γ/δ >> α/β
Angioimmunoblastic T-cell lymphoma#	+	+	–	+(–)	–(+)	–	–	–	α/β#
Extranodal NK/T-cell lymphoma	S –, C +	–	–(+)	–(+)	–	–	–/+	+	–
Enteropathy-associated T-cell lymphoma	+	+	+	–(+)	+(–)	+(–)	–	+	α/β >> γ/δ
Adult T-cell leukemia/lymphoma&	+	+	–	+(–)	–(+)	+(–)	–	–	α/β

+ = > 90% positive; +(-) = > 50% positive; -(+) = < 50% positive; - = < 10% positive; ALCL = anaplastic large cell lymphoma; C = cytoplasmic; LGL = large granular lymphoproliferative; NK = natural killer; PLL = prolymphocytic leukemia; S = surface; TCR = T-cell-rearranged (molecular)

* Approximately 15% to 20% of LGL cases arise from a NK lineage; they are typically CD56+ and CD16-negative.

^ The anaplastic lymphoma kinase (ALK) protein is expressed in 50% to 60% of cases.

Expanded follicular dendritic cell clusters (CD21+) are present around proliferated venules; Epstein-Barr virus (EBV) genomes are detected in most cases (eg, EBER) and may be present in either T or B cells; in addition, TCR may be negative or oligoclonal in 20% to 25% of cases, whereas B-cell immunoglobulin may be rearranged in 10% of cases.

& Adult T-cell leukemia/lymphoma cases are always associated with the presence of HTLV-I; further, CD25 is expressed in the majority of cases.

TABLE 4: WHO classification of the mature B-cell, T-cell, and NK-cell neoplasms (2008)

Mature B-cell neoplasms

- Chronic lymphocytic leukemia/small lymphocytic lymphoma
- B-cell prolymphocytic leukemia
- Splenic marginal zone lymphoma
- Hairy cell leukemia
- *Splenic lymphoma/leukemia, unclassifiable*
  - *Splenic diffuse red pulp small B-cell lymphoma**
  - Hairy cell leukemia-variant*
- Lymphoplasmacytic lymphoma
- Waldenström macroglobulinemia
- Heavy chain diseases
  - Alpha heavy chain disease
  - Gamma heavy chain disease
  - Mu heavy chain disease
- Plasma cell myeloma
- Solitary plasmacytoma of bone
- Extraosseous plasmacytoma
- Extranodal marginal zone lymphoma of mucosa-associated lymphoid tissue (MALT lymphoma)
- Nodal marginal zone lymphoma
- *Pediatric nodal marginal zone lymphoma*
- Follicular lymphoma
- *Pediatric follicular lymphoma*
- Primary cutaneous follicular center lymphoma
- Mantle cell lymphoma
- Diffuse large B-cell lymphoma (DLBCL), NOS
  - T-cell/histiocyte-rich large B-cell lymphoma
  - *EBV+ DLBCL of the elderly*
  - *DLBCL associated with chronic inflammation*
  - Lymphomatoid granulomatosis
- Primary mediastinal (thymic) large B-cell lymphoma
- Intravascular large B-cell lymphoma
- *Primary cutaneous DLBCL, leg type*
- ALK+ large B-cell lymphoma
- Plasmablastic lymphoma
- *Large B-cell lymphoma arising in HHV-8–associated multicentric Castleman disease*
- Primary effusion lymphoma
- Burkitt lymphoma
- *B-cell lymphoma, unclassifiable, with features intermediate between DLBCL and Burkitt lymphoma*
- B-cell lymphoma, unclassifiable, with features intermediate between DLBCL and classic Hodgkin lymphoma

Mature T-cell and NK-cell neoplasms

- T-cell prolymphocytic leukemia
- T-cell large granular lymphocytic leukemia
- Chronic lymphoproliferative disorder of NK cells*
- Aggressive NK cell leukemia
- *Systemic EBV+ T-cell lymphoproliferative disease of childhood*
- Hydroa vacciniforme-like lymphoma
- Adult T-cell leukemia/lymphoma
- Extranodal NK/T-cell lymphoma, nasal type
- Enteropathy-associated T-cell lymphoma
- Hepatosplenic T-cell lymphoma
- Subcutaneous panniculitis-like T-cell lymphoma
- Mycosis fungoides
- Sézary syndrome
- Primary cutaneous CD30+ T-cell lymphoproliferative disorders
  - Lymphomatoid papulosis
  - Primary cutaneous anaplastic large cell lymphoma
- *Primary cutaneous gamma-delta T-cell lymphoma*
- *Primary cutaneous CD8+ aggressive epidermotropic cytotoxic T-cell lymphoma**
- *Primary cutaneous CD4+ small/medium T-cell lymphoma**
- Peripheral T-cell lymphoma, NOS
- Angioimmunoblastic T-cell lymphoma
- Anaplastic large cell lymphoma, ALK+
- *Anaplastic large cell lymphoma, ALK−**

Hodgkin lymphoma

- Nodular lymphocyte-predominant Hodgkin lymphoma
- Classic Hodgkin lymphoma
  - Nodular sclerosis classic Hodgkin lymphoma
  - Lymphocyte-rich classic Hodgkin lymphoma
  - Mixed cellularity classic Hodgkin lymphoma
  - Lymphocyte-depleted classic Hodgkin lymphoma

Posttransplantation lymphoproliferative disorders (PTLDs)

- Early lesions
- Plasmacytic hyperplasia
- Infectious mononucleosis-like PTLD
- Polymorphic PTLD
- Monomorphic PTLD (B and T/NK-cell types)†
- Classic Hodgkin lymphoma type PTLD†

*Provisional entities for which the WHO Working Group thought there was insufficient evidence to recognize as distinct diseases at this time.

†These lesions are classified according to the leukemia or lymphoma to which they correspond. Diseases shown in italics were newly included in the 2008 WHO classification.

> **J**ohnson et al studied the mean fluorescence intensity of CD20 on 272 diagnostic DLBCL samples. R-CHOP–treated patients with dim CD20 expression had significantly inferior outcomes (3-year overall survival, ~50%) compared with bright CD20 expression (3-year overall survival, ~80%). Interestingly, this finding was similarly apparent in the pre-rituximab era (ie, CHOP-treated; *Johnson NA et al: Blood 113:3773–3780, 2009).*

STAGING AND PROGNOSIS

Determining the extent of disease in patients with NHL provides prognostic information and is useful in treatment planning. However, histologic subclassification (WHO classification) is the primary determinant of survival and potential for cure. Compared with patients with limited disease, those with extensive disease usually require different therapy, and certain extranodal sites of involvement, such as the CNS and testes, require specific treatment modalities.

Ann Arbor system Although initially devised for Hodgkin lymphoma, the Ann Arbor system has been routinely applied to NHL (Table 5). Because Hodgkin lymphoma commonly spreads via contiguous lymph node groups, this system is based primarily on the distribution of lymphatic involvement with respect to the diaphragm and the presence of extralymphatic organ involvement. The Ann Arbor system does not reflect the noncontiguous nature of disease spread in NHL, does not discriminate well between stages III and IV disease, and fails to account for tumor bulk or number of extranodal sites.

Some trials in Burkitt and Burkitt-like lymphoma use the St. Jude/Murphy staging system, in part to more completely describe the extent of extranodal disease. Unlike the current WHO classification, this staging system recognizes Burkitt leukemia as a separate entity. Moreover, this system was developed when surgery was used for diagnostic and therapeutic purposes. Patients are also typically stratified into two risk groups, with low-risk patients defined as having a normal LDH level and a single focus of disease measuring less than 10 cm and all others considered to be high risk.

Prognostic factors Histology and morphology remain the major determinants of treatment outcome and prognosis, but gene expression signatures are likely to be the principal determinants in the future. Some patients with slow-growing low-grade lymphoma may remain well for many years with minimal or no initial therapy, whereas survival of patients with some types of high-grade lymphoma is measured only in weeks unless aggressive treatment is initiated promptly. The biologic and clinical behaviors of these disorders vary among the different histologic subtypes.

The International Prognostic Index (IPI) was developed by 16 institutions and cooperative groups in the United States, Europe, and Canada as a prognostic factor model for aggressive NHL treated with doxorubicin-containing regimens. The IPI clinical features, which have been shown to be independently predictive of survival, are provided in Table 6.

This index appears to be a useful guide for selecting treatment for patients with aggressive DLBCL, by identifying subsets of patients in whom intensified primary or novel therapy may be warranted. Because younger and older patients have markedly different prognoses and younger patients are more likely to be considered for more intensive investigational regimens, an age-adjusted model for patients ≤ 60 years old has been proposed. In younger patients, stage (III or IV), high LDH level, and

TABLE 5: Ann Arbor staging classification for NHL[a]

Stage	Area of involvement
I	One lymph node region
IE	One extralymphatic organ or site
II	Two or more lymph node regions on the same side of the diaphragm
IIE	One extralymphatic organ or site (localized) in addition to criteria for stage II
III	Lymph node regions on both sides of the diaphragm
IIIE	One extralymphatic organ or site (localized) in addition to criteria for stage III
IIIS	Spleen in addition to criteria for stage III
IIISE	Spleen and one extralymphatic organ or site (localized) in addition to criteria for stage III
IV	One or more extralymphatic organs with or without associated lymph node involvement (diffuse or disseminated); involved organs should be designated by subscript letters (P, lung; H, liver; M, bone marrow)

[a]Class A patients experience no symptoms; class B patients experience unexplained fever of ≥ 101.5°F; unexplained, drenching night sweats; or loss of > 10% body weight within the previous 6 months.

nonambulatory performance status are independently associated with decreased survival. Notably, the IPI has remained a valid prognostic index for R-CHOP (rituximab [Rituxan]-cyclophosphamide, hydroxydaunorubicin, vincristine [Oncovin], prednisone)–treated DLBCL. In the post-rituximab era, persons with no risk factors have a predicted 5-year overall survival of 94%, compared with 55% for high-risk patients with three to five risk factors.

The IPI also appears to be useful in predicting outcome in patients with relapsed or refractory DLBCL undergoing autologous stem cell transplantation (SCT).

A prognostic factor model has been devised based on a study of 919 cases of follicular lymphoma, known as the Follicular Lymphoma IPI (FLIPI; Table 7). Multivariate analysis showed that age, Ann Arbor stage, number of nodal sites, LDH level, and hemoglobin level were predictors of overall survival.

TABLE 6: International Prognostic Index

Parameter	Adverse factor
Age	> 60 years
Ann Arbor stage	III or IV
Serum LDH level	Above normal
Number of extranodal sites of involvement	≥ 2
Performance status	≥ ECOG 2 or equivalent

ECOG = Eastern Cooperative Oncology Group; LDH = lactate dehydrogenase
From International non-Hodgkin's Lymphoma Prognostic Factors Project: N Engl J Med 329:987–994, 1993.

Geisler et al applied the MCL International Prognostic Index (MIPI) to 158 patients treated in the Nordic MCL2 trial of first-line intensive immunochemotherapy followed by autologous stem cell transplantation. The simplified MIPI (s-MIPI) predicted survival significantly better (*P* < .001) than the International Prognostic Index (*P* < .004; *Geisler CH et al: Blood 115:1530–1533, 2010*).

An analysis of the FLIPI in the post-rituximab era has been reported (FLIPI-2). Multivariate analysis showed that elevated beta2-microglobulin, longest nodal diameter over 6 cm, bone marrow involvement, anemia, and age over 60 years independently predicted survival. Including all patients (n = 832) with 0, 1–2, or 3–5 factors, the 3-year progression-free survival was 91%, 69%, and 51% (*P* = .00001), whereas the 5-year progression-free survival was 79%, 51%, and 20%, respectively (*P* = .00001). Among patients treated with rituximab-containing regimens only (n = 559), the FLIPI-2 remained predictive of outcome (3-year progression-free survival of 89%, 73%, and 57%, respectively; *P* = .001). The MCL International Prognostic Index (MIPI) was created from 455 advanced-stage MCL patients treated within three German clinical trials. It consisted of several clinical factors. The simplified MIPI (s-MIPI) is the sum of increasing points for grouped values of age, performance status, LDH level > the upper limit normal, and leukocyte count and is scored as low (0–3 points), intermediate (4–5 points), and high risk (> 5 points; Table 8). Patients with low or intermediate risk according to the sMIPI had a 5-year overall survival > 75% to 80% compared with 38% for patients with high risk (> five factors).

Immunobiologic factors Various immunobiologic factors have been suggested as predictors of outcome in NHL.

Immunophenotype Several studies have suggested that patients with aggressive T-cell NHL have a higher relapse rate and decreased overall survival than do patients with B-cell disease, especially in the post-rituximab era.

Tumor cell proliferation Studies using the Ki-67 antibody, a marker of nuclear proliferation, have shown that increased tumor cell proliferation is a poor prognostic factor in DLBCL and MCL.

Cytogenetic abnormalities and oncogene expression Mutations of *p53* are associated with histologic transformation in follicular NHL, which is a phenomenon frequently

TABLE 7: Follicular lymphoma International Prognostic Indices

FLIPI-1	FLIPI-2
Age > 60 years	Age > 60 years
Stage III or IV	Bone marrow involvement
Hemoglobin level < 120 g/L	Hemoglobin level < 120 g/L
LDH > ULN	Beta2-microglobulin > ULN
Number of nodal sites > 4	Largest nodal diameter > 6 cm

LDH = lactate dehydrogenase; ULN = upper limit of normal

From Solal-Celigny P, Roy P, Colombat P, et al: Follicular Lymphoma International Prognostic Index. Blood 104:1258–1265, 2004; Federico M, Bellei M, Marcheselli L, et al: J Clin Oncol 27:4555–4562, 2009.

TABLE 8: Simplified MCL International Prognostic Index (sMIPI)

Points	Age, y	ECOG performance status	LDH ULN	WBC, 10^9/L
0	< 50	0–1	< 0.67	< 6.70
1	50–59	–	0.67–0.99	6.7–9.9
2	60–69	2–4	1.0–1.49	10.0–14.9
3	≥ 70	–	≥ 1.5	≥ 15

ECOG = Eastern Cooperative Oncology Group; LDH = lactate dehydrogenase; MCL = mantle cell lymphoma; ULN = upper limit of normal; WBC = white blood cell count; y = years
From Hoster E, Dreyling M, Klapper W, et al: Blood 111:558-565, 2008.

associated with a poor prognosis. Expression of *bcl*-2 in DLBCL has also been associated with inferior survival, whereas *bcl*-6 expression is a marker of germinal center derivation, a predictor of a favorable outcome with CHOP-like therapy. Dual expression of *bcl*-2 and *c-myc* in B-cell lymphomas is also a poor prognostic sign.

Molecular profiling DNA microarray technology for gene expression profiling has identified distinct prognostic subgroups in DLBCL and follicular NHL. Studies in DLBCL have characterized patients into the following subgroups: germinal center B-like DLBCL, activated B-like DLBCL, and a heterogeneous subgroup termed type-3 DLBCL. In the pre-rituximab era, patients with germinal center B-like DLBCL had a significantly improved overall survival compared with the other molecular profiles. Although in the post-rituximab era, this prognostic difference is less apparent. Studies in follicular NHL have identified two gene expression signatures that also predicted survival: immune-response 1 and immune-response 2. Interestingly, the genes that defined the prognostic signatures were not expressed in the tumor cells but were expressed by the nonmalignant tumor-infiltrating cells (primarily T cells, macrophages, and dendritic cells). A variety of immunologically active cell types, including specific T-cell subsets and tumor-associated macrophages, have been associated with prognosis in some studies. Similar data are available in DLBCL regarding gene-expressing studies of the surrounding (nonmalignant) microenvironment. Lenz et al showed that the stromal-1 signature (composed of extracellular-matrix deposition and histiocytic infiltration) was associated with a significantly improved outcome compared with stromal-2 (tumor blood-vessel density) in CHOP and R-CHOP treated populations.

TREATMENT

The therapeutic approach for NHL differs for each subtype. Chemotherapy remains the most important modality (Tables 9 and 10). However, in select instances, radiation therapy or, rarely, surgical resection plays a critical role. Biologic approaches, including interferons, monoclonal antibodies (Table 11), and recombinant toxins, have shown significant activity and are now incorporated into treatment paradigms. Autologous and allogeneic SCTs, traditionally reserved for recurrent or refractory disease, are being evaluated as part of initial therapy in high-risk settings. This section will be organized by NHL subtype to best illustrate the biologic characteristics and

TABLE 9: Chemotherapeutic regimens for NHL

Regimen	Dose	Route and frequency
CVP ± rituximab		
Cyclophosphamide	750–1,000 mg/m²	IV on day 1
Vincristine	1.4 mg/m²	IV on day 1 (maximum, 2 mg)
Prednisone	100 mg or 100 mg/m²	PO on days 1–5
Rituximab	375 mg/m²	IV on day 1
Repeat treatment every 21 days.		
CHOP ± rituximab		
Cyclophosphamide	750 mg/m²	IV on day 1
Doxorubicin	50 mg/m²	IV on day 1
Oncovin (vincristine)	1.4 mg/m²	IV on day 1 (maximum, 2 mg)
Prednisone	40 mg/m² or 100 mg/d or 100 mg/m²/d	PO on days 1–5
Rituximab	375 mg/m²	IV on day 1
Repeat treatment every 21 days or every 14 days (with granulocyte colony-stimulating factor).		
FCR		
Fludarabine	25 mg/m²	IV on days 1–3
Cyclophosphamide	300 mg/m²	IV on days 1–3
Rituximab	375 mg/m²	IV on day 1
Repeat treatment every 28 days.		
FCM + R		
Fludarabine	25 mg/m²	IV on days 1–3
Cyclophosphamide	200 mg/m²	IV on days 1–3
Mitoxantrone	6 mg/m²	IV on day 1
Rituximab	375 mg/m²	IV on day 0
Repeat treatment every 28 days.		
R-B		
Rituximab	375 mg/m²	
Bendamustine	90 mg/m²	IV on days 1 and 2
Repeat treatment every 28 days.		

therapeutic considerations that determine the management strategy for individual patients. Common NHLs will be covered in depth, whereas less frequent entities will be described in limited detail.

FOLLICULAR LYMPHOMA

Follicular lymphoma comprises 22% of all NHLs; only DLBCL is more common. The clinical presentation may be nodal or extranodal, and bone marrow involvement occurs in the majority of cases. Extensive intra-abdominal adenopathy without peripheral node enlargement is not uncommon. Clinical behavior is variable, reflecting the heterogeneity of the underlying biology; some patients survive decades, whereas others progress rapidly to resistant disease or transform to a more aggressive histology. There are rare spontaneous remissions. Transformation is common, occurring in 3% to 6% of patients each year and ultimately 30% to 50% of all patients. Although generally responsive to treatment, the clinical course of follicular lymphoma is characterized by repeated relapses. Although there was no improvement in survival for patients with follicular lymphoma for many years, there is now evidence that outcomes are improving. Median survival has reached 10 or more years. It is likely that this is, in part, attributable to use of rituximab in combination with chemotherapy, but survival was already improving before the approval of rituximab.

It is crucial to distinguish between reactive follicular hyperplasia and follicular lymphoma, as the former is a benign condition. Morphologic features as well as the absence of Bcl-2 staining within the follicle and the absence of CD10 and/or Bcl-6 protein expression in the interfollicular areas help to distinguish reactive follicular hyperplasia from follicular lymphoma. Follicular lymphoma is graded according to the number of admixed centroblasts within the neoplastic follicles. Grade 3 follicular lymphoma, previously known as follicular large cell lymphoma, is now subdivided into two subtypes: Grade 3a is characterized by a mixture of centrocytes and centroblasts within the follicle, whereas grade 3b has only sheets of centroblasts with no

TABLE 10: Commonly used salvage regimens for NHL

Regimen	Dose	Route and frequency
EPOCH[a]		
Etoposide	50 mg/m²/d	Continuous 96-h IV infusion on days 1–4
Oncovin (vincristine)	0.4 mg/m²/d	Continuous 96-h IV infusion on days 1–4
Doxorubicin	10 mg/m²/d	Continuous 96-h IV infusion on days 1–4
Cyclophosphamide	750 mg/m²	IV on day 5
Prednisone	60 mg	PO on days 1–5
Repeat treatment every 21 days. Doses of etoposide, doxorubicin, and cyclophosphamide are adjusted 20% each cycle to achieve an absolute neutrophil count below 0.5 × 10⁹/L.		
DHAP[a]		
Platinol (cisplatin)	100 mg/m²	Continuous 24-h IV infusion on day 1
Cytarabine	2 g/m²	3-h IV infusion q12h for 2 doses on day 2
Dexamethasone	40 mg	IV on days 1–4
Repeat treatment every 21–28 days depending on hematologic recovery.		
ESHAP[a]		
Etoposide	40 mg/m²	1-h IV infusion on days 1–4
Solu-Medrol (MPS)	250–500 mg	15-min IV infusion on days 1–5
Cytarabine	2 g/m²	2-h IV infusion on day 5
Platinol (cisplatin)	25 mg/m²	Continuous 96-h IV infusion on days 1–4 (total dose, 100 mg/m²)
GEMOX[a]		
Gemcitabine	1,000 mg/m²	IV on day 1
Oxaliplatin	100 mg/m²	IV on day 1
Repeat treatment every 14–21 days depending on hematologic recovery.		
ICE[a]		
Ifosfamide	5,000 mg/m²	Continuous IV × 24 h on day 2
Mesna	5,000 mg/m²	Continuous IV × 24 h on day 2
Carboplatin	AUC 5 mg/mL/min	IV on day 2
Etoposide	100 mg/m²	IV on days 1–3

[a] ± Rituximab

AUC = area under the curve; MPS = methylprednisolone

TABLE 11: Monoclonal antibodies for lymphoid malignancies

Antigen	Antibody	Type	Investigational status
CD20	Rituximab	Chimeric	FDA approved
	Ibritumomab	Y-90-murine	FDA approved
	Tositumomab	I-131 murine	FDA approved
	Ofatumumab	Human	Phase III planned
	Ocrelizumab	Humanized	Phase I/II
	Afutuzumab	Humanized	Phase III
CD52	Alemtuzumab	Humanized	FDA approved
CD22	Epratuzumab	Humanized	Phase II/III
CD80	Galiximab (IDEC-114)	Primatized	Phase II
CD23	Lumiliximab (IDEC-152)	Primatized	Phase I
CD30	SGN-30	Chimeric	Phase II

residual centrocytes. The neoplastic lymphocytes in follicular lymphoma express the pan-B markers CD19, CD20, CD22, and CD79a and antigens of the germinal center (including CD10 and Bcl-6). Most follicular lymphomas express Bcl-2 protein, which is highly correlated with the t(14;18)(q32;q21). This translocation results in the juxtaposition of the *bcl*-2 oncogene into the immunoglobulin H heavy-chain locus on chromosome 14, resulting in its constitutive expression. Follicular lymphoma grade 3b with *bcl-6* rearrangement but no t(14;18)(q32;21) may be more closely related to DLBCL than to other follicular lymphomas.

As previously mentioned, the FLIPI is a prognostic index designed specifically for follicular lymphomas based on five adverse prognostic factors (Table 7). Age is the most important factor. Three risk categories have been defined, each consisting of approximately one-third of patients. More than two-thirds of low-risk patients but only one-third of high-risk patients survive 10 years. A new prognostic scoring system, the FLIPI2, is based on prospectively collected data from the rituximab-era (Table 7), and has progression-free survival rather than overall survival as its principal endpoint. Among patients receiving rituximab-containing therapy, it is a robust predictor of clinical outcome. Whereas clinical parameters are surrogates for biologic characteristics, biologic correlates such as gene expression signatures may soon supersede clinical prognostic indicators.

As noted before, investigators from the NCI have described two gene-expression signatures associated with vastly different clinical outcomes in follicular lymphoma. These two signatures represent the expression of immunoregulatory genes in the nonmalignant cells infiltrating the malignant lymphoma at the time of diagnosis. Others have reported that the number of tumor-associated macrophages, or specific T-cell subsets was an independent predictor of overall survival in follicular lymphoma, also underscoring the importance of host response in follicular lymphoma.

Treatment of early-stage disease

For the relatively small number of patients with stage I or II follicular lymphoma, radiotherapy continues to be the recommended approach because of the potential for long-term disease-free survival and possible cure. Results from the Princess Margaret Hospital's series of involved-field radiotherapy (IFRT) for early-stage disease show cumulative relapse rates of 54% and 56% at 15 and 25 years, with only a 2% risk of relapse beyond 15 years. A recently published analysis of the SEER database for adults with stage I or II follicular lymphoma diagnosed between 1973 and 2004 showed improved disease-specific survival and overall survival with upfront IFRT, compared with all other approaches. Combined-modality therapy has also resulted in excellent disease control, and a randomized trial comparing IFRT with combined-modality therapy is ongoing.

Despite the excellent outcomes associated with radiotherapy, the National Lymphocare Study revealed that the majority of patients in the United States are either observed or treated with rituximab alone or in combination with chemotherapy, foregoing the potential for cure, even in young patients. Use of functional imaging with PET may improve the results of IFRT by more accurately identifying patients with truly localized disease.

For clinical stages I and IIA low-grade follicular lymphoma, irradiation alone is directed to the entire involved lymphoid region, as defined by Kaplan and coworkers, or the involved region plus one additional uninvolved region on each side of the involved nodes. Radiation to the intra-abdominal or pelvic area is associated with increased morbidity and thus may be a location to avoid. The recommended dose is approximately 30 Gy for nonbulky disease showing prompt regression and 36 Gy for bulky or slowly regressive disease, in 1.75 to 2.0 Gy daily fractions. As the majority of subsequent relapses occur outside previous radiation fields, often in adjacent or distal lymph nodes, extended-field or total lymphoid irradiation has been used to try to improve cure rates. Clinical series have shown improvement in freedom from relapse only, with no significant difference in long-term survival.

Treatment of advanced-stage disease

Watch and wait The standard management of asymptomatic patients with follicular lymphoma has been a "watch-and-wait" approach. Treatment is delayed until symptoms or cytopenias intervene or there is impending compromise of vital organs. In the pre-rituximab era, multiple phase III randomized trials comparing immediate chemotherapy with observation for asymptomatic patients with advanced-stage follicular lymphoma have shown no difference in outcome. In fact, for patients older than age 70, the chances of not requiring chemotherapy were 40% at 10 years in a recently published trial. The median time to first systemic therapy for patients randomized to the observation arm was 2.6 years. Complete remission rates, however, were higher in the patients treated immediately after diagnosis than in those who were observed and later treated (63% vs 27%). The achievement of a complete remission may prove to be important if the ultimate goal is to administer postremission therapy (eg, vaccine) that is likely to be most effective in the presence of minimal residual disease. A phase III trial comparing the watch-and-wait approach with rituximab therapy for asymptomatic advanced-stage disease is ongoing in Europe.

At the same time, an American intergroup trial comparing two different rituximab dosing regimens in patients with low tumor burden indolent lymphoma who are asymptomatic has met accrual, but the results are not yet available.

Irradiation Radiation is not typically used in conjunction with systemic therapy. However, radiation may be effective when used locally for palliation of symptomatic sites of disease. Abbreviated fractionated schedules (25 to 30 Gy in 2.5 to 3 Gy daily fractions, respectively) are often used. A low-dose regimen of 4 Gy in 2 fractions has been shown to be effective, with an overall response rate of approximately 80% in the palliation of symptoms, and is well tolerated. Total-body irradiation, usually consisting of 12 Gy in 2 Gy fractions twice a day, is used as part of preparative regimens for bone marrow transplantation.

Rituximab For patients with symptoms or other reasons for treatment, there are many treatment options, including single or multiagent chemotherapy, monoclonal antibodies or radioimmunoconjugates, combinations of chemotherapy and immunotherapy with anti-idiotype vaccines, and new agents such as bortezomib (Velcade) or bendamustine (Treanda). Treatment with rituximab results in overall response rates of nearly 50%, with a median response duration of approximately 1 year, in relapsed or refractory indolent lymphomas. In previously untreated patients, however, the overall response rate was 80%, and the median progression-free survival is 18 months in one trial from France. Of note, 28% of all treated patients and 34% of all complete and partial responders maintained their responses for 5 or more years. Similar results have been reported by the US NCCTG.

To improve on response rates and duration of response, additional doses of rituximab have been administered as "maintenance therapy." The median event-free survival is prolonged with this approach, especially for previously untreated patients. In previously treated patients, the total duration of benefit from rituximab appears to be the same whether patients receive maintenance rituximab on a scheduled basis or reinduction with rituximab only at the time of disease progression. A confirmatory trial (ECOG 4402) in asymptomatic untreated patients with a low tumor burden has met accrual, and the results are eagerly awaited. Maintenance regimens have varied, and the impact of the frequency of administration on the duration of response is unknown.

Among previously untreated patients with follicular lymphoma who responded to immunochemotherapy (R-CVP, R-CHOP, or R-FCM), rituximab (Rituxan) maintenance resulted in a significant improvement in progression-free survival over observation (2-year, 82% vs 66%; *P* < .0001). The most common grade 3/4 adverse events were infection (22% for rituximab maintenance and 16% for observation). Whether this approach will impact overall survival will require further follow-up *(Salles GA et al: J Clin Oncol 28: abstract 8004, 2010).*

Rituximab maintenance also impacts progression-free survival among patients treated with chemotherapy alone and those receiving rituximab plus chemotherapy. Compared with observation, maintenance rituximab improved progression-free survival in previously untreated patients with follicular lymphoma who responded to cyclophosphamide, vincristine, and prednisone (3-year progression-free survival, 64% vs 33%). Among relapsed/refractory patients treated with CHOP or rituximab-CHOP (R-CHOP) maintenance, rituximab also improved progression-free survival. Whether these results will translate into an overall survival benefit remains to be seen. Questions also remain regarding the impact of maintenance rituximab on the quality of life and the cost of care. Compared with observation, maintenance rituximab has been associated with an increased risk of infectious complications.

Interferon-α The use of interferon (IFN)-α in follicular lymphoma has been extensively investigated both in combination with chemotherapy and as maintenance therapy, with varying results. In most studies, IFN-α was associated with a prolongation of remission but not overall survival. A notable exception was the GELF86 trial, in which overall survival was prolonged. The SWOG reported the results of a large phase III trial in which patients with indolent lymphomas were randomized to receive IFN-α or observation following induction with an intensive anthracycline-containing regimen and in some cases radiotherapy. Postremission therapy did not prolong progression-free or overall survival. Although these results, along with the toxicities associated with IFN-α, have led many physicians to abandon its use altogether, a large phase III study is currently ongoing in Germany comparing standard vs intensive dose maintenance.

Chemotherapy with and without rituximab Studies comparing single-agent chemotherapy with multiagent therapy in patients with advanced-stage follicular lymphoma have not shown meaningful differences in outcomes. Fludarabine, identified in the 1980s as an active agent in follicular lymphoma, has been incorporated into combination regimens with high response rates (including molecular remissions) but has not been shown to prolong the duration of remission when compared with other multiagent regimens. Secondary myelodysplastic syndromes and acute leukemias have now been associated with the fludarabine, mitoxantrone (Novantrone), dexamethasone (FND) regimen. High response rates and durable remissions have resulted when rituximab was combined with CHOP chemotherapy in a small number of patients with follicular lymphoma, some of whom were treatment-naive. These encouraging results led to four phase III trials comparing combinations of chemotherapy and rituximab with chemotherapy alone in previously untreated patients. Overall response rates and either median time to treatment failure or event-free survival were superior in the chemoimmunotherapy arm in every series. An overall survival benefit has been demonstrated in three of the four trials and in the high-risk subset of the fourth study.

Radioimmunotherapy The anti-CD20 radioimmunoconjugates Y-90 ibritumomab (Zevalin) and I-131 tositumomab (Bexxar) both deliver ionizing radiation to target cells and their neighbors and have proven to be relatively easy to administer, safe, and effective. Response rates are higher and remissions more durable when radioimmunoconjugates are used early in the clinical course. Both agents are likely to have their greatest impact when used in previously untreated patients.

In previously treated patients, Y-90 ibritumomab, a high-energy beta-emitter, yielded an overall response rate of 80% for relapsed or refractory follicular or transformed CD20+ B-cell NHL, with a median duration of response of 14 months. For patients whose disease is refractory to rituximab, response rates with Y-90 ibritumomab are high (74% overall response rate), but the median duration of response is relatively short (6.4 months; range, 0.5–25+ months). The dose-limiting feature of this approach is hematologic toxicity. Short-lived myelosuppression occurs 7 to 9 weeks posttreatment. Dosing is based on weight (0.4 mCi/kg), with a reduction (0.3 mCi/kg) for those with mild thrombocytopenia (< 100,000/μL). When used to consolidate first partial or complete remission, Y-90 ibritumomab prolonged progression-free survival from 13.5 to 37 months. However, only 14% of the 414 patients enrolled on this randomized phase III trial received a rituximab-containing regimen for induction. Now that the addition of rituximab to chemotherapy has become standard of care based on demonstrated improvement in progression-free and overall survival rates, the benefit of consolidation with radioimmunotherapy will need to be evaluated in large numbers of patients treated first with chemoimmunotherapy.

I-131 tositumomab is both a gamma- and beta-emitter and is individually dosed on the basis of dosimetry to deliver 75 cGy of total-body irradiation. Similar to Y-90 ibritumomab, it is effective in both heavily pretreated relapsed and refractory patients. Heavily pretreated patients with refractory low-grade or transformed NHL had an overall response rate of 65% (20% complete response rate), with a median duration of response of 6.5 months. These rates were notable in view of a response rate of only 28% in the preceding chemotherapy regimen. Like Y-90 ibritumomab, I-131 tositumomab is associated with predictable myelosuppression. Secondary myelodysplasia and leukemia have occurred in patients treated with radioimmunotherapy, but only in patients previously treated with chemotherapy and thereby already at risk. In previously untreated patients, the complete response rate was 75%, with a 5-year progression-free survival of 59%. These data must be interpreted carefully, as this study enrolled a relatively young patient population (median age, 49 years), with low-bulk disease, a group that some physicians would choose to observe rather than treat.

I-131 tositumomab has been used to consolidate responders following induction with CHOP chemotherapy. In a phase II trial of previously untreated patients with follicular lymphoma, the percentage of complete response/unconfirmed complete response increased from 39% following CHOP chemotherapy to 69% following consolidation with I-131 tositumomab. With a median follow-up of 5.1 years, 66% of patients are alive and disease-free. Based on these phase II results and the encouraging outcome of patients treated with R-CHOP, the American intergroup has completed a phase III trial comparing CHOP followed by I-131 tositumomab with R-CHOP in treatment-naive patients. The results of this study will be forthcoming in the near future.

Anti-idiotype vaccines Lymphoma-specific idiotypes serve as tumor-specific antigens in follicular lymphoma and constitute the basis for vaccine therapy. In early vaccine trials, immunized patients who generated an anti-idiotype response experienced longer remissions than those who failed to mount a response. In phase I trials, vaccination resulted in tumor shrinkage in some patients, and in a phase II trial, anti-idiotype vaccine eliminated minimal residual disease detectable only by PCR after intensive chemotherapy.

Based on these encouraging results, a phase III randomized trial comparing vaccination plus KLH (keyhole limpet hemocyanin, a nonspecific immunostimulant) to KLH alone in previously untreated patients who achieved a complete remission with intensive anthracycline-containing combination chemotherapy was conducted. Patients receiving the vaccine experienced a statistically significant prolongation of cancer-free survival. In contrast, two other placebo-controlled trials of anti-idiotype vaccination have shown no benefit. Compared with placebo, vaccination following induction chemotherapy with cyclophosphamide, vincristine, prednisone, or induction immunotherapy with rituximab did not impact progression-free or overall survival. Differences in study design are likely responsible for the differences in outcomes among the trials. New directions in vaccination include Id-pulsed dendritic cell and membrane proteoliposomal vaccines.

Novel agents New agents targeting specific molecular targets such as the ubiquitin-proteasome pathway, histone deacetylase, the mammalian target of rapamycin (mTOR), the microenvironment, and Bcl-2 have shown promise in the treatment of follicular lymphoma. In recently reported phase II trials, bortezomib has shown activity in follicular lymphoma as well as in MCL. New combinations including bortezomib are now being investigated. Bendamustine is a novel alkylator with activity in both rituximab-refractory and rituximab-sensitive indolent NHL that has recently been approved by the FDA for relapsed disease that is refractory to rituximab. New agents such as bendamustine, bortezomib, and lenalidomide (Revlimid) in combination with rituximab provide many potential options for treatment.

Novel antibody approaches to follicular lymphoma include new and improved anti-CD20s, antibodies that bind to alternative targets, and chemoimmuno- and radioimmunoconjugates.

SCT The natural history of follicular lymphoma is characterized by response to therapy but repeated relapses and progressively shorter and shorter remissions, ultimately resulting in death from progressive disease. Autologous and allogeneic SCTs are alternative strategies often associated with durable remissions that may impact overall survival. Unfortunately, immediate and long-term toxicities are significant and must be considered when assessing the appropriate role of transplantation in the overall treatment plan for individual patients. The only phase III trial to address the role of autologous SCT in patients with relapsed follicular lymphoma closed prematurely because of poor accrual. Nonetheless, progression-free and overall survival rates were significantly longer with high-dose chemotherapy (HDCT) and autologous SCT (with purged or unpurged autografts) than with conventional alkylator therapy. Whether any of the new therapeutic strategies will prove to be as effective as autologous SCT in the relapsed setting remains to be seen.

Several groups have investigated the role of autologous SCT as consolidation therapy for patients in first complete or partial remission. Although progression-free survival may be prolonged, an impact on survival has not been demonstrated consistently. An increased incidence of secondary myelodysplasia following autologous SCT in first remission has reduced enthusiasm for this approach. Contemporary trials evaluating the role of autologous SCT for follicular lymphoma in first remission induced

Bendamustine (Treanda) plus rituximab (Rituxan) proved more effective than R-CHOP as first-line therapy in previously untreated patients with follicular, indolent, and mantle cell lymphomas, resulting in significantly longer median progression-free survival (54.8 months vs 34.8 months; *P* = .0002). In a multicenter, randomized phase III trial that enrolled 549 patients, bendamustine plus rituximab was less myelosuppressive than R-CHOP and resulted in fewer infections, less peripheral neuropathy, and fewer episodes of stomatitis *(Rummel MJ et al: Blood 114: abstract 405, 2009).*

with rituximab-containing regimens are needed. The results of a GLSG trial comparing IFN maintenance with myeloablative chemotherapy with autologous SCT after induction with CHOP or R-CHOP are awaited.

An alternative approach to consolidating complete and partial remissions achieved with conventional induction therapy is the use of a sequential HDCT program, which culminates in an autologous SCT. The Italian cooperative groups have reported results of a phase III randomized trial comparing R-CHOP for 6 cycles with sequential HDCT with autologous SCT. Again, there was a significant difference in event-free survival but no difference in overall survival.

Single-institution studies as well as analysis of registry data suggest that a tumor-free graft is an important determinant of outcome in follicular lymphoma. Administration of rituximab during stem cell mobilization provides an "in vivo" purge, reducing contamination of the autograft with malignant lymphocytes. The long-term benefit of such an approach has not yet been demonstrated.

Allogeneic SCT has been investigated primarily in young patients with HLA-identical sibling donors and extensive disease and/or marrow involvement. Low relapse rates suggest that this approach is potentially curative but is associated with treatment-related morbidity and mortality. Reduced-intensity transplantation is based on the assumption that a graft-vs-lymphoma effect is operative and has the potential to cure follicular lymphoma. Whether this approach will reduce toxicity while maintaining the low relapse rates associated with standard myeloablative allotransplants remains to be established. A randomized trial comparing this strategy with autologous SCT in relapsed follicular lymphoma has been initiated in the United States.

Overall treatment strategy

Whereas treatment choices were once limited to single or combination alkylator-based treatment, we now are faced with choosing among a wide variety of strategies. There are many unanswered questions that can only be addressed through well-designed clinical trials. Hence, whenever possible, every patient with follicular lymphoma should be enrolled in prospective clinical studies. In the absence of symptoms or other indications for treatment, patients should be observed. A combination of rituximab and chemotherapy is recommended in the absence of a clinical trial for those who require treatment. Selected patients with comorbidities may be best served with rituximab alone. Radioimmunotherapy is a good option at the time of relapse, with transplantation reserved for selected patients in first or subsequent relapse.

CHRONIC LYMPHOCYTIC LEUKEMIA/SMALL LYMPHOCYTIC LYMPHOMA

CLL/SLL is a malignancy of small, round, B lymphocytes involving peripheral blood, bone marrow, and lymph nodes. The term "SLL" is reserved for cases in which there are no circulating malignant lymphocytes. SLL generally presents with lymph node and splenic involvement. Involvement of the bone marrow and peripheral blood may develop later in the course of disease. At the time of presentation, patients may be asymptomatic, complain of only fatigue, or have symptoms related to cytopenias (including autoimmune hemolytic anemia, lymphadenopathy, or splenomegaly).

The immunophenotype helps to distinguish CLL/SLL from other B-cell leukemias/lymphomas, including mantle cell and leukemic forms of follicular lymphoma. Typically, the malignant lymphocytes stain weakly with surface immunoglobulin, CD20, CD22, and CD79b; they are CD5+, CD23+, and FMC7–. Cytogenetic abnormalities are detected in the majority of cases when fluorescence in situ hybridization (FISH) analysis is used. Trisomy 12, deletions at 13q14, and deletions at 11q22-23 are common. Many molecular markers of prognosis have been studied in CLL, including Zap-70, but their value in SLL is unknown.

Given the relatively small numbers of patients with SLL, they have generally been included in clinical trials of "indolent lymphoma." Conventional alkylator-based regimens with rituximab as well as purine analogues and combinations including the recently approved agent bendamustine have been used when patients become symptomatic. Anthracyclines have not been shown to benefit patients with CLL/SLL. When compared with follicular lymphoma, CLL/SLL is less likely to respond to rituximab as a single agent. Alemtuzumab (Campath), a potent therapy for CLL, is less effective in treating nodal disease than peripheral blood and bone marrow involvement. SCT, both autologous and allogeneic, has been studied in selected patient populations but should be reserved for relapsed young patients with a good performance status.

SPLENIC MARGINAL ZONE LYMPHOMA

Splenic marginal zone lymphoma (SMZL) is a rare disorder comprising less than 1% of NHLs. Clinically, this lymphoma most often presents as splenomegaly with splenic hilar node involvement but without peripheral adenopathy. The bone marrow is commonly involved, and malignant villous lymphocytes may be detected in the peripheral blood. Cytopenias are a common presenting feature, often related to hypersplenism and less frequently to an autoimmune process or marrow replacement. Sometimes confused with CLL or MCL, SMZL may be distinguished by its immunophenotype. Typically, cells are CD20+, CD79a+, CD5–, CD10–, CD23–, and CD43–. Staining for cyclin D1 is negative, excluding MCL. The absence of CD103 helps to exclude hairy cell leukemia. Complex karyotypes are common. The clinical course is indolent. Cytopenias respond to splenectomy with long-lasting remissions. High response rates have been reported with rituximab, but the longevity of those responses remains to be determined. Transformation to more aggressive histologies may occur. Fludarabine alone or with rituximab appears to be more effective than alkylators but may be associated with significant toxicity.

NODAL MARGINAL ZONE LYMPHOMA

Nodal marginal zone lymphoma (NMZL) is a primary nodal B-cell disorder that resembles lymph nodes involved by marginal zone lymphomas of extranodal or splenic origin without extranodal or splenic involvement. Lymphadenopathy (either localized or generalized) is the presenting complaint in most cases. Extranodal lymphoma may be uncovered in the evaluation of many cases of suspected NMZL. The clinical course is usually indolent, similar to that of other marginal zone lymphomas.

EXTRANODAL MARGINAL ZONE B-CELL LYMPHOMA OF MALT TYPE

MALT lymphomas comprise only 7% to 8% of B-cell lymphomas but nearly 50% of all gastric lymphomas. Although the GI tract is most often involved, other common sites include the lungs, head and neck, ocular adnexae, skin, thyroid, and breasts. There often is an associated history of autoimmune disorders, such as Sjögren syndrome or Hashimoto thyroiditis or chronic inflammatory processes secondary to infectious agents (*Helicobacter pylori*, *Borrelia burgdorferi*, or *Chlamydophila psittaci*). A form of MALT involving the small bowel (immunoproliferative small intestinal disease, previously known as α-heavy chain disease) has been associated with *Campylobacter jejuni*. The majority of patients present with stage I or II disease. The frequency of bone marrow involvement appears to differ depending on the primary site of involvement. Multiple extranodal sites may be involved at the time of presentation. Transformation to a high-grade lymphoma may occur in approximately 8% of cases.

The malignant lymphocytes of MALT lymphoma are typically CD20+, CD79a+, CD5–, CD10–, and CD23–. The t(11;18)(q21;q21) is characteristic of MALT lymphomas, particularly those involving the stomach or lungs. The translocation creates a fusion between the *MALT-1* gene, which is an essential regulator of *bcl-10*–mediated NF (nuclear factor)-kB signaling, and the *API2* gene, which inhibits apoptosis. This genetic abnormality is a marker of MALT lymphomas that do not respond to antibiotic therapy for *H pylori* infection, are associated with a more advanced stage, and do not transform into more aggressive NMZLs, SMZLs nodal or splenic MZLs or other types of lymphoma. Additional characteristic translocations have been discovered (Table 1), but their clinical significance is uncertain at this time.

Treatment of *H pylori* infection with triple therapy (eg, omeprazole [Prilosec], metronidazole, and clarithromycin [Biaxin]) results in regression in the majority of early lesions. However, tumors invading beyond the submucosa and lesions with t(11;18) are associated with a failure to respond to *H pylori* eradication, deep penetration, and distant spread.

Localized MALT gastric lymphoma that does not respond to antibiotics may be cured with local irradiation, with a field including the stomach and perigastric lymph nodes. This treatment is safe, extremely effective, and preserves the stomach. A single-institution experience reported a 96% complete response rate and a 90% freedom-from-treatment-failure rate, at a median follow-up of 4 years. If local irradiation fails, chemotherapy or rituximab, and in some instances surgery, can be used. Alkylator-based therapy or purine analogues have been used with success for persistent or disseminated disease. The typical dose of radiotherapy is 30 Gy in 20 fractions directed to the stomach and perigastric lymph nodes. Localized nongastric MALT lymphomas also respond well to local radiotherapy.

LYMPHOPLASMACYTIC LYMPHOMA/WALDENSTRÖM'S MACROGLOBULINEMIA

Lymphoplasmacytic lymphoma/Waldenström's macroglobulinemia is a disorder of small B lymphocytes; plasmacytoid lymphocytes; and plasma cells, typically involving the bone marrow, lymph nodes, and spleen. It is usually associated with a serum monoclonal protein (usually IgM) with associated hyperviscosity or cryoglobulinemia. The clinical presentation is usually related to hyperviscosity with visual symptoms, stroke, or congestive heart failure. Peripheral neuropathies occur in approximately 10% of patients related to reactivity of IgM with myelin-associated glycoprotein or gangliosides. An association with HCV infection has been demonstrated. Characteristically, the immunophenotypic analysis reveals surface and cytoplasmic immunoglobulin, usually IgM type, and B-cell–associated antigens (such as CD19, CD20, CD22, and CD79a). The malignant cells are CD5–, CD10–, and CD23–.

The clinical course is generally indolent. Asymptomatic patients may be observed. Plasmapheresis may be appropriate first therapy for those who present with hyperviscosity. The clinical status of the patient, not the level of the protein, determines when treatment is initiated. Choice of therapy depends on many individual factors, including age, comorbidities, and the particular indication for therapy. Rituximab and nucleoside analogues (cladribine and fludarabine) as well as the traditional oral alkylators have shown efficacy, whereas anthracyclines are not beneficial. Rituximab monotherapy may not be associated with a rapid rise in IgM levels associated with increased serum viscosity requiring plasmapheresis. Combinations of these agents are also under study. Bortezomib, thalidomide (Thalomid), and alemtuzumab have shown activity in Waldenström's macroglobulinemia. SCT, both autologous and allogeneic, is being investigated in younger patients with relapsed or refractory disease.

DIFFUSE LARGE B-CELL LYMPHOMA

Clinical presentation DLBCL makes up about one-third of the cases of NHL and is classified as a mature peripheral B-cell neoplasm by WHO. The clinical presentation is variable, but generally patients present with either peripheral lymphadenopathy (neck, axillae) or enlarged nodes in the mediastinum, the mesenteric region, or the retroperitoneum. These sites predict symptoms, which may include chest pain; facial swelling and suffusion of the eyelids (superior vena cava [SVC] syndrome from mediastinal disease); abdominal discomfort, ascites (mesenteric), or back pain; or renal obstruction (retroperitoneal presentations). More than 30% of patients present with disease in extranodal sites, such as the GI tract (including Waldeyer's ring), skin, bone marrow, sinuses, GU tract, thyroid, and CNS. B symptoms, consisting of fever, sweats, and weight loss, are more common in DLBCL than in the indolent lymphomas and occur in about 30% of patients. The median age at presentation is 60 years.

Once the diagnosis is clearly established, staging studies are carried out to determine treatment and define parameters for follow-up. Generally, imaging studies of the chest, abdomen, and pelvis are obtained, and CT scans provide the most accurate anatomic information. Recently, functional imaging using PET scans (which have largely replaced gallium scans) has shown promise as a means of distinguishing between residual scar and active disease after treatment. Further, some investigators have shown that early response by PET scan (after 2 to 3 cycles) is a good prognostic indicator. In addition to CT and PET scans, bone marrow aspirate and biopsy, serum LDH level, and serum beta2-microglobulin level have been described as important predictors of outcome.

TABLE 12: Outcome according to International Prognostic Index (IPI) factors in 365 DLBCL patients treated with R-CHOP in British Columbia

Risk group	No. of IPI factors	% of patients	4-year PFS	4-year OS
Very good	0	10%	94%	94%
Good	1, 2	45%	80%	79%
Poor	3, 4, 5	45%	53%	55%

Pathology/Immunology The diagnosis should be made by incisional or excisional biopsy of an available lymph node, with adequate tissue for immunologic studies, such as flow cytometry or immunohistochemistry (IHC), to identify the characteristic B-cell clonality (kappa or lambda restriction). In many cases of DLBCL, CD10 is present, indicating a germinal center origin. The CD20 antigen is present in almost all cases. In addition, markers for *bcl*-2 and *bcl*-6 offer prognostic information and are part of most diagnostic evaluations of DLBCL. The use of FNA or core biopsy should be discouraged and is acceptable only when tissue cannot be safely obtained by other means and only if flow cytometry is used to help classify the disease and distinguish it from epithelial malignancies that can masquerade as lymphoma.

Prognostic factors Clinical predictors of response have been identified and are now widely used to help design therapeutic plans and clinical trials. These predictors include patient age (< or > age 60), performance status (0, 1 vs 2–4), number of extranodal sites (more than two), Ann Arbor stage (I or II vs III or IV), and serum LDH level (> normal; Table 6). Older patients, higher stage, poorer performance status, higher number of extranodal sites, and higher LDH level all predict a worse outcome, and this model has been validated in more than 3,000 patients. These parameters have been called the IPI; this index is used to plan therapy and clinical trials in the United States and abroad and may be used to predict survival (Table 12).

More recently, genomics have been used to help predict outcome based on molecular signature (see subsection on Molecular profiling). This molecular system provides prognostic information independent of the IPI. Several investigators using similar statistical methodologies have yielded comparable results, and recently these analyses have been extended to other lymphomas.

Treatment Prior to the 1970s, most patients with stage I/II large cell lymphoma (intermediate grade in the Working Formulation) were treated with irradiation alone, with overall cure rates of 40% to 50%. Patients with pathologically favorable stage I/II disease had even better outcomes, but relapse rates, even in these patients, were still 20% to 30%. Pathologic staging, therefore, selected a group suitable for irradiation alone. This approach is no longer appropriate, in view of the success of combined chemotherapy and irradiation in clinically staged patients.

Coiffier et al found that the addition of rituximab improved results in elderly patients with DLBCL, and recent data confirm these observations for younger patients as well. For patients with clinical stage I or II disease (by the Ann Arbor criteria), most studies suggest that chemotherapy (CHOP, and most would add rituximab) for 3 to 4 cycles followed by localized radiation therapy is preferred. Excellent local and systemic tumor control is obtained with combined-modality therapy.

In an ECOG phase III trial, Horning et al showed that 8 cycles of CHOP and irradiation produced a 10-year disease-free survival rate of 57%, compared with 46% with CHOP alone ($P = .04$). Overall survival was 64% vs 60%, respectively ($P = .23$), and time to disease progression was 73% vs 63%, respectively ($P = .07$).

Miller et al showed that CHOP (3 cycles of CHOP and irradiation) produced a progression-free survival at 5 years of 77%, vs 64% for 8 cycles of CHOP alone ($P = .03$). Overall survival at 5 years was 82% vs 72%, respectively ($P = .02$). A recent update of this SWOG study was reported by Miller et al, with an 8.2-year median follow-up. The 5-year estimates for CHOP (3 cycles plus irradiation) vs CHOP (for 8 cycles) remained unchanged. Kaplan-Meier estimates now show overlapping curves at 7 years for failure-free survival and 9 years for overall survival. The treatment advantage for CHOP (for 3 cycles plus irradiation) for the first 7 to 9 years was diminished because of excess late relapses and NHL deaths occurring between 5 and 10 years. Patients with good IPI risk factors had a 5-year overall survival of 94%; patients with one adverse risk factor had an overall survival of 70%; those with three adverse risk factors had a 5-year survival of 50%.

These results were confirmed by a single-arm (doxorubicin-containing chemotherapy) approach followed by IFRT conducted by the British Columbia Cancer Agency. However, two reports from European investigators question the value of consolidation irradiation in early-stage disease. These studies did not use rituximab or FDG-PET staging, and details on the irradiation technique used were not available. The necessity of consolidation radiation therapy after complete response to R-CHOP chemotherapy is now being tested in a randomized study in Germany.

Until further studies define the optimal therapy for stages IA to IIA DLBCL (non-bulky), many investigators consider 3 to 4 cycles of R-CHOP and IFRT the initial treatment of choice. For patients with bulky disease, a minimum of 6 cycles of R-CHOP is typically administered. Irradiation doses of 30 to 36 Gy, delivered in 1.75 to 1.8 Gy over 3 to 4 weeks after completion of systemic therapy, appear to be adequate. Radiation fields usually include involved lymph node sites or an involved extranodal site and its immediate lymph node drainage areas. Furthermore, the disease should be easily encompassed in a radiation field with acceptable toxicity.

Disease site or potential toxicities may influence the treatment plan:

- Lymphomas of the head and neck may be managed with chemotherapy alone to avoid the acute mucositis and long-term xerostomia associated with radiation therapy fields that are large and include both parotid glands. Alternatively, precise radiation therapy techniques can be employed with intentional sparing of salivary glands, using intensity-modulated radiation therapy (IMRT).
- Fully resected gastric or small intestinal lymphoma may be treated with chemotherapy alone. Patients at high risk of perforation or life-threatening hemorrhage may require surgical resection. Alternatively, chemotherapy followed by local irradiation allows gastric preservation and is preferred in most patients.

For patients with more advanced stage (III or IV) disease, CHOP has been the standard (now with rituximab) for 6 to 8 cycles or 2 cycles beyond remission. Recent data suggest an advantage to "dose-dense" therapy, shortening the interval between cycles from 3 to 2 weeks with growth factor support. More data are needed to validate these results. Many studies now suggest an advantage to the addition of immunotherapy in the form of rituximab, and in almost every study, the combination of rituximab and chemotherapy has improved the response rate and disease-free survival. There appears to be no advantage to maintenance therapy with rituximab in this setting, however, as long as rituximab is included in the induction. Responses are seen in upward of 80% of patients, and approximately 50% to 60% achieve a complete remission. It appears that 50% of these patients (30% to 50% overall) are likely cured.

For patients who either do not have a complete remission or who relapse, alternative therapies are possible, but long-term responses have been seen mostly with autologous or allogeneic SCT. Patients who do not have responsive disease prior to SCT generally do poorly. The IPI has been used to predict outcome for transplantation in DLBCL. The role of autologous SCT for high-risk patients remains open to debate. A randomized clinical trial of early vs delayed high-dose therapy for patients with high- and high-intermediate risk diffuse aggressive lymphoma conducted by the US Intergroup is just completing accrual. If this trial confirms the benefit of early SCT in poor-risk patients with chemosensitive diffuse aggressive NHL, subsequent studies will focus on increasing the number of patients who become eligible for transplant consolidation. Investigational treatments include novel antibodies, radioimmunotherapy, and single-agent chemotherapy drugs. Nonmyeloablative SCT is being evaluated in patients with recurrent or refractory disease.

Some investigators believe that irradiation for stages III and IV (advanced or extensive) DLBCL may be added after the completion of definitive chemotherapy if there is localized residual disease, to improve local tumor control. Irradiation may also be delivered after chemotherapy to areas of initially bulky disease, again to enhance local tumor control. These recommendations are based on the observation that when DLBCL relapses after definitive chemotherapy, it usually does so in initially involved or bulky areas of disease. The benefits and potential side effects of irradiation should be weighed against the use of alternative chemotherapy salvage regimens.

MANTLE CELL LYMPHOMA

Clinical presentation By comparison with low-grade NHL, patients with MCL are older (median age is 64 years), mostly male (75%), and more likely to have peripheral blood involvement (about 30%) and extranodal involvement (mostly the GI tract and CNS, as discussed below). The clinical course in MCL is characterized by the worst features of the aggressive lymphomas (an aggressive course) and the indolent lymphomas (frequent recurrences). The disease is often widespread at diagnosis, and marrow involvement and splenomegaly are common. GI tract involvement is also common, and many centers suggest evaluation of the GI tract at the time of diagnosis. CNS recurrences are frequent

Recently, Zhao et al found that microRNA (mRNA) expression predicts outcome in MCL. They found that *MIR-29* downregulation predicted short survival compared with patients who had high *MIR-29* expression and this was comparable to the MCL International Prognostic Index (MIPI). *MIR-29* also inhibited CDK6 proteins (regulated by cyclin D1) and mRNA levels by direct binding to the 3'-untranslated region, linking *MIR-29* to the prognosis and pathogenesis of MCL *(Zhao JJ et al: Blood 115:2630–2639, 2009).*

(up to 20%), but isolated CNS disease is a rare occurrence. Leukemic presentations are not uncommon, especially in patients with "blastic" MCL.

Pathology/Immunology This disorder was originally classified as diffuse, small, cleaved lymphoma by the REAL classification and represents less than 10% of all NHLs. In this disease, a homogeneous population of small lymphoid cells with irregular nuclear borders arises from and expands the mantle zone surrounding the germinal centers of the lymph nodes, spreading diffusely through the node as the germinal centers are overrun. The lymphocytes express IgM or IgD, as in CLL, but in much greater density. It was recognized that the cells carry a translocation of the long arms of chromosomes 11 and 14, notated as t(11;14)(q13;q23). This molecular event juxtaposes the *bcl-1* gene on chromosome 11 to the immunoglobulin heavy-chain gene on chromosome 14, leading to overexpression of *bcl-1*. This gene encodes the cell-cycle regulatory protein cyclin D1, which is believed to play a role in checkpoint control in DNA synthesis. The immunophenotype is characteristic, and MCLs are usually CD5+, CD20+, CD10–, CD23–, and FMC7+. This immunophenotype is similar to that seen with CLL/SLL, except that CD23 is most often expressed in CLL/SLL but usually is not expressed in MCL. The key to the diagnosis is the demonstration in tumor tissue or peripheral blood of the t(11;14) by FISH or the cyclin D1 protein by IHC. Inactivation of the *ATM* gene has been described in MCL. Recent data show that MCL cells express high levels of CXCR4, CXCR5, and VLA-4 (CD49d), suggesting a relationship with the stromal environment.

Treatment Responses to aggressive chemotherapy (CHOP or R-CHOP) are seen, but patients relapse frequently, and median survival is short. Recent data suggest an advantage to SCT while patients are in remission, but more data are required to validate these results. Patients who have relapsed after autologous SCT have been "rescued" by allogeneic SCT.

The NCCN guidelines recommend clinical trials for patients with MCL (there is no "standard" therapy), and ongoing trials are investigating a short course of R-CHOP followed by radioimmunotherapy with ibritumomab. The complete response/unconfirmed complete response rate is 55% after R-CHOP plus ibritumomab, compared with 13% after R-CHOP alone; however, further follow-up is needed. Investigators have found that aggressive hyperfractionated chemotherapy with rituximab (R-hyper-CVAD) may result in long-term responses in patients with MCL (Table 13). Anti-idiotype vaccine studies are also under way in this disease, and novel chemotherapy regimens/agents designed to take advantage of the molecular biology of this disease (flavopiridol, bortezomib, cladribine) are being tested. In addition, recent data suggest that a combination of rituximab and the novel hybrid alkylating agent bendamustine produces high response rates in patients with recurrent MCL.

Recently, the Nordic group presented data that suggest it is possible to achieve long-term disease-free survival in patients with MCL. They compared their prior experience (1996–2000) using a high-dose CHOP regimen for 4 cycles followed by an autologous SCT with BEAM (carmustine [BiCNU], etoposide, cytarabine [Ara-C], methotrexate) or BEAC (carmustine [BiCNU], etoposide, cytarabine [Ara-C], cyclophosphamide) conditioning with a newer regimen (2000–2006). With the newer regimen, patients received Ara-C in between cycles of CHOP, and then rituximab was added starting at week 10. This regimen was followed by an autologous SCT with BEAM or BEAC.

TABLE 13: Hyper-CVAD/Ara-C–MTX for mantle cell lymphoma, lymphoblastic lymphoma, and acute lymphoblastic leukemia

Agent	Dose and frequency
Cyclophosphamide	300 mg/m^2 infused over 3 h q12h × 6 doses (days 1–3) with mesna
Doxorubicin	50 mg/m^2/d on day 4
Vincristine	1.4 mg/m^2 (max 2 mg) IV on days 4 and 11
Dexamethasone	40 mg/d days 1–4 and 11–14
	Alternate every 21 days with
Methotrexate (MTX)	1 g/m^2 continuous infusion over 24 h (day 1)
Ara-C (cytarabine)	3 g/m^2 over 2 h q12h × 4 doses (days 2 and 3)
Leucovorin rescue	50 mg PO at the end of MTX infusion and then 25 mg PO q6h × 48 h

Aggressive supportive care, including administration of cytokines, fluconazole (Diflucan), acyclovir, and trimethoprim-sulfamethoxazole, is strongly recommended.

Patients were then followed using molecular markers by PCR (t[11;14]); those who showed molecular recurrence were treated with rituximab preemptively. Only morphologic relapse was considered a "relapse" for the purposes of this trial.

The results of the two trials were compared and showed that 5-year event-free survival improved from 15% to 41% and overall survival, from 63% to 75%. These data suggest that there may be a plateau in the curve in MCL and that the addition of Ara-C and rituximab may have contributed to that improvement. Further studies are needed to verify these data. Recently, Martin et al from Cornell have suggested that patients with MCL can be observed without treatment. Better performance status and lower-risk IPI scores were characteristic of the patients who could be observed. This finding suggests that a deferred approach to treatment is acceptable in a select group of patients with MCL.

In addition, new agents such as lenalidomide, nutlin-3, romidepsin (Istodax), and belinostat have been found to have activity in preclinical studies in MCL.

An update and summary of the GMCLG group have recently been published, and these data suggest that overall, the outlook for patients with this disease has improved.

BURKITT AND BURKITT-LIKE LYMPHOMA

Clinical presentation These diseases present as three distinct clinical entities: endemic, sporadic, and immunodeficiency-related types. Endemic Burkitt lymphoma most often presents in young children or adolescents with large nodes in the neck, often involving the maxilla or mandible. These cases are most often seen in equatorial Africa and follow the distribution of endemic malaria, hence its designation as "endemic Burkitt lymphoma." In American, or sporadic, Burkitt or Burkitt-like lymphomas, the disease presents in the abdomen and extranodal sites, especially in the GI tract. Sporadic Burkitt lymphoma accounts for 1% to 2% of all adult lymphomas in Western Europe and the United States. The immunodeficiency type is seen in the setting of HIV infection but can be seen in patients with CD4 cell counts > 200 cells/μL. In both endemic and sporadic Burkitt and Burkitt-like lymphomas, males are affected more often than females.

The LDH level is often elevated, owing to the high turnover rate of these cells and the bulk of disease. The bone marrow and CNS are often involved, and if not involved initially, they are at risk, so CNS prophylaxis is needed. A staging system for Burkitt and Burkitt-like lymphomas has been developed by Murphy and associates.

Pathology/Immunology These lymphomas are the most rapidly proliferating NHLs. Under the microscope, it is difficult to distinguish Burkitt from Burkitt-like lymphomas and from the B-cell French-American-British (FAB) L3 variant of acute lymphoblastic leukemia. Indeed, the WHO classification recognizes the lymphoma and leukemic phases as a single entity, a mature B-cell neoplasm. The disease is characterized by medium-sized cells with an abundant basophilic cytoplasm with lipid vacuoles. There are round nuclei with clumped chromatin and multiple nucleoli; a diffuse pattern of infiltration is seen and is classic for Burkitt lymphoma. The numerous macrophages that are usually seen in the lymph node biopsy specimens give rise to the so-called starry-sky appearance.

The proliferative rate of this tumor is high, and there are frequent apoptotic cells. In the Burkitt-like variant, there is greater pleomorphism in nuclear size and shape, and the nuclei have fewer nucleoli. There is a low level of concordance among pathologists (about 53%) when they attempt to distinguish Burkitt from Burkitt-like lymphomas, and even by clinical criteria, that distinction is difficult. The cells express surface IgM, CD19, CD20, CD22, CD10, and CD79a and do not express CD5, CD23, and TdT. Bcl-6, a zinc finger protein, is usually expressed. The major consideration in the differential diagnosis is precursor B-cell lymphoma/leukemia, which in contrast expresses TdT; surface immunoglobulin is mostly negative. CD20 may also be negative in this disorder. In Burkitt lymphoma, the expression of CD10 and Bcl-6 protein suggests that these cells originate from the germinal center, and indeed, this is confirmed by sequence analysis of the immunoglobulin variable heavy-chain and light-chain genes. Somatic hypermutation of these genes has been described.

Genetics The almost constant genetic abnormality in Burkitt lymphoma is overexpression of the c-*myc* oncogene; in 80% of cases, this abnormality results from a balanced translocation between chromosomes 8 and 14, notated as t(8;14), where the c-*myc* oncogene on chromosome 8 is juxtaposed to immunoglobulin heavy-chain enhancer elements on chromosome 14.

In the remaining 20% of cases, there are other translocations, including t(2;8)(p12;q24) and t(8;22)(q24;q11). There have been different breakpoints identified in Burkitt lymphoma, and they have been associated with the sporadic and immunodeficiency subtypes.

EBV One cannot discuss these highly aggressive NHLs without discussing the role of EBV. This virus, a member of the herpesvirus family, has the ability to infect resting B cells and transform

> **In a retrospective analysis, LaCasce et al showed that R-CHOP followed by high-dose therapy and autologous stem cell rescue or R-hyper-CVAD with no transplant was superior to R-CHOP alone as measured by overall and progression-free survival *(LaCasce A et al: Blood 114: abstract 403, 2009).***

TABLE 14: Cyclophosphamide, vincristine, doxorubicin, high-dose methotrexate (CODOX-M) regimen

Day	Drug	Dose	Method	Time
1	Cyclophosphamide	800 mg/m^2	IV	–
	Vincristine	1.5 mg/m^2 (max 2 mg)	IV	–
	Doxorubicin	40 mg/m^2	IV	–
	Cytarabine	70 mg/m^2	IT	–
2–5	Cyclophosphamide	200 mg/m^2	IV	Daily
3	Cytarabine	70 mg	IT	–
8	Vincristine	1.5 mg/m^2 (max 2 mg)	IV	–
10	Methotrexate	1,200 mg/m^2	IV	Over 1 h
		240 mg/m^2	IV	Each hour over 23 h
11	Leucovorin	192 mg/m^2	IV	At hour 36
		12 mg/m^2	IV	Every 6 h until methotrexate level is < 5 × 10^{-8} M
13	G-CSF	5 µg/kg (or 1 × 263 µg ampule)	SC	Daily until AGC 1 × 10^9/L
15	Methotrexate	12 mg	IT	–
16	Leucovorin	15 mg	PO	24 h after IT methotrexate
Ifosfamide, etoposide, and high-dose cytarabine (IVAC) regimen[a]				
1–5	Etoposide	60 mg/m^2	IV	Daily over 1 h
	Ifosfamide	1,500 mg/m^2	IV	Daily over 1 h
	Mesna	360 mg/m^2 (mixed with ifosfamide)	IV	Over 1 h
		then 360 mg/m^2	IV	3 h (7 doses/ 24 h)
1 & 2	Cytarabine	2 g/m^2	IV	Over 3 h, 12 hourly (total of four doses)
5	Methotrexate	12 mg	IT	–
6	Leucovorin	15 mg	PO	24 h after IT methotrexate
7	G-CSF	5 µg/kg	SC	Daily until AGC > 1.0 × 10^9/L

[a] Commence next cycle (CODOX-M) on the day that the unsupported AGC is > 1.0 × 10^9/L, with an unsupported platelet count of > 75 × 10^9/L.

AGC = absolute granulocyte count; G-CSF = granulocyte colony-stimulating factor; IT = intrathecal; IV = intravenous; PO = oral; SC = subcutaneous them into proliferating blasts, most likely by bypassing antigens on lymphocytes and activating signaling molecules. By contrast, certain viruses (HCV) and bacteria (*H pylori*) may cause lymphoma by activating lymphocytes in an antigen-specific manner. EBV infection results in a polyclonal proliferation of lymphoblasts that are latently infected with the virus, as opposed to the infection seen in infectious mononucleosis, which is a lytic infection. This process is regulated by the expression of up to nine latent viral proteins, which are under the control of the transcription factor EBV nuclear antigen 2 (EBNA-2). It appears that the type and result of EBV infection in lymphoid tissue are controlled by various "growth programs," each causing expression of different viral proteins, which then determine the fate of the infected cell. These in vitro events are different from what occurs in healthy carriers of EBV (up to 90% of the population have been exposed), where the viral proteins are not expressed because all of the latently infected cells are resting memory B cells. It is in the germinal center of the lymph node, however, that virally infected cells can transform into memory B cells, as the viral proteins are expressed within the B cells of the germinal center.

Although EBV was found in patients with Burkitt lymphoma over 40 years ago, the role of EBV in the disease still remains uncertain. The exact role of c-*myc* overexpression in the pathogenesis of the disease is also not known, but c-*myc* is known to play a role in cell-cycle progression and cellular transformation. EBV is found in over 95% of cases of "endemic Burkitt lymphoma," which occurs in Africa, but its role in the pathogenesis of the disease is still not clear. The reason therapy with antiviral agents (ganciclovir or acyclovir) cannot be used to treat EBV-associated lymphomas is that the required thymidine kinase gene is not expressed in latent EBV infection. Recent studies using the small molecule arginine butyrate, to upregulate the thymidine kinase gene and protein expression, with concomitant antiviral antibiotics have met with some success.

Treatment Patients must be treated quickly after diagnosis, which should be made on a full biopsy so that adequate tissue is obtained. Tumor lysis syndrome occurs most often with Burkitt lymphoma, and attempts to reduce uric acid production with allopurinol or to degrade it with the enzyme rasburicase (Elitek) should be part of the management, as should aggressive hydration. Patients should be managed in a facility with access to support such as urgent dialysis, because it may be necessary if tumor lysis syndrome occurs.

Treatment includes aggressive chemotherapy, with anthracyclines and cyclophosphamide as the cornerstone. Regimens incorporating hyperfractionated cyclophosphamide such as hyper-CVAD, developed by Murphy and adopted by the M. D. Anderson group, have been used. Other published regimens include CODOX-M/IVAC (cyclophosphamide, vincristine, doxorubicin, high-dose methotrexate/ifosfamide, etoposide, and high-dose Ara-C; Table 14) and the French regimen, which incorporate intensive therapy given weekly in various combinations and intrathecal chemotherapy, and systemic high-dose methotrexate or high-dose Ara-C to facilitate CNS penetration. In children, the results are excellent, and about 80% of patients can be cured. In adults, the outcome is not as favorable, but with newer more intensive regimens 40% to 60% of patients survive 5 years without disease. New approaches using rituximab and early SCT are being investigated, as are new agents (flavopiridol and an analogue of resveratrol) with unique mechanisms of action, which may have relevance to Burkitt and Burkitt-like lymphoma. Addition of rituximab to hyper-CVAD has resulted in marked improvement in outcome in adults with Burkitt lymphoma. Recent data have suggested excellent outcomes in patients treated with DA-EPOCH-R (dose-adjusted etoposide, prednisone, Oncovin [vincristine], cyclophosphamide, hydroxydaunorubicin-rituximab).

PRIMARY MEDIASTINAL LARGE B-CELL LYMPHOMA

Clinical presentation Primary mediastinal large B-cell lymphoma (PMLBCL) occurs most often in young women (female:male ratio is 2:1) who present with mediastinal masses only. These masses are usually bulky and often invade surrounding structures, such as the pleura, lungs, pericardium, and chest wall, but disease is infrequently found outside the chest cavity. At recurrence, however, extranodal sites such as the lungs, adrenal glands, liver, or kidneys may be involved. Because of the location and bulk of the disease, patients complain of chest pain, cough, and shortness of breath and are often found to have SVC syndrome. This can be subtle, with unexplained breast enlargement the only symptom in some cases. The diagnosis can be delayed if the clinician does not recognize the signs and symptoms of SVC. This clinical presentation is similar to classic Hodgkin lymphoma, and indeed, that is the primary differential diagnostic consideration when these patients are evaluated.

Pathology/immunology The pathology is characterized by a diffuse proliferation of large cells with clear cytoplasm, often accompanied by extensive sclerosis. The cells are mostly of B-cell origin and express CD20 and other B-cell markers but do not express surface immunoglobulin (Ig). Indeed, the discordant expression of CD79a and Ig expression are distinguishing features of PMLBCL. There are data that describe gains of chromosomal material in tissue specimens, most often 2p, 9p, 12q, and Xq. The *rel*, *mal*, and *fig1* (interleukin-4 [IL-4] gene) oncogenes are overexpressed in tissue specimens. *Ig* genes have a high level of somatic hypermutation. All of these observations suggest that this entity is unique, especially compared with B-cell lymphomas that arise in peripheral nodes. IL-13 expression and downstream effectors of IL-13 signaling pathways are overexpressed, along with tumor necrosis factor (TNF) family members and TNF receptor–associated factor-1.

The overexpression of the *rel* oncogene, previously described, has been associated almost exclusively with the nucleus, consistent with NF-κB pathway activation, and *mal* gene overexpression has been confirmed in gene array studies. These data help us to reorder our thinking about these clinically unique lymphomas and to begin to build a molecular story that is consistent with the clinical observation that PMLBCL is more like classic Hodgkin lymphoma than like DLBCL. Further, the observations that certain signaling pathways are involved provide a rationale to attack these pathways specifically in a targeted approach.

Treatment The clinical course is variable; some report a poor outcome with conventional, CHOP-based chemotherapy regimens and irradiation, and some report an excellent outcome. It seems clear that bulk of disease and LDH level are important prognostic factors and that prediction of the outcome by the IPI is useful. A variety of chemotherapy regimens have been evaluated, including CHOP and MACOP-B/VACOP-B (methotrexate or etoposide, Adriamycin, [doxorubicin], cyclophosphamide, Oncovin, [vincristine], prednisone, bleomycin), and more recently rituximab has been incorporated into the management. Usually, radiation therapy is a part of the initial treatment; however, recent data suggest that radiation therapy may not be necessary in all patients. Indeed, data from the NCI have suggested that patients with PMBCL may be treated with DA-EPOCH-R with no radiation, with excellent outcomes (see sidebar). In general, in 2010, patients receive anthracycline-containing chemotherapy with rituximab, and after 4 to 6 courses, radiation therapy may be given to patients with bulky disease. There are no randomized trials comparing radiation therapy versus no radiation therapy in this setting. PET scanning may influence the use of consolidation radiation therapy in the future.

Recently, Dunleavy et al found that 35 patients with primary mediastinal B-cell lymphoma treated with dose-adjusted EPOCH-R (DA-EPOCH-R) had 100% progression-free and overall survival rates, with 4 years of median follow-up with no consolidation radiation therapy. Patients with grey zone lymphoma had a worse outcome *(Dunleavy K et al: Blood 114: abstract 106, 2009).*

PERIPHERAL T-CELL LYMPHOMA, UNSPECIFIED

PTCL, unspecified is predominantly a nodal lymphoma that represents the most common T-cell lymphoma subtype in Western countries, comprising approximately 50% to 60% of T-cell lymphomas and 5% to 7% of all NHLs. PTCL usually affects male adults (1.9:1 male-to-female ratio) with a median age of 61 years (range, 17–90), with 25% of patients presenting in stage I or IIE; 12%, in stage III; and 63%, in stage IV. Patients with PTCL from this study commonly presented with unfavorable characteristics, including B symptoms (40%), elevated LDH level (66%), bulky tumor ≥ 10 cm (11%), nonambulatory performance status (29%), and extranodal disease (56%), leading to the majority of patients (53%) falling into the unfavorable IPI category (score of 3 to 5).

Most T-cell NHL patients are treated in the same manner as aggressive B-cell patients, with anthracycline-based combination chemotherapy such as CHOP. Randomized trials comparing CHOP with other combination regimens confirmed CHOP as a standard regimen for aggressive B-cell NHL; unfortunately, these trials do not allow for subset analysis of T-cell patients. Rituximab should not be included in the treatment of PTCL (unless other conditions such as immune thrombocytopenic purpura exist), as CD20 is not expressed. Other therapeutic agents being tested in T-cell NHL include purine and pyrimidine analogues, denileukin diftitox (Ontak), and a retinoic acid/IFN-α combination.

Denileukin diftitox is a novel recombinant fusion protein consisting of peptide sequences for the enzymatically active and membrane translocation domains of diphtheria toxin with recombinant IL-2 (CD25 receptor); it has been studied mostly in cutaneous T-cell NHL, although clinical benefit has been reported in other T-cell NHL patients. Recently, the histone deacetylase inhibitors suberoylanilide hydroxamic acid (SAHA), romidepsin, and depsipeptide have shown activity against PTCL.

Using gene expression profiling, Iqbal et al constructed robust molecular classifying signatures for multiple T-cell lymphoma subtypes, including PTCL NOS, ALCL, AITL, and ATLL. In addition, within PTCL NOS and AITL, they were able to identify unique molecular subgroups with distinctly different survival rates *(Iqbal J et al: Blood 115:1026–1036, 2010).*

In addition, the US FDA has approved the novel antifolate pralatrexate (Folotyn) for the treatment of patients with relapsed or refractory PTCL (see sidebar below). The histone acetylase inhibitor romidepsin has also shown activity in this clinical setting.

ANGIOIMMUNOBLASTIC T-CELL LYMPHOMA

Angioimmunoblastic T-cell lymphoma (AITL), also known as angioimmunoblastic lymphadenopathy with dysproteinemia, is one of the more common T-cell lymphomas, accounting for 15% to 20% of cases and 3% to 4% of all lymphomas. Pathologically, AITL has distinct features, with a diffuse polymorphous infiltrate, prominent arborizing blood vessels, perivascular proliferation of follicular dendritic cells, and the presence of large B-cell blasts often infected with EBV. The malignant cells are mature follicular helper CD4 α β T cells. The mean age at presentation is 57 to 65 years, with a slight male predominance, and the majority of patients present with stage III or IV disease. AITL is commonly a systemic disease with nodal involvement with various associated disease features, such as organomegaly, B symptoms (50% to 70%), skin rash, pruritus, pleural effusions, arthritis, eosinophilia, and varied immunologic abnormalities (positive Coombs' test, cold agglutinins, hemolytic anemia, antinuclear antibodies, rheumatoid factors, cryoglobulins, and polyclonal hypergammaglobulinemia).

Spontaneous disease regression is seen on rare occasions, although AITL typically follows an aggressive clinical course. Treatment with anthracycline-based combination chemotherapy results in complete remission rates of 50% to 70% of AITL patients, although only 10% to 30% of patients are long-term survivors.

One prospective, nonrandomized multicenter study treated newly diagnosed "stable" AITL patients with single-agent prednisone and combination chemotherapy for relapsing/refractory patients or initially if "life-threatening" disease was present at diagnosis. The complete remission rate was 29% with single-agent prednisone, whereas the complete remission rate for relapsed/refractory patients or patients treated initially with combination chemotherapy was 56% and 64%, respectively. With a median follow-up of 28 months (range, 7 to 53), the overall and disease-free survival rates were 40.5% (CI: 24%–56%) and 32.3% (CI: 17%–47%), respectively, although the median overall survival was 15 months.

O'Connor and colleagues reported results using the novel antifolate pralatrexate (Folotyn), for the treatment of relapsed/refractory lymphoma. The overall response rate (ORR) was 31%, including a 17% complete remission (CR) rate. The ORR was higher in T-cell compared with B-cell lymphomas (54% vs 10%, respectively), and all CRs were seen in T-cell lymphoma patients *(O'Connor OA et al: J Clin Oncol 27:4357–4364, 2009).*

There are anecdotal reports of relapsed AITL patients who have responded to immunosuppressive therapy, such as low-dose methotrexate/prednisone, as well as reported responses to purine analogue treatment. Furthermore, cyclosporine has demonstrated activity in relapsed AITL patients in case reports, and the ECOG is evaluating this agent in a prospective study. There are anecdotal reports of responses to thalidomide plus steroid in AITL.

ANAPLASTIC LARGE-CELL LYMPHOMA, T-/NULL-CELL, PRIMARY SYSTEMIC TYPE

Anaplastic large cell lymphoma (ALCL), primary systemic type, is a CD30-positive T-cell lymphoma that accounts for approximately 2% to 3% of all NHLs. This disease mainly involves lymph nodes, although extranodal sites may be involved (not exclusively the skin; see subsection on ALCL, CD30+ cutaneous type). This disease may be divided in part based on the expression of the tyrosine kinase anaplastic lymphoma kinase (ALK), created from a balanced chromosomal translocation t(2;5) and other less common translocations involving 2p23 (see Table 1). When heterogeneous patient populations are analyzed, the prevalence of ALK positivity in primary systemic ALCL cases is 50% to 60%. ALK-positive ALCL is typically diagnosed in men prior to age 35 (male-to-female ratio, 1.7:1), with frequent systemic symptoms and extranodal and advanced-stage disease. ALK-negative patients are usually older (median age, 61 years), with a male-to-female ratio of 1.5:1, with a similar high incidence of extranodal disease.

In addition to the prognostic importance of ALK positivity, the IPI has been identified as an independent prognostic factor within the group of ALK-positive ALCL patients, with a reported 5-year overall survival of 94% vs 41% for IPI 0 or 1 and 2 to 4, respectively. This better prognosis is apparent despite the fact that ALK-positive patients more commonly present with a poorer performance status and more advanced-stage disease compared with ALK-negative patients.

Therapy for pediatric ALCL is often based on prognostic risk factors, with treatment regimens modeled after high-grade B-cell NHL protocols. Following a brief cytoreductive prephase, short, intensified polyagent chemotherapy is administered, with the number of cycles dependent on the stage of disease. Therapy for adult ALCL, primary systemic type, has commonly included anthracycline-based regimens such as CHOP. Autologous hematopoietic SCT in first complete remission for ALK-negative ALCL has been advocated by some groups, although this approach warrants prospective validation. Both naked anti-CD30 monoclonal antibodies (SGN-30) and immunoconjugate such as brentuximab vedotin (SGN-35) anti-CD30–directed antitubulin have shown activity against this disease.

HEPATOSPLENIC T-CELL LYMPHOMA

Hepatosplenic T-cell lymphoma (HSTCL) is an uncommon T-cell lymphoma that is seen mainly in young males (median age, 35) presenting with B symptoms, prominent hepatosplenomegaly, mild anemia, neutropenia, thrombocytopenia (commonly severe), significant peripheral blood lymphocytosis, and rare lymphadenopathy. It is associated with an aggressive clinical course (median survival, 12 to 14 months).

The tumor cells are usually negative for CD4 and CD8 (85%); positive for CD2, CD3, and CD7 (negative for CD5); and express CD56 in 70% to 80% of cases. TIA-1 is present in almost all cases, but commonly granzyme B and perforin are not present, an indication of a nonactivated cytotoxic T-cell phenotype. Cells usually express the γ/δ T-cell receptor (Vd1+/Vd2–/Vd3–) but are negative for EBV.

Historically, patients with HSTCL have been treated with CHOP-like regimens. Early autologous SCT has been favored by some investigators based on anecdotal cases;

however, if feasible, an allogeneic transplant may be more appropriate. A recent report described activity with the purine analogue pentostatin in relapsed HSTCL patients. Approximately 10% to 20% of HSTCL cases arise in immunocompromised patients, predominantly in the solid-organ transplant setting.

EXTRANODAL NK/T-CELL LYMPHOMA, NASAL-TYPE

Extranodal NK/T-cell lymphoma, nasal-type, formerly known as angiocentric lymphoma, is rare in Western countries, being more prevalent in Asia and Peru. The disease commonly presents in men at the median age of 50 years. This entity is associated with EBV and is typically characterized by extranodal presentation and localized stage I/II disease but with angiodestructive proliferation and an aggressive clinical course. These tumors have a predilection for the nasal cavity and paranasal sinuses ("nasal"), although the "nasal-type" designation encompasses other extranodal sites of NK/T-cell lymphomatous disease (skin, GI, testis, kidneys, upper respiratory tract, and rarely orbit/eyes).

Combined-modality therapy incorporating doxorubicin-based chemotherapy (minimum of 6 cycles for patients with stage III or IV disease) and IFRT (minimum 50 Gy), is recommended for patients with extranodal NK/T-cell lymphoma, nasal type, although the benefit of the addition of chemotherapy to radiation therapy has not been confirmed for limited-stage disease.

Patients with systemic disease have poor long-term survival (5-year overall survival, 20% to 25%), with high locoregional (over 50%) and systemic failure rates (over 70%). Asparaginase (Elspar) has been shown to have significant activity against this lymphoma.

ENTEROPATHY-ASSOCIATED T-CELL LYMPHOMA

Enteropathy-associated T-cell lymphoma (EATL; also known as intestinal T-cell lymphoma) is a rare T-cell lymphoma of intraepithelial lymphocytes that commonly presents with multiple circumferential jejunal ulcers in adults with a brief history of gluten-sensitive enteropathy. EATL accounts for less than 1% of NHLs, according to the ILSG, and has been recognized to have a poor prognosis, with reported 5-year overall and disease-free survival rates of 20% and 3%, respectively. This finding is in part related to many patients presenting with a poor performance status and varied complications of locally advanced disease by the time a diagnosis of EATL has been confirmed.

EATL may present without an antecedent celiac history, but most patients have abdominal pain and weight loss. Evidence of celiac serologic markers such as positive antigliadin antibodies and/or HLA types such as DQA1*0501/DQB1*0201/DRB1*0304 may be present at diagnosis of EATL. Moreover, these genotypes may represent celiac patients at higher risk for development of EATL. Small bowel perforation or obstruction, GI bleeding, and enterocolic fistulae are recognized complications of this disease. The immunophenotype consists of pan–T-cell antigens, usually CD8+, and the mucosal lymphoid antigen CD103 is often expressed.

Following diagnosis of EATL, doxorubicin-based combination chemotherapy should be considered for each patient, and aggressive nutritional support with parenteral or enteral feeding is critical in the care of these patients. Patients with known celiac disease should adhere to a gluten-free diet.

ADULT T-CELL LEUKEMIA/LYMPHOMA

The retrovirus HTLV-1 has been documented to be critical to the development of ATLL. HTLV-1 is known to cause diseases other than ATLL, including tropical spastic paraparesis/HTLV-1–associated myelopathy, infective dermatitis, and uveitis. In endemic areas in Japan, approximately 10% to 35% of the population is infected with HTLV-1. Among these carriers, the overall risk of ATLL is approximately 2.5% in patients who live to age 70. Of the Caribbean population, 2% to 6% are HTLV-1 carriers, whereas less than 1% of the population in lower-risk areas, such as the United States and Europe, are seropositive. HTLV-1 is transmitted through sexual intercourse, transfused blood products (products containing white blood cells, not fresh frozen plasma), shared needles, breast milk, and vertical transmission. Transfusion of HTLV-1–contaminated blood products results in seroconversion in approximately 30% to 50% of patients, at a median of 51 days.

The clinical features of 187 ATLL patients included a median age at onset of 55 years, lymphadenopathy (72%), skin lesions (53%), hepatomegaly (47%), splenomegaly (25%), and hypercalcemia (28%) present at diagnosis. The differential diagnosis between cutaneous ATLL and mycosis fungoides is often difficult. ATLL is separated into four subtypes divided by clinicopathologic features and prognosis: acute, lymphoma, chronic, and smoldering. Shimoyama and colleagues reported on the characteristics of 818 ATLL patients. Patients with acute-type ATLL present with hypercalcemia, leukemic manifestations, and tumor lesions and have the worst prognosis, with a median survival of approximately 6 months. Patients with lymphoma-type ATLL present with low circulating abnormal lymphocytes (< 1%) and nodal, liver, splenic, CNS, bone, and GI disease; the median survival is 10 months. Patients with chronic-type ATLL present with > 5% abnormal circulating lymphocytes and have a median survival of 24 months, whereas the median survival of patients with smoldering-type ATLL has not yet been reached.

ATLL is an aggressive neoplasm with resistance to conventional chemotherapy, in part due to the viral protein Tax-mediated resistance to apoptosis and overexpression of *p*-glycoprotein (the product of the multidrug resistance-1 gene). Patients may initially respond to combination chemotherapy, but unfortunately, response durations are brief (5 to 7 months). El-Sabban and colleagues combined arsenic trioxide (Trisenox) with IFN-α, which induced cell-cycle arrest and apoptosis. Response rates of 70% to 90% to combination IFN-α and zidovudine therapy have been demonstrated in ATLL, with associated increased median survival rates compared with those of historic controls. The Japanese Clinical Oncology Group Study (JCOGS) randomized untreated aggressive ATLL to VCAP-AMP-VECP vincristine, cyclophosphamide, Adriamycin [doxorubicin], prednisone-Adriamycin [doxorubicin], MCNU [ranimustine], prednisone-vindesine, etoposide, carboplatin, prednisone) chemotherapy vs biweekly CHOP. They reported a higher complete remission rate and improved survival rates with VCAP-AMP-VECP, although treatment-related toxicity was high. Allogeneic SCT has been successfully employed in select patients.

Other agents with anecdotal activity in ATLL include irinotecan and the purine analogues (pentostatin and 2-chlorodeoxyadenosine, although pentostatin did not appear to improve outcomes when added to combination chemotherapy). Future research should include the investigation of recombinant toxins and antibodies, such as denileukin diftitox and alemtuzumab. Allogeneic SCTs have also been incorporated into the treatment strategies.

CUTANEOUS T-CELL LYMPHOMAS

Cutaneous T-cell lymphomas (CTCLs) constitute a group of cutaneous NHLs with clonal expansion of T lymphocytes into the skin. Several entities are recognized by the combined EORTC and WHO classification, which is based on morphologic, histopathologic, and molecular features (Table 15). The frequency and disease-specific survival rates differ for each entity.

MYCOSIS FUNGOIDES/SÉZARY SYNDROME

Mycosis fungoides and its variants represent the most common type of CTCL, comprising 50% of CTCLs, with a male predominance of approximately 2:1 and a predominance of African-American patients of 1.6:1. It has a yearly incidence of 0.36 cases per 100,000 population that has remained constant over the past decade. Clinical and histologic diagnosis of mycosis fungoides has proved to be difficult, because in early stages, it may resemble other dermatoses such as eczematous dermatitis, psoriasis, and parapsoriasis.

Clinically, mycosis fungoides is characterized by erythematous patches, evolving into plaques or tumors; however, the progress is variable. It is classified as an indolent lymphoma by the EORTC. The neoplastic cells have a mature CD3+, CD4+, CD45RO+, CD8– memory T-cell phenotype. Sézary syndrome is the aggressive, leukemic, and erythrodermic form of CTCL, which is characterized by circulating, atypical, malignant T lymphocytes with cerebriform nuclei (Sézary cells), and lymphadenopathy. Circulating Sézary cells also have a mature memory T-cell phenotype with loss of CD7 and CD26. For staging purposes, the tumor node metastasis (TNM) system is most commonly used (Table 16).

Investigative and recently approved options that have shown activity against mycosis fungoides/Sézary syndrome include the histone deacetylase inhibitors vorinostat (Zolinza, FDA approved), romidepsin (FDA approved), and panobinostat; the novel antifolate pralatrexate; the proteasome inhibitor bortezomib; and monoclonal antibodies targeting CD4 (zanolimumab), CD2 (siplizumab), and CD30 (SGN-30).

Treatment of early-stage disease

At present, CTCLs are regarded as incurable. In early CTCL, the cell-mediated immune response is usually normal. Therefore, the majority of these cases can be treated successfully with topical modalities. Early aggressive therapy does not improve the prognosis of patients with CTCL. The skin-targeted modalities include psoralen plus ultraviolet A (PUVA); narrow-band–ultraviolet B (NB-UVB); skin electron-beam radiation therapy; spot radiation therapy; as well as topical preparations of steroids, retinoids, carmustine, or nitrogen mustard (Table 17). Radiation therapy

TABLE 15: The WHO–EORTC consensus classification for primary cutaneous lymphomas with relative frequency and 5-year survival

WHO–EORTC	Frequency	5-year survival
Cutaneous T-cell and NK-cell lymphomas		
Indolent		
Mycosis fungoides (MF)	44%	88%
· Follicullar MF	4%	80%
· Pagetoid reticulosis	< 1%	100%
· Granulomatous slack skin	< 1%	100%
CD30+ lymphoproliferative disorders		
· Anaplastic large cell lymphoma	8%	95%
· Lymphomatoid papulosis	12%	100%
Subcutaneous panniculitis-like T-cell lymphoma	1%	82%
CD4+ small/medium pleomorphic T-cell lymphoma	2%	72%
Aggressive		
Sézary syndrome	3%	24%
Cutaneous peripheral T-cell lymphoma, unspecified	2%	16%
· Cutaneous aggressive CD8+ T-cell lymphoma	< 1%	18%
· Cutaneous γ/δ T-cell lymphoma	< 1%	–
Cutaneous NK/T-cell lymphoma, nasal type	< 1%	–
Cutaneous B-cell lymphomas		
Indolent		
Primary cutaneous follicular center lymphoma	11%	95%
Marginal zone lymphoma	7%	99%
Intermediate clinical behavior		
Primary cutaneous diffuse large B-cell lymphoma, leg type	4%	55%
Cutaneous diffuse large B-cell lymphoma, other	< 1%	50%
Intravascular large B-cell lymphoma	< 1%	65%

NK = natural killer

prescriptions may be similar to those for other lymphomas or may be delivered at high doses in limited fractions.

Treatment of advanced-stage disease

A limited number of patients progress to more aggressive and advanced disease with either cutaneous or extracutaneous tumor manifestations. Treatment goals in advanced stages should be to reduce the tumor burden, relieve symptoms, and decrease the risk of transformation into aggressive lymphoma. Established treatment options include mono- or polychemotherapy including COP (cyclophosphamide, vincristine [Oncovin], prednisone) or CHOP regimens, extracorporeal photopheresis, interferons, retinoids and rexinoids (bexarotene [Targretin] capsules), histone deacetylase inhibitors (vorinostat and romidepsin), novel antifolates (pralatrexate), monoclonal antibodies (alemtuzumab), and recombinant toxins (denileukin diftitox). Combinations are frequently used (Table 17). Select patients with progressive and recalcitrant disease have been cured with an allogeneic SCT.

TABLE 16: Stage classification for mycosis fungoides and Sézary syndrome

Stage	T	N	NP	M
IA	1	0	0	0
IB	2	0	0	0
IIA	1/2	1	0	0
IIB	3	0/1	0	0
III	4	0/1	0	0
IVA	1–4	0/1	1	0
IVB	1–4	0/1	0/1	1

T (Skin)	
T1	Limited patch/plaque (< 10% of BSA)
T2	Generalized patch/plaque (> 10% of BSA)
T3	Tumors
T4	Generalized erythroderma
N (Nodes)	
N0	No clinically abnormal peripheral lymph nodes
N1	Clinically abnormal peripheral lymph nodes
NP0	Biopsy performed, not CTCL
NP1	Biopsy performed, CTCL
LN0	Uninvolved
LN1	Reactive lymph node
LN2	Dermatopathic node, small clusters of convoluted cells (< 6 cells per cluster)
LN3[a]	Dermatopathic node, large clusters of convoluted cells (> 6 cells per cluster)
LN4[a]	Lymph node effacement
M (Viscera)	
M0	No visceral metastasis
M1	Visceral metastasis
B (Blood)	
B0	Atypical circulating cells not present (< 5%)
B1	Atypical circulating cells present (> 5%)

[a]Pathologically involved lymph nodes

BSA = body surface area; CTCL = cutaneous T-cell lymphoma; M = viscera; N = node; NP1 = biopsy performed, not cutaneous T-cell lymphoma; NP2 = biopsy performed, cutaneous T-cell lymphoma; T = tumor; TNMB = tumor, node, metastasis, blood

TABLE 17: Treatment options for cutaneous T-cell lymphoma by stage

Stage	Clinical features	Treatment options
IA	Limited patch, plaque (< 10% BSA)	Topical steroids, nitrogen mustard or BiCNU, bexarotene gel,[a] spot electron-beam irradiation, PUVA
IB–IIA	Extensive patch, plaque (> 10% BSA)	Topical nitrogen mustard or BiCNU, PUVA, bexarotene gel,[a] total skin electron-beam irradiation, methotrexate, IFN, PUVA + IFN, bexarotene capsules, PUVA + bexarotene capsules, vorinostat, romidepsin, pralatrexate
IIB	Tumors	Spot electron-beam irradiation, PUVA ± IFN, methotrexate, bexarotene capsules, denileukin diftitox, vorinostat, romidepsin, pralatrexate
III	Erythroderma without Sézary cells	PUVA, total skin electron-beam irradiation, topical Sézary cells, nitrogen mustard, or BiCNU, bexarotene capsules, IFN, PUVA + IFN or bexarotene capsules, alemtuzumab, methotrexate, purine analogue, photopheresis, vorinostat, romidepsin, pralatrexate
III	Erythroderma with Sézary cells	Extracorporeal photopheresis, PUVA + IFN, bexarotene capsules ± PUVA, methotrexate, purine analogues, denileukin diftitox, alemtuzumab, vorinostat, romidepsin, pralatrexate
IV	Lymph node or visceral organ	Bexarotene capsules, IFN, denileukin, diftitox, purine analogue, visceral involvement cytotoxic hemotherapy ± skin-directed therapies, vorinostat, romidepsin, pralatrexate

[a]Topical bexarotene may cause irritation if applied to a large body surface area.
BiCNU = carmustine; BSA = body surface area; IFN = interferon; PUVA = psoralen plus ultraviolet A

PRIMARY CUTANEOUS CD30-POSITIVE LYMPHOPROLIFERATIVE DISORDERS

Primary cutaneous CD30-positive lymphoproliferative disorders are the second most common group of CTCL, representing approximately 30% of CTCLs. This spectrum of diseases includes lymphomatoid papulosis, ALCL CD30+ cutaneous type, and borderline cases. The distinction between these entities can be challenging and is often made based on clinical behavior.

LYMPHOMATOID PAPULOSIS

Lymphomatoid papulosis is most commonly associated with mycosis fungoides, CD30+ large T-cell lymphoma, and Hodgkin lymphoma. Three histologic types have been identified, characterized as types A, B, and C. Types A and C consist of large lymphocytes resembling Reed-Sternberg cells. Type A cells are embedded in a dense inflammatory background, whereas type C cells form large sheets imitating CD30+ large T-cell lymphoma. Type B simulates classic features of mycosis fungoides, with epidermotropism and a dermal band-like infiltrate composed of small to medium cells. Lymphomatoid papulosis lesions occasionally exhibit clonal gene rearrangements.

Lymphomatoid papulosis represents a benign, chronic recurrent, self-healing, papulonodular, and papulonecrotic CD30+ skin eruption. However, 10% to 20% of patients may develop a lymphoid malignancy, but the prognosis for patients with lymphomatoid papulosis is otherwise excellent, with a 5-year survival of 100%. There is no curative treatment available. Lymphomatoid papulosis is managed by observation, intralesional steroid injection, topical bexarotene, ultraviolet light therapy, or low-dose methotrexate.

ANAPLASTIC LARGE CELL LYMPHOMA, CD30+ CUTANEOUS TYPE

Primary systemic CD30+ ALCL and primary cutaneous CD30+ ALCL represent identical morphologic entities, but they are clinically distinct diseases.

The neoplastic cells of primary cutaneous CD30+ ALCL are of the CD4+ helper T-cell phenotype with CD30 expression. It represents 9% of CTCLs and typically presents with solitary or localized nodules. This tumor has an excellent prognosis, as confirmed in several studies, in contrast to the transformation of mycosis lymphoma to a CD30– large cell variant. It shows histologic and immunophenotypic overlap with lymphomatoid papulosis. In most cases, tumor cells show anaplastic features, less commonly a pleomorphic or immunoblastic appearance. However, there is no difference in the prognosis and survival rate. Primary CD30+ ALCL rarely carries the t(2;5) translocation and is usually ALK-negative. These lesions may undergo spontaneous regression, as do the lesions of lymphomatoid papulosis. The mechanism of tumor regression remains unknown.

Spot radiation therapy or surgical excision is the preferred treatment, with systemic chemotherapy reserved for cases with large tumor burden and extracutaneous involvement. More recently, there has been reported efficacy of recombinant IFN-γ-1b (Actimmune) and combined treatment with bexarotene and IFN-α-2a (Roferon-A). Naked anti-CD30 monoclonal antibodies (SGN-30) and immunoconjugates (SGN-35–targeting tubulin) have shown promising activity against this lymphoma.

SUBCUTANEOUS PANNICULITIS-LIKE T-CELL LYMPHOMA

Subcutaneous panniculitis-like T-cell lymphoma (SCPTCL) is a rare T-cell lymphoma that infiltrates the subcutaneous fat without dermal and epidermal involvement, causing erythematous to violaceous nodules and/or plaques. Systemic symptoms are frequent and include weight loss, fever, and fatigue. The disease may be complicated by the hemophagocytic syndrome. SCPTCL may be preceded by a benign-appearing panniculitis for years. The infiltrate is pleomorphic and associated with inflammation and necrosis. The T-cell phenotype is α/ß+ with CD4(+/–), CD8+, and CD56(–/+). Standard treatment has historically included CHOP-like chemotherapy. However, recent data suggest patients can be controlled for long periods with local radiation treatment and/or steroids. Five-year survival rates exceed 80%.

CUTANEOUS γ/δ T-CELL LYMPHOMA

Cutaneous γ/δ T-cell lymphoma is a rare panniculitis presenting with disseminated (ulcerated) plaques, nodules, or tumors. Involvement of mucosal or extranodal sites is common. Systemic symptoms, including weight loss, fever, and fatigue, are almost always present. The hemophagocytic syndrome is often noted. The γ/δ+ T cells are characteristically CD2+, CD3+, CD4–, CD5–, CD7(–/+), CD8(–/+), and CD56+. Aggressive chemotherapy is indicated, with consideration of autologous or allogeneic SCT incorporated into the initial treatment schema. The median survival is less than 2 years.

PLEOMORPHIC T-CELL LYMPHOMAS WITH SMALL/MEDIUM CELLS

The small/medium pleomorphic CTCL type appears clinically with single erythematous to violaceous nodules or tumors and accounts for less than 3% of CTCL cases. Most cases have an unfavorable prognosis, with a median survival of ≤ 24 months; however, the CD3+, CD4+, CD8–, CD30– subtype with limited lesions might be associated with a better prognosis, with a reported 45% 5-year survival rate.

The optimal therapy for pleomorphic T-cell lymphomas with small/medium cells has not been defined. Localized lesions have been treated with radiation therapy or surgical excision. Only short-term outcome has been reported. Patients with generalized skin disease or progression have been treated effectively with systemic treatments, including multiagent chemotherapy, retinoids, interferons, and monoclonal antibodies.

CUTANEOUS B-CELL LYMPHOMAS

Primary cutaneous B-cell lymphomas (CBCLs) are rare entities. They constitute up to 25% of all cutaneous lymphomas. However, the incidence of CBCLs has been underestimated due to the absence of immunologic and molecular markers. In addition, their terminology and classification remain controversial, with until recently separate and distinct terminology promoted by WHO and EORTC. Primary CBCLs are distinct from nodal lymphomas, and the majority of them have an excellent prognosis. Several types are recognized, with the most common types being follicular center lymphoma and marginal zone lymphoma.

Primary cutaneous follicular center lymphoma (PCFCL) is defined as a proliferation of centrocytes (small to large cleaved cells) and centroblasts (large round cells with prominent nuclei), showing a nodular or diffuse infiltrate in the majority of cases and presenting only rarely a true follicular pattern. PCFCL is the most common subtype, comprising 40% of CBCLs. PCFCL shows a predilection for the head, neck, and trunk in elderly patients, with a median age of 60 years and a male predominance of approximately 1.5:1. The clinical course is usually indolent, with an excellent overall survival of up to 97%. However, relapses occur frequently. The large round cell morphology might be associated with a higher rate of disease progression and poorer prognosis.

Small centrocytes predominate in low-grade PCFCL, whereas an increased number of large cells occurs in high-grade PCFCL; however, lesions with pure high-grade disease may behave indolently and should not by themselves drive the treatment administered. In contrast to their nodal counterpart, *bcl*-2 is usually not expressed in neoplastic cells, and the t(14;18) translocation is rarely detected. More recently, low rates of *bcl*-2 expression have been reported. In addition to CD10+ and *bcl*-6+ expression, PCFCL also has an aberrant expression of CD45 RA and CD43 and thus

EORTC and ISCL consensus recommendations for the management of CBCLs were recently published *(Senff NJ et al: Blood 112:1600–1609, 2008).*

provides a helpful clue to distinguish it from pseudolymphomas. Radiation therapy is often the preferred therapy for solitary or localized group lesions. Surgical excision can be considered for small lesions. Chemotherapy, though effective, rarely results in cure. Rituximab has proven to be effective for palliation. Observation is a reasonable alternative in many instances.

Primary cutaneous marginal zone lymphoma (PCMZL) is a recently recognized low-grade lymphoma and represents the second most common subtype of CBCLs. It predominantly occurs on the upper and lower extremities. The median age at presentation is 55 years, and females are affected more often than males. The reported survival rates are 97% to 100%, although relapses commonly occur. Histologically, PCMZL has features of MALT lymphomas and shows a nodular or diffuse dermal infiltrate with a heterogeneous cellular infiltrate of small lymphocytes, lymphoplasmacytoid cells, plasma cells, intranuclear inclusions (Dutcher bodies), and reactive germinal centers that may be infiltrated by neoplastic cells. Diagnosis can be difficult, because of the variable composition of the infiltrate that may be interpreted as a reactive process or as PCFCL. In contrast to PCFCL, marginal zone lymphoma is negative for *bcl*-6 and CD10. In 50% of cases, CD43 is highly expressed. Large cell transformation and a head and neck presentation may be associated with a worse prognosis. Therapeutic alternatives are similar to those described for PCFCL.

PRIMARY CUTANEOUS DIFFUSE LARGE B-CELL LYMPHOMA, LEG TYPE

Primary cutaneous diffuse large B-cell lymphoma, leg type (PCLBCL, LT) forms a separate category in the WHO–EORTC classification, as a more aggressive type seen in elderly patients, with a median age of 76 years at diagnosis and a female predominance of 7:2. Most cases have a follicle center cell origin, and histologic evaluation shows a diffuse dermal infiltrate with predominance in large B cells with multilobulated nuclei, comprised of centroblasts and immunoblasts, with the presence of small, cleaved cells and a minor admixed infiltrate component. Eosinophilic intranuclear (Dutcher body) or intracytoplasmic (Russell body) inclusions of immunoglobulin are common. Unlike PCFCL, PCLBCL, LT consistently express *bcl*-2, although it is not associated with the t(14;18) translocation.

The prognosis is less favorable for PCLBCL, LT than for other CBCLs, with a 5-year survival rate of 50% to 60%. Prognostic factors identified with a poor outcome include the predominance of round cells (centroblasts/immunoblasts) over cleaved cells (centrocytes) in the tumor infiltrate, MUM-1 expression, and multiple lesions at presentation. The use of an IPI-based model is required to investigate whether PCLBCL, LT is associated with a poorer prognosis. These lymphomas should be treated as systemic DLBCLs with anthracycline-based chemotherapy. In patients presenting with a single, small skin tumor, radiotherapy is a consideration. Rituximab has also been incorporated into combination regimens.

Intravascular large B-cell lymphoma WHO and EORTC have proposed intravascular large B-cell lymphoma (IVLBCL) or angiotropic B-cell lymphoma as a provisional entity. This subtype is rare and corresponds to the proliferation of malignant lymphocytes within lumina of small vessels, involving most frequently the skin and CNS. It was previously considered a vascular tumor and referred to as malignant angioendotheliomatosis. Although the majority of cases are of B-cell origin, few cases of T-cell lineage have been reported. The reason for intravascular localization is not clear, but association with an unknown surface receptor or dysfunction of lymphocyte-endothelial interaction affecting adhesion molecules has been suspected.

IVLBCL is clinically characterized by tender erythematous, purpuric, indurated patches and plaques located on the trunk and thighs, where it can resemble panniculitis. Cases of generalized telangiectasia over normal skin have been reported. Cytomorphology reveals intravascular occlusion of small vessels, filled with large atypical centroblast-like B lymphocytes. IHC shows CD19, CD20, CD45, and CD79a expression. Genotypic analysis has demonstrated clonality, although it may not be positive in every case. Generally, the prognosis of this aggressive type of lymphoma is poor despite the use of combination chemotherapy, because of the initial or secondary CNS involvement. Prognosis appeared better in some reports, if isolated cutaneous involvement was present. However, no large series permitting a precise prognosis to be determined are available.

CD4+/CD56+ HEMATODERMIC NEOPLASM (BLASTIC NK-CELL LYMPHOMA)

The CD4+/CD56+ hematodermic neoplasm commonly presents in the skin, with nodular and extracutaneous systemic involvement. This rare disorder appears to be derived from a plasmacytoid dendritic cell precursor. T-cell receptor genes are in germline configuration. This entity causes a dismal prognosis (median survival, 14 months) despite intensive chemotherapy.

PLASMACYTOMA

Primary cutaneous involvement of plasmacytoma is uncommon and generally develops as a consequence of direct spread from an underlying multiple myeloma. It represents 4% of extramedullary plasmacytomas and affects predominantly elderly men, with a median age of 60 years at diagnosis. It is characterized by a monoclonal proliferation of mature plasma cells. Cutaneous plasmacytomas are potentially curable, with a 5-year survival rate of > 90%. However, the presentation of multiple lesions is an important adverse prognostic factor. Histopathology shows a dense monomorphous dermal infiltrate of plasma cells with a varying degree of maturation and atypia, admixed with few lymphocytes and histiocytes. Neoplastic plasma cells express clonal immunoglobulin, CD38, and CD79a but are negative for CD20. Rarely, amyloid deposition within the tumor is demonstrated, which is more common in secondary cutaneous involvement of plasmacytoma. A recent organized workshop on plasma cell dyscrasias questioned whether these cases are true cutaneous plasmacytomas, represent reactive B-cell infiltrates associated with an infectious etiology, or represent a variant of marginal zone lymphoma with a predominant population of plasma cells. Diagnosis may rely on demonstration of monoclonality by restriction of Ig light-chain expression. Excision or radiation treatment is most commonly used.

HIV-RELATED LYMPHOMAS

Most lymphomas seen in patients who have HIV infection are of an aggressive histology and advanced stage at presentation. Extranodal disease is common, with unusual sites of presentation, including the GI tract, CNS, and multiple soft-tissue masses. Some patients present with primary CNS lymphoma. Poor-risk factors include a high LDH level, large tumor bulk, extranodal disease, and low CD4 cell counts (< 100 cells/μL). Because of their increased risk of opportunistic infections and impaired hematologic reserve, historically many patients with HIV-related lymphomas have been unable to tolerate aggressive chemotherapy regimens. Current antiviral medications have allowed for the use of more traditional regimens, including R-CHOP and EPOCH-R,with results comparable to those of other NHL patients with similar histologies and presentations.

CNS prophylaxis with intrathecal chemotherapy is necessary to prevent meningeal dissemination. (For a more detailed discussion of HIV-related NHL, see chapter 24.)

POSTTRANSPLANTATION NHL

Posttransplantation lymphoproliferative disorders (PTLDs) remain a morbid complication associated with solid organ transplantation (SOT). The incidence varies from 1% to 2% in renal transplant recipients to 12% to 14% in heart transplant recipients; the latter require more potent immunosuppressive therapy.

The pathologic spectrum of PTLD is heterogeneous, comprising a spectrum ranging from hyperplastic-appearing lesions to frank aggressive lymphoma. The most frequent subtype seen is monomorphic, of which the most common histology is akin to DLBCL. PTLDs are fully depicted in the updated WHO classification (see Table 4).

Historically, PTLDs were reported to occur at a median of 6 months from SOT, although recent data suggest this interval may be longer (ie, median 40 to 60 months). Early PTLD cases (ie, < 12 months after SOT) more often express EBV, whereas late-onset cases are typically EBV-negative.

Overall survival rates have been poor, with mortality rates ranging from 50% to 70% in most studies. However, recent evidence suggests improved outcomes in the modern era.

Treatment for PTLD initially involves the reduction of immunosuppression (usually by at least 50%), especially for early EBV-positive cases. EBV-negative PTLD will respond to immunosuppression reduction but less frequently (15% to 25%) than EBV-positive cases (50% to 65%). In addition, the status of the transplanted organ will in part dictate the amount of immunosuppression safely allowable to avoid organ rejection. The exact role of rituximab in B-cell PTLD is not well defined. Single-agent rituximab was evaluated in two phase II studies for patients who failed RI reduction in immune suppression, with reported overall response rates of 42% and 73% and modest survival rates. However, a recent retrospective series using frontline rituximab-based therapy, in conjunction with reduced immunosuppression, was associated with significantly improved survival compared with prior reports.

The decision of initially treating with rituximab alone vs rituximab with chemotherapy (eg, R-CHOP) is often determined on a patient-by-patient basis. Factors in small studies associated with lower response to rituximab in PTLD include EBV-negative disease and elevated LDH levels. In addition, chemotherapy may be needed as initial therapy for patients who have a large tumor burden warranting rapid response of disease. Of note, during chemotherapy, immunosuppressant medication doses should be either significantly reduced or carefully stopped completely, in part to avoid infectious complications. Carefully selected patients with relapsed/refractory monomorphic PTLD are able to receive HDCT followed by autologous SCT, with long-term survival noted in some reports.

Anecdotal reports have described the activity of thymidine kinase inhibitor antiviral therapies such as ganciclovir and acyclovir to prevent and/or treat PTLD, although the data are not convincing. This finding is not surprising, as EBV survives as an episome outside the lymphocyte genome, and these drugs do not eradicate latently infected B cells. However, one group has shown that arginine butyrate was able to induce EBV tyrosine kinase activity in EBV-immortalized B cells and convert patient-derived latently infected B-cell lymphoma tumor cells that were resistant to ganciclovir to a sensitive phenotype. A phase I/II study with encouraging clinical results was reported. In hematopoietic SCT-related PTLD, EBV-specific cytotoxic T lymphocytes (CTLs) have been utilized. In a recent report, 11 of 13 patients treated with CTLs achieved complete remission, which was associated with long-term persistence of functional CTLs.

PRIMARY CNS LYMPHOMA

Primary CNS lymphoma is a rare form of NHL, arising within and confined to the CNS. Histologically, primary CNS lymphomas are indistinguishable from systemic NHLs. More than 40% of patients have evidence of leptomeningeal dissemination, and 15% have ocular disease at presentation. Thus, examination of the eyes for lymphoma (slit lamp) at diagnosis is important, as is MRI of the entire neurospinal axis, to rule out multifocal disease. A stereotactic needle biopsy is the procedure of choice for diagnosis. Resection does not appear to improve survival.

The two most important prognostic factors in primary CNS lymphoma are age (> 50 years) and poor performance status (Karnofsky Performance Score < 70). Retrospective studies have documented that treatment of primary CNS lymphoma with whole-brain radiotherapy (WBRT) alone (with or without corticosteroids) results in a median survival of 10 to 15 months, with a 5-year survival of 3% to 4%. Current standard therapy for newly diagnosed primary CNS lymphoma is systemic chemotherapy, including high-dose intravenous methotrexate-based therapy (at least 2,500 to 3,500 mg/m^2 per cycle) commonly combined with agents that penetrate the CNS (vincristine, procarbazine [Matulane], and high-dose

In an international multicenter prospective study, Trappe et al studied 104 PTLD patients with sequential single-agent rituximab (Rituxan) followed by CHOP chemotherapy. The initial 64 patients received 4 weeks of rituximab followed by 4 cycles of CHOP, whereas the subsequent 40 patients only proceeded to CHOP if complete remission was not obtained following the initial single-agent rituximab. Two-year time to disease progression (TTP) in the former group was 74%, whereas 2-year TTP was > 80% in the latter risk-stratified group *(Trappe R et al: Blood 114: abstract 100, 2009).*

cytarabine). This regimen results in median survival rates of 50 to 60 months. The most important component in the treatment of primary CNS lymphoma is the use of high-dose methotrexate therapy (at least 2,000 mg/m^2 and up to doses of 8,000 mg/m^2). WBRT had been considered a standard component following chemotherapy; however, long-term neurotoxicity remains a major concern, especially for patients older than 60 years.

A recent study reported encouraging results for primary CNS lymphoma patients who achieved complete remission following 5 to 7 cycles of high-dose methotrexate-based chemoimmunotherapy and subsequently received reduced-dose WBRT (23.4 Gy) compared with the standard WBRT of 45 Gy. Long-term survival data are available using autologous or allogeneic SCT for relapsed/refractory primary CNS lymphoma, although an important factor is control of CNS disease immediately prior to transplant.

TUMOR LYSIS SYNDROME

Tumor lysis syndrome is a common complication after treatment of high-grade, bulky NHLs (due to their exquisite sensitivity to therapy and high proliferative capacity). The syndrome is characterized by renal failure, hyperkalemia, hyperphosphatemia, and hypocalcemia.

Measures to prevent this complication include aggressive hydration; allopurinol; alkalinization of the urine; and frequent monitoring of electrolytes, uric acid, and creatinine. Dialysis is sometimes required. Rasburicase, a recombinant urate-oxidase enzyme, is now available for the prevention and treatment of hyperuricemia. (For a more comprehensive discussion of the tumor lysis syndrome, see chapter 38.)

FOLLOW-UP OF LONG-TERM SURVIVORS

Relapse The most important risk to patients with NHL is relapse. Among patients with diffuse aggressive lymphomas, most recurrences are seen within the first 2 years after the completion of therapy, although later relapses may occur. Physical examination and laboratory testing at 2- to 3-month intervals and follow-up CT scans (with or without PET scan) at 6-month intervals for the first 2 years following diagnosis are recommended. However, it is recognized that upon relapse of disease, the patient usually presents with symptoms rather than the relapse being diagnosed purely on the basis of surveillance scans or routine clinic visits.

Early detection of recurrent disease is important because these patients may be candidates for potentially curative high-dose therapy and SCT. Patients with advanced low-grade NHL are at a constant risk of relapse, and late recurrence of disease may be seen, sometimes after more than a decade-old remission.

Secondary malignancies Long-term survivors are at increased risk of second cancers. In a survey of 6,171 patients with NHL who survived 2 or more years, nearly 1,000 patients lived 15 or more years after diagnosis. Second cancers were reported in 541 subjects, with significant excesses seen for all solid tumors; acute myeloid leukemia; melanoma; Hodgkin lymphoma; and cancers of the lungs, brain, kidneys, and bladder. The actuarial risk of developing a second malignancy at 3 to

20 years after diagnosis of NHL was 21%, compared with a population-expected cumulative risk of 15%.

Treatment complications There has been a more selective use of irradiation as part of the initial therapy for NHL; therefore, the risk of certain radiation-induced complications has been reduced or eliminated in more recently diagnosed patients. Nevertheless, total-body irradiation may be used as a component of myeloablative conditioning regimens. Also, transplant recipients are at increased risk of secondary myelodysplasia and acute myeloid leukemia, regardless of whether they received a radiation-containing conditioning regimen. All individual chemotherapy agents have their own potential long-term morbidity.

Long-term survivors need continued follow-up for possible treatment-related complications. Some of these toxicities may still be unknown. Careful documentation of late complications will be important in the design of future treatment strategies aimed at preserving or improving response rates and the duration of remission while reducing toxicity.

SUGGESTED READING

Al-Tourah AJ, Gill KK, Chhanabhai M, et al: Population-based analysis incidence and outcome of transformed non-Hodgkin's lymphoma. J Clin Oncol 26:5165–5169, 2008.

Au WY, Weisenburger DD, Intragumtornchai T, et al: Clinical differences between nasal and extranasal natural killer/T-cell lymphoma: A study of 136 cases from the International Peripheral T-Cell Lymphoma Project. Blood 113:3931–3937, 2009.

Bachy E, Brice P, Delarue R, et al: Long-term follow-up of patients with newly diagnosed follicular lymphoma in the prerituximab era: Effect of response quality on survival--A study from the groupe d'etude des lymphomes de l'adulte. J Clin Oncol 28:822–829, 2010.

Bernstein SH, Unger JM, Leblanc M, et al: Natural history of CNS relapse in patients with aggressive non-Hodgkin's lymphoma: A 20-year follow-up analysis of SWOG 8516—the Southwest Oncology Group. J Clin Oncol 27:114–119, 2009.

Booth CM, Le Maître A, Ding K, et al: Presentation of nonfinal results of randomized controlled trials at major oncology meetings. J Clin Oncol 27:3938–3944, 2009.

Carson KR, Evens AM, Richey EA, et al: Progressive multifocal leukoencephalopathy after rituximab therapy in HIV-negative patients: A report of 57 cases from the Research on Adverse Drug Events and Reports project. Blood 113:4834–4840, 2009.

Chadburn A, Chiu A, Lee JY, et al: Immunophenotypic analysis of AIDS-related diffuse large B-cell lymphoma and clinical implications in patients from AIDS malignancies consortium clinical trials 010 and 034. J Clin Oncol 27:5039–5048, 2009.

Cheson BD, Pfistner B, Juweid ME, et al: Revised response criteria for malignant lymphoma. J Clin Oncol 25:579–586, 2007.

Ci W, Polo JM, Cerchietti L, et al: The BCL6 transcriptional program features repression of multiple oncogenes in primary B cells and is deregulated in DLBCL. Blood 113:5536–5548, 2009.

de Jong D, Koster A, Hagenbeek A, et al: Impact of the tumor microenvironment on prognosis in follicular lymphoma is dependent on specific treatment protocols. Haematologica 94:70–77, 2009.

Dunleavy K, Little RF, Pittaluga S, et al: The role of tumor histogenesis, FDG-PET, and short-course EPOCH with dose-dense rituximab (SC-EPOCH-RR) in HIV-associated diffuse large B-cell lymphoma. Blood 115:3017–3024, 2010.

Evens AM, David KA, Helenowski I, et al: Multicenter analysis of 80 solid organ transplantation recipients with post-transplantation lymphoproliferative disease: Outcomes and prognostic factors in the modern era. J Clin Oncol 28:1038–1046, 2010.

Evens AM, Sehn LH, Farinha P, et al: Hypoxia-inducible factor-1 {alpha} expression predicts superior survival in patients with diffuse large B-cell lymphoma treated with R-CHOP. J Clin Oncol 28:1017–1024, 2010.

Federico M, Bellei M, Marcheselli L, et al: Follicular lymphoma international prognostic index 2: A new prognostic index for follicular lymphoma developed by the international follicular lymphoma prognostic factor project. J Clin Oncol 27:4555–4562, 2009.

Fernàndez V, Salamero O, Espinet B, et al: Genomic and gene expression profiling defines indolent forms of mantle cell lymphoma. Cancer Res 70:1408–1418, 2010.

Freedman A, Neelapu SS, Nichols C, et al: Placebo-controlled phase III trial of patient-specific immunotherapy with Mitumprotimut-T and GM-CSF after rituximab in patients with follicular lymphoma. J Clin Oncol 27:3036–3043, 2009.

Gerami P, Wickless SC, Rosen S, et al: Applying the new TNM classification system for primary cutaneous lymphomas other than mycosis fungoides and Sezary syndrome in primary cutaneous marginal zone lymphoma. J Am Acad Dermatol 59:245–254, 2008.

Ghobrial IM, Gertz M, Laplant B, et al: Phase II trial of the oral mammalian target of rapamycin inhibitor everolimus in relapsed or refractory Waldenstrom macroglobulinemia. J Clin Oncol 28:1408–1414, 2010.

Herrmann A, Hoster E, Zwingers T, et al: Improvement of overall survival in advanced stage mantle cell lymphoma. J Clin Oncol 27:511–518, 2009.

Heslop HE, Slobod KS, Pule MA, et al: Long-term outcome of EBV-specific T-cell infusions to prevent or treat EBV-related lymphoproliferative disease in transplant recipients. Blood 115:925–935, 2010.

Hess G, Herbrecht R, Romaguera J, et al: Phase III study to evaluate temsirolimus compared with investigator's choice therapy for the treatment of relapsed or refractory mantle cell lymphoma. J Clin Oncol 27:3822–3829, 2009.

Hochster H, Weller E, Gascoyne RD, et al: Maintenance rituximab after cyclophosphamide, vincristine, and prednisone prolongs progression-free survival in advanced indolent lymphoma: Results of the randomized phase III ECOG 1496 study. J Clin Oncol 27:1607–1614, 2009.

Johnson NA, Boyle M, Bashashati A, et al: Diffuse large B-cell lymphoma: Reduced CD20 expression is associated with an inferior survival. Blood 113:3773–3780, 2009.

Johnson NA, Savage KJ, Ludkovski O, et al: Lymphomas with concurrent BCL2 and MYC translocations: The critical factors associated with survival. Blood 114:2273–2279, 2009.

Kchour G, Tarhini M, Kooshyar MM, et al: Phase 2 study of the efficacy and safety of the combination of arsenic trioxide, interferon alpha, and zidovudine in newly diagnosed chronic adult T-cell leukemia/lymphoma (ATL). Blood 113:6528–6532, 2009.

Kurtora AV, Tamayo AT, Ford RJ, et al: Mantle cell lymphoma cells express high levels of CXCR4, CXCR5, and VLA-4 (CD49d): Importance for interactions with the stromal environment and specific targeting. Blood 113:4604–4613, 2009.

Kyriakou C, Canals C, Finke J, et al: Allogeneic stem cell transplantation is able to induce long-term remissions in angioimmunoblastic T-cell lymphoma: A retrospective study from the lymphoma working party of the European group for blood and marrow transplantation. J Clin Oncol 27:3951–3958, 2009.

Leich E, Salaverria I, Bea S, et al: Follicular lymphomas with and without translocation t(14;18) differ in gene expression profiles and genetic alterations. Blood 114:826–834, 2009.

Lenz G, Wright G, Dave SS, et al: Stromal gene signatures in large B-cell lymphomas. N Engl J Med 359:2313–2323, 2008.

Malumbres R, Sarosiek KA, Cubedo, et al: Differentiation stage-specific expression of microRNAs in B lymphocytes and diffuse large B-cell lymphomas. Blood 113:3754–3764, 2009.

Martin P, Chadburn A, Christor P, et al: Outcome of deferred initial therapy in mantle-cell lymphoma. J Clin Oncol 27:1209–1213, 2009.

Martin PJ, Counts GW Jr, Appelbaum FR, et al: Life expectancy in patients surviving more than 5 years after hematopoietic cell transplantation. J Clin Oncol 28:1011–1016, 2010.

Morschhauser F, Radford J, Van Hoof A, et al: Phase III trial of consolidation therapy with yttrium-90-ibritumomab tiuxetan compared with no additional therapy after first remission in advanced follicular lymphoma. J Clin Oncol 26:5156–5164, 2008.

Moskowitz CH, Schöder H, Teruya-Feldstein J, et al: Risk-adapted dose-dense immunochemotherapy determined by interim FDG-PET in advanced-stage diffuse large B-cell lymphoma. J Clin Oncol 28:1896–1903, 2010.

Morton LM, Wang SS, Cozen W, et al: Etiologic heterogeneity among non-Hodgkin lymphoma subtypes. Blood 112:5150–5160, 2008.

Pfreundschuh M, Schubert J, Ziepert M, et al: Six versus eight cycles of bi-weekly CHOP-14 with or without rituximab in elderly patients with aggressive CD20+ B-cell lymphomas: A randomised controlled trial (RICOVER-60). Lancet Oncol 9:105–116, 2008.

Pugh TJ, Ballonoff A, Newman F, et al: Improved survival in patients with early stage low-grade follicular lymphoma treated with radiation. Cancer 116:3843–3851, 2010.

Querfeld C, Kuzel TM, Guitart J, et al: Primary cutaneous CD30+ lymphoproliferative disorders: New insights into biology and therapy. Oncology (Williston Park) 21:689–700, 2007.

Relander T, Johnson NA, Farinha P, et al: Prognostic factors in follicular lymphoma. J Clin Oncol 28:2902–2913, 2010.

Salles G, Mounier N, de Guibert S, et al: Rituximab combined with chemotherapy and interferon in follicular lymphoma patients: Results of the GELA-GOELAMS FL2000 study. Blood 112:4824–4831, 2008.

Savage KJ, Harris NL, Vose JM, et al: ALK-anaplastic large-cell lymphoma is clinically and immunophenotypically different from both ALK+ and ALCL and peripheral T-cell lymphoma, not otherwise specified: Report from the International Peripheral T-Cell Lymphoma Project. Blood 111:5496–5504, 2008.

Savage KJ, Johnson NA, Ben-Neriah S, et al: MYC gene rearrangements are associated with a poor prognosis in diffuse large B-cell lymphoma patients treated with R-CHOP chemotherapy. Blood 114: 3533–3537, 2009.

Sebban C, Brice P, Delarue R, et al: Impact of rituximab and/or high-dose therapy with autotransplant at time of relapse in patients with follicular lymphoma: A GELA study. J Clin Oncol 26:3614–3620, 2008.

Sharkey RM, Press OW, Goldenberg DM: A re-examination of radioimmunotherapy in the treatment of non-Hodgkin lymphoma: Prospects for dual-targeted antibody/radioantibody therapy. Blood 113:3891–3895, 2009.

Suzumiya J, Ohshima K, Tamura K, et al: The International Prognostic Index predicts outcome in aggressive adult T-cell leukemia/lymphoma: Analysis of 126 patients from the International Peripheral T-Cell Lymphoma Project. Ann Oncol 20:715–721, 2009.

Trautinger F, Knobler R, Willemze R, et al: EORTC consensus recommendations for the treatment of mycosis fungoides/Sézary syndrome. Eur J Cancer 42:1014–1030, 2006.

Tsukasaki K, Hermine O, Bazarbachi A, et al: Definition, prognostic factors, treatment, and response criteria of adult T-cell leukemia-lymphoma: A proposal from an international consensus meeting. J Clin Oncol 27:453–459, 2009.

van de Schans SA, Steyerberg EW, Nijziel MR, et al: Validation, revision and extension of the Follicular Lymphoma International Prognostic Index (FLIPI) in a population-based setting. Ann Oncol 20:1697–1702, 2009.

van Leeuwen MT, Grulich AE, Webster AC, et al: Immunosuppression and other risk factors for early and late non-Hodgkin lymphoma after kidney transplantation. Blood 114:630–637, 2009.

van Oers MH, Van Glabbeke M, Giurgea L, et al: Rituximab maintenance treatment of relapsed/resistant follicular non-Hodgkin's lymphoma: Long-term outcome of the EORTC 2098/phase III randomized intergroup study. J Clin Oncol 28:2853–2858, 2010.

Willemze R, Jaffe ES, Burg G: WHO-EORTC classification for cutaneous lymphomas. Blood 105:3768–3785, 2005.

Winter JN, Inwards DJ, Spies S, et al: Yttrium-90 ibritumomab tiuxetan doses calculated to deliver up to 15 Gy to critical organs may be safely combined with high-dose BEAM and autologous transplantation in relapsed or refractory B-cell non-Hodgkin's lymphoma. J Clin Oncol 27:1653–1659, 2009.

Winter JN, Li S, Aurora V, et al: Expression of p21 protein predicts clinical outcome in DLBCL patients older than 60 years treated with R-CHOP but not CHOP: A prospective ECOG and Southwest Oncology Group correlative study on E4494. Clin Cancer Res 16:2435–2442, 2010.

Witzig TE, Wiernick PH, Moore T, et al: Lenalidomide oral monotherapy produces durable responses in relapsed or refractory indolent non-Hodgkin's lymphoma. J Clin Oncol 27:5404–5409, 2009.

Abbreviations in this chapter

ACS = American Cancer Society; ECOG = Eastern Cooperative Oncology Group; EORTC = European Organisation for Research and Treatment of Cancer; GELF = Group d'Etude des Lymphomes Folliculaires; GLSG = German Lymphoma Study Group; GMCLG = German Mantle Cell Lymphoma Group; ILSG = International Lymphoma Study Group; ISCL = International Society for Cutaneous Lymphomas; JCOGS = Japanese Clinical Oncology Group Study; NCCN = National Comprehensive Cancer Network; NCI = National Cancer Institute; NCCTG = North Central Cancer Treatment Group; REAL = Revised European-American Lymphoma Classification; SEER = Surveillance, Epidemiology, and End Results; SWOG = Southwest Oncology Group

CHAPTER 28

Multiple myeloma and other plasma cell dyscrasias

Sundar Jagannath, MD, Paul Richardson, MD, and Nikhil C. Munshi, MD

MULTIPLE MYELOMA

Multiple myeloma is a disseminated malignancy of monoclonal plasma cells that accounts for 15% of all hematologic cancers. In 2010, an estimated 20,180 new cases will be diagnosed in the United States, and 10,650 Americans will die of this disease. Incidence rates for myeloma (5.3 in men and 3.5 in women) and mortality rates (3.7 in men and 2.5 in women) per 100,000 population have remained stable for the past decade, although median survivial is now improving to between 5 to 7 years.

EPIDEMIOLOGY

Gender

Men are affected more frequently than women (1.4:1 ratio).

Age

The median age at presentation is 70 years, according to most tumor registries, although the median age reported in some studies is approximately 66 years.

Race

The annual incidence per 100,000 population is 6.6 among white men and 4.1 among white women. Among black men and women, the frequency doubles to 14.3 and 10.0, respectively, per 100,000 population. This racial difference is not explained by socioeconomic or environmental factors and is presumably due to unknown genetic factors.

Geography

There is no clear geographic distribution of multiple myeloma. In Europe, the highest rates are noted in the Nordic countries, the United Kingdom, Switzerland, and Israel. France, Germany, Austria, and Slovenia have a lower incidence, and developing countries have the lowest incidence. This higher relative incidence in more developed countries probably results from the combination of a longer life expectancy and more frequent medical surveillance.

Survival

The relative survival rate measures the survival of the cancer patients in comparison to the general population to estimate the effect of cancer. The overall 5-year relative survival rate was 37.1% for 1999–2005, and has further improved in the last 5 years.

ETIOLOGY AND RISK FACTORS

No predisposing factors for the development of multiple myeloma have been confirmed.

Environment

Some causative factors that have been suggested include radiation exposure (radiologists and radium dial workers), occupational exposure (agricultural, chemical, metallurgical, rubber plant, pulp, wood and paper workers, and leather tanners), and chemical exposure to formaldehyde, epichlorohydrin, Agent Orange, hair dyes, paint sprays, and asbestos. None of these associations has proven to be statistically significant, and some have been contradicted by negative correlations. The initial report that survivors of the atomic bombings in Japan had an increased risk of developing myeloma has been refuted by longer follow-up.

> Interactions between multiple myeloma cells and their microenvironment (the extracellular matrix and the bone marrow stroma), allow multiple myeloma cells to survive, grow, migrate, and resist apoptosis induced by traditional chemotherapies. These effects are partially mediated through adhesion-mediated signalling and partly through various cytokines, including IL-6, vascular endothelial growth factor, insulin-like growth factor 1 (IGF-1), and TNF-α. The molecular signals mediating the proliferative effects include the RAS/RAF/mitogen activated protein kinase (MAPK) pathway, whereas the P13 kinase (P13K/AKT) pathway provides cell survival and drug resistance signals. Improved understanding of these interactions and the molecular mechanisms mediating them has now allowed us to evaluate novel therapies that directly target multiple myeloma cells as well as act on the bone marrow microenvironment.

Viruses

A preliminary report in a limited number of patients noted the presence of herpesvirus 8 in the dendritic cells of patients with multiple myeloma. However, further evaluation by a number of investigators has failed to confirm this result. Patients with myeloma also do not appear to have a significant immune response against this virus.

Cytogenetics

Karyotypic abnormalities in myeloma are complex, with both numeric and structural abnormalities. DNA aneuploidy is observed in more than 90%; these are predominantly hyperdiploid, with less than 10% being hypodiploid, and carry a poor prognosis. Recurrent nonrandom structural abnormalities have been identified and linked to the pathogenesis and prognosis of myeloma. The immunoglobulin (Ig) heavy-chain gene at 14q32 is frequently involved in translocations with partner chromosomes 4, 6, 8,

TABLE 1: The location and oncogenes involved in multiple myeloma

Locus	Oncogene	Incidence
11q13	*CCND1*	15%–20%
6p21	*CCND3*	5%
4p16.3	*FGFR3* and *WHSC1*	12%
16q23	*MAF*	5%–10%
8q24	*MYC*	< 10%
6p25	*MUM1/IRF4*	5%
20q11	*MAFB*	5%
1q21-34	*BCL9, IL6R, MCL1*	Frequent

11, and 16. The location and oncogenes involved are shown in Table 1. Translocations involving chromosomes 4, 14, and 16 as well as del17p13 (*TP53*) have been associated with a poor prognosis. Del13q or monosomy 13 is observed in 15% to 20% of patients with conventional cytogenetics and also carries a poor prognosis across both standard and high-dose therapies but not certain novel agents. Interphase fluorescence in situ hybridization (FISH) with a specific probe for chromosome 13q34 (retinoblastoma gene, *[RB1]*) identifies this abnormality in up to 50% of patients, with a less clear prognostic implication.

Genetic factors

Multiple myeloma is not an inherited disease, but there have been numerous reports of multiple cases in the same family. However, a case-control study revealed no significant increase in its incidence among relatives of patients who had multiple myeloma, other hematologic malignancies, or other cancers.

Monoclonal gammopathy of unknown significance (MGUS)

Patients with MGUS develop myeloma, macroglobulinemic lymphoma, or amyloidosis at a rate of 1% per year. Recent studies indicate that the diagnosis of symptomatic multiple myeloma is always preceded by monoclonal gammopathy for 2 or more years.

SIGNS AND SYMPTOMS

The clinical features of multiple myeloma are variable. Findings that suggest the diagnosis include lytic bone lesions, anemia, azotemia, hypercalcemia, and recurrent infections. Approximately 30% of patients are free of symptoms and are diagnosed on routine physicals with abnormal laboratory studies, including elevation of serum protein.

Bone disease

Bone pain, especially from compression fractures of the vertebrae or ribs, is the most common symptom. At diagnosis, 70% of patients have lytic lesions, which are due to accelerated bone resorption. These changes are due to pathological imbalance between osteoblast (bone formation) and osteoclast (bone resorption) activity in the bone marrow microenvironment induced by the presence of myeloma cells. Factors inducing osteoclastic activity include interleukin (IL)-1beta, tumor necrosis factor (TNF)-α, and IL-6 as well as newly identified factors such as osteoprotogerin, TNF-related activation-induced cytokine (TRANCE), macrophage inflammatory protein (MIP)-1 α, and receptor activator of nuclear factor kappa B (RANK) ligand.

Osteoblastic activity is inhibited due to production of a soluble factor Dickkopf homolog 1 (DKK-1) by multiple myeloma cells, and overexpression of Activin-A by bone marrow stromal cells.

Anemia

Normocytic, normochromic anemia is present in 60% of patients at diagnosis. It is due primarily to the decreased production of red blood cells by marrow, infiltration with plasma cells, and the suppressive effect of various cytokines. Patients with renal failure may also have decreased levels of erythropoietin, which can worsen the degree of anemia.

Hypercalcemia

Among newly diagnosed patients, 20% have hypercalcemia (corrected serum calcium level > 11.5 mg/dL) secondary to progressive bone destruction, which may be exacerbated by prolonged immobility. Hypercalcemia should be suspected in patients with myeloma who have nausea, fatigue, confusion, polyuria, or constipation. It may suggest high tumor burden. It should be considered an oncologic emergency and requires prompt treatment with aggressive hydration and use of bisphosphonates, calcitonin, and antimyeloma therapy.

Renal failure

Approximately 20% of patients present with renal insufficiency and another 20% to 40% develop this complication in later phases of the disease. Light-chain cast nephropathy is the most common cause of renal failure. Additional causes include hypercalcemia, dehydration, and hyperuricemia. Less commonly, amyloidosis, light-chain deposition disease, nonsteroidal anti-inflammatory agents taken for pain control, intravenous radiographic contrast administration, and calcium stones may contribute to renal failure. More recently, bisphosphonate therapy has been associated with azotemia.

Infections

Many patients with myeloma develop bacterial infections that may be serious, and infectious complications remain the most common cause of death in myeloma patients. In the past, gram-positive organisms (eg, *Streptococcus pneumoniae*, *Staphylococcus aureus*) and *Haemophilus influenzae* were the most common pathogens. More recently, however, infections with gram-negative organisms, anaerobes, and fungi have become frequent. The increased susceptibility of patients with multiple myeloma to bacterial infections, specifically with encapsulated organisms, has been attributed to impairments of host-defense mechanisms, such as hypogammaglobu-

TABLE 2: Common laboratory features of plasma cell dyscrasias

Multiple myeloma
Marrow plasmacytosis ≥ 10%
Clonal immunoglobulin peak (usually > 3.0 g/dL)
Suppressed uninvolved immunoglobulins
Presence of Bence-Jones protein
Lytic bone lesions and/or diffuse osteopenia
Related organ or tissue impairment
Smoldering myeloma
Monoclonal immunoglobulin level > 3.0 g/dL and/or bone marrow plasma cells > 10%
No symptoms due to plasma cell dyscrasia
No lytic bone disease
Normal calcium and renal function
No anemia
Solitary plasmacytoma of bone
Solitary bone lesion due to plasma cell tumor
Normal skeletal survey and MRI of the skull, spine, and pelvis
Normal bone marrow plasmacytosis
No anemia, hypercalcemia, or renal disease
Preserved levels of uninvolved immunoglobulins
Monoclonal gammopathy of unknown significance (MGUS)
Monoclonal immunoglobulin level < 3.0 g/dL
Bone marrow plasma cells < 10%
No bone lesions
No symptoms due to plasma cell dyscrasia
Usually preserved levels of uninvolved immunoglobulins
No related organ or tissue impairment
Amyloidosis without myeloma
Same as MGUS plus evidence of amyloidosis on biopsy

linemia, granulocytopenia, decreased cell-mediated immunity, and the prolonged use of steroids.

SCREENING AND DIAGNOSIS

No screening measures for multiple myeloma have demonstrated any benefit.

The diagnosis usually requires the presence of bone marrow plasmacytosis and a monoclonal protein in the urine and/or serum (Table 2), along with end-organ damage. One immunoglobulin class is produced in excess, whereas the other classes are usually depressed.

Initial workup

The initial workup for patients suspected of having a plasma cell dyscrasia should include:

- CBC with differential count and platelet count
- Routine serum chemistry panel (to include calcium, blood urea nitrogen, creatinine)

- Bone marrow aspirate and biopsy to assess clonal plasmacytosis
- Serum protein electrophoresis and immunofixation to quantitate and define protein type
- Serum free light chain
- 24-hour urine protein, electrophoresis, and immunofixation
- Quantitative serum Ig levels
- Skeletal survey (bone scans contribute little since isotope uptake is often low in purely lytic bone disease)
- Cytogenetics, including FISH on bone marrow cells.

The recently available serum free light chain assay is useful especially in patients with light-chain–only disease, oligo- or nonsecretory myeloma, patients with renal failure, and amyloidosis.

MRI is an excellent tool for evaluation of spinal cord compression/impingement. In addition, MRI identifies generalized marrow signal abnormalities and focal lesions that can be monitored after therapy. Whole-body ^{18}F-fluorodeoxyglucose (FDG) positron emission tomography (PET)/CT scan is becoming more widely used, as it provides details of axial and appendicular skeletal involvement but also identifies extramedullary soft-tissue plasmacytomas presenting as macrofocal lesions. Both MRI and PET/CT are especially useful in staging oligo- or nonsecretory disease.

In addition, additional useful data may be obtained by analysis of such prognostic factors as plasma cell labeling index, ploidy, and analysis of beta-2-microglobulin, serum albumin, C-reactive protein (CRP), and lactate dehydrogenase (LDH) levels.

LABORATORY AND PATHOLOGIC FEATURES

Peripheral blood

The peripheral blood smear may reveal a normocytic, normochromic anemia with rouleaux formation. Plasma cells may also be seen.

Bone marrow

Bone marrow examination usually reveals an increased number of plasma cells. These cells are strongly positive for CD38, CD138, and a single class of cytoplasmic immunoglobulin (cIg). The majority of myeloma cells also express CD40 and CD56. Myeloma cells are negative for CD5, CD19, and surface Ig (sIg) expression. CD20 may be expressed in a subset of myeloma patients often presenting with the t(11;14) translocation. CD10 expression is generally negative but has sometimes been noted in advanced disease. Monoclonality may be demonstrated by immunoperoxidase staining with κ and λ antibodies.

The pattern of bone marrow involvement in plasma cell myeloma may be macrofocal. As a result, plasma cell count may be normal when an aspirate misses the focal aggregates of plasma cells that are better visualized radiographically or on direct needle biopsy.

Monoclonal proteins

The types of monoclonal protein produced are IgG (60%), IgA (20%), IgD (2%), IgE (< 0.1%), or light-chain κ or λ only (18%). Biclonal elevations of myeloma proteins occur in < 1% of patients, and < 5% of patients are considered to have nonsecretory disease, because their plasma cells do not secrete detectable levels of monoclonal Ig.

STAGING AND PROGNOSIS

Patients with symptomatic myeloma should be staged using either the Durie-Salmon system at diagnosis or the International Staging System (ISS), which is determined at the time systemic therapy is begun. These two systems are compared in Table 3. The Durie-Salmon staging system better provides information on tumor burden, whereas the ISS staging system better serves as a prognostic indicator. The ISS is easier to use, and it classifies patients correctly regardless of their geographic origin (ie, North America, Europe, or Asia), age (ie, ≥ 65 years vs younger age), or type of treatment

TABLE 3: Durie-Salmon and International Staging System for multiple myeloma

Stage	Durie-Salmon system[a]	International Staging System
I	*All* of the following: · Hemoglobin level > 10 mg/dL	Serum β_2-microglobulin level < 3.5 mg/L
	· Serum calcium level normal or 12 mg/dL	Serum albumin level ≥ 3.5 g/d
	· On x-ray, normal bone structure (scale 0) or solitary bone plasmacytoma only	
	· Low M-component production rates:	
	Immunoglobulin (Ig) -G value < 5 g/dL	
	IgA value < 3 g/dL	
	Bence-Jones protein level < 4 g/24 h	
II	Fitting neither stage I nor stage III	Not stage I or III[b]
III	*One or more* of the following: · Hemoglobin level < 8.5 mg/dL	Serum β_2-microglobulin level ≥ 5.5 mg/L
	· Serum calcium level > 12 mg/dL	
	· Advanced lytic bone lesions (scale 3)	
	· High M-component production rates:	
	IgG value > 7 g/dL	
	IgA value > 5 g/dL	
	Bence-Jones protein level > 12 g/24 h	

[a]Subclassification: A = relatively normal renal function (serum creatinine (Scr) value < 2.0 mg/dL); B = abnormal renal function (Scr ≥ 2.0 mg/dL)

[b]For stage II, there are two categories: serum β_2-microglobulin level < 3.5 mg/L, but serum albumin level < 3.5 mg/dL; or serum β_2-microglobulin level of 3.5 to < 5.5 mg/L, irrespective of the serum albumin level.

Ig = immunoglobulin

Adapted from Durie BG, Salmon SE: Cancer 36:842–854, 1975; and Greipp PR, San Miguel J, Durie BG, et al: J Clin Oncol 23:3412–3420, 2005.

(ie, conventional chemotherapy vs high-dose therapy followed by autologous stem cell transplantation). More recent studies have provided evidence that the ISS is reliable in patients managed with thalidomide (Thalomid), bortezomib (Velcade), or lenalidomide (Revlimid).

Prognosis

Prognostic indicators may help guide treatment strategy, but the presence of poor prognostic features should not result in initiation of therapy in patients with asymptomatic myeloma. Prognostic factors for risk stratification are well established for conventional chemotherapy. Use of bortezomib and, to some extent, lenalidomide may be able to overcome some features of poor risk.

Cytogenetic abnormalities

Cytogenetic abnormalities detected by conventional karyotyping, especially loss of whole chromosome 13 (monosomy) or deletions of parts of chromosome 13 (13q), with hypodiploidy have been associated with inferior survival after both standard chemotherapy and high-dose therapy. Primary translocations involving 14q32 and 4p16 (fibroblast growth factor receptor 3 [*FGFR3*]), 16q23 (*c-maf* proto-oncogene), and del17p13 (*TP53*) detected by FISH in multivariate analysis have been shown to be important predictors of poor survival. These cryptic translocations are best detected using FISH.

Beta-2-microglobulin

Serum beta-2-microglobulin level is an important and convenient prognostic indicator. When cytogenetic changes are not studied, beta-2-microglobulin is consistently the most important prognostic indicator on multivariate analysis. As beta-2-microglobulin is excreted by the kidneys, high levels are observed in patients with renal failure; even in this setting, elevated serum β-2 microglobulin is associated with poor outcome.

LDH

High LDH levels also have been associated with plasmablastic disease, extramedullary tumor, plasma cell leukemia, plasma cell hypodiploidy, drug resistance, and shortened survival.

Other indicators

Other indicators of shortened survival include elevated CRP, DNA hypodiploidy, high plasma cell labeling indices, and plasmablastic histology. Patients with DNA hypodiploidy are also less likely to respond to chemotherapy.

TREATMENT RESPONSE CRITERIA

Because the criteria for treatment response in patients with multiple myeloma have varied among institutions, response rates have been difficult to compare in the past. In responders, the Bence-Jones protein level is reduced more rapidly than is serum myeloma protein because of the rapid renal clearance of light chains.

The CIBMT/EBMT response criteria follow:

Complete response requires all of the following:

- No serum/urine M protein by immunofixation electrophoresis for ≥ 6 weeks
- < 5% plasma cells in bone marrow aspirate
- No increase in the size or number of lytic bone lesions
- Disappearance of soft-tissue plasmacytomas.

Partial response requires all of the following:

- ≥ 50% reduction in serum M protein > 6 weeks
- ≥ 90% reduction in 24-hr urinary light-chain excretion
- ≥ 50% reduction in soft-tissue plasmacytomas.

Minimal response (but ≤ 49%) requires:

- ≥ 25% reduction in serum M protein for > 6 weeks
- ≥ 50%–89% reduction in 24-hour urinary light-chain excretion
- No increase in the size or number of lytic bone lesions.

The more recent Uniform Criteria for response proposed by the IMWG have sought to further refine these criteria by describing a stringent complete response and a very good partial response (> 90% reduction in the serum paraprotein level), as well as further defining progressive disease. Near complete response is another modification of the criteria and has been applied to the EBMT as part of a number of prospective studies.

TREATMENT

Exciting advances in the understanding of tumor biology and microenvironment—and their potential interaction—have helped to identify unique targets for rational therapeutic intervention to enhance outcome, which has not improved with conventional chemotherapy over the past 3 decades. Until recently, only 5% to 10% of patients with multiple myeloma lived longer than 10 years, which has now dramatically improved with the novel therapies; however cure remains elusive.

Newly diagnosed patients

Chemotherapy

Dexamethasone/thalidomide Thalidomide has been employed alone and in combination with dexamethasone as initial therapy in newly diagnosed patients. When employed alone, response (50% reduction in paraprotein) was observed in 36% of patients; when it was used along with dexamethasone, the response rate was higher (72% and 64% in two studies), including a 16% complete response rate in one study. The results of a randomized ECOG trial showed that the combination of thalidomide and dexamethasone was superior to use of dexamethasone alone (63% vs 41%; $P = .001$). This combination does not damage stem cells and allows adequate stem-cell collection. A definite increase in thrombotic episodes has been observed with this combination, prompting prophylactic administration of aspirin, coumadin, or low-molecular-weight heparin.

VAD or VDD (vincristine, liposomal doxorubicin [Doxil], and dexamethasone) regimens were widely used in the past as induction therapy before high-dose therapy. Recent randomized trials have confirmed the inferiority of VAD when compared with both thalidomide- and bortezomib-based regimens, making this an increasingly less appealing combination.

Pulse dexamethasone alone as initial therapy no longer is recommended. However, brief therapy with pulse dexamethasone may be warranted under special clinical circumstances (eg, renal failure, hypercalcemia, cord compromise requiring radiation therapy, cytopenia) (Table 4).

MP The combination of melphalan (Alkeran) and prednisone has been used over the past 40 years, and other combinations of multiple alkylating agents have not been found to be superior to MP. Approximately 40% of patients respond to the MP regimen, with a median remission duration of 18 months and an overall median survival of 3 years. The MP regimen should be avoided in patients considered to be transplant candidates. Currently, MP should be combined with a novel agent, as noted in this chapter.

MP and thalidomide (MPT) In two large, prospective, randomized trials in patients older than age 65, and a third randomized trial in patients over 75 years of age, MPT has been shown to be superior to MP for response rate as well as progression-free and overall survival. Side effects (including constipation, deep vein thrombosis [DVT], and peripheral neuropathy) were more commonly encountered with thalidomide but were found to be manageable. MPT offers a possible alternative for older people who generally are not candidates for high-dose therapy.

MP and Velcade (bortezomib; MPV) Bortezomib is a first-in-class, potent, selective, and reversible small-molecule inhibitor of the proteasome. In a large international, randomized clinical trial, MPV was shown to be superior to MP for response as well as survival endpoints. MPV induced complete remissions in one-third of the patients, with an overall response rate of 71% and a 2-year overall survival of > 80%. Such high complete responses previously were never seen in this population of patients, where one- third of the patients were over age 75 years. Adverse side effects (eg, peripheral neuropathy, asthenia, fatigue, diarrhea, and constipation) were more frequently encountered on the bortezomib arm. However, the treatment was well tolerated by most patients, with treatment discontinuation due to toxicity noted in only 14% of patients in both arms, and a treatment-related mortality of 1% with MPV (vs 2% in the MP group). The use of weekly bortezomib with this combination has reduced its neurotoxicity substantially, without significant impact on response.

Rd (lenalidomide [Revlimid], low-dose dexamethasone) and VD (bortezomib [Velcade], dexamethasone) combinations Combinations of novel agents with dexamethasone have now been extensively investigated to provide high response rates in newly diagnosed patients.

A randomized study performed by ECOG compared lenalidomide with high-dose dexamethasone (RD; 40 mg/d on days 1 to 4, 9 to 12, and 17 to 20) versus lenalidomide with low-dose dexamethasone (Rd; 40 mg once a week). In this study, the Rd

TABLE 4: Proposed initial treatments for multiple myeloma

Candidates for high-dose therapy	
Dexamethasone	40 mg PO on days 1–4, 9–12, and 17–20 every 35 days or on days 1–4 every 2 weeks
TD	
Thalidomide	Up to 200 mg/d PO
Dexamethasone	40 mg PO once a week or at a higher dose (as above)
VD	
Bortezomib (Velcade)	1.3 mg/m^2 IV on days 1, 4, 8, and 11 every 3 weeks
Dexamethasone	40 mg PO on the day of and the day after bortezomib
Rd	
Lenalidomide (Revlimid)	25 mg/d PO on days 1–21 every 28 days for 4 cycles
Dexamethasone	40 mg/d PO once a week
RVD	
Lenalidomide (Revlimid)	25 mg/d PO for 2 weeks
Bortezomib (Velcade)	1.3 mg/m^2 IV on days 1, 4, 8, and 11 every 3 weeks
Dexamethasone	20 mg PO on the day of and the day after bortezomib
VTD	
Bortezomib (Velcade)	1.3 mg/m^2 IV on days 1, 4, 8, and 11 every 3 weeks
Thalidomide	200 mg/d PO for 2 weeks
Dexamethasone	40 mg PO on the day of and the day after bortezomib
BDox	
Bortezomib (Velcade)	1.3 mg/m^2 IV on days 1, 4, 8, and 11 every 3 weeks
Liposomal doxorubicin (Doxil)	30 mg/m^2 IV on day 4
HDM 200	
Melphalan (high-dose)	200 mg/m^2 IV and stem cell transplant following induction therapy
Clinical trials	Examples of certain combinations currently under study include: Bortezomib, cyclophosphamide, and dexamethasone for 3 courses; VTD for 3 courses Bortezomib, lenalidomide, cyclophosphamide, and dexamethasone Lenalidomide, cyclophosphamide, and dexamethasone
Not candidates for high-dose therapy	
MPV	
Melphalan	9 mg/m^2/d PO on days 1–4 every 6 weeks for 12 cycles
Prednisone	100 mg/d PO on days 1–4 every 6 weeks for 12 cycles
Bortezomib (Velcade)	1.3 mg/m^2 IV on days 1, 4, 8, and 11 and 22, 25, 29, and 32[a]
MPT	
Melphalan	9 mg/m^2/d PO on days 1–4 every 5–6 weeks for 12 cycles
Prednisone	100 mg/d PO on days 1–4 every 5–6 weeks for 12 cycles
Thalidomide	100 mg/d PO monthly for 18 months
Rd	
Lenalidomide (Revlimid)	25 mg/d PO on days 1–21 every 28 days until progression
Dexamethasone	40 mg PO once a week

[a]Consider lower doses and weekly dosing in elderly patients (aged 75 years and older).

arm had significantly fewer toxicities than did the RD arm, including a lower rate of early mortality (5% vs 0.5%, respectively) and a reduced incidence of DVT (24% vs 9%, respectively). Responses were superior in the RD arm; however, the times to progression (27 months) and the overall survivals at 3 years (79%) were identical between the two arms. A select group of patients proceeding to transplant after 4 cycles also had excellent outcomes. Thus, lenalidomide and dexamethasone can be an induction therapy whether or not the patient is likely to undergo high-dose therapy. Stem-cell collection requires use of chemotherapy mobilization.

Bortezomib-containing regimens have also been evaluated in newly diagnosed patients. Using the combination of bortezomib and dexamethasone, Jagannath et al have reported a complete response rate of 18% and an overall response rate of 88% in a phase II study in newly diagnosed patients. Two large, randomized trials have shown that bortezomib plus dexamethasone or VTD (bortezomib [Velcade], thalidomide, and dexamethasone) is an excellent induction regimen pretransplant. These regimens induce rapid tumor cytoreduction; responses attained pretransplant are additive posttransplant, and patients at risk have had better outcomes following their use. Currently, the combination of RVD (lenalidomide [Revlimid], bortezomib [Velcade], and dexamethasone) is under investigation in newly diagnosed patients (Table 5); its use has been promising, leading to response rates in 100% of high-risk patients and very manageable toxicity.

High-dose therapy following induction therapy

High-dose therapy employed after induction therapy improves the response rate as well as event-free and overall survival. The impressive improvement in event-free (median, 28 vs 18 months) and overall survival (57 vs 42 months) reported in a randomized trial (IFM 90) has been confirmed by another large, randomized trial (median overall survival, 54.8 vs 42.3 months; MRC VII). Most of these studies enrolled patients < 65 years old. Older individuals (< age 70) may tolerate high-dose therapy with peripheral stem cell support well and without excess mortality. Moreover, outcome, in terms of event-free and overall survival, is comparable to that in matched cohorts < 65 years old, making older individuals (≥ 65 years old) also candidates for high-dose therapy. More recently, older patients (> 70 years of age) receiving intermediate-dose melphalan (100 mg/m^2) with stem cell support have had a better outcome than have matched controls receiving conventional therapy.

A high-dose alkylating agent, most commonly melphalan at 200 mg/m^2 with peripheral blood stem cell support, is a standard conditioning regimen. Addition of total-body irradiation (TBI) does not improve the outcome but increases morbidity and results in higher mortality. Interestingly, in a randomized study, Fermand et al have confirmed an equivalent survival benefit between up-front high-dose therapy versus high-dose therapy as a salvage regimen at relapse following initial induction therapy.

Tandem transplants The improved outcome reported after tandem transplants in large cohorts of patients in single-institution studies has been confirmed in one mature, randomized study. Seven years after initiation of therapy, the event-free (42% vs 21%) and overall survival (20% vs 10%) rates were superior for patients receiving tandem transplants than for those given single transplants, respectively (IFM 94). Another randomized trial with a shorter follow-up has confirmed the

TABLE 5: Other treatment options for multiple myeloma

RVD	
Lenalidomide (Revlimid)	25 mg/d PO for 2 weeks[a]
Bortezomib (Velcade)	1.3 mg/m^2 IV on days 1, 4, 8, and 11 every 3 weeks[a]
Dexamethasone	20 mg PO on the day of and the day after bortezomib
Clinical trials	Examples of other novel combinations currently under study include: RVD plus vorinostat, and MPV plus CNTO 328 (anti-interleukin-6 monoclonal antibody)
Relapsed myeloma	
Novel agent combinations	TD, RD, VD, RVD, VTD, and BDox (see Table 4)
Conventional chemotherapy	Alkylating agent combinations (MP [melphalan and prednisone]) and DCEP (dexamethasone, cyclophosphamide, etoposide, and cisplatin [Platinol]), typically combined with novel agents (eg, thalidomide, bortezomib)
HDM 200	
Melphalan (high-dose) therapy	200 mg/m^2 IV and stem cell transplant following induction (either as a second transplant if the first SCT was more than or equal to 2–3 years or after successful salvage at 1st relapse)
Clinical trials	Pomalidomide (a new immunomodulatory drug) Carfilzomib (a new proteasome inhibitor) Bortezomib and vorinostat (Zolinza; an inhibitor of histone deacetylase) Bortezomib and perifosine (an AKT inhibitor) Bortezomib and panobinostat (a histone deacetylase inhibitor) Bortezomib and tanespimycin (a HSP90 inhibitor) Lenalidomide, dexamethasone, and elotuzumab (a novel monoclonal antibody targeting CS1, a marker specific to MM)

[a]Consider lower doses and weekly dosing in elderly patients (aged 75 years and older).

superior event-free survival (median, 34 vs 25 months) for patients receiving tandem transplants when compared with those given single transplants but not in overall survival. Moreover, the added benefit of the second transplant was not seen in a subset of patients with a complete response or a very good partial response (> 90% paraprotein reduction) after the first transplant in either study. With the advent of novel therapies, the use of tandem transplant has undergone re-evaluation and the need for a second transplant in patients responding to novel agent–based therapy and single transplant appears to have diminished, making this approach less attractive than, for example, a delayed transplant after subsequent relapse.

Radiotherapy

Higher doses of radiotherapy (40–50 Gy) are employed for local control and cure of solitary plasmacytoma involving bone and extramedullary sites. Lower doses (20–30 Gy) may be employed for palliation of local bone pain from tumor infiltration, pathologic fractures, and spinal cord compression. It should be emphasized that excellent pain relief may be obtained by prompt institution of high-dose corticosteroid therapy, especially in newly diagnosed patients.

Radiotherapy should be employed sparingly, as irradiation of multiple sites may impair stem-cell mobilization in patients who are candidates for high-dose therapy. Employment of high doses of radiation to the spine may preclude the subsequent use of TBI as a conditioning regimen for high-dose therapy.

Remission maintenance

Maintenance therapy been shown to prolong remission duration after initial treatment with or without high-dose therapy and has become an intense area of clinical research.

Thalidomide

Patients responding to thalidomide and achieving maximal response have received lower-dose thalidomide (50–100 mg) with or without added dexamethasone (40 mg for 4 days every month) as maintenance therapy. In the MPT regimen, continued administration of thalidomide prolonged the duration of remission. Three large randomized trials have shown the prolonged remission and improved survival following thalidomide maintenance therapy after autologous stem cell transplantation.

Lenalidomide

Typically lenalidomide-dexamethasone induction therapy is followed by continuation of lenalidomide with or without steroids until progression. Continuation of lenalidomide after MPR regimen has been shown to improve remission duration compared to MP or MPR alone without maintenance. The French group (IFM 2005-002) and CALGB study have completed trials using lenalidomide as maintenance post transplantation. The preliminary results presented for both the studies confirm significant prolongation of event-free survival with lenalidomide maintenance.

Bortezomib

Bortezomib is currently under study as a maintenance strategy. In the APEX study, bortezomib administered weekly proved efficacious and was well tolerated in responding patients who had successfully completed initial treatment. In another study by the Spanish myeloma group (PETHEMA), following a bortezomib-based induction regimen for patients ineligible for transplantation, maintenance with bortezomib–thalidomide was shown to be superior to bortezomib–prednisone.

Interferon-α

Twenty-four randomized trials have investigated interferon-α as maintenance therapy and neither consistent nor significant benefits have been seen. A large Intergroup trial also reported no benefit of interferon maintenance therapy after conventional therapy and autotransplantation.

Alkylating agents

Maintenance therapy with alkylating agents has not prolonged survival when compared with no maintenance therapy. This approach is no longer recommended.

Steroids for maintenance

Two large, randomized trials have shown that glucocorticoid maintenance prolongs the duration of remission and improves life expectancy although side effects are a concern, particularly with long-term use. The SWOG used prednisone (50 mg) every other day, whereas the maintenance regimen in the NCI Canada trial contained dexamethasone (40 mg) daily for 4 days every 4 weeks.

Refractory and relapsed, refractory disease

The majority of patients progress after initial remission lasting between 18 months and 5 years. Rapid progress is being made in the management of relapsed disease and many drugs are being introduced in clinical trials.

Conventional chemotherapy

Alkylating agents, alone or in combination, have been effective in approximately one-third of patients with VAD-refractory disease. Patients relapsing after novel agents only often have responded to alkylating agent therapy. Patients presenting with high LDH and soft tissue plasmacytoma respond to combination chemotherapy with cyclophosphamide, etoposide, cisplatin, and dexamethasone (DCEP) with or without doxorubicin, bortezomib, or thalidomide (VDT-PACE).

Thalidomide

Thalidomide has an established role in therapy for refractory/relapsed multiple myeloma, with 30% of patients achieving at least 50% reduction in paraprotein levels. Remissions obtained are durable. In a large cohort of patients with multiple myeloma receiving thalidomide, 2-year event-free survival rates of ~25% have been observed. Initially, thalidomide was employed in a dose-escalating schedule, starting at 200 mg and achieving a maximal dose of 800 mg. Recently, lower doses have been employed in combination with steroids as well as with other agents (Table 4).

High-dose chemotherapy

High-dose melphalan and stem cell rescue should be offered to patients who have deferred the transplant initially. A randomized trial on early versus late transplantation has shown that an equivalent survival is conferred on patients undergoing salvage, compared with early transplantation.

Novel agents

Lenalidomide

Lenalidomide has greater potency than does thalidomide in preclinical studies and is better tolerated, with less neurotoxicity, somnolence, and constipation.

Two large, multicenter, phase III trials of lenalidomide (25 mg daily for 3 weeks with 1 week off) compared dexamethasone with dexamethasone and placebo in patients with relapsed multiple myeloma. In one study, there was significant improvement in response rate (partial response, 59% vs 21%, respectively) and time to disease progression (11.1 vs 4.7 months, respectively) in the cohort receiving the lenalidomide combination; the results of the second study were almost identical. Similar responses were seen in patients relapsing after prior bortezomib or thalidomide exposure. Prophylaxis against DVT and monitoring for myelosuppression are recommended.

Proteasome inhibitors

A large, multi-institution, phase II trial of the proteasome inhibitor bortezomib (given IV at a dose of 1.3 mg/m^2 on days 1, 4, 8, and 11 every 21 days) demonstrated remarkable activity in a heavily treated population of patients with relapsed or refractory multiple myeloma, including patients relapsing after transplantation or not responding to thalidomide, with durable responses noted in about 35% (with 10% complete response). Side effects related to the drug were predominantly gastrointestinal (GI) in nature, with neuropathy, fatigue, and reversible cytopenias also noted. Toxicities were generally manageable with supportive care and dose reduction. Patients who did not respond to bortezomib monotherapy (progressive disease after 2 cycles or stable disease after the first 4 cycles) were permitted to receive combination bortezomib and dexamethasone. Combination therapy induced additional responses in 18% of patients (13 of 74).

The large, randomized, phase III APEX trial of bortezomib monotherapy compared with high-dose dexamethasone enrolled 669 patients with relapsed multiple myeloma. This trial showed significant improvement in the median time to disease progression (6.5 vs 3.6 months, respectively; $P < .0001$) and median overall survival (29.8 vs 23.7 months, respectively; $P = .027$). Response rates to bortezomib as a single agent were impressive at 43%. The most commonly reported adverse events for bortezomib were GI events, fatigue, pyrexia, and thrombocytopenia; for dexamethasone, they were fatigue, insomnia, and anemia. Neuropathy was also an important issue with bortezomib, but it proved generally manageable with dose reduction and schedule change. DVT was very rare, and efficacy in patients with significant renal dysfunction was noted. Finally, encouraging responses were noted in patients with adverse cytogenetics as well as in patients with advanced bone disease.

Bortezomib has synergistic activity when combined with pegylated liposomal doxorubicin, thalidomide, melphalan, and lenalidomide and showed impressive disease control in refractory myeloma. In a randomized, phase III, multicenter, international study in patients with relapsed refractory myeloma, the combination of bortezomib (1.3 mg/m^2 days 1, 4, 8, and 11) and pegylated liposomal doxorubicin (30 mg/m^2 on day 4) was reported to be superior to bortezomib alone in terms of both overall response (50% vs 42%, respectively; $P = .05$) and time to disease progression (9.3 months vs 6.5 months, respectively; $P < .0001$). When bortezomib (1.0 or 1.3 mg/m^2) was administered with thalidomide (in doses ranging from 50 to 200 mg starting at cycle 2), 86% of patients with relapsed or refractory disease achieved a complete or partial response. A phase II study combining bortezomib with lenalidomide and dexamethasone has shown remarkable activity with minimal toxicity.

Promising drugs in clinical trials

Pomalidomide (CC 4047) is a new immunomodulatory molecule that has shown activity in patients with relapsed and refractory myeloma. In a phase II trial of 60 patients on pomalidomide and low-dose dexamethasone, complete response was noted in 5% of patients, very good partial responses in 28% of patients, and partial

TABLE 6: Supportive therapies for multiple myeloma

Problem	Therapy
Chronic anemia (especially with renal impairment)	Erythropoietin
Prolonged neutropenia with infection	G-CSF
Recurrent infections with IgG < 400 mg/dL	IVIG
Osteoporosis	Bisphosphonates

G-CSF = granulocyte colony-stimulating factor; IgG = immunoglobulin G; IVIG = IV γ globulin

responses in 30% of the patients. Responses were noted in patients with tumors refractory to thalidomide or lenalidomide, and/or bortezomib.

Carfilzomib is a new proteasome inhibitor that does not seem to have significant neurotoxicity. This drug has also been shown to be effective in the treatment of relapsed multiple myeloma as a single agent and in clinical trials with other agents.

Several HDAC inhibitors are currently in phase III clinical trials in multiple myeloma. Both vorinostat (Zolinza) and panobinostat (LBH589) have shown minimal single-agent activity. However, they have shown to have synergistic activity when combined with bortezomib or lenalidomide.

Allogeneic stem cell transplantation

For younger patients with resistant relapse or poor-prognosis disease (eg, with deletion of chromosome 13), allogeneic transplantation may be an important option. The role of allogeneic transplant in myeloma should still be considered investigational. High-dose myeloablative therapy with allogeneic stem cell rescue has been abandoned in light of high transplant-related mortality. A nonmyeloablative regimen is ineffective in tumor cytoreduction and, consequently, is related to a high relapse rate. Thus, uniquely in multiple myeloma, high-dose melphalan and stem cell transplant is followed by a nonmyeloablative regimen and allogeneic stem cell transplantation. Two large, randomized trials from France and Italy that compared tandem autologous transplantation with autologous transplantation followed by allogeneic transplantation from matched sibling donors had different outcomes. French investigators noted no improvement in progression-free or overall survival when inclusion criteria were restricted to a high-risk group, whereas Italian investigators noted better event-free and overall survival when no such restriction for patient entry to the study were in place. In addition, chronic graft-versus-host disease inflicts considerable morbidity in excess of 50% of patients post-allograft.

Supportive therapy

Various supportive therapies may be beneficial in patients with multiple myeloma (Table 6).

Chronic anemia

The use of erythropoietic-stimulating agents (ESAs) in myeloma should generally be restricted to patients who are anemic due to concomitant chemotherapy or moderate-to-severe renal failure. The combined use of ESA and immunomodulatory agents is associated with an increased incidence of venous thromboembolism, but this is not seen with bortezomib. For additional information about the use of ESAs in patients with cancer visit www.fda.gov/Drugs/DrugSafety/PostmarketDrugSafetyInformationforPatientsandProviders/ucm109375.htm

Infection

Serious infection with encapsulated organisms is encountered by patients with myeloma due to their inability to mount successful antibody production (and lack of opsonization). Prompt institution of antibiotics is therefore recommended in the face of systemic infection. Antibiotic prophylaxis is also recommended whenever high-dose glucocorticoids are used for treatment. Patients with recurrent serious infections may benefit from monthly IVγ globulin. Shingles is not uncommon in these patients, and prophylaxis following transplantation and during bortezomib therapy is advised.

Bone pain or imminent fracture

Therapy with bisphosphonates, such as pamidronate, alendronate (Fosamax), or zoledronic acid (Zometa), may prevent or delay bone pain or recurrent or imminent pathologic fracture in patients with stage III disease and at least one bone lesion. Pamidronate administered over the long term (21 monthly treatments) to patients with stage III multiple myeloma with at least one lytic lesion reduces skeletal events and decreases the need for irradiation. Moreover, patients without lytic lesions also show a decrease in bone mineral density, and this decrease persists despite chemotherapy. These patients may also benefit from therapy with pamidronate. Several clinical and preclinical studies suggest that pamidronate may have an antimyeloma effect.

Zoledronic acid, a more potent bisphosphonate, has comparable efficacy and safety to pamidronate in preventing skeletal lesions. The ease of administration of a 4-mg dose, which reduces the infusion time to 15 minutes as compared with 2 hours for pamidronate, has led to approval of zoledronic acid by the FDA for prevention of bone-related complications in myeloma. Caution should be exercised with long-term use of bisphosphonates, as renal impairment and osteonecrosis of the jaw bones have been reported.

Percutaneous vertebroplasty provides pain relief that is not only rapid but sustained, and it also strengthens the vertebral bodies. Kyphoplasty is a safer procedure that involves insertion of a balloon followed by injection of polymethyl methacrylate, the principal component of bone cement, into the balloon. It is performed with the patient under local anesthesia. Transient worsening of pain and fever that may occur is responsive to nonsteroidal anti-inflammatory agents.

SMOLDERING MYELOMA

Smoldering, or asymptomatic, myeloma is characterized by the presence of monoclonal Ig > 3 g/dL and/or bone marrow plasmacytosis in excess of 10%. The diagnosis is often made by a chance finding of an elevated serum protein level during a screening examination.

Laboratory features

Features of low tumor mass are usually present, without renal disease, hypercalcemia, or lytic bone lesions (Table 2). Marrow plasma cytosis occurs in less than 30% of patients, and anemia, if present, is mild (hemoglobin value > 10.5 g/dL).

Treatment

Chemotherapy should be withheld until the patient becomes symptomatic. The role of bisphosphonates and lenalidomide in this setting is under investigation, although a series of studies have suggested benefit from reducing the incidence of bone complications and increasing the time to progression with bisphosphonate use. An MRI finding of multifocal plasmacytomas or FDG-PET/CT findings of multifocal osseous lesions would be considered to be evidence of end-organ damage and would warrant initiation of systemic therapy.

Prognostic factors Smoldering myeloma generally progresses to multiple myeloma at the rate of 10% per year for the first 5 years, 3% per year for the next 5 years, and then 1% for the last 10 years. The initial concentration of serum monoclonal protein > 3.0 g/dL, bone marrow plasmacytosis > 10%, and abnormal serum free light chain ratio are significant predictors of progression to symptomatic myeloma.

OTHER PLASMA CELL DYSCRASIAS

Other plasma cell dyscrasias include MGUS, solitary plasmacytoma of bone (SPB), solitary extramedullary plasmacytoma, Waldenström's macroglobulinemia, amyloidosis, POEMS (polyneuropathy, organomegaly, endocrinopathy, monoclonal gammopathy, and skin changes) syndrome, and heavy-chain diseases.

MONOCLONAL GAMMOPATHY OF UNKNOWN SIGNIFICANCE

MGUS occurs in 1% of normal individuals > 40 years old, and its frequency rises progressively with age. Recent studies indicate that the diagnosis of symptomatic multiple myeloma is always preceded by monoclonal gammopathy for 2 or more years.

Laboratory features

Common laboratory features of MGUS are listed in Table 2.

Treatment

Approximately 25% of patients with this disorder develop multiple myeloma, macroglobulinemia, or non-Hodgkin lymphoma over 20 years. The initial concentration of serum monoclonal protein > 1.5 g/dL, non–IgG-type paraprotein, and abnormal serum free light-chain ratio are significant predictors of disease progression at 20 years. The long period of stability supports annual monitoring with serum electrophoresis and blood counts and suggests that chemotherapy may be withheld until there is evidence of progression to myeloma.

SOLITARY PLASMACYTOMA OF BONE

Approximately 3% of patients with myeloma have solitary plasmacytoma of bone (SPB).

Laboratory features

All patients have either no myeloma protein or very low levels in serum or urine (Table 2). MRI may reveal abnormalities not detected by bone survey and may upstage patients to multiple myeloma. Persistence of monoclonal protein for more than 1 year after irradiation predicts early disease progression to multiple myeloma.

Treatment

Management of SPB consists of radiation therapy (at least 45 Gy). Multiple myeloma becomes evident in most patients over time, so only 20% of patients remain free of disease for more than 10 years. The median time for disease progression is approximately 2 to 3 years.

SOLITARY EXTRAMEDULLARY PLASMACYTOMA

In contrast to SPB, solitary extramedullary plasmacytoma is often truly localized and can be cured in up to 50% of patients with localized radiation therapy (45–50 Gy) and/or resection. Careful observation after treatment is nonetheless warranted.

WALDENSTRÖM'S MACROGLOBULINEMIA

This uncommon disease is characterized by lymphoplasmacytic bone marrow and tissue infiltrate in addition to elevated IgM production. The mutation pattern analysis suggests that final transformation occurs in the postgerminal center IgM memory B cell. Corresponding with variation in cell morphology, there is variation in the immunophenotype. Mature plasma cells exhibit CD38 antigen; however, lymphoid cells are typically positive for CD19, CD20, and CD22.

Waldenström's macroglobulinemia usually affects people in the fifth to seventh decades of life and can cause symptoms due to tumor infiltration (marrow, lymph nodes, and/or spleen), circulating IgM (hyperviscosity, cryoglobulinemia, and/or cold agglutinin hemolytic anemia), and tissue deposition of IgM (neuropathy, glomerular disease, and/or amyloidosis). Neuropathy may be due to the IgM antibody reacting with myelin-associated glycoprotein.

Hyperviscosity syndrome

With hyperviscosity syndrome, patients may have visual symptoms, dizziness, cardiopulmonary symptoms, decreased consciousness, and a bleeding diathesis.

Therapy for hyperviscosity consists of plasmapheresis followed by chemotherapy to control the malignant proliferation. Patients with poor performance status and elderly patients who are unable to tolerate chemotherapy may be maintained with periodic plasmapheresis.

Treatment

Alkylating agents used in combination with steroids or purine analogs remain the mainstay of therapy. Alkylating agents alone or in combination with steroids effect a 50% reduction in paraprotein in about half of patients, and the median survival time is around 5 years. The purine analogs fludarabine (Fludara) and cladribine (Leustatin) elicit a more rapid response than other agents, with a response rate of more than 75% observed in a small series of patients. Preliminary results of a large, American multi-institution evaluation of fludarabine reported partial responses in only 33% of patients.

Purine analog therapy may result in significant myelosuppression in later cycles of therapy and prolonged immunosuppression with increased opportunistic infections. Purine analogs are effective salvage options in patients refractory to or relapsing following alkylator therapy. Patients refractory to one purine analog are rarely salvaged by a different purine analog. Patients with resistant relapse are less likely to benefit from purine analogs (response rate, 18%) and should be considered for more intensive intervention, including high-dose therapy.

Other treatment options

Rituximab (Rituxan), an anti-CD20 monoclonal antibody, is effective in Waldenström's macroglobulinemia, because the CD20 antigen is usually present on the lymphoid cell component of macroglobulinemia. Preliminary results indicate that about 30% of previously treated patients (refractory or relapsing off therapy) may benefit from rituximab.

Striking activity of thalidomide in multiple myeloma has prompted its use in Waldenström's macroglobulinemia. In a series of 20 patients receiving thalidomide, 25% achieved a 50% reduction in paraprotein. Higher doses of thalidomide were not well tolerated in an elderly cohort of patients. Interestingly, preliminary results of bortezomib-based therapy in relapsed Waldenström's macroglobulinemia have been promising.

High-dose therapy with autologous bone marrow or blood stem cell rescue has been effective in achieving 50% reduction in paraprotein in almost all patients in small pilot trials.

AMYLOIDOSIS

Amyloidosis occurs in 10% of patients with multiple myeloma. This infiltrative process results from organ deposition of amyloid fibrils, which consist of the NH2 terminal amino acid residues of the variable portion of the light-chain Ig molecule. The abnormal protein is produced by clonal plasma cells.

Clinical features

These include the nephrotic syndrome, cardiomyopathy, hepatomegaly, neuropathy, macroglossia, carpal tunnel syndrome, and periorbital purpura.

Laboratory features

Serum and urine immunofixation studies show a monoclonal Ig in approximately 80% of patients. Measurement of serum free light chain may provide a marker to evaluate response to therapy. The light chain is more frequently of the λ than κ type. Diagnosis can be made by the presence of apple-green birefringence on polarized light examination of subcutaneous fat aspirates stained with Congo red. Elevated serum B-type natriuretic peptide levels may indicate cardiac involvement, which, in the majority of patients, may be confirmed with echocardiography.

Treatment of primary amyloidosis (AL; monoclonal protein–associated)

Survival of patients with amyloidosis is variable. Patients with congestive heart failure have a median survival of only 4 months. Oral MP extends the median survival to 17 months, as compared with 13 months in untreated patients. Complete hematologic response is rare; similarly, reversal of organ damage is uncommon.

In a large cohort of patients receiving high-dose melphalan with stem cell support, a complete hematologic response was observed in 47% of patients with at least 1 year of follow-up. However, the transplant-related mortality is high with high-dose therapy (14% to 37%). Complete hematologic response was associated with improved clinical response (improved organ function) and survival. Complete hematologic response in the absence of cardiac involvement predicted excellent outcome (1-year survival, 91%). Preliminary studies have also shown encouraging results with bortezomib as well as lenalidomide.

Patients with the overlap syndrome of myeloma and AL amyloidosis should be treated aggressively for myeloma; response can be seen in terms of both myeloma and resolution of amyloid symptoms.

POEMS SYNDROME

Clinical features and course

The POEMS syndrome is a rare plasma cell dyscrasia that presents with peripheral, usually sensorimotor, neuropathy; monoclonal gammopathy (IgA λ being more common); sclerotic bone lesions, noted in nearly all patients; and organomegaly, endocrinopathy, and skin changes.

Other features include hyperpigmentation, hypertrichosis, thickened skin, papilledema, lymphadenopathy, peripheral edema, hepatomegaly, splenomegaly, and hypothyroidism. Diabetes mellitus is not part of this syndrome.

Compared with patients with symptomatic myeloma, individuals with POEMS syndrome are younger (median age, 51 years) and live longer (median, 8 years). The clinical course is commonly characterized by progressive neuropathy.

Treatment

Plasmapheresis does not appear to be of benefit in POEMS syndrome, and patients are often treated similarly to those with myeloma. Patients presenting with isolated sclerotic lesions may have substantial resolution of neuropathic symptoms after local therapy for plasmacytoma with surgery and/or radiotherapy. Autologous stem cell transplantation has been pursued in selected patients and has been associated with prolonged progression-free survival.

HEAVY-CHAIN DISEASES

Heavy-chain diseases are rare plasma cell dyscrasias characterized by the production of heavy-chain Ig molecules that lack light chains (IgG, IgA, IgM).

α Heavy-chain disease

This condition results from lymphocyte and plasma cell infiltration of the mesenteric nodes and small bowel and has features of malabsorption, such as diarrhea, weight loss, abdominal pain, edema, and nail clubbing. The heavy-chain molecule may be detected in serum, jejunal secretions, and urine. There is an association with infection with *Campylobacter jejuni* and α heavy-chain disease. Large proportions of patients can benefit from antibiotic therapy directed at this infection.

γ Heavy-chain disease

Patients with γ heavy-chain disease may present with fever, weakness, lymphadenopathy, hepatosplenomegaly, and involvement of Waldeyer's ring. Eosinophilia, leukopenia, and thrombocytopenia are common. Treatment with regimens similar to those used for non-Hodgkin lymphoma may be effective.

μ Heavy-chain disease

This condition is seen exclusively in patients with chronic lymphocytic leukemia (CLL). Vacuolated plasma cells are common in the marrow, and many patients have κ light chains in the urine. Therapy is similar to that used for CLL (see chapter 31).

SUGGESTED READING

ON MULTIPLE MYELOMA

Attal M, Harousseau JL, Facon T, et al: Single versus double autologous stem-cell transplantation for multiple myeloma. N Engl J Med 349:2495–2502, 2003.

Attal M, Harousseau JL, Leyvraz S, et al: Maintenance treatment with thalidomide after autologous transplantation for myeloma: Final analysis of a prospective randomized study of the "Intergroupe Francophone du Myelome." Blood 106:1148, 2005.

Barlogie B, Desikan R, Eddlemon P, et al: Extended survival in advanced and refractory myeloma after single-agent thalidomide: Identification of prognostic factors in a phase II study of 169 patients. Blood 98:492–494, 2001.

Bruno B, Rotta M, Patriarca F, et al: Nonmyeloablative allografting for newly diagnosed multiple myeloma: The experience of the Gruppo Italiano Trapianti di Midollo. Blood 113:3375–3382, 2009.

Dimopoulos M, Spencer A, Attal M, et al: Lenalidomide plus dexamethasone for relapsed or refractory multiple myeloma. N Engl J Med 357:2123–2132, 2007.

Facon T, Avet-Losieau H, Guillerm G, et al: Chromosome 13 abnormalities identified by FISH analysis and serum β_2-microglobulin produce a powerful myeloma staging system for patients receiving high-dose therapy. Blood 97:1566–1571, 2001.

Fermand JP, Ravaud P, Chevret S, et al: High-dose therapy and autologous peripheral blood stem cell transplantation in multiple myeloma: Up-front or rescue treatment? Results of a multicenter sequential randomized clinical trial. Blood 92:3131–3136, 1998.

Hideshima T, Richardson P, Chauhan D, et al: The proteasome inhibitor PS-341 inhibits growth, induces apoptosis, and overcomes drug resistance in human multiple myeloma cells. Cancer Res 61:3071–3076, 2001.

Jagannath S, Durie BG, Wolf J, et al: Bortezomib therapy alone and in combination with dexamethasone for previously untreated symptomatic multiple myeloma. Br J Haematol 129:776–783, 2005.

Kyle RA, Rajkumar SV: Multiple myeloma. N Engl J Med 351:1860–1873, 2004.

Munshi NC, Hideshima T, Carrasco D, et al: Identification of genes modulated in multiple myeloma using genetically identical twin samples. Blood 103:1799–1806, 2004.

Rajkumar SV, Blood E, Vesole D, et al: Phase III clinical trial of thalidomide plus dexamethasone compared with dexamethasone alone in newly diagnosed multiple myeloma: A clinical trial coordinated by the Eastern Cooperative Oncology Group. J Clin Oncol 24:431–436, 2006.

Rajkumar SV, Hayman S, Lacy MQ, et al: Combination therapy with lenalidomide plus dexamethasone (Rev/Dex) for newly diagnosed myeloma. Blood 106:781, 2005.

Rajkumar SV, Jacobus S, Callander NS, et al: Lenalidomide plus high-dose dexamethosone versus lenalidomide plus low-dose dexamethasone as initial therapy for newly diagnosed multiple myeloma: An open-label randomised controlled trial. Lancet Oncol 11:29–37, 2010.

Richardson PG, Sonneveld P, Schuster M, et al: Extended follow-up of a phase 3 trial in relapsed multiple myeloma: Final time-to-event results of the APEX trial. Blood 110:3557–3560, 2007.

Richardson PG, Sonneveld P, Schuster MW, et al: for the Assessment of Proteasome Inhibition for Extending Remissions (APEX) Investigators: Bortezomib or high-dose dexamethasone for relapsed multiple myeloma. N Engl J Med 352:2487–2498, 2005.

Richardson PG, Weller E, Lonial S, et al: Lenalidomide, bortezomib, and dexamethasone combination therapy in patients with newly diagnosed multiple myeloma. Blood 116:679–686, 2010.

Rosen LS, Gordon D, Antonio BS, et al: Zoledronic acid vs pamidronate in the treatment of skeletal metastases in patients with breast cancer or osteolytic lesions of multiple myeloma: A phase III, double-blind, comparative trial. Cancer J 7:377–387, 2001.

San Miguel JF, Schlag R, Khuageva NK, et al: Bortezomib plus melphalan and prednisone for initial treatment of multiple myeloma. N Engl J Med 359:906–917, 2008.

Spencer A, Prince HM, Roberts AW, et al: Consolidation therapy with low-dose thalidomide and prednisolone prolongs the survival of multiple myeloma patients undergoing a single autologous stem-cell transplantation procedure. J Clin Oncol 27:1788–1793, 2009.

Weber DM, Chen C, Niesvizky R, et al: Lenalidomide plus dexamethasone for relapsed multiple myeloma in North America. N Engl J Med 357:2133–2142, 2007.

ON OTHER PLASMA CELL DYSCRASIAS

Dhodapkar MV, Jacobson JL, Gertz MA, et al: Prognostic factors and response to fludarabine therapy in Waldenström's macroglobulinemia: Results of US intergroup trial (Southwest Oncology Group S9003). Blood 98:41–48, 2001.

Dimopoulos MA, Zomas A, Viniou NA, et al: Treatment of Waldenström's macroglobulinemia with thalidomide. J Clin Oncol 19:3596–3601, 2001.

Sanchorawala V, Wright DG, Seldin DC, et al: An overview of the use of high-dose melphalan with autologous stem-cell transplantation for the treatment of AL amyloidosis. Bone Marrow Transplant 28:637–642, 2001.

Weber D, Treon SP, Emmanouilides C, et al: Uniform response criteria in Waldenstrom's macroglobulinemia: Consensus panel recommendations for the Second International Workshop on Waldenstrom's macroglobulinemia. Semin Oncol 30:127–131, 2003.

Abbreviations in this chapter

APEX = Assessment of Proteasome Inhibtion for Extending Remissions; CIBMTR = Center for International Bone Marrow Transplant Registry; ECOG = Eastern Cooperative Oncology Group; EBMTR = European Bone Marrow Transplant Registry; FDA = US Food and Drug Administration; IFM = Intergroupe Francophone du Myélome; IMWG = International Myeloma Working Group; MRC = Medical Research Coucil; NCI = National Cancer Institute; PETHEMA = Programa para el Estudio de la Terapéutica en Hemopatía Maligna; SWOG = Southwest Oncology Group

CHAPTER 29

Acute leukemias

Margaret R. O'Donnell, MD

Hematopoietic malignancies account for 6% to 8% of new cancers diagnosed annually. In the year 2010, an estimated 43,050 new cases of leukemia were diagnosed, and 21,840 deaths were attributable to leukemias of all types. The total age-adjusted incidence of leukemia, including both acute and chronic forms, is 9.6 per 100,000 population; the incidence of acute lymphoblastic leukemia (ALL) is 1.5 per 100,000 and of acute myelogenous leukemia (AML) is 2.7 per 100,000 population.

EPIDEMIOLOGY

Gender

The incidence of both ALL and AML is slightly higher in males than in females.

Age

The age-specific incidence of AML is similar to that of other solid tumors in adults, with an exponential rise after age 40. With regard to ALL, 60% of cases are seen in children, with a peak incidence in the first 5 years of life and a subsequent drop in incidence until age 60, when a second peak emerges.

Race and ethnicity

The incidence of acute leukemia is slightly higher in populations of European descent. Also, a report from the University of Southern California indicates that acute promyelocytic leukemia (APL) is more common in Hispanic populations than in other ethnic groups.

ETIOLOGY AND RISK FACTORS

There is wide diversity in the behavior of the various subsets of acute leukemias. Thus, it is unlikely that there is one common etiology for these aberrant cellular proliferations. There are, however, some accepted risk factors for leukemogenesis.

Chemical exposure

The increased incidence of AML and myelodysplasia (preleukemia) has been reported in persons with prolonged exposure to benzene and petroleum products. The interval between exposure and the onset of leukemia is long (10–30 years). Chromosomal damage is common.

Pesticide exposure also has been linked to some forms of AML. The incidence of AML is beginning to rise in developing countries, as industrialization and pollution increase.

Other environmental exposures

Exposure to hair dyes, smoking, and nonionic radiation may also increase the risk of leukemia.

Prior chemotherapy or irradiation

Use of alkylating agents, such as cyclophosphamide and melphalan (Alkeran), in the treatment of lymphomas, myelomas, and breast and ovarian cancers has been associated with the development of AML, usually within 3 to 5 years of exposure and often preceded by a myelodysplastic phase. Cytogenetic abnormalities, particularly monosomy 5, 7, 11, and 17, are common. Concurrent radiation exposure slightly increases the risk of leukemogenesis posed by alkylating agents.

Topoisomerase II inhibitors (etoposide, teniposide [Vumon]), doxorubicin and its derivatives, and mitoxantrone, used to treat ALL, myeloma, testicular cancer, and sarcomas, as well as taxanes used to treat breast cancer, have also been implicated in leukemogenesis. These agents, in contrast to alkylators, are associated with a short latency period without antecedent myelodysplasia and with cytogenetic abnormalities involving chromosome 11q23 or 21q22 in the malignant clone.

Genetic disorders

An increased incidence of AML is seen in patients with Down syndrome, Bloom syndrome, or Fanconi's anemia, as well as in individuals with ataxia-telangiectasia or Wiskott-Aldrich syndrome. In identical twins younger than age 10, if one child develops leukemia (usually ALL), there is a 20% chance that the other twin will develop leukemia within a year; subsequently, the risk falls off rapidly and joins that of nonidentical siblings, which is three to five times that of the general population.

SIGNS AND SYMPTOMS

Effects on hematopoiesis

Leukemia manifests symptomatically by its impact on normal hematopoiesis. Thus, easy fatigability, bruising, and bleeding from mucosal surfaces, fever, and persistent infection are all reflections of the anemia, thrombocytopenia, and decrease in functional neutrophils associated with marrow replacement by malignant cells. Bone pain is common in children with ALL (occurring in 40% to 50%) but is less common in adults (5% to 10%).

Whereas a marked elevation in WBC count is the classic hallmark of leukemia, pancytopenia is more common, particularly in patients of all ages with ALL or in elderly patients with AML, who may have had preexisting marrow dysfunction (myelodysplasia). Only 10% of newly diagnosed patients with either AML or ALL present with leukocyte counts > 100,000/µL. These patients, however, constitute a poor prognostic group and are at increased risk of CNS disease, tumor lysis syndrome, and leukostasis due to impedance of blood flow from intravascular clumping of blasts, which are "stickier" than mature myeloid or lymphoid cells.

Leukostasis may manifest as an alteration in mental status; intermittent or persistent cranial nerve palsies, particularly those involving extraocular muscles; priapism; dyspnea; or pleuritic chest pain, due to small leukemic emboli in the pulmonary vasculature.

Physical findings

Physical findings in AML are usually minimal. Pallor, increased ecchymoses or petechiae, retinal hemorrhage, gingival hypertrophy, and cutaneous involvement are more common with monocytic (M4 or M5) variants of AML than with other variants of AML.

Mild hepatosplenomegaly and lymphadenopathy are seen in many cases, particularly in childhood ALL. Massive hepatosplenomegaly occurs infrequently and should raise the suspicion of a leukemia evolving from a prior hematologic disorder, such as chronic myelogenous leukemia (CML) or myelodysplasia. Mediastinal adenopathy is seen in 80% of cases of T-cell ALL, is less common in other ALLs, and is rare in AML.

Visceral involvement is also rare, occurring as an initial manifestation of AML in < 5% of cases, but it may be more frequent during subsequent relapses. These focal collections of blasts, called chloromas or granulocytic sarcomas, can present as soft-tissue masses, infiltrative lesions of the small bowel and mesentery, or obstructing lesions of the hepatobiliary or genitourinary system.

CNS involvement is uncommon at presentation in adult AML (< 1%) and adult ALL (3%–5%). In most instances, CNS involvement is detected by screening lumbar puncture in high-risk patients who are asymptomatic at the time of the puncture. Symptoms, when they do occur, include headache, diplopia, cranial nerve palsies, radicular pain, and/or weakness in a particular nerve root distribution. CNS involvement usually is restricted to leptomeninges; parenchymal mass lesions are uncommon.

Like the CNS, the testes appear to be a "sanctuary" for isolated relapses in pediatric but not adult ALL. Signs of testicular involvement include painless, asymmetric enlargement.

Metabolic effects

Metabolic effects of acute leukemia relate primarily to the rate of cell death.

Hyperuricemia

Hyperuricemia with possible interstitial or ureteral obstruction is seen predominantly in AML with moderate leukocytosis, and ALL with bulky adenopathy; this condition may be exacerbated by a rapid response to chemotherapy and the "tumor lysis syndrome" (hyperuricemia with renal insufficiency, acidosis, hyperphosphatemia, and hypocalcemia), which may occur within the first 24 to 48 hours after initiating chemotherapy. To prevent this complication, all patients should receive allopurinol and urine alkalinization before marrow-ablative chemotherapy is initiated. In patients with a high tumor burden, renal insufficiency, or acidosis prior to initiation of chemotherapy, rasburicase (Elitek) may offer a more rapid treatment for hyperuricemia.

Coagulopathies

Coagulopathies can also complicate the hemostatic defects associated with thrombocytopenia. Disseminated intravascular coagulation (DIC) is most often seen in APL due to release of procoagulants from the abnormal primary granules, which activate the coagulation cascade, leading to decreased factors II, V, VIII, and X, and fibrinogen, as well as rapid platelet consumption. Lysozyme released from monoblasts in M4 and M5 subtypes of AML with monocytic differentiation can also trigger the clotting cascade. Finally, DIC can occur following L-asparaginase (Elspar) chemotherapy for ALL.

DIAGNOSIS

Abnormalities of the CBC raise the possibility of leukemia. The diagnosis is substantiated pathologically by a bone marrow examination.

All patients should have cytochemistry, immunophenotyping by fluorescent-activated cell sorter using monoclonal antibodies directed at leukemia-specific antigens, and cytogenetic analysis of the marrow or peripheral blood blasts at diagnosis. Samples of marrow should also be collected and preserved for subsequent analysis for molecular mutations. Several of these mutations are helping to define risk groups in patients with normal cytogenetics. Other tests used to evaluate metabolic abnormalities (electrolytes, creatinine, and liver function tests) and coagulopathies are also needed at diagnosis. A lumbar puncture should be performed at diagnosis in all pediatric patients with ALL and in all patients with neurologic symptoms regardless of age and pathology.

Pathology and cytogenetics

Acute leukemias comprise a group of clonal disorders of maturation at an early phase of hematopoietic differentiation. Morphology and cytochemical stains designed to detect intracellular myeloperoxidase or esterases have been the traditional methods used to classify acute leukemias into either myeloid or lymphoid derivations.

Coupling these traditional methods with cytogenetic analysis and highly specific monoclonal antibodies directed against cell-surface antigens has led to the detection of new prognostic factors and has provided an approach to detect minimal residual disease.

In 1997, a panel of hematopathologists under the aegis of the WHO met to update the FAB classification of hematologic malignancies, which was based on morphology and cytochemistry alone. The classification incorporated immunophenotyping, cytogenetics, and clinical disease features such as prior myelodysplasia and treatment related to AML. The updated 2008 WHO classification (Tables 1 and 2) also has incorporated provisional categories for inclusion of molecular markers, such as mutations of *NPM1* and *CEBPA*, in AML.

Myeloid leukemias

The WHO classification retained the morphologic subgroups of the FAB system in the subgroup of "AML not otherwise specified" but has created new categories that recognize the importance of certain cytogenetic translocations as predictors of response to therapy. In this category are AML with t(8;21)(q22;q22), AML with abnormal eosinophils and inv(16)(p13;q22) or t(16;16)(p13;q11), AML with 11q23 mixed-lineage leukemia abnormalities, and APL with t(15;17)(q22;q11-12) or variants (Table 1). They have also included for the first time two molecular genetic mutations that appear to favorably impact outcome.

The WHO classification also attempts to deal with the evidence that, in many older patients, marrow dysfunction antedates the onset of acute leukemia. These

TABLE 1: 2008 WHO classification of acute myelogenous leukemia (AML)

AML with recurrent genetic abnormalities
AML with t(8;21)(q22;q22); *RUNX1-RUNX1T1*
AML with inv(16)(p13,1q22) or t(16;16)(p13.1;q22); *CBFB-MYH11*
AML with t(15;17)(q22;q12); *PML-RARA*
AML with t(9;11)(p22;q23); *MLLT3-MLL*
AML with t(6;9)(p23;q34); *DEK-NUP214*
AML with inv(3)(q21q26.2) or t(3;3)(q21;q26.2); *RPN1-EVI1*
AML (megakaryoblastic) with t(1;22)(p13;q13); *RBM15-MKL1*
Provisional entity: AML with mutated *NPM1*
Provisional entity: AML with mutated *CEBPA*
AML with myelodysplasia-related changes
Therapy-related myeloid neoplasms
AML, not otherwise specified
AML with minimal differentiation
AML without maturation
AML with maturation
Acute myelomonocytic leukemia
Acute monoblastic/monocytic leukemia
Acute erythroid leukemias
Pure erythroid leukemia
Erythroleukemia, erythroid/myeloid
Acute megakaryoblastic leukemia
Acute basophilic leukemia
Acute panmyelosis with myelofibrosis
Myeloid sarcoma

WHO = World Health Organization

Swerdlow SH, Campo E, Harris NL, et al (eds): WHO classification of tumours of haematopoietic and lymphoid tissues. Lyon, France: IARC Press; 109–138, 2009.

myelodysplastic syndromes (MDSs) are characterized by ineffective hematopoietic production and disrupted maturation of one or more cell lines. These abnormalities are often accompanied by loss of chromosomal material, particularly −5 or −5q, −7 or −7q, and −3 or −20. As the bone marrow becomes more dysfunctional, increasing numbers of blasts are seen in the marrow.

In the FAB classification, the demarcation line between myelodysplasia and AML was 30% marrow blasts. However, patients with 20% to 29% blasts (previously classified as refractory anemia with excess blasts in transition [RAEB-t]) have a biologic behavior and poor survival similar to those of patients with AML. WHO lowered the threshold for the diagnosis of AML to 20% marrow blasts and deleted the FAB category of RAEB-t. In addition, patients with 5% to 20% blasts who have t(15;17), t(18;21), or inv(16) are considered to have AML rather than MDS and should receive AML treatment.

The WHO system further subdivided the AML patients with dysplastic maturation into those with or without antecedent cytopenias (usually 3 months prior to diagnosis had been the arbitrary cutoff point) and those with a history of exposure to chemotherapy agents (alkylating agents, epipodophyllotoxins, or others).

TABLE 2: WHO 2008 classification of acute lymphoblastic leukemia (ALL)

Precursor lymphoid neoplasms
B-cell lymphoblastic leukemia/lymphoma, not otherwise specified
B-cell lymphoblastic leukemia/lymphoma with recurrent genetic abnormalities
B-cell lymphoblastic leukemia/lymphoma with t(9;22)(q34;q11.2); *BCR-ABL1*
B-cell lymphoblastic leukemia/lymphoma with t(v;11q23); *MLL* rearranged
B-cell lymphoblastic leukemia/lymphoma with t(12;21)(p13;q22); *TEL-AML1 (ETV6-RUNX1)*
B-cell lymphoblastic leukemia/lymphoma with hyperploidy
B-cell lymphoblastic leukemia/lymphoma with hypoploidy (hypodiploid ALL)
B-cell lymphoblastic leukemia/lymphoma with t(5;14)(q31;q32); *IL3-IGH*
B-cell lymphoblastic leukemia/lymphoma with t(1;19)(q23;p13.3); *E2A-PBX1 (TCF3-PBX1)*
T-cell lymphoblastic leukemia/lymphoma

WHO = World Health Organization

Swerdlow SH, Campo E, Harris NL, et al (eds): WHO classification of tumours of haematopoietic and lymphoid tissues. Lyon, France: IARC Press; 109–138, 2009.

The genetic profile of malignant cells has been found to vary widely from normal, with many genes being either overexpressed or suppressed. DNA microarray techniques allow the simultaneous analysis of thousands of genes that are being studied in AML and ALL for their predictive ability to define cohorts of patients with similar outcomes; this process may in turn allow the selection of candidate genes that can be used as therapeutic targets in the future.

Lymphoblastic leukemias

Lymphoblastic leukemias can arise from either B-cell or T-cell progenitors that arrest at an early stage of maturation and then proliferate. Marrow involvement of > 25% lymphoblasts is used as the demarcation line between lymphoblastic lymphoma, in which the preponderance of tumor bulk is in nodal structures, and ALL. Approximately 75% of adult ALLs are B cell in derivation and 25% are T cell.

B-cell ALL Most B-cell leukemias are early or "pre-B" cell, expressing CD19 and CD10 (the common acute leukemia antigen [cALLa]) but lacking surface or cytoplasmic immunoglobulin. Chromosomal rearrangements juxtaposing an oncogene with a promoter region are often seen in this disease category (Table 2).

A small fraction (2%) of patients with precursor B-cell ALL lacks CD10 expression. Patients with CD10-negative disease have a high incidence of *MLL* gene expression (83%) and a very poor disease-free survival (DFS; 12%) at 2 years.

Mature B-cell ALL The more mature B-cell ALL, or Burkitt-cell leukemia, is associated with translocations of the c-*MYC* gene on chromosome 8 and the immunoglobulin heavy-chain gene on chromosome 14q32 in 80% of cases or with the light-chain genes of chromosome 2p11 or 22q11 in the other 20%. Burkitt-cell leukemia has been removed from the leukemia category by the WHO 2008 classification and is now listed with high-grade B-cell lymphoma.

T-cell ALL is frequently associated with translocations of T-cell receptor genes on chromosome 14q11 or 7q34 with other gene partners. T-cell ALL had been associated with a poor prognosis when treated with conventional ALL regimens but now is associated with a better prognosis if treated with aggressive antimetabolite therapy.

Infection with human T-cell leukemia virus-1 (HTLV-1) should be looked for in patients with T-cell ALL presenting with hypercalcemia and lytic bone lesions. HTLV-1 infection is endemic in southern Japan, the southern Pacific basin, the Caribbean basin, and sub-Saharan Africa. High infection rates are also seen in parts of Iran, India, and Hawaii. Recent immigrants from endemic areas retain a risk of infection similar to that of their point of origin. However, fewer than 0.1% of persons carrying HTLV-1 will develop T-cell leukemia.

ALL with myeloid antigen expression vs undifferentiated leukemia

A subset of patients with leukemia exhibits features of both myeloid and lymphoid differentiation. These patients were originally classified as having mixed-lineage leukemia. Patients with a leukemic clone that expresses two or more ALL antigens and one myeloid antigen comprise 20% of adult ALL cases. Although expression of myeloid antigen is considered to be a poor-risk feature in children, it does not constitute a distinct poor-risk feature in adults.

Immunophenotyping has also helped define a group of patients with undifferentiated myeloid leukemia (M0) who previously were likely to be treated as if they had ALL. These leukemias have a primitive morphology and lack myeloperoxidase. On immunophenotyping, they express at least one early myeloid antigen, usually CD13 or CD33, and no T- or B-cell markers. Based on immunophenotyping, undifferentiated leukemias are now recommended to be treated in the same manner as myeloid malignancies.

ALL prognostic factors

Factors known to have an impact on the ability to achieve and maintain remission in ALL include age, lineage derivation, elevated WBC count, and cytogenetic abnormality. In children, rapid early response (< 25% marrow blasts on day 7 from start of therapy) also is strongly associated with better outcome such that patients with slow responses are now treated with intensified regimens postinduction. The cure rate for children aged 2 to 12 is over 80%, and recent pediatric studies that included augmented postinduction therapy using additional vincristine, pegasparaginase, and high-dose methotrexate reported a 5-year DFS of 50% to 70% for patients 16 to 21 years of age. Risk factors for relapse were use of nonintensive therapy postinduction in rapid responders, WBC count = 750,000 cells/mm^3 in B-cell ALL, and cytogenetics. The 5-year DFS rates have been 40% to 60% in most large adult trials for patients 21–40 years of age and < 30% for those involving patients over 60 years of age. Poorer outcomes in adults have been attributed to a higher proportion of patients with poor-risk karyotypes, particularly t(9;22) or the Philadelphia chromosome (Ph), as well as poorer tolerance to chemotherapy, especially L-asparaginase and high-dose methotrexate.

The recent 1,500 patient MRC XII/ECOG adult ALL trial reconfirmed that age (> 35 years), elevated WBC count, B-cell lineage, and karyotypic abnormalities are significant independent risk factors for DFS and overall survival (OS) in adults. In addition to the previously reported poor-risk karyotypes of t(9;22), t(4;11), and t(8;14), this trial also identified complex (≥ 5) abnormalities and low hypodiploid/near-triploid as new poor-risk features.

In a recent Italian study, minimal residual disease detected at 16 to 22 days from the start of induction therapy proved to be a high predictor of relapse, with a 5-year relapse-free survival of only 15% as compared with 71% for patients with no detectable markers for immunoglobulin or T-cell receptor gene rearrangements at that time.

Philadelphia chromosome

The most common cytogenetic abnormality in ALL is the translocation of the *ABL* gene from chromosome 9 to the breakpoint cluster region on chromosome 22, forming a new gene product *(BCR-ABL)* with tyrosine kinase activity. This translocation, referred to as the Philadelphia chromosome (Ph), is found in 95% of cases of CML and in 20% to 30% of newly diagnosed adults with ALL.

The fusion protein produced by the *BCR-ABL* translocation in Ph+ ALL (p190) differs from the product seen in CML (p210); the p190 product is a smaller protein than the p210 product and has higher tyrosine kinase activity. Use of polymerase chain reaction (PCR) techniques that target only the p210 product will significantly underestimate the incidence of Ph+ ALL. In a recent update of the German ALL trials, 37% of patients were Ph+, with 77% showing the p190 product vs 23% showing the p210 product.

Although patients with Ph+ ALL may attain a morphologic remission with conventional chemotherapy (82%), almost all such patients will have persistent molecular evidence of disease on PCR. Patients who do achieve a molecular remission have a longer duration of remission than those who continue to express p190 or p210 activity (30 vs 12 months).

GIMEMA, the Italian oncologic cooperative group, published outcomes data of a large trial of adult patients with ALL in which both cytogenetic data and molecular probes for specific gene products were combined to define prognostic groups. The molecular abnormalities that were evaluated were t(9;22) *BCR-ABL*, t(4;11)/ *MLL-AFA*, t(1;19) *E2A-PBX1*, 9p/p15-p16 deletions, and 6q deletions. Categories based primarily on classic karyotypes were normal, hyperdiploid, and miscellaneous structural abnormalities of uncertain significance.

The use of molecular probes was particularly informative in patients with failed karyotypic analysis or normal cytogenetics. The use of the *BCR-ABL* probe increased the number of cases with a t(9;22) abnormality from 64 to 104 (26% of patients in the trial); more than 50% of add(9p)/p15-p16 abnormalities were detected only by molecular testing. Patients with t(4;11) and t(1;19) had disease-free intervals of 0.4 to 0.6 years, whereas those with del(6q), hyperdiploid, or pseudodiploid karyotypes had intermediate DFS of 1.3 to 1.6 years; those with a normal karyotype or del(9p)/p15-p16 had better outcomes (2.9 and 4 years, respectively). Disease-free survival for patients with *BCR-ABL* was also poor in this study (0.6 years) which antedated the addition of tyrosine kinase inhibitors (TKIs) such as imatinib (Gleevec) to chemotherapy, a change that has improved outcomes. A small subgroup of high-risk ALL patients has been identified as having a gene expression profile similar to *BCR-ABL* fusion with a deletion in the Ikaros family zinc finger (*IKZF1*) region.

Recently, activating mutations of *NOTCH1*, a gene that regulates normal T-cell development, has been identified in the majority of T-cell ALLs.

Other translocations

Translocations involving the mixed-lineage leukemia gene at chromosome 11q23 are partnered with several other chromosomes, including 4q21, 9q22, and 19q13. Translocations involving chromosome 11q23 are frequently seen in secondary leukemias, particularly those arising after chemotherapy with etoposide or teniposide. Although most of these translocations are associated with AML, ALL has also arisen in this setting. All the 11q23 translocations, as well as the (1;19) translocation, are associated with poorer outcomes when compared with similar immunophenotypes coupled with normal cytogenetics.

TREATMENT

Treatment for patients with ALL and AML can be subdivided into two or three phases. Induction chemotherapy is the initial treatment designed to clear the marrow of overt leukemia. This phase usually involves multiple drugs that cause pancytopenia for 2 to 3 weeks.

The purpose of consolidation therapy is to further reduce the residual leukemic burden in patients who are in morphologic remission. Molecular markers of residual disease can often be detected after induction chemotherapy, which indicates the need for further treatment. The intensity of consolidation therapy varies, depending on the risk of relapse (based primarily on cytogenetic or molecular risk groups) and patient age, or comorbid conditions.

Maintenance chemotherapy using low-dose oral chemotherapy for 18 to 24 months has been shown to prolong relapse-free survival in pediatric patients with ALL and in adults with APL. Its value is less clear in adults with ALL; maintenance is used much less frequently in AML.

ALL

Induction therapy

The initial goal of therapy is to rapidly reduce the leukemic burden to a level undetectable by conventional methods of light microscopy and flow cytometry, a state that is deemed a complete remission (CR). Two standard induction regimens have been used in adults with ALL—the Hoelzer regimen, developed by the BFM multicenter group, and the Larson regimen, developed by the CALGB. Along with the standard induction schemas, two newer regimens, the Hyper-CVAD (high-dose cyclophosphamide, vincristine, Adriamycin [doxorubicin], dexamethasone) regimen from M. D. Anderson and the Linker regimen (2002 version), which have an induction drug dosing similar to that of the older regimens but include much higher doses of antimetabolites (cytarabine [Ara-C] and methotrexate) and etoposide for dose-dense consolidations, are outlined in Table 3 along with the standard induction schemas. All of these induction regimens consist of treatment with one cycle each of two regimens with differing mechanisms of cytotoxicity. Overall, CRs are obtained in 80% to 94% of adults younger than age 60 treated with any of these regimens. The incidence of death during induction therapy for these trials was low (2%–9%).

TABLE 3: ALL induction and consolidation therapy

Induction	Consolidation	CNS prophylaxis	Maintenance
BERLIN-FRANKFURT-MUNSTER (BFM) REGIMEN			
Phase I	**Phase I**[a]	**Weeks 5–8**	6-MP 60 mg/m² PO on weeks 10–18 and 29–130
VCR 2 mg IV on days 1, 8, 15, 22	VCR 2 mg IV on days 1, 8, 15, 22	MTX 10 mg IT on days 31, 38, 45, 52	
DNR 25 mg/m² IV on days 1, 8, 15, 22	Adria 25 mg/m² IV on days 1, 8, 15, 22		
PSE 60 mg/m² PO on days 1–28	DEX 10 mg/m² PO on days 1–28	Cranial RT[b] 2,400 cGy (given along with phase II induction)	MTX 20 mg PO or IV weekly on weeks 10–18 and 29–130
L-Asp 5,000 IU/m² IV on days 1–14			
Phase II	**Phase II**		
CTX 650 mg/m² IV on days 29, 43, 57 (maximum, 1,000 mg)	CTX 650 mg/m² IV on day 29		
Ara-C 75 mg/m² IV on days 31–34, 38–41, 45–48, 52–55	Ara-C 75 mg/m² IV on days 31–34, 38–41		
6-MP 60 mg/m² IV on days 29–57	6-TG 60 mg/m² PO on days 29–42		

Adria = Adriamycin (doxorubicin); ALL = acute lymphoblastic leukemia; Ara-C = cytarabine; CTX = cyclophosphamide; DEX = dexamethasone; DNR = daunorubicin; DOX = doxorubicin; IT = intrathecally; L-Asp = L-asparaginase; 6-MP = mercaptopurine; MTX = methotrexate; PSE = prednisone; RT = radiation therapy; 6-TG = thioguanine; VCR = vincristine

[a] Begin week 20

[b] Cranial RT dose for prophylaxis is reduced to 1,800 cGy if patient is being considered for allogeneic BMT while in first complete remission.

TABLE 3: ALL induction and consolidation therapy *(continued)*

CALGB REGIMEN (Larson Regimen)

Course I: Induction (4 wk)		**Course III: CNS prophylaxis and interim maintenance[e] (12 wk)**		**Course IV: Late intensification[f] (8 wk)**		**Course V: Prolonged maintenance[g]**	
CTX	1,200 mg/m^2 IV on day 1[c]	Cranial RT	2,400 cGy on days 1–12	DOX	30 mg/m^2 IV on days 1, 8, 15	VCR	2 mg IV on day 1 of q4wk
DNR	45 mg/m^2 IV on days 1–3[c]	MTX	15 mg IT on days 1, 8, 15, 22, 29	VCR	2 mg IV on days 1, 8, 15	PSE	60 mg/m^2/d on days 1–5 of q4wk
VCR	2 mg IV on days 1, 8, 15, 22	6-MP	60 mg/m^2/d PO on days 1–70	DEX	10 mg/m^2/d PO on days 1–14	MTX	20 mg/m^2 PO on days 1, 8, 15, 22
PSE	60 mg/m^2/d PO/IV on days 1–21[c]	MTX	20 mg/m^2 PO on days 36, 43, 50, 57, 64	CTX	1,000 mg/m^2 IV on day 29	6-MP	80 mg/m^2/d PO on days 1–28
L-Asp	6,000 IU/m^2 SC on days 5, 8, 11, 15, 18, 22			6-TG	60 mg/m^2/d PO on days 29–42		
	or			Ara-C	75 mg/m^2/d SC on days 29, 32, 36–39		
Peg-Asp	2,000 IU SC on day 15						
Course II: Early intensification[d] (4 wk; repeat once)							
MTX	15 mg IT on day 1						
CTX	1,000 mg/m^2 IV on day 1						
6-MP	60 mg/m^2/d PO on days 1–14						
Ara-C	75 mg/m^2/d SC on days 1–4, 8–11						
VCR	2 mg IV on days 15, 22						
L-Asp	6,000 IU/m^2 SC on days 15, 18, 22, 25						
	or						
Peg-Asp	2,000 IU on day 15						

ALL = acute lymphoblastic leukemia; Ara-C = cytarabine; CTX = cyclophosphamide; DEX = dexamethasone; DNR = daunorubicin; DOX= doxorubicin; L-Asp = L-asparaginase; 6-MP = mercaptopurine; MTX = methotrexate; Peg-Asp = pegaspargase; PSE = prednisone; RT = radiation therapy; 6-TG = thioguanine; VCR = vincristine

[c]For patients > 60 years old, modify doses as follows: CTX, 800 mg/m^2 on day 1; DNR, 30 mg/m^2 on days 1–3; PSE, 60 mg/m^2 on days 1–7
[d]Weeks 5–12 [e]Weeks 13–25 [f]Begin week 26 [g]Until 24 months from diagnosis

TABLE 3: ALL induction and consolidation therapy *(continued)*

Induction/consolidation	Dosage
LINKER REGIMEN	
Induction 1A (DVPAsp)	
DNR	60 mg/m^2 IV on days 1–3 (and day 15 if day 14 bone marrow had residual leukemia)
VCR	1.4 mg/m^2 IV on days 1, 8, 15, and 22 (capped at 2.0 mg if age > 40 years)
PSE	60 mg/m^2 PO on days 1–28
L-Asp	6,000 IU/m^2 SC on days 17–28 or Peg-Asp 2,000 IU/m^2 SC on day 15
Consolidation 1B, 2B (HDAC/etoposide)	
Ara-C	2,000 mg/m^2 IV over 2 h on days 1–4
Etoposide	500 mg/m^2 IV over 3 h on days 1–4
Consolidation 2A (DVPAsp)	
DNR	60 mg/m^2 IV on days 1–3
VCR	1.4 mg/m^2 IV on days 1, 8, and 15 (capped at 2.0 mg if age > 40 years)
PSE	60 mg/m^2 PO on days 1–21
L-Asp	6,000 IU/m^2 SC 6 doses over 2 weeks (alternate days beginning day 2) or Peg-Asp 2,000 IU/m^2 SC on day 15
Consolidation 1C, 2C, 3C (HDMTX/6-MP)	
MTX	220 mg/m^2 IV bolus, then 60 $mg/m^2/h \times 36$ h on days 1–2, 15–16
Leucovorin	50 mg/m^2 IV every 6 h for 3 doses, then oral leucovorin until methotrexate < 0.05 µmol/L
6-MP	75 mg/m^2 PO on days 1–28
Maintenance[h]	
MTX	20 mg/m^2 weekly
6-MP	75 mg/m^2 daily

ALL = acute lymphoblastic leukemia; Ara-C = cytarabine; DEX = dexamethasone; DNR = daunorubicin; DVPAsp = daunorubicin, vincristine, prednisone, and L-asparaginase; HDAC = high-dose cytarabine + Ara-C; HDMTX = high-dose methotrexate; L-Asp = L-asparaginase; 6-MP = mercaptopurine; MTX = methotrexate; PSE = prednisone; VCR = vincristine

[h]Beginning after hematologic recovery from cycle 3C and continuing until 30 months from complete response

Patients are intended to receive 4 courses of each regimen (4A + 4B) before starting maintenance therapy.

TABLE 3: ALL induction and consolidation therapy *(continued)*

Induction/consolidation	Dosage
M. D. ANDERSON (HYPER-CVAD) REGIMEN	
CTX	300 mg/m^2 infused over 3 h q12h × 6 doses (days 1–3)
DOX	25 mg/m^2/d continuous infusion over 24 h × 2 days to begin 12 h after last CTX dose (days 4 and 5)
VCR	1.4 mg/m^2 (max 2 mg) IV on days 4 and 11
DEX	40 mg/d on days 1–4 and 11–14
Alternate q21d with	
MTX	1 g/m^2 continuous infusion over 24 h (day 1)
Ara-C	3 g/m^2 over 2 h q12h × 4 doses (days 2 and 3)
Leucovorin rescue	50 mg PO at end of MTX infusion and then 25 mg PO q6h × 48 h
Methylprednisolone	50 mg IV twice daily (days 1–3)

All patients received a minimum of 4 doses of intrathecal methotrexate for CNS prophylaxis. All patients received maintenance therapy twice a year with 6-MP (150 mg/d), MTX (20 g/m^2 oral weekly), VCR (2 mg/month IV), and PSE (200 mg oral daily for 5 days along with VCR).

ALL = acute lymphoblastic leukemia; Ara-C = cytarabine; CTX = cyclophosphamide; DEX = dexamethasone; DOX = doxorubicin; 6-MP = mercaptopurine; MTX = methotrexate; PSE = prednisone; VCR = vincristine

Cytokines (such as filgrastim [Neupogen]) may be used to shorten the period of cytopenia during ALL therapy.

L-asparaginase has been a major agent in pediatric trials in both induction and consolidation therapies. Although L-asparaginase is used during induction therapy in adults younger than age 50 with ALL (except in the M. D. Anderson Hyper-CVAD regimen), it is rarely used in consolidation therapy. The potential importance of this drug was emphasized by observations on L-asparaginase depletion during induction therapy in the most recent CALGB trial, which showed a median survival of 31 months in patients who were depleted vs 13 months for those who were not depleted. They also showed improved depletion using the pegylated form of L-asparaginase (pegaspargase [Oncaspar]), which has a longer half-life. In most clinical trials, a single dose of pegasparaginase (2,000 IU/m^2) is now used to replace multiple doses of L-asparaginase.

Assessment of outcomes for young adults (< 30 years) treated on either pediatric or adult regimens has shown comparable remission rates but significant differences in long-term disease-free survival. As a rule, the pediatric regimen contains higher and more frequent doses of L-asparaginase as well as stricter adherence to a tight dose schedule. All three US adult cooperative groups are now collaborating on a trial using the most recent COG high-risk arm for adult patients (18–40 years) to see if results comparable to those reported by COG can be achieved. Toxicities may differ and are age-dependent. As an example, in the COG trial, the incidence of avascular necrosis was 20% in patients 16 to 21 years of age, 10% in patients 10 to 15 years old, and 1% in those under 10 years of age.

A recent Canadian study using a modified pediatric regimen with weekly high-dose L-asparaginase for 30 weeks during intensification in adults aged 18 to 60 years showed an overall survival of 63% and a disease-free survival of 71% at 5 years. Adverse predictors of outcome included age > 35 years, *MLL* gene rearrangement, high WBC count, and < 80% planned L-asparaginase dose. The regimen was associated with significant morbidity, however, including infections (47%), avascular necrosis of major joints (32%), thromboembolic events (23%), and peripheral neuropathy (22%).

T-cell ALL There is evidence that patients with T-cell ALL may benefit from early treatment with Ara-C and cyclophosphamide. Pharmacologic studies show high levels of Ara-C triphosphate accumulation in T lymphoblasts and synergy between cyclophosphamide and Ara-C in cell lines of T-cell malignancies. T lymphocytes also have a lower expression of polyglutamate synthetase than pre-B blasts. Randomized trials in children with T-cell ALL showed that the use of high-dose methotrexate (up to 5 g/m^2) also improved outcome.

Adults with T-cell ALL treated on the recent MRC UKALL XII/ECOG 2993 trial had a 94% CR rate and a 48% 5-year survival. Patients with complex cytogenetics, however, had a very poor outcome of 19% at 5 years.

Mature B-cell ALL Patients with the more mature B-cell ALL (Burkitt-cell leukemia) experienced an improvement in survival when high doses of cyclophosphamide, methotrexate, and Ara-C were incorporated early in the treatment course (HyperCVAD regimen; Table 3). The probability of leukemia-free survival improved from 35% with standard ALL induction to 60% to 70% with these newer regimens.

Rituximab (Rituxan) is also being added in patients whose blasts express CD20.

Ph+ ALL The development of imatinib, a selective BCR-ABL protein kinase inhibitor, provided a potent new agent in the treatment of Ph+ ALL. As a single agent, it produced CRs in 30% of patients with relapsed Ph+ disease. Several centers have reported improved remission rates of 90% to 95% when imatinib (600 mg/d) was added to initial induction therapy (usually in regimens lacking L-asparaginase) without additional toxicity. With continuation of imatinib through consolidation therapy, 50% to 60% of patients will achieve a molecular remission by 60 days post induction. Patients who achieve a molecular remission and continue on imatinib therapy have an improved disease-free survival of 62% at 3 years, compared with 14% at 1 year in the pre-imatinib era. Clinical trials are being designed to incorporate new, more potent TKIs (eg, dasatinib [Sprycel], nilotinib [Tasigna]); both of these agents have shown activity in the relapse setting.

Consolidation therapy

The BFM, CALGB, Linker (2002), and Hyper-CVAD COG regimens for ALL are outlined in Table 3. There is a CALGB Intergroup Study regimen for adults age 30 or younger which uses more dose-intensive consolidation with asparaginase usage (for more information about this, visit www.ClinicalTrials.gov and search for trial NCT 00558519). As yet, no randomized trials have compared these regimens. However, in sequential studies from Memorial Sloan-Kettering Cancer Center, BFM group, and the Linker study, use of multiple cycles of non–cross-resistant drugs for 3 to 8 cycles after remission followed by maintenance with methotrexate and mercaptopurine (Purinethol) resulted in overall long-term DFS rates of 38% to 52%.

Long-term outcome data of 282 patients treated with Hyper-CVAD showed an 81% CR rate after cycle 1A and a 92% rate after receiving both cycles 1A and 1B (see Table 3); a 5% overall death rate during induction was noted, although treatment-related mortality reached 15% in patients older than age 60 despite the use of G-CSF (granuolocyte colony-stimulating factor). At a median follow-up of 63 months, the 5-year DFS was 38%, similar to that reported in the BFM and CALGB trials. In this series, adverse prognostic factors for DFS were age ≥ 45 years, poor performance status, WBC count > 50,000/μL, Ph+ cytogenetics, more than 1 cycle to achieve a CR, or > 5% residual blasts at day 14. Patients with none or one of these factors had a 52% 5-year DFS rate, vs 37% for patients with two or three factors and only 10% for patients with at least four risk factors.

In the 2002 Linker trial, which intensifies the consolidation with alternating cycles of higher-dose Ara-C (HDAC) and etoposide alternating with cycles of high-dose methotrexate, the 5-year relapse-free survival rate was 52% overall and 60% for patients with standard-risk features. Prognostic features that were associated with a poor outcome in this study included pre-B ALL with > 100,000/μL WBC count at diagnosis, cytogenetic abnormalities involving chromosome 11q23 or t(9;22), and time to remission > 30 days. Without either allogeneic or autologous transplantation, all high-risk patients relapsed within a short time (1 to 9 months). A recent update of the Ph– pre-B ALL subgroup showed a 3-year DFS rate of 60% and an overall survival rate of 50%.

The French LALA-94 trial of 922 patients was designed to look at postremission therapy that was stratified by risk of relapse. The standard-risk patients who achieved CR with 1 cycle of induction therapy were randomized to receive either conventional cyclophosphamide, Ara-C, and mercaptopurine or early intensification with intermediate-dose Ara-C (1 g/m^2 × 8 doses) and mitoxantrone.

In this study, there was no difference in 5-year DFS (33% conventional vs 37% early intensification, with an OS at 5 years of 44%). High-risk patients included those with defined cytogenetic risks (excluding Ph+), WBC count > 30,000/μL, and CNS disease at diagnosis or who required more than 35 days to achieve CR. Patients with a sibling donor received allogeneic transplant in CR, with the remainder randomized to receive either the early intensification chemotherapy or autologous transplant. The 5-year DFS was 45% for those receiving allogeneic transplant and 23% for those without a donor. There was no significant difference in OS with chemotherapy vs autologous transplant, but there was a different pattern of relapse, with fewer late relapses in the autologous patients.

High-risk patients Although the BFM regimen is now standard therapy for standard-risk patients (aged 30 to 55 years), high-risk patients are being selected for dose-intensive therapies, including HDAC and methotrexate or etoposide, high-dose methotrexate, L-asparaginase, or TKIs such as imatinib in the case of Ph+ ALL. Patients with high-risk features including Ph+ have DFS of 50%–60% when allogeneic stem cell transplant is performed in CR1 (or first CR) for adults.

The presence of minimal residual disease using PCR-based probes at end of double induction in pediatric series or at 16 to 22 weeks from the start of therapy in adults has been the strongest predictor of relapse and should inform choices regarding intensified therapy or allogeneic transplant.

Allogeneic hematopoietic transplantation (HCT)

Myeloablative allogeneic HCT combines dose-intensive chemotherapy and radiation therapy with the immunotherapeutic aspects of graft-vs-leukemia effect from donor antitumor surveillance. Relapse rates following allogeneic HCT for high-risk patients are significantly lower (15% to 20% vs 50% to 65%) for nontransplant recipients, but transplant-related mortality is also high (20% to 30%) and increases with age. Several studies have shown improved survival for high-risk patients receiving allogeneic transplants in first CR. Results from the ECOG/MRC trial also showed improved disease-free survival (62% vs 52%) at 5 years for standard-risk patients transplanted from a sibling donor. Three sequential French ALL trials as well as the ECOG/MRC trial failed to show any survival advantage for autologous HCT compared with 2.5 to 3 years of consolidation and maintenance chemotherapy.

For patients with Ph+ ALL, imatinib has provided a means to achieve molecular remission in approximately half of these very high-risk patients; this has allowed physicians more time to identify an unrelated donor. Studies that will assess the impact of molecular remission pre-HCT on the risk of relapse are in progress. Imatinib (at 400 mg/day orally) is also studied in the post-HCT phase. Patients who remain molecularly positive or revert to a positive state are at high risk of relapse and should be considered for treatment with second-generation TKIs such as dasatinib or nilotinib. (See CML chapter for further details.)

CNS prophylaxis

CNS relapse occurs at a much higher frequency in patients with ALL than in those with AML. The rate of CNS relapse was 20% in the first year in a pediatric ALL trial in which the CNS therapy was attenuated to a subtherapeutic level.

Patients with ALL require preemptive therapy for occult CNS disease with either (1) intrathecal methotrexate and/or Ara-C combined with cranial irradiation or (2) high-dose systemic Ara-C or methotrexate combined with intrathecal therapy. Specific use of intrathecal liposomal Ara-C should not be used concomitantly with high-dose systemic chemotherapy such as Ara-C, methotrexate, or etoposide, which cross the blood-brain barrier, due to a high risk (15%–20%) of serious neurotoxicity (seizures, cauda equina syndrome, and encephalitis).

Maintenance therapy

Maintenance therapy with daily mercaptopurine and weekly methotrexate for 18 to 24 months beyond consolidation remains the standard of care for children with ALL. In adults, the benefit of maintenance therapy is less certain. In low-risk adults, who may have an outcome more similar to that in the pediatric population, maintenance therapy would appear to be justified (see Table 3 for maintenance regimens). In individuals who have mature B-cell ALL, it is unlikely that maintenance therapy has any effect. In other high-risk adult populations, more than half of patients relapse while on maintenance therapy, indicating the need for other strategies to eradicate minimal residual disease.

Treatment of relapse

Treatment of relapsed adult ALL is a major challenge. Because most protocols for initial treatment incorporate 6 to 11 agents with different cytotoxic mechanisms, a selection process for drug resistance has occurred. The overall remission rate for relapse therapy is 30% to 40%, with a median duration of remission of 6 months. In the MRC/ECOG trial, the 5-year overall survival for adults who relapsed was 7% in the absence of allogeneic transplant.

Salvage strategies include reinduction with the initial regimen in patients with late relapse or high-dose antimetabolites (Ara-C or methotrexate [see Hyper-CVAD regimen, Table 3]) in those who relapse early. Recent experimental approaches include monoclonal antibodies directed against leukemia-specific antigens conjugated to either radionuclides or toxins, TKIs, allogeneic or autologous transplantation, or new agents.

Clofarabine (Clolar) has been approved for treatment of relapsed refractory ALL in children. Of 61 patients, 12 achieved CR, including children who had relapsed following allogeneic transplantation. The maximum tolerated dose was 52 mg/m^2 infused over 2 hours daily for 5 days. Significant toxic effects include febrile neutropenia, anorexia and nausea, capillary leak syndrome, hepatotoxicity, and skin rash. A small, phase I trial combined clofarabine, etoposide, and cyclophosphamide in patients with relapsed ALL (n = 20) or AML (n = 5). Nine of 13 pre-B-cell ALL patients achieved CR, as compared with 1 of 5 of those with T-cell ALL. Four patients developed severe liver toxicity, including veno-occlusive disease of the liver in patients with prior stem cell transplant or hepatitis. Liposomal vincristine also has been explored in combination with dexamethasone for relapsed ALL. In one trial, 7 of 36 patients achieved CR. A rate-limiting toxicity was neuropathy.

In individuals with Ph+ ALL or CML in lymphoid blast crisis, imatinib (400 to 800 mg orally daily) can induce remissions in up to 30% of patients. These remissions are short-lived but may control the leukemia long enough for a donor to be identified, thus providing an option for an allogeneic transplant in second remission. Nilotinib, which has been recently approved by the FDA, is an imatinib analog with high binding affinity to BCR-ABL. It has been shown to overcome imatinib resistance in approximately 30% of Ph+ ALL patients.

Dasatinib, which is a kinase inhibitor of multiple targets including BCR-ABL, c-Kit, SRC, and PDGFR (platelet-derived growth factor receptor), can provide short-term salvage therapy for patients whose disease progresses while receiving combinations of imatinib and chemotherapy. Dasatinib has a higher propensity for complications related to serositis, with significant pleural and peritoneal effusion. There is some evidence of CNS penetration for dasatinib compared with imatinib. Patients with Ph+ ALL who develop active CNS disease should be switched to dasatinib in conjunction with intrathecal chemotherapy.

Nelarabine (Arranon) has been approved for the treatment of T-cell lymphoblastic disease. In a recommended dose of 1,500 mg/m^2 on days 1, 3, and 5, this agent has produced response rates of 30% to 50% in heavily pretreated patients. Vinorelbine has produced remission in 50% of adults with relapsed ALL in a small pilot study.

AML

Although the chemotherapeutic agents used in the initial therapy for AML have not changed much in the past 30 years, our knowledge of the biology of leukemia has increased. The identification of prognostic factors can provide more realistic expectations of response to standard treatment and can define the population for whom investigational therapy is appropriate early in the course of disease.

Prognostic factors

Cytogenetic abnormalities are the major predictors of remission and risk of relapse for patients with AML. Patients with translocation of genetic material involving core binding regions [t(15;17), t(8;21) inv(16), or t(16;16)] have a good prognosis, with remission rates of 88% and 5-year DFS rates of 55% to 80%, whereas patients with loss of genetic material from chromosome 5 or 7 (−5 or −5q, −7 or −7q) and complex karyotypic abnormalities (defined as more than five abnormalities) have lower rates of CR (30% to 40%) and DFS (5%) at 5 years. Patients with either normal or intermediate cytogenetic abnormalities have a CR rate of 67% and a 5-year DFS rate of 25% to 30%, based on data from a large CALGB trial using HDAC-based consolidation therapy.

Another poor-risk karyotype is t(3;3)(q21;q23), which is correlated with ecotropic viral integration site 1 *(EVI1)* expression. *EVI1* expression also occurs in about 4% of patients with a normal karyotype and about half of those with the *MLL* gene rearrangement. In patients with the *EVI1* gene rearrangement, the median survival is 10.3 months with 0% 5-year relapse-free survival.

With more detailed genetic mapping of leukemia cells, new molecular markers are being identified, which may explain some of the initiation events in transforming cells from normal to leukemic. Internal duplication of *FLT3* can be found in one-third of patients with normal cytogenetics or in patients with t(15;17) (APL) but is uncommon in either poor-risk karyotypes or non-APL translocations. This abnormality does not appear to have an impact on remission, but it is a predictor for relapse (74% relapse rate in patients with a normal karyotype with an isolated *FLT3* mutation vs 46% for patients with wild-type *FLT3*). In patients with otherwise favorable cytogenetic abnormalities [t(8;21) or inv(16)], the presence of c-*KIT* mutation increases the risk of relapse.

Mutations of nucleophosmin (nucleolar phosphoprotein B23, numatrin; *NPM1*) which shuttles nucleic acids and proteins from the nucleus to the cytoplasm as well as binding *TP53*, are also a commonly reported abnormality, present in 47% of patients with a normal karyotype. Although there is frequent overlap with *FLT3* mutations, patients with an isolated *NPM1* mutation and a normal karyotype have a 60% DFS vs 40% for those with either wild-type or mutations of both *FLT3* and *NPM1* and 20% for those with an isolated *FLT3* mutation. Other molecular mutations in patients with normal cytogenetics that have been reported to favorably impact relapse-free survival are CCAAT enhancer binding protein alpha *(CEBPA)* and neuroblastoma RAS viral (v-ras) oncogene homolog *(NRAS),* while *MLL* partial tandem duplication carries an unfavorable implication.

Poor-risk cytogenetics, antecedent MDS, and a high incidence of ATP-binding cassette, subfamily B (MDR/TAP), member 1 (ABCB1) protein are found more commonly in patients older than age 60, which has been used to explain the lower CR rates (30%–55%) seen in older individuals compared with their younger counterparts (60%–80%). Many older patients with preexisting MDS may clear marrow blasts with antileukemic treatment but may still have impaired hematopoiesis and persistent cytopenias, since they may have no residual normal stem cells to repopulate the marrow.

Induction therapy

Ara-C and an anthracycline such as daunorubicin or idarubicin have been the standard drugs used for AML induction chemotherapy for 30 years (Table 4). Depending on the prognostic groups, remission rates of 60% to 80% are seen in younger (< age 60) patients and of 35% to 55% in patients older than age 60. Recent studies have focused on optimizing anthracycline dosing. In 2009, the ECOG published results of a phase III trial comparing the prior standard

The French ALFA 9801 study compared 80 mg/m² of daunorubicin for 3 days with 12 mg/m² of idarubicin given for 3 or 4 days along with standard infusion of cytarabine in 468 AML patients between the ages of 50 and 70 years. After two consolidation courses based on intermediate cytarabine doses, patients in continuous remission were randomly assigned to receive or not receive maintenance therapy with recombinant interleukin (IL)-2 for 12 months. CR rates were 70% for those using daunorubicin, 83% for those using idarubicin for 3 days, and 78% for those using idarubicin for 4 days. There was no difference in relapse incidence, event-free survival, or OS. At 2 years, event-free survival was 23.5%, and OS was 38%. Neither intensification of anthracycline doses nor maintenance with recombinant IL-2 impacted the course of AML significantly. This implies that idarubicin at 12 mg/m² for 3 days should produce response equivalent to 90 mg/m² of daunorubicin for 3 days *(Pautas C et al: J Clin Oncol 28:808–814, 2010).*

TABLE 4: AML induction and consolidation therapies

Induction		Consolidation	
AML			
Ara-C	200 mg/m^2 IV as continuous infusion × 7 d	Ara-C[b]	3 g/m^2 q12h IV as 2- to 3-h infusion on days 1, 3, and 5; repeat q28d × 4 cycles
IDA[a]	12 mg/m^2 IV on days 1–3		
or			
Daun	60–90 mg/m^2 on days 1–3		
ALSG regimen			
Ara-C[b]	3 g/m^2 IV q12h as 2- to 3-h infusion on days 1, 3, 5, and 7 (8 doses)	Ara-C	100 mg/m^2 IV as continuous infusion × 5 d
		Daun	50 mg/m^2 IV × 2 d
Daun	45–60 mg/m^2 IV on days 1–3	VP-16	75 mg/m^2 IV × 5 d
VP-16	75 mg/m^2 IV × 7 d		

ALSG = Australian Leukemia Study Group; AML = acute myelogenous leukemia; Ara-C = cytarabine; Daun = daunorubicin; IDA = idarubicin; VP-16 = etoposide

[a] Idarubicin has been substituted for daunorubicin, 45 mg/m^2, which had been the prevalent anthracycline used in clinical trials prior to 1993. Mitoxantrone, 10 mg/m^2 × 5 days, has also been used as an alternative.

[b] For patients < 60 years of age

dose of daunorubicin (45 mg^2) with 90 mg/m^2, both given on days 1 to 3 along with 7 days of infused cytarabine (100 mg/m^2/d). CR rates were higher for the group using high-dose daunorubicin than for those using the standard dose (71% vs 53%, respectively), and median survival was also improved (23.7 vs 15.7 months) in patients up to 60 years of age. A large European consortium study by Löwenberg et al compared the same doses in patients over 60 years of age; after the first remission, an improved CR rate in the high-dose daunorubicin group (52%) when compared with the lower-dose group (35%) was reported. The 30-day mortality was 11% and 12%, respectively. Patients 60 to 65 years of age benefitted most and exhibited a higher event-free survival (29% vs 14%) and OS (38% vs 23%).

Previous attempts to improve outcomes in patients under age 60 focused on dose escalation of cytarabine in induction and/or consolidation. Both the ALSG and the SWOG compared standard Ara-C and daunorubicin (and etoposide in the ALSG trial) with HDAC in patients < 50 years (Table 4). The CR rates were 71% and 74% for standard vs high-dose therapy in the ALSG study and 55% vs 58% in the SWOG trial. In both studies, there was a significantly higher DFS for the high-dose arm at 5 years (48% vs 25% for ALSG and 33% vs 22% for SWOG) but no difference in OS due to increased early toxicity.

Subgroups of patients may benefit from HDAC. In the SWOG trial, patients with CD34+ blasts had a low CR rate of 36% with standard Ara-C but an equivalent rate in those with CD34– blasts (58%) when treated with HDAC. There was a strong correlation between CD34 positivity and expression of ABCB1, the transporter protein associated with intracellular clearance of drugs, in this cohort, leading to the inference that HDAC might help overcome drug resistance.

However, a 1,700-patient German trial showed no difference in DFS when 2 cycles of HDAC and mitoxantrone (HAM) were compared with 1 cycle of the standard Ara-C–containing regimen followed by HAM. The overall DFS was 40% for both arms in patients younger than age 60 and 29% for those older than age 60; 80% of young patients received both cycles, whereas only one-third of patients over 60 received cycle 2 irrespective of dose intensity of the initial cycle. Other agents such as mitoxantrone and etoposide also have antileukemic activity, but no significant increase in remission rates or relapse-free survival has been seen when mitoxantrone was substituted for an anthracycline or etoposide was added to infusional Ara-C and daunorubicin.

Therapy-related AML has a particularly poor prognosis. At best, only 50% of patients will achieve a remission, usually of brief duration (median, 5 months), despite the use of aggressive drug combinations. Allogeneic or unrelated-donor transplants appear to offer the only curative option in these patients, achieving a 3-year DFS rate of 25% in two studies of allogeneic transplantation.

Gemtuzumab ozogamicin (Mylotarg), an anti-CD33 antibody conjugated to calicheamicin, was originally given accelerated approval by the FDA in 2000 for the treatment of relapsed AML in older patients after showing a 16% to 23% remission rate when used as a single agent. However, a large, randomized, phase III study conducted in the United States failed to show any improvement in remission rate when combined with cytarabine and daunorubicin in initial induction for patients under age 60. In addition, early mortality during induction was higher in the gemtuzumab arm (5.7%) than in the standard therapy arm (1.4%). The drug was withdrawn from the commercial market as of October 2010. It has shown benefit in treating APL and in initial high-risk APL when combined with arsenic trioxide (Trisenox) and all-trans retinoic acid (ATRA, Tretinoin, Vesanoid).

INITIAL TREATMENT OF AML IN OLDER PATIENTS

The majority of AML patients are older than age 60 and constitute a group whose disease has a higher prevalence of unfavorable cytogenetics. Many also have poor marrow regenerative characteristics due to prior myelodysplasia. These patients are frequently burdened with comorbid conditions, which make them poor candidates for conventional Ara-C/anthracycline-based chemotherapy. Cytogenetics and performance status were the two most important predictive factors in this age group, followed by age in 5-year increments and secondary AML.

Mitoxantrone and etoposide were compared with Ara-C and daunorubicin as induction for patients older than age 55 in SWOG trials; CR rates were 44% for Ara-C and daunorubicin and 33% for mitoxantrone and etoposide, and median survival was 8 and 6 months, respectively. Older patients (> 65 years) with poor-risk cytogenetics have a CR rate of < 30% with standard induction chemotherapy, whereas those with a normal or favorable karyotype have a CR rate of 45% to 50%.

Thus, before initiating chemotherapy for older patients, it may be helpful to await the results of cytogenetic and molecular mutational profiles before choosing conventional chemotherapy in those "fit" for such therapy. Recent trials from the GLSG showed a benefit to chemotherapy in patients older than age 60 using Ara-C, idarubicin, and etoposide in those with either favorable cytogenetics or normal karyotypes with

NPM1-positive/*FLT3*-negative mutational status, with a CR rate over 60% and a remission duration of 1,125 days. In other subgroups, the remission rates were 42%, with a remission duration of 440 days, and only 210 days for those who were *FLT3*-positive. Given these underwhelming outcomes combined with 30-day mortality in excess of 15% in many trials of Ara-C–based chemotherapy, new agents are being assessed as initial therapy for patients with abnormal karyotypes.

Given that 25% to 35% of older patients have a history of cytopenias or chemotherapy for a prior malignancy, trials of hypomethylation agents such as azacitidine (Vidaza) or decitabine (Dacogen) have been reasonable starting places. The original phase III trials of azacitidine for treatment of high-risk MDS included over 100 patients who would now be classified as having AML (20%–30% blasts in marrow). The 2-year OS for this group was 50% for those treated with azacitidine versus 16% for those treated with supportive care. Trials of decitabine (20 mg/m^2 IV over 1 hour daily for 5 days) reported a CR rate of 26% when used alone or 49% when given at the same dose for 10 days combined with valproic acid. Clinical trials combining decitabine with a histone deacetylating agent, such as vorinostat (Zolinza), are now in progress.

Clofarabine is also being evaluated as a single agent for older patients with AML. In phase II trials using a dose of 30 mg/m^2 IV for 5 days for induction therapy, CR was achieved in 38% of patients older than age 60 (median, 71 years). Patients achieving remission received a maximum of 6 cycles of consolidation therapy (at 20 mg/m^2 for 5 days). The median DFS was 37 weeks, with a median survival of 59 weeks for those achieving CR or complete pathologic response. The 30-day mortality was 10% for those older than age 70. A British trial in a similar population also had a CR of 32% with an additional 16% CR with incomplete count recovery. Mortality at 30 days was higher (18%). The median OS was 19 weeks and 5 weeks for those not achieving CR. At the present time, the FDA has not approved the use of clofarabine for older AML patients pending the outcome of ongoing phase III comparative induction trials.

Farnesyl transferase inhibitors such as tipifarnib (Zarnestra) and tandutinib are being evaluated as initial therapy for patients over age 70 with newly diagnosed AML. The CR rate for tipifarnib as a single agent was 15% in several phase I/II trials. As tipifarnib did not have significant enough activity to use alone for induction therapy, it is currently being evaluated as maintenance therapy post standard induction chemotherapy.

Consolidation therapy

Once remission of AML is attained, consolidation chemotherapy is required to achieve a durable remission or cure. Standard consolidation regimens are listed in Table 4.

In a CALGB study, 596 patients in CR were assigned to receive 4 courses of postremission Ara-C in one of three dosages: 100 mg/m^2 as a continuous infusion for 5 days, 400 mg/m^2 as a continuous infusion for 5 days, or 3 g/m^2 as a 3-hour infusion every 12 hours on days 1, 3, and 5. For patients ≤ 60 years old, the percentage of patients in CR at 4 years was significantly higher in the HDAC group (44%) than in either the 400-mg/m^2 or 100-mg/m^2 group (29% and 24%, respectively). For patients > 60 years old, consolidation dose intensity had no impact on DFS, with all groups plateauing at a rate of 16% by 2 years. However, more recent information suggests that for the small subset of patients with favorable cytogenetic or molecular markers, modified HDAC (1.5 to 2 g/m^2) may improve outcomes in patients 60 to 70 years of age.

Other approaches to consolidation therapy include 1 to 3 cycles of consolidation followed by autologous or allogeneic hematopoietic stem cell transplantation (HSCT). Historically, both of these approaches also tend to be limited to patients < 60 years old and have produced long-term DFS rates of 45% to 60% in several studies. Long-term DFS is strongly influenced by cytogenetic and molecular abnormalities present at diagnosis. Transplant options should be considered for patients with high-risk features while in first remission, due to poor outcomes with conventional chemotherapy. However, patients with t(8;21), inv(16), or isolated *NPM1* mutations can expect a 60% relapse-free survival following 3 to 4 cycles of HDAC. For these patients, HSCT should be reserved for relapse or CR2. Molecular mutations are being used to identify patients with normal karyotypes with a high risk (≥ 50%) of relapse for whom multiple cycles of HDAC consolidation therapy will not be sufficient to prevent relapse.

Reduced-intensity conditioning regimens are being employed as treatment options in older patients and in those with comorbidity that would otherwise preclude full-dose allogeneic transplantation. Preliminary results from several centers have shown 1- and 2-year DFS rates of 50% for patients aged 55 to 70 years receiving reduced-intensity allogeneic transplantation for consolidation of first remission.

CNS prophylaxis

CNS prophylaxis is not routinely recommended for adult patients with AML. Exceptions for which a screening lumbar puncture should be considered following remission induction therapy include those at high risk for CNS recurrence, ie, patients with a WBC count > 50,000/μL at presentation or those with myelomonocytic or monocytic AML (FAB M4 or M5). Patients receiving HDAC (≥ 2 g/m^2) for induction or consolidation therapy achieve therapeutic drug levels in the cerebrospinal fluid, obviating the need for intrathecal therapy. Patients given conventional Ara-C doses may be treated with intrathecal methotrexate (12 mg IT) or Ara-C (30 mg IT). Both agents can be combined with hydrocortisone (30 mg IT) for patients with active CNS disease.

Treatment of Refractory or Relapsed AML

Patients who do not respond to initial therapy or who relapse within 6 months of attaining CR, as well as those with antecedent myelodysplasia or therapy-related AML, are considered to have relatively resistant disease.

Efforts to overcome drug resistance have focused on (1) HDAC-containing regimens, (2) new agents, and (3) targeted therapy using leukemia-specific monoclonal antibodies conjugated with radionuclides or toxins.

HDAC

High doses of Ara-C (2–3 g/m^2 for 8–12 doses) paired with mitoxantrone, etoposide, methotrexate, or fludarabine have produced short-lived CRs in 40% to 60% of relapsed patients with AML (see Table 5 for dosage regimens). Response rates were higher in patients who had received standard-dose Ara-C for induction therapy and

TABLE 5: AML relapse therapy

Ara-C	2–3 g/m² IV q12h as 3-h infusion × 8 doses	plus	Mitox	12 mg/m² IV on days 1–3[a] or
			Daun	60 mg/m² IV on days 5 and 6 or
			VP-16	100 mg/m² IV daily × 5 d[a]
Ara-C	2 g/m²/d IV × 5 d	plus	FdURD	300 mg/m²/d × 5 d + G-CSF[a] ± Ida 10 mg/m²/day on days 1–3
Mitox	10 mg/m² IV	plus	VP-16	100 mg/m² IV as 2-h infusion daily × 5 d

AML = acute myelogenous leukemia; Ara-C = cytarabine; Daun = daunorubicin; FdURD = fludarabine; G-CSF = granulocyte colony-stimulating factor; Ida = idarubicin; Mitox = mitoxantrone; VP-16 = etoposide

[a] Also used for relapsed acute lymphoblastic leukemia

who had subsequently relapsed than in those in whom induction therapy had failed. The median duration of remission was 4 to 6 months.

Combinations of mitoxantrone and etoposide have been reported to produce a 40% to 50% CR rate in patients who had relapsed or for whom standard-dose Ara-C and anthracycline had failed, again with a median duration of remission of 4 to 6 months. Combinations of intermediate-dose Ara-C (1 g/m²/day for 6 days) with mitoxantrone and etoposide produced CR rates of 79% in relapsed patients and 46% in those who did not respond to induction therapy or had AML evolving from MDS, with a median CR duration of 8 months.

New agents

Nucleoside analogs, such as cladribine (2-CdA) and fludarabine, showed activity in pediatric AML. A British trial reported a 61% CR rate for a combination of fludarabine, Ara-C, G-CSF, and idarubicin, with a median CR duration of 7 months. Clofarabine showed a 16% remission rate in a phase I/II trial in patients with relapsed AML as a single agent and a 38% remission rate when combined with Ara-C (1 g/m²).

Targeted therapy

Sorafenib (Nexavar), a small molecule kinase inhibitor, has shown activity in *FLT3*-positive AML. Sorafenib was combined with 1.5 g/m² of cytarabine plus idarubicin in a phase I/II trial of relapsed refractory AML. CRs were achieved in 14 of 15 *FLT3*-positive patients and 24 of 36 unmutated patients with a 1-year OS of 74%, but 10 of 14 of the *FLT3*-positive had relapsed.

Transplantation for relapsed disease

Although none of the previous options currently offers more than a 10% to 15% chance of long-term DFS, they do provide temporary cytoreduction sufficient to permit further allogeneic HCT from sibling or unrelated donors. Allogeneic HCT achieves a 30% to 40% DFS rate at 5 years in patients transplanted during first relapse or second remission. Autologous bone marrow transplantation also has curative potential for patients beyond first CR, with most large series reporting DFS rates of 30% to 35% in selected patients (usually those with good-risk cytogenetics or initial CR duration longer than 1 year).

New methods of hematopoietic cell purging and post-transplant immune stimulation also are being explored to decrease relapse-related mortality.

APL

APL represents a uniquely homogeneous subset of AML defined by its cytogenetic abnormality, t(15;17), which results in fusion of the retinoic acid receptor *(RARA)* gene on chromosome 17 with the promyelocytic leukemia (*PML)* gene on chromosome 15. This abnormality yields the PML/RARA fusion protein, detectable by PCR techniques, which is useful for both diagnosis and evaluation of minimal residual disease. Most patients (80%) with APL have characteristic hypergranular blasts; laboratory evidence of DIC is present in 70% to 90% of patients at diagnosis or shortly after. Hemorrhagic events contribute 10% to 15% excess mortality during induction chemotherapy for APL compared with other AML subtypes.

Because of the unique biology and specific clinical features of APL, induction and consolidation regimens for APL differ from strategies used for other pathologic subgroups.

Involvement of the *RARA* gene in the pathogenesis of APL suggested the use of retinoids as therapy. A study from Shanghai showed CR rates of 85% with single-agent ATRA and offered the advantages of a shorter neutropenic period (2 weeks) and slightly faster resolution of DIC (4 vs 7 days), as compared with standard chemotherapy with Ara-C and daunorubicin. Normalization of marrow morphology and cytogenetics requires 30 to 60 days of ATRA.

Initial treatment options

The backbone of APL induction therapy includes an anthracycline and ATRA (Table 6). The French and North American APL trials have also included standard-dose Ara-C as an integral part of induction and consolidation therapies. All three groups report CR rates in excess of 90% in patients with an initial WBC count < 10,000 /μL.

Based on data from the Spanish PETHEMA Group trials, a stratification schema of risk of relapse was constructed using WBC and platelet counts at presentation. Patients with a WBC count < 10,000/μL and a platelet count > 40,000/mL have a DFS of 97%; those with a WBC count < 10,000/μL and a platelet count < 40,000/mL have a DFS of 86%; those with a WBC count > 10,000/μL have a DFS of 78%.

In a comparison of the outcomes from the Spanish LAP 99 trial and the French APL 2000 trial, the CR rates and 3-year survival rates were similar for the low- and intermediate-risk groups, with a lower rate of relapse (4% vs 14%) and fewer days in the hospital (50 vs 72 days) for the group that did not receive Ara-C. In patients with elevated WBC counts ≥ 10,000 μL, Ara-C during induction significantly increased CR rates (95% vs 83%). Survival at 3 years was also higher for the group receiving Ara-C (92% vs 81%), and relapse was lower (9.9% vs 18.8%). In the LAP 99 trial, the use of ATRA along with anthracycline in consolidation significantly decreased the relapse rate among the low- and intermediate-risk groups.

TABLE 6: APL induction and consolidation therapies

Induction	Consolidation	Maintenance
PETHEMA LPA 99 (Sanz, et al)		
ATRA 45 mg/m²/d PO daily in 2 divided doses until hematologic remission (max 90 days)	**Cycle 1** IDA 5 mg/m²/d IV on days 1–4 ATRA 45 mg/m²/d PO on days 1–15 (for intermediate/high)	6-MP 50 mg/m²/d PO on days 1–15 ATRA 45 mg/m²/d PO on days 1–15 MTX 15 mg/m² 1M on days 1, 8 and 15 } q 3m × 24 m
IDA 12 mg/m²/d IV days 2, 4, 6, 8 (omit day 8 if patient > age 70)	**Cycle 2** Mitox 10 mg/m²/d IV on days 1–5 ATRA 45 mg/m²/d PO on days 1–15 (for intermediate/high)	
	Cycle 3 IDA 12 mg/m² on day 1 IV + ATRA 45 mg/m² PO on days 1–12	
French APL 2000 (Ades, et al)		
ATRA 45 mg/m²/d PO DNR 60 mg/m² IV days 1–3 Ara-C 200 mg/m² CI days 1–7	**Cycle 1** DNR 60 mg/m² IV on days 1–3 Ara-C 200 mg/m² CI on days 1–7	Same as LPA 99
	Cycle 2 DNR 45 mg/m² IV on days 1–5 Ara-C 1 g/m² IV over 3 h q12h 8 doses (2 g for patients < 60 years with WBC count > 10,000/μL prophylactically) All patients with a WBC ≥ 10,000 receive 5 doses of intrathecal Ara-C for CNS prophylaxis	

APL = acute promyelocytic leukemia; Ara-C = cytarabine; ATRA = all-trans retinoic acid; CI = continuous infusion; CNS = central nervous system; DNR = daunorubicin; IDA = idarubicin; Mitox = mitoxantrone; MTX = methotrexate; 6-MP = mercaptopurine; WBC = white blood cell

TABLE 6: APL induction and consolidation therapy *(continued)*

Induction		Consolidation		Maintenance
MDA (Ravandi, et al)				
ATRA	45 mg/m^2/d PO in 2 divided doses; day 1–hematologic response	ATO	0.15 mg/kg IV M–F weeks 1–4, 9–12, 17–20, 25–28, 33–36, and 42–46	Treatment for differentiation syndrome Stop ATRA ± ATO Methylprednisolone 45–60 mg IV every day × 7
		ATRA	45 mg/m^2/d PO × 7 days each month (weeks 1, 5, 9, 13, 17, 21, 25, 29, 33, 37, 42)	
ATO	0.15 mg/kg IV over 1 h daily; day 10–until CR (marrow every wk beginning day 25 until < 5% blasts and no abnormal promyelocytes; median time to CR day 28) (19–48)			

APL = acute promyelocytic leukemia; ATO = arsenic trioxide; ATRA = all-trans-retinoic acid; CI = continuous infusion; CR = complete response; M–F= Monday to Friday

The most recent North American Intergroup trial showed improved relapse-free survival when 2 cycles of arsenic trioxide were used as the initial component of consolidation. All three groups were monitored for molecular remission at the end of consolidation and at frequent intervals during 2 years of maintenance chemotherapy. Relapse rates are lower than 5% for low-risk patients, and new trials will evaluate the need for maintenance therapy for this group.

Small single-institution series have reported favorable remission and DFS rates in patients induced with arsenic trioxide alone (CR of 86%) or combined with ATRA (95% for low- and intermediate-risk patients). High-risk patients had poorer response rates (CR of 75%) despite the addition of gemtuzumab ozogamicin (9 mg/m^2) on day 1 of induction therapy.

APL syndrome Approximately 25% of patients with APL develop "differentiation syndrome" (formerly known as ATRA syndrome). Symptoms of this syndrome are fever, respiratory distress with pulmonary infiltrates or pleural effusions, and cardiovascular collapse. Temporary pseudotumor cerebri is a fairly common (10%) side effect of ATRA. Although these symptoms most often correlate with leukocytosis (WBC count > 10,000/μL), many patients develop symptoms with WBC counts between 5,000/μL and 10,000/μL. The syndrome is seen in patients treated with arsenic trioxide as well as in those treated with ATRA.

Treatment of this syndrome involves prompt use of high-dose steroids, initiation of conventional Ara-C/daunorubicin chemotherapy to control leukocytosis, and temporary discontinuation of ATRA or arsenic trioxide.

Relapse therapy Arsenic trioxide is now the standard reinduction therapy for patients with APL who are refractory to, or have relapsed from, retinoid and anthracycline chemotherapy. As a single agent, arsenic trioxide has produced CR in 34 of 40 patients (85%) with relapsed APL, with 86% of patients achieving molecular remission. Relapsed patients who achieved a molecular remission with arsenic trioxide alone had a median relapse-free survival of 18 months; those who received arsenic trioxide followed by autologous transplantation have had relapse-free survivals in excess of 70% at 2 years. Allogeneic transplantation should be reserved for those who do not achieve a molecular remission.

Although liver toxicity was reported with the use of arsenic trioxide in the original Chinese studies, the most significant toxicities in the US multicenter trial were the "APL syndrome," ventricular arrhythmia in patients with prolongation of the AT/QTc interval on electrocardiogram, and peripheral neuropathy. It is important to monitor potassium, magnesium, and calcium levels closely, almost daily, during arsenic trioxide therapy; maintaining these levels near the upper range of normal is important in preventing arrhythmia.

Gemtuzumab ozogamicin is also an effective agent for patients with relapsed APL. In a small series, 91% of patients with a molecular relapse of APL achieved a molecular remission following two doses of gemtuzumab ozogamicin (6 mg/m^2). Although this drug is no longer commercially available, efforts are in progress to maintain access to the drug for patients with relapsed APL.

Monitoring response to therapy Reverse-transcriptase PCR for the PML/RARA fusion protein can be used to follow response to therapy. The marker clears slowly, with many patients still testing positive following induction therapy. However, patients with persistence of PML/RARA fusion protein at the end of consolidation therapy are at high risk of relapse, as are those with reemergence of the marker following a period without detectable protein. Salvage chemotherapy should be considered for patients with persistent or recurrent confirmed molecular relapse.

SUGGESTED READING

ON ALL

Bassan R, Spinelli O, Oldani E, et al: Improved risk classification for risk-specific therapy based on molecular study of minimal residual disease in adult acute lymphoblastic leukemia. Blood 113:4153–4162, 2009.

Gruber F, Mustjoki S, Porkka K: Impact of tyrosine kinase inhibitors on patient outcomes in Philadelphia chromosome-positive acute lymphoblastic leukemia. Br J Haematol 145:581–597, 2009.

Huguot F, Leguay T, Raffoux E, et al: Pediatric inspired therapy in adults with Philadelphia chromosome-negative acute lymphoblastic leukemia: The GRAALL-2003 study. J Clin Oncol 27:911–918, 2009.

Moorman AV, Harrison CJ, Buck GA, et al: Karyotype is an independent prognostic factor in adult acute lymphoblastic leukemia (ALL): Analysis of cytogenetic data from patients treated on the Medical Research Council (MRC) UKALLXII/Eastern Cooperative Oncology Group (ECOG) 2993 trial. Blood 109:3189–3197, 2007.

Stock W, La M, Sanford B, et al: What determines outcomes for adolescents and young adults with acute lymphoblastic leukemia treated on cooperative group protocols? A comparison of Children's Cancer Group and Cancer and Leukemia Group B studies. Blood 112:1646–1654, 2008.

Storring JM, Minden MD, Kao S, et al: Treatment of adults with BCR-ABL negative acute lymphoblastic leukemia with a modified paediatric regimen. Br J Haematol 146:76–85, 2009.

Thomas DA, O'Brien S, Faderl S, et al: Chemoimmunotherapy with a modified hyper-CVAD and rituximab regimen improves outcome in de novo Philadelphia chromosome-negative precursor B-lineage acute lymphoblastic leukemia. J Clin Oncol 28:3880–3889, 2010.

ON AML

Cashen AF, Schiller GJ, O'Donnell MR, et al: Multicenter phase II study of decitabine for the first-line treatment of older patients with acute myeloid leukemia. J Clin Oncol 28:556–561, 2010.

Fenaux P, Mufti GJ, Hellström-Lindberg E, et al: Azacitidine prolongs overall survival compared with conventional care regimens in elderly patients with low bone marrow blast count acute myeloid leukemia. J Clin Oncol 28:562–569, 2010.

Fernandez HF, Sun Z, Yao X, et al: Anthracycline dose intensification in acute myeloid leukemia. N Engl J Med 361:1249–1259, 2009.

Kantarjian HM, Erba HP, Clayton D, et al: Phase II study of clofarabine monotherapy in previously untreated older adults with acute myeloid leukemia and unfavorable prognostic factors. J Clin Oncol 28:549–555, 2010.

Lowenberg B, Ossenkoppele GJ, van Putten W, et al: High-dose daunorubicin in older patients with acute myeloid leukemia. N Engl J Med 361:1235–1248, 2009.

Pantas C, Merabet F, Thomas X, et al: Randomized study of intensified anthracycline doses for induction and recombinant interleukin 2 for maintenance in patients with acute myeloid leukemia age 50–70 years: Results of the ALFA 9801 study. J Clin Oncol 28:808–819, 2010.

Schlenk RF, Döhner K, Krauter J, et al: Mutations and treatment outcome in cytogenetically normal acute myeloid leukemia. N Engl J Med 358:1909–1918, 2008.

Vardiman JW, Thiele J, Arber DA, et al: The 2008 revision of the World Health Organization classification of myeloid neoplasms and acute leukemia: Rationale and important changes. Blood 114:937–951, 2009.

ON APL

Adès L, Guerci A, Raffoux E, et al: Very long-term outcome of acute promyelocytic leukemia after treatment with all trans-retinoic acid and chemotherapy: The European APL Group experience. Blood 115:1690–1696, 2010.

Adès L, Sanz MA, Chevret S, et al: Treatment of newly diagnosed acute promyelocytic leukemia (APL): A comparison of French-Belgian-Swiss and PETHEMA results. Blood 111:1078–1084, 2008.

Ravandi F, Estey E, Jones D, et al: Effective treatment of acute promyelocytic leukemia with all-trans-retinoic acid, arsenic trioxide, and gemtuzumab ozogamicin. J Clin Oncol 27:504–510, 2009.

Abbreviations in this chapter

ALSG = Australian Leukemia Study Group; BFM = Berlin-Frankfurt-Munster; CALGB = Cancer and Leukemia Group B; COG = Children Oncology Group; ECOG = Eastern Cooperative Oncology Group; FAB = French-American-British Cooperative Group; GLSG = German Leukemia Study Group; MRC = Medical Research Council; PETHEMA = Programa para el Estudio de la Terapeutica en Hemopatia Maligna; SWOG = Southwest Oncology Group; WHO = World Health Organization

CHAPTER 30

Chronic myeloid leukemia

Jorge E. Cortes, MD, Richard T. Silver, MD, and Hagop Kantarjian, MD

CML

Chronic myeloid leukemia (CML) is a clonal myeloproliferative disorder resulting from the neoplastic transformation of the primitive hematopoietic stem cell. The disease is monoclonal in origin, affecting myeloid, monocytic, erythroid, megakaryocytic, B-cell, and, sometimes, T-cell lineages. Bone marrow stromal cells are not involved.

CML accounts for 15% of all leukemias in adults. Approximately 4,870 new cases of CML will be diagnosed in 2010, with an estimated 440 deaths. The incidence is 1.1 per 100,000 population. With imatinib (Gleevec) therapy, the annual mortality has been reduced significantly (less than 2% to 3% per year).

EPIDEMIOLOGY

Gender

The male-to-female ratio is 1.1:1 to 1.4:1.

Age

According to SEER and MRC data, the median age of patients with CML is 66 years. However, most patients who are admitted to medical therapy studies are 50 to 60 years old, (median: approximately 53 years). Patients in bone marrow transplantation (BMT) studies are even younger, (median age: approximately 40 years). Age differences must be considered in all studies, because this variable may affect results.

ETIOLOGY AND RISK FACTORS

The etiology of CML is unclear. Some associations with genetic and environmental factors have been reported, but, in most cases, no such factors can be identified.

Genetic factors

There is little evidence linking genetic factors to CML. Offspring of parents with CML do not have a higher incidence of CML than does the general population.

TABLE 1: Criteria for accelerated-phase CML according to MDACC, IBMTR, and WHO

Characteristic	MDACC	IBMTR	WHO
Blasts	15%–29%	10%–29%	10%–19%[a]
Blasts + promyelocytes	≥ 30%	≥ 20%	NA
Basophils	≥ 20%	≥ 20%[b]	≥ 20%
Platelets ($\times 10^9$/L)	< 100	Unresponsive ↑ or persistent ↓	< 100 or > 1,000 unresponsive
Cytogenetics	CE	CE	CE not at diagnosis
WBC	NA	Difficult to control or doubling in < 5 days	NA
Anemia	NA	Unresponsive	NA
Splenomegaly	NA	Increasing	NA
Other	NA	Chloromas, myelofibrosis	Megakaryocyte proliferation, fibrosis

[a] Blast phase > 20% blasts (> 30% for MDACC and IBMTR)
[b] Basophils + eosinophils
CE = clonal evolution; CML = chronic myeloid leukemia; IBMTR = International Bone Marrow Transplant Registry; MDACC = M. D. Anderson Cancer Center; NA = not applicable; WBC = white blood cell; WHO = World Health Organization

Environmental factors

Nuclear and radiation exposures, including therapeutic radiation, have been associated with the development of CML. Exposure to chemicals has not been consistently associated with greater risk.

SIGNS AND SYMPTOMS

CML usually runs a biphasic or triphasic course. This process includes an initial chronic phase and a terminal blastic phase, which is preceded by an accelerated phase in 60% to 80% of patients.

Chronic phase

If untreated, chronic-phase CML is associated with a median survival of 3.5 to 5.0 years. During the chronic phase, CML is asymptomatic in 25% to 60% of all cases; in these cases, the disease is discovered on a routine blood examination.

In symptomatic patients, the most common presenting signs and symptoms are fatigue, left upper quadrant pain or mass, weight loss, and palpable splenomegaly. Occasionally, patients with very high WBC counts may have manifestations of hyperviscosity, including priapism, tinnitus, stupor, visual changes from retinal hemorrhage, and cerebrovascular accidents.

Patients in chronic-phase CML do not have an increased risk for infection. Splenomegaly is documented in 30% to 70% of patients. The liver is enlarged in 10% to 20% of cases.

Accelerated phase

This is an ill-defined transitional phase. The criteria used in all the studies with tyrosine kinase inhibitors include the presence of 15% to 29% blasts, at least 30% blasts and promyelocytes, or at least 20% basophils in the peripheral blood or a platelet count $< 100 \times 10^9$/L unrelated to therapy. Cytogenetic clonal evolution is also a criterion for acceleration. Other classifications include more subjective criteria (Table 1) and have not been clinically validated. The classification used may affect the expected outcome for a group of patients defined as accelerated phase. With imatinib therapy, the estimated 4-year survival rate exceeds 50%.

The accelerated phase is frequently symptomatic, including the development of fever, night sweats, weight loss, and progressive splenomegaly.

Blastic phase

The blastic phase morphologically resembles acute leukemia. Its diagnosis requires the presence of at least 30% of blasts in the bone marrow or peripheral blood. The WHO has proposed to consider blast phase with at least 20% blasts, but this classification has not been validated, and recent evidence suggests that patients with 20% to 29% blasts have a significantly better prognosis than do those having at least 30% blasts. In some patients, the blastic phase is characterized by extramedullary deposits of leukemic cells, most frequently in the CNS, lymph nodes, skin, or bones.

Patients in blastic phase usually die within 3 to 6 months. Approximately 70% of patients in blastic phase have a myeloid phenotype, 25% have a lymphoid phenotype, and 5% have an undifferentiated phenotype. Prognosis is slightly better for a lymphoid blastic phase than for myeloid or undifferentiated cases (median survival: 9 vs 3 months).

Patients in the blastic phase are more likely to experience symptoms, including weight loss, fever, night sweats, and bone pain. Symptoms of anemia, infectious complications, and bleeding are common. Subcutaneous nodules or hemorrhagic tender skin lesions, lymphadenopathy, and signs of CNS leukemia may also occur.

LABORATORY FEATURES

Peripheral blood

The most common feature of CML is an elevated WBC count, usually exceeding 25×10^9/L and frequently exceeding 100×10^9/L, occasionally with cyclic variations. The finding of unexplained, persistent leukocytosis (eg, $> 12–15 \times 10^9$/L) in the absence of infections or other causes of WBC count elevation should prompt a workup for CML.

The WBC differential usually shows granulocytes in all stages of maturation, from blasts to mature, morphologically normal granulocytes. Basophils are elevated, but only 10% to 15% of patients have ≥ 7% basophils in the peripheral blood. Frequently, eosinophils are also mildly increased. The absolute lymphocyte count is elevated at the expense of T lymphocytes.

The platelet count is elevated in 30% to 50% of patients and is higher than $1{,}000 \times 10^9$/L in a small percentage of patients with CML. When thrombocytopenia occurs, it usually signals disease acceleration.

Some patients have mild anemia at diagnosis.

Neutrophil function is usually normal or only mildly impaired, but natural killer (NK) cell activity is impaired. Clonal expansion of T-cell lymphocytes is detected in some patients at the time of diagnosis and may increase during therapy with dasatinib (Sprycel). Platelet function is frequently abnormal but usually has no clinical significance.

Bone marrow

The bone marrow is hypercellular, with cellularity of 75% to 90%. The myeloid-to-erythroid ratio is usually 10:1 to 30:1. All stages of maturation of the WBC series are usually seen, but the myelocyte predominates.

Megakaryocytes are increased in number early in the disease and may show dysplastic features. They are usually smaller than the typical normal megakaryocytes. Fibrosis may be evident at diagnosis, but it is more common with disease progression and is usually an adverse prognostic finding.

Other laboratory findings

Leukocyte alkaline phosphatase activity is reduced at diagnosis. Serum levels of vitamin B_{12} and transcobalamin are increased, sometimes up to 10 times normal values. Serum levels of uric acid and lactate dehydrogenase (LDH) are also frequently elevated.

CYTOGENETIC AND MOLECULAR FINDINGS

Philadelphia (Ph) chromosome

CML is characterized by the Ph chromosome, which represents a balanced translocation between the long arms of chromosomes 9 and 22, t(9;22)(q34;q11.2). The *ABL1* proto-oncogene located in chromosome 9q34 encodes for a nonreceptor protein tyrosine kinase expressed in most mammalian cells. In chromosome 22, the breakpoint occurs within the *BCR* gene and usually involves an area known as the major breakpoint cluster region *(m-BCR),* located either between exons b3 and b4 or between exons b2 and b3. Therefore, two different fusion genes can be formed, both of them joining exon 2 of *ABL1* with either exon 13, e13a2 (b2a2) or exon 14, e14a2 of *BCR* (b3a2). Among the 5% to 10% of patients who do not have the Ph chromosome detected by karyotyping, 30% to 40% have the molecular rearrangement identified by fluorescent in situ hybridization (FISH)/polymerase chain reaction (PCR). Those patients without this rearrangement are considered to have "atypical CML," a unique entity having a different natural history, prognosis, and treatment.

Upon translation, a new protein with a molecular weight of 210 kd ($p210^{BCR\text{-}ABL}$) is synthesized, which, when compared with the normal *ABL1*, has markedly increased kinase activity and can transform transfected cells and induce leukemia in transgenic mice. Occasionally, the breakpoint can occur in other areas (m-*BCR* and μ-*BCR*), leading to different transcripts (eg, $p190^{BCR\text{-}ABL}$ and $p230^{BCR\text{-}ABL}$, respectively). The mechanism of oncogenesis of $p210^{BCR\text{-}ABL}$ is unclear, but, upon phosphorylation, it can activate several intracellular pathways, including the Ras and the mitogen-activated protein kinase pathway, the Jak-Stat pathway, the PI3 kinase pathway, and the MYC pathway. Ultimately, this process leads to altered adhesion to extracellular matrix and stroma, constitutive activation of mitogenic signals, and inhibition of apoptosis.

STAGING AND PROGNOSIS

Staging systems

Several characteristics of CML affect the prognosis, including age; spleen size; WBC and platelet counts; and percentage of blasts, eosinophils, and basophils in the peripheral blood. Deletions of the derivative chromosome 9 are identified in 10% to 15% of patients and have been associated with an adverse prognosis with most treatment modalities. Imatinib may overcome the adverse prognosis associated with del der(9). These factors have been incorporated into several staging systems.

Sokal's classification

A frequently used risk classification is Sokal's prognostic risk system. In this system, the hazard ratio function is derived from the following formula: $\lambda_i(+)/\lambda_o(t)$ = Exp 0.0116 (age – 43.4) + 0.0345 (spleen – 7.51) + 0.188 [(platelets/700)^2 – 0.563] + 0.0887 (blasts – 2.10).

This risk classification defines three prognostic groups with hazard ratios of < 0.8, 0.8–1.2, and > 1.2 (ie, low-, intermediate-, and high-risk).

The Hasford classification has been suggested to separate more clearly and without overlap risk groups among patients treated with interferon therapy. The Hasford score is derived from the formula (0.6666 × age [0 when age < 50 years; 1, otherwise] + 0.0420 × spleen size [cm below costal margin] + 0.0584 × blasts [%] + 0.0413 × eosinophils [%] + 0.2039 × basophils [0 when basophils < 3%; 1, otherwise] + 1.0956 × platelet count [0 when platelet count < 1,500 × 10^9/L; 1, otherwise]) × 1,000. Based on the score, patients can be classified into three risk groups: low (score ≤ 780), intermediate (score > 780 and ≤ 1,480), and high (score ≥ 1,480). This classification may be less predictive in the imatinib era. Both the Sokal and Hasford classifications predict the probability of achieving a response to tyrosine kinase inhibitors.

TREATMENT

Chronic phase

Conventional chemotherapy

Busulfan (Busulfex, Myleran) and hydroxyurea were the chemotherapeutic agents used most frequently in CML until the development of imatinib. Busulfan is now rarely used.

Hydroxyurea is most frequently used to control the WBC while confirming the diagnosis of CML. The dose can be adjusted individually to control the WBC count. In some instances, a dose of 10 to 12 g/d may be needed.

Neither busulfan nor hydroxyurea significantly reduces the percentage of cells bearing the Ph chromosome, and, therefore, the risk of transformation to the blastic phase is unchanged. Their use should be limited to temporary control of hematologic manifestations before definitive therapy (eg, imatinib, stem cell transplantation) is instituted. Once the diagnosis of CML is confirmed, imatinib should be initiated immediately. There is usually no need for or benefit to initially "debulking" with hydroxyurea.

TABLE 2: Response definitions in CML

Response	Category	Criteria
Hematologic remission	Complete	Normalization of WBC counts with normal differential; normalization of platelet counts to $< 450 \times 10^9$/L; disappearance of all signs and symptoms of disease
Cytogenetic response[a]	Complete[b]	No Ph chromosome–positive metaphases
	Partial[b]	5%–35% of Ph chromosome–positive metaphases
	Minor	36%–95% of Ph chromosome–positive metaphases
	None	Persistence of Ph chromosome in all analyzable metaphases

[a] Response is assessed on routine cytogenetic analysis with at least 20 metaphases counted.
[b] Major cytogenetic response includes complete and partial cytogenetic responses.
CML = chronic myeloid leukemia; Ph = Philadelphia; WBC = white blood cell

Interferon

Interferon-α can induce a complete hematologic response (Table 2) in 70% to 80% of patients with CML, and with some degree of suppression of Ph chromosome-positive cells (ie, cytogenetic response) in 40% to 60% of patients, which is complete in up to 20% to 25% of patients. Randomized studies have documented a survival advantage for patients treated with interferon-α who achieved a major, and particularly a complete, cytogenetic response.

Patients who achieve a complete cytogenetic response have a 10-year survival rate of 75% or more, compared with less than 40% for those having a partial response and less than 30% for individuals having a lesser or no response.

Interferon and cytarabine (Ara-C) The combination of interferon-α and low-dose Ara-C induced a higher (ie, 40% to 50%) response rate, and possibly a survival advantage, when compared with interferon-α alone.

Approximately 30% of those achieving complete cytogenetic remission with interferon-α may achieve a sustained molecular remission and are probably cured. Among the others, 40% to 60% remain free of disease after more than 10 years despite the presence of minimal residual disease. This has been called "operational cure."

Formulations of interferon-α attached to polyethylene glycol (PEG) have a longer half-life that allows for weekly administration and may have decreased toxicity.

Imatinib is a potent inhibitor of the tyrosine kinase activity of BCR-ABL and a few other tyrosine kinases, such as PDGF-R (platelet-derived growth factor-receptor) and KIT. It has demonstrated significant activity in patients with CML in all phases of the disease, whether they have received prior therapy or not. Among patients with chronic-phase CML who failed to respond to for whom prior interferon-α therapy, 55% to 85% of patients achieved a major cytogenetic remission, including 45% to 80% with a complete cytogenetic remission. The estimated rate of survival free of transformation to accelerated with blast phase is 69% at 60 months. Among patients treated in early chronic-phase CML who had not received prior therapy, the rate of complete cytogenetic response is 83%, with an overall survival rate at 96 months of 85%, and an event-free survival of 81%.

Overall and event-free survival rates with imatinib therapy are significantly better than those seen with other therapies. Thus, imatinib has become the standard therapy for CML (Figure 1). The proper management of patients receiving imatinib is important.

Dose The standard dose of imatinib is 400 mg/d for the chronic phase and 600 mg for the accelerated and blastic phases. Dose reductions may be needed in some patients because of toxicity, but doses less than 300 mg/d are not recommended. Available data from the phase I study show a clear decrease in the probability of response with doses lower than 300 mg/d.

Toxicity Imatinib is well tolerated. However, several patients develop grade 1–2 adverse events, including nausea, peripheral or periorbital edema, muscle cramps, diarrhea, skin rashes, weight gain, and fatigue. These events frequently are minor and either do not require therapy or respond to adequate early intervention. Fluid retention responds to diuretics when indicated; diarrhea can be managed with loperamide or other agents; nausea usually responds to prochlorperazine, promethazine, or other agents; muscle cramps can be managed with tonic water or quinine; skin rash may be managed with antihistamines and/or corticosteroids (topical and/or systemic).

Myelosuppression is the most common grade 3–4 adverse event. Neutropenia can be seen in up to 45% of patients; thrombocytopenia in up to 25% of patients; and anemia in 10% of patients. Treatment is held for grade ≥ 3 neutropenia (neutrophil count < 10^9/L) or thrombocytopenia (platelet count < 50 × 10^9/L) and restarted when counts recover above these levels. If the recovery takes longer than 2 weeks, the dose may be reduced. Treatment interrup-

Preliminary results of a randomized phase III study comparing 400 mg and 800 mg of imatinib (Gleevec) daily as initial therapy for patients in chronic phase suggested a higher rate of response at earlier time points for patients treated with 800 mg, with a lower rate of transformation by 18 months of follow-up (3.2% vs 1.9%; *Cortes JE et al: J Clin Oncol 28:424–430, 2010*). An update of this same study after 24 months of follow-up showed no difference in the rate of complete cytogenetic response, major molecular response, event-free survival, or progression-free survival between the two cohorts. This result may have been explained in part by the high rate of dose reductions and treatment discontinuation, particularly in the high-dose group. Patients who had two dose interruptions or more had a significantly worse outcome, and patients who maintained a dose intensity throughout the study of at least 600 mg had a significantly higher rate of major molecular response (*Baccarani M et al: Blood 114: abstract 337, 2009*). Another randomized study exploring 400 mg and 800 mg of imatinib or imatinib combined with interferon as initial therapy for patients with CML in chronic phase showed an improvement in the time to complete cytogenetic response and major molecular response for patients treated with 800 mg, compared with the other two arms. This result translated into an improved 5-year progression-free survival (94%), compared with those treated with standard-dose imatinib (87%) or with imatinib plus interferon (91%). The long-term benefit in this study might be due to the fact that dose intensity was maintained at a higher level (*Hehlmann R et al: Blood 114: abstract 339, 2009*).

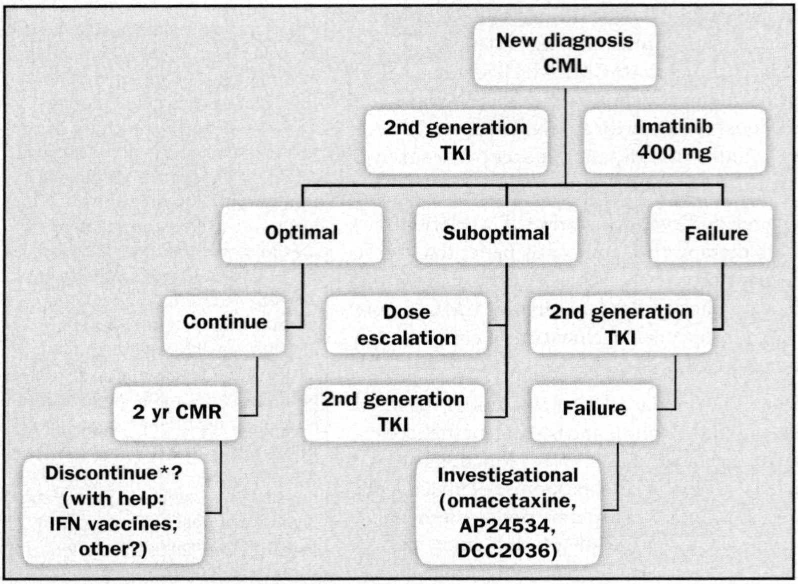

Figure 1: Treatment algorithm for chronic-phase CML. Options marked with a question mark define investigational approaches that cannot be considered standard at this time.

TKI = tyrosine kinase inhibitor; 2 yr CMR = sustained complete molecular response for 2 years; IFN = interferon-alpha; HHT = omacetaxine (homoharringtonine); * treatment discontinuation can only be recommended in the setting of clinical trials

tions and dose reductions are not usually recommended for anemia. Myelosuppression is much more likely to occur during the first 2 to 3 months of therapy and is best managed with treatment interruption and close monitoring. Hematopoietic growth factors (granulocyte colony-stimulating factor [G-CSF, filgrastim, (Neupogen)], oprelvekin [Neumega], and erythropoietin) have been used successfully to manage prolonged or recurrent myelosuppression, but the long-term safety of this approach needs to be assessed.

Monitoring The treatment objective has evolved from hematologic responses (hydroxyurea) to cytogenetic responses (interferon-α), to molecular responses in the imatinib era. All patients have to be evaluated with cytogenetic analysis before the start of therapy, and a baseline quantitative PCR analysis is useful. Conventional cytogenetic analysis is important at baseline and for follow-up, because it provides valuable information about the entire karyotype (ie, clonal evolution, cytogenetic abnormalities in Ph chromosome-negative cells) that cannot be obtained with FISH or PCR and has prognostic implications. A cytogenetic analysis every 3 to 6 months during the first year and every 12 to 24 months thereafter is recommended. Quantitative PCR is recommended every 3 to 6 months. It is inappropriate not to follow patients with cytogenetics and real-time PCR.

Duration of therapy At this time, the duration of therapy is unclear. A minority of patients have reached undetectable levels of disease by PCR. Few have discontinued therapy which has usually resulted in relapse. Thus, unless patients are included in clinical trials investigating treatment discontinuation, patients should continue therapy indefinitely.

Imatinib failure The most frequently identified mechanism of resistance to imatinib is the development of mutations at the *ABL* kinase domain. Mutations are identified in 40% to 60% of patients with imatinib resistance, with the most frequent occurring in the P-loop. Not all mutations confer the same level of resistance to imatinib, and some may be overcome by increased concentrations of imatinib. The most resistant mutation is *T315I*. P-loop mutations have been reported to be linked to a poor prognosis, but this theory has not been confirmed in all studies, and it is probably more appropriate to consider individual mutations rather than group them by location.

Changing therapy based on failure to achieve or losing a molecular response cannot be justified in most instances at the present time. Even when patients who have not achieved a major molecular response after 18 months of therapy have an inferior prognosis compared with those with at least a major molecular response, they still have an 86% probability of event-free survival at 7 years (provided they have a complete cytogenetic response), and, in most instances, the event only represents a loss of cytogenetic response. If the proposed alternative treatment option has any significant risk of mortality or morbidity, the risk may be unnecessary. The clinical significance of the presence of mutations only in patients with an adequate response is still unclear. Thus, mutations should be investigated in patients with clinical evidence of failure. In this setting, a change of therapy is indicated whether a mutation is indicated or not, but, in some instances, specific mutations may guide the selection of therapy.

Preliminary results of a randomized trial of imatinib (Gleevec) vs nilotinib (Tasigna, 400 mg twice daily [BID] or 300 mg BID) as initial therapy for patients with CML in chronic phase were recently reported. With a median follow-up of less than 14 months, the rate of complete cytogenetic response at 12 months was significantly superior for patients treated with nilotinib (78% with 400 mg and 80% with 300 mg) compared with those treated with imatinib (65%). A similar advantage in major molecular response was seen (rates at 12 months, 43%, 44%, and 22%, respectively). Most important, the rate of transformation at the time of the initial report was significantly lower for patients treated with nilotinib (< 1% for each arm) than for those treated with imatinib (4%; *Saglio G et al: Blood 114: abstract LBA-1, 2009*). A similar study comparing dasatinib 100-mg daily to imatinib 400-mg daily as initial therapy reported an improved cumulative rate of complete cytogenetic response (83% vs 72%) and major molecular response (46% vs 28%) by 12 months of therapy. This also translated into an improved rate of transformation with dasatinib compared to imatinib (1.8% vs 3.5%; *Kantarjian H et al: J Clin Oncol 28: abstract LBA6500, 2010*). Results of a third study, comparing bostutinib to imatinib in the same setting, are expected by the end of 2010. With these results, second-generation tyrosine kinase inhibitors might become standard initial therapy for patients with CML in early chronic phase.

The European LeukemiaNet has established criteria for failure and suboptimal response that have become standard (Table 3). These criteria emphasize the response achieved and the time to such response. Patients who meet criteria for failure should be offered therapy with a second-generation tyrosine kinase inhibitor. For patients with suboptimal responses, there are no available data indicating what the optimal management may be, although imatinib dose escalation is usually recommended.

A French study called STIM (Stop Imatinib) investigated the impact of imatinib (Gleevec) discontinuation among patients with CML who had sustained a complete molecular remission for at least 2 years while on imatinib. Thirty-five of the 69 patients reported had not received prior imatinib. The projected probability of survival without relapse at 12 months was 47% for patients with prior exposure to interferon-alpha and 34% for those with no prior exposure. All relapses occurred within the first 7 months after discontinuation of imatinib. These results suggest that a subset of patients may maintain a molecular remission after discontinuation of imatinib therapy, but the risk of relapse is high. The recommendation today is still to continue imatinib uninterrupted. However, exploring options that may allow treatment discontinuation with minimal risk of relapse will dominate research in CML in years to come *(Mahon FX et al: Blood 114: abstract 859, 2009).*

Second-generation tyrosine kinase inhibitors A second-generation of tyrosine kinase inhibitors has been developed to overcome resistance to imatinib. Two of these agents have gained regulatory approval (dasatinib and nilotinib [Tasigna]), and others are being developed (bosutinib, SKI-606). Both agents have been shown to inhibit both the wild type *BCR-ABL* and nearly all of the clinically significant mutants of *BCR-ABL*, except for the *T315I* mutation. The results from the initial clinical trials have demonstrated significant clinical activity with both agents.

Dasatinib Dasatinib is structurally unrelated to imatinib and can bind both the inactive and active configurations of BCR-ABL. In addition, dasatinib is a dual inhibitor that blocks Src and ABL and that is two orders of magnitude more potent than is imatinib.

The initial phase II trials of dasatinib used a dose of 70 mg twice daily. Significant clinical activity was seen in patients in all stages of the disease after imatinib resistance or intolerance, with complete cytogenetic responses in 53% in chronic phase, 33% in accelerated phase, 27% in myeloid blast phase, and 46% in lymphoid blast phase. Duration of response correlates with the stage of disease, with progression-free survival of 80% at 24 months for those in chronic phase and 46%, in accelerated phase. In contrast, the median progression-free survival was 5.6 and 3.1 months, respectively, for those in the myeloid and lymphoid blast phases.

Some of the most significant adverse events include myelosuppression (grade 3–4 neutropenia and thrombocytopenia in nearly 50% each), pleural effusion, and gastrointestinal hemorrhage (particularly in the advanced stages). Alternative schedules may improve the toxicity profile. In a randomized study, dasatinib administered as 100 mg once daily was associated with significantly less myelosuppression and pleural effusion when compared with 70 mg twice daily (and to 50 mg twice daily or 140 mg once daily). The response to therapy was identical, with a trend toward improved progression-free survival with use of 100 mg once daily.

TABLE 3: European LeukemiaNet criteria for failure and suboptimal response

	Response	
Time (mo)	**Failure**	**Suboptimal**
3	No HR	No CHR
6	No CHR 100% Ph+	≥ 35% Ph+
12	≥ 35% Ph+	≥ 5% Ph+
18	≥ 5% Ph+	No MMR (< 3-log ↓ *BCR-ABL/ABL*)
Any	Loss of CHR Loss of CCgR Mutation	Clonal evolution Loss of MMR Mutation

CCgR = complete cytogenetic response; CHR = complete hematologic response; HR = hematologic response; MMR = major molecular response; Ph+ = Philadelphia chromosome-positive

Dasatinib is approved for treatment of patents with CML in all phases of the disease who have experienced resistance or intolerance to imatinib. The standard dose for patients in chronic phase is 100 mg once daily; 140 mg once daily is recommended for patients in advanced stages.

Nilotinib Nilotinib was designed based on the imatinib structure and modified to improve its binding to BCR-ABL and to increase its selectivity. These modifications result in an agent at least one order of magnitude more potent than imatinib against BCR-ABL.

Significant activity has been documented in patients treated after imatinib failure with nilotinib (400 mg twice daily) in phase II studies. The rate of complete cytogenetic response for patients treated in chronic phase after imatinib resistance or intolerance was 44% and for those treated in accelerated phase, 19%. Responses have been durable, with a sustained major cytogenetic response at 18 months in 84% of patients treated in the chronic phase. In the accelerated phase, progression-free survival is 57% at 12 months. The most significant toxicities reported have been myelosuppression (grade 3–4 neutropenia or thrombocytopenia in approximately 30%, each), and biochemical abnormalities (elevation of indirect bilirubin, lipase, and glucose) that have been usually transient and asymptomatic.

A prognostic model has been developed to predict the probability of response and event-free survival after treatment with second-generation tyrosine kinase inhibitors (dasatinib [Sprycel] and nilotinib [Tasigna]) after imatinib failure. Among 123 patients treated with these agents, a multivariate analysis identified two factors as being significantly and independently associated with long-term outcome: performance status (adverse feature, ≥ 1) and cytogenetic response with prior imatinib therapy (adverse feature, no prior cytogenetic response). Patients with no, one, and two adverse features had event-free survival probabilities at 24 months of 78%, 49%, and 20%, respectively *(Jabbour E et al: Blood 114: abstract 509, 2009).*

Bosutinib is another second-generation tyrosine kinase inhibitor being investigated for use after imatinib failure. Like dasatinib, bosutinib is a potent inhibitor of the Src family of kinases in addition to inhibiting ABL, but in contrast to all other available inhibitors, bosutinib has no significant inhibitory activity against PDGF receptor or c-kit. Among 294 patients who received bosutinib after imatinib resistance or intolerance, 47% achieved a complete cytogenetic response (59% for imatinib intolerant, 43% for imatinib resistant). Responses have been durable and are observed across a wide range of mutations, except *T315I*. The main adverse event is diarrhea and rash (grade 3 in 9% each, leading to treatment discontinuation in 2% and 1%, respectively). *(Cortes J et al: J Clin Oncol 28: abstract 6502, 2010).*

There is also the potential for QTc prolongation (a class effect for all tyrosine kinase inhibitors), although less than 3% of patients have had significant prolongation, most frequently asymptomatic.

Nilotinib is currently approved for treatment of patients in chronic or accelerated phase of the disease who have experienced resistance or intolerance to imatinib, and the standard dose is 400 mg twice daily. Recently, nilotinib has also been approved as initial therapy for CML in chronic phase, with the standard dose for this indication being 300mg twice daily. Nilotinib should be taken on an empty stomach, as food may significantly increase the absorption.

Other agents Other investigational agents are being developed for patients who fail to respond to imatinib therapy. Bosutinib is another Src and ABL inhibitor with activity against most mutants of *BCR-ABL*. Early results suggest significant activity among patients who fail to respond to imatinib therapy. Bosutinib has minimal or no activity against PDGF-R and KIT, which could lead to decreased toxicity (eg, pleural effusions and myelosuppression); however, this drug has activity against LYN and ABL and has also shown activity in patients who have failed to respond to imatinib and other tyrosine kinase inhibitors. Several agents are being developed to treat patients with the *T315I* mutation that is resistant to all available agents. They include omacetaxine (homoharringtonine), MK-0457, XL 228, PHA-739358, DCC-2036, and AP24534. Early results from these trials suggest activity in some patients.

Allogeneic BMT

Allogeneic BMT is potentially curative in CML, although relapses and mortality from complications such as chronic graft-vs-host disease (GVHD) may occur many years after transplantation. Results are better for patients in the chronic phase than for those in either the accelerated or blastic phase. Long-term survival rates of 50% to 80% and disease-free survival rates of 30% to 70% can be achieved in the chronic phase. The role of BMT is now changing in view of the results obtained with imatinib.

Predictors of response Early BMT within the first 1 to 3 years after diagnosis may be associated with a better outcome than is BMT performed later in the course of disease. Younger patients also have a better outcome than do older patients, with those younger than age 20 to those 30 years of age having the best prognosis. The use of the EBMT score helps to separate those patients who may have a better outcome from those who may not.

Conditioning regimens, including total-body irradiation (TBI), have been traditionally used, but non–TBI-containing regimens (eg, with busulfan and cyclophosphamide) have produced similar results. More recently, conditioning regimens using pharmacologic targeting of busulfan have been associated with decreased regimen-related toxicity while preserving efficacy. Also, nonmyeloablative conditioning regimens frequently containing purine analogs (mini-BMT) have been tested recently to expand the use of transplants to older patients or to those with medical conditions that preclude conventional BMT.

GVHD The major morbidity from BMT is GVHD. T-cell depletion of the graft can reduce the incidence of this complication, but at the expense of higher relapse and graft failure rates. (For a full discussion of GVHD, see chapter 33.)

Alternatives to matched-related donors For patients who do not have a matched-related donor, matched-unrelated donor transplants are reasonable alternatives. The 9-year experience from the National Marrow Donor Program in 1,432 patients reported a 3-year survival rate of 37.5%. Early transplantation results in better outcome, with patients transplanted in the chronic phase having a 3-year disease-free survival of 63%. The outcome of patients transplanted during the accelerated, blastic, or second chronic phase is inferior.

None of the currently available kinase inhibitors has significant activity against CML with *T315I* mutation. Omacetaxine (Omapro, homoharringtonine) has been shown to have preclinical activity against cells carrying this mutation. In a phase II study of 81 patients with CML resistant to imatinib (Gleevec) with *T315I* mutation, complete hematologic responses have been reported in 86% of patients treated in chronic phase (complete hematologic response in all), 35% of those in accelerated phase, and 47% of patients in blast phase. Cytogenetic responses occurred in 41% of patients treated in chronic phase and 6% of those in accelerated phase. There was a reduction in the *T315I* clone in 57% of all patients, and it became undetectable in 9%. Thus, omacetaxine offers a good treatment option for patients with this mutation *(Cortes J et al: Blood 114: abstract 644, 2009).*

Relapse after BMT Donor leukocyte infusions are the most effective strategy to treat patients who relapse after BMT. With this strategy, 70% to 80% of patients can achieve a cytogenetic complete response; the best results are achieved when patients are treated during cytogenetic or molecular relapse. Imatinib has also been effective for patients who relapse after BMT. A complete hematologic response in more than 70% of patients, and a cytogenetic response in 58% have been reported, with the best responses obtained in patients relapsing in chronic phase.

Treatment recommendations

The long-term results of imatinib are excellent, with an overall survival of nearly 90% at 8 years. Thus, all patients in chronic phase should be offered standard-dose imatinib or second-generation tyrosine kinase inhibitors nilotinib or dasatinib as initial therapy. Patients should be followed closely to determine that the expected results are met at the specified times (Table 3). If this is the case, treatment should continue uninterrupted indefinitely. For patients having a suboptimal response, dose escalation is recommended. For patients who fail to respond to imatinib, a change in therapy to one of the second-generation tyrosine kinase inhibitors is indicated.

The role of allogeneic stem cell transplant in CML has changed, and it is considered mostly a second- or third-line treatment option currently. For patients who fail imatinib therapy, transplant, or an initial trial with a second-generation tyrosine kinase inhibitor should be considered in most patients. Adequate response at early time points is important, particularly for young patients with a transplant option. If there is no cytogenetic response at 6 months or no major cytogenetic response by 12 months, transplant should be considered. Patients with a *T315I* mutation or who have failed to respond to two or more tyrosine kinase inhibitors should be considered for stem cell transplantation if adequate candidates. Otherwise, they should be included in clinical trials.

Accelerated and blastic phases

Imatinib

Imatinib is also effective for patients with CML in transformation. Seventy-one percent of patients in accelerated phase treated with 600 mg/d of imatinib had a hematologic response. The major cytogenetic response rate was 24%, with 67% having a time to disease progression of 12 months. These results are significantly superior to those achieved using 400 mg/d, making 600 mg/d the standard dose for patients in accelerated phase. In blast phase, 52% of patients achieved a hematologic remission, and 31% achieved a sustained remission lasting at least 4 weeks with imatinib. However, the median response duration is only 10 months, even when considering only patients with sustained remission (ie, lasting at least 4 weeks). Patients with clonal evolution have a lower probability of response and a shorter survival than do patients without clonal evolution when treated with imatinib.

Nilotinib and dasatinib also have significant clinical activity in patients with advanced-stage disease. In accelerated phase, complete hematologic response rates of 26% and 50% have been reported, respectively, and corresponding rates of complete cytogenetic response were 19% and 33%. In blast phase, complete hematologic response was reported in 11% to 13% and 26% to 29% with nilotinib and dasatinib, respectively, and complete cytogenetic responses, in 27% to 46% and 29% to 32%, respectively. Their use should be considered for patients who have failed to respond to prior therapy, including imatinib. Both agents are approved for patients in accelerated phase, but only dasatinib is currently approved for blast phase. However, responses are of shorter duration in patients in advanced stages, particularly among those in the blast phase. Combined use of these agents with other drugs (eg, standard chemotherapy) is being investigated to improve outcomes.

BMT

Compared with results in patients in the chronic phase, results with allogeneic BMT are worse in patients in the accelerated or blast phase, with 4-year survival rates of only 10% to 30%. Patients in the accelerated phase (determined on the basis of clonal evolution only) who undergo BMT less than 1 year after diagnosis have a 4-year probability of survival of 74%. Patients in the blast phase who respond to therapy with a second-generation tyrosine kinase inhibitor should be offered a BMT in the second chronic phase if an adequate donor is available.

SUGGESTED READING

Apperley JF: Part I: Mechanisms of resistance to imatinib in chronic myeloid leukaemia. Lancet Oncol 8:1018–1029, 2007.

Baccarani M, Cortes J, Pane F, et al: Chronic myeloid leukemia: An update of concepts and management recommendations of European LeukemiaNet. J Clin Oncol 27:6041–6051, 2009.

Cortes JE, Baccarani M, Guilhot F, et al: Phase III, randomized, open-label study of daily imatinib mesylate 400 mg versus 800 mg in patients with newly diagnosed, previously untreated chronic myeloid leukemia in chronic phase using molecular end points: Tyrosine kinase inhibitor optimization and selectivity study. J Clin Oncol 28:424–430, 2010.

Cortes JE, Jones D, O'Brien S, et al: Nilotinib as front-line treatment for patients with chronic myeloid leukemia in early chronic phase. J Clin Oncol 28:392–397, 2010.

Cortes JE, Jones D, O'Brien S, et al: Results of dasatinib therapy in patients with early chronic-phase chronic myeloid leukemia. J Clin Oncol 28:398–404, 2010.

Cortes JE, Egorin MJ, Guilhot F, et al: Pharmacokinetic/pharmacodynamic correlation and blood-level testing in imatinib therapy for chronic myeloid leukemia. Leukemia 23:1537–1544, 2009.

Jemal A, Siegel R, Xu J, et al: Cancer statistics, 2010. CA Cancer J Clin 60:277–300, 2010.

Kantarjian H, Cortes J, Kim DW, et al: Phase 3 study of dasatinib 140 mg once daily versus 70 mg twice daily in patients with chronic myeloid leukemia in accelerated phase resistant or intolerant to imatinib: 15-month median follow-up. Blood 113:6322–6329, 2009.

Kantarjian H, Pasquini R, Lévy V, et al: Dasatinib or high-dose imatinib for chronic-phase chronic myeloid leukemia resistant to imatinib at a dose of 400 to 600 milligrams daily: Two-year follow-up of a randomized phase 2 study (START-R). Cancer 115:4136–4147, 2009.

Kantarjian H, Schiffer C, Jones D, Cortes J: Monitoring the response and course of chronic myeloid leukemia in the modern era of BCR-ABL tyrosine kinase inhibitors: Practical advice on the use and interpretation of monitoring methods. Blood 111:1774–1780, 2008.

Kantarjian H, Shah NP, Hochhaus A, et al: Dasatinib versus imatinib in newly diagnosed chronic-phase chronic myeloid leukemia. NEJM 362: 2260–2270; 2010.

Kantarjian HM, Shan J, Jones D, et al: Significance of increasing levels of minimal residual disease in patients with Philadelphia chromosome-positive chronic myelogenous leukemia in complete cytogenetic response. J Clin Oncol 27:3659–3663, 2009.

Khoury HJ, Guilhot F, Hughes TP, et al: Dasatinib treatment for Philadelphia chromosome-positive leukemias: Practical considerations. Cancer 115:1381–1394, 2009.

le Coutre P, Ottmann OG, Giles F, et al: Nilotinib (formerly AMN107), a highly selective BCR-ABL tyrosine kinase inhibitor, is active in patients with imatinib-resistant or -intolerant accelerated-phase chronic myelogenous leukemia. Blood 111:1834–1839, 2008.

Marin D, Bazeos A, Mahon FX, et al: Adherence is the critical factor for achieving molecular responses in patients with chronic myeloid leukemia who achieve complete cytogenetic responses on imatinib. J Clin Oncol 28:2381–2388, 2010.

Quintas-Cardama A, Cortes J: Molecular biology of bcr-abl1-positive chronic myeloid leukemia. Blood 113:1619–1630, 2009.

Quintas-Cardama A, Cortes JE, O'Brien S, et al: Dasatinib early intervention after cytogenetic or hematologic resistance to imatinib in patients with chronic myeloid leukemia. Cancer 115:2912–2921, 2009.

Quintas-Cardama A, Kantarjian H, Jones D, et al: Delayed achievement of cytogenetic and molecular response is associated with increased risk of progression among patients with chronic myelogenous leukemia in early chronic phase receiving high-dose or standard-dose imatinib therapy. Blood 113:6315–6321, 2009.

Redaelli S, Piazza R, Rostagno R, et al: Activity of bosutinib, dasatinib, and nilotinib against 18 imatinib-resistant BCR/ABL mutants. J Clin Oncol 27:469–471, 2009.

Rosti G, Palandri F, Castagnetti F, et al: Nilotinib for the frontline treatment of Ph(+) chronic myeloid leukemia. Blood 114:4933–4938, 2009.

Saglio G, Kim DW, Issaragrisil S, et al: Nilotinib versus imatinib for newly diagnosed chronic myeloid leukemia. NEJM 362: 2251–2259; 2010.

Velev N, Cortes J, Champlin R, et al: Stem cell transplantation for patients with chronic myeloid leukemia resistant to tyrosine kinase inhibitors with BCR-ABL kinase domain mutation T315I. Cancer 116:3631–3637, 2010.

White DL, Dang P, Engler J, et al: Functional activity of the OCT-1 protein is predictive of long-term outcome in patients with chronic-phase chronic myeloid leukemia treated with imatinib. J Clin Oncol 28:2761–2767, 2010.

Abbreviations in this chapter

EBMT = European Bone Marrow Transplant; MRC = Medical Research Council; SEER = Surveillance, Epidemiology and End Results; WHO = World Health Organization

CHAPTER 31

Chronic lymphocytic leukemia and hairy-cell leukemia

Nicole Lamanna, MD, Mark A. Weiss, MD,
and Kieron Dunleavy, MD

CLL

CHRONIC LYMPHOCYTIC LEUKEMIA

Chronic lymphocytic leukemia (CLL) is a clonal malignancy that results from expansion of the mature lymphocyte compartment. This expansion is a consequence of prolonged cell survival, despite a varied cell. The affected lymphocytes are of B-cell lineage in 95% of cases, and the remaining cases involve T lymphocytes, representing a distinct disorder.

CLL is the most common leukemia in adults in Western countries, accounting for approximately 25% to 30% of all leukemias. The proportion of cases diagnosed with the early stages of the disease (Rai stage 0) has risen from 10% to 50%, probably because of earlier diagnosis (routine automated blood counts).

EPIDEMIOLOGY

The incidence of CLL in the general population is 4.2:100,000 population, with an estimated death rate of 1.1:100,000 population. It was estimated that there were 14,990 patients diagnosed with CLL in 2010 in the United States.

Gender

The male-to-female ratio is 2:1. There is little change with age, as the male-to-female ratio is 2.1:1 for patients < 65 years old, compared with 1.9:1 for those ≥ 65 years old.

Age

The median age at diagnosis is 72 years, and 70% of patients are > 65 years of age at diagnosis. CLL is rarely seen in younger patients, with $< 2\%$ being younger than 45 years old at the time of diagnosis.

CLL

Race

In the American population, the incidence of CLL is similar in different races. However, the incidence is much lower in Asia (Japan, Korea, and China), Latin America, and Africa than in the United States and Western Europe.

ETIOLOGY AND RISK FACTORS

The etiology of CLL is unclear. However, some factors associated with CLL have been identified.

Genetic factors

There is a familial risk for CLL, with family members of patients with CLL having a twofold to sevenfold higher risk of developing the disease. CLL with a familial association tends to occur in younger individuals with subsequent generations, perhaps because of increased screening. Association with certain human lymphocyte antigen (HLA) patterns has not been consistent, and ongoing studies are attempting to identify susceptibility genes for CLL.

Environmental factors

There is no documented association of CLL with exposure to radiation, alkylating agents, or known leukemogenic chemicals. However, exposure to some chemicals used in agriculture may increase the risk of developing CLL.

Viral infections

Associations between CLL and several viruses, including human T-cell lymphotrophic viruses I and II (HTLV-I and HTLV-II) and Epstein-Barr virus, have been suggested. However, no conclusive evidence of a causal relationship exists. Adult T-cell leukemia/lymphoma, a T-cell disorder that can resemble CLL, is caused by HTLV-I.

Monoclonal B lymphocytosis

Recent studies suggest that over 4% of the population over 40 years of age harbor a population of clonal B cells with the phenotype of CLL or another B-cell malignancy, a condition now called monoclonal B-cell lymphocytosis (MBL). These asymptomatic individuals have no clinical evidence of disease and do not fulfill diagnostic criteria for CLL. All cases of CLL appear to be preceded by MBL, but most patients with MBL will not develop a hematologic malignancy.

In one study, 5.1% of patients > age 62 in the general population had monoclonal CLL-phenotype B cells. These asymptomatic individuals did not have lymphocytosis or clinical evidence of disease and did not fulfill diagnostic criteria for CLL. Whether or not these individuals will eventually develop diagnostic criteria or symptomatic disease is unknown. In that same study, patients with lymphocytosis (> 4,000 lymphocytes/μL), CLL requiring treatment developed at the rate of 1.1% per year.

SIGNS AND SYMPTOMS

In the majority of patients, CLL is asymptomatic at diagnosis and is discovered on a routine blood examination. When symptoms are present, they are nonspecific and include fatigue, weakness, and malaise and, in fact, may not even be attributable to CLL.

Constitutional B symptoms

Constitutional B symptoms (ie, fever, weight loss, and night sweats) are not common at diagnosis but may signal disease transformation. Patients frequently notice enlarged lymph nodes or abdominal distention related to mesenteric lymphadenopathy and/or splenomegaly.

Patients with CLL have an increased susceptibility to infections, which may be the presenting complaint.

Lymphadenopathy

Lymphadenopathy is common at diagnosis. Lymph nodes are usually symmetric, mobile, and nontender.

Splenomegaly and hepatomegaly

The spleen and, less frequently, the liver may be enlarged. Splenomegaly may be massive in advanced cases. Only occasionally is splenomegaly found in the absence of lymphadenopathy, but recognition of such patients may identify a group that may benefit from splenectomy.

Other organs

In advanced disease, other organs may be involved, including the GI mucosa, prostate, lungs, pleura, and bones. Rarely is such involvement clinically important unless (Richter's) transformation has occurred.

TABLE 1: Diagnostic criteria for CLL according to the National Cancer Institute (NCI) and International Workshop on CLL (IWCLL)

Cells	NCI	IWCLL
Lymphocytes	$\geq 5 \times 10^9$/L + $\geq$ 1 B-cell marker (CD19, CD20, CD23) + CD5, monoclonal	$\geq 10 \times 10^9$/L + B-cell phenotype or bone marrow involvement
Atypical cells (eg, prolymphocytes)	< 55%	Not stated
Bone marrow lymphocytes	$\geq$ 30%	> 30%

LABORATORY FEATURES

Peripheral blood

The most consistent feature of CLL is lymphocytosis, with median values of 30% to 50% × 10^9/L. The lymphocytes are small and mature-appearing, with little cytoplasm and clumped chromatin. Smudge cells are frequently seen; when present in a high proportion, they may predict for a more indolent course. A few larger nucleolated cells, which represent prolymphocytes, usually constitute < 10% of the total lymphocytes. Diagnostic criteria for CLL defined by the NCI and IWCLL are presented in Table 1.

A positive Coombs' test is seen in as many as 30% of patients at some time during the disease course, although it is uncommon (< 5%) during early stages. Autoimmune phenomena are relatively frequent, with hemolytic anemia (lifetime risk, approximately 10%–20%) and thrombocytopenia (lifetime risk, approximately 5% to 10%) occurring most commonly. Autoimmune neutropenia and other autoimmune sequelae are infrequent but more common than in the general population.

Bone marrow

The bone marrow is usually hypercellular but can be normocellular. The most characteristic feature is the presence of at least 30% mature lymphocytes. The lymphocyte infiltration can be interstitial, nodular, mixed interstitial and nodular, or diffuse. Diffuse lymphocyte infiltration is associated with a poor prognosis.

Other laboratory findings

Progressive hypogammaglobulinemia is seen in > 50% of patients with CLL, usually affecting IgA first, followed by IgM and IgG. However, 5% to 10% of patients may have a small monoclonal peak. Paraproteinemia is more common at disease transformation.

Elevated serum levels of B_2-microglobulin (β2M) have been associated with a poor prognosis. Elevation of serum lactate dehydrogenase (LDH) levels is found in < 10% of patients at diagnosis and may indicate autoimmune hemolytic anemia or (Richter's) transformation to large-cell lymphoma (LCL).

Immunophenotyping

More than 95% of all cases of CLL have a B-cell phenotype with monoclonality by light chain restriction. In these patients, CD19 and/or CD20 are essentially always coexpressed with CD5, which normally is expressed on T cells and a subset of normal B cells. Other markers, such as CD21 and CD22, may also be expressed. Expression of CD23 helps to differentiate CLL from mantle cell lymphoma, in which cells coexpress CD19 and CD5 but lack CD23. Furthermore, the monoclonal antibody FMC7 (which recognizes an epitope on CD20) rarely reacts with CLL cells but frequently binds the cells of patients with mantle cell lymphoma.

Expression of surface immunoglobulin is usually weak and is lower than in normal B lymphocytes or most other B-cell lymphomas. Expression of CD38 on the surface of CLL cells portends a worse prognosis than that for patients whose cells do not express CD38.

CYTOGENETIC AND MOLECULAR FINDINGS

Chromosomal abnormalities

A number of recurrent cytogenetic abnormalities have been identified in CLL. Most have not been associated with a specific gene defect or abnormality; however, their detection is prognostically important, and work continues toward identifying the associated gene or genes.

Using interphase fluorescent in situ hybridization (FISH), cytogenetic abnormalities can be identified in > 80% of CLL cases. Because of the low mitotic rate in CLL, traditional karyotypic methods frequently fail, and FISH has increased the detection of clonal genetic abnormalities in patients with CLL.

In a landmark study, Dohner et al evaluated 325 patients with CLL. Using a variety of fluorescent probes, they identified chromosomal aberrations in 82%. Among these findings was the recognition that some subtypes (17p del and 11q del) had markedly shorter time to initiate chemotherapy and shorter overall survival than did other types. In this study, the most frequent change was a deletion in 13q14 (55% of patients). Other typical abnormalities included deletion 11q22–23 (18%), trisomy 12q13 (16%), and deletion 17p13 (7%).

These genetic abnormalities help explain some of the clinical variations seen in CLL. For example, patients with 13q deletions tend to have modest or absent lymphadenopathy, whereas patients with deletion 11q frequently have bulky adenopathy.

Disease progression also is heavily influenced by the underlying genetic abnormality. Time from diagnosis to treatment averaged only 9 months for patients with 17p abnormalities, compared with 92 months for patients with 13q deletions.

These chromosomal abnormalities were potent predictors of outcome with the following median survivals: deletion 17p, 32 months; deletion 11q, 79 months; trisomy 12, 114 months; and deletion 13q, 133 months.

Molecular abnormalities

No single gene has been implicated in the pathogenesis of CLL. However, several genetic abnormalities have biologic and/or prognostic implications.

The *TP53* gene is located on the short arm of chromosome 17 and is deleted in the leukemia clone of up to 10% of patients with CLL. Mutations of *TP53* occur in a similar proportion of CLL cases, usually in association with *TP53* deletion in the other *TP53* allele. The 17p deletion involving *TP53* is considered the most significant negative cytogenetic prognostic factor in CLL. The *TP53* protein normally responds to DNA damage by inducing cell cycle arrest and facilitating DNA repair. It can also induce apoptosis in cells with damaged DNA and in this way mediates the cytotoxicity of many anticancer agents. Resistance to treatment is a particular characteristic of *TP53* deletion and has been observed for agents including purine analogs. Further investigation of the common 13q deletion has revealed the detection of specific micro-RNA genomic sequence abnormalities expressed in patients with CLL. Further analysis suggests a micro-RNA signature profile may be associated with *ZAP-70* expression and mutational status of IgV_H (immunoglobulin heavy-chain

TABLE 2: Staging systems for CLL

RAI SYSTEM

Rai stage	Modified Rai stage (risk)	Clinical characteristics	Median survival (yr)
0	Low	Lymphocytosis in peripheral blood and bone marrow only	> 10
I	Intermediate	Lymphocytosis and enlarged lymph nodes	6
II		Lymphocytosis and enlarged spleen and/or liver	
III	High	Lymphocytosis and anemia (hemoglobin < 11 g/dL)	2
IV		Lymphocytosis and thrombocytopenia (platelets < 100 × 10^9/L)	

BINET SYSTEM

Binet stage	Clinical characteristics	Median survival (yr)
A	Hemoglobin level ≥ 10 g/dL, platelet count ≥ 100 × 10^9/L, and < 3 areas involved	> 7
B	Hemoglobin level ≥ 10 g/dL, platelet count ≥ 100 × 10^9/L, and ≥ 3 areas involved	< 5
C	Hemoglobin level < 10 g/dL, platelet count < 100 × 10^9/L, or both (independent of areas involved)	< 2

variable) as well as disease progression. Though the exact significance of this finding is not known with certainty, the specific micro-RNA signature may be relevant to the pathogenesis of CLL. In addition, germline mutations affecting these micro-RNAs may be a predisposing factor in familial CLL.

Overexpression of *BCL2*

Abnormalities of the long arm of chromosome 14 frequently involve region 14q32, the site encoding for the immunoglobulin heavy-chain gene. However, gene translocations such as t(11;14)(q13;q32) and t(14;18)(q32;q21), which juxtapose genes *CCND1* and *BCL2* to the heavy-chain immunoglobulin gene, are not typical and should prompt consideration of alternative diagnoses (mantle cell or follicular lymphoma). Nevertheless, increased expression of *BCL2* mRNA and protein is common in CLL. Because overexpression of *BCL2* inhibits apoptosis, it is possible that this gene participates in the pathogenesis of CLL.

STAGING AND PROGNOSIS

Staging systems

Two staging systems of CLL are commonly used: one proposed and later modified by Rai and the other proposed by Binet (Table 2). Both systems include three categories of low, intermediate, and high risk, with median survival durations of approximately 10, 6, and 2 years, respectively.

Other prognostic factors

Stage of disease has been considered the main prognostic indicator for CLL. However, other factors have prognostic implications, such as chromosomal aberrations, serum level of β2M, pattern of bone marrow infiltration, the lymphocyte doubling time, and serum levels of soluble CD23.

Somatic hypermutation (SHM) normally occurs in germinal centers of lymphoid tissues and is a process that introduces mutations in the variable region of immunoglobulin genes. It is responsible for affinity maturation, the process of producing B cells with high-affinity antibody. CLL can be divided into two distinct prognostic groups based on the extent to which the expressed IgV_H gene has undergone SHM. CLL cases with an IgV_H gene with < 98% homology to germline are considered mutated and those with an IgV_H gene with ≥ 98% homology to germline are considered unmutated.

CLL cases with an unmutated IgV_H gene generally have rapid progression and an unfavorable prognosis, whereas CLL cases with a mutated IgV_H gene generally have slowly progressive disease and a favorable prognosis. Patients with unmutated IgV_H genes have a median survival of 8 years, compared with 24 years for those with mutated IgV_H genes. The biologic differences between these groups are also reflected in the association of unmutated IgV_H genes with other poor prognostic features, such as expression of CD38, and unfavorable cytogenetic abnormalities. These results need to be interpreted carefully in light of the fact that the study population was not representative of the epidemiology of CLL, for which median survival for all patients is approximately 5 years.

The immunoglobulins expressed by CLL cells can be polyreactive autoantibodies. It follows that the cell that gives rise to the CLL B cell may experience persistent antigen stimulation, which contributes to malignant transformation. The role of antigen selection is implicated by the overrepresentation of certain IgV_H genes in CLL. In addition, there is also a biased distribution of these genes between the mutated and unmutated subgroups. The *VH3* and *VH4* families of genes are frequently found in the subgroup with mutated IgV_H genes, whereas the *VH1* family, particularly *VH1-69*, is more common in the subgroup with unmutated IgV_H genes. Specific genes, such as *VH3-21*, have also been associated with a poor prognosis, independent of IgV_H mutation status.

ZAP-70 encodes a protein tyrosine kinase normally expressed by T cells and involved in intracellular signaling initiated by T-cell receptor ligation. Expression of *ZAP-70* by CLL B cells (> 20% of CLL cells are *ZAP-70*–positive) is associated with unmutated IgV_H genes, shorter time to initial treatment, and inferior survival compared with CLL cells that are *ZAP-70*–negative (< 20% cases). Detection of the ZAP-70 protein by flow cytometry or immunohistochemistry may provide a useful prognostic marker for patients with CLL.

TREATMENT

Treatment recommendations

Traditionally, the initial therapy for CLL has been chlorambucil (Leukeran) with or without prednisone. However, accumulating data suggest that fludarabine has significantly greater activity than these agents. This agent produces higher overall and complete remission (CR) rates and provides a longer remission duration than chlorambucil. Newer data suggest that combination chemotherapy, particularly a nucleoside analog combined with an alkylating agent, produces higher response rates, and the addition of monoclonal antibodies to such regimens appears to increase CR rates. However, to date, a survival advantage has not been demonstrated for administering these regimens as initial therapy.

The development of nonmyeloablative transplants has provided the possibility of allogeneic transplantation for CLL, where the median age of patients is near 70 years, but this new technique should only be performed in the context of a clinical trial. An effort should be made to enroll patients in clinical trials that offer them the possibility of receiving some of the new alternatives, which may eventually achieve the goal of curing CLL.

Early-stage disease

Since patients with early-stage CLL have a good long-term prognosis, and early therapy has not changed the outcome of the disease, patients in the early stages should not be treated unless specific indications exist. Randomized trials comparing chlorambucil vs no therapy have documented no advantage for patients with early-stage CLL who received immediate therapy with chlorambucil. New alternatives for treatment of high-risk early-stage CLL (*ZAP-70*–positive, unmutated *IgH* status) are being investigated.

A recent study by Eichhorst et al randomized patients > 65 years of age to monotherapy with either fludarabine or chlorambucil. More responses, including CRs, were seen in patients randomized to fludarabine therapy. Despite this improvement in response, there was no difference in progression-free survival (fludarabine, 19 months; chlorambucil, 18 months). However, median survival appeared to favor the chlorambucil arm (fludarabine, 53 months; chlorambucil, not reached), although this result did not reach statistical significance *(P = .07; Eichhorst BF et al: Blood 114:3382–3391, 2009).*

Conventional chemotherapy

Single-agent chemotherapy

Historically, the initial agent used for CLL has been chlorambucil, given as either 0.1 mg/kg daily or 20 to 40 mg/m^2 every 2 to 4 weeks. Therapy is continued until the signs or symptoms requiring therapy are controlled.

Chlorambucil is frequently combined with oral prednisone (30–100 mg/m^2/day), although there is no clear evidence that the combination improves responses or overall survival over chlorambucil alone. Prednisone is of value, however, in the management of autoimmune cytopenias.

Cyclophosphamide is an alternative to chlorambucil. The usual dose is 0.5 to 1 g/m^2 every 3 to 4 weeks alone or together with vincristine

TABLE 3: Response criteria in CLL according to the IWCLL

Complete response

Resolution of lymphadenopathy, splenomegaly, hepatomegaly, and constitutional symptoms

Normalization of blood counts:

- Neutrophils $> 1.5 \times 10^9/L$
- Platelets $> 100 \times 10^9/L$
- Lymphocytes $< 4 \times 10^9/L$

Normalization of bone marrow

- $< 30\%$ lymphocytes[a]
- Nodular focal infiltrates[b]

Partial response

Downstaging (from Binet stages C to A or B and from B to A)[b]

or

$> 50\%$ decrease in absolute lymphocyte count, splenomegaly, lymphadenopathy, hepatomegaly

- Neutrophils $\geq 1.5 \times 10^9/L$
- Platelets $\geq 100 \times 10^9/L$
- Hemoglobin > 11 g/dL
- $> 50\%$ improvement in peripheral blood counts[a]

[a] National Cancer Institute (NCI) criteria; [b] International Workshop on CLL (IWCLL) criteria

and steroids (eg, COP [cyclophosphamide, Oncovin (vincristine), and prednisone] regimen).

Combination chemotherapy

Various drug combinations have been used in CLL, mostly in patients with advanced-stage disease. Historically, the most frequently employed combinations have been COP and these three drugs plus doxorubicin (CHOP). The dose of doxorubicin used is usually low (25 mg/m^2). A higher dose of doxorubicin (50 mg/m^2) has been employed in some regimens, such as CAP (cyclophosphamide, doxorubicin [Adriamycin], and prednisone).

Response rates have been 40% to 85% with these combinations. In randomized studies, COP was no better than chlorambucil plus prednisone. Although CHOP initially achieved better survival than COP (in patients with Binet stage C disease) or chlorambucil plus prednisone, longer follow-up has not confirmed this survival advantage.

Nucleoside analogs

Fludarabine, now frequently the drug of choice for treating CLL, has been demonstrated to be more effective than chlorambucil for the treatment of CLL in

> Recently, the GCLLSG presented a prospective randomized trial of FCR vs FC for previously untreated patients with CLL. Overall response, complete response, and progression-free survival rates were improved with FCR *(Hallek M et al: Blood 112: abstract 325, 2008)*. With additional follow-up, this is the first randomized trial to demonstrate a benefit in overall survival with the addition of rituximab to FC (FCR arm, 84%; FC arm, 79%; *P* = .01; *Hallek M et al: Blood 114:535, 2009)*.

younger patients. When given to previously treated patients at a dose of 25 to 30 mg/m^2/day for 5 days every 3 to 4 weeks, this nucleoside analog produced responses in 20% to 50% of patients, with 5% to 15% of patients achieving CR and an additional 5% to 20% achieving a "nodular partial response (PR)," ie, a CR but with the presence of lymphoid nodules in the bone marrow (Table 3). In previously untreated patients, the response rate was 63% to 80%, with 8% to 35% of patients achieving a CR.

The addition of prednisone or chlorambucil to fludarabine therapy did not improve the response rate and is associated with an increased incidence of opportunistic infections and other toxicities. A large randomized study comparing fludarabine, CAP, and CHOP demonstrated an increased response rate with fludarabine but no difference in survival. Randomized trials of fludarabine vs chlorambucil in previously untreated younger patients showed improvements in response rate (overall and CR), duration of response, and disease progression–free survival with fludarabine but no survival advantage.

Cladribine (2-chlorodeoxyadenosine, 2-CdA) is also active in CLL when given at doses of 0.1 mg/kg/daily (or 4 mg/m^2/day) for 7 days. At therapeutic doses, this agent appears to be associated with more myelosuppression, particularly thrombocytopenia, than fludarabine.

The third purine analog active against CLL is pentostatin (Nipent). Previously, toxicity limited its use as an antineoplastic agent. More recently, the recognition that safe use of this drug requires concomitant hydration and close attention to renal function (it is both toxic to and cleared by the kidneys) has renewed interest in clinical evaluation with this agent. The group at Memorial Sloan-Kettering Cancer Center has studied pentostatin combined with cyclophosphamide and demonstrated responses in > 70% of previously treated patients (including those whose disease is refractory to fludarabine) with acceptable toxicity.

Combination chemotherapy

To improve the frequency of response achieved with single-agent purine nucleoside analogs, a variety of combination regimens have been developed. Initial studies of fludarabine and cyclophosphamide (FC), pentostatin and cyclophosphamide (PC), cladribine and cyclophosphamide (CC), as well as fludarabine and rituximab (Rituxan, FR) suggested an increased frequency of overall response and CR rates but at the price of added myelotoxicity and infectious complications. Three prospective clinical trials for chemotherapy-naive patients with CLL have randomized patients to receive monotherapy with fludarabine or combination therapy with FC. All three studies reported an increased frequency of overall response and CR rates and a longer progression-free survival with FC combination therapy than with monotherapy. These studies included ECOG 2997, BMRC CLL 4 trial, and GCSG CLL 4 trials. Despite improvement in overall response, CR, and progression-free survival rates, none of these studies demonstrated a survival advantage for patients receiving combination therapy.

Because of the success of two-drug combinations, several groups started exploring triple-drug therapy in CLL. Three published trials have evaluated the combination of fludarabine, cyclophosphamide, and rituximab as up-front treatment of CLL. These three studies used variations in dose and schedule, but all achieved excellent results in a cohort of primarily younger, healthier patients (Table 4). Despite the encouraging results in younger patients, these combinations are not recommended for most older patients (over age 65–70) with CLL.

Because of the concern about toxicity with these regimens, some groups looked at an alternative purine analog to maintain efficacy in a more tolerable regimen. Building on the positive results of combination pentostatin, cyclophosphamide, and rituximab (PCR) in previously treated patients, Kay et al reported on the use of this regimen in patients with untreated CLL. Responses occurred in 91% of patients, with 63% achieving a CR or a nodular response. More important, a subset analysis demonstrated that PCR treatment was equally effective in patients over the age of 70 as in younger individuals.

Two other monoclonal antibodies that may have potent activity in CLL are ofatumumab (Arzerra) and GA101 (RO5072759). Ofatumumab has good efficacy as a single agent in relapsed and refractory CLL; it recently was combined with fludarabine and cyclophosphamide and showed high activity in patients with previously untreated CLL. In 61 patients assessable for response (31 at the 500-mg dose level), overall response and complete response rate were 77% and 32%, respectively. At the 1,000-mg dose level, overall response and complete response rates were 73% and 50% *(Wierda et al: Blood 114: abstract 207, 2009)*. RO5072759 is the first humanized and glycoengineered type II monoclonal anti-CD20 antibody to enter clinical trials. In a phase I study in relapsed and refractory CLL, of 13 evaluable patients, 62% had a response, and the response duration ranged from 3.5 to 8 months *(Morschhauser et al: Blood 114: abstract 884, 2009)*.

Monoclonal antibody–targeted therapy

Monoclonal antibodies have been used in patients with CLL to exploit antibody-mediated cytotoxicity. Alemtuzumab (Campath) has been approved by the FDA for the treatment of refractory CLL. In a pivotal trial in patients with fludarabine-refractory disease, alemtuzumab resulted in an overall response rate of 33%.

TABLE 4: Comparison of sequential F→C→R, FCR, and FCR lite

	Response rate		
Patient characteristic	**F→C→R**	**FCR**	**FCR lite**
Complete response	61%	70%	79%
Response duration	43 months	NR	22 months
High-risk disease	61 months	33%	16%

FCR = fludarabine, cyclophosphamide, and rituximab; NR = not reported

Ferrajoli et al combined lenalidomide with rituximab for relapsed and refractory CLL patients. They achieved an overall response frequency of 68%, with responses seen across all prognostic groups, including patients with deletion 17p. Not only did the combination appear to be more active than did single-agent lenalidomide, but, by acting as a "debulking" agent, rituximab reduced the toxicity associated with lenalidomide therapy (ie, flare reactions, tumor lysis; *Ferrajoli A et al: Blood 114:206, 2009*).

Rituximab also has been investigated and is active both as a single agent and in combination with chemotherapy. Because rituximab has demonstrated improvement in survival when given with chemotherapy, it currently is being used in most treatment regimens for patients with CLL.

The combination of alemtuzumab and rituximab has been evaluated in patients with relapsed or refractory lymphoid malignancies. Alemtuzumab was given twice weekly at 30 mg IV for 4 weeks. Rituximab (375 mg/m^2) was given concurrently weekly for the 4 weeks. Responses were reported for 48 patients, 32 with CLL, 9 with CLL/PLL (prolymphocytic leukemia), 1 with PLL, 4 with mantle cell lymphoma, and 2 with Richter's transformation. The overall response rate was 52%; CR was noted in 8%, nodular PR in 4%, and PR in 40% of treated patients. Toxicities included infusion-related reactions. Infections occurred in 52% of patients, with cytomegalovirus reactivation occurring in 27% of patients. Overall, this was a well-tolerated combination for relapsed patients with CLL. Recently, early results of a randomized study of FCR vs FCR-alemtuzumab were reported in 165 patients. There was excessive toxicity in the alemtuzumab arm leading to premature cessation of the study. In March 2008, the FDA approved bendamustine (Treanda) for CLL. In a randomized, multicenter study of 319 treatment-naive patients with CLL, those treated with bendamustine had a significantly higher overall response than those treated with chlorambucil (68% vs 31%; $P < .0001$). Eight percent of the bendamustine group had a CR, compared with less than 1% of the chlorambucil group. In addition, patients who received bendamustine had a longer progression-free survival than those who received chlorambucil (21.6 months vs 3 months, $P < .0001$). Reportedly, the most common adverse events in the trial were myelosuppression, fever, nausea, and vomiting.

Recently, bendamustine plus rituximab was evaluated as initial therapy for patients with CLL. In a group of 117 patients (median age, 64 years), the overall response frequency was 91%, with 33% achieving a CR. First-line use of this combination continues to be investigated in patients with advanced CLL.

Ofatumumab (Arzerra) is an anti-CD20 antibody that differs from rituximab in that it binds to the "small loop epitope" of CD20. Recent studies of ofatumumab in patients with CLL who were refractory to fludarabine or alemtuzumab (or were inappropriate candidates for alemtuzumab because of bulky adenopathy) demonstrated an impressive response frequency (51% and 44% overall response rates, respectively). This trial led to the approval of ofatumumab by the FDA for selected patients with CLL. In a pilot study evaluating ofatumumab with fludarabine and cyclophosphamide as initial therapy, CR frequencies of 32% (low-dose ofatumumab arm) and 50% (higher-dose ofatumumab arm) were achieved.

Lumiliximab is an anti-CD23 monoclonal antibody. A phase I study in patients with relapsed or refractory CLL demonstrated an acceptable toxicity profile but revealed no responses. Recently, the results of a phase I/II dose-escalation study of lumiliximab added to fludarabine, cyclophosphamide, and rituximab (FCR) in previously untreated CLL patients was reported. Two different doses of lumiliximab were combined with FCR for 6 cycles, and the overall response rate was 65% with 52% of patients achieving a CR.

In a phase I study, a pharmacokinetically derived hybrid schedule of flavopiridol showed promising activity in CLL, even in patients with high-risk features. Recently, the results of a phase II study of this hybrid schedule in relapsed and refractory CLL was published. A total of 64 patients (median age, 60 years; median prior therapies, 4) were enrolled. In all, 53% of patients achieved a PR or CR, and the median PFS among responders was 10 to 12 months across all cytogenetic risk groups *(Lin TS et al: J Clin Oncol 27:6012–6018, 2009).*

Immunomodulatory drugs

Lenalidomide (Revlimid) has recently been investigated and shown to be active in patients with relapsed or refractory CLL. It is reported to modulate an immune effector cell response through activation of the T and natural killer cells and to directly induce apoptosis in tumor cells. Initial studies by Chanan-Khan et al in patients with relapsed or refractory CLL demonstrated an overall response rate of 47% (CR in 9%) in patients with relapsed or refractory CLL. Lenalidomide was administered orally at 25 mg on days 1 through 21 of a 28-day cycle. Myelosuppression led to a dose reduction to 10 mg.

Ferrajoli et al also evaluated lenalidomide in patients with relapsed or refractory CLL utilizing a low-dose daily schedule starting at 10 mg on a 28-day cycle (with a 5-mg incremental increase to a maximum of 25 mg daily if no significant toxicities were observed). Most patients were treated with 5 or 10 mg daily. Reponses were obtained in 14 of 44 evaluable patients (3 CRs, 1 no response, and 10 PRs). Eleven patients had disease improvement without fulfilling the criteria for PR and were able to continue on treatment. Notable toxicities with this agent include myelosuppression, tumor lysis syndrome, and tumor flare.

Lenalidomide has also been evaluated in patients with previously untreated CLL. Chen et al evaluated the drug in 25 patients with CLL starting at 2.5 mg (days 1–21) with a dose escalation of 5 mg with each cycle. All patients achieved stable disease or better, including 11 PRs and 6 cases of stable disease. Ferrajoli et al also reported the use of low-dose lenalidomide as initial treatment of "elderly" patients with CLL (median age, 72 years). All patients received continuous lenalidomide, starting at 5 mg for the first 56 days. Thereafter, the drug could be titrated up by 5-mg increments every 28 days to a maximum of 25 mg. A total of 47% of patients achieved a hematologic CR, and 38% achieved a hematologic PR.

Achieving minimal residual disease-free status

The current formal criteria to assess response are based on physical examination, blood counts, and microscopic evaluation of bone marrow (Table 3). Minimal residual disease (MRD) can be evaluated by more sensitive methods such as polymerase chain reaction (PCR) for the IgV_H gene or 4-color flow cytometry. In a study of 91 previously treated patients who received alemtuzumab (30 mg thrice weekly for up to 16 weeks), 36% achieved CR, and the overall response rate was 54%. Of the 91 patients, 18 achieved MRD-free status by flow-cytometry evaluation of their bone marrow. Survival was significantly longer for patients who achieved MRD-free status. Overall survival for the 18 patients with MRD-free remission was 84% at 5 years.

Another study demonstrated the utility of an MRD-negative state. Lamanna et al found that patients who achieved an MRD-negative complete response had a superior response duration when compared with those who were in CR but MRD-positive ($P = .007$).

Stem cell transplantation

Both allogeneic and autologous stem-cell transplantations (SCTs) have been tested in patients with CLL.

Allogeneic SCT is a viable option for younger patients with CLL, particularly if they have not responded to alkylating agents and/or nucleoside analogs and are in an advanced stage of disease. The series reported to date, including a majority of patients with advanced refractory disease, has documented a CR rate in excess of 70%. The response is sustained in most patients, although reported follow-up is typically short. SCT using nonablative conditioning regimens has produced encouraging results and should be considered in the setting of a clinical trial, particularly for patients > 60 years.

Since the median age of patients with CLL is usually higher than the age considered acceptable for allogeneic SCT, autologous transplants using purged marrow have also been investigated. In general, results have been disappointing, with the best results seen in patients with responsive disease and low tumor burdens—a group that might have fared well without a transplant.

Splenectomy

Splenectomy may be beneficial for cytopenias caused by hypersplenism (particularly in patients without significant lymphadenopathy) or for palliation when splenomegaly is symptomatic and refractory to chemotherapy. Cytopenias frequently respond to splenectomy. Perioperative mortality varies widely and is largely related to the experience of the surgeon in performing splenectomy in these patients. In experienced hands, splenectomy can be performed with minimal mortality, even in patients with end-stage disease.

COMPLICATIONS

Infections

Patients with CLL are prone to multiple infections, and infectious complications are a leading cause of death in patients with CLL. Hypogammaglobulinemia plays a central role in the predisposition of patients to this problem, and prophylactic IV administration of immunoglobulin preparations may reduce the incidence of infections. Cytotoxic therapy further weakens the immune system and may increase the risk of opportunistic infections.

Autoimmune cytopenias

These frequently complicate CLL and may be precipitated or aggravated by therapy (eg, fludarabine) for CLL. Autoimmune hemolytic anemia can be treated successfully with prednisone in the majority of patients. Combinations of cyclophosphamide with rituximab are beneficial in cases refractory to prednisone, splenectomy, or cyclosporine. Similar approaches may be useful for autoimmune thrombocytopenia. In a study from The University of Texas M. D. Anderson Cancer Center, 31 patients with CLL and autoimmune anemia or thrombocytopenia received cyclosporine (300 mg/day). Sixty-three percent of patients responded, with a median duration of response of 10 months. No grade 3/4 toxicity was seen.

Pure red cell aplasia and the less commonly amegakaryocytic thrombocytopenia are infrequent complications of CLL, which are mediated by immune mechanisms. Therapy with cyclosporine (3 to 6 mg/kg/day) is frequently effective.

Transformation

LCL

CLL transforms into LCL in 3% to 10% of patients. This phenomenon, known as Richter's transformation, has an aggressive presentation with fever and other B symptoms and progressive lymphadenopathy. Extranodal involvement occurs in approximately 40% of patients. Paraproteinemia, hypercalcemia, and a sharp rise in serum LDH levels can be frequently seen.

The prognosis of patients whose disease progresses to LCL is variable and depends in part on the degree of prior treatment used for the underlying CLL. In treatment-naive patients with LCL, standard therapy with CHOP and rituximab may offer long-term control of the transformed component. In patients who have had significant prior therapy, the disease is often refractory, and combination chemotherapy including SCT is frequently ineffective.

PLL

More rarely, CLL can transform into PLL, characterized by a > 55% increase in prolymphocytes. The transformation is frequently accompanied by progression of splenomegaly, cytopenias, and refractoriness to therapy.

Other diseases Anecdotal cases of CLL evolving into acute lymphocytic leukemia, myeloma, low-grade lymphoma, and Hodgkin lymphoma have been reported. The rarity of these reports makes a true causal connection less likely.

HAIRY-CELL LEUKEMIA

Hairy-cell leukemia (HCL) is an infrequent B-cell malignancy usually associated with pancytopenia and splenomegaly. About 600 cases are reported yearly in the United States. Despite its relative rarity, there are a disproportionate number of highly effective therapies available.

EPIDEMIOLOGY AND ETIOLOGY

The male-to-female ratio of HCL is 4:1. The median age at presentation is 50 years. The etiology is unknown.

DIFFERENTIAL DIAGNOSIS

HCL can be confused with malignant lymphomas, splenic lymphoma with villous lymphocytes (SLVLs), CLL, other non-Hodgkin lymphomas in leukemic phase, and occasionally even myelodysplastic syndromes.

TREATMENT

The indications for treatment of HCL are an absolute neutrophil count (ANC) < 1,000/μL, a platelet count < 100×10^3/μL, or a hemoglobin level < 10 g/dL; leukemic phase of HCL; symptomatic splenomegaly; recurrent infections; or autoimmune complications.

Response criteria

The criteria for a CR are normalization of the complete blood cell (CBC) count, with an ANC > 1,500/μL, a platelet count > 100,000/μL, and a hemoglobin level > 12 g/dL; regression of organomegaly to normal; and bone marrow and peripheral blood free of hairy cells. PRs require reduction of the hairy cells in the bone marrow to < 50%, < 5% hairy cells in peripheral blood, > 50% reduction in organomegaly, and normalization of the CBC count.

Splenectomy

This procedure is reserved for patients with splenic rupture, infarcts, a massively enlarged spleen, severe hypersplenism, or failure to respond to systemic chemotherapy.

Interferon-alfa

Interferon-alfa, at a dose of 3 mU/daily administered by IM or SC injection for 6 months followed by 3 mU/daily three times weekly for 12 or 24 months, induces a CR in 8% to 10% of patients and a PR in 74%. The median time to response was 6 months in patients achieving a PR and 14 months in those achieving a CR. Patients frequently relapse between 12 and 24 months after discontinuation of therapy. The superiority of purine analog therapy (discussed later) has essentially led most clinicians to abandon the use of interferon for this disease.

Purine analogs

The recommended dose of pentostatin is 4 mg/m^2 by IV bolus every other week until a CR is obtained. Usually, patients require a median of 8 courses (range, 4–15). The CR rate varies between 59% and 89% in different studies, and the PR rate varies between 4% and 37%. Responses can last for many years, and patients who relapse often respond to retreatment with pentostatin. In an update of a large randomized trial comparing pentostatin and interferon-alfa, Flinn et al reported that in 241 patients with HCL treated with pentostatin, the 10-year overall survival rate was 81%, with only two deaths (1%) attributable to HCL.

Cladribine shows activity in treating HCL similar to that of pentostatin. Due to this finding and the fact that cladribine is given as 1 cycle of a 7-day continuous infusion or a 5-day bolus, this agent usually is the preferred treatment of this disorder. Piro et al treated 144 HCL patients with cladribine, 0.1 mg/kg/daily by continuous IV infusion for 7 days. A total response rate of 97% was obtained, with 85% CRs and 12% PRs. Response was independent of previous treatment with interferon or splenectomy, and three patients whose disease was refractory to pentostatin responded to cladribine. Recovery of CBC counts occurred on average by day 61 (range, 11–268 days).

The largest series reporting long-term follow-up results on patients with HCL treated with cladribine was from the Scripps group. A total of 349 patients, with a median duration of response follow-up of 59 months, were evaluated. Twenty-six percent had relapsed at a median of 29 months, but most of them were patients who had achieved only a PR. The time-to-treatment failure rate at 48 months was only 16% in complete responders.

Else et al reported on a large series of 219 patients with HCL, comparing their experience with pentostatin and cladribine. Treatment results were similar in terms of frequency of CR, relapse, and overall survival. Though the results are excellent, with more than 95% of patients alive at 10 years, the disease-free survival curves do not plateau, indicating these drugs are not curative in HCL.

Immunotoxin

The NCI evaluated a recombinant immunotoxin containing an anti-CD22 variable domain fused to a truncated Pseudomonas exotoxin; it was given by IV infusion every other day for a total of three doses. Sixteen patients whose disease was resistant to cladribine were treated; 2 achieved a PR and 11 achieved a CR. Of the 11 patients, 3 who had a CR relapsed and were retreated; all of these patients achieved a second CR.

SUGGESTED READING

Byrd JC, Kipps TJ, Flinn IW, et al: Phase I/II study of lumiliximab combined with fludarabine, cyclophosphamide, and rituximab in patients with relapsed or refractory chronic lymphocytic leukemia. Blood 115:489–495, 2010.

Byrd JC, Peterson BL, Morrison VA, et al: Randomized phase II study of fludarabine with concurrent vs sequential treatment with rituximab in symptomatic, untreated patients with B-cell chronic lymphocytic leukemia: Results from Cancer and Leukemia Group B 9712 (CALGB 9712). Blood 101:6–14, 2003.

Calin GA, Ferracin M, Cimmino A, et al: A MicroRNA signature associated with prognosis and progression in chronic lymphocytic leukemia. N Engl J Med 353:1793–1801, 2005.

Catovsky D, Richards S, Matutes E, et al: Assessment of fludarabine plus cyclophosphamide for patients with chronic lymphocytic leukaemia (the LRF CLL4 Trial): A randomised controlled trial. Lancet 370:230–239, 2007.

Chanan-Khan A, Miller KC, Musial L, et al: Clinical efficacy of lenalidomide in patients with relapsed or refractory chronic lymphocytic leukemia: Results of a phase II study. J Clin Oncol 24:5343–5349, 2006.

Crespo M, Bosch F, Villamor N, et al: ZAP-70 expression as a surrogate for immunoglobulin-variable-region mutations in chronic lymphocytic leukemia. N Engl J Med 348:1764–1775, 2003.

Damle RN, Wasil T, Fais F, et al: Ig V gene mutation status and CD38 expression as novel prognostic indicators in chronic lymphocytic leukemia. Blood 94:1840–1847, 1999.

Eichhorst BF, Busch R, Hopfinger G, et al: Fludarabine plus cyclophosphamide versus fludarabine alone in first-line therapy of younger patients with chronic lymphocytic leukemia. Blood 107:885–891, 2006.

Else M, Ruchlemer R, Osuji N, et al: Long remissions in hairy cell leukemia with purine analogs. Cancer 104:2442–2448, 2005.

Ferrajoli A, Lee BN, Schlette EJ, et al: Lenalidomide induces complete and partial remissions in patients with relapsed and refractory chronic lymphocytic leukemia. Blood 111:5291–5297, 2008.

Flinn IW, Neuberg DS, Grever MR, et al: Phase III trial of fludarabine plus cyclophosphamide compared with fludarabine for patients with previously untreated chronic lymphocytic leukemia: US Intergroup Trial E2997. J Clin Oncol 25:793–798, 2007.

Foon KA, Boyiadzis M, Land SR, et al: Chemoimmunotherapy with low-dose fludarabine and cyclophosphamide and high-dose rituximab in previously untreated patients with CLL. J Clin Oncol 27:498–503, 2009.

Hillmen P, Skotnicki AB, Robak T, et al: Alemtuzumab compared with chlorambucil as first-line therapy for chronic lymphocytic leukemia. J Clin Oncol 25:5616–5623, 2007.

Jemal A, Siegel R, Xu J, et al: Cancer statistics 2010. CA Cancer J Clin 60:277–300, 2010.

Kay NE, Geyer SM, Call TG, et al: Combination chemoimmunotherapy with pentostatin, cyclophosphamide, and rituximab shows significant clinical activity with low accompanying toxicity in previously untreated B chronic lymphocytic leukemia. Blood 109:405–411, 2007.

Keating MJ, O'Brien S, Albitar M, et al: Early results of a chemoimmunotherapy regimen of fludarabine, cyclophosphamide, and rituximab as intital therapy for chronic lymphocytic leukemia. J Clin Oncol 23:4079–4088, 2005.

Knauf WU, Lissichkov T, Aldaoud A, et al: Phase III randomized study of bendamustine compared with chlorambucil in previously untreated patients with chronic lymphocytic leukemia. J Clin Oncol 27:4378–4384, 2009.

Lamanna N, Kalaycio M, Maslak P, et al: Pentostatin, cyclophosphamide, and rituximab is an active, well-tolerated regimen for patients with previously treated chronic lymphocytic leukemia. J Clin Oncol 24:1575–1581, 2006.

Landgren O, Albitar M, Ma W, et al: B-cell clones as early markers for chronic lymphocytic leukemia. N Engl J Med 60: 659–667, 2009.

Lin KI, Tam CS, Keating MJ, et al: Relevance of the immunoglobulin VH somatic mutation status in patients with chronic lymphocytic leukemia treated with fludarabine, cyclophosphamide and rituximab (FCR) or related chemoimmunotherapy regimens. Blood 113:3168–3171, 2009.

Lin TS, Ruppert AS, Johnson AJ, et al: Phase II study of flavopiridol in relapsed chronic lymphocytic leukemia demonstrating high response rates in genetically high-risk disease. J Clin Oncol 27: 6012–6018, 2009.

Lundin J, Kimby E, Bjorkholm M, et al: Phase II trial of subcutaneous anti-CD52 monoclonal antibody alemtuzumab (Campath-1H) as first-line treatment for patients with B-cell chronic lymphocytic leukemia (B-CLL). Blood 100:768–773, 2002.

Moreton P, Kennedy B, Lucas G, et al: Eradication of minimal residual disease in B-cell chronic lymphocytic leukemia after alemtuzumab therapy is associated with prolonged survival. J Clin Oncol 23:2971–2979, 2005.

Rai KR, Peterson BL, Appelbaum FR, et al: Fludarabine compared with chlorambucil as primary therapy for chronic lymphocytic leukemia. N Engl J Med 343:1750–1757, 2000.

Wierda W, O'Brien S, Wen S, et al: Chemoimmunotherapy with fludarabine, cyclophosphamide, and rituximab for relapsed and refractory chronic lymphocytic leukemia. J Clin Oncol 23:4070–4078, 2005.

Wierda WG, Kipps TJ, Mayer J, et al: Ofatumumab as single-agent CD20 immunotherapy in fludarabine-refractory chronic lymphocytic leukemia. J Clin Oncol 28:1749–1755, 2010.

Abbreviations in this chapter

BMRC = British Medical Research Council; ECOG = Eastern Cooperative Oncology Group; FDA = US Food and Drug Administration; GCSG = German CLL Study Group; IWCLL = International Workshop on CLL; NCI = National Cancer Institute

CHAPTER 32

Myelodysplastic syndromes

Guillermo Garcia-Manero, MD, Alan List, MD, Hagop Kantarjian, MD, and Jorge E. Cortes, MD

Myelodysplastic syndromes (MDS) are a group of hematologic malignancies of the pluripotent hematopoietic stem cells. These disorders are characterized by ineffective hematopoiesis, including abnormalities in proliferation, differentiation, and apoptosis. The overall clinical phenotype is peripheral cytopenias in the setting of a normocellular or hypercellular bone marrow and an increased risk for transformation to acute leukemia.

The incidence of MDS approximates 3 to 4 cases per 100,000 population per year, with 30 cases per 100,000 population per year in patients > 70 years old. It is estimated that approximately 10,000 to 15,000 new cases are diagnosed annually in the United States. Data on the epidemiology of MDS are now starting to emerge.

EPIDEMIOLOGY

Gender

The overall incidence of MDS is slightly higher in males than in females (1.5 to 2:1).

Age

The incidence of MDS increases with age, with a median age at diagnosis of about 70 years. MDS is rare in children; childhood cases are more frequently associated with monosomy of chromosome 7.

ETIOLOGY AND RISK FACTORS

MDS is a clonal disorder of bone marrow stem cells. The vast majority of cases (80% to 90%) occur de novo, whereas 10% to 20% of cases are secondary. The etiology of de novo MDS is unclear. Exposure to radiation and/or cytotoxic agents is a recognized etiologic factor in secondary disease forms. Cumulative exposure to environmental toxins, genetic differences in leukemogen susceptibility and metabolism, and genomic senescence may contribute to disease pathogenesis in de novo cases.

Genetic factors

It has been suggested that a genetic insult causes an irreversible alteration in the structure and function of the stem cell, with disruption of a multistep process involving control of cell proliferation, maturation, and interactions with growth factors; mutations of tumor-suppressor genes and proto-oncogenes; and deregulation of apoptosis.

Constitutional childhood disorders, such as Fanconi's anemia, Shwachman-Diamond syndrome, Down's syndrome, neurofibromatosis, and mitochondrial cytopathies, have been associated with MDS and monosomy of chromosome 7. Recently, heritable mutations of the *RUNX1* gene have been linked to familial cases of adult MDS.

Environmental factors

Exposure to benzene and its derivatives may result in karyotypic abnormalities often seen in MDS and acute myelogenous leukemia (AML). Persons chronically exposed to insecticides and pesticides may have a higher incidence of MDS than the general population.

An increased incidence of MDS has been reported among smokers and ex-smokers, possibly linked to associated exposures to polycyclic hydrocarbons and radioactive polonium present in tobacco smoke.

An association of MDS with magnetic fields, alcohol, or occupational exposure to other chemicals has not been demonstrated.

Antineoplastic drugs

Therapy-related myelodysplasia and therapy-related AML are recognized long-term complications of chemotherapy and radiotherapy. Therapy-related MDS usually develops 3 to 7 years after exposure to chemotherapy and is most frequently related to complete or partial loss of chromosomes 5 or 7 in patients previously treated with alkylating agents. Approximately 80% of cases of AML occurring after exposure to antineoplastic drugs, particularly alkylating agents, are preceded by MDS.

More than 85% of patients who develop chemotherapy-related leukemia or MDS have been exposed to alkylating agents. Patients exposed to nitrosoureas have a relative risk of developing MDS or AML of 14.4 and a 6-year actuarial risk of 4%. The mean cumulative risk of leukemia in patients exposed to epipodophyllotoxins (eg, etoposide and teniposide [Vumon]) is about 5% at 5 years. Most of these therapy-related leukemias are not preceded by a dysplastic phase and are associated with abnormalities in chromosome 11q23.

Autologous bone marrow transplantation (BMT)

BMT has also been associated with a 5-year actuarial risk of MDS of 15% (95% CI, 3.4%–16.6%). Fluorescent in situ hybridization analyses of pretreatment bone marrow specimens for informative cytogenetic markers indicate that these secondary myeloid malignancies derive from clones demonstrable before the transplant procedure. Prior therapy with fludarabine, older age, low CD34+ dose, and prolonged platelet reconstitution have been associated with the development of MDS or AML in patients with lymphoid malignancies after autologous stem cell transplantation (SCT).

CLASSIFICATION

In 1982, the French-American-British (FAB) group proposed a classification system for MDS that consists of five subgroups, based on the percentage of blast cells in

TABLE 1: Main features of MDS according to the FAB classification

FAB subgroup	BM blasts (%)	Ringed sideroblasts (%)	PB monocytes ($\times 10^9$/L)	Chromosomal abnormalities (%)	Frequently associated karyotype	Rate of leukemic progression (%)	Median survival (mo)
RA	< 5	< 15	< 1	30	5q-, -7, +8, 20q-	12	32
RARS	< 5	≥ 15	< 1	20	+8, 5q-, 20q-	8	42
RAEB	5–20	Variable	< 1	45	-7, 7q-, -5, 5q-, +8	44	12
RAEB-t	21–30	Variable	Variable	60	-7, 7q-, -5, 5q-, +8	66	5
CMML	1–20	Variable	≥ 1	30	-7, +8, t(5;12), 7q-, 12q-	14	20

BM = bone marrow; CMML = chronic myelomonocytic leukemia; FAB = French-American-British; MDS = myelodysplastic syndromes; PB = peripheral blood; RA = refractory anemia; RAEB = refractory anemia with excess blasts; RAEB-t = refractory anemia with excess blasts in transformation; RARS = refractory anemia with ringed sideroblasts the peripheral blood and bone marrow, the presence of ringed sideroblasts in the bone marrow, and the monocyte count in the peripheral blood (Table 1). The five subgroups are:

- refractory anemia (RA)
- refractory anemia with ringed sideroblasts (RARS)
- refractory anemia with excess blasts (RAEB)
- refractory anemia with excess blasts in transformation (RAEB-t)
- chronic myelomonocytic leukemia (CMML).

The presence of Auer rods in granulocyte precursors classifies a patient as having RAEB-t, even if blasts comprise < 20% of bone marrow cells. The presence of > 30% blast cells in the bone marrow or peripheral blood establishes the diagnosis of AML rather than MDS.

More recently, the WHO has proposed a modified classification of hematologic malignancies (Table 2). The following changes were proposed, based on the effect of cytogenetics and the number of dysplastic lineages on clinical behavior:

- The FAB classification of RAEB-t is eliminated.
- The blast percentage that defines AML is changed to ≥ 20%.
- RA and RARS are defined by dysplasia restricted to the erythroid lineage either with or without ringed sideroblasts, respectively.
- RA and single lineage dysplasias limited to the myeloid or megakaryocyte lineage are included in the category of refractory cytopenia with unit lineage dysplasia (RCUD).
- The presence of dysplasia in erythroid and nonerythroid lineages (multilineage dysplasia with or without ringed sideroblasts) and MDS with isolated deletion 5q are regarded as separate entities of MDS.
- RAEB is divided into two categories distinguished by marrow blast percentage (ie, RAEB-1: 5%–9%; RAEB-2: 10%–19%) or the presence of Auer rods (RAEB-2).
- Two new provisional categories were introduced in the 2008 proposal:

  (a) RARS with thrombocytosis (RARS-T), ie, ≥ 450,000 μL platelet count

  (b) MDS with minimal cytogenetic criteria, ie, absence of dysplasia in the presence of a clonal cytogenetic abnormality characteristic of MDS.
- CMML is included in a separate category of myelodysplastic/myeloproliferative neoplasms that also includes atypical CML and juvenile myelomonocytic leukemia. CMML is further classified into CMML-1 (≤ 9% blasts), CMML-2 (10%–19% blasts), and CMML-Eos (eosinophils ≥ 1,500 μL).

This proposal represents a step ahead, but there are some aspects that still need to be addressed. For example, some biologic features that have been associated with MDS, such as the presence of spontaneous apoptosis, increased angiogenesis, and pres-

TABLE 2: Criteria for myelodysplastic syndromes (MDS) according to the WHO classification

Disease	Blood findings	Bone marrow findings
Refractory anemia (RA); refractory neutropenia (RN); refractory thrombocytopenia (RT)	Unicytopenia or bicytopenia No or rare blasts	Unilineage dysplasia < 5% blasts < 15% ringed sideroblasts
Refractory anemia with ringed sideroblasts (RARS)	Anemia No blasts	Erythroid dysplasia only ≥ 15% ringed sideroblasts < 5% blasts
Refractory cytopenia with multilineage dysplasia (RCMD)	Cytopenia(s) No or rare blasts No Auer rods $< 1 \times 10^9$/L monocytes	Dysplasia in ≥ 10% of cells in 2 or more myeloid cell lines, including erythroids < 5% blasts in marrow No Auer rods < 15% ringed sideroblasts
Refractory anemia with excess blasts-1 (RAEB-1)	Cytopenias < 5% blasts No Auer rods $< 1 \times 10^9$/L monocytes	Unilineage or multilineage dysplasia 5%–9% blasts No Auer rods
Refractory anemia with excess blasts-2 (RAEB-2)	Cytopenias 5%–19% blasts Auer rods ± $< 1 \times 10^9$/L monocytes	Unilineage or multilineage dysplasia 10%–19% blasts Auer rods ±
MDS unclassified (MDS-U)	Cytopenias < 1% blasts	Unequivocal dysplasia in < 10% of cells in 1 or more cell lines when accompanied by a cytogenetic abnormality < 5% blasts
MDS associated with isolated del(5q)	Anemia Platelets normal or increased No or rare blasts	Normal to increased megakaryocytes with hypolobulated nuclei < 5% blasts Isolated del(5q) No Auer rods

WHO = World Health Organization

ence of specific mutations such as *TET2* or *RPS14* may define better specific subsets, and the WHO classification does not incorporate unfavorable cytogenetic patterns.

SIGNS AND SYMPTOMS

Nearly 50% of patients with MDS are asymptomatic at the time of initial diagnosis. Signs and symptoms relate to hematopoietic failure, leading to anemia, thrombocytopenia, or leukopenia.

Symptoms related to anemia

These may range from fatigue to exertional dyspnea that may exacerbate angina or cause congestive heart failure.

Infection

Approximately one-third of patients report recurrent localized or systemic infections as a result of granulocytopenia or dysfunctional granulocytes and monocytes.

Bleeding manifestations

Bleeding manifestations such as petechiae or gross hemorrhage, can occur with thrombocytopenia or platelet dysfunction. However, < 10% of patients present with serious bleeding.

Organomegaly and lymphadenopathy

Splenomegaly and/or hepatomegaly may be found in 5% to 25% of patients. A large spleen is more frequently seen in CMML.

Acute neutrophilic dermatosis (Sweet's syndrome) and pyoderma gangrenosum

These may be observed, particularly in patients with CMML or advanced MDS.

Paraneoplastic syndromes

Diabetes insipidus, vasculitis, and other rare paraneoplastic syndromes have been described in patients with MDS.

Laboratory features

Peripheral blood

Anemia is the most frequent abnormality in MDS, with > 80% of patients presenting with hemoglobin concentrations < 10 g/dL. The anemia is usually normocytic or macrocytic, but the mean corpuscular volume rarely exceeds 120 μm^3.

Other RBC abnormalities Hypochromic changes and red-shape abnormalities are frequent, including poikilocytosis, anisocytosis, elliptocytosis, macro-ovalocytosis, and sometimes stomatocytes. Stippled and nucleated RBCs can be observed in 10% of cases. Reticulocyte counts are usually reduced.

WBC abnormalities The peripheral WBC count may be normal or low in MDS but is frequently elevated in CMML. The proportion of monocytes may be increased, and a circulating monocyte count of $\geq 1 \times 10^9$/L defines CMML.

Neutropenia is seen in about 50% of patients with MDS at diagnosis, often associated with pseudo–Pelger-Huët anomaly (neutrophils have condensed chromatin and unilobed or bilobed nuclei with a pince-nez shape), ring-shaped nuclei, hypogranulation, and hypolobulation or other signs of dysgranulopoiesis.

Granulocytes frequently disclose reduced myeloperoxidase activity, increased α-naphthyl acetate esterase activity, and other functional abnormalities.

Chemotactic and bactericidal capability is impaired, which can potentiate the risk of infection, even in the presence of normal WBC counts.

Patients frequently have a decreased number of natural killer cells and helper T lymphocytes.

Platelet abnormalities Thrombocytopenia is present at diagnosis in approximately 30% of patients.

Platelets may be abnormally large; have poor granulation; or have large, fused central granules. Decreased platelet aggregation is observed when platelets of patients with MDS are challenged with collagen or epinephrine. Thrombocytosis may be seen in association with the 5q- syndrome and in those with RARS-t.

Bone marrow

Bone marrow aspiration and biopsy should be performed in every patient suspected of having MDS or unexplained persistent cytopenias. The bone marrow is normocellular or hypercellular in 85% to 90% of patients with MDS but may be hypocellular for the patients' age in as many as 10% to 15%.

Trilineage dyspoiesis The main morphologic feature of MDS is hematopoietic dyspoiesis, although myelodysplastic features do not always involve all three lineages. Cytologic dysplasia must be detected in ≥ 10% of the affected lineages.

Dyserythropoiesis Erythroblasts usually have a megaloblastoid appearance. Iron may be abnormally deposited in mitochondria and is easily stained with Prussian blue, producing a ring-shaped staining pattern around the nucleus. Pathologic sideroblasts have five or more granules/cell.

Dysgranulopoiesis The characteristic findings in dysgranulopoiesis are hypogranulation and hyposegmentation with nuclear morphologic abnormalities.

Excess bone marrow blasts Bone marrow blasts > 5% but < 30% are seen in 30% to 50% of patients with MDS; in the context of myelodysplasia, this finding is a feature of MDS.

The FAB group distinguishes three types of blasts on the basis of the maturation as assessed by morphology. Type I blasts have an uncondensed nuclear chromatin, one to three nucleoli, and basophilic cytoplasm without a Golgi zone. Cytoplasmic granules and Auer rods are absent. In type II blasts, the nuclear/cytoplasm ratio is lower than in type I blasts, and few primary granules are seen. Type III blasts have 20 or more azurophilic granules without a Golgi zone.

Dysmegakaryocytopoiesis At least 10 megakaryocytes should be evaluated. Micromegakaryocytes are small cells with a diameter two times smaller than the normal megakaryocyte (< 80 µm). Multiple, dispersed, small nuclei or mononucleated forms, as well as hypogranulated megakaryocytes, also can be found.

Other abnormalities An increase in reticulin and collagen fibers in the bone marrow may be seen in some patients.

Angiogenesis Increased marrow vascularity and increased levels of angiogenic cytokines such as vascular endothelial growth factor (VEGF) and basic fibroblast growth factor have been described in patients with MDS.

Other laboratory findings

Serum iron, transferrin, and ferritin levels may be elevated. As a result of ineffective hematopoiesis, lactate dehydrogenase (LDH) and uric acid concentrations are frequently increased. Monoclonal gammopathy, polyclonal hypergammaglobulinemia, and hypogammaglobulinemia are found occasionally but may be detected in up to 15% of patients with CMML.

Cytogenetic and molecular findings

Chromosomal abnormalities

Clonal cytogenetic abnormalities are found at diagnosis in 50% to 60% of patients with de novo MDS and 75% to 85% of those with secondary MDS or AML. An interesting feature that distinguishes MDS from AML is the high incidence of complete or partial chromosomal loss or, less frequently, chromosomal gain and the relative rarity of translocations. Among the translocations, unbalanced translocations leading to a loss of chromosomal material are most frequent.

Common cytogenetic abnormalities are listed in Table 1. None of them is specific for MDS, since all can be found in other myeloid disorders.

Some of the most frequent abnormalities are interstitial deletion of the long arm of chromosome 5 (5q-), monosomy of chromosome 7, trisomy of chromosome 8, 20q-, and loss of the Y chromosome. "Complex" cytogenetic abnormalities involving three or more chromosomes occur in approximately 15% of de novo MDS cases and 50% of secondary MDS cases.

Therapy-related MDS Loss of chromosome 7 and/or 7q- has been reported in as many as 50% of patients previously exposed to chemotherapy for other malignancies, most frequently in association with prolonged use of alkylating agents. Other abnormalities commonly associated with prior exposure to alkylating agents include -5 and/or del(5q) in 25% of cases and involvement of chromosomes 17p and 21 in 10% to 15%. Complex chromosomal abnormalities may be found in nearly 50% of patients.

Cytogenetics and FAB classification

RA and RARS Approximately 15% to 30% of patients with RA and RARS have abnormal karyotypes. The most frequent abnormality in patients with RA is 5q, whereas the most common abnormalities in patients with RARS are 5q-, +8, and 20q- (each occurring in 20% of patients).

RAEB and RAEB-t Nearly 60% of patients with RAEB and RAEB-t have cytogenetic abnormalities, with 5q-, -7, 7q-, and +8 being the most frequent.

CMML Chromosomal abnormalities are found in 25% to 30% of patients with CMML; the predominant abnormalities include -7, 7q-, +8, 12q-, and t(5;12). Interestingly, 5q- is seen in < 1 % of cases of CMML.

Monosomy of chromosome 7 is found in up to 25% of children with MDS, most frequently as an isolated abnormality. In contrast, older patients most often have monosomy of chromosome 7 associated with other chromosomal abnormalities.

5q- syndrome

The isolated interstitial deletion characteristic of the 5q- syndrome involves a variable segment length that includes a 1.5-megabase segment critical deleted region extending between bands 5q31 and 5q32, a region known to contain genes coding for numerous growth factors and receptors. However, the critical gene deletion involved in this syndrome may be a ribosomal protein processing gene, *RPS14*, haploinsufficiency of which limits erythroid differentiation and survival in laboratory models.

Clinical features The 5q- syndrome represents a subset of MDS with isolated chromosome 5q deletion that has characteristic clinical features, including older age, female predominance, diagnosis of RA without excess (< 5%) blasts in 75% of cases, macrocytosis with severe anemia, erythroblastopenia, normal leukocyte counts, normal or increased platelet counts, and hypolobulated megakaryocytes in the bone marrow.

Progression to AML is infrequent (< 20%), and the prognosis is usually good. However, not every patient with del(5q) has this syndrome and its associated good prognosis. Additional cytogenetic abnormalities or the presence of ≥ 5% blasts in the peripheral blood or bone marrow is inconsistent with this diagnosis.

Molecular findings

The *RAS* family and *TET2* genes are most frequently altered in MDS, although other abnormalities involving *NF1, CSF1R, TP53, ETV6, MECOM, AXL, TEC, HCK, c-MPL, RPS14,* and other genes have also been described. Recently, inactivating mutations of *TET2* were found in 20%–30% of MDS cases, which is believed to contribute to increased genomic methylation.

Mutations in *RAS* Mutations in the *RAS* family occur in approximately 20% to 40% of patients with MDS but are most frequently found in those with CMML. Mutations in *ras* are more common in codons 12, 13, and 61. Mutations in *NRAS* are more common than those in *KRAS* or *HRAS*.

A difference in the surface expression of phosphatidylserine (a marker of apoptosis) on cell membranes among de novo AML, MDS, and secondary AML and normal bone marrow cells has been found (increased in MDS and secondary AML). Epigenetic silencing of the *CDKN2B* tumor-suppressor gene by promoter hypermethylation occurs particularly among patients with high-risk MDS and is associated with a poor prognosis. *FLT3* mutations or internal tandem duplications are more rare in MDS (usually < 5%) than in AML.

STAGING AND PROGNOSIS

Prognostic factors

FAB and WHO classifications

The FAB classification has a long history of use to evaluate survival and risk for AML transformation (Table 1). The WHO classification has similar prognostic implications, based primarily upon the prognostic impact of blast percentage and the number of dysplastic lineages.

Cytogenetics

Patients with complex karyotypes and abnormalities in chromosome 7 have a poor prognosis, whereas those with a normal karyotype, -Y, 5q-, or 20q- have a favorable prognosis.

TABLE 3: International Prognostic Scoring System (IPSS) for MDS

Characteristic	Value	Score
Bone marrow blasts (%)	< 5	0
	5–10	0.5
	11–20	1.5
	21–30	2.0
Karyotype[a]	Good	0
	Intermediate	0.5
	Poor	1.0
Cytopenias	0–1	0
	2–3	0.5
Risk group	**Sum of score**	
Low	0	
Intermediate 1	0.5–1.0	
Intermediate 2	1.5–2.0	
High	≥ 2.5	

[a] Good = diploid, -Y, del(5q), del(20q); Poor = chromosome 7 abnormalities or complex (≥ 3) abnormalities; Intermediate = all others

Peripheral cytopenias

(hemoglobin level < 10 g/dL, absolute neutrophil count [ANC] < 1.8×10^9/L, and platelet count < 100×10^9/L) have a cumulative adverse effect on prognosis.

Other prognostic factors

Other parameters associated with a poor outcome include CD34 cell expression, high serum LDH, abnormal localized immature myeloid precursors, *RAS* mutations, severe thrombocytopenia, *CDKN2B* inactivation, *TP53* mutations, and extent of genomic methylation. However, it is unclear whether these factors have independent prognostic value.

International Prognostic Scoring System (IPSS)

An International MDS Risk Analysis Workshop has proposed a system that combines clinical, morphologic, and cytogenetic data to generate a consensus prognostic system.

By multivariate analysis, the most significant independent variables were percentage of bone marrow blasts, cytogenetics, and number of cytopenias (Table 3). It is important to keep in mind, however, that other variables (eg, age and prior therapy) not included in this system may alter the prognosis and influence the results of therapy among patients in similar IPSS groups. Still, this may be the most valuable risk classification for treatment planning.

Other scoring systems

The IPSS and WHO classifications have limitations in assessing the risk of patients with MDS: excess weight toward percentage of blasts, lack of discrimination of patients with lower-risk disease, and other clinical characteristics.

TABLE 4: Multivariate analysis parameters and assigned score for patients with low/int-1 disease

Adverse factor	Assigned score
Unfavorable cytogenetics[a]	1
Age ≥ 60 years	2
Hgb < 10 (g/dL)	1
Plt < 50 × 10^9 per L	2
50–200 × 10^9 per L	1
BM blasts ≥ 4%	1

BM = bone marrow; Hgb = hemoglobin; Plt = platelets

[a] In this analysis, diploid and 5q only were favorable cytogenetics, all others were considered as unfavorable cytogenetics.

Recently, several newer models have been developed to address these issues, such as the WHO classification-based prognostic scoring system and the M. D. Anderson low-risk model.

In one study, investigators found it possible to use the M. D. Anderson low-risk model to identify patients with lower-risk MDS and a poor prognosis who may benefit from early intervention (Tables 4 and 5). The implementation of this model may have significant implications for clinical trial design and eventually treatment decisions for patients with lower-risk MDS.

TREATMENT

The treatment of MDS is dictated by the risks imposed by the disease, age, and patient preference. Suggested guidelines are outlined in Table 6 and discussed later in this chapter.

TABLE 5: Estimated survival outcomes within each score range and proposed risk categories

Score	No. of patients	Median (month)	Four-year survival (%)
0	11	NR	78
1	58	83	82
2	113	51	51
3	185	36	40
4	223	22	27
5	166	14	9
6	86	16	7
7	13	9	NA

NA = not assessable; NR = not reached

Supportive care

The use of transfusions affords temporary benefits and is an alternative that can be considered in patients with lower-risk MDS or that otherwise can be used in conjunction with more definitive therapy. To delay or prevent end-organ complications, chelation therapy could be considered when RBC transfusions exceed 25 U or ferritin levels > 1,000 to 2,500 ng/mL. Recent reports suggest that the use of chelation or growth factors may be associated with improved survival but this needs confirmation in randomized clinical trials.

G-CSF and GM-CSF Granulocyte colony-stimulating factor (G-CSF, filgrastim, [Neupogen]) or granulocyte-macrophage colony-stimulating factor (GM-CSF) may improve neutropenia and decrease infections in up to 70% of patients with MDS, but the effect is usually transient. No increase in the probability of developing AML has been demonstrated with extended use of these cytokines.

Other alternatives

Antithymocyte globulin (ATG) has been associated with response (defined as independence from transfusions) in 34% of patients, which was sustained for a median of 36 months in 81% of them. Also, 48% had sustained platelet improvement and 55% had an increase in neutrophils. Younger patients are more likely to respond than older patients.

A simple method for predicting response to immunosuppressive therapy in MDS has been proposed. It is based on the age of the patient, the duration of RBC transfusion dependence, and the HLA (human lymphocyte antigen)-DR15 status. Younger patients with a shorter duration of transfusion requirements have a higher predicted probability of response (40% to 100%), particularly when their status is positive for HLA-DR15. A subsequent validation study showed that age < 60 years is the most powerful predictor for response to ATG.

Cyclosporine significantly increases cell–colony growth in laboratory studies of hypoplastic RA. Responses have been reported in a limited number of patients.

Lenalidomide Lenalidomide (Revlimid) is a thalidomide analog that belongs to the immunomodulatory family of drugs. Lenalidomide has numerous properties that make it attractive for the management of neoplastic and inflammatory conditions, including the inhibition of production of cytokines such as tumor necrosis factor-α (TNF-α), IL-1, IL-6, IL-10, and IL-12. Lenalidomide is markedly more potent than thalidomide (Thalomid) in inhibiting the secretion of TNF-α. In addition, lenalidomide may potentiate erythropoietin-induced signaling in erythroid progenitors and stimulate stem–cell differentiation to erythroid cells.

Lenalidomide has been approved for the treatment of patients with MDS with abnormalities in the long arm of chromosome 5 (5q- abnormalities), whether they are isolated or present together with other cytogenetic abnormalities. In a study of patients with transfusion-dependent MDS with 5q- abnormalities, 75% of patients responded, with 66% of the total population becoming transfusion independent. The response rate was similar regardless of whether the cytogenetic abnormality was isolated or seen in conjunction with other cytogenetic abnormalities, and more than half of the responses were durable for more than 1 year. In addition, a cytogenetic

TABLE 6: Suggested approach to the treatment of MDS

IPSS risk group	Treatment
Low, intermediate 1	Observation (particularly if mild cytopenia) Supportive care (transfusions, hematopoietic growth factors, iron chelation) Lenalidomide (for patients with 5q- abnormalities) Hypomethylating agents (azacitidine, decitabine) ATG for patients with hypoplastic MDS New (investigational) approaches, such as p38 MAPK, GST inhibitors, HDAC inhibitors
High, intermediate 2	Hypomethylating agents (azacitidine, decitabine) SCT (particularly for young patients with HLA-identical siblings; front-line vs in remission?) New (investigational) agents, such as topoisomerase inhibitors (topotecan, rubitecan), HDAC inhibitors, combination of hypomethylating agents and HDAC inhibitor clofarabine

ATG = antithymocyte globulin; HDAC = histone deacetylase; HLA = human lymphocyte antigen; IPSS = International Prognostic Scoring System; MDS = myelodysplastic syndromes; SCT = stem-cell transplantation

response was observed in 70% of patients. Lenalidomide has also been investigated for patients with MDS without 5q- abnormalities. Erythroid responses were seen in over 40%, with 27% of the total population becoming transfusion independent.

Azacitidine (Vidaza) and 5-Aza-2'-deoxycytidine (Dacogen, DAC, decitabine) are hypomethylating agents that have shown activity in MDS. In a randomized trial, 191 patients with MDS (63% RAEB or RAEB-t) were treated with azacitidine or supportive care. Responses were observed in 60% of those treated with azacitidine (complete response [CR]: 6%; partial response [PR]: 10%; hematologic improvement: 47%) compared with 5% with supportive care. There was a significant improvement in probability of transformation to AML and overall survival when the confounding effect of early crossover to azacitidine was eliminated.

Azacitidine is approved by the FDA for the treatment of patients with all types of MDS. The standard dose is 75 mg/m^2/d subcutaneously for 7 days every 4 weeks for as long as the patient benefits. Responses occur after a median of 3 to 4 cycles, so it is recommended to continue therapy for at least 4 to 6 cycles, unless there is significant toxicity or progression of disease. The dose may be increased to 100 mg/m^2/d after 2 cycles if no improvement has occurred. Myelosuppression may occur but is not a reason to discontinue therapy. Rather, patients should be supported during myelosuppression and should continue therapy to give them the best opportunity of response. In a post-approval phase III trial, treatment with azacitidine significantly improved survival by a median of 9 months (median survival, 25 months vs 15 months) compared with a conventional care arm that included supportive care, low-dose cytarabine, and conventional leukemia induction and consolidation therapy.

Decitabine is approved by the FDA for the treatment of patients with all types of MDS. In a multicenter phase II study, 66 patients (73% RAEB or RAEB-t) were treated with decitabine. The overall response rate was 49% (CR: 20%; PR: 4%; improvement: 24%). The actuarial median response duration was 31 weeks, and median survival

> **A** randomized phase III study of azacitidine, (n = 179) vs conventional care (n = 179); (supportive care, low-dose cytarabine or "7 + 3" induction chemotherapy) has been conducted. It demonstrated that treatment with azacitidine was associated with a significant improvement in overall survival (hazard ratio = 0.58; *P* = .0001), translating into a doubling of survival at 24 months. The median number of courses of azacitidine administered was 9 and the overall response rate was 78% *(Fenaux P et al: Lancet Oncol 10:223–232, 2009).*

was 22 months. In addition, 31% of patients with cytogenetic abnormalities presented before treatment achieved a cytogenetic response. Cytogenetic response conferred a survival advantage to these patients.

Recently, several studies combining decitabine or azacitidine with valproic acid (a histone deacetylase [HDAC] inhibitor) have shown success in MDS and AML but this needs to be demonstrated in randomized clinical trials.

Steroids, androgens, and pyridoxine are rarely effective, although they are often used clinically.

Chemotherapy

The rationale for this strategy stems from the concepts that MDS is a clonal disorder and that MDS and AML are overlapping illnesses with an arbitrary frontier defined by the WHO and FAB classifications (ie, a 20%–30% blast threshold).

The CALGB treated 874 patients with AML and 33 patients with MDS with AML-like chemotherapy. The CR rate was 79% for patients with MDS vs 68% for patients with AML (*P* = .37), median CR duration was 11 vs 15 months (*P* = .28), and median survival was 13 vs 16 months. The authors concluded that the FAB distinction between MDS (RAEB and RAEB-t) and AML has minimal therapeutic implications.

Estey et al treated 372 patients with AML, 52 with RAEB, and 106 with RAEB-t with AML-type chemotherapy. CR rates were 62% for patients with RAEB, 66% for those with RAEB-t, and 66% for those with AML (*P* = .79). Event-free survival was significantly better for patients with AML/RAEB-t than for patients with RAEB. However, when cytogenetics and other prognostic variables were considered in a multivariate analysis, no difference in outcome could be identified among FAB subgroups.

These findings suggest that the prognosis is determined more by cytogenetics and other prognostic features than by the percentage of blasts or FAB classification. However, this finding does not necessarily mean that MDS and AML are biologically equivalent entities.

Combination regimens Different combination chemotherapy regimens have been investigated. The combination of cytarabine (Ara-C) and anthracycline is the cornerstone of intensive chemotherapy, leading to CRs in 40% to 60% of patients. However, despite the fact that cytogenetic remissions frequently accompany hematologic CRs, the median remission duration and survival times are brief, rarely exceeding 1 year. The death rate during induction therapy is 5% to 20%.

Myeloblasts in RAEB-t and secondary AML commonly express the multidrug exporter Pgp, which extrudes anthracyclines and limits their activity. A randomized, controlled trial performed by the SWOG reported a twofold improvement in survival for patients treated with an anthracycline- and Ara-C–containing induction and consolidation regimens with the Pgp antagonist cyclosporine added. It is possible that certain chemotherapeutic agents may be particularly useful in MDS.

SCT

Allogeneic SCT can be of benefit in a subset of patients with MDS. However, most series have concentrated on younger patients, who constitute a minority of patients with MDS and frequently have favorable cytogenetics and therefore a better prognosis. The best results to date have been reported in patients with a better prognosis (ie, those with RA/RARS). In most series, allogeneic SCT is associated with a long-term remission rate of approximately 40%, a relapse rate of 30%, and a rate of transplant-related death of 30%.

The timing of transplantation remains controversial. Runde et al reported on a group of 131 patients (median age, 33 years; range: 2–55 years) who underwent allogeneic SCT as front-line therapy without prior induction chemotherapy. The 5-year disease-free survival rate was 34%, overall survival rate was 41%, and transplant-related mortality was 38%. The actuarial probability of relapse at 5 years was 39%, with better results observed in the RA/RARS subgroup.

Patients with adverse cytogenetics have a poor outcome with other treatment modalities, and SCT can be considered for such patients during first CR. However, the long-term outcome for these patients after SCT has not proved to be superior to that after any other approach, although the procedure may prove to be curative in a small percentage of patients. SCT should be considered particularly in the setting of a clinical trial.

New applications for allogeneic SCT (eg, nonmyeloablative) to make this option available to the typical patient with MDS (who is frequently older and has other associated medical problems), as well as for matched-unrelated donor SCT, should be investigated further.

Autologous SCT In the majority of patients with MDS, lymphocytes do not appear to be part of the clone, suggesting the presence of normal nonclonal stem cells. De Witte et al described 79 patients with MDS or secondary AML who underwent autologous SCT during first CR. The 2-year survival, disease-free survival, and relapse rates were 39%, 34%, and 64%, respectively. The 2-year survival rate for the MDS group was 40%, and treatment-related mortality was 9%. The best outcome was seen among patients with RA/RARS.

> Stem cell transplantation is a treatment option for some patients with MDS, although its timing remains controversial. An International Bone Marrow Transplant Registry analysis used a Markov model to examine three transplantation strategies for newly diagnosed MDS: transplantation at the time of diagnosis, transplantation at the time of progression to leukemia, and transplantation at an interval from diagnosis but prior to leukemic progression. Although transplantation at diagnosis may be superior for patients with intermediate-2 and high-risk IPSS scores, delayed transplantation was associated with improved life expectancy *(Cutler CS et al: Blood 104:579–585, 2004).*

Treatment recommendations

Treatment of patients with MDS is an evolving and controversial issue, and enrollment in a clinical trial should be encouraged. Treatment can be considered according to the IPSS.

Patients with low or intermediate-1 IPSS scores can frequently be treated with supportive measures. Agents such as ATG and cyclosporine could be used alone or in combination. Patients with 5q- benefit from lenalidomide, particularly in terms of erythroid response, and this should be considered the treatment of choice in these patients. Some patients with MDS without the 5q- abnormality may also benefit from lenalidomide, but its use in this setting is still being investigated. Azacitidine should be considered for all patients in view of its effect on survival. Decitabine is another possible option for patients with MDS, although a recent study did not reveal a survival benefit.

Patients with high or intermediate-2 IPSS scores have a significant risk of mortality from cytopenias or AML evolution. They should be considered for treatment options with the intention to cure, extend survival, or delay the progression of AML. In view of the survival effect of azacitidine, it should be considered as first-line therapy for patients with higher-risk disease. Preliminary results of a similar survival study with decitabine administered in the European 3-day schedule compared with best supportive care showed no survival benefit. Intensive chemotherapy did not appear to improve survival in an EORTC study.

SCT is an alternative for younger patients with higher-risk MDS and an HLA-identical donor, particularly patients with adverse cytogenetic abnormalities. However, the best results to date have been reported in patients with a better prognosis (ie, younger patients and those with RA/RARS). Therefore, allogeneic transplantation and other transplant alternatives should be considered preferentially in a research setting (eg, mixed-unrelated donor and minitransplants) or in patients who have failed to respond to other therapies.

SUGGESTED READING

Fenaux P, Mufti GJ, Hellstrom-Lindberg E, et al: Efficacy of azacitidine compared with that of conventional care regimens in the treatment of higher-risk myelodysplastic syndromes: A randomised, open-label, phase III study. Lancet Oncol 10:223–232, 2009.

Garcia-Manero G, Kantarjian HM, Sanchez-Gonzalez B, et al: Phase 1/2 study of the combination of 5-aza-2'-deoxycytidine with valproic acid in patients with leukemia. Blood 108:3271–3279, 2006.

Garcia-Manero G, Shan J, Faderl S, et al: A prognostic score for patients with lower risk myelodysplastic syndrome. Leukemia 22:538–543, 2008.

Garcia-Manero G, Yang H, Bueso-Ramos C, et al: Phase I study of the histone deacetylase inhibitor vorinostat (suberoylanilide hydroxamic acid, SAHA) in patients with advanced leukemias and myelodysplastic syndromes. Blood 111:1060–1066, 2007.

Greenberg P, Cox C, LeBeau MM, et al: International scoring system for evaluating prognosis in myelodysplastic syndromes. Blood 89:2079–2088, 1997.

Kantarjian H, Issa JP, Rosenfeld CS, et al: Decitabine improves patient outcomes in myelodysplastic syndromes: Results of a phase III randomized study. Cancer 106:1794–1803, 2006.

Kantarjian H, Oki Y, Garcia-Manero G, et al: Results of a randomized study of 3 schedules of low-dose decitabine in higher-risk myelodysplastic syndrome and chronic myelomonocytic leukemia. Blood 109:52–57, 2007.

List A, Dewald G, Bennett J, et al: Lenalidomide in the myelodysplastic syndrome with chromosome 5q deletion. N Engl J Med 355:1456–1465, 2006.

Malcovati L, Germing U, Kuendgen A, et al: Time-dependent prognostic scoring system for predicting survival and leukemic evolution in myelodysplastic syndromes. J Clin Oncol 25:3503–3510, 2007.

Rollison DE, Howlader N, Smith MT, et al: Epidemiology of myelodysplastic syndromes and chronic myeloproliferative disorders in the United States, 2001-2004, using data from the NAACCR and SEER programs. Blood 112:45–52, 2008.

Silverman LR, Demakos EP, Peterson BL, et al: Randomized controlled trial of azacitidine in patients with the myelodysplastic syndrome: A study of the cancer and leukemia group B. J Clin Oncol 20:2429–2440, 2002.

Soriano AO, Yang H, Faderl S, et al: Safety and clinical activity of the combination of 5-azacytidine, valproic acid, and all-trans retinoic acid in acute myeloid leukemia and myelodysplastic syndrome. Blood 110:2302–2308, 2007.

Steensma DP, Baer MR, Slack JL, et al: Preliminary results of a phase II study of decitabine administered daily for 5 days every 4 weeks to adults with myelodysplastic syndrome (MDS). Blood 110:1450, 2007.

WijerMans P, Suciu S, Baila L, et al: Low dose decitabine versus best supportive care in elderly patients with intermediate or high risk MDS not eligible for intensive chemotherapy: Final results of the randomized phase III study (06011) of the EORTC Leukemia and German MDS Study Groups. Blood 112:226, 2008.

Abbreviations in this chapter

CALGB = Cancer and Leukemia Group B; EORTC = European Organisation for Research and Treatment of Cancer; SWOG = Southwest Oncology Group; WHO = World Health Organization

CHAPTER 33

Hematopoietic cell transplantation

Stephen J. Forman, MD

Hematopoietic cell transplantation (HCT) is the IV infusion of hematopoietic stem and progenitor cells designed to establish marrow and immune function in patients with a variety of acquired and inherited malignant and nonmalignant disorders. These include hematologic malignancies (eg, leukemia, lymphoma, and myeloma), nonmalignant acquired bone marrow disorders (aplastic anemia), and genetic diseases associated with abnormal hematopoiesis and function (thalassemia, sickle cell anemia, and severe combined immunodeficiency). HCT also is used in the support of patients undergoing high-dose chemotherapy for the treatment of certain solid tumors for whom hematologic toxicity would otherwise limit drug administration (germ-cell, soft-tissue sarcomas, and neuroblastoma).

TYPES OF TRANSPLANTATION

Since the advent of HCT in the 1960s, several different methods of transplantation have evolved. At present, the hematopoietic cells used for HCT are obtained from either bone marrow or peripheral blood. The decision to use a certain type of HCT is dictated by the patient's age, disease and condition, and the availability of a donor. In some cases, more than one approach is possible. Table 1 summarizes the advantages and disadvantages of each stem-cell source.

Allogeneic BMT, match related

This method involves procurement of bone marrow from a human leukocyte antigen (HLA)-identical sibling of the patient. In some cases, a partially matched sibling or family donor (one antigen mismatch) can be used for bone marrow transplantation (BMT).

Allogeneic BMT, match unrelated

Given that there are a limited number of alleles of the HLA system, typing of large numbers of individuals has led to the observation that full molecular matches for patients exist in the general population. Tissue typing is performed on the patient's blood, and a search of the computer files of various international registries is made to determine whether a patient has a match with an unrelated individual.

TABLE 1: Stem cell sources for allogeneic BMT

Type	Advantages	Disadvantages
Allogeneic		
Sibling donor 10/10 HLA match or 9/10	Match able to be identified rapidly (2 weeks) Low rate of graft rejection (2%–5%)	GVHD (25%–40%) for non–T-cell-depleted marrow grafts Only 30% of patients will have sibling donor
Matched unrelated donor	Extends donor availability (60%–70% of patients will have potential match) Greater graft-versus-tumor effect	Takes time to find donor (6 weeks to > 6 months) Higher graft failure rates (5%–10%) Higher GVHD rates (50%–60%)
Umbilical cord donor	Lesser degrees of match can be used Much lower rate of GVHD (10%–20%) despite one and two antigen mismatches	Limited number of cells (reduced applicability to large recipient) Slower engraftment Higher rate of graft failure (10%) No chance for second infusion for graft failure or DLI for relapse
Haploidentical family donor	Almost all patients have a sibling, parent, or child who is haploidentical. These donors can be used if patients have relapsed or there is refractory disease and no better donor has been identified	Needs much more profound immunosuppression (T-cell depletion of donor product included) to achieve engraftment High risk of infectious complications Graft failure rate of 10%–15%
Syngeneic Identical twin	No need for immunosuppression No GVHD	No graft-versus-tumor effect

BMT = bone marrow transplantation; DLI = donor lymphocyte infusion; GVHD = graft-versus-host disease

Haploidentical transplantation

This technique usually involves the transplantation of large numbers of T-cell–depleted stem cells from a donor, usually a sibling or a parent, who is half matched to the patient. Although these are the most difficult transplantations to perform successfully, there is great interest in this approach, because most patients will have a donor in their family who is at least a 50% HLA match. Most transplants will engraft, and few patients will have significant graft-versus-host disease (GVHD). However, the relapse rate is high, and the process of immune reconstitution is slow, with patients often having troublesome infections for a long time after transplantation.

Autologous BMT

This form of transplantation is not utilized anymore, but entails the use of the patient's own bone marrow, which is harvested and then cryopreserved prior to administration of chemotherapy and/or high-dose radiation therapy. Following completion of therapy, the marrow cells are then thawed and reinfused into the patient to reestablish hematopoiesis.

Autologous peripheral blood stem-cell transplantation

With the recognition that the marrow stem cells circulate in the peripheral blood, methods have been devised to augment the number of these cells in the patient's circulation. The blood is then collected on a cell separator and frozen in a manner similar to that of autologous marrow, to be used after high-dose chemotherapy and/or radiation therapy. This is now the most common source of stem cells used in the autologous setting.

Syngeneic transplantation

In this form of transplantation, marrow or peripheral blood stem cells are procured from an individual who is a genetic identical twin to the patient.

Donor leukocyte infusion

This method involves the infusion of mononuclear cells from the marrow donor into the recipient to treat relapse after transplantation. The cells can mediate an antitumor effect, known as a graft-versus-tumor effect (often in association with concomitant GVHD), and can achieve remission of the malignancy.

Nonmyeloablative or reduced-intensity transplantation

This approach uses lower doses of chemotherapy, with or without total-body irradiation (TBI) and immunosuppression, to facilitate engraftment of donor stem cells. Donor stem cells obtained from either the peripheral blood or marrow are then infused into the patient, leading to hematopoietic engraftment. The major therapeutic effect that results from this type of transplantation is a graft-versus-tumor effect, as the nonmyeloablative regimen has limited long-term antitumor efficacy. Some disorders, such as chronic myelogenous leukemia (CML), acute myelogenous leukemia (AML), low-grade lymphoma, and multiple myeloma, are particularly sensitive to this approach. This type of transplant allows older patients to undergo the procedure, as transplant-related mortality is greatly reduced with this approach.

Cord blood transplantation

The blood in the umbilical cord of newborn babies contains large numbers of stem cells, which have been shown to be capable of long-term engraftment in children and some adults after transplantation. Similar to unrelated-donor registries, cord blood banks have been developed to store cord blood cells that can be used for unrelated-donor transplantation. Given the immunologic immaturity of cord blood cells, these transplants can be accomplished even when there are disparities (mismatching) in the HLA typing between the donor and recipient. Cord blood transplants are generally used in situations where the patient does not have a sibling donor and an unrelated adult donor cannot be identified through the international registries.

ALLOGENEIC TRANSPLANTATION

HLA typing

Finding a related donor

As noted previously, matched related allogeneic BMT involves a donor who is an HLA-matched sibling of the recipient. The formula for calculating the chances of a particular person having an HLA-matched sibling is $1 - (0.75)^N$, where N denotes the number of potential sibling donors. In general, a patient with one sibling has a 25% chance of having a match. The average American family size usually limits the success of finding a family donor to approximately 30% of patients.

HLA typing is performed on blood samples or from buccal smears obtained from the patient and potential donor. Molecular methods are now used for more refined matching of both class I and class II antigens. A match is noted when the major class I antigens (A and B loci), as well as class II antigens (DR), are the same as those of the donor. Each sibling receives one set of antigens (A, B, DR) from each parent (chromosome 6). Genotypic identity can be confirmed by testing the parents and determining the inheritance of each set of antigens.

Finding an unrelated donor

In cases in which the patient needs an allogeneic transplant and a donor cannot be found within the family, the identification of a matched-unrelated donor is accomplished by searching the computer files of the National Marrow Donor Program, as well as other international registries. As there are multiple alleles of any given HLA locus, serologic identity does not necessarily imply genotypic identity, such as is the case among sibling donor-recipient pairs. The development of oligonucleotide probes has greatly increased the precision of HLA typing and has allowed for more specific selection of bone marrow donors by matching molecular alleles of the class I and II antigens.

Advantages and disadvantages

The major advantages of an allogeneic graft include the absence of malignant cells contaminating the graft; the potential for an immunologic anticancer graft-versus-tumor effect; and the ability to treat malignant and nonmalignant disorders of the bone marrow, including genetic and immunologic diseases.

The disadvantages of an allogeneic transplant include the difficulty in finding an appropriate HLA-matched donor and the development of GVHD after HCT, which contributes to the morbidity and mortality of the procedure.

Reduced-intensity transplantation has allowed older patients up to age 70 to undergo this type of transplant to treat their disease when clinically indicated.

AUTOLOGOUS TRANSPLANTATION

Advantages and disadvantages

In autologous transplantation, the reinfused stem cells come from either the patient's own bone marrow or peripheral blood. These cells do not cause GVHD, and, thus,

TABLE 2: Comparison of allogeneic versus autologous stem cell transplantation

Allogeneic	
Advantages	
No tumor contamination of the graft and no prior marrow injury from chemotherapy (less risk of later myelodysplasia)	
Graft vs tumor effect	
Can be used for patients with marrow involvement by tumor or with bone marrow dysfunction, such as aplastic anemia, hemoglobinopathies, or prior pelvic irradiation	
Disadvantages	
Dose-intensive regimen limited by toxicity (usually limited to patients < age 55)	
Time needed to identify donor if no sibling donor available/limited availability of donor for some ethnic groups	
Higher early treatment-related mortality from GVHD and infectious complications (20%–40% depending upon age and donor source)	
Autologous	
Advantages	
No need to identify donor if peripheral blood marrow is uninvolved by tumor at the time of collection	
No immunosuppression = less risk of infections	
No GVHD	
Dose-intensive therapy can be used for older patients (usually up to age 70)	
Low early treatment-related mortality (2%–5%)	
Disadvantages	
Not feasible if peripheral blood stem cells/marrow involved	
Possible marrow injury leading to late myelodysplasia (either from prior chemotherapy or transplant regimen)	
No graft-versus-tumor effect	
Not all patients can be mobilized to give adequate cell doses for reconstitution	

GVHD = graft-versus-host disease

autologous transplantation is associated with less morbidity and mortality than is allogeneic BMT and increases in the number of patients who can undergo the procedure and in the upper age limit.

The disadvantages of autologous BMT include the likelihood of tumor cell contamination within the graft in many diseases, which can cause relapse; the lack of a significant therapeutic graft-versus-tumor effect; and the limited ability to use autologous stem cells to treat patients not in remission or with inherited nonmalignant lymphohematopoietic diseases. Table 2 summarizes the advantages and disadvantages of these two approaches.

MODIFICATIONS OF THE STEM CELL GRAFT

The disadvantages of both allogeneic and autologous transplantations have led to the modifications of the stem cell graft.

Removing T cells from donor marrow

With regard to allogeneic BMT, contaminating T cells from the donor mediate the onset and persistence of acute and chronic GVHD. T cells have been removed from the donor marrow to prevent the development of severe GVHD. However, this approach has increased the incidence of both graft rejection and relapse of malignancy. Some investigators are exploring planned return of donor T cells after hematopoietic recovery to help prevent relapse and to improve immunologic recovery.

Primed peripheral blood stem cells

Primed peripheral blood stem cells from marrow donors have reduced transplant-related complications by faster recovery of hematopoiesis without substantially increasing the incidence of acute GVHD. Thus far, data show that this approach induces more rapid engraftment. Most studies have reported an increase in chronic GVHD.

Eliminating tumor cells from autologous grafts

Although autologous peripheral blood stem cell transplantation has led to more rapid restoration of hematopoiesis, it is associated with a higher relapse rate than is allogeneic BMT. Attempts to deplete the autologous graft of tumor cells have included in vivo purging with chemotherapy and monoclonal antibodies, in vitro purging with monoclonal antibodies, and the enrichment of stem cells over various separation columns.

Post-transplantation immunomodulation

For patients undergoing autologous transplantation, several post-transplantation immunomodulating strategies, such as administration of rituximab (Rituxan) after autologous transplantation for B-cell lymphoma, are being tested to determine whether they will decrease relapse by augmenting immunologic antitumor responses following transplantation. In some diseases, such as myeloma, post-transplant treatment with medication such as dexamethasone and thalidomide (Thalomid) or lenalidomide (Revlimid) helps in prolonging remission.

Although busulfan-based regimens are most commonly used worldwide for allogeneic transplantation, the oral administration of busulfan leads to unpredictable absorption, which has been correlated with relapse (low absorption) and increased toxicity (increased absorption). Studies with an IV formulation of the drug have shown much more predictable pharmacokinetics, less toxicity, and good survival when used in the transplantation regimen.

COLLECTION OF THE GRAFT

Allogeneic bone marrow cells

Current techniques for harvesting bone marrow involve repeated aspirations from the posterior iliac crests that are designed to obtain adequate numbers of cells that can lead to hematopoiesis. While the donor is under general or spinal anesthesia, between 1 × 10^8 cells/kg to 3 × 10^8 cells/kg of the recipient's body weight are procured. The procedure has no long-term side effects and poses little risk if care is taken to ensure that the donor has no confounding medical conditions. In most cases of ABO incompatibility, the marrow can be treated to remove RBCs to prevent lysis after infusion.

Autologous peripheral stem cells

Collection of circulating peripheral blood progenitor cells is performed via an apheresis technique. Although this procedure can be accomplished in an individual with a baseline blood count, the number of cells and the efficiency of collection are increased if the cells are procured during WBC recovery following chemotherapy or after the administration of hematopoietic growth factors.

The most effective strategy appears to be the collection of cells after the administration of both chemotherapy and growth factors. In most circumstances, adequate numbers of cells can be collected using granulocyte colony-stimulating factor (G-CSF, filgrastim [Neupogen]) to prime the patient prior to one to three apheresis procedures. In particular, in patients for whom this is not successful, the use of plerixafor (Mozobil) may be effective.

Currently, the adequacy of the number of hematopoietic stem cells is assessed by determining the number of cells that have the CD34 antigen (stem cell) marker. Usually, a minimum of 2 × 10^6 CD34 cells/kg of body weight is required to ensure engraftment.

The use of autologous stem cells continues to undergo refinement. Approaches under study include ex vivo expansion to augment the number of progenitor cells, as well as techniques that separate hematopoietic cells from any potential contaminating tumor cells. In addition, hematopoietic stem cells are the usual targets of marrow-based gene therapy using viral vectors for transduction of cells prior to cryopreservation.

INDICATIONS FOR TRANSPLANTATION

The expanded methods of stem cell transplantation have complicated transplantation choices for patients and their physicians. Therefore, the decision requires evaluation of the patient and the disease involved. In general, for disorders that require replacement of an abnormally functioning hematopoietic system, such as thalassemia and aplastic anemia, an allogeneic transplantation is performed. However, as genetic therapy for hematopoietic stem cells becomes more of a reality, even patients with these diseases may be candidates for autologous transplantation after gene modification (adenosine deaminase deficiency, chronic granulomatous disease).

Hematologic malignancies

The most common use of allogeneic BMT has been for the eradication of hematologic malignancies, such as leukemia and non-Hodgkin lymphoma. For some disorders (eg, aplastic anemia, myelodysplasia, leukemia in relapse, CML), allogeneic transplantation is the only significant therapeutic option, whereas for other diseases (eg, AML in remission, lymphoma, Hodgkin lymphoma, multiple myeloma), either autologous or allogeneic marrow grafting may be possible.

TABLE 3: Disease sensitivity to a graft-versus-malignancy effect

Most sensitive	
Chronic myelogenous leukemia	
Low-grade lymphoma	
Mantle cell lymphoma	
Chronic lymphocytic leukemia	
Intermediately sensitive	
Acute myelogenous leukemia	
Hodgkin lymphoma	
Intermediate-grade lymphoma	
Multiple myeloma	
Least sensitive	
Acute lymphoblastic leukemia	
High-grade lymphoma	
Renal cell carcinoma	

The worldwide study of nonmyeloablative or reduced-intensity transplantation approaches has facilitated transplantation for many people who otherwise would not have been candidates due to concomitant medical problems or older age. The results indicate that slower-growing malignancies are the most responsive. Thus, patients with low-grade lymphoma, AML, myeloma, myelodysplasia, and CML are probably good candidates for this type of allogeneic transplantation, whereas those with advanced disease (eg, leukemia in relapse, high-grade lymphoma) benefit less, as the allogeneic antitumor effect requires time to develop and achieve remission of the disease. Table 3 shows the relative sensitivity of different hematologic malignancies to a graft-versus-malignancy effect that could be mediated by a nonmyeloablative transplant.

Solid tumors

In general, only autologous transplantation is used for some solid tumors, such as germ-cell, soft-tissue sarcomas, and neuroblastoma. Allogeneic transplant studies in patients with renal cell cancer suggest that a graft-versus-tumor effect can be elicited against this tumor, but the results are inconsistent.

TIMING OF TRANSPLANTATION

The Goldie-Coldman model proposes that the probability that a tumor contains treatment-resistant cells is a function of its size and inherent mutation rate. This finding suggests that the likelihood of cure is greatest when marrow transplantation is performed early in the natural history of an inherently chemosensitive tumor. Studies to date indicate that patients undergoing transplantation late in their disease course have inferior disease-free survival when compared with those who undergo transplantation early.

PHASES OF TRANSPLANTATION

Preparative phase

In the first phase of marrow transplantation, the preparative phase, patients receive high-dose chemotherapy and/or radiation therapy (sometimes referred to as a conditioning regimen).

Allogeneic transplantation

The conditioning regimen used in the allogeneic setting has both a therapeutic component designed to eliminate tumor cells and an immunosuppressive component to prevent host immune responses from rejecting the transplanted donor graft. The doses of radiation therapy and chemotherapy employed take advantage of the steep dose-response curve that exists for many malignancies. These doses have been established based on the limitations of other nonhematopoietic organs, such as the liver and lungs.

Typically, preparative regimens for full allogeneic BMT consist of TBI and/or chemotherapeutic agents (cyclophosphamide, busulfan [Busulfex, Myleran], and etoposide). The most commonly used regimens are (1) TBI (1,200–1,400 cGy administered in multiple fractions over a period of days) and cyclophosphamide (60 mg/kg for 2 days); (2) fractionated TBI and etoposide (60 mg/kg); and (3) busulfan (16 mg/kg over 4 days) and cyclophosphamide (60 mg/kg for 2 days).

Reduced Intensity Allogeneic Transplantation

This type of transplant is utilized primarily for patients who are older or who have comorbid conditions that might increase the risk of a fully ablative transplant. The most common regimens utilize fludarabine combined with either melphalan or busulfan or with a single fraction of TBI, followed by infusion of either donor bone marrow or peripheral blood-derived stem cells. All patients still require post-transplant immunosuppression similar to all other patients undergoing non–T-cell-depleted transplants. For patients receiving either a matched sibling or fully matched unrelated transplant, the engraftment of donor cells after reduced-intensity transplant is usually 100% by day 30–60 after transplant, and the immunosuppressive medications are tapered over a few months. Although the chemotherapy does have antitumor activity in this type of transplant, the major factor in eliminating the malignancy is the donor immune system, and is, as in the fully ablative transplant setting, influenced by the presence or absence of GVHD.

Autologous transplantation

For patients undergoing autologous transplantation, stem cells are reinfused following high-dose therapy to reestablish hematopoiesis as rapidly as possible. The regimens used for autologous BMT depend upon the disease being treated. High-dose melphalan (Alkeran; 200 mg/m^2) is the most commonly used regimen for myeloma, and BEAM (BiCNU [carmustine], etoposide, cytarabine [Ara-C], and melphalan) or CBV (cyclophosphamide, BiCNU [carmustine], and etoposide [VePesid]) are the two most commonly used regimens for lymphoma. Recent trials have incorporated radioimmunotherapy into the high-dose chemotherapy regimens in the treatment

TABLE 4: Acute and long-term toxicities of common preparative agents used for HCT

Agent	Acute toxicity	Long-term toxicity
Total-body irradiation	Nausea, vomiting, enteritis, mucositis	Cataracts, sterility, pneumonitis, myelodysplasia
Cyclophosphamide	Nausea, vomiting, hemorrhagic cystitis, cardiac toxicity	Sterility, leukemia
Etoposide	Skin rash, hypotension, acidosis, mucositis	Leukemia
Carmustine	Seizures, nausea, vomiting, headaches	Interstitial pneumonitis
Busulfan	Seizures, nausea, vomiting, veno-occlusive disease	Alopecia, pulmonary fibrosis
Cisplatin	Renal impairment, hearing loss, tinnitus	Hearing loss, tinnitus, neuropathy
Thiotepa	Nausea, vomiting, CNS changes, veno-occlusive disease	—
Paclitaxel	Allergic reactions	Neuropathy
Fludarabine	Hemolytic anemia, CNS changes	Prolonged immune suppression, EBV related lympho-proliferative disorder
Melphalan	Nausea, pulmonary toxicity	Peripheral neuropathy

BMT = bone marrow transplantation; CNS = central nervous system; EBV = Epstein-Barr virus

of B-cell lymphoma (Bexxar, Zevalin), with promising results especially in the treatment of recurrent large B-cell lymphoma.

Toxicities of preparative regimens

The acute toxicities of irradiation and chemotherapy include nausea and vomiting, which can be managed by prophylactic use of antiemetics, particularly serotonin antagonists. Busulfan can cause seizures; prophylactic phenytoin is effective in preventing this complication. Both cyclophosphamide and etoposide require forced hydration to reduce toxicities. Table 4 lists the acute and long-term toxicities of the major agents used in BMT preparative regimens.

Transplant phase

After completion of the preparative regimen, there is a day or more wait before reinfusion of marrow or peripheral blood stem cells. This delay allows for elimination of any active drug metabolites so that the reinfused cells are not injured by any remaining drug.

Minimal toxicities are associated with the infusion. They include headache, nausea, and dizziness. This dizziness is related more to the cryoprotectant dimethyl sulfoxide used to store cells from most patients undergoing autologous transplantation than to the infusion.

SUPPORTIVE CARE PHASE

Following administration of the preparative regimen and during and after marrow transplantation, all patients require strict attention to infectious disease–related complications secondary to neutropenia. The duration of neutropenia following transplantation increases the risk of complicating infections. Patients undergoing full allogeneic transplantation usually require more stringent isolation, whereas patients undergoing autologous transplantation need less rigorous protection. With the availability of more effective antiemetics (eg, ondansetron [Zofran], granisetron [Kytril]), portions of the transplantation can now be performed in the outpatient setting.

Following allogeneic transplantation, various complications may develop that require treatment. For some complications, prophylactic measures can be instituted to prevent their occurrence.

Neutropenic sepsis

Nearly all patients undergoing transplantation will develop fever, often with positive blood cultures, within 7 days of becoming neutropenic. Sepsis usually is caused by enteric bacteria or those found on the skin, and antibiotic choices are based on initial assessment and the results of blood cultures. The antibiotics chosen are continued until the neutrophil count begins to rise (> 500 k/μL).

Prevention of fungal infections For patients who are expected to have prolonged neutropenia, various methods of antifungal prophylaxis are used, including PO fluconazole (Diflucan; 200 mg bid) or voriconazole (Vfend; 200 mg IV or PO bid). The use of liposomal amphotericin B (AmBisome, Abelcet) or caspofungin (Cancidas) formulations has improved the safety and lowered the toxicity of antifungal therapy and is particularly worthwhile in patients with renal compromise.

Mucositis, nausea, and anorexia

Regimen-related toxicity often results in severe oral mucositis, nausea, and anorexia. Patients often require supplemental parenteral nutrition to maintain adequate caloric intake during this period. Because of the mucositis, enteral feedings are usually not employed, and total parenteral nutrition is maintained until patients are able to eat. Studies are exploring novel agents that could prevent severe mucositis or accelerate healing with recombinant keratinocyte growth factor (palifermin), which has been shown to decrease this complication following TBI-based autologous transplant regimens.

Oral herpes simplex virus (HSV) reactivation

Nearly all patients who are seropositive for HSV will have a reactivation of the virus, which can accentuate the pain and oral discomfort following BMT. To prevent this problem, most transplant programs use acyclovir at a dose of 250 mg/m^2 tid during the neutropenic phase.

TABLE 5: Clinical classification of acute GVHD according to organ injury

Stage key	0	1	2	3	4
Skin	No rash	Maculopapular rash, less than 25% of body surface	Maculopapular rash, 25%–50% of body surface	Rash on greater than 50% of body surface or generalized erythroderma	Generalized or erythroderma with bullous formation and/or desquamation
Lower GI (diarrhea)	≤ 500 mL/d or < 280 mL/m^2	> 500 but ≤ 1,000 mL/d or 280–555 mL/m^2	> 1,000 but ≤ 1,500 mL/d or 556–833 mL/m^2	> 1,500 mL/d or > 833 mL/m^2	Severe abdominal pain with or without ileus or stool with frank blood or melena
Upper GI	No protracted nausea and vomiting	Persistent nausea, vomiting, or anorexia plus biopsy showing GVHD of the stomach or duodenum			
Liver (total bilirubin)	< 2.0 mg/dL	2.0–3.0 mg/dL	3.1–6.0 mg/dL	6.1–15.0 mg/dL	> 15 mg/dL

Overall clinical grading of severity of acute GVHD–1994 Keystone Consensus Criteria

Grade	Skin		Liver		Gut		KPS
I	1–2	&	0	&	0		
II	3	or	1	or	1		
III	0–4	or	2–3	or	2–4		
IV	4	or	4	or	0–4	or	KPS score ≤ 30 or decrease ≥ 40% from baseline KPS score

GI = gastrointestinal; GVHD = graft-versus-host disease; KPS = Karnofsky Performance Status scale

Transfusion

All patients will require both RBCs and platelets in proportion to the duration of the pancytopenia. Platelet levels are kept over 10,000 to 20,000/μL because of complicating bleeding from mucositis, although, in some instances, a lower threshold is feasible. Patients no longer receive granulocyte transfusions unless they have uncontrolled sepsis with positive blood cultures. For patients who are negative for cytomegalovirus (CMV) and who have a CMV-negative donor, CMV-negative cell support is generally provided (see "CMV infection" section).

All blood products are irradiated to prevent engraftment of lymphoid cells and are often filtered to reduce CMV or alloimmunization and febrile reactions. Most patients receive single-donor platelet pheresis products, which may need to be HLA-matched if patients show evidence of refractoriness to the transfusion (ie, if platelet levels fail to rise after transfusion).

Sinusoidal obstruction syndrome (veno-occlusive disease)

In the first few weeks after BMT, sinusoidal obstruction syndrome, characterized by hepatomegaly, jaundice, and fluid retention, develops in 5% to 20% of patients. It is caused by damaged endothelial cells, sinusoids, and hepatocytes and is related to the intensity of the cytoreductive therapeutic regimen.

The diagnosis of sinusoidal obstruction syndrome is usually made on clinical grounds, based on the occurrence (usually within 8 to 10 days after starting the cytoreductive regimen) of the triad of hepatomegaly, weight gain, and jaundice. Patients also exhibit renal sodium retention, and the prognosis is related to the degree of liver and kidney dysfunction and the level of bilirubin. The use of regimens that contain busulfan has been associated with the highest incidence of veno-occlusive disease, which has decreased with targeted oral or IV busulfan dosing.

Treatment Once veno-occlusive disease has occurred, treatment is primarily supportive, consisting of careful management of fluid overload, kidney dysfunction, and other attendant complications. In a few cases, the early use of thrombolytic agents can reverse established veno-occlusive disease. Based on early phase II studies, defibrotide is now being tested in phase III trials as an agent that can help reverse the syndrome.

Acute GVHD

GVHD is a clinical syndrome that results from the infusion of immunocompetent lymphocytes accompanying the marrow graft that are capable of recognizing minor HLA-related antigens in the host and initiating an immunologic reaction. This syndrome may arise after allogeneic transplantation or rarely after transfusion of cellular blood products in patients who are immunodeficient and share HLA loci that allow engraftment of transfused cells. For unknown reasons, the primary organs affected by acute GVHD are the skin, liver, and GI tract.

The syndrome usually occurs within 15 to 60 days after transplantation and can vary in severity. Table 5 shows a commonly used grading system for GVHD. This system has both therapeutic and prognostic importance.

Prophylaxis All patients undergoing non–T-cell-depleted transplantation require some form of GVHD prophylaxis. The most common regimens involve a combination of methotrexate and cyclosporine or tacrolimus [Prograf]. The combination of tacrolimus and sirolimus (Rapamune) has been studied and appears to be an effective approach for the prevention of GVHD. These medications, in the absence of GVHD, are tapered over 6 to 12 months after BMT. The regimens of sirolimus and tacrolimus are tapered in a similar manner. Side effects of tacrolimus and cyclosporine include renal toxicity, hypertension, magnesium wasting, seizures, and microangiopathy. Sirolimus, an oral agent, can cause hemolytic uremic syndrome in association with tacrolimus and requires careful dose and drug level monitoring. It can also raise blood triglyceride levels.

Treatment Despite prophylaxis, many allogeneic transplant recipients still develop some degree of GVHD and require increasing doses of prednisone (1–2 mg/kg/d). For patients who do not respond to steroids, antithymocyte globulin (Atgam; 10 mg/kg/d for 5–10 days) has been used. Daclizumab (Zenapax; 1 mg/kg on days 1, 4, 8, 15, and 22), pentostatin (Nipent), and etanercept (Enbrel), or mycophenolate mofetil (CellCept) likely are more effective agents than antithymocyte globulin. Studies are being conducted to determine whether the addition of CellCept to prednisone will improve the response rate of initial treatment of acute GVHD.

Chronic GVHD

Chronic GVHD may occur within 3 to 6 months in patients who have undergone allogeneic HCT. It is often preceded by acute GVHD that may or may not have resolved. Although chronic GVHD is also related to infusion of T cells with the graft, it resembles other autoimmune connective tissue diseases, such as scleroderma, Sjögren syndrome, biliary cirrhosis, and bronchiolitis obliterans. Patients with chronic GVHD often have accompanying cytopenias and immune deficiency as well as abnormalities of the oral mucosa, conjunctiva, and gastrointestinal tract.

Treatment Chronic GVHD is generally treated with prolonged courses of steroids, cyclosporine, tacrolimus, and, occasionally, azathioprine and other modalities, such as psoralen-ultraviolet A light for skin and mouth GVHD. Thalidomide, mycophenolate mofetil, sirolimus, and photopheresis have also been employed, with varying response rates. Like that for acute GVHD, the prognosis for chronic GVHD is related to the extent of organ compromise and response to treatment.

GVHD and relapse Although, in general, GVHD has contributed to significant morbidity and mortality in patients undergoing allogeneic BMT, it is also associated with reduced relapse rates, primarily in patients with hematologic malignancies.

Late infections

Late infections after BMT are caused by impaired cellular and humoral immunity. The most common late pathogens include *Pneumocystis carinii*, varicella zoster, and encapsulated bacteria.

***P carinii* prophylaxis** All patients undergoing allogeneic transplantation require prophylaxis against *P carinii* infection. This can be accomplished with one double-strength trimethoprim-sulfamethoxazole tablet bid twice a week once hematopoiesis has been restored. Alternatively, atovaquone (Mepron; 750 mg bid) has been used.

Treatment of herpes zoster Approximately 40% of patients will develop herpes zoster infection (either dermatomal or disseminated), which is often treated with oral or IV acyclovir. A patient may complain of severe localized pain for several days before the rash develops. The use of valacyclovir (Valtrex) for 1 year after BMT can reduce or delay the risk of reactivation of herpes zoster after allogeneic BMT.

Bacterial prophylaxis Many patients with chronic GVHD develop an accompanying severe immunodeficiency syndrome that leaves them susceptible to infection with encapsulated bacteria, primarily in the sinuses and lungs. In some cases, prolonged prophylaxis with trimethoprim-sulfamethoxazole or penicillin is necessary, as well as immunoglobulin (Ig) replacement.

CMV infection

Historically, CMV interstitial pneumonia has been responsible for approximately 15% to 20% of patient deaths following allogeneic BMT. CMV pneumonia occurs 7 to 10 weeks after BMT and is due to reactivation of latent CMV or is acquired from donor marrow or transfusions. Active CMV infection, GVHD, and the inability to develop a virus-specific immune response that limits viral infection are risk factors for CMV pneumonia.

Diagnosis Infection is diagnosed by the combination of an abnormal chest x-ray, hypoxemia, and the detection of CMV in bronchoalveolar lavage or lung biopsy specimens, as well as the absence of other pathogens.

Treatment The only consistent treatment has been the combination of ganciclovir, 5 mg/kg bid for 3 weeks, and IV Ig, given every other day. Although the reason for the synergy between these agents is unclear, neither one alone is effective in reversing pneumonia once it has developed.

Prevention in CMV-seronegative patients The most successful means of preventing CMV infection in CMV-seronegative patients who have a seronegative donor is to limit their exposure to the virus by providing CMV-negative blood and platelet support. As most patients who undergo marrow transplantation are CMV-seropositive, this strategy has limited application. However, the presence of leukocytes in blood products increases the transmission of CMV. Thus, the use of CMV-seronegative blood products in CMV-seronegative recipients decreases the incidence of primary CMV infection. Also, CMV status should be determined in all patients prior to BMT to plan for post-transplantation transfusion strategies.

Prevention in CMV-seropositive patients The most effective strategy for preventing reactivation of CMV infection in patients who are CMV-seropositive is the preemptive use of ganciclovir, either prophylactically in all CMV-seropositive patients or more commonly at the first sign of CMV after transplantation (as indicated by blood culture, shell viral culture, or antigen or polymerase chain reaction detection of the virus). The duration of prophylaxis is somewhat controversial for CMV, but is usually for at least 2 weeks after the CMV polymerase chain reaction becomes negative.

Ganciclovir has been the most effective agent for both strategies, as it significantly reduces both viral reactivation and associated disease. However, if one waits until after viral reactivation to initiate ganciclovir therapy, there are a subset of patients who will not benefit from a prophylactic strategy, namely those in whom reactivation occurs simultaneously with disease. Ganciclovir has many side effects, including neutropenia and elevated creatinine levels, and thus exposes a large number of patients to potential toxicity. For those patients with ganciclovir-induced cytopenia or resistant virus, foscarnet (Foscavir) is utilized with careful attention to renal function.

The required duration of ganciclovir treatment is also unclear, but it appears that several weeks is necessary to protect the patient from viral reactivation and the development of pneumonitis within the first 3 months after BMT. Monitoring of all patients for CMV infection after completion of antiviral therapy is necessary, as some patients, particularly those with GVHD, or who have undergone cord blood or T-cell–depleted transplant, are at risk for infection due to an inadequate immune response against CMV. Some patients have developed late CMV pneumonia after drug discontinuation, which is probably related to ganciclovir inhibition of the development of CMV-specific cytolytic T cells. Nevertheless, the use of ganciclovir has reduced the problems related to CMV pneumonia and should be a part of every management strategy for preventing complications following allogeneic transplantation. Currently, newer antiviral drugs such as maribavir are being tested and appear to have good antiviral activity with less toxicity.

POST-TRANSPLANTATION THERAPIES

Growth factors

Growth factors have found their most significant use in the acceleration of hematopoietic recovery after autologous reinfusion of stem cells. Clinical trials in allogeneic transplantation have not yet shown an advantage to their use, probably due to the immunosuppressive medications such as methotrexate used to prevent GVHD. Studies do support the use of G-CSF or granulocyte-macrophage colony-stimulating factor (GM-CSF; sargramostim [Leukine, Prokine]) after autologous hematopoietic cell transplantation, although the impact of these growth factors on acceleration of hematopoietic recovery, beyond that achieved with the use of primed autologous stem cells, is not clear.

Erythropoietic agents

Epoetin alfa (Epogen, Procrit) or darbepoetin alfa (Aranesp) is sometimes used effectively in patients who have persistent anemia after transplantation.

MANAGEMENT OF RELAPSE

Despite the intensity of the preparative regimen, some patients relapse after receiving an allogeneic BMT. For patients with CML, withdrawal of immunosuppression to allow for an augmented graft-versus-tumor effect sometimes leads to remission. Other patients with CML may respond to post-transplantation interferon or reintroduction of drugs such as imatinib (Gleevec) or dasatinib (Sprycel), which appears to be a useful approach. Intriguingly, infusion of donor lymphoid cells into patients with CML is an effective means of inducing hematologic and cytogenetic responses in those who have relapsed after transplantation; this approach has led to complete and durable remissions.

Some patients with AML have responded to either infusion of donor stem cells or the combination of chemotherapy and donor stem cells. Patients with acute lymphoblastic leukemia have had the lowest response rate to this strategy. Patients who develop myelodysplasia after autologous transplantation can sometimes be successfully treated with reduced-intensity allogeneic transplant to restore normal hematopoiesis and cure the myelodysplastic syndrome.

Long-term problems

For patients undergoing autologous stem cell transplantation, the major long-term problem is the risk of relapse and myelodysplasia, but changes in libido, sexual dysfunction, and infertility also should be addressed to help patients achieve good long-term quality of life. Patients undergoing allogeneic transplantation have similar long-term issues but also have major long-term effects related to chronic GVHD and the complications related to immunosuppression, especially infection. In addition, patients undergoing allogeneic transplantation are at higher risk for second malignancies, and, thus, aggressive screening studies should be part of the care of all long-term survivors of transplantation.

SECOND MALIGNANCY AFTER HCT

Patients undergoing transplantation are at risk for developing a second cancer. For those undergoing autologous transplantation, particularly for treatment of lymphoma and Hodgkin lymphoma, the most common cancer is myelodysplasia/AML, which occurs in up to 10% of patients, usually within 3 to 7 years after transplantation.

Risk factors for the development of myelodysplasia/AML after transplantation include the number of prior chemotherapy and radiation therapy treatments, specific drugs such as alkylating agents or topoisomerase inhibitors, difficulty in mobilizing stem cells, persistent cytopenias after transplantation, and use of TBI in the transplant preparative regimen. All patients should undergo cytogenetic screening of the marrow prior to stem cell collection and should be followed for this complication after recovery from transplantation.

Patients undergoing either autologous or allogeneic transplantation are also at risk for the development of solid tumors up to 20 years after transplantation. The risk is greater in patients receiving an allogeneic transplant. The most common tumors are related to the skin, but both common (breast, lung, and colon) and less common (sarcoma) tumors have been seen. As part of their long-term follow-up, all patients require screening for this complication to diagnose the cancer in its earliest stage.

SUGGESTED READING

Appelbaum FR, Forman SJ, Negrin RS, et al (eds): Hematopoietic Cell Transplantation, 4th ed. Malden, Massachusetts, Blackwell Science, 2009.

Brunstein CG, Gutman JA, Weisdorf DJ, et al: Allogeneic hematopoietic cell transplantation for hematological malignancy: Relative risks and benefits of double umbilical cord blood. Blood 2010 Aug 4. [Epub ahead of print]

Cutler C, Kim HT, Ayanian S, et al: Prediction of veno-occlusive disease using biomarkers of endothelial injury. Biol Blood Marrow Transplant 16:1180–1185, 2010.

Deeg HJ, Sandmaier BM: Who is fit for allogeneic transplantation? Blood 2010 Aug 11. [Epub ahead of print]

de Lima M, Giralt S: Allogeneic transplantation for the elderly patient with acute myelogenous leukemia or myelodysplastic syndrome. Semin Hematol 43:107–117, 2006.

Fung HC, Cohen S, Rodriguez R, et al: Reduced-intensity allogeneic stem cell transplantation for patients whose prior autologous stem cell transplantation for hematologic malignancy failed. Biol Blood Marrow Transplant 9:649–656, 2003.

Geisler CH, Kolstad A, Laurell A, et al: Long-term progression-free survival of mantle cell lymphoma after intensive front-line immunochemotherapy with in vivo-purged stem cell rescue: A nonrandomized phase 2 multicenter study by the Nordic Lymphoma Group. Blood 112:2687–2693, 2008.

Harousseau JL, Moreau P: Evolving role of stem cell transplantation in multiple myeloma. Clin Lymphoma Myeloma 6:89–95, 2005.

Hertzberg M, Grigg A, Gottlieb D, et al: Reduced-intensity allogeneic haemopoietic stem cell transplantation induces durable responses in patients with chronic B-lymphoproliferative disorders. Bone Marrow Transplant 37:923–928, 2006.

Ho VT, Aldridge J, Kim HT, et al: Comparison of Tacrolimus and Sirolimus (Tac/Sir) versus Tacrolimus, Sirolimus, and mini-methotrexate (Tac/Sir/MTX) as acute graft-versus-host disease prophylaxis after reduced-intensity conditioning allogeneic peripheral blood stem cell transplantation. Biol Blood Marrow Transplant 15:844–850, 2009.

Ito JI, Kriengkauykiat J, Dadwal SS, et al: Approaches to the early treatment of invasive fungal infection. Leuk Lymphoma 51:1623–1631, 2010.

Krishnan A, Nademanee A, Fung HC, et al: Phase II trial of transplantation regimen of yttrium-90 ibritumomab tiuxetan and high-dose chemotherapy in patients with non-Hodgkin's lymphoma. J Clin Oncol 26:90–95, 2008.

Laughlin MJ, Eapen M, Rubinstein P, et al: Outcomes after transplantation of cord blood or bone marrow from unrelated donors in adults with leukemia. N Engl J Med 351:2265–2275, 2004.

Lavoie JC, Connors JM, Phillips GL, et al: High-dose chemotherapy and autologous stem cell transplantation for primary refractory or relapsed Hodgkin lymphoma: Long-term outcome in the first 100 patients treated in Vancouver. Blood 106:1473–1478, 2005.

Lokhorst H, Einsele H, Vesole D, et al: International Myeloma Working Group consensus statement regarding the current status of allogeneic stem-cell transplantation for multiple myeloma. J Clin Oncol 2010 Aug 9. [Epub ahead of print]

Loren AW, Chow E, Jacobsohn DA, et al: Pregnancy after hematopoietic-cell transplantation: A report from the late effects working committee of the center for international blood and marrow transplant research (CIBMTR). Biol Blood Marrow Transplant 2010 Jul 23. [Epub ahead of print]

Maloney DG, Molina AJ, Sahebi F, et al: Allografting with nonmyeloablative conditioning following cytoreductive autografts for the treatment of patients with multiple myeloma. Blood 102:3447–3454, 2003.

Martin PJ, Counts GW Jr, Appelbaum FR, et al: Life expectancy in patients surviving more than 5 years after hematopoietic cell transplantation. J Clin Oncol 28:1011–1016, 2010.

Michallet M, Ito JI: Approaches to the management of invasive fungal infections in hematologic malignancy and hematopoietic cell transplantation. J Clin Oncol 27:3398–3409, 2009.

Nademanee A, Forman S, Molina A, et al: A phase 1/2 trial of high-dose yttrium-90-ibritumomab tiuxetan in combination with high-dose etoposide and cyclophosphamide followed by autologous stem cell transplantation in patients with poor-risk or relapsed non-Hodgkin lymphoma. Blood 106:2896–2902, 2005.

Oliansky DM, Czuczman M, Fisher RI, et al: The role of cytotoxic therapy with hematopoietic stem cell transplantation in the treatment of diffuse large b-cell lymphoma: Update of the 2001 evidence-based review. Biol Blood Marrow Transplant 2010 Jul 22. [Epub ahead of print]

Paczesny S, Choi SW, Ferrara JL: Acute graft-versus-host disease: New treatment strategies. Curr Opin Hematol 16:427–436, 2009.

Richardson PG, Soiffer RJ, Antin JH, et al: Defibrotide for the treatment of severe hepatic veno-occlusive disease and multiorgan failure after stem cell transplantation: A multicenter, randomized, dose-finding trial. Biol Blood Marrow Transplant 16:1005–1017, 2010.

Rodriguez R, Nakamura R, Palmer JM, et al: A phase II pilot study of tacrolimus/sirolimus GVHD prophylaxis for sibling donor hematopoietic stem cell transplantation using 3 conditioning regimens. Blood 115:1098–1105, 2010.

Snyder DS, Palmer J, Gaal K, et al: Improved outcomes using tacrolimus/sirolimus for graft-versus-host disease prophylaxis with a reduced-intensity conditioning regimen for allogeneic hematopoietic cell transplant as treatment of myelofibrosis. Biol Blood Marrow Transplant 16:281–286, 2010.

Sun CL, Francisco L, Kawashima T, et al: Prevalence and predictors of chronic health conditions after hematopoietic cell transplantation: A report from the Bone Marrow Transplant Survivor Study. Blood 2010 Jul 23. [Epub ahead of print]

Syrjala KL, Langer SL, Abrams JR, et al: Late effects of hematopoietic cell transplantation among 10-year adult survivors compared with case-matched controls. J Clin Oncol 23:6596–6606, 2005.

Tauro S, Craddock C, Peggs K, et al: Allogeneic stem-cell transplantation using a reduced-intensity conditioning regimen has the capacity to produce durable remissions and long-term disease-free survival in patients with high-risk acute myeloid leukemia and myelodysplasia. J Clin Oncol 23:9387–9393, 2005.

Tuthill M, Chen F, Paston S, et al: The prevention and treatment of cytomegalovirus infection in haematopoietic stem cell transplantation. Cancer Immunol Immunother 58:1481–1488, 2009.

Wagner JE, Gluckman E: Umbilical cord blood transplantation: the first 20 years. Semin Hematol 47:3–12, 2010.

CHAPTER 34

Pain management

Sharon M. Weinstein, MD, and Alan W. Yasko,* MD

Most patients with advanced cancer, and up to 60% of patients with any stage of the disease, experience significant pain. The WHO estimates that 25% of all cancer patients die with unrelieved pain.

The cause of cancer pain should be treated whenever possible. By doing so, one can frequently achieve rapid, lasting pain relief and may prevent the problems associated with untreated progressive disease, such as spinal cord compression and pathologic fracture. Also, the need for pain medications may be diminished, thus reducing side effects and drug interactions.

Although pain can be relieved adequately in most cancer patients, it is undertreated for a multitude of reasons. The problem is not trivial, as unrelieved pain is known to be a risk factor for suicide in cancer patients. Current efforts are being directed toward standardizing pain treatment and separating issues of pain treatment from those of substance abuse.

The effective management of cancer patients with pain is best accomplished with coordination of the services of multidisciplinary professionals, community volunteers, and the family.

PATHOPHYSIOLOGY

Pathophysiologic classification of pain forms the basis for therapeutic choices. Pain states may be broadly divided into those associated with ongoing tissue damage (nociceptive) and those resulting from nervous system dysfunction in the absence of ongoing tissue damage (non-nociceptive or neuropathic).

Damage to the nervous system may result in pain in an area of altered sensation. Such pain is typically described as burning or lancinating. Patients may report bizarre complaints, such as painful numbness, itching, or crawling sensations. The postamputation phenomenon of phantom pain (pain referred to the lost body part) may be disabling.

Psychological factors

Psychological factors may affect the reporting of pain. Chronic unrelieved pain has psychological consequences, but this does not support a psychiatric basis for the

*Dr. Alan W. Yasko, 1958–2010. The editors of *Cancer Management: A Multidisciplinary Approach*, would like to acknowledge the significant contributions that Dr. Yasko has made to the book and express our sadness at his passing.

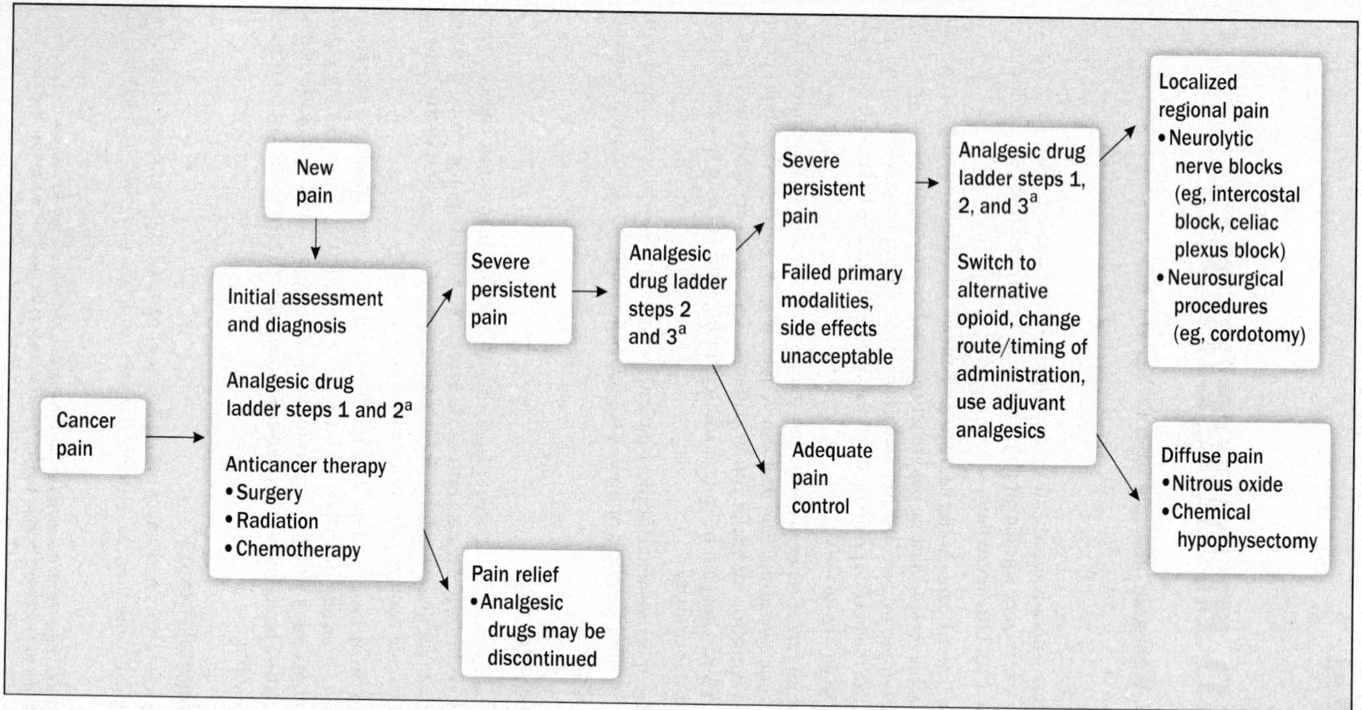

FIGURE 1: Algorithm for the integration of pharmacologic management approaches to cancer pain.
[a]Step 1 – Nonopioid ± adjuvant; Step 2 – Opioid + nonopioid ± adjuvant; Step 3 – Strong opioid ± nonopioid ± adjuvant
Adapted from Foley KM, Arbit E, in DeVita VT, Hellman S, Rosenberg SA (eds): Cancer: Principles & Practice of Oncology, 3rd ed, vol 2, pp 2064–2087. Philadelphia, JB Lippincott, 1989.

TABLE 1: Features of the pain history—"PQRST"

P	Provocative factors, palliative factors
Q	Quality (characteristics)
R	Region, pattern of radiation, referral
S	Severity, intensity (use pain rating scales [Figure 2])
T	Temporal factors: onset, duration, time to maximum intensity, frequency, daily variation

pain complaint. "Psychogenic pain" or somatoform pain disorder is rare in cancer patients.

Pain syndromes

Cancer pain syndromes vary by tumor type and are related to patterns of tumor growth and metastasis. Pain may also be related to antineoplastic therapy or may be unrelated to either the neoplasm or its treatment.

ELEMENTS OF MANAGEMENT

Elements of cancer pain management include a proper medical evaluation, psychosocial assessment, formulation of the pain "diagnosis," and consideration of pharmacologic and nonpharmacologic treatments. Ongoing care is needed to monitor the efficacy of analgesics and the evolution of different symptoms during treatment or disease progression.

The steps in medical decision-making are to:

- determine whether primary antineoplastic therapy is indicated for palliation,
- tailor pharmacologic analgesic therapy to individual needs,
- consider concurrent nonpharmacologic analgesic methods, and
- monitor response and modify treatment accordingly (Figure 1).

The patient is the focus of care, although family members and others often participate in treatment decisions and require emotional support.

Medical evaluation

Pain history

The medical evaluation should begin with a thorough history. As there are no objective means with which to verify the presence of pain, one must believe a patient's complaint. The physiologic signs of acute pain—elevated blood pressure and pulse rate—are unreliable in subacute or chronic pain.

Most cancer patients report more than one site of pain. A detailed history of each type of pain should be elicited (Table 1). As the chief complaint resolves, what was initially a secondary problem may require attention.

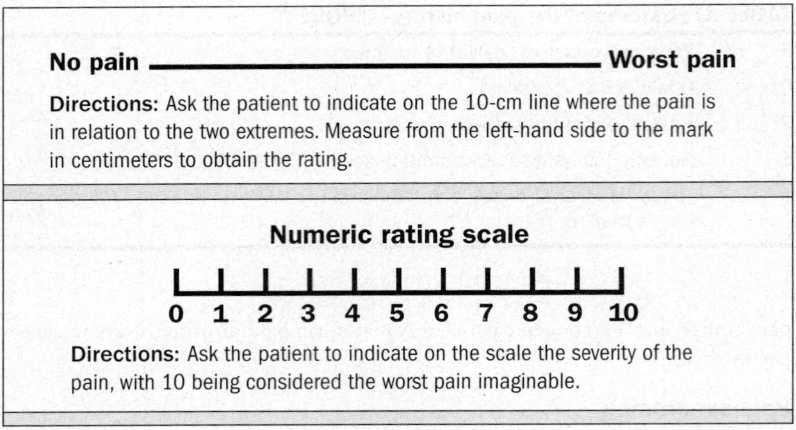

No pain
Worst pain
Directions: Ask the patient to indicate on the 10-cm line where the pain is in relation to the two extremes. Measure from the left-hand side to the mark in centimeters to obtain the rating.
Numeric rating scale
0 1 2 3 4 5 6 7 8 9 10
Directions: Ask the patient to indicate on the scale the severity of the pain, with 10 being considered the worst pain imaginable.

FIGURE 2: Pain rating scale used to establish a baseline against which treatment results are judged; the numeric scale is also administered verbally.

Pain rating scales

Such scales should be used to establish a baseline against which the success of treatment may be judged (Figure 2). Behavioral observations may be used to assess patients who are unable to communicate. There are standardized tools that can be used for preverbal children and impaired adults. It is sometimes necessary to treat pain presumptively.

Physical examination

This includes careful neurologic testing, especially if neuropathic pain is suspected. Pain in an area of reduced sensation, allodynia (ie, when normal stimuli are reported as painful), and hyperpathia or summation of painful stimuli indicate a neuropathic process. The assessment should evaluate the putative mechanisms that may underlie the pain.

Review of disease extent and current conditions

The extent of disease and current medical conditions must be understood.

Diagnostic tests

Diagnostics should be reviewed and supplemented as necessary.

Treatment and drug history

Cancer treatment and prior analgesic interventions, along with their outcomes, should be recorded. Psychological dependency on any drug, including alcohol, must be identified.

Psychosocial assessment

To establish trust, the evaluating clinician should explore with the patient the significance of the pain complaint. The impact of pain and other symptoms on functional status must be understood to establish treatment goals. Suffering may be attributable to many factors besides physical complaints. The clinician should ask about such psychological factors as financial worries, loss of independence, family problems, social isolation, and fear of death. Often, cancer patients meet diagnostic criteria for the psychiatric diagnosis of adjustment disorder with anxiety and/or depressed mood.

Subgrouping of patients

To help define therapeutic goals, the patient's age and prognosis may be considered. Adjustments in drug doses are usually needed for elderly patients, who are more sensitive to analgesics and their side effects. Adolescents may require relatively larger doses of opioids. Pain in children is underreported and should be specifically elicited using age-appropriate assessment tools.

Pharmacologic treatment

The WHO has devised a three-step analgesic ladder outlining the use of non-opioid analgesics, opioid analgesics, and adjuvant medications for progressively severe pain. According to this schema, a nonopioid analgesic, with or without an adjuvant agent, should be tried first (step 1). If pain persists or increases on this regimen, the patient should be switched to an opioid plus a nonopioid agent, with or without an adjuvant medication (step 2). If pain continues or intensifies despite this change in therapy, a more potent dose of opioid analgesic should be prescribed, with or without a nonopioid and/or an adjuvant agent (step 3). This basic approach remains clinically useful.

Nonopioid analgesics

Nonopioid analgesics are associated with ceiling effects, and exceeding the maximum dose ranges can result in organ toxicity. Potential side effects, such as hematologic, renal, and gastrointestinal reactions, may be of clinical concern in cancer patients (Table 2). Cyclo-oxygenase (COX)-2 inhibitors are many times more potent against COX-2 than COX-1. Clinicians are advised to watch the emerging literature regarding the safety of these agents.

Opioid analgesics

General guidelines for opioid therapy are outlined in Table 3.

Dosage Opioid agonists do not exhibit ceiling effects. Dosing is guided by efficacy and limited by side effects (Table 4). Dosages of tablets combining a nonsteroidal anti-inflammatory drug (NSAID) or acetaminophen and an opioid are limited according to the nonopioid component.

Routes of administration The oral route should be used when possible, although some patients may express a preference for an alternative route. If so, or if the oral route is not feasible or systemic side effects are uncontrollable, alternative routes

TABLE 2: Nonopioid analgesics and NSAIDs useful for treating cancer pain

Generic name (usual dosage range)	Maximum dose/day	Adverse effects/ comments
Acetaminophen (325–975 mg q4–6h)	4,000 mg	Hepatic and renal impairment
Acetylsalicylic acid (aspirin, ASA) (325–975 mg q4–6h)	4,000 mg	Dyspepsia and GI ulceration, antiplatelet effect, bleeding
Celecoxib	400 mg	See note[a]
Choline magnesium trisalicylate (500–1,500 mg q8–12h)	4,500 mg	Dyspepsia, reduced antiplatelet effect, hypermagnesemia in renal failure
Choline salicylate (435–870 mg q3–4h)	5,220 mg	Dyspepsia, reduced antiplatelet effect
Magnesium salicylate (300–600 mg q4h)	4,800 mg	Same as choline salicylate
Salsalate (1,000–1,500 mg q8–2h)	4,000 mg	Same as choline salicylate
Sodium salicylate (325–650 mg q3–4h)	5,200 mg	Same as choline salicylate
Ibuprofen (200–800 mg q4–6h)	2,400 mg	[b]Dermatitis +
Ketoprofen (25–75 mg q6–8h)	300 mg	[b]Headache +++
Ketorolac tromethamine (oral: 10 mg q4–6h; parenteral: 60 mg, then 15–30 mg q6h)	Oral: 40 mg Parenteral: 120 mg	[b]Limit duration of therapy; headache +++, GI bleeding [b]Limit therapy to 5 days; headache +++, GI bleeding
Meclofenamate sodium (50–100 mg q4–6h)	400 mg	[b]Headache +, dermatitis +
Mefenamic acid (250 mg q6h)	1,000 mg	[b]Limit therapy to 7 days
Naproxen sodium (220–550 mg q8–12h)	1,375 mg	[b]Headache +
Naproxen (250–500 mg q8–12h)	1,500 mg	[b]Headache +

[a] Monitor emerging literature regarding safety concerns.

[b] Minor adverse reactions include dyspepsia, heartburn, nausea, vomiting, anorexia, diarrhea, constipation, flatulence, bloating, epigastric pain, abdominal pain, dizziness, and drowsiness. Major adverse reactions that may appear at any time include renal failure, hepatic dysfunction, bleeding, and gastric ulceration.

+ Each plus sign represents a 5% incidence of the reported adverse effect.

GI = gastrointestinal; NSAIDs = nonsteroidal anti-inflammatory drugs

Adapted with permission from American Pain Society: Principles of Analgesic Use in the Treatment of Acute Pain and Cancer Pain, 5th ed. Skokie, Illinois, American Pain Society, 2003.

TABLE 3: Guidelines for the use of opioid analgesics

Start with an analgesic with the potential to provide relief

Know the essential pharmacology of the analgesic:

- Analgesic type
- Pharmacokinetics
- Influences of coadministered drugs, disease, or age on analgesic disposition and response
- Equianalgesic starting dose for the drug and route to be used
- Route of administration and a dosage form to fit the patient's needs

Individualize/titrate the dosage

Administer analgesics regularly after the initial dose titration

Provide for breakthrough pain

Use drug combinations that enhance analgesia

Recognize and treat side effects

Make conversions from one route to another or from one agent to another using known equianalgesic doses

Manage physical dependence (ie, prevent withdrawal)

Adapted with permission from Inturrisi C: Cancer 63(suppl):2308–2320, 1989.

TABLE 4: Opioid-agonist analgesics for mild-to-moderate pain

Drug	Equianalgesic dose to 650 mg of aspirin[a]	Dose interval	Half-life (h)	Comments
Codeine	32–65 mg	q4–6h	2–3	See notes[b, c]
Hydrocodone	—	q3–4h	4	See note[b]
Oxycodone	2.5 mg	q3–6h	2–3	See note[b]

[a] The equianalgesic dose should not be interpreted as the starting, standard, or maximum dose but rather as a guide for switching drugs or changing routes of administration.

[b] Doses of products containing aspirin or acetaminophen should be monitored for safety.

[c] Doses above 65 mg provide diminished incremental analgesia with increasing doses, but side effects may worsen.

Adapted with permission from American Pain Society: Principles of Analgesic Use in the Treatment of Acute Pain and Cancer Pain, 3rd ed. Skokie, Illinois, American Pain Society, 1992.

TABLE 5: Opioid agonist analgesics for severe pain

Drug	Equianalgesic dose to 10 mg of IV morphine: Oral	Parenteral	Half-life (h)	Comments
Fentanyl, oral transmucosal	See[a]	NA	See note[a]	For breakthrough cancer pain
Fentanyl, transdermal	NA	NA	—	[b,c]Patch sizes of 12, 25, 50, 75, 100 μg/h; slow onset to effect, necessitating "breakthrough" analgesics
Hydromorphone	7.5 mg	1.5 mg	2–3	See note[b]
Levorphanol	4 mg	2 mg	12–16	See note[b]
Methadone	3–20 mg	10 mg	15–50	[b,d]Risk of delayed toxicity due to accumulation; reduce dose or lengthen dose interval if oversedation occurs after 4–5 days; may schedule as prn initially
Morphine sulfate, controlled release	30 mg	NA	3	[b]Mg-for-mg-conversion from immediate-release form; do not crush or chew tablets
Morphine sulfate, immediate release	30 mg	10 mg	3	See note[b]
Oxycodone, controlled release	15 mg	NA	—	See notes[b,e]
Oxycodone, immediate release	15 mg	NA	2–3	See note[b]

(eg, transdermal, transmucosal, rectal, and neuraxial infusion) are indicated. Such alternative routes of administration of certain opioid agonists (see Table 5) may improve patients' quality of life and may be particularly useful for treating certain types of cancer pain.

Side effects of opioids can usually be anticipated and treated. In particular, with regular opioid dosing, laxatives should be prescribed for constipation.

Physical dependence and tolerance to some effects develop with chronic opioid use. Tolerance to respiratory depression, sedation, and nausea is likely. Tolerance to analgesia is not a major clinical problem and can usually be managed by changing the dose or substituting another agent.

Most current definitions of addiction imply a behavioral syndrome of compulsive, harmful use but do not require the existence of physical dependence or tolerance.

TABLE 5: Opioid agonist analgesics for severe pain, *continued*

Drug	Equianalgesic dose to 10 mg of IV morphine: Oral	Parenteral	Half-life (h)	Comments
Oxymorphone	10 mg	1 mg	2–3	See note[b]
Oxymorphone, controlled release	10 mg	NA	—	

IV = intravenous; NA = not available; prn = as needed

[a] See package insert for dosing instructions. Available in lozenge and effervescent tablets.

[b] Common side effects include constipation, nausea, and sedation. Uncommon side effects include itching, dry mouth, and urinary retention. Rare side effects are hypotension and inappropriate antidiuretic hormone secretion.

[c] Patch duration = 72 hours, but may be 48 hours for some patients.

Equianalgesic conversion for fentanyl:

Parenteral morphine dose (mg/24 h)	Transdermal fentanyl (μg/h)
8–22	25
23–37	50
38–52	75
53–67	100
68–82	125
83–97	150

[d] Consult pain expert if converting to/from methadone in high-dose patients. Unique cardiac toxicity.

[e] Available alone and in combination with aspirin or acetaminophen; at higher doses, use as a single agent.

Adapted with permission from American Pain Society: Principles of Analgesic Use in the Treatment of Acute Pain and Cancer Pain, 5th ed. Skokie, Illinois, American Pain Society, 2003.

Aberrant drug-taking is not likely to occur in patients without a history of substance abuse. However, compliance should always be monitored.

Precautions during chronic therapy During chronic opioid therapy, certain precautions should be observed:

- Normeperidine is a toxic metabolite of meperidine that accumulates with repetitive dosing; thus, use of meperidine for chronic pain should be limited. Propoxyphene is also relatively contraindicated due to accumulation of norpropoxyphene.
- Placebo use is discouraged, as it does not help distinguish the pathophysiology of pain.
- Physical withdrawal symptoms can be avoided by tapering doses.
- A change in mental status should not be attributed to opioid therapy until medical and neurologic factors have been fully evaluated.
- Mixed agonist-antagonist drugs and partial agonist drugs are not recommended for cancer pain.
- Methadone has unique pharmacokinetics. Inexperienced practitioners should consult a pain medicine expert before prescribing methadone. See FDA warnings.

TABLE 6: Adjuvant drug therapy for cancer pain

Antidepressants
Anticonvulsants
Anxiolytics
Muscle relaxants
Topical local anesthetics and other agents
Amphetamines
Phenothiazines
Bisphosphonates
Corticosteroids

Adjuvant medications Neuropathic pain may be less responsive to standard analgesics alone. Adjuvants, such as antidepressants, anticonvulsants, benzodiazepines, local anesthetics, neuroleptics, psychostimulants, antihistamines, corticosteroids, levodopa, calcitonin, and bisphosphonates, are useful for particular indications (Table 6). These agents may be administered via oral and other routes. Administration of topical local anesthetics, NSAIDs and other preparations (Table 7), and neurolytic blocks (Table 8) should also be considered.

TABLE 7: Anesthetic/neurosurgical approaches for controlling cancer pain

Procedure	Usual indication(s)	Examples
Local anesthetic blocks with or without steroids	Diagnostic blocks Prognostic blocks Acute pain, muscle spasm Premorbid chronic pain Postsurgical syndromes Herpes zoster	Trigger point injection Intercostal block Epidural steroids
Neurolytic/neuroablative blocks and ablative neurosurgery	Localized refractory pain that is expected to persist, usually in the presence of a short life expectancy; pain localized to a region that is associated with a low risk of neurologic complications	Alcohol celiac plexus block Phenol intercostal block Percutaneous cordotomy Midline myelotomy
Spinal analgesics	Refractory pain, usually in the lower body but may be widespread or diffuse	Externalized epidural catheter Intrathecal catheter with fully implanted pump

TABLE 8: Neurolytic procedures[a] that may be considered early in certain pain situations

Procedure	Indication
Celiac plexus neurolysis	Abdominal pain, back pain
Superior hypogastric plexus neurolysis	Pelvic pain
Phenol saddle block	Perineal pain with urinary diversion
Thoracic subarachnoid neurolysis	Focal chest wall pain
Intercostal neurolysis	Focal chest wall pain
Lumbar subarachnoid neurolysis	Unilateral leg pain

[a] The risk-benefit ratio of these procedures in the specified settings is sufficiently favorable and well established to warrant early consideration.

Surgery for bone metastasis

Surgical intervention is warranted for bone metastases to stabilize a pathologic fracture or preempt an impending fracture. The objectives of surgery are to palliate pain, reduce patient anxiety, improve patient mobility and function, facilitate nursing care, and control local tumors when nonsurgical therapies fail. In general, surgery involves excision of all gross tumor followed by stabilization of the bone before or after fracture by means of an internal fixation or prosthetic device.

There are no clearly defined criteria for the presence of an impending fracture of a long bone. Current guidelines derived from retrospective clinical studies include lytic lesions > 2.5 cm in diameter, cortical destruction > 50%, and pain despite local irradiation. In the proximal femur, an avulsion fracture of the lesser trochanter places the hip at high risk for fracture, and operative intervention should be considered.

Indications

No strict criteria have been established for surgical treatment. Clinical parameters, such as the patient's general medical condition, performance status, nature of the primary tumor, effectiveness of other therapies, extent of extraskeletal disease, and degree of osseous involvement, as well as the patient's life expectancy, must be considered before surgery.

Fracture and long bone pain In general, the presence of a pathologic fracture, an impending fracture, or a painful lesion in a long bone despite radiotherapy should be considered to be indications for surgery. A pathologic fracture can result from structural insufficiency and can develop in the absence of a viable tumor following treatment with irradiation and/or systemic therapy.

Other considerations Patients deemed to be candidates for surgery should have an expected longevity of > 1 month. All patients should be medically able to withstand the planned surgical procedure. The surgical goals should be achievable with reasonable certainty, and the potential benefits should outweigh the operative risks. All surgical interventions should be performed with the intent to provide benefit that will outlast the patient's anticipated survival.

Lesion site Major long bones (femur, tibia, and humerus), the vertebrae, and periacetabular regions demand specific attention, as optimal patient function and mobility are predicated on a stable, painless extremity. Osseous destruction sufficient to compromise the mechanical integrity of these bones should be addressed surgically. Lesions in the weight-bearing bones of the lower extremity (femur and tibia) are particularly vulnerable to fracture.

Lesions in the humerus should be treated surgically when the upper extremities serve a weight-bearing function (eg, assisted ambulation using a walker, crutches, or cane). Early surgical intervention, aggressive rehabilitation, and vigilant postoperative surveillance may optimize patient outcome.

The treatment of metastatic spine disease is mostly palliative. Minimally invasive techniques, such as kyphoplasty and vertebroplasty, are very promising options for treatment in selected patients. Different techniques for performing vertebral body augmentation in patients with symptomatic fractures associated with malignant spinal lesions are being refined.

Radiation therapy

Cancer pain can often be relieved by radiation therapy delivered by localized external-beam irradiation (also known as involved-field irradiation), wide-field external-beam irradiation (eg, hemibody irradiation), or systemic treatment with radioactive isotopes (eg, strontium-89 chloride [Metastron], samarium-153 lexidronam [Quadramet], phosphorus-32, and iridium-131). Because the most common cause of cancer pain is bone metastasis, this discussion will focus on the use of irradiation in its treatment. Other examples of cancer pain due to primary or metastatic cancer that are amenable to irradiation include headache from CNS involvement, pain due to localized neural involvement (eg, brachial plexus or sciatic nerve), visceral pain (eg, liver or adrenal), pain due to effusions (eg, pericardial or pleural), and pain due to obstruction (eg, urethral, esophageal).

Systemic radiotherapy

Strontium-89 is a systemic radionuclide that has clinical efficacy in the palliation of pain from bone metastases. Reduction of pain due to bone metastases has been observed most frequently in patients with metastases from prostate cancer.

The primary toxicity of strontium-89 is myelosuppression, particularly thrombocytopenia. Therefore, it should not be administered to patients with thrombocytopenia or significant bone marrow suppression. Strontium-89 levels in bone are regulated much like calcium, and strontium-89 has less hematologic toxicity than phosphorus-32.

Samarium-153 is a β-emitting radioisotope that is bound to a phosphonate that preferentially localizes in active bone, specifically in sites of metastatic disease. Mild-to-moderate myelosuppression was noted in the samarium-153 group, yet use of samarium-153 is associated with a lower incidence and severity of hematologic toxicity than is strontium-89.

Physical treatments

Cancer patients may benefit from formal rehabilitation, evaluation, and treatment. Physical modalities, such as massage, ultrasonography, hydrotherapy, transcutaneous electrical nerve stimulation, electroacupuncture, and trigger-point manipulation, are indicated for musculoskeletal pain. Also, any of these techniques may enhance exercise tolerance in a patient undergoing rehabilitation. Skillful soft-tissue manipulation probably is underused. Electrical stimulation may also be applied to the peripheral nerves, spinal cord, and even deep brain structures.

Management of psychological, sociocultural, and spiritual factors

The appropriate treatment of cancer pain must extend beyond the physical complaint. Psychological, sociocultural, and spiritual factors significantly affect the patient's quality of life. Thus, the clinician must always care for the whole person. A multimodal approach to pain management recognizes the complexity of the human being, especially one with a terminal illness.

Although the physician's initial therapeutic goal is to cure the disease, cancer can be incurable. Caring entails recognizing the whole person as a physical, intellectual, social, emotional, and spiritual being. Empathic caring helps the patient perceive the value in life despite the gravity of the situation. Palliative care is meant to prevent and relieve suffering, and this supportive care can be integrated throughout the course of illness.

Psychiatric diagnoses

Psychiatric conditions, such as anxiety and depression, and psychological factors must be thoroughly addressed, as revealed by emerging evidence from the disciplines of psycho-oncology and psychoneuroimmunology. Attitude and state of mind affect the individual's perception of pain and response to it in myriad ways and may affect the duration of survival. In addition, patients may regain a much needed sense of control by using psychological techniques, such as imagery, hypnosis, relaxation, biofeedback, and other cognitive or behavioral methods.

Sociocultural influences

These factors affect the patient's experience and expression of pain. This is especially true for the patient whose cancer does not respond to therapy and progresses to end-stage disease.

Pain may be an unwelcome reminder of the presence and progression of cancer. Concomitant fear, anger, frustration, disappointment, and other negative emotions may hold the patient hostage to physical pain.

Existential distress

This may bridge an undesirable transition from hopeful coping with pain to hopeless suffering from it. As patients are confronted with personal mortality, the limits of their life spans move from an abstract concept to a real issue. Self-image changes, and patients may develop emotional and psychic turmoil, which may compromise their medical condition and treatment.

Achieving relief of psychic suffering may enable the patient to transcend physical pain, enhancing the effects of pain medications and other treatments. Prayer, meditation, counseling, clergy visits, and support groups may all be beneficial.

Relieving suffering means allowing the patient and family to realize improved quality of life and even find contentment or peace in the face of failing health and imminent death. Palliative care of the family includes bereavement counseling in anticipation of and after the loss of a loved one.

Ongoing care

The goals of pain management must be frequently reviewed and integrated into the overall management plan. Communication among the professional staff, patient, and family is essential. A sensitive, frank discussion with the patient regarding his or her wishes should guide medical decision-making during all phases of the illness.

SUGGESTED READING

ON CANCER PAIN MANAGEMENT

American Pain Society: Principles of Analgesic Use in the Treatment of Acute Pain and Cancer Pain, 6th ed. Skokie, Illinois, American Pain Society, 2008.

Breitbart W: Suicide, in Holland J, Rowland J (eds): Handbook of Psychooncology. New York, Oxford University Press, 1999.

Chochinov HM, Breitbart W (eds): Ethical and Spiritual Issues: Handbook of Psychiatry in Palliative Medicine, Part VI, pp 337–396. New York, Oxford University Press, 2000.

Doyle D, Hanks G, Cherny NI, et al (eds): Oxford Textbook of Palliative Medicine, 3rd ed. New York, Oxford University Press, 2005.

World Health Organization: Cancer Pain Relief and Palliative Care in Children. Geneva, Switzerland, World Health Organization, 1998.

ON ANESTHETIC AND SURGICAL APPROACHES

Georgy BA: Vertebroplasty technique in metastatic disease. Clin N Am 20:169–177, 2010.

Quraishi NA, Gokasian ZL, Boriani S: The surgical management of metastatic epidural compresssion of the spinal cord. J Bone Joint Surg Br 92:1054–1060, 2010.

Weinstein SM: Management of spinal cord and cauda equina compression, in Berger A, Levy MH, Portenoy RK, Weissman DE (eds): Principles and Practice of Palliative Care and Supportive Oncology, 3rd ed. Philadelphia, JB Lippincott, 2006.

ON RADIATION THERAPY IN CANCER PAIN MANAGEMENT

Gaze MN, Kelly CG, Kerr GR, et al: Pain relief and quality of life following radiotherapy for bone metastases: A randomized trial of two fractionation schedules. Radiother Oncol 45:109–116, 1997.

Rose CM, Kagan AR: The final report of the expert panel for the radiation oncology bone metastasis work group of the American College of Radiology. Int J Radiat Oncol Biol Phys 40:1117–1124, 1998.

Abbreviations in this chapter

FDA = US Food and Drug Administration; WHO = World Health Organization

CHAPTER 35

Management of nausea and vomiting

Steven M. Grunberg, MD, Nathan B. Adams, and Richard Gralla, MD

Although marked progress in controlling chemotherapy-induced emesis has occurred over the past 25 years, nausea and vomiting remain among the most distressing side effects of cancer chemotherapy. With the increased use of chemotherapy in primary and adjuvant treatment settings, the need for improved control of emesis remains an important consideration in both medical oncology and supportive care.

Several major oncology groups have published consensus reports or guidelines on the prevention of chemotherapy-induced emesis. However, the introduction of several new agents may change these paradigms. In addition, an understanding of the neuropharmacology of this problem is useful in planning patient care.

PATHOPHYSIOLOGY OF EMESIS

Although the mechanism by which cancer chemotherapy induces emesis is still not completely understood, a physiologic basis for our current understanding of this complex problem has now emerged.

STIMULATION OF NEUROTRANSMITTER RECEPTORS

The emetic reflex arc is activated by stimulation of receptors in the central nervous system (CNS) and/or gastrointestinal (GI) tract. These receptor areas relay information to the vomiting center in the medulla, which then coordinates the act of vomiting. The chemoreceptor trigger zone (CTZ), also located in the medulla, serves as a "chemosensor" and is exposed to blood and cerebrospinal fluid (CSF). These areas are rich in a variety of neurotransmitter receptors.

Dopamine For many years, the dopamine receptors were the main focus of interest in antiemetic research. Available antiemetics, such as phenothiazines (chlorpromazine and prochlorperazine) and substituted benzamides (metoclopramide), were known to affect these receptors, as were butyrophenones (haloperidol and droperidol).

Serotonin The role of the neurotransmitter serotonin (5-hydroxytryptamine [5-HT]) has also been elucidated. The improved antiemetic activity of higher doses of metoclopramide was not explained by its dopamine-binding properties but by the fact that it also affects serotonin receptors. This finding led to the development of several highly specific compounds that interact solely with serotonin receptors, specifically the type 3, or 5-HT_3, receptor subtype. Four compounds (ondansetron, granisetron, dolasetron [Anzemet], palonosetron [Aloxi]) from this family are currently available in the United States. The 5-HT_3 receptor, which is found in both the GI tract and CNS, is an important mediator of the emetic reflex arc. Recent work has suggested that mutation of the 5-HT_{3B} receptor subunit may affect antiemetic efficacy.

Substance P Tachykinins, such as substance P, play an important role in emesis, as well as in pain and a variety of inflammatory conditions. These neurotransmitters are 11–amino acid molecules that bind to specific receptors. Substance P binds to the neurokinin type 1, or NK_1, receptor.

Several NK_1 receptor antagonists have been synthesized and used both preclinically and in clinical trials in patients receiving cancer chemotherapy. Results indicate that these agents are effective against a broad range of causes of emesis, particularly delayed emesis. One member of this family, aprepitant (Emend), has been approved for clinical use.

EMETIC PROBLEMS

EMESIS RELATED TO CHEMOTHERAPY

Both nausea and vomiting are seen in patients receiving cancer chemotherapy. Nausea occurs at a higher frequency than vomiting and is more difficult to control. The control of vomiting is strongly correlated with the control of nausea, although some patients experience nausea without vomiting.

The three most common emetic patterns in patients receiving chemotherapy are outlined below.

Acute chemotherapy-induced emesis is defined as nausea or vomiting that occurs within the initial 24 hours of chemotherapy administration. The time of greatest risk is from 1 to 6 hours after chemotherapy with most agents.

Delayed emesis is emesis that begins ≥ 24 hours after chemotherapy. Delayed emesis is particularly likely to occur in patients who have received cisplatin, carboplatin, or cyclophosphamide. Recent data indicate that this problem may begin somewhat earlier than 24 hours in some patients.

Anticipatory emesis is defined as a conditioned vomiting response following inadequate antiemetic protection with prior courses of chemotherapy.

EMESIS UNRELATED TO CHEMOTHERAPY

Patients receiving anticancer drugs may also develop emesis for other reasons. Emesis can be induced by concomitant medications (such as analgesics, anti-infectives, or bronchodilators) or by tumor-related complications (such as intestinal obstruction or brain metastases). In these instances, adjustment of medication or treatment of tumor-related complications is more important than selecting an antiemetic agent.

PATIENT CHARACTERISTICS AND EMESIS

History of poor emetic control Poor control of emesis with past courses of chemotherapy predisposes a patient to unsatisfactory antiemetic results with any subsequent treatment, regardless of the emetic stimulus or antiemetic employed. Both delayed and conditioned anticipatory emesis are more likely to occur in these patients, and there is likely to be greater difficulty in controlling acute emesis.

History of alcohol intake Emesis is easier to control in patients with a history of chronic, high alcohol intake (> 100 g/d of alcohol [approximately five alcohol units or drinks]). In a prospective evaluation of 52 patients receiving high-dose cisplatin and an effective combination antiemetic regimen, 93% of those with a history of high alcohol intake had no emesis, as opposed to 61% of those without such a history. This difference in emesis control is independent of the patient's current alcohol intake.

Age Most trials have found that it is easier to control emesis in older patients than in younger ones. Younger patients have a predilection for developing acute dystonic reactions when dopamine-blocking antiemetics are administered (see section on "Antiemetic agents for high–emetic-risk chemotherapy"). Younger patients also have a greater tendency to develop anticipatory emesis than do older patients.

Gender It is more difficult to control emesis in women than in men given the same chemotherapy and antiemetic regimen.

Motion sickness Patients with a history of motion sickness are more likely to develop chemotherapy-induced nausea and vomiting than are those without such a history.

The above predisposing factors appear to be additive. One can identify patients at particularly high risk of emesis, such as younger women without a history of high alcohol intake. Awareness of these factors is helpful in monitoring individual patients and interpreting the results of clinical trials.

CHEMOTHERAPEUTIC AGENTS AND EMESIS

Emetic potential The most accurate predictor of the risk of emesis is the chemotherapeutic agent that a patient is receiving. Several different classifications of commonly used chemotherapy agents have been devised. Table 1 is based on the consensus report of the MASCC as updated in March 2008.

The emetic potential of a chemotherapeutic combination is determined by identifying the most emetic agent in the combination. Other agents in a combination may also increase the risk.

In general, agents associated with the highest *incidence* of emesis also induce the most *severe* emesis. Differences occur among patients and even between identical treatment courses in the same patient. The dose, route, and schedule of administration of the chemotherapeutic agent can affect the incidence of nausea and vomiting.

Time of onset of emesis In patients receiving initial chemotherapy of high emetic risk, nausea or vomiting typically begins between 1 to 2 hours after chemotherapy. Cyclophosphamide and carboplatin may be associated with a late onset of emesis (ie, 8 to 18 hours following chemotherapy administration).

TABLE 1: Emetic potential of chemotherapy agents

Level	Frequency of emesis (%)[a]	Agent
High	> 90	Carmustine Cisplatin Cyclophosphamide (≥ 1,500 mg/m^2) Dacarbazine Hexamethylmelamine Mechlorethamine Procarbazine Streptozocin
Moderate	30–90	Carboplatin Cyclophosphamide (< 1,500 mg/m^2) Cytarabine (> 1,000 mg/m^2) Daunorubicin Doxorubicin Epirubicin Idarubicin Ifosfamide Irinotecan Oxaliplatin Temozolomide
Low	10–30	Bortezomib Capecitabine Cetuximab Cytarabine (≤ 100 mg/m^2) Docetaxel Etoposide Fluorouracil Gemcitabine Methotrexate Mitomycin Mitoxantrone Paclitaxel Pemetrexed Topotecan Trastuzumab
Minimal	< 10	Bevacizumab Bleomycin Busulfan Chlorambucil 2-Chlorodeoxyadenosine Fludarabine Hydroxyurea Melphalan Thioguanine Vinblastine Vincristine Vinorelbine

[a] Proportion of patients experiencing emesis in the absence of effective antiemetic prophylaxis

ANTIEMETIC AGENTS FOR HIGH–EMETIC-RISK CHEMOTHERAPY

Careful antiemetic research has shown that numerous agents are safe and effective. Dosage and administration schedules for some of these agents are given in Table 2. Antiemetic therapy is commonly administered either PO or IV.

Among the best-studied agents are ondansetron, granisetron, dolasetron, palonosetron, metoclopramide, haloperidol, dexamethasone, aprepitant, lorazepam, dronabinol (Marinol), prochlorperazine, and chlorpromazine.

The combination of a single prechemotherapy dose of a 5-HT_3 antagonist and dexamethasone is the most commonly used therapy to prevent emesis in patients receiving chemotherapy of high emetic risk (both cisplatin and noncisplatin) as listed in Table 1. Addition of aprepitant may increase the rate of antiemetic protection.

SEROTONIN ANTAGONISTS: ONDANSETRON, GRANISETRON, DOLASETRON, AND PALONOSETRON

Ondansetron, granisetron, dolasetron, and palonosetron are highly selective 5-HT_3 receptor antagonists. All are effective in controlling emesis induced by a variety of chemotherapeutic agents. Oral and IV routes of administration available for ondansetron, granisetron, dolasetron, and palonosetron are effective, as demonstrated in large randomized trials. Granisetron is also now available as a transdermal patch (Sancuso). Single-dose regimens given before chemotherapy appear to be as effective as more cumbersome multiple- or continuous-dose regimens.

All four serotonin receptor antagonists are similar with regard to efficacy and side effects, although palonosetron has a significantly longer half-life of approximately 40 hours and may exhibit more noncompetitive binding. Doses of these agents are given in Table 2.

Side effects Ondansetron, granisetron, dolasetron, and palonosetron have all demonstrated excellent safety characteristics over a large dosing range. Toxicities have been minor and have included headache, mild transient elevation of hepatic enzyme levels, constipation, and, with some agents, minor prolongation of cardiac conduction intervals.

Ginger, in combination with a 5-HT_3 receptor–antagonist antiemetic, may significantly reduce chemotherapy-related nausea in patients with cancer, according to data from an NCI-funded phase II/III randomized, placebo-controlled, double-blind clinical trial. A total of 644 patients who had previously experienced nausea with chemotherapy were randomly assigned to receive a placebo or ginger capsules (0.5, 1.0, or 1.5 g per day in divided doses) for 6 days, starting 3 days before the first day of a chemotherapy cycle. In addition all patients received standard antiemetics to manage chemotherapy-related vomiting. Administration of ginger significantly reduced nausea compared with placebo (*P* = .003), but the largest reduction in nausea occurred with ginger given at the 0.5-g and 1.0-g daily doses. Researchers concluded that ginger supplementation at a daily dose of 0.5 to 1.0 g significantly aids in reducing nausea during the first day of chemotherapy *(Ryan JL et al: J Clin Oncol 27[15S]: abstract 9511, 2009).*

TABLE 2: Dosage and administration schedules of antiemetic agents for acute emesis for chemotherapy of high emetic risk

	Dosage[a]	
Antiemetic agent	**Oral**	**Intravenous**
Dolasetron	100 mg once	100 mg (1.8 mg/kg) once
Granisetron	1 or 2 mg once	1 mg (0.01 mg/kg) once
Ondansetron	16–24 mg once or 8 mg bid	8 mg (0.15 mg/kg) once
Palonosetron	0.5 mg once[b]	0.25 mg once
Dexamethasone	20 mg once	20 mg once over 5 min
Metoclopramide	Not recommended	2–3 mg/kg q2h
Haloperidol	1–2 mg q4–6h	1–3 mg q4–6h
Dronabinol	5 mg/m^2 q4h	Not available
Nabilone	1–2 mg bid	Not available
Prochlorperazine	Not recommended	10–20 mg q3–4h
Lorazepam[c]	0.5–2.0 mg	0.5–2.0 mg q4–6h
Aprepitant	125 mg	115 mg

[a] All agents are to be administered prior to chemotherapy, usually 30 minutes beforehand, although the serotonin antagonists can be effective if administered as late as immediately before the start of chemotherapy. Recommended dosages have been found to be effective in clinical trials and may vary from those given in package inserts.

[b] Registered

[c] Lorazepam is indicated only as an adjunct to antiemetics in this setting.

Dystonic reactions and akathisia (restlessness), which may be treatment-limiting with antiemetic agents known to block dopamine receptors, are not seen with serotonin antagonists, even when given on consecutive days. This finding is of particular importance for younger patients, in that several regimens used to treat malignancies in this age group utilize a schedule of daily chemotherapy.

Efficacy The serotonin antagonists have been reported to achieve complete control of emesis in 30% to 50% of patients receiving cisplatin. These agents have also proved to be at least as effective against all other chemotherapeutic agents, with complete control rates of about 70%.

Many trials have examined the benefit of adding corticosteroids to a serotonin antagonist. Typically, the complete control of emesis is improved by 10% to 20% in patients receiving highly emetic chemotherapy. Both the ASCO and MASCC guidelines recommend that a corticosteroid be added whenever a serotonin antagonist is indicated (ie, in all patients receiving chemotherapy of high emetic risk).

DEXAMETHASONE

The antiemetic mechanism of action of dexamethasone remains unclear. Several randomized trials and a meta-analysis have all confirmed its effectiveness in controlling emesis and its safety. Other corticosteroids are also effective; however, dexamethasone is the most widely studied steroid and is available in oral and parenteral dosage forms as an inexpensive generic product. Dexamethasone is an excellent agent for use in combination antiemetic regimens and as a single agent for patients receiving chemotherapy of low emetic risk (< 30% incidence).

Dose Dexamethasone doses have generally ranged from 4 to 20 mg/d. In a randomized trial in patients receiving chemotherapy of high emetic risk, a single 20-mg dose was superior in completely controlling both nausea and vomiting. Thus, the 20-mg dose is recommended in this setting. For patients receiving chemotherapy of moderate emetic risk, a single 8-mg dose may be sufficient.

Side effects Toxicities associated with short courses of dexamethasone used for antiemetic therapy have been mild and generally consist of insomnia and mild epigastric burning. Care using this agent in patients with diabetes is particularly warranted.

METOCLOPRAMIDE

Metoclopramide has proven to be safe and effective when given in high IV doses. Metoclopramide was thought to function as an antiemetic through blockade of dopamine receptors. However, high concentrations of this agent effectively block 5-HT_3 receptors as well.

Efficacy High-dose metoclopramide is a second-choice agent, after the serotonin antagonists, in patients receiving cisplatin.

Side effects Commonly observed side effects with metoclopramide include mild sedation, dystonic reactions, akathisia, anxiety, and depression. Dystonic reactions are age-related and route-related. In a report summarizing the experience of nearly 500 patients receiving metoclopramide, the incidence of trismus or torticollis was only 2% in those older than age 30; in contrast, a 27% occurrence was reported in younger patients. Also, such reactions are more common when metoclopramide is administered by the oral route or is given over several consecutive days.

Acute dystonic reactions are not allergic in nature. In general, dystonic reactions and akathisia can be prevented or easily controlled by administering diphenhydramine, benztropine (Cogentin), or a benzodiazepine. These reactions should not be viewed as a contraindication to further use of dopamine-blocking drugs.

HALOPERIDOL

Haloperidol exerts its antiemetic action through dopaminergic blockade. A formal study comparing haloperidol with metoclopramide in patients receiving cisplatin found both agents to be effective, although metoclopramide afforded better emetic control.

Dose Haloperidol doses of 1 to 3 mg given IV q4–6h have been used.

Side effects Toxicities of haloperidol include sedation, dystonic reactions, akathisia, and occasional hypotension.

BENZODIAZEPINES

Although lorazepam and other benzodiazepines are potent anxiolytic agents that can be useful additions to antiemetic therapy, they should not be used as single agents for chemotherapy-induced emesis. Lorazepam has been shown to achieve a high degree of patient acceptance and subjective benefit but only minor objective antiemetic activity. However, the anxiolytic properties of benzodiazepines may be particularly useful in the treatment of anticipatory nausea and vomiting.

Dose Lorazepam is usually given in doses of 0.5 to 1.5 mg/m^2 IV or 1 to 2 mg PO. These doses, especially the higher IV administrations, can be associated with marked sedation lasting for several hours.

CANNABINOIDS

Many trials have tested the antiemetic effects of dronabinol (delta-9-tetrahydrocannabinol [THC]; Marinol), a component of marijuana. Dronabinol has modest antiemetic activity, similar to that seen with oral prochlorperazine, but it may have a greater effect against nausea.

Semisynthetic cannabinoids (such as nabilone [Cesamet]) have been tested but appear to have no clear advantage over dronabinol. The modest antiemetic activity and significant toxicity of cannabinoids make them a second choice for the control of chemotherapy-related emesis.

Dose Dronabinol has been tried in many doses and schedules. The most useful doses have ranged from 5 to 10 mg/m^2 PO every 3 to 4 hours. The usual dose of nabilone is 1 to 2 mg PO twice daily.

Side effects are frequently associated with cannabinoids and are particularly bothersome in older adults. They include dry mouth, sedation, orthostatic hypotension, ataxia, dizziness, euphoria, and dysphoria.

PHENOTHIAZINES

Although phenothiazines were the first effective antiemetics, the results of antiemetic trials with this class of agents against highly emetogenic chemotherapy have been poor. Randomized trials have found standard-dose prochlorperazine, given orally or intramuscularly, to be less effective than metoclopramide or dexamethasone and equivalent to or less effective than dronabinol. IV administration is more effective than oral administration but can rarely cause profound hypotension (unlike serotonin antagonists or metoclopramide). Phenothiazines are seldom used as first-line antiemetic agents for highly or moderately emetogenic chemotherapy.

Side effects of phenothiazines include sedation, akathisia, hypotension, and dystonic reactions.

TABLE 3: Antiemetic regimens for acute emesis, by emetic risk

Risk level	Recommended antiemetic regimen[a]
High (cisplatin)	Serotonin antagonist
	plus
	Dexamethasone (12 mg)
	plus
	Aprepitant (125 mg)
High/moderate	Serotonin antagonist
	plus
	Dexamethasone (20 mg)
Low	Single agent, such as a corticosteroid or serotonin antagonist
Minimal	No preventive agent is recommended for general use

[a] See Table 2 for doses.

NK_1 antagonists

Aprepitant is the first NK_1-antagonist antiemetic, although others are in development. NK_1 antagonists have demonstrated activity against a wide range of emetogenic stimuli. Although less effective than serotonin antagonists as single agents against acute emesis, NK_1 antagonists have shown superior activity against delayed emesis, suggesting the value of combination therapy.

In a multicenter, randomized, double-blind, phase III trial, 866 breast cancer patients being treated with cyclophosphamide with or without doxorubicin or epirubicin were randomized to receive either a regimen of aprepitant (125 mg), ondansetron (8 mg bid), and dexamethasone (12 mg) on day 1 with aprepitant (80 mg/d) on days 2 to 3 or a standard regimen of ondansetron (8 mg bid) on days 1 to 3 and dexamethasone (20 mg) on day 1. Of the 857 evaluable patients, 50.8% in the aprepitant arm, versus 42.5% (P = .015) in the standard regimen arm, achieved a complete response. In addition, more patients in the aprepitant arm achieved a complete response during both acute (75.7% vs 69.0%; P = .034) and delayed (55.4% vs 49.1%; P = .064) phases. Both treatments were generally well tolerated.

COMBINATION ANTIEMETIC REGIMENS

Table 3 summarizes recommended antiemetic regimens, according to the emetic potential of the chemotherapy regimen.

Serotonin antagonist plus dexamethasone Combinations of a 5-HT_3 antagonist and dexamethasone form the basis of the most effective regimens for controlling acute chemotherapy-induced emesis. Use of these two agents combined has proved to be more effective than either agent alone. Addition of an NK_1 antagonist (aprepitant) results in increased activity against acute cisplatin-induced emesis. However, inhibition by aprepitant of the CYP3A4 metabolic pathway may require a decrease in the dose of concomitantly administered dexamethasone.

TREATMENT OF EMESIS

ACUTE EMESIS

A management strategy to prevent acute chemotherapy-induced emesis is outlined in Table 3. All patients should receive education and reassurance, as well as antiemetics tailored to the chemotherapy regimen. For regimens that commonly cause emesis (> 30%), antiemetic combinations are recommended; for regimens of low risk (10% to 30% incidence), a single agent will usually suffice. As stated in Table 3, chemotherapy of minimal risk typically does not require preventive treatment.

DELAYED EMESIS

Delayed emesis is defined as nausea or vomiting beginning or persisting ≥ 24 hours after chemotherapy administration. The pathophysiology of this problem is unclear, but it is particularly common after high-dose cisplatin (≥ 50 mg/m^2), carboplatin (≥ 300 mg/m^2), cyclophosphamide (≥ 600 mg/m^2), or doxorubicin (≥ 50 mg/m^2).

In one natural history study, 89% of patients experienced some delayed emesis from 24 to 120 hours after receiving high-dose cisplatin, with a peak incidence occurring between 48 and 72 hours. With anthracyclines or cyclophosphamide, the rate of delayed emesis without preventive antiemetics is about 30%.

Some observations suggest that delayed emesis may begin earlier. When combination antiemetic regimens for acute emesis "fail," the initial emetic episode is often at 17 to 23 hours following chemotherapy. In some trials, antiemetics to prevent delayed emesis have been initiated at 16 to 17 hours.

Treatment options The combination of oral dexamethasone and metoclopramide has been found to be superior to dexamethasone alone or placebo in a double-blind, randomized trial. The combination of dexamethasone and aprepitant has demonstrated efficacy. Activity of palonosetron may also continue for several days. The recommended doses and schedules for the prevention of delayed emesis are given in Table 4.

ANTICIPATORY EMESIS

This problem is defined as nausea or vomiting beginning before the administration of chemotherapy in patients with poor emetic control during previous chemotherapy. As this problem is a conditioned response, the hospital environment or other treatment-related associations may trigger the onset of emesis unrelated to chemotherapy. Strong emetic stimuli combined with poor emetic control increase the likelihood that anticipatory emesis will occur.

Treatment approach Behavioral therapy involving systematic desensitization can be helpful in managing anticipatory emesis. Also, benzodiazepines appear to be useful.

TABLE 4: Treatment regimens for prevention of delayed emesis

Risk level	Duration	Agent	Dose and schedule
High	Days 2–4	Aprepitant	80 mg PO qd × 2
		plus	
		Dexamethasone	8 mg PO qd × 3
		Serotonin antagonist	
		Ondansetron	8 mg PO bid
		Dolasetron	100 mg PO bid
		Granisetron	1 mg PO bid
		Palonosetron[a]	0.25 mg IV on day 1 only
		plus	
		Dexamethasone	8 mg PO bid
		Metoclopramide	30–40 mg PO bid
		plus	
		Dexamethasone	8 mg PO bid
Moderate	Days 2–3	Serotonin antagonist, dexamethasone, metoclopramide, or aprepitant as single agent or in combination at dose and schedule above	
Low		No preventive regimen is recommended for general use	
Minimal		No preventive regimen is recommended for general use	

[a] Palonosetron has only been studied when given on day 1 with a single dose of dexamethasone (20 mg IV).

However, the best approach to anticipatory emesis is prevention, which underscores the need to provide the most effective and appropriate antiemetic regimens with the initial course of emesis-producing chemotherapy.

SUGGESTED READING

Gralla R, Lichinitser M, Van Der Vegt S, et al: Palonosetron improves prevention of chemotherapy-induced nausea and vomiting following moderately emetogenic chemotherapy: Results of a double-blind randomized phase III trial comparing single doses of palonosetron with ondansetron. Ann Oncol 14:1570–1577, 2003.

Koeller JM, Aapro MS, Gralla RJ, et al: Antiemetic guidelines: Creating a more practical treatment approach. Support Care Cancer 10:519–522, 2002.

Kris MG, Gralla RJ, Clark RA, et al: Incidence, course, and severity of delayed nausea and vomiting following the administration of high-dose cisplatin. J Clin Oncol 3:1379–1384, 1985.

Poli-Bigelli S, Rodrigues-Pereira J, Carides AD, et al: Addition of the neurokinin 1 receptor antagonist aprepitant to standard antiemetic therapy improves control of chemotherapy-induced nausea and vomiting: Results from a randomized, double-blind, placebo-controlled trial in Latin America. Cancer 97:3090–3098, 2003.

Rojas C, Stathis M, Thomas AG, et al: Palonosetron exhibits unique molecular interactions with the 5-HT3 receptor. Anesth Analg 107:469–478, 2008.

Saito M, Aogi K, Sekine I, et al: Palonosetron plus dexamethasone versus granisetron plus dexamethasone for prevention of nausea and vomiting during chemotherapy: A double-blind, double-dummy, randomised, comparative phase III trial. Lancet Oncol 10:115–124, 2009.

Tremblay PB, Kaiser R, Sezer O, et al: Variations in the 5-hydroxytryptamine type 3B receptor gene as predictors of the efficacy of antiemetic treatment in cancer patients. J Clin Oncol 21:2147–2155, 2003.

Warr DG, Hesketh PJ, Gralla RJ, et al: Efficacy and tolerability of aprepitant for the prevention of chemotherapy-induced nausea and vomiting in patients with breast cancer after moderately emetogenic chemotherapy. J Clin Oncol 23:2822–2830, 2005.

Abbreviations in this chapter

ASCO = American Society of Clinical Oncology; MASCC = Multinational Association of Supportive Care in Cancer

CHAPTER 36

Fatigue and dyspnea

Sriram Yennurajalingam, MD, and Eduardo Bruera, MD

Fatigue and dyspnea are two of the most common symptoms associated with advanced cancer. Fatigue is also commonly associated with cancer treatment and occurs in up to 90% of patients undergoing chemotherapy. Both symptoms have many possible underlying causes. In most patients, the etiology of fatigue or dyspnea is multifactorial, with many contributing interrelated abnormalities. In one study of patients with advanced cancer, fatigue was found to be significantly correlated with the intensity of dyspnea. This chapter will discuss the mechanisms, clinical features, assessment, and management of both of these troublesome and often undertreated symptoms in cancer patients.

FATIGUE

Cancer-related fatigue is defined by the NCCN as "a distressing, persistent, subjective sense of tiredness or exhaustion related to cancer or cancer treatment that is not proportional to recent activity and interferes with usual functioning." In cancer patients, fatigue is often severe; has a marked anticipatory component; and results in lack of energy, malaise, lethargy, and diminished mental functioning that profoundly impairs quality of life. It may be present early in the course of the illness, may be exacerbated by treatments, and is present in almost all patients with advanced cancer.

Fatigue is sometimes referred to as asthenia, tiredness, lack of energy, weakness, and exhaustion. Not all these terms have the same meaning to all patient populations. Moreover, different studies of fatigue and asthenia have looked at different outcomes, ranging from physical performance to the purely subjective sensation.

MECHANISM

The mechanisms of cancer-related fatigue are not well understood. Substances produced by the tumor are postulated to induce fatigue. Blood from a fatigued subject when injected into a rested subject has produced manifestations of fatigue. The host production of cytokines in response to the tumor can also have a direct fatigue-inducing effect. Muscular or neuromuscular junction abnormalities are a possible cause of chemotherapy- or radiotherapy-induced fatigue. In summary, fatigue is the result of many syndromes—not just one. Multiple mechanisms are involved in causing fatigue in most patients with advanced cancer.

CLINICAL FEATURES

The causes of fatigue in an individual patient are often multiple, with many interrelated factors. Figure 1 summarizes the main contributors to fatigue in cancer patients.

Cachexia

Cancer cachexia results from a complex interaction of host and tumor products. Host cytokines such as tumor necrosis factor, interleukin-1 (IL-1), and IL-6 are capable of causing decreased food intake, loss of body weight, a decrease in synthesis of both lipids and proteins, and increased lipolysis. The metabolic abnormalities involved in the production of cachexia and the loss of muscle mass resulting from progressive cachexia may cause profound weakness and fatigue. However, many abnormalities described in Figure 1 are capable of causing profound fatigue in the absence of significant weight loss.

Immobility

Decreased physical activity has been shown to cause deconditioning and decreased endurance to both exercise and normal activities of daily living. On the other hand, overexertion is a frequent cause of fatigue in noncancer patients. It should also be considered in younger cancer patients who are undergoing aggressive antineoplastic treatments such as radiation therapy and chemotherapy and who are nevertheless trying to maintain their social and professional activities.

Psychological distress

In patients without cancer who present with fatigue, the final diagnosis is psychological (eg, depression, anxiety, and other psychological disorders) in almost 75% of patients. The frequency of major psychiatric disorders in cancer patients is low.

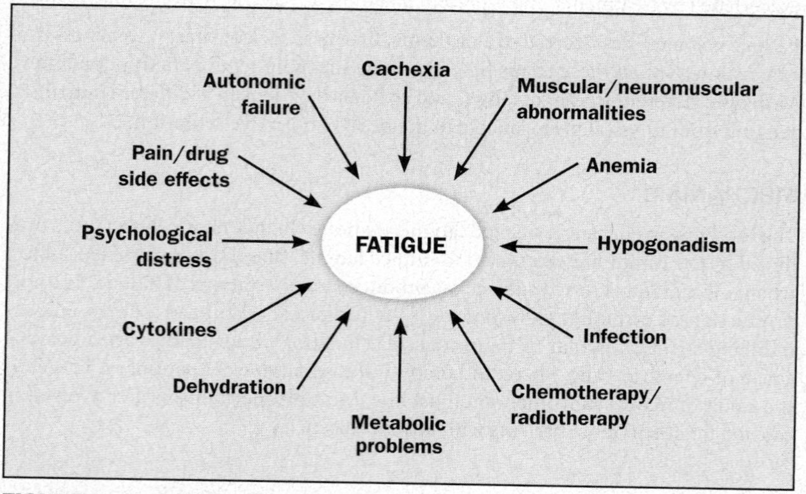

FIGURE 1: Contributors to fatigue in cancer patients.

However, symptoms of psychological distress or adjustment disorders with depressive or anxious moods are much more frequent. Patients with an adjustment disorder or a major depressive disorder can have fatigue as their most prevalent symptom.

Anemia

Low red blood cell count related to advanced cancer or chemotherapy has been associated with fatigue, and its treatment results in improvement of fatigue and quality of life in these patients. In terminally ill patients with advanced cancer, treatment of anemia may not resolve fatigue adequately due to the multifactorial nature of its etiology. Fatigue may be the result of the more intense nature of the other contributory factors.

Autonomic failure

Autonomic insufficiency is a frequent complication of advanced cancer. Autonomic failure has also been documented in patients with a subset of severe chronic fatigue syndrome. Although the association between fatigue and autonomic dysfunction has not been established in cancer patients, it should be suspected in patients with severe postural hypotension or other signs of autonomic failure.

Hypogonadism

Both intrathecal and systemic opioid therapies, as well as cachexia and some antineoplastic therapies, can result in hypogonadotropic hypogonadism. This condition can lead to fatigue, depression, and reduced libido.

Chemotherapy/radiotherapy

Chemotherapy and radiotherapy treatments are common causes of fatigue in cancer patients. The pattern of fatigue reported by patients with cancer who receive myelosuppressive chemotherapy is cyclical. It begins within the first few days after therapy is started, peaks around the time of the white blood cell nadir, and diminishes in the week thereafter, only to recur again with the next cycle of chemotherapy. Fatigue tends to worsen with subsequent cycles of chemotherapy, which suggests a cumulative dose-related toxic effect. Compared with women with no history of cancer, former patients with breast cancer who had received adjuvant chemotherapy reported more fatigue and worse quality of life due to this symptom. Similar results have been noted in breast cancer patients who have been treated with high-dose chemotherapy and autologous stem-cell support and in patients treated for lymphoma.

Radiation therapy tends to cause a different pattern of fatigue. It is often described as a "wave" that starts abruptly within a few hours after treatment and subsides shortly thereafter. Fatigue has been noted to decrease in the first 2 weeks after localized treatment for breast cancer but then to increase as radiation therapy persists into week 4. It then decreases again 3 weeks after radiation therapy ceases. The mechanism for fatigue in these situations is not well understood.

Administration of chemotherapy and radiotherapy for malignancy causes a specific fatigue syndrome. Combined therapy with the two modalities appears to cause worse fatigue than does either modality given alone.

TABLE 1: Assessment of fatigue

Functional capacity	
	Treadmill performance (time, speed)
	Number of errors (eg, driving, pilots)
	Six-minute walk test
	Hand-grip strength test
Task-related fatigue (eg, treadmill, driving)	
	VAS (visual analog scales), numerical scale
	Pearson and Byars Fatigue Feeling Checklist
Performance status	
	Eastern Cooperative Oncology Group
	Karnofsky Performance Status scale
	Edmonton Functional Assessment Tool
Subjective assessment of fatigue	
	VAS, numeric scale
	Edmonton Symptom Assessment Scale–Fatigue (0 to 10 scale; 0 = no fatigue, 10 = worst fatigue)
	Brief Fatigue Inventory
	Piper Fatigue Self-Report Scale
	Functional Assessment of Cancer Therapy–Fatigue subscale

Surgery

Surgery is another common cause of fatigue in patients with cancer. In addition, commonly used medications such as opioids and hypnotics may cause sedation and fatigue.

Other

Comorbid conditions not necessarily related to cancer, such as renal failure or congestive heart failure, may coexist and contribute to the problem. Other conditions include the chronic stress response (possibly mediated through the hypothalamic-pituitary axis), disrupted sleep or circadian rhythms, and hormonal changes (eg, premature menopause and androgen blockade secondary to cancer treatment).

ASSESSMENT

Since fatigue is essentially a subjective sensation, it is by nature difficult to assess. There is agreement that self-assessment should be the "gold standard." Due to the complex nature of the symptoms of fatigue, an effort to identify a set of diagnostic criteria similar to those for depression has been attempted. This syndromal approach has been useful to assess the presence or absence of the clinical syndrome of fatigue.

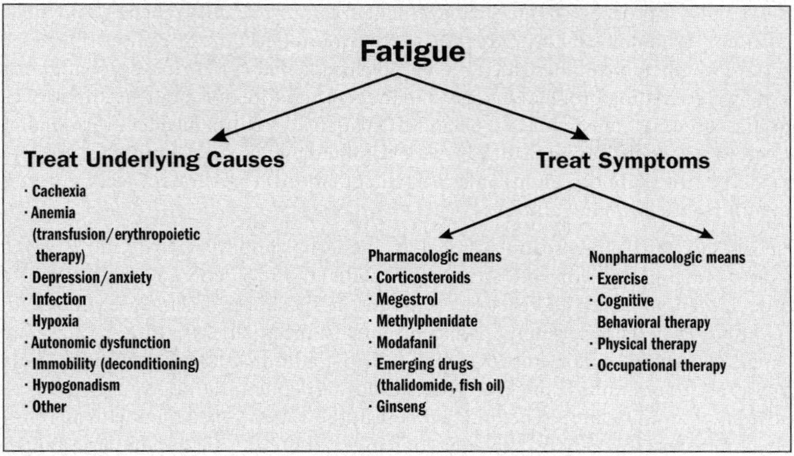

FIGURE 2: Therapeutic approach to managing fatigue.

Table 1 summarizes the four most common measurable indices to assess fatigue. The first category in Table 1 looks at the objective function that the patient is capable of performing when subjected to a standard task. These functional tasks have limited value in cancer care, however, as they are very difficult for the advanced cancer patient to perform.

The second category in Table 1 attempts to assess the subjective effects of standard tasks.

The third category in Table 1 has been the most commonly used in oncology. The two most common scales, ECOG and Karnofsky Performance Status, consist of a physician's rating of the patient's functional capabilities after a regular medical consultation. A physical therapist completes the Edmonton Functional Assessment Tool and attempts to determine the functional status, as well as all the obstacles to clinical performance, of these patients.

The fourth category in Table 1 is the most relevant for both clinical management and clinical trials in fatigue. Visual analog scales, numerical scales, the Brief Fatigue Inventory, and the Piper Fatigue Self-Report Scale have been validated. In addition, there are validated functional assessments in most quality-of-life questionnaires.

In addition to the assessment of the intensity of fatigue, the clinical assessment of these patients requires clinicians to determine the impact of all factors on the presence of fatigue.

MANAGEMENT

To treat fatigue optimally, it is vital to identify and prioritize the different underlying factors in the individual patient. Thorough records, including recent treatment history, physical examination, and medication review, in addition to simple laboratory investigations will help identify possible underlying causes. Figure 2 outlines a therapeutic approach to fatigue management in cancer patients. Whenever possible, an attempt should be made to treat these contributing factors. It is impossible to be certain whether one of these identified problems is a major contributor to fatigue or simply a coexisting problem in a given patient. Therefore, it is of great importance to measure the intensity of fatigue and the patient's performance before and after treating any contributing factor. If the level of fatigue does not improve after correction of these abnormalities, it is clear then that further treatment will not result in improvement in the future.

In patients with cancer treatment–related fatigue, it is important to exclude specific causes, such as hypothyroidism, hypogonadism, and anemia, and to consider other potential adverse effects of treatment. If specific problems are identified, they should be appropriately managed. For instance, patients with anemia may experience symptomatic improvement with the administration of erythropoietic therapy (epoetin alfa [Epogen, Procrit] and darbepoetin alfa [Aranesp]) at the dose and administration schedule that best fit the patient's need. Epoetin alfa may be administered weekly by subcutaneous injection; darbepoetin alfa has a longer half-life, requiring less frequent dosing. Dosages and schedules of both agents may be increased if necessary. (For up-to-date information about the safety and use of erythropoiesis-stimulating agents, go to www.fda.gov/Drugs/DrugSafety/PostmarketDrugSafetyInformationForPatientsandProviders/ucm109375.htm)

In most patients, there will be no identified reversible causes. A number of effective pharmacologic and nonpharmacologic symptomatic treatments are available for these patients.

Pharmacologic treatments

Corticosteroids

There is substantial evidence that corticosteroids can reduce fatigue and other symptoms in cancer patients. They are probably best retained for short-term use. Their beneficial effects generally last between 2 and 4 weeks, and longer-term use carries the risk of serious adverse effects. Most studies have used the equivalent of 40 mg/d of prednisone.

Progestational agents

In recent studies of terminally ill patients, megestrol (60–480 mg/d) has been shown to have a rapid (less than 1 week) beneficial effect on appetite, fatigue, and general well-being.

Psychostimulants

Psychostimulants (eg, methylphenidate, 5–10 mg in the morning and at noon or 5 mg as needed) may be of use in treating fatigue in patients with advanced cancer. The safety and efficacy of long-term methylphenidate use for fatigue have not been established. Recently, Morrow et al found modafanil (Provigil) therapy to be beneficial in mitigating fatigue, especially when used in cancer patients with severe baseline fatigue who were on cytotoxic therapy.

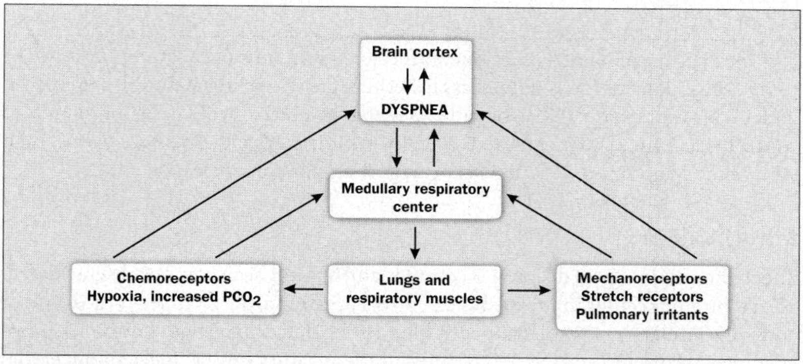

FIGURE 3: Mechanisms of dyspnea. PCO_2 = partial pressure of carbon dioxide.

In addition to these agents, a number of other drugs have been tried in preliminary studies in patients with fatigue. Early positive results have been observed with both thalidomide (Thalomid) and fish oils.

In a recent double-blind, randomized, controlled trial by the NCCTG, 282 patients with cancer reported improvement of cancer-related fatigue on treatment with American ginseng (*Panax quinquefolius*) vs placebo.

In a randomized, controlled study of 142 patients with advanced cancer conducted by Bruera et al, donepezil (Aricept) was not significantly superior to placebo in the treatment of cancer-related fatigue.

Nonpharmacologic treatment

Physical therapy and occupational therapy

Physical therapy may encourage increased activity, where appropriate, and provide active range of motion to prevent painful tendon retraction. Recent evidence suggests that aerobic exercise may reduce fatigue during chemotherapy. Assessment of the home environment by an occupational therapist can be useful. The provision of ramps, walkers, wheelchairs, elevated toilets, and hospital beds may allow the patient to remain at home in a safe environment. Education regarding the pattern of fatigue during treatment has been helpful. Counseling (more specifically, cognitive behavioral therapy) for stress management, depression, and anxiety may reduce distress and fatigue as well as improve mood.

Segal et al recently studied the effect of exercise on the fatigue experienced by prostate cancer patients receiving radiation therapy. Over 24 weeks, 40 patients initiating radiotherapy with or without androgen deprivation took part in resistance exercise, 40 participated in aerobic exercise, and 41 received usual care. Results of the FACIT-F subscale showed that when compared with usual care, resistance exercise resulted in both short- and long-term improvement in fatigue and aerobic exercise resulted in short-term improvement *(Segal RJ et al: J Clin Oncol 27:344–351, 2009).*

DYSPNEA

Dyspnea has been defined as an uncomfortable awareness of breathing. It is a subjective sensation and does not necessarily correlate with clinical findings in a given patient. It occurs in up to 75% of patients with advanced cancer, and good symptom control is less frequently achieved, even by experienced palliative care teams, than with other symptoms of terminal cancer, such as pain or nausea.

MECHANISMS

The pathophysiology of dyspnea is complex and has not been completely elucidated. The respiratory center in the medulla controls breathing, but dyspnea is the result of cortical stimulation. Abnormalities of blood gases detected by both lung and central chemoreceptors and stimulation of lung and respiratory muscle mechanoreceptors stimulate the respiratory center. Mechanoreceptors respond to stretch and irritants and also have a demonstrated effect on the brain cortex, causing dyspnea. In addition, it is possible that both the chemoreceptors and the medullary respiratory center stimulate the cerebral cortex, directly contributing to the sensation of dyspnea. Figure 3 summarizes the mechanisms of dyspnea.

CLINICAL FEATURES

In patients with advanced cancer, there are many causes of dyspnea, such as pulmonary embolism, lung metastasis, pleural effusion, congestive heart failure, anemia, psychological distress, pneumonia, muscle weakness, and preexisting pulmonary disease.

Direct tumor effects

Dyspnea may be the result of direct primary or metastatic tumor effects such as airway obstruction, atelectasis, parenchymal lung involvement, phrenic nerve palsy, carcinomatous lymphangitis, or superior vena caval obstruction.

TABLE 2: Management of specific causes of dyspnea in cancer patients

Cause	Treatment
Airway obstruction by tumor	Corticosteroids (eg, dexamethasone 6–8 mg qid), radiation therapy
Pleural or pericardial effusion	Drain if effusion is significant
Pneumonia	Antibiotics (oral route preferred)
Carcinomatous lymphangitis	Corticosteroids (eg, dexamethasone 6–8 mg qid)
Congestive heart failure	Diuretic therapy (eg, furosemide 10–20 mg IV/SC) and ACE inhibitors
Underlying asthma, COPD	Optimize bronchodilators, corticosteroids if required
Anemia	Transfuse packed red blood cells, erythropoietic therapy

ACE = angiotensin-converting enzyme; COPD = chronic obstructive pulmonary disease, IV = intravenous; SC = subcutaneous

Indirect tumor effects

Indirect cancer effects include pneumonia, anemia, pleural effusion, and pulmonary embolism. Cardiac complications of cancer, such as congestive heart failure, pericarditis, or pericardial effusion, may contribute to the problem. Intra-abdominal disorders, such as gross ascites or hepatomegaly, may cause elevation of the diaphragm and may interfere with respiratory function. Generalized muscle weakness due to cachexia or fatigue may exacerbate breathlessness. Preexisting lung diseases, including asthma or chronic obstructive pulmonary disease (COPD), may contribute to the problem.

Treatment side effects

Contributing treatment side effects include pneumonitis or fibrosis following chemotherapy or radiotherapy.

Psychological conditions

Anxiety, depression, or somatization will alter a patient's perception of dyspnea. Anxiety has been found to be an independent correlate of the intensity of dyspnea in cancer patients with moderate to severe dyspnea. Any of these factors may occur in isolation or in combination, and care is needed during assessment, as there are often many contributors in an individual patient.

ASSESSMENT

Dyspnea is a subjective sensation, and researchers have found much variability in the expression of dyspnea in individuals with similar levels of functional abnormalities. In addition, patients' perception of dyspnea can be influenced by their beliefs and intrapsychic and cultural factors. The presence or absence of physical signs such as tachypnea, wheezing, or use of accessory muscles is not a reliable indicator of the degree of distress felt by patients. The intensity of dyspnea can be easily assessed using verbal, numeric, or visual analog scales similar to those used in pain or nausea. A descriptive study by Henoch et al examined dyspnea in correlation with other symptoms, as well as personal and health factors in 105 patients with advanced lung cancer. More than 50% of patients had perceived dyspnea. The intensity of dyspnea and the occurrence of activity-related dyspnea correlated with the presence of anxiety, depression, fatigue, and cough. A lower coping capacity was associated with a greater likelihood of dyspnea.

Recently, maximal inspiratory pressure has been found to be an independent correlate of the intensity of dyspnea. Physical examination, chest x-ray, and pulse oximetry should be performed. Other investigations, such as complete blood count, echocardiography, or pulmonary function tests, may be indicated.

MANAGEMENT

Specific causes

Underlying specific causes will require treatment as indicated in Table 2.

Symptomatic management

The three modalities of symptomatic treatment in cancer-related dyspnea are oxygen therapy, drug therapy, and counseling.

> In patients with advanced malignant and nonmalignant disease, Bausewein et al found breathing training, walking aids, neuroelectrical muscle stimulation, and chest wall vibration to be effective to relieve dyspnea *(Bausewein C et al: Cochrane Database Syst Rev [2]:CD005623, 2010).*

Oxygen therapy

In hypoxemic cancer patients with dyspnea, oxygen has been shown to provide significant symptomatic relief. Oxygen (O_2) can be administered by nasal cannula at 2–6 L/min or by mask and titrated to maintain an O_2 saturation at > 90%. Care must be taken in patients with COPD. Oxygen is not useful in patients with dyspnea and an O_2 saturation > 90%.

Drug therapy

There is substantial evidence that systemic opioids have a beneficial effect on cancer-related dyspnea. This is possible without inducing respiratory depression. The optimal type, dose, and mode of administration have not been determined. If the patient is already on opioids, the breakthrough dose can be used to manage dyspnea as well as pain. If not, morphine can be started at 5–10 mg PO (or 2.5–5.0 mg SC) q4h with additional prn doses of 2.5–5.0 mg PO (or 2.5 mg SC) every hour for breakthrough dyspnea. Nebulized opiates are not recommended, as there is insufficient evidence to support their use.

Benzodiazepines have not been found to be effective in the general management of dyspnea, but they may be useful for treatment of episodes associated with anxiety attacks. Regular use of benzodiazepines should be avoided where possible to limit side effects, such as confusion or falls.

> In a recent Cochrane review, Simon et al recently found no evidence of beneficial effect from benzodiazepines given to treat dyspnea in patients with advanced cancer and COPD *(Simon ST et al: Cochrane Database Syst Rev [1]:CD007354, 2010).*

Conditions that cause dyspnea in cancer patients and that respond to corticosteroid medication include superior vena caval obstruction, carcinomatous lymphangitis, and COPD. However, corticosteroids may adversely affect muscle function, and the diaphragm may be more susceptible than other muscles. This may be of importance because of the frequency of muscle weakness and fatigue in patients with advanced cancer.

Counseling

Dyspnea is a variable symptom and is exacerbated by physical activities. Patients and families should be educated so they can identify factors likely to worsen dyspnea. Devices such as bathroom aids and wheelchairs can help reduce physical activity, and the addition of portable oxygen can enable the patient to remain active and autonomous. For symptomatic relief, medication such as opioids can be administered 30–45 minutes prior to dyspnea-causing maneuvers. The family should be educated that dyspnea is subjective and that tachypnea and use of accessory muscles do not necessarily indicate that the patient is suffering. The aim of treatment is to relieve the patient's subjective dyspnea, not to abate physical signs of respiratory distress.

SUGGESTED READING

ON FATIGUE

Bruera E, Driver L, Barnes EA, et al: Patient-controlled methylphenidate for the management of fatigue in patients with advanced cancer: A preliminary report. J Clin Oncol 21:4439–4443, 2003.

Bruera E, El Osta B, Valero V, et al: Donepezil for cancer fatigue: A double-blind, randomized, placebo-controlled trial. J Clin Oncol. 25:3475–3481, 2007

Bruera E, Strasser F, Shen L, et al: The effect of donezepil on sedation and other symptoms in patients receiving opioids for cancer pain: A pilot study. J Pain Symptom Manage 26:1049–1054, 2003.

Cleary J: The reversible causes of asthenia in cancer patients, in Portenoy R, Bruera E (eds): Topics in Palliative Care, vol 2, pp 183–202. New York, Oxford University Press, 1998.

Dimeo F, Stieglitz R, Novelli-Fischer U, et al: Effects of physical activity on the fatigue and psychological status of cancer patients during chemotherapy. Cancer 85:2273–2277, 1999.

Hann DM, Garovoy N, Finkelstein B, et al: Fatigue and quality of life in breast cancer patients undergoing autologous stem-cell transplantation: A longitudinal comparative study. J Pain Symptom Manage 17:311–319, 1999.

Henoch I, Bergman B, Gustafsson M, et al: Dyspnea experience in patients with lung cancer in palliative care. Eur J Oncol Nurs 12:86–96, 2007.

Howell SJ, Radford JA, Adams JE, et al: Randomized placebo-controlled trial of testosterone replacement in men with mild Leydig cell insufficiency following cytotoxic chemotherapy. Clin Endocrinol 55:315–324, 2001.

Munch TN, Zhang T, Willey J, et al: The association between anemia and fatigue in patients with advanced cancer receiving palliative care. J Palliat Med 8:1144–1149, 2005.

Neuenschwander H, Bruera E: Pathophysiology of cancer asthenia, in Portenoy R, Bruera E (eds): Topics in Palliative Care, vol 2, pp 171–181. New York, Oxford University Press, 1998.

Sadler IJ, Jacobsen PB, Booth-Jones M, et al: Preliminary evaluation of a clinical syndrome approach to assessing cancer-related fatigue. J Pain Symptom Manage 23:406–416, 2002.

Seidenfeld J, Piper M, Flamm C, et al: Epoetin treatment of anemia associated with cancer therapy: A systematic review and meta-analysis of controlled clinical trials. J Natl Cancer Inst 93:1204–1214, 2001.

ON DYSPNEA

Allard P, Lamontagne C, Bernard P, et al: How effective are supplementary doses of opioids for dyspnea in terminally ill cancer patients? A randomized continuous sequential clinical trial. J Pain Symptom Manage 17:256–265, 1999.

Bruera E, Schmitz B, Pither J, et al: The frequency and correlates of dyspnea in patients with advanced cancer. J Pain Symptom Manage 19:357–362, 2000.

Currow DC, Agar M, Smith J, et al: Does palliative home oxygen improve dyspnoea? A consecutive cohort study. Palliat Med 23:309–316, 2009.

Mancini I, Body JJ: Assessment of dyspnea in advanced cancer patients. Support Care Cancer 7:229–232, 1999.

Reddy SK, Parsons HA, Elsayem A, et al: Characteristics and correlates of dyspnea in patients with advanced cancer. J Palliat Med 12:29–36, 2009.

Ripamonti C, Fulfaro F, Bruera E: Dyspnea in patients with advanced cancer: Incidence, causes, and treatments. Cancer Treat Rev 42:60–80, 1998.

Simon ST, Higginson IJ, Booth S, et al: Benzodiazepines for the relief of breathlessness in advanced malignant and non-malignant diseases in adults. Cochrane Database Syst Rev (1):CD007354, 2010.

Xue D, Abernethy A: Management of dyspnea in advanced lung cancer: recent data and emerging concepts. Curr Opin Support Palliat Care 4:85–91, 2010.

Abbreviations in this chapter

ECOG = Eastern Cooperative Oncology Group; FACIT-F = Functional Assessment of Chronic Illness Therapy–Fatigue; NCCN = National Comprehensive Cancer Network; NCCTG = North Central Cancer Treatment Group

CHAPTER 37

Anorexia and cachexia

Aminah Jatoi, MD

Many patients with advanced cancer undergo a wasting syndrome associated with cancer anorexia/cachexia and asthenia. In defining these terms a bit further, anorexia is associated with a marked loss of appetite and/or an aversion to food. Cachexia is a wasting syndrome associated with loss of body mass, including lean body mass, associated with a disease. In a study that assessed symptoms in cancer patients being entered into a palliative care service, anorexia/cachexia and asthenia were more common problems than were pain or dyspnea. Patients who exhibit such symptoms generally have a short survival time, respond poorly to cytotoxic agents, and suffer from increased toxicity from these agents.

In addition, cancer anorexia/cachexia often is associated with weakness, fatigue, and a poor quality of life. This problem not only affects the patient but also frequently has an impact on family members, as the patient is no longer able to participate fully in eating as a social activity.

ANOREXIA

DIAGNOSTIC CRITERIA

Cancer cachexia is not difficult to identify. In North Central Cancer Treatment Group (NCCTG) research trials involving more than 2,500 patients, simple criteria for anorexia/cachexia have been used:

- a 5-lb weight loss in the preceding 2 months and/or an estimated daily caloric intake of < 20 calories/kg
- a desire by the patient to increase his or her appetite and gain weight
- the physician's opinion that weight gain would be beneficial for the patient.

Recently, other investigators have attempted to provide more detailed or comprehensive definitions of cachexia. These definitions are important in stimulating further discussion of this entity and its pathophysiology.

> **Artoun and others found that over time, cancer patients treated with a well-tolerated intervention (eg, sorafenib) can manifest a notable degree of muscle wasting. Sorafenib-treated patients manifested an 8% decrease in lean tissue at 1 year *(Artoun S et al: J Clin Oncol 28:1054–1060, 2010).***

MANAGEMENT

Nutritional counseling

Nutritional counseling, as provided by written materials, dietitians, physicians, and nurses,

A recent meta-analysis investigating the effect of dietary counseling on clinical outcomes in cancer patients revealed a trend suggesting an improvement in quality of life. The authors noted that nutritional counseling in cancer patients merits further study *(Haldanarson TR et al: J Support Oncol 6:234–237, 2008).*

has been recommended, although its value has not been well demonstrated. Recommendations typically include eating frequent, small meals (as opposed to large meals), consuming larger quantities of food in the morning than in the evening, and avoiding spicy foods. Patients may do better if they are not exposed to the aroma of cooking. Although the benefits of such nutritional counseling are clearly limited, it does appear reasonable to provide.

Recent trials have led to further interest in studying dietary counseling. Ravasco and others observed improvements in treatment-related side effects and quality of life among colorectal cancer patients who had received dietary counseling as part of a randomized controlled trial. Similar findings from this same group were observed among head and neck cancer patients. These findings require confirmation.

Appetite stimulants

Corticosteroids

Corticosteroids were the first agents to undergo placebo-controlled, double-blind evaluation for possible use in cancer cachexia. The first such trial, conducted in the 1970s by Moertel and colleagues at the Mayo Clinic, demonstrated that corticosteroids can stimulate appetite in patients with advanced, incurable cancer. Several subsequent placebo-controlled trials, using various steroid preparations and doses, have confirmed these results.

Dexamethasone (3 to 8 mg/d) is a reasonable option for clinical use. Known detriments to corticosteroid use include the well-known toxicities associated with chronic administration, including myopathy, peptic ulcer disease, infection, and adrenal suppression. Many patients with advanced cancer anorexia and cachexia, however, do not survive long enough to suffer from these toxicities.

Progestational agents

Several placebo-controlled, double-blind clinical trials have demonstrated that progestational agents, such as megestrol and medroxyprogesterone, can lead to appetite stimulation and weight gain in patients with anorexia and cachexia. These trials also demonstrated that the effect of these drugs is seen in a matter of days and that they are effective antiemetics.

Although high doses of progestational agents can cause adrenal suppression because of their mild corticosteroid-type activity (a phenomenon not well understood by many clinicians), they do not appear to cause many of the side effects attributable to classic corticosteroids (such as peptic ulcer disease, myopathy, and opportunistic infections). In lieu of this adrenal suppression, however, stress doses of corticosteroids may be necessary in patients with trauma or infection or in surgical patients while on progestational agents. On the other hand, progestational agents increase the risk of thromboembolic phenomena—a side effect not seen with classic corticosteroids.

A dose-response study with megestrol demonstrated a positive correlation between appetite stimulation and increased megestrol doses, as doses ranged from 160 to 800 mg/d. Nonetheless, given that appetite stimulation has been demonstrated with megestrol acetate doses as low as 240 mg/d, much lower doses are used by many physicians, based primarily upon cost considerations.

Navari and Brenner evaluated 80 patients with cancer, randomizing them to megestrol acetate or to megestrol acetate and olanzapine. The latter group showed greater rates of weight gain and improvement in appetite. These results suggested that this combination merits further testing *(Navari RM, Brenner MC: Support Care Cancer 18:951–956, 2010).*

In the United States, a liquid formulation of megestrol is considerably less expensive than the tablet form, and, milligram for milligram, the liquid preparation is more bioavailable. It is reasonable to start with 400 mg/d of liquid megestrol, titrating this dose upward (maximum, 800 mg/d) or downward based upon clinical response or the emergence of side effects.

A randomized, prospective clinical trial comparing the utility of megestrol (800 mg/d) with dexamethasone (0.75 mg qid) demonstrated similar effects of these medications on patients' appetites but different toxicity profiles. Whereas megestrol was associated with a higher incidence of thromboembolic phenomena, dexamethasone was associated with more myopathy, cushingoid body changes, and peptic ulcers.

Other agents

Various other drugs have been evaluated definitively for the treatment of cancer anorexia and cachexia and have demonstrated little or no benefit. These drugs include fluoxymesterone, pentoxifylline, hydrazine sulfate, dronabinol, cyproheptadine, eicosapentaenoic acid (EPA), and etanercept (Enbrel). Of note, however, the antiserotonergic drug cyproheptadine does appear to be a relatively strong appetite stimulant in patients with the carcinoid syndrome, presumably because it directly counteracts the large amounts of serotonin secreted in these patients.

EPA has been tested extensively for cancer anorexia and cachexia. Although preliminary studies had claimed improvement in appetite, body composition, and survival with EPA, these favorable findings have not been borne out in subsequent phase III trials. Three phase III trials have shown that EPA does relatively little for cancer anorexia and cachexia when tested in the setting of either EPA versus placebo or EPA versus megestrol.

A number of other drugs have been evaluated in a pilot fashion for the treatment of cancer anorexia and cachexia. They include branched-chain amino acids, thalidomide (Thalomid), metoclopramide, oxandrolone (Oxandrin), insulin, and adenosine triphosphate. It is hoped that new information will be available in the near future to shed light on the possible therapeutic roles of these agents.

Even more recently, exciting data have arisen from a preliminary study of ghrelin, an endogenous ligand for the growth hormone secretagogue receptor. A study of 21 patients demonstrated the safety of this substance, allowing for the possibility of its further testing in the future.

> Montavani and others recently conducted a 332-patient trial that examined the effect of medroxyprogesterone or megesterol acetate, eicosapentanoic acid, L-carnitine, or thalidomide or a combination of all of these agents for 4 months on cancer cachexia–lean body mass, resting energy expenditure, and fatigue plus secondary endpoints. A preliminary investigation found that combination therapy was most beneficial and suggested that further study of combination approaches be performed *(Montavani G et al: Oncologist 15:200–211, 2010).*

Enteral or parenteral nutrition

Despite the demonstrated efficacy of corticosteroids and progestational agents in patients with cancer anorexia and cachexia, these drugs do not have a major long-term impact on the vast majority of such patients. Consequently, other treatment approaches, such as enteral or parenteral nutritional methods, have been studied extensively. Several randomized trials failed to demonstrate that these nutritional approaches improve either quantity or quality of life. As a result, experts generally agree that the routine use of parenteral or enteral nutrition cannot be justified in patients with advanced cancer anorexia and cachexia.

There are, however, relatively rare circumstances in which parenteral nutrition may play a role in patients with advanced cancer. Such circumstances have been documented by case reports and small case series and have included patients with GI insufficiency due to surgery, radiation therapy, or abdominal carcinomatosis (without impending failure of other organs). The decision to initiate parenteral nutrition under these circumstances typically requires a multidisciplinary approach with extensive discussions between healthcare providers and family members.

Prophylactic therapy

Given the positive impact of corticosteroids and progestational agents on cancer anorexia and cachexia and the fact that many patients with advanced cancer die with, and/or of, inanition, the potential prophylactic use of these agents was evaluated. A double-blind trial was conducted in which patients with newly diagnosed, extensive-stage small-cell lung cancer were randomized to receive megestrol or placebo along with standard chemoradiation therapy. This trial was unable to demonstrate any beneficial effect of megestrol on treatment response, quality of life, or survival.

Thus, patients should not be treated prophylactically for cancer anorexia and cachexia outside of a clinical trial. Rather, such treatment should be reserved for patients in whom anorexia and cachexia are patient-determined, symptomatic clinical problems.

NUTRITION AS IT RELATES TO END-OF-LIFE CARE

Anorexia and cachexia are major problems for many oncology patients as they approach the final stage of life. Family members are generally more distressed than the patients if/when appetite stimulants do not provide relief. Questions commonly arise about giving enteral or parenteral nutrition or "forcing" patients to consume more calories in the belief that they would feel better, get stronger, and live longer. A small measure of appropriate education, noting that the intake of more calories does not appear to have a clinical benefit, provides substantial relief. It is worthwhile to note that patients randomized to receive total parenteral nutrition or appetite stimulants (such as megestrol) do not live any longer than do control patients and that "force-feeding" is not in patients' best interests.

SUGGESTED READING

Bozzetti F, Mariani L: Defining and classifying cancer cachexia: A proposal by the SCRINIO Working Group. JPEN J Parenter Enteral Nutr 33:361–367, 2009.

Evans WJ, Morley JE, Argilés J, et al: Cachexia: A new definition. Clin Nutr 27:793–799, 2008.

Halfdanarson TR, Thordardottir E, West CP, et al: Does dietary counseling improve quality of life in cancer patients? A systematic review and meta-analysis. J Support Oncol 6:234–237, 2008.

Jatoi A, Dakhil SR, Nguyen PL, et al: A placebo-controlled double blind trial of etanercept for the cancer anorexia/weight loss syndrome: Results from N00C1 from the North Central Cancer Treatment Group. Cancer 110:1396–1403, 2007.

Jatoi A, Rowland K, Loprinzi CL, et al: An eicosapentaenoic acid supplement versus megestrol acetate versus both for patients with cancer-associated wasting: A North Central Cancer Treatment Group and National Cancer Institute of Canada collaborative effort. J Clin Oncol 22:2469–2476, 2004.

Jatoi A, Windschitl HE, Loprinzi CL, et al: Dronabinol vs megestrol acetate vs both for cancer-associated anorexia: A North Central Cancer Treatment Group Study. J Clin Oncol 20:567–573, 2002.

Loprinzi CL, Kugler JW, Sloan JA, et al: Randomized comparison of megestrol acetate versus dexamethasone versus fluoxymesterone for the treatment of cancer anorexia/cachexia. J Clin Oncol 17:3299–3306, 1999.

Lundholm K, Körner U, Bunnebo L, et al: Insulin treatment in cancer cachexia: Effects on survival, metabolism, and physical functioning. Clin Cancer Res 13:2699–2706, 2007.

Mann M, Koller E, Murgo A, et al: Glucocorticoid-like activity of megestrol. Arch Intern Med 157:1651–1656, 1997.

Moertel CG, Schutt AJ, Reitemeier RJ, et al: Corticosteroid therapy of preterminal gastrointestinal cancer. Cancer 33:1607–1609, 1974.

Ravasco P, Monteiro-Grillo I, Marques Vidal P, et al: Impact of nutrition on outcome: A prospective randomized controlled trial in patients with head and neck cancer undergoing radiotherapy. Head Neck 27:659–668, 2005.

Ravasco P, Monteiro-Grillo I, Vidal PM, et al: Dietary counseling improves patient outcomes: A prospective, randomized controlled trial in colorectal cancer patients undergoing radiotherapy. J Clin Oncol 23:1431–1438, 2005.

Rock CL: Dietary counseling is beneficial for the patient with cancer. J Clin Oncol 23:1348–1349, 2005.

Strasser F, Lutz TA, Maeder MT, et al: Safety, tolerability and pharmacokinetics of intravenous ghrelin for cancer-related anorexia/cachexia: A randomised, placebo-controlled, double-blind, double-crossover study. Br J Cancer 98:300–308, 2008.

Abbreviations in this chapter

NCCTG = North Central Cancer Treatment Group; SCRINIO = Screening the Nutritional Status in Oncologic Patients

Dermatologic toxicities associated with targeted therapies

Mario E. Lacouture, MD

Improved cancer therapies have brought about unprecedented improvements in survival along with decreased hematopoietic toxicities, when compared with cytotoxic chemotherapy. Therefore, other components of the cancer experience have come forward, such as supportive care and psychological well-being. Most notably, dermatologic toxicities have gained considerable attention due to their high frequency, appearance in functional and cosmetically sensitive areas, and association with symptoms of pain and pruritus—all of which lead to decreased quality of life and inconsistent dose intensity. In turn, clinical outcome may be affected with dose modifications in response to these untoward events.

Therapies targeting specific pathways or proteins in cancer cells are especially noted for dermatologic toxicities, which affect up to 90% of treated patients. These toxicities are generally a class effect, and will occur with the use of monoclonal antibodies or small-molecule kinase inhibitors with similar targets. Epidermal growth factor receptor (EGFR) inhibitors, ie, erlotinib (Tarceva), cetuximab (Erbitux), and panitumumab (Vectibix), will lead to a papulopustular eruption, xerosis, pruritus, paronychia, alopecia, and hypertrichosis of the face with trichomegaly of the eyelashes. These effects will occur at different times during therapy, and not all patients will develop most toxicities. In a similar fashion, a number of dermatologic side effects have been associated with the small-molecule multikinase inhibitors sunitinib (Sutent) and sorafenib (Nexavar), including hand-foot skin reaction (HFSR), xerosis, rash, and subungual splinter hemorrhages.

On the following pages a number of photographs are provided to depict the various types of dermatologic reactions that may occur in patients receiving these agents.

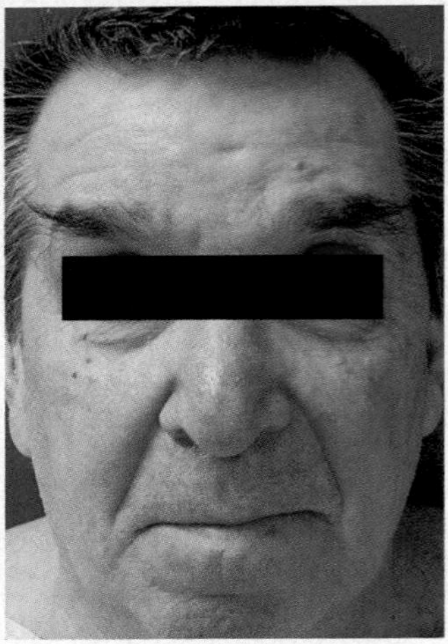

FIGURE 1: Sensory disturbance (first) stage: Within the first few days of EGFR inhibitor drug initiation, a sensation of sunburn, associated with edema, occurs in the central face.

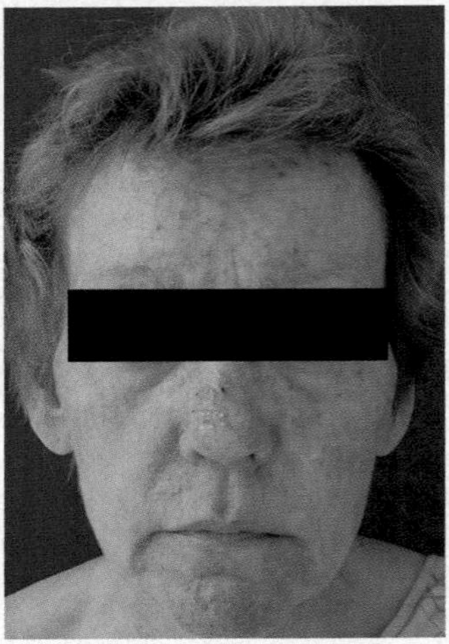

FIGURE 2: Pustular (second) stage: Papules and pustules which may be tender or pruritic appear in weeks 1–3.

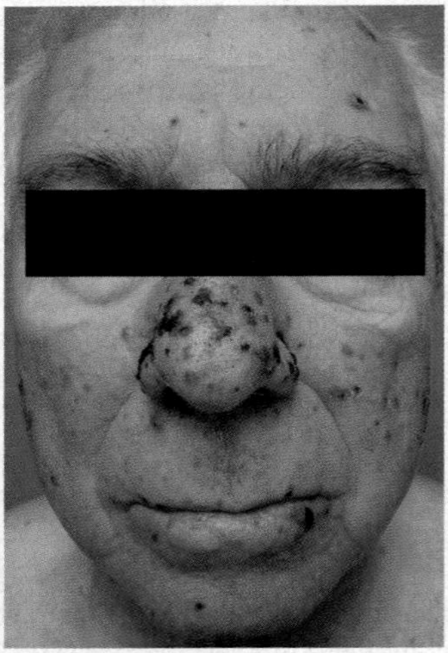

FIGURE 3: Papulopustular crust (third) stage: Crusting of papulopustules usually indicates resolving eruption from exposure to EGFR inhibitors.

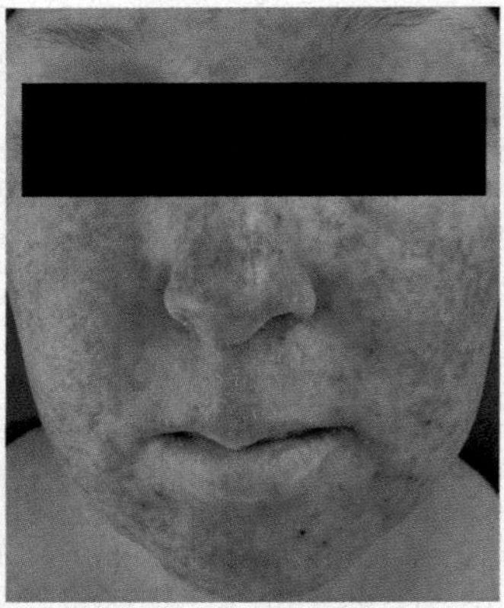

FIGURE 4: Erythematous (fourth) stage: Upon resolution of the papulopustules and crusting, postinflammatory erythema or hyperpigmentation is a common sequela, which may persist for several months.

Papulopustular (Acneiform) Eruption, Phases 1–4 — Treatment of papulopustular eruption from exposure to EGFR inhibitors and multikinase inhibitors consists of a tetracycline antibiotic (tetracycline 500 mg bid, minocycline 100 mg qd, or doxycycline 100 mg bid). Topical corticosteroids of medium to low potency have also shown benefit.

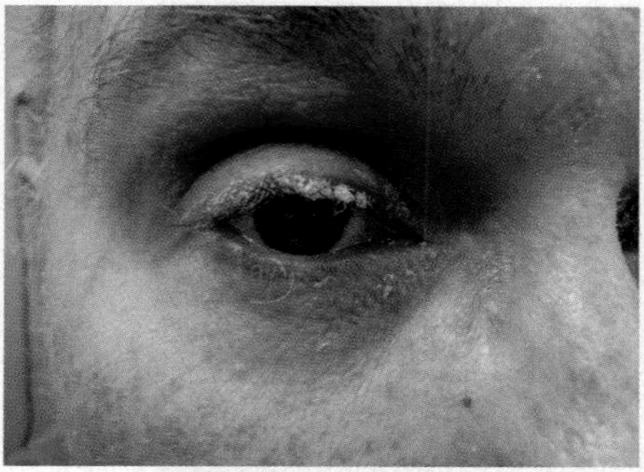

FIGURE 5: Eyelash trichomegaly: Increased thickness and waviness of eyelashes and facial hair occurs in up to 33% of patients after 3–4 months of EGFR inhibitor therapy. Eyelashes may need to be trimmed, as they may grow inward causing corneal erosions or ulcerations.

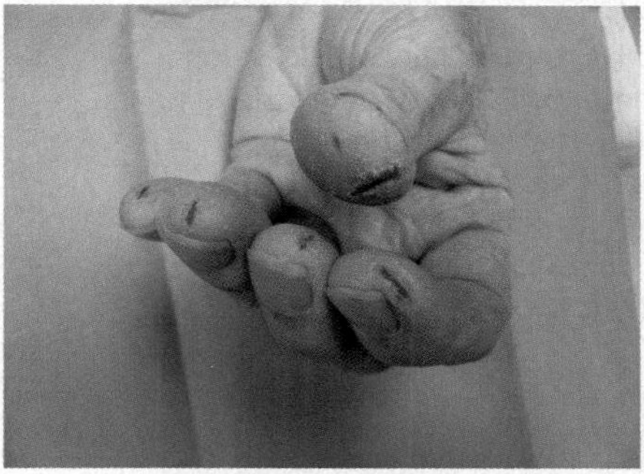

FIGURE 6: EGFR inhibitor fissures: Fissures associated with tenderness in the fingertips and heels are a manifestation of severe xerosis in response to EGFR inhibitors. Treatment consists of liquid bandages and topical zinc oxide (20%–30%).

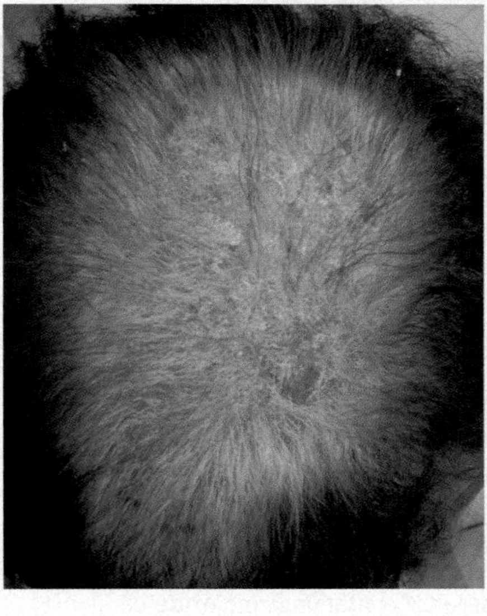

FIGURE 7: EGFR inhibitor inflammatory alopecia: Alopecia on the scalp as a result of EGFR inhibitor therapy induced follicular inflammation/superinfection. Treatment consists of topical steroid foams or solutions and oral antibiotics if infection is evidenced or suspected.

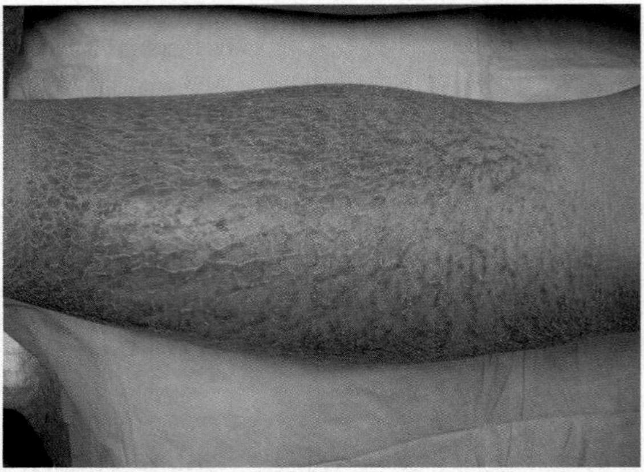

FIGURE 8: EGFR inhibitor xerosis: Dry skin develops in up to 58% of patients on EGFR inhibitor therapy, and usually occurs after the second month of drug initiation. Depending on the severity, treatment with topical creams/ointments, ammonium lactate, and topical steroids is usually effective.

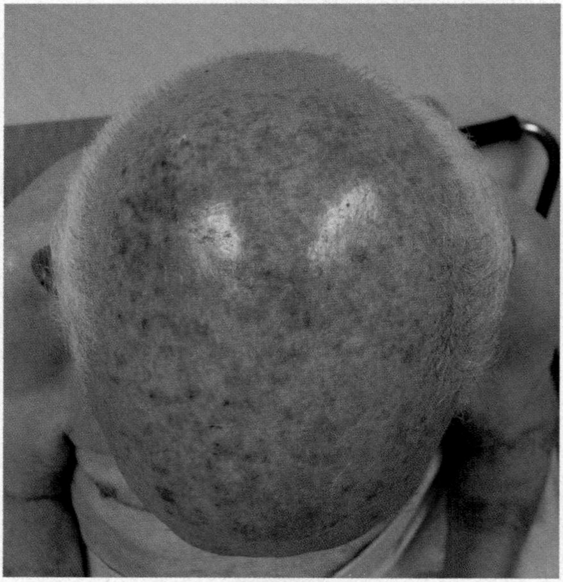

FIGURE 9: EGFR inhibitor photosensitivity: Increased sensitivity to ultraviolet radiation, manifested as sunburn, may occur when patients are receiving EGFR inhibitors. Therefore, it is critical for patients to apply broad spectrum sunscreens (containing zinc oxide or titanium dioxide) with an SPF >30.

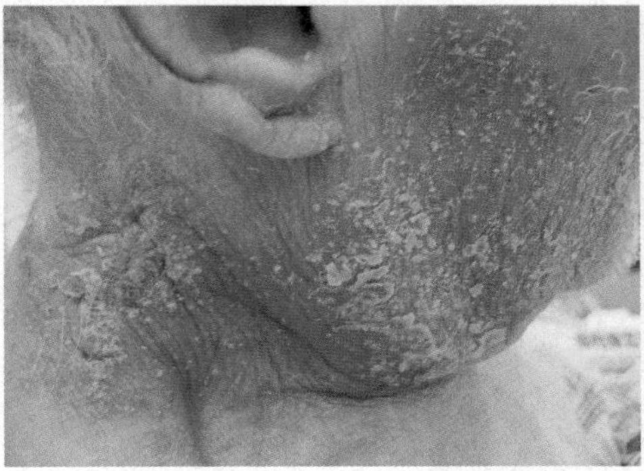

FIGURE 10: EGFR inhibitor plus radiotherapy radiation dermatitis: Concurrent administration of EGFR inhibitors and radiation increases the risk of severe in-field radiation dermatitis. Prophylactic treatment of patients with high potency topical steroids (mometasone 0.1% cream) has shown benefit.

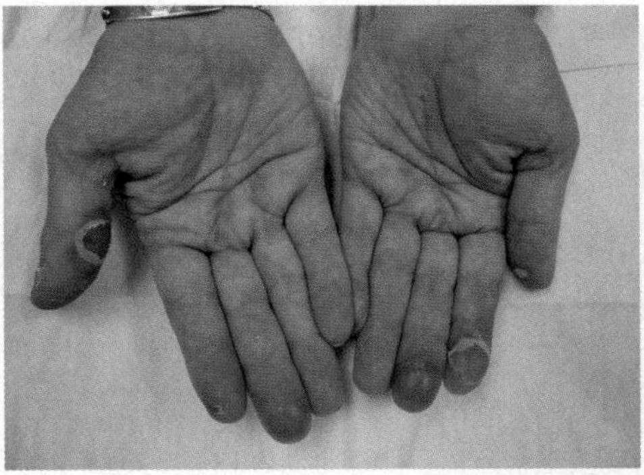

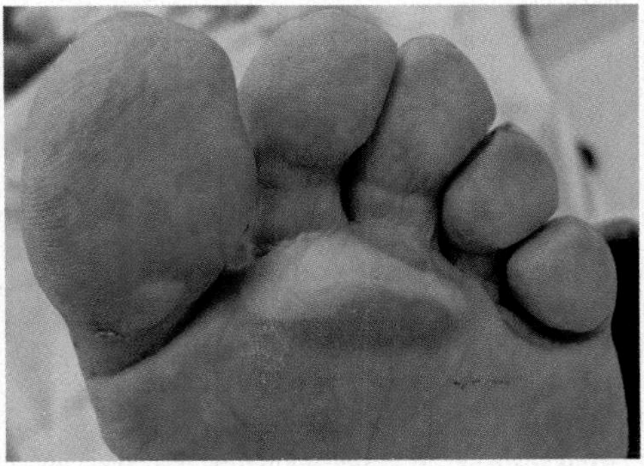

FIGURES 11A and 11B: Hand-foot skin reaction: Hand-foot skin reaction to the multikinase inhibitors sorafenib and sunitinib occurs in 30% of patients. Usually it develops within the first 2 weeks, and it is associated with blisters or hyperkeratosis overlying areas of pressure, which may impair activities of daily living in up to 10% of patients. Treatment with topical clobetasol and 40% urea, and pain control with nonsteroidal anti-inflammatories or gabapentin/pregabalin, may be necessary.

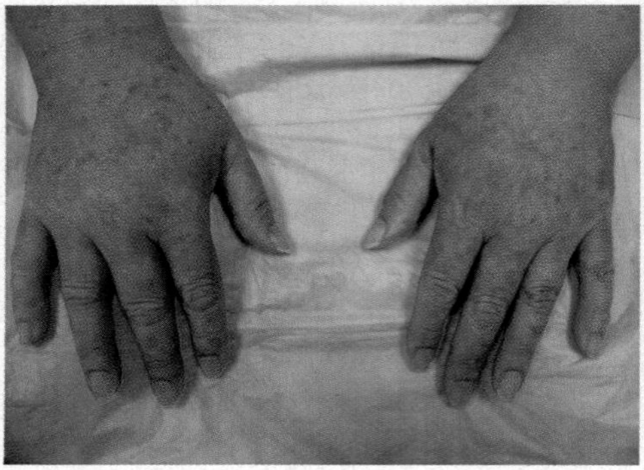

FIGURE 12: Docetaxel Periarticular thenar erythema with onycholysis (PATEO) syndrome: Docetaxel-induced tender or pruritic erythema in dorsum of the hands, along with subungual hemorrhages leading to nail separation and infection in up to 30% of treated patients. Therapy consists of high-potency topical steroids for erythematous areas, cold gloves used during infusion, antiseptic soaks, and antibiotics for the nail changes and infection.

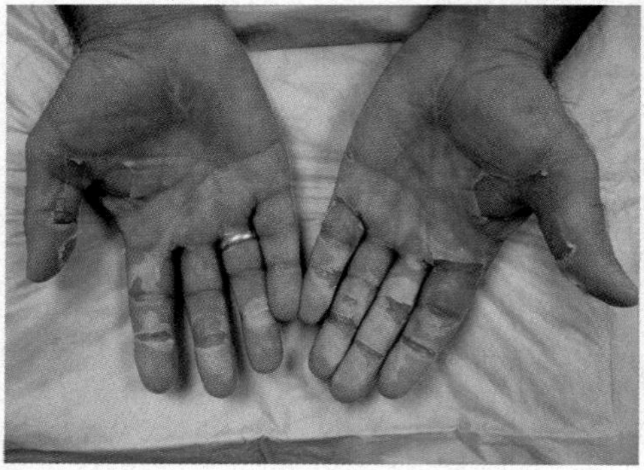

FIGURE 13: Pegylated doxorubicin and capecitabine hand-foot syndrome: Painful erythema, edema, and sensation of tightness and cracking in the palms and soles occurs in up to 30% of patients. Treatment consists of topical ammonium lactate 12%, and topical/oral steroids (dexamethasone at 8 mg bid for 5 days from day 1, followed by 4 mg bid for day 1, then 4 mg qd for 1 day).

SUGGESTED READING

Jatoi A, Rowland K, Sloan JA, et al: Tetracycline to prevent epidermal growth factor receptor inhibitor-induced skin rashes: Results of a placebo-controlled trial from the North Central Cancer Treatment Group (N03CB). Cancer 113:847–853, 2008.

Lacouture ME: Mechanisms of cutaneous toxicities to EGFR inhibitors. Nat Rev Cancer 6:803–812, 2006.

Lacouture ME, Wu S, Robert C, et al: Evolving strategies for the management of hand-foot skin reaction associated with the multitargeted kinase inhibitors sorafenib and sunitinib. Oncologist 13:1001–1011, 2008.

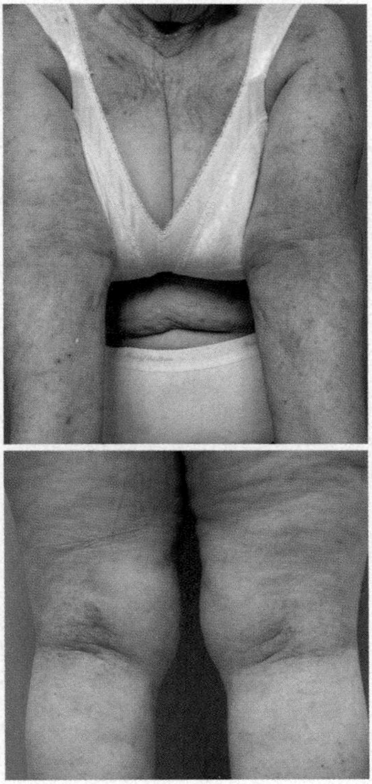

FIGURE 14: Temsirolimus and everolimus-induced rash: A pruritic rash in the trunk and extremities develops in approximately 45% and 25% of patients, respectively. Usually mild in severity and responds to topical corticosteroid creams (ie, clobetasol, fluocinonide bid). Temsirolimus and everolimus have also been associated with peripheral edema and mucositis ***(Photos from Gandhi M, Kuzel T, Lacouture M: Eosinophilic Rash Secondary to Temsirolimus. Clin Genitourin Cancer 7:E34–E36, 2009).***

Lacouture ME, Mitchell EP, Shearer H, et al: A phase II, open-label trial of skin toxicity (ST) evaluation (STEPP) in metastatic colorectal cancer (mCRC) patients (pts) receiving panitumumab (pmab) + FOLFIRI or irinotecan-only chemotherapy (CT as 2nd-line treatment (tx): Interim analysis. J Clin Oncol 28:1351–1357, 2010.

Scotte F, Tourani JM, Banu E, et al: Multicenter study of a frozen glove to prevent docetaxel-induced onycholysis and cutaneous toxicity of the hand. J Clin Oncol 23:4424–4429, 2005.

Scope A, Agero AL, Dusza SW, et al: Randomized double-blind trial of prophylactic oral minocycline and topical tazarotene for cetuximab-associated acne-like eruption. J Clin Oncol 25:5390–5396, 2007.

von Moos R, Thuerlimann BJ, Aapro M, et al: Pegylated liposomal doxorubicin-associated hand-foot syndrome: Recommendations of an international panel of experts. Eur J Cancer 44:781–790, 2008.

CHAPTER 38

Oncologic emergencies and paraneoplastic syndromes

Carmen P. Escalante, MD, Ellen Manzullo, MD, and Mitchell Weiss, MD

SUPERIOR VENA CAVA SYNDROME

Superior vena cava syndrome (SVCS) is a common occurrence in cancer patients and can lead to life-threatening complications such as cerebral or laryngeal edema. Although most commonly resulting from external compression of the vena cava by a tumor, SVCS can also stem from nonmalignant causes in cancer patients.

ETIOLOGY

Malignant causes

Primary intrathoracic malignancies are the cause of SVCS in approximately 87% to 97% of cases. The most frequent malignancy associated with the syndrome is lung cancer, followed by lymphomas and solid tumors that metastasize to the mediastinum.

Lung cancer SVCS develops in approximately 3% to 15% of patients with bronchogenic carcinoma, and it is four times more likely to occur in patients with right- versus left-sided lesions.

Metastatic disease Breast and testicular cancers are the most common metastatic malignancies causing SVCS, accounting for > 7% of cases. Metastatic disease to the thorax is responsible for SVCS in ~3% to 20% of patients.

Nonmalignant causes

Thrombosis The most common nonmalignant cause of SVCS in cancer patients is thrombosis secondary to venous access devices.

Other nonmalignant causes include cystic hygroma, substernal thyroid goiter, benign teratoma, dermoid cyst, thymoma, tuberculosis, histoplasmosis, actinomycosis, syphilis, pyogenic infections, radiation therapy, silicosis, and sarcoidosis. Some cases are idiopathic.

SIGNS AND SYMPTOMS

Classic symptoms

Patients with SVCS most often present with complaints of facial edema or erythema, dyspnea, cough, orthopnea, or arm and neck edema. These classic symptoms are seen most commonly in patients with complete obstruction, as opposed to those with mildly obstructive disease.

Other associated symptoms

These may include hoarseness, dysphagia, headaches, dizziness, syncope, lethargy, and chest pain. The symptoms may be worsened by positional changes, particularly bending forward, stooping, or lying down.

Common physical findings

The most common physical findings include edema of the face, neck, or arms; dilatation of the veins of the upper body; and plethora or cyanosis of the face. Periorbital edema may be prominent.

Other physical findings

These include laryngeal or glossal edema, mental status changes, and pleural effusion (more commonly on the right side).

DIAGNOSIS

It is important to establish the diagnosis and underlying etiology of SVCS, because some malignancies may be more amenable to specific treatment regimens than others. In the majority of cases, the diagnosis of SVCS is evident based on clinical examination alone.

The following diagnostic procedures may aid in establishing the diagnosis of SVCS and its etiology: chest x-ray, bronchoscopy, limited thoracotomy or thoracoscopy, contrast and radionuclide venography, Doppler ultrasonography, CT (especially contrast-enhanced spiral CT), and MRI.

PROGNOSIS

The prognosis of SVCS depends on the etiology of the underlying obstruction. A review by Schraufnagel showed the average overall survival after the onset of SVCS to be 10 months, but there was wide variation (± 25 months) depending on the underlying disease, with an average survival of 7.6 months. This duration was not significantly different from the survival duration of 12.2 months in patients presenting with SVCS as the primary manifestation of the disease. Thoracic malignancy, the most common cause of SVCS, had a poor prognosis of < 5 months' survival.

TREATMENT

Treatment includes radiotherapy, chemotherapy, thrombolytic therapy and anticoagulation, expandable wire stents, balloon angioplasty, and surgical bypass.

Most patients derive sufficient relief from obstructive symptoms when treated with medical adjuncts, such as diuretics and steroids (see section on "Adjunctive medical therapy"), so they can tolerate a workup to determine the etiology of SVCS. In some instances, it is appropriate to delay treatment for 1 to 2 days if necessary to establish a firm tissue diagnosis.

Radiotherapy and chemotherapy

Both radiotherapy and chemotherapy are treatment options for SVCS, depending on the tumor type. The specific drugs and doses used are those active against the underlying malignancy.

Life-threatening symptoms, such as respiratory distress, are indications for urgent radiotherapy. A preliminary determination of the treatment goal (potentially curative or palliative only) is necessary prior to the initiation of treatment, even in the emergent setting.

Radiation therapy is the standard treatment of non–small-cell lung cancer (NSCLC) with SVCS. Recent studies suggest that chemotherapy may be as effective as radiotherapy in rapidly shrinking small-cell lung cancer (SCLC). Chemoradiation therapy may result in improved ultimate local control over chemotherapy alone in SCLC and non-Hodgkin lymphoma. Retrospective reviews of patients with SCLC have reported equivalent survival in patients with or without SVCS treated definitively with chemoradiation therapy.

Reasonable palliative courses can range from 2,000 cGy in 1 week to 4,000 cGy in 4 weeks. Curative regimens can range from 3,500 to 6,600 cGy based on histology. If indicated, more rapid palliation may be achieved by delivering daily doses of 400 cGy up to a dose of 800 to 1,200 cGy, after which the remainder of the appropriate total dose can be given in more standard daily fractions of 180 to 200 cGy. Some European investigators have used doses as high as 600 cGy 1 week apart in elderly patients.

Anticoagulation and thrombolysis

Anticoagulation for SVCS has become increasingly important due to thrombosis related to intravascular devices. In certain situations, the device remains in place. Both streptokinase and urokinase have been used for thrombolysis, although urokinase has been more effective in lysing clots in this setting. Urokinase is given as a 4,400-U/kg bolus followed by 4,400 U/kg/h, whereas streptokinase is administered as a 250,000-U bolus followed by 100,000 U/h. The use of thrombolytic therapy is controversial for catheter-related thrombosis, however.

Stenting

Placement of an expandable wire stent across the stenotic portion of the vena cava is an appropriate therapy for palliation of SVCS symptoms when other therapeutic modalities cannot be used or are ineffective. Use of stents is limited when intraluminal thrombosis is present. The Institut Catala d'Oncologia in Barcelona, Spain, published its results using endovascular stent insertion for the treatment of malignant SVCS. Stenting was performed in all 52 patients with lung cancer. Phlebographic resolution of the obstruction was achieved in 100% of cases, and symptomatic improvement was achieved in more than 80% of patients. There was one major complication due to bleeding during anticoagulation. Reobstruction of the stent occurred in 17% of cases, mostly due to disease progression. Improvement of the obstruction allowed for delivery of full-dose systemic therapy for patients for whom this approach was indicated.

Other interventional treatments

Balloon angioplasty and surgical bypass have also been used in appropriate patients but are rarely indicated. Balloon angioplasty may be considered in patients with SVCS, significant clinical symptoms, and critical superior vena cava obstruction demonstrated by angiography. Surgical bypass is usually limited to patients with benign disease; however, for a select group of patients with SVCS, bypass may be an important aspect of palliative treatment. Other palliative efforts may be considered prior to bypass in this patient population.

Adjunctive medical therapy

Medications that may be used as adjuncts to the treatments described above include diuretics and steroids.

Diuretics may provide symptomatic relief of edema that is often immediate although transient. The use of diuretics is not a definitive treatment, and resulting complications may ensue, such as dehydration and decreased blood flow. Loop diuretics, such as furosemide, are often used. Dosage depends on the patient's volume status and renal function.

Steroids may be useful in the presence of respiratory compromise. They are also thought to be helpful in blocking the inflammatory reaction associated with irradiation.

Dosage depends on the severity of clinical symptoms. For severe and significant respiratory symptoms, hydrocortisone, 100 to 500 mg IV, may be administered initially. Lower doses every 6 to 8 hours may be continued. Tapering of the steroid dosage should begin as soon as the patient's condition has stabilized. Prophylactic gastric protection is advised during steroid administration.

VENOUS THROMBOEMBOLIC COMPLICATIONS OF CANCER

Deep vein thrombosis (DVT) and pulmonary embolism (PE) are common and potentially serious clinical challenges. In the United States, the estimated incidence of DVT and PE is approximately 450,000 and 355,000 cases per year, respectively. The actual incidence is likely much higher than presently documented due to often vague complaints and symptoms. PE may be associated with increased mortality and contributes to approximately 240,000 deaths annually in the United States.

Armand Trousseau noted the association between thrombosis and cancer more than 125 years ago. The risk of venous thromboembolism (VTE) in cancer patients depends upon the type and extent of the malignancy; the type of cancer treatment; the existence and nature of comorbidities; and changes in hemostasis of the blood, which have been noted in more than 90% of cancer patients. The prevalence of clinically noted venous thrombosis in cancer patients is 15%; patients undergoing surgery, hormonal therapy, and chemotherapy have the highest risk. Venous thrombosis is the second leading cause of death in cancer patients.

ETIOLOGY OF VTE IN CANCER PATIENTS

The etiology of VTE in cancer patients may be attributed to several factors, including hypercoagulable states, surgical interventions, chemotherapy, indwelling central venous catheters, and prolonged immobilization.

The mechanisms by which tumors cause a hypercoagulable state are not completely understood, but they may be attributed to abnormalities of blood composition (increased plasma levels of clotting factors, cancer procoagulant A, tissue factor, and cytokines) and increased release of plasminogen activator. Postoperative VTE was more common in patients with malignant disease (36%) than in those patients with benign disease (20%), according to recent analyses of several clinical trials in surgical patients.

Patients undergoing chemotherapy are at increased risk of venous thrombosis secondary to endothelial cell damage from drug toxicity. In the ATAC trial, the aromatase inhibitor anastrozole (Arimidex) was compared with tamoxifen for 5 years in 9,366 postmenopausal women with localized breast cancer. Forty-eight patients (1.6%) receiving anastrozole developed DVT events, compared with 74 patients (2.4%) in the tamoxifen arm ($P = .02$). Anastrozole was associated with significant reductions in DVT events and should be considered for initial treatment in this population.

Indwelling central venous catheters predispose patients to upper-extremity thrombosis and thrombosis of the axillary/subclavian vein. The catheters are also prone to occlusion. Increased venous stasis owing to immobility also promotes blood pooling into the intramuscular venous sinuses of the calf and may lead to thrombosis formation.

TUMOR TYPE ASSOCIATED WITH VTE

Several tumor types have been associated with higher rates of VTE, including those arising from the pancreas, lungs, and other mucin-secreting tumors. In general, tumor types associated with an increased incidence of thromboembolic events reflect the frequency of the tumors in the general population: In women, the most common tumors are breast, lung, gynecologic, and GI tumors; in men, prostate, lung, and GI tumors are most common. However, hematologic malignancies (multiple myeloma, lymphoma, and leukemia) also have significant rates of VTE.

TREATMENT

Several classes of agents have been used for prevention and treatment of VTE. Nonpharmacologic approaches to prophylaxis may include intermittent pneumatic compression and elastic stockings. Commonly used pharmacologic agents for thromboprophylaxis and treatment of VTE include unfractionated heparin (UFH; standard, low-dose, or adjusted-dose), oral anticoagulants such as warfarin, and low molecular weight heparin (LMWH). The preferred and recommended anticoagulant for treatment of VTE is LMWH (ASCO guidelines). UFH may be needed if the patient has a planned procedure or is on dialysis. If LMWHs are not accessible, consider switching to warfarin after 5 days of LMWH therapy.

Initial treatment of DVT and PE includes inpatient LMWH and, outpatient LMWH for low-risk patients with VTE.

The LMWH treatment and prophylaxis doses for VTE are variable. The most common LMWHs utilized in the US are dalteparin, enoxaparin, and tinzaparin. If UFH is utilized, it is administered as a bolus of 5,000 U followed by a continuous drip, usually initiated between 750 to 1,000 U/h. A baseline partial thromboplastin time (PTT) and prothrombin time (PT) are drawn prior to the initiation of treatment. PTT is then rechecked approximately 4 to 6 hours after treatment is begun, and the UFH is titrated to approximately 1.5 to 2 times control in most patients.

For patients without accessibility to LMWHs, or if such therapy is contraindicated, warfarin is usually begun on day 1 or 2 of treatment; therapy is monitored to maintain an international normalized ratio (INR) between 2.0 and 3.0. (Patients with prosthetic valves require a higher INR if UFH is utilized.) It is standard practice to maintain UFH for 4 to 5 days while the warfarin is titrated to therapeutic levels. Most patients are maintained on warfarin for a minimum of 6 months depending upon underlying risk factors. Patient response to warfarin depends on numerous factors, such as age, diet, alcohol consumption, and liver and GI function, as well as concomitant medications. Patients with active cancer should continue anticoagulation, preferably LMWH, for as long as the cancer remains active. Patients with recurrent VTE are usually maintained on anticoagulants for the rest of their lives.

Recent studies have demonstrated the safety and efficacy of LMWH in the treatment and management of VTE. Several studies have demonstrated no appreciable differences in recurrent thromboembolism and an increased risk of bleeding with UFH and LMWHs. Because LMWHs do not require a continuous drip and frequent serum testing, low-risk patients are now treated as outpatients. Both ASCO and NCCN recommend LMWHs as the preferable agents for treatment of VTE in cancer patients.

LMWH doses vary by product and are not equivalent. Enoxaparin is generally administered once or twice a day for treatment of VTE, whereas the indications for tinzaparin and dalteparin are for once-daily dosing. The commonly administered dose for treatment of DVT with enoxaparin is 1 mg/kg SC every 12 hours. Tinzaparin is given via SC injection at a dose of 175 IU/kg body weight once daily, and the dalteparin dose is 200 IU/kg SC once daily for the first month, followed by 150 IU/kg SC daily thereafter. Therapy with LMWH is continued for a minimum of 5 days during the acute phase of treatment. Generally, laboratory monitoring is unnecessary, although for individuals with renal insufficiency or those with < 50 kg body weight or obesity, plasma anti–factor Xa concentrations may need to be monitored.

In an international study comparing the long-term treatment benefits of dalteparin vs warfarin in cancer patients with VTE, long-term dalteparin substantially reduced the rate of recurrent VTE, compared with warfarin therapy, without an increase in bleeding. Based on this trial, cancer patients requiring VTE treatment should continue dalteparin (or possibly another LMWH) during the chronic phase of treatment instead of switching to warfarin. Cost issues may require patients to remain on warfarin.

Inpatient cancer patients should all be assessed for VTE prophylaxis and appropriately prophylaxed with pharmacologic agents. If these are contraindicated then mechanical alternatives (graduated compression stockings, intermittent pneumatic compression) should be considered. Early ambulation as tolerated should be encouraged. Prophylaxis doses for VTE should include: UFH 5,000 units SC every 8 hours; dalteparin 5,000 units SC daily; enoxaparin 40 mg SC daily; fondaparinux 2.5 mg SC daily (for patients allergic to heparin products).

DIFFICULTIES IN ANTICOAGULATION

Often, therapeutic challenges arise in patients on anticoagulation therapy for VTE who require surgical interventions and, therefore, temporary discontinuation of their anticoagulation treatment.

Preoperative guidelines

The timing of discontinuation of anticoagulation depends upon the type of treatment and the surgical intervention planned. For patients on continuous-drip heparin, the drip may be discontinued 4 to 6 hours prior to the procedure. A PTT should be drawn prior to the procedure to check for total reversal of the treatment. In cases in which only partial reversal is noted or an emergency arises, fresh frozen plasma may be administered for rapid reversal.

Patients on warfarin may be advised to discontinue their medication 3 to 5 days prior to the planned procedure. This approach allows for a gradual reduction in the anticoagulation effect. An INR should be checked prior to the procedure. If partial reversal is noted or an emergency arises, vitamin K and/or fresh frozen plasma may be administered for acute reversal.

Postoperative guidelines

Timing of postoperative therapy depends on the type of procedure undertaken and its associated risk of bleeding. Direct communication between the surgeon and the physician managing the anticoagulation treatment is necessary. When the surgeon believes that the risk of bleeding is at an acceptable level, anticoagulation should be restarted. It may be prudent to utilize UFH or LMWH prior to the initiation of warfarin, especially if a substantial risk of bleeding remains.

High-risk patients

For high-risk patients (with prosthetic valves, recurrent VTE), it may be reasonable to switch from warfarin to either UFH or LMWH, with appropriate discontinuation prior to the procedure. Both UFH and LMWH have shorter reversal times than does warfarin, although LMWHs are not fully reversible. Another option is to continue warfarin until shortly before the procedure, reversing treatment with vitamin K and/or fresh frozen plasma. The risk/benefit ratio should be considered when reviewing the options for the individual patient.

Surgery has long been known to be a risk factor for VTE. The nature of surgery in part determines the relative risk: Patients undergoing orthopedic surgery are at a particularly high risk. The risk is modified by the presence of other factors, such as underlying malignancy, age, obesity, and history of previous thromboembolism. Meta-analyses of clinical trials have shown there is a high overall risk of DVT during general surgery, based on rates observed in control subjects; there is a confirmed incidence of DVT of 25% noted by the fibrinogen uptake test. The risk is even higher (29%) in surgical patients with malignancy. Risk is also increased in those individuals with multiple risk factors (eg, age > 65 years, obesity, bed rest > 5 days). A comparison of commonly used prophylaxis in 160 clinical trials indicates that overall, low-dose UFH and LMWH are the most effective agents in reducing the incidence of DVT after general surgery. A higher dosage of the prophylactic agent may be needed for adequate prevention in patients with malignant disease.

Treatment alternatives for recurrence

There are several treatment options for patients with recurrent VTE. Patients who develop recurrence of thrombosis while on therapeutic doses of anticoagulation should be considered for inferior vena cava filter placement. The filter will not prevent new clots from forming, but it does provide a physical barrier to prevent propagation of clots to the pulmonary bed. Alternatively, an inferior vena cava filter can be placed to avoid the need for long-term anticoagulant therapy if there are contraindications to anticoagulation. Alternately, another LMWH may be utilized prior to placement of an inferior vena cava filter, because there may be other complications related to filter placement (ie, postphlebitis syndrome, clotting of the filter).

Depending upon patient prognosis and tumor factors, other comorbidities, and propensity for bleeding, continued therapy with an anticoagulant may also be considered in addition to filter placement.

SPINAL CORD COMPRESSION

Spinal cord compression develops in 1% to 5% of patients with systemic cancer. It should be considered an emergency, as treatment delays may result in irreversible paralysis and loss of bowel and bladder function.

ETIOLOGY

Compression of the spinal cord is due predominantly to extradural metastases (95%) and usually results from tumor involvement of the vertebral column. A tumor may occasionally metastasize to the epidural space without bony involvement.

Site of involvement

The segment most often involved is the thoracic spine (70%), followed by the lumbosacral (20%) and cervical spine (10%).

Most common malignancies

Spinal cord compression occurs in a variety of malignancies; the most common are lung, breast, unknown primary, prostate, and renal cancers.

SIGNS AND SYMPTOMS

Early signs

More than 90% of patients present with pain localized to the spine or radicular in nature (ie, not due to bony involvement but rather to neural compression). Pain, which is usually secondary to bony involvement, is often exacerbated with movement, recumbency, coughing, sneezing, or straining. The majority of patients experience pain for weeks to months before neurologic symptoms appear.

Intermediate signs

If cord compression goes untreated, weakness often develops next. It may be preceded or accompanied by sensory loss.

Late signs

Symptoms of autonomic dysfunction, urinary retention, and constipation are late findings. Once autonomic, motor, or sensory findings appear, spinal cord compression usually progresses rapidly and may result in irreversible paralysis in hours to days if untreated.

Physical findings

These may include tenderness to palpation or percussion over the involved spine, pain in the distribution of the involved nerve root, muscle weakness, spasticity, abnormal muscle stretch reflexes and extensor plantar responses, and sensory loss. Sensory loss occurs below the involved cord segment and indicates the site of compression. In patients with autonomic dysfunction, physical findings include a palpable bladder or diminished rectal tone.

DIAGNOSIS

The first step in the diagnosis of spinal cord compression is an accurate neurologic history and examination.

X-rays

More than 66% of patients with spinal cord compression have bony abnormalities on plain radiographs of the spine. Findings include erosion and loss of pedicles, partial or complete collapse of vertebral bodies, and paraspinous soft-tissue masses. Normal spine films are not helpful for excluding epidural metastases.

MRI

The standard for diagnosing and localizing epidural cord compression is MRI. Gadolinium-enhanced MRI has been especially helpful in assessing cord compression secondary to spinal epidural abscesses, as gadolinium enhances actively inflamed tissues and defines anatomic boundaries. An abnormal signal within the disk space suggests the possibility of infection.

Primary or secondary neoplasms involving the vertebral bodies generally demonstrate a long T1, resulting in decreased signal intensity on a T1-weighted image, and a long T2, with increased signal intensity on the T2-weighted image.

CT and myelography

If MRI is unavailable, a CT scan and/or myelogram may be used to diagnose and localize epidural cord compression.

PROGNOSIS

Treatment outcome correlates with the degree and duration of neurologic impairment prior to therapy. In a prospective analysis of 209 patients treated for spinal cord compression with radiotherapy and steroids, Maranzano and Latini reported that of patients who were ambulatory, nonambulatory, or paraplegic prior to treatment, 98%, 60%, and 11%, respectively, were able to ambulate following therapy. Treatment outcome in the most radiosensitive malignancies (eg, lymphoma) was superior to that in the less sensitive cancers (renal cell carcinoma). Almost all ambulatory patients treated with either irradiation alone or laminectomy followed by postoperative irradiation remained ambulatory after treatment, whereas ~10% of patients whose lower extremities were paralyzed could walk after treatment.

TREATMENT

The goals of treatment of spinal cord compression are recovery and maintenance of normal neurologic function, local tumor control, stabilization of the spine, and pain control. Choice of treatment depends on clinical presentation, availability of histologic diagnosis, rapidity of the clinical course, type of malignancy, site of spinal involvement, stability of the spine, and previous treatment.

In general, radiation therapy has been the treatment of choice for these patients. This is based upon the belief that radiotherapy is as effective as surgery in terms of pain relief and maintaining neurologic function. In other words, the potential complications and convalescence associated with surgery can be avoided in this group of patients with a limited life expectancy.

This approach has been further investigated in a randomized clinical trial reported by Patchell et al. A total of 101 patients with spinal cord compression caused by metastatic cancer were randomized to undergo either surgery followed by adjuvant radiation therapy (n = 50) or radiation therapy alone (n = 51). Radiotherapy for both groups consisted of 10 fractions of 300 cGy each. The primary endpoint was the ability to walk.

The study was stopped after an interim analysis of the 101 patients revealed that 42 of 50 patients (84%) in the surgery group were able to walk after treatment, compared with 29 of 51 patients (57%) in the radiotherapy group (P = .001). Additionally, patients treated with surgery retained the ability to walk significantly longer than those patients treated with radiation therapy alone (median, 122 days vs 13 days;

P = .003). Of the 32 patients who entered the trial unable to walk, 10 of 16 (62%) in the surgery arm regained the ability to walk, compared with 3 of 16 (19%) in the radiotherapy arm (P = .01). Based on the results of this trial, decompressive surgery followed by adjuvant radiation therapy should be considered in the treatment of patients with spinal cord compression.

The ability to regain ambulatory function after surgery had been recognized prior to this study. This finding represented the rationale for strong consideration of surgery in this group of patients. The authors advocated the wider use of surgery in most patients with spinal cord compression. Still, there are reasons to consider radiotherapy alone as appropriate initial treatment. They include the disappointing results in the radiotherapy-alone arm in this study compared with the experiences of previous studies and the possible reluctance to consider spinal surgery by patients and/or physicians (based upon limited life expectancy). These issues should, of course, be thoroughly reviewed during the process of informed consent.

Patchell et al have recently reexamined the role of age in determining outcomes of surgery vs radiation therapy. Secondary data analysis of the randomized trial with age stratification demonstrated a strong interaction between age and treatment outcomes. Multivariate modeling and Kaplan-Meier curves revealed that for patients 65 years or older, there was no difference in the preservation of ambulation between the surgery and radiotherapy-alone arms. However, for patients younger than age 65, surgery still resulted in prolonged ambulation (P = .002).

Steroids

Dexamethasone should be administered if the patient's history and neurologic examination suggest spinal cord compression. There is controversy as to whether an initial high dose of IV dexamethasone (100 mg) followed by 10 mg of dexamethasone every 6 hours is necessary. Some studies have suggested lower doses are just as effective.

Radiation therapy

Radiation therapy alone is still usually the standard initial treatment for most patients with spinal cord compression due to a radiosensitive malignancy. Treatment outcome is contingent upon both the relative radiosensitivity of the malignancy and the neurologic status of the patient at the time radiotherapy is initiated.

Radiation portal In general, the treatment volume should include the area of epidural compression (as determined by MRI or myelography) plus two vertebral bodies above and below. Consideration should be given to including adjacent areas of abnormalities if feasible. Careful matching techniques should be employed in patients treated to adjacent vertebral levels, a situation that is not uncommon.

Radiation dose and fractionation The chosen regimen should take into account such factors as field size and normal tissue tolerance. Smaller fields are appropriately treated to 2,000 to 3,000 cGy over 1 or 2 weeks, respectively. Larger fields may occasionally necessitate longer courses, such as 4,000 cGy over 4 weeks, to minimize side effects.

Investigators from the University Hospital Hamburg reported their results on five fractionation schemes of radiation therapy for spinal cord compression. In this retrospective review, 1,304 patients were treated from January 1992 through December 2003. Radiation schedules included 1 × 8 Gy (n = 261), 5 × 4 Gy (n = 279), 10 × 3 Gy (n = 274), 15 × 2.5 Gy (n = 233), and 20 × 2 Gy (n = 257). Improvement in motor function was noted in 26% (1 × 8 Gy), 28% (5 × 4 Gy), 27% (10 × 3 Gy), 31% (15 × 2.5 Gy), and 28% (20 × 2 Gy). Motor function improvement and posttreatment ambulatory rates were not significantly different throughout all groups.

On multivariate analysis, age, performance status, pretreatment ambulatory status, and length of time motor deficits were present prior to the initiation of radiotherapy were all significantly associated with improved functional outcome, whereas the schedule of radiation therapy was not a significant indicator. Recurrence rates at 2 years were 24%, 26%, 14%, 9%, and 7%, respectively. There was mild acute toxicity and no late toxicity. The authors concluded that shorter fractionation schemes should be considered for those patients with poor predicted survival.

The ability to maintain local control in a patient with spinal cord compression has been recently reported. Rades et al conducted a prospective nonrandomized study evaluating recurrence rates in short-course vs long-course radiotherapy. A total of 231 patients received radiation therapy for spinal cord compression: 114 patients received short-course radiation therapy (1 × 8 Gy or 5 × 4 Gy), and 117 patients received long-course radiation therapy (10 × 3 Gy, 15 × 2.5 Gy, or 20 × 2 Gy). This study showed an improvement in progression-free survival at 12 months (72% vs 55%) for long-course radiation therapy compared with short-course radiation therapy ($P = .034$). Additionally there was improvement in local control in favor of the long-course group (77% vs 61%; $P = .032$). However, there was no difference in functional outcome or overall survival.

In another study, the University Hospital Hamburg reported its prospective evaluation of 10 vs 20 fractions of radiation therapy for metastatic spinal cord compression. A total of 214 patients were irradiated with 30 Gy in 10 fractions (n = 110) or 40 Gy in 20 fractions (n = 104). Motor function improved in 43% of patients treated with 30 Gy and in 41% of patients treated with 40 Gy ($P = .799$). There was no significant difference in posttreatment ambulatory rates (60% and 64%, respectively; $P = .708$). As expected, being ambulatory prior to the initiation of treatment was associated with better functional outcome after irradiation ($P = .035$). Acute toxicity was mild, and no late toxicity was observed during the 12-month follow-up.

Retreatment may be entertained, particularly when no effective alternative exists. Usually, doses of 2,000 cGy over 2 weeks can be used for retreatment. It is important, however, to counsel the patient regarding the risk of radiation neuropathy. Furthermore, only those patients who had a lasting response to the initial treatment should be reirradiated, as tumors that were refractory to the first course or that recur within 3 months are unlikely to respond to subsequent courses.

Surgery

Vertebral body resection for a tumor anterior to the cord and posterior laminectomy for a tumor posterior to the cord may be appropriate treatment options for relieving spinal cord compression in patients who require spinal stability, have undergone previous radiotherapy in the area of the compression, require a tissue diagnosis of malignancy, or experience progression of the cord compression despite optimal treatment with steroids and irradiation.

In general, surgical decompression should be strongly considered in patients whose cord compression is caused by a relatively radioresistant cancer and who have a severe neurologic deficit (such as bowel or bladder dysfunction). Unfortunately, many patients in this situation are not candidates for aggressive surgery. In these cases, radiotherapy is offered, albeit with limited expectations for neurologic recovery.

Chemotherapy

Chemotherapy may be an effective treatment of spinal cord compression in select patients with a chemosensitive metastatic tumor. It also may be considered in combination with other treatment modalities, such as radiotherapy, or as an alternative if those modalities are not suitable options for relieving spinal cord compression.

HYPERCALCEMIA

Hypercalcemia is the most common metabolic emergency seen in individuals with cancer, occurring in an estimated 10% to 20% of patients.

ETIOLOGY

The malignancies most commonly associated with hypercalcemia include myeloma, lung cancer (epidermoid tumors more often than small-cell tumors), and renal cancer. In some cases, the pathogenesis of hypercalcemia may relate to the release of parathyroidlike hormones, prostaglandins, and osteoclast-activating factor.

SIGNS AND SYMPTOMS

Symptoms of hypercalcemia may involve various organ systems, including the central nervous, cardiac, GI, and renal systems (Table 1).

Bony metastasis vs paraneoplastic syndrome

The signs and symptoms of hypercalcemia secondary to bony metastases are often indistinguishable from those of hypercalcemia as a paraneoplastic syndrome. The laboratory findings may vary. A tumor secreting an immunoreactive parathyroid hormone (iPTH)-like substance will have increased levels of cyclic adenosine monophosphate, low levels of serum phosphorus, and variable levels of iPTH, depending on the specificity of the assay. Many patients with bony metastases also exhibit features consistent with "ectopic" hyperparathyroidism.

DIAGNOSIS

An accurate history and physical examination are often the most helpful diagnostic tools to exclude correctable nonmalignant causes of hypercalcemia. Hypercalcemia in association with occult malignancies is rare. The presence of weight loss, fatigue, or muscle weakness should increase clinical suspicion of malignancy as the cause of hypercalcemia.

TABLE 1: Symptoms associated with hypercalcemia by organ system

General	CNS	Cardiac	GI	Renal
Dehydration	Weakness	Bradycardia	Nausea and vomiting	Polyuria
Anorexia	Hypotonia	Short QT interval	Constipation	Nephrocalcinosis
Pruritus	Proximal myopathy	Prolonged PR interval	Ileus	–
Weight loss	Mental status changes	Wide T wave	Pancreatitis	–
Fatigue	Seizure Coma	Atrial or ventricular arrhythmia	Dyspepsia	–

Laboratory findings

In patients with hypercalcemia of malignancy, serum iPTH levels, determined by a double-antibody method, are extremely low or undetectable; levels of inorganic phosphorus are low or normal; and levels of 1,25-dihydroxyvitamin D are low or normal.

Use of additional tests to identify the underlying malignancy responsible for the hypercalcemia often depends on the history and physical findings.

TREATMENT

Asymptomatic patients with minimally elevated calcium levels (< 12.0 mg/dL) may be treated as outpatients, with close monitoring of calcium levels and symptoms. Encouragement of oral hydration, mobilization, and elimination of drugs that contribute to hypercalcemia are essential. Patients who are symptomatic or have calcium levels ≥ 12.0 mg/dL should be considered for inpatient management if medically appropriate. An algorithm for the acute and chronic treatment of hypercalcemia of malignancy is shown in Figure 1.

Volume expansion (eg, lactated Ringer's solution, 0.9% NaCl)

Volume expansion and natriuresis increase renal blood flow and enhance calcium excretion secondary to the ionic exchange of calcium for sodium in the distal tubule. The volume required depends on the extent of hypovolemia, as well as the patient's cardiac and renal function. Often, infusion rates of 250 to 500 mL/h are needed. Typically, the onset of action is 12 to 24 hours.

Loop diuretics

There is much controversy over the effectiveness of loop diuretics in the treatment of hypercalcemia. In theory, furosemide-induced natriuresis should enhance urinary

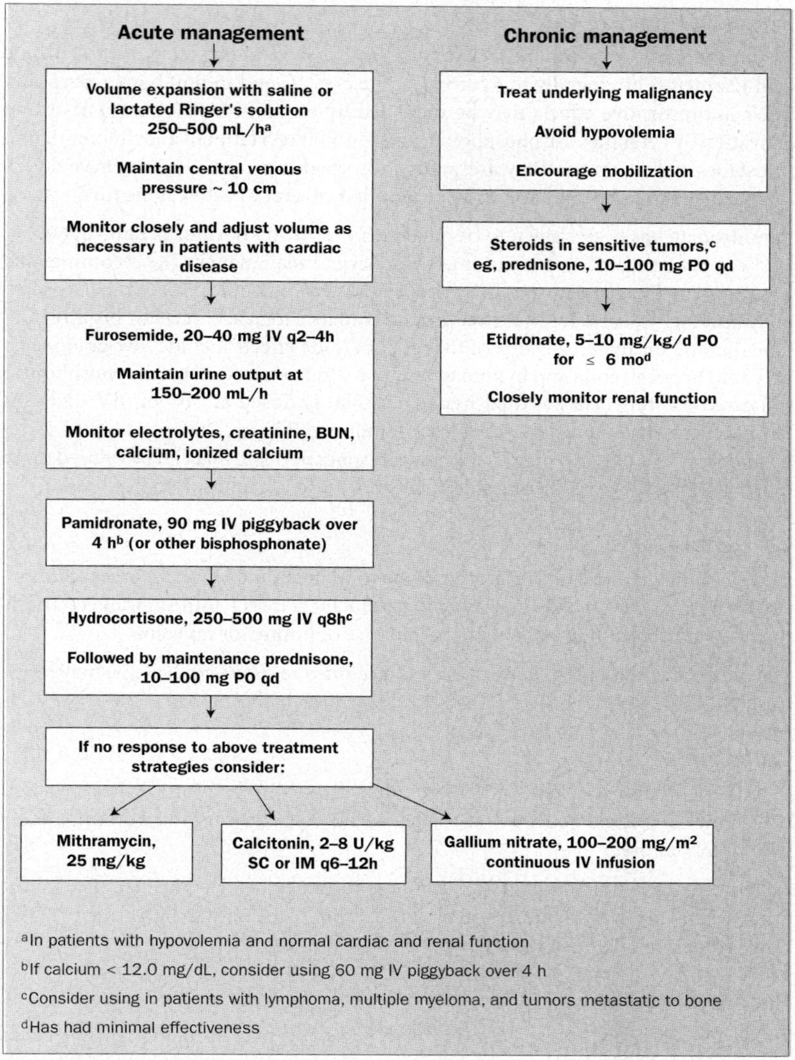
Acute management
Volume expansion with saline or lactated Ringer's solution 250–500 mL/h[a]
Maintain central venous pressure ~ 10 cm
Monitor closely and adjust volume as necessary in patients with cardiac disease
Furosemide, 20–40 mg IV q2–4h
Maintain urine output at 150–200 mL/h
Monitor electrolytes, creatinine, BUN, calcium, ionized calcium
Pamidronate, 90 mg IV piggyback over 4 h[b] (or other bisphosphonate)
Hydrocortisone, 250–500 mg IV q8h[c]
Followed by maintenance prednisone, 10–100 mg PO qd
If no response to above treatment strategies consider:
Mithramycin, 25 mg/kg
Calcitonin, 2–8 U/kg SC or IM q6–12h
Gallium nitrate, 100–200 mg/m2 continuous IV infusion
Chronic management
Treat underlying malignancy
Avoid hypovolemia
Encourage mobilization
Steroids in sensitive tumors,[c] eg, prednisone, 10–100 mg PO qd
Etidronate, 5–10 mg/kg/d PO for ≤ 6 mo[d]
Closely monitor renal function
[a]In patients with hypovolemia and normal cardiac and renal function
[b]If calcium < 12.0 mg/dL, consider using 60 mg IV piggyback over 4 h
[c]Consider using in patients with lymphoma, multiple myeloma, and tumors metastatic to bone
[d]Has had minimal effectiveness

FIGURE 1: Algorithm for the treatment of hypercalcemia of malignancy.

calcium excretion. However, in most cases of significant hypercalcemia, hypovolemia is present. Thus, once euvolemia has been achieved with saline infusion, diuretics may be useful in preventing hypervolemia. Diuretic dosages depend on the patient's underlying renal function, and the dosing frequency should be based on hourly urine output. In patients with normal renal function, furosemide, 20 to 40 mg IV, may be initiated after volume expansion is achieved, with subsequent doses given when urine output is < 150 to 200 mL/h.

Bisphosphonates

Bisphosphonates (etidronate, clodronate [Bonefos], pamidronate, and zoledronic acid [Zometa]) bind avidly to hydroxyapatite crystals and inhibit bone resorption. Their antiresorptive effects may be mediated by the inhibition of osteoclasts and activation by cytokines. Bisphosphonates also inhibit recruitment and differentiation of osteoclast precursors. They are poorly absorbed from the GI tract, have a very long half-life in bone, and appear to accumulate at sites of active bone turnover.

Pamidronate has been shown to be effective in restoring normocalcemia in 60% to 100% of patients with hypercalcemia secondary to malignancy. The recommended dose is 90 mg IV over 4 hours. The single IV dose over 4 hours, lack of renal toxicity, and superiority over etidronate make pamidronate a logical choice for bisphosphonate therapy for hypercalcemia of malignancy. Side effects include low-grade fever and mild hypocalcemia and hypomagnesemia. Clodronate, another bisphosphonate indicated for cancer-associated hypercalcemia, is dosed at 300 mg IV daily for 5 consecutive days (infused over at least 2 hours) or 800 to 3,200 mg/d orally. Zoledronic acid (Zometa, at 4 mg IV) is a newer bisphosphonate that can be infused more quickly and has fewer systemic side effects than other bisphosphonates.

Corticosteroids

In certain malignancies, such as lymphomas and hormone-sensitive breast cancers, corticosteroids may be of some value in producing a direct antitumor effect. In the majority of solid tumors, however, steroids are of limited or no value.

The onset of action is 3 to 5 days. Doses of prednisone (or its equivalent) may range from 10 to 100 mg/d.

Calcitonin

This drug inhibits bone degradation by binding directly to receptors on the osteoclast. It has few serious side effects (rare hypersensitivity) and can be given to patients with organ failure.

Calcitonin's onset of action is 2 to 4 hours, but its hypocalcemic effect is of short duration and peaks at 48 hours. There is little response to continued treatment. Doses range from 2 to 8 U/kg SC or IM every 6 to 12 hours.

Plicamycin (Mithracin)

This drug has direct osteoclast-inhibitory effects and may also block the effects of vitamin D or parathyroid hormone. It reportedly is effective in ~80% of patients with hypercalcemia secondary to malignancy.

The onset of action of plicamycin is 24 to 48 hours. The duration of normocalcemia varies, but retreatment is required in 72 to 96 hours in most patients. The usual dose is 25 μg/kg (range: 10–50 μg/kg).

Significant toxicity increases with multiple injections and includes renal and liver toxicity. Thrombocytopenia is a common side effect.

Gallium nitrate (Ganite)

Gallium nitrate directly inhibits osteoclasts and increases bone calcium without producing cytotoxic effects on bone cells. It successfully restores normocalcemia in 75% to 85% of patients.

Gallium nitrates's onset of action is 24 to 48 hours. The dose range is 100 to 200 mg/m^2 given by continuous IV infusion for 5 days.

A study by Bertheault-Cvitkovic et al suggested that gallium nitrate may be superior to pamidronate for the acute normalization of cancer-related hypercalcemia. In other comparative trials, gallium nitrate proved to be more effective than both calcitonin and etidronate in patients with hypercalcemia that is secondary to malignancy.

There are some disadvantages to gallium nitrate therapy, including the need for inpatient care and daily IV infusions and potential nephrotoxicity. It has been recommended that the drug not be used in patients with creatinine levels > 2.5 mg/dL.

HYPERURICEMIA

Compared with hypercalcemia, hyperuricemia is a less common metabolic emergency in cancer patients.

ETIOLOGY AND RISK FACTORS

Hyperuricemia occurs most often in patients with hematologic disorders, particularly leukemias, high-grade lymphomas, and myeloproliferative diseases (polycythemia vera). It may occur secondary to treatment of the malignancy.

Drugs

Hyperuricemia is also associated with certain cytotoxic agents (eg, tiazofurin and aminothiadiazoles). Various other drugs can contribute to hyperuricemia by increasing uric acid production or decreasing its excretion. Diuretics (thiazides, furosemide, and ethacrynic acid [Edecrin]) cause acute uricosuria, and hyperuricemia may occur secondary to volume contraction. Antituberculous drugs, such as pyrazinamide and ethambutol, as well as nicotinic acid (niacin) are also associated with hyperuricemia.

Extensive or aggressive tumors

Patients with extensive, anaplastic, or rapidly proliferating tumors are at greatest risk for hyperuricemia. These patients include those with bulky lymphomas and sarcomas, those with chronic myelocytic leukemia or chronic lymphocytic leukemia and extreme leukocytosis, and those undergoing remission-induction chemotherapy for acute leukemia.

Renal impairment

Individuals with preexisting renal impairment are also at risk of becoming hyperuricemic.

SIGNS AND SYMPTOMS

Patients with clinical syndromes caused by hyperuricemia present with significant elevations of serum uric acid. Gouty arthritis may be seen occasionally, but the most significant complication is renal dysfunction, particularly acute renal failure. Clinical symptoms associated with renal dysfunction vary depending on the degree of dysfunction and the timing of its development. In patients with acute renal failure, clinical symptoms may include abnormal mental status, nausea and vomiting, fluid overload, pericarditis, and seizures.

DIAGNOSIS

The diagnosis of hyperuricemia is based on laboratory findings of high serum uric acid levels, hyperuricosuria, and increased serum creatinine and urea nitrogen levels.

PROGNOSIS

Prognosis often depends on the etiology of the hyperuricemia.

TREATMENT

Prophylactic measures

Prophylactic measures against the development of hyperuricemia should be undertaken prior to the initiation of chemotherapy. Drugs that increase serum urate levels or produce acidic urine (eg, thiazides and salicylates) should be discontinued if possible. Alkalinization of the urine should be initiated to maintain a urine pH > 7.0. Usually, sodium bicarbonate solution (50–100 mmol/L) is added to IV fluids and then adjusted so that an alkaline urinary pH is maintained. The carbonic anhydrase inhibitor acetazolamide may be used to increase the effects of alkalinization. It is important to remember that alkalinization is secondary to the overall goal of decreasing urinary uric acid concentration by increasing urinary volume.

Allopurinol

This xanthine oxidase inhibitor is the mainstay of drug treatment and may be started 1 to 2 days prior to cytotoxic treatment. Dosages range from 300 to 600 mg/d, and therapy is usually continued for 1 to 2 weeks or until the danger of hyperuricemia has passed.

Rasburicase (Elitek) is an antihyperuricemia drug. It has been approved by the FDA for malignancy-associated hyperuricemia in pediatric patients but is also used in adults. The usual pediatric dose is 0.15 or 0.2 mg/kg IV over 30 minutes for 5 days. The usual adult dosage is 0.15 to 0.2 mg/kg/d in limited studies.

Acute oliguria

In patients who develop acute oliguria, ureteral obstruction by urate calculi should be considered. This condition should be evaluated by ultrasonography or CT. Administration of IV contrast agents for pyelography should be avoided, as they may increase the risk of acute tubular necrosis.

Dialysis

Patients with advancing renal insufficiency and subsequent renal failure may benefit from peritoneal dialysis or hemodialysis. Dialysis has been shown to be effective in reversing renal failure caused by urate deposition.

TUMOR LYSIS SYNDROME

Tumor lysis syndrome occurs due to the rapid release of intracellular contents into the bloodstream, leading to life-threatening concentrations. If the resulting metabolic abnormalities remain uncorrected, patients may develop renal failure and sudden death.

ETIOLOGY AND RISK FACTORS

Tumor lysis syndrome most commonly develops during the rapid growth phase of high-grade lymphomas and leukemia in patients with high leukocyte counts; it is less common in patients with solid tumors. The syndrome is often iatrogenic, caused by cytotoxic chemotherapy. Because of clinicians' increased awareness of the tumor lysis syndrome during the past decade and the use of adequate prophylaxis prior to the initiation of chemotherapy, there are fewer cases currently. Occasionally, the syndrome occurs following treatment with irradiation, glucocorticosteroids, tamoxifen, or interferon.

The typical patient at risk for tumor lysis syndrome tends to be young (< 25 years of age) and male and has an advanced disease stage (often with abdominal disease) and a markedly elevated lactate dehydrogenase level.

Other predisposing factors include volume depletion, concentrated acidic urine pH, and excessive urinary uric acid excretion rates.

SIGNS AND SYMPTOMS

The syndrome is characterized by hyperuricemia, hyperkalemia, hyperphosphatemia, hypocalcemia, and often, oliguric renal failure.

DIAGNOSIS

The diagnosis of tumor lysis syndrome is based on the development of increased levels of serum uric acid, phosphorus, and potassium; decreased levels of serum calcium; and renal dysfunction following chemotherapy.

PROGNOSIS

The prognosis varies depending on the adequate correction of metabolic abnormalities and the underlying etiology of tumor lysis.

TREATMENT

Prophylactic measures

Patients at risk for tumor lysis syndrome should be identified before the initiation of chemotherapy and should be adequately hydrated and given agents to alkalinize the urine. Treatment with allopurinol (IV or oral) may be instituted to minimize hyperuricemia. The recommended dosage of IV allopurinol ranges from 200 to 400 mg/m^2/d. This regimen should be started 24 to 48 hours before the initiation of cytotoxic treatment. The dose may be equally divided into 6-, 8-, or 12-hour increments, but the final concentration should not exceed 6 mg/mL. (For oral dosages of allopurinol and IV doses of rasburicase, see the section on hyperuricemia treatment earlier in this chapter.)

Serum electrolytes, uric acid, phosphorus, calcium, and creatinine levels should be checked repeatedly for 3 to 4 days after chemotherapy is initiated, with the frequency of monitoring dependent upon the clinical condition and the risk profile of the patient.

Established tumor lysis

Once tumor lysis is established, treatment is directed at vigorous correction of electrolyte abnormalities, hydration, and hemodialysis (as appropriate in patients with renal failure).

SYNDROME OF INAPPROPRIATE SECRETION OF ANTIDIURETIC HORMONE

The syndrome of inappropriate secretion of antidiuretic hormone (SIADH) is a paraneoplastic condition that is associated with malignant tumors (particularly SCLC), CNS disease (eg, infection, intracerebral lesions, head trauma, and subarachnoid hemorrhage), and pulmonary disorders (eg, tuberculosis, pneumonia, and abscess).

SIGNS AND SYMPTOMS

Hyponatremia

Hyponatremia is the most common presenting sign of SIADH. Patients who experience a rapid fall in plasma sodium levels are usually the most symptomatic.

Other presentations

Patients with SIADH can also experience malaise, altered mental status, seizures, coma, and occasionally, death. Focal neurologic findings can occur in the absence of brain metastases.

DIAGNOSIS

To make a diagnosis of SIADH, certain criteria must be met (Table 2). In addition to those criteria, patients should have normal renal, adrenal, and thyroid function, along with normal extracellular fluid status.

TABLE 2: Criteria for the diagnosis of SIADH

Criterion	Definition
Hyponatremia	Serum sodium level < 135 mEq/L
Hyperosmotic plasma	Plasma osmolality < 280 mOsm/kg
Hyperosmotic urine	Urinary osmolality > 500 mOsm/kg
Hypernatremic urine	Urinary sodium level > 20 mEq/L (without diuretic therapy)

SIADH = syndrome of inappropriate secretion of antidiuretic hormone

Drug history

It is important to obtain a full list of the medications that the patient is taking, because certain drugs can impair free water excretion either by acting on the renal tubule or by inducing pituitary arginine vasopressin expression. These drugs include morphine, cyclophosphamide, vincristine, chlorpropamide, amitriptyline, and clofibrate.

TREATMENT

The major focus of treatment for SIADH related to malignancy is successful treatment of the underlying cancer.

Acute treatment

Acute treatment is indicated in patients who are symptomatic and who have severe hyponatremia (eg, serum sodium level < 125 mEq/L). The goals of therapy in these patients are to initiate and maintain rapid diuresis with IV furosemide (1 mg/kg body weight) and to replace the sodium and potassium lost in the urine. Usually, the latter goal can be achieved by administering 0.9% saline with added potassium.

This rapid correction should not exceed a 20-mEq/L rise in serum sodium concentration during the first 48 hours. Patients who experience too rapid a rise in serum sodium concentration may suffer neurologic damage and central pontine myelinolysis.

Chronic treatment

The mainstay of chronic therapy is water restriction to 500 to 1,000 mL/d. When this measure alone is unsuccessful, demeclocycline, 300 to 600 mg orally bid, may be used in patients without liver disease. The onset of action may be > 1 week.

LAMBERT-EATON SYNDROME

The Lambert-Eaton syndrome is strongly associated with SCLC. It is caused by antibodies that interfere with the release of presynaptic acetylcholine at the neuromuscular junction.

SIGNS AND SYMPTOMS

This syndrome is characterized by fatigue and proximal muscle weakness, particularly of the pelvic girdle and thighs.

Many patients with this disorder have autonomic symptoms, one of the most common of which is dry mouth.

Other possible symptoms include diplopia or blurred vision, ptosis, dysarthria, dysphagia, and paresthesias.

DIAGNOSIS

Patients with the Lambert-Eaton syndrome show an improvement in muscle strength with exercise.

Electromyographic (EMG) studies

These studies are helpful in making the diagnosis. They reveal an increase in the muscle action potential, with repeated nerve stimulation at rates faster than 10 per second.

Edrophonium test

In addition, in contrast to individuals with myasthenia gravis, patients with the Lambert-Eaton syndrome have a poor response to the edrophonium test.

TREATMENT

Chemotherapy

This is the first line of treatment, as 90% of patients with SCLC will respond to this measure. In fact, recovery from the Lambert-Eaton syndrome has been noted in some patients treated with chemotherapy.

Other therapies

For patients in whom chemotherapy fails to improve symptoms or control the tumor, guanidine has been reported to be useful, as has 3,4-diaminopyridine.

Guanidine is taken orally, beginning with a dosage of 5 to 10 mg/kg/d divided throughout the waking hours. The dosage may be increased to a maximum of 30 mg/kg/d on the basis of the patient's clinical response. However, side effects may be severe at dosages > 1 g/d. Also, the dose of guanidine should not be increased more often than every 3 days, because the maximum response to a dose may not be seen for 2 to 3 days. At dosages of 5 to 25 mg three to four times per day, 3,4-diaminopyridine can significantly improve symptoms. Side effects of this drug include perioral and acral paresthesias, insomnia, and epigastric distress.

In addition, plasmapheresis, steroids, immunosuppression, and IV gamma globulin are all of potential benefit.

POLYMYOSITIS/DERMATOMYOSITIS

The relationship between polymyositis/dermatomyositis and malignancy was established long ago. The most commonly associated malignancies are breast, lung, and ovarian cancers. An increased incidence of cancer patients with dermatomyositis (10%) has been observed, but the association of cancer with polymyositis is less clear.

SIGNS AND SYMPTOMS

Muscle weakness

Patients with this syndrome typically experience proximal muscle weakness that progresses over weeks to months. Weakness in the hips, thighs, and shoulder girdle may cause patients to have difficulties in getting out of a chair, climbing stairs, or combing their hair. Patients also may experience dysphagia as well as weakness of the flexor muscles of the neck.

In the majority of cases, the distal muscles of the extremities are not involved. Also, most patients do not have involvement of the extraocular muscles.

Rashes

Patients with dermatomyositis can have involvement of the eyelids, forehead, cheeks, chest, elbows, knees, and knuckles, with the classic heliotrope rash. A more diffuse rash may also occur.

DIAGNOSIS

Patients with polymyositis/dermatomyositis usually have an elevation in their serum muscle enzyme levels and erythrocyte sedimentation rate.

In addition, EMG tracings are abnormal, and muscle biopsies reveal minimal inflammatory changes, along with muscle fiber necrosis, in patients with polymyositis/dermatomyositis.

TREATMENT

Steroids

In addition to treatment of the underlying malignancy, patients with polymyositis or dermatomyositis are treated with high-dose oral steroids (eg, prednisone, 60 to 80 mg/d). Other supportive measures, such as range-of-motion exercises, are also prescribed.

Immunosuppressives

In patients who do not respond to steroid therapy, immunosuppressive therapy is often added. This type of therapy needs to be tailored to the individual patient, and consultation with a rheumatologist should be considered.

Therapy for skin disease

The skin disease of dermatomyositis can be treated with a variety of measures, such as topical corticosteroids, antimalarials, photoprotection, and, at times, low-dose methotrexate.

SUGGESTED READING

ON SUPERIOR VENA CAVA SYNDROME

Nguyen NP, Borok TL, Welsh J, et al: Safety and effectiveness of vascular endoprosthesis for malignant superior vena cava syndrome. Thorax 64:174–178, 2009.

ON VENOUS THROMBOEMBOLIC COMPLICATIONS

Nalluri SR, Chu D, Kerestes R, et al: Risk of venous thromboembolism with the angiogenesis inhibitor bevacizumab in cancer patients: A metanalysis. JAMA 300:2277–2285, 2008.

Wagman LD, Baird MF, Bennett CL, et al: Venous thromboembolic disease. NCCN. Clinical practice guidelines in oncology. J Natl Compr Cancer Netw 6:716–753, 2008.

ON SPINAL CORD COMPRESSION

Chi JH, Gokaslan Z, McCormick P, et al: Selecting treatment for patients with malignant epidural spinal cord compression—does age matter?: Results from a randomized clinical trial. Spine 34:431–435, 2009.

Rades D, Lange M, Veninga T, et al: Preliminary results of spinal cord compression recurrence evaluation (score-1) study comparing short-course versus long-course radiotherapy for local control of malignant epidural cord compression. Int J Radiat Oncol Biol Phys 73:228–234, 2009.

ON HYPERCALCEMIA

Kikuchi A, Kigasawa H, Tsurusawa M, et al: A study of rasburicase for the management of hyperuricemia in pediatric patients with newly diagnosed hematologic malignancies at high risk for tumor lysis syndrome. Int J Hematol 90:492–500, 2009.

ON HYPERURICEMIA/TUMOR LYSIS SYNDROME

Tosi P, Barosi G, Lazzaro C, et al: Consensus conference on the management of tumor lysis syndrome. Haematologica 93:1877–1885, 2008.

ON SYNDROME OF INAPPROPRIATE SECRETION OF ANTIDIURETIC HORMONE

Flombaum CD: Metabolic emergencies in the cancer patient. Semin Oncol 27:322–334, 2000.

Raftopoulos H: Diagnosis and management of hyponatremia in cancer patients. Support Care Cancer 15:1341–1347, 2007.

ON LAMBERT-EATON SYNDROME

Titulaer MJ, Wirtz PW, Kuks JB, et al: The Lambert-Eaton myasthenic syndrome 1988–2008: A clinical picture in 97 patients. J Neuroimmunol 201–202:153–158, 2008.

ON POLYMYOSITIS/DERMATOMYOSITIS

Andras C, Ponyi A, Constantin T, et al: Dermatomyositis and polymyositis associated with malignancy: A 21-year retrospective study. J Rheumatol 35:438–444, 2008.

Fardet L, Dupuy A, Gain M, et al: Factors associated with underlying malignancy in a retrospective cohort of 121 patients with dermatomyositis. Medicine (Baltimore) 88:91–97, 2009.

Abbreviations in this chapter

ASCO = American Society of Clinical Oncology; ATAC = Arimidex, Tamoxifen, Alone or in Combination; NCCN = National Comprehensive Cancer Network

CHAPTER 39

Infectious complications

Sanjeet Dadwal, MD, Jane Kriengkauykiat, PharmD, and James Ito, MD

Infections are among the most common, potentially serious complications of cancer and its treatment. This chapter discusses infections from a syndromic approach: that is, infections present as a complex of signs and symptoms to the clinician. The syndromes addressed include febrile neutropenia, pneumonia, catheter-associated infections, and gastrointestinal infections (*Clostridium difficile*–associated diarrhea and typhlitis). Special sections focus on fungal and viral infections.

INFECTION DURING FEBRILE NEUTROPENIA

It has long been recognized that the incidence of infection is high in patients who develop a fever during neutropenia and that empiric antimicrobial therapy is warranted in such patients.

DEFINITIONS

Fever is usually defined as a temperature ≥ 38.3°C.

Neutropenia is defined as a neutrophil count of < 500/µL, although patients with a neutrophil count between 500 and 1,000/µL in whom a decrease is anticipated are considered to be neutropenic. Patients with a neutrophil count < 100/µL are at greatest risk for infection, as are those with a rapid decrease in neutrophil count and those with protracted neutropenia.

ETIOLOGY

Bacteria Infections occurring during episodes of febrile neutropenia are caused predominantly by aerobic gram-negative bacilli (especially *Escherichia coli, Klebsiella pneumoniae,* and *Pseudomonas aeruginosa*) and gram-positive cocci (coagulase-negative staphylococci, β-hemolytic streptococci, viridans streptococci, enterococci, and *Staphylococcus aureus*). In recent years, multidrug-resistant organisms have become more prominent.

Fungi Fungal infections usually occur after a patient has received broad-spectrum antimicrobial therapy and/or steroids. The most common fungal pathogens are *Candida* species (predominantly C *albicans* and C *tropicalis*) and *Aspergillus* species.

Less common are *Fusarium*, *Scedosporium*, and *Zygomycetes* infections (see also section on "Fungal infections").

Viruses Viral infections occurring during neutropenia are caused predominantly by herpesviruses and respiratory viruses. The herpesviruses include herpes simplex virus (HSV), varicella zoster virus (VZV), cytomegalovirus (CMV), and Epstein-Barr virus (EBV). The respiratory viruses include adenovirus, respiratory syncytial virus, parainfluenza virus, influenza A and B viruses, metapneumovirus, and rhinovirus (see also section on "Viral infections").

SIGNS AND SYMPTOMS

The most remarkable aspect of the febrile, neutropenic patient is the lack of physical findings. This is due to the neutropenia and the absence of an inflammatory response at the infection site. The patient may have only a fever with or without chills or rigors. Even if the patient has pneumonia, there may be few respiratory symptoms. Likewise, a perirectal abscess may be relatively asymptomatic.

DIAGNOSIS

An initial evaluation and diagnostic workup of any fever in a neutropenic patient should begin immediately but should not delay the initiation of empiric therapy. A complete history (exposures, past infections, rashes, cough, abdominal pain, diarrhea) should be taken and a physical examination (skin lesions, exit site and tunnel of right atrial catheter, oropharynx, abdomen, perineum) should be performed.

Diagnostic workup should include:

- at least two sets of blood cultures: one from a peripheral vein and one from each port of a central venous catheter. If fever persists in the face of negative cultures, blood cultures for fungi and acid-fast bacilli should be considered.
- culture of any drainage from a catheter exit site
- stool examination for *C difficile* and other bacterial/protozoal agents
- urine culture and urinalysis
- chest radiograph
- aspiration or biopsy of any skin lesions.

CT If indicated by signs or symptoms, CT scans of the brain (followed by lumbar puncture), chest, abdomen, and pelvis can be performed.

Laboratory tests Determination of serum transaminases, CBC, and serum creatinine is also recommended. Other useful serologies include *Aspergillus galactomannan*, beta-D-glucan, *Coccidioides* antibody panel, and histoplasmosis antigen, depending on the region.

TREATMENT

INITIAL EMPIRIC ANTIBIOTIC THERAPY

Initial antibacterial therapy in the febrile, neutropenic patient should be broad-spectrum and should be based on the prevalence and susceptibility of bacterial isolates seen in the individual hospital setting (Figure 1). When choosing an antibiotic, the clinician also should take into consideration the patient's allergies, renal and hepatic function, and other drugs he or she is receiving that may interact with the empiric antimicrobial agent.

The choice of initial empiric antibiotic therapy for the febrile, neutropenic patient is dictated in part by the susceptibility pattern of blood isolates seen at a particular cancer center. If the prevalence of extended-spectrum beta-lactamase (ESBL) gram-negative bacteria is high, for example, one probably would not want to use a third-generation cephalosporin such as ceftazidime as initial empiric monotherapy. Some data suggest that prolonged use of ceftazidime monotherapy in this setting promotes the emergence of ESBL bacteria. City of Hope has been using ceftazidime as initial monotherapy for the past 15 years, however, without a significant rise in the incidence of resistant gram-negative infections, and this experience has been shared by other centers. Finally, any special circumstance, such as the suspicion of an indwelling IV catheter-associated infection, may influence the antibiotic choice.

Either single antibiotics or antibiotic combinations can be used for initial empiric therapy (see Table 1 for dosage regimens).

Monotherapy

Ceftazidime, cefepime (Maxipime), imipenem-cilastatin (Primaxin), or meropenem (Merrem), when used as monotherapy, avoids the potential for nephrotoxicity. However, none of these antibiotics covers coagulase-negative staphylococci, methicillin-resistant *S aureus* (MRSA), vancomycin-resistant or vancomycin-susceptible enterococci, some strains of penicillin-resistant *Streptococcus pneumoniae*, and viridans streptococci. Also, ceftazidime does not cover anaerobes well, and imipenem-cilastatin may have CNS toxicity at high doses.

Duotherapy

Aminoglycoside plus antipseudomonal β-lactam The aminoglycoside could be gentamicin, tobramycin, or amikacin (Amikin). The β-lactam could be ticarcillin (Ticar) or piperacillin (Pipracil), either alone or with a β-lactamase inhibitor (piperacillin/tazobactam [Zosyn]); ceftazidime; cefepime; or a carbapenem.

Advantages of the combination of an aminoglycoside and an antipseudomonal β-lactam include possible synergistic effects against gram-negative bacilli and decreased emergence of resistant strains. The major disadvantages of the combination are potential nephrotoxicity, ototoxicity, hypokalemia, and the need to monitor drug levels of the aminoglycoside. Also, gram-positive coverage is not ideal.

Vancomycin plus one or two drugs The use of vancomycin as part of the initial regimen is controversial. Certainly, a majority of documented bacteremias in

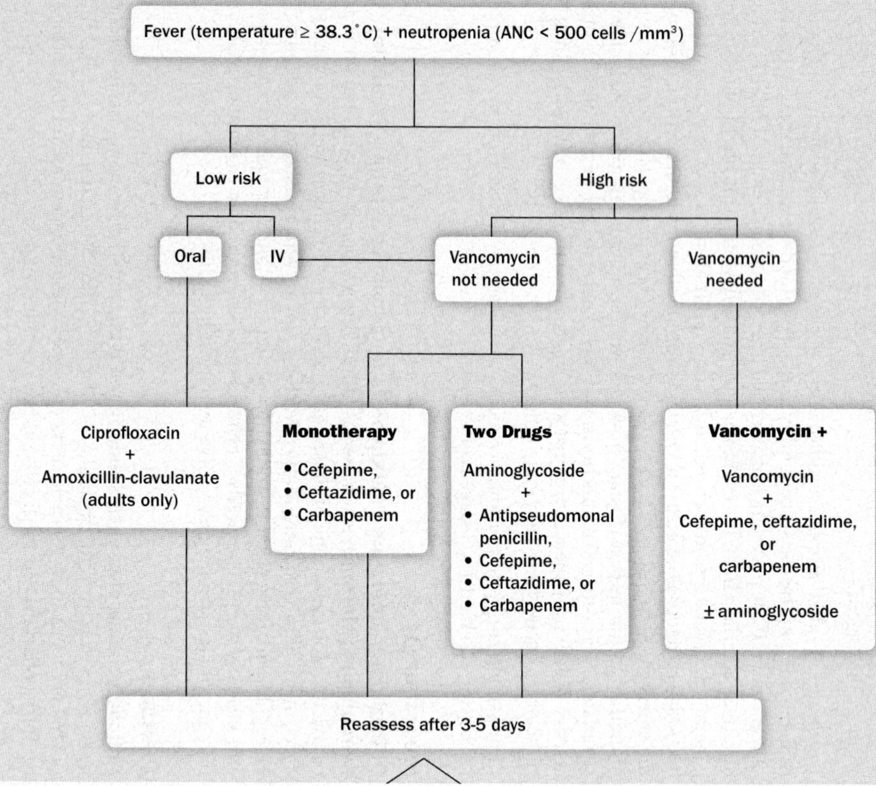
Fever (temperature ≥ 38.3˚C) + neutropenia (ANC < 500 cells /mm³)
Low risk
High risk
Oral
IV
Vancomycin not needed
Vancomycin needed
Ciprofloxacin + Amoxicillin-clavulanate (adults only)
Monotherapy
• Cefepime,
• Ceftazidime, or
• Carbapenem
Two Drugs
Aminoglycoside +
• Antipseudomonal penicillin,
• Cefepime,
• Ceftazidime, or
• Carbapenem
Vancomycin +
Vancomycin + Cefepime, ceftazidime, or carbapenem
± aminoglycoside
Reassess after 3-5 days

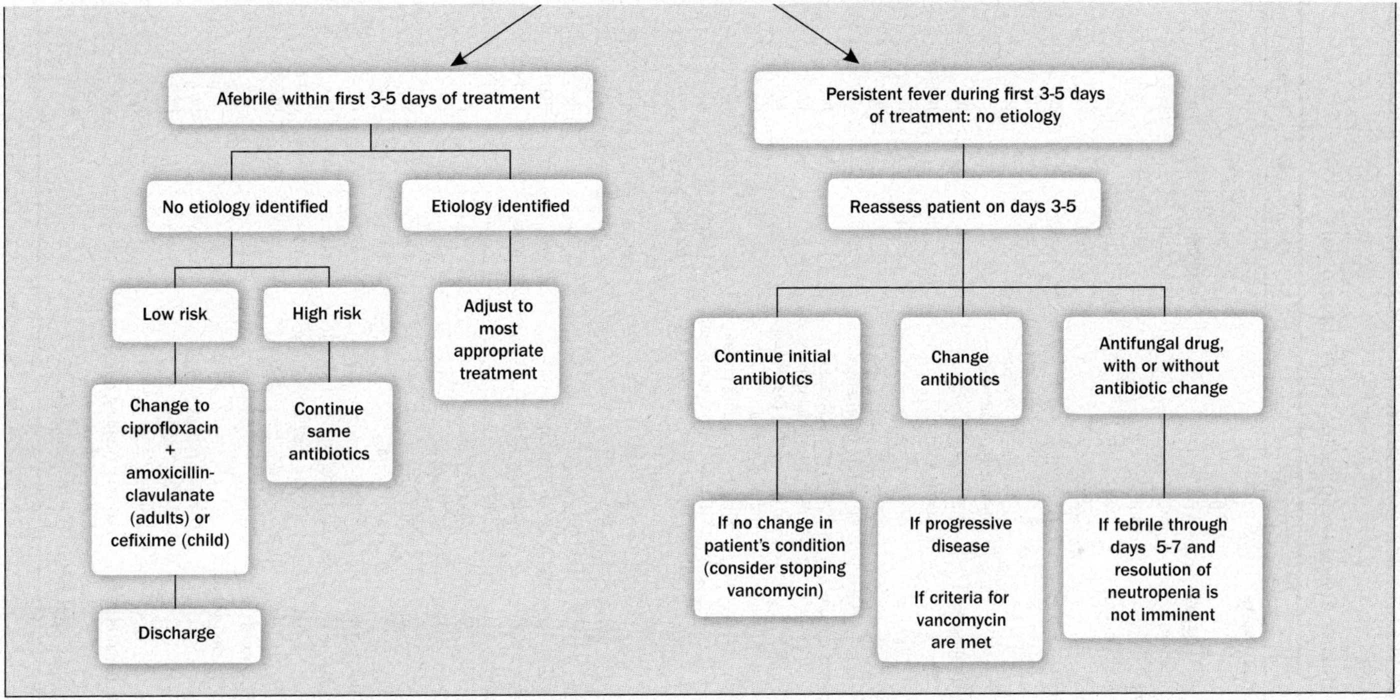

FIGURE 1: Guide to the initial management of the febrile neutropenic patient.

Adapted, with permission, from Hughes WT, et al: 2002 guidelines for the use of antimicrobial agents in neutropenic patients with cancer. Clin Infect Dis 34:730–751, 2002.

TABLE 1: Dosing schedules of selected antimicrobials

Drug	Dose	Frequency	Route
Antibacterial agents			
Ceftazidime	2 g	q8h	IV
Cefepime	2 g	q8h	IV
Imipenem-cilastatin	500 mg	q6h	IV
Meropenem	1 g	q8h	IV
Piperacillin/tazobactam	4.5 g	q6h	IV
Aztreonam	2 g	q8h	IV
Vancomycin	15 mg/kg	q12h	IV
	7.5 mg/kg	q6h	IV
	125 mg (for *C difficile*–associated diarrhea)	q6h	PO
Quinupristin/dalfopristin	7.5 mg/kg	q8h	IV
Linezolid	600 mg	q12h	IV/PO
Daptomycin	4–6 mg/kg	q24h	IV
Tigecycline	100 mg (loading dose)	× 1	IV
	50 mg (maintenance)	q12h	IV
Gentamicin/tobramycin	2 mg/kg (loading dose)		IV
	1.5 mg/kg (maintenance)	q8	IV
	or 5–7 mg/kg (extended-interval dose)	q24h	IV
Amikacin	8 mg/kg (loading dose)		IV
	7.5 mg/kg (maintenance)	q12h	IV
	or 15–20 mg/kg (extended-interval dose)	q24h	IV
Cefazolin	2 g	q8h	IV
Nafcillin	2 g	q4h	IV
Ciprofloxacin	400 mg	q12h	IV
	500–750 mg	bid	PO
Levofloxacin	750 mg	q24h	IV/PO
Metronidazole	500 mg	q6h	IV/PO
Clindamycin	900 mg	q8h	IV
TMP-SMZ	15 mg/kg/d	q6h	IV
Amoxicillin/clavulanate	500 mg	q8h	PO
	or 875 mg	bid	PO
Ampicillin/sulbactam	3 g	q6h	IV
Clarithromycin	500 mg	bid	PO
Azithromycin	500 mg (day 1), 250 mg	q24h	IV/PO
	500 mg	q24h	IV/PO
Antifungal agents			
Amphotericin B deoxycholate			
Therapy	0.5–1.0 mg/kg	daily	IV
Prophylaxis	0.1–0.2 mg/kg	daily	IV
Fluconazole	400 mg	daily	IV or PO
Itraconazole capsules	200 mg (loading dose)	tid × 4 d	PO
	200 mg (maintenance)	bid	PO
Itraconazole oral solution	(see capsules above)		

TABLE 1: Dosing schedules of selected antimicrobials, *continued*

Drug	Dose	Frequency	Route
Amphotericin B			
Lipid complex	5 mg/kg	daily	IV
Cholesteryl sulfate	3–6 mg/kg	daily	IV
Liposome	3–5 mg/kg	daily	IV
Prophylaxis	1 mg/kg	daily	IV
Caspofungin	70 mg (loading dose)		IV
	50 mg (maintenance)	daily	IV
Voriconazole	6 mg/kg (loading dose)	× 2 q12h	IV
	4 mg/kg (maintenance)	q12h	IV/PO
Prophylaxis	200 mg for > 40 kg	q12h	PO
	100 mg for ≤ 40 kg	q12h	PO
Micafungin	50 mg (for prophylaxis)	q24h	IV
	100 mg (treatment)	q24h	IV
Anidulafungin	200 mg (loading dose)		IV
	100 mg (maintenance)	daily	IV
Posaconazole	200 mg (prophylaxis)	tid	PO
	400 mg (treatment)	bid	PO
Antiviral agents			
Acyclovir			
For HSV	5 mg/kg	q8h	IV
For VZV	10 mg/kg	q8h	IV
For HSV encephalitis	10–12 mg/kg	q8h	IV
Ganciclovir	5 mg/kg (induction)	q12h	IV
	5 mg/kg (maintenance)	daily	IV
Valganciclovir	900 mg (induction)	q12h	PO
Foscarnet	60 mg/kg (induction)	q8h	IV for 14 d
	90 mg/kg (maintenance)	daily	IV
Cidofovir	5 mg/kg	q wk × 2	IV
	then	q2wk	
	or 1 mg/kg	qod	IV
Amantadine, rimantadine	100 mg	bid	PO
Zanamivir	10 mg	bid	inhalation
Oseltamivir	75 mg	bid	PO

HSV = herpes simplex virus; TMP-SMZ = trimethoprim-sulfamethoxazole; VZV = varicella zoster virus

neutropenic febrile patients are caused by gram-positive organisms, and most of them are due to coagulase-negative staphylococci. Also, vancomycin is probably the preferred drug for viridans streptococcal sepsis and the drug of choice for MRSA and *Corynebacterium* infections. On the other hand, there is concern for the overuse of vancomycin and the emergence of vancomycin-resistant enterococci (and now *S aureus*). A study by the EORTC and the NCIC did not support the use of vancomycin in initial empiric therapy.

It should be noted that the CDC advises against the use of vancomycin in initial empiric therapy for a febrile, neutropenic patient "unless initial evidence indicates that the patient has an infection caused by gram-positive microorganisms (eg, at an inflamed exit site of a Hickman catheter) and the prevalence of infections caused by MRSA in the hospital is substantial."

Thus, it is recommended (in the 2002 guidelines for the use of antimicrobial agents in neutropenic patients with unexplained fever developed by the IDSA) that vancomycin be added to the initial regimen (eg, with ceftazidime) in selected patients, including:

- patients with clinically obvious, serious catheter-related infections
- patients undergoing intensive chemotherapy that produces substantial mucosal damage (ie, high-dose cytarabine [Ara-C], which increases the risk of penicillin-resistant streptococcal infections, particularly those due to viridans streptococci)
- patients receiving prophylaxis with quinolones before the onset of the febrile episode
- patients who have known colonization with pneumococci that are resistant to penicillin and cephalosporins or MRSA
- patients with a blood culture positive for gram-positive bacteria before final identification and susceptibility testing
- patients with hypotension or other evidence of cardiovascular impairment.

Double β-lactam therapy usually consists of a third-generation cephalosporin (ceftazidime or cefoperazone [Cefobid]) and a ureidopenicillin (piperacillin, ticarcillin, or mezlocillin [Mezlin]). The advantages of this regimen are low toxicity (mainly renal) and theoretical synergism. However, it is more costly (compared with monotherapy) and has the possibility of antagonism.

CHANGES IN INITIAL THERAPY

Defervescence If the fever subsides after 3 days of empiric therapy and a specific organism is identified, broad-spectrum antibiotic coverage can be modified to provide optimal treatment. Antibiotics can be discontinued after 7 days if all evidence of infection has been eradicated and if neutropenia has resolved.

If no organism is isolated, treatment with the initial regimen should be continued for a minimum of 7 days. If the patient is clinically well, the regimen can be switched to an oral antibiotic, such as cefixime (Suprax) or a quinolone.

Persistent, unresponsive fever If the fever persists after 3–5 days of antibiotic therapy, reassessment is recommended. If no infectious etiology is determined, a change in or addition to the antibiotic regimen is recommended.

If vancomycin was not part of the initial empiric regimen, many physicians would consider adding it. However, because of the recommendation by the CDC against empiric vancomycin use, it probably should not be added unless there is a strong clinical or microbiologic reason to do so. Instead, cefazolin or nafcillin could be added for better gram-positive coverage. If the initial regimen did not provide anaerobic coverage, metronidazole could be added. Finally, if fever and neutropenia persist despite ≥ 4 days of antibiotic therapy, an antifungal agent (caspofungin [Cancidas], liposomal amphotericin B [AmBisome], amphotericin B lipid complex [Abelcet],

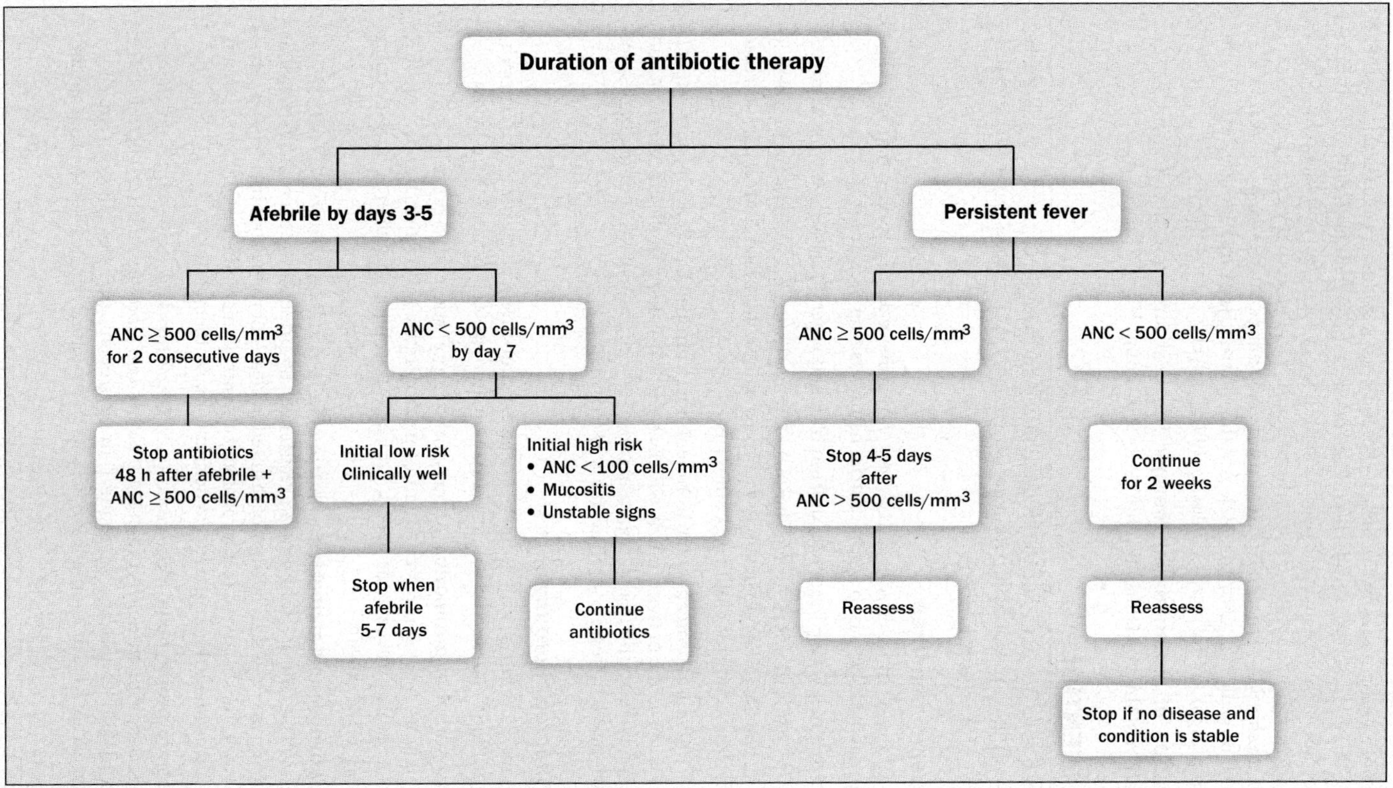

FIGURE 2: Duration of antibiotic therapy ANC = absolute neutrophil count

Adapted, with permission, from Hughes WT, et al: 2002 guidelines for the use of antimicrobial agents in neutropenic patients with cancer. Clin Infect Dis 34:730–751, 2002.

itraconazole [Sporanox], voriconazole [Vfend]), or even fluconazole (Diflucan, if the risk of mold infection is low) should be added. If the patient is already on antifungal prophylaxis with an azole or echinocandin, a polyene (an amphotericin B lipid formulation) should be started. If the patient is receiving a polyene as prophylaxis, the dose should be escalated, or, alternatively, a change can be made to an extended-spectrum azole (eg, voriconazole). Another alternative is to add an echinocandin (caspofungin) to the increased dosage of the polyene.

Duration of antimicrobial therapy The most important determinant of the duration of therapy is the absolute neutrophil count (Figure 2).

PREVENTION

Attempts to prevent infection in the neutropenic host focus on two broad areas: preventing acquisition of pathogenic organisms and suppressing or eradicating endogenous microbial flora.

Hygienic measures

The simplest, most effective, and least expensive way to prevent acquisition of potential pathogens is to institute strict hand-washing precautions.

A cooked diet with elimination of fresh fruit and vegetables is also recommended.

Water purification systems (to eliminate *Legionella* organisms) and high-efficiency particulate air (HEPA) filtration systems (to eliminate fungal spores) can decrease the rates of acquisition of these pathogens.

The use of more "protective" environments for neutropenic patients is controversial. The total protective environment, which consists of a totally sterile environment and an aggressive antimicrobial regimen, can reduce the rate of infection but does not contribute to increased survival and is also costly.

Antibacterial prophylaxis

Prophylactic antibacterial therapy generally falls into three categories: oral nonabsorbable antibiotics, selective decontamination regimens, and systemic prophylaxis.

Nonabsorbable antibiotics Although the use of oral nonabsorbable antibiotics has demonstrated some reduction in infection rates, this option has become less popular due to its cost, side effects, unpalatability, poor compliance, and selection of resistant organisms.

Selective decontamination with trimethoprim-sulfamethoxazole (TMP-SMZ), ie, establishment of "colonization resistance" by preserving anaerobic flora while reducing aerobic bacteria, has not resulted in clear-cut reductions in infection rates. Moreover, the disadvantages of prolonged neutropenia and emergence of resistant organisms make this regimen less desirable than others.

Systemic prophylaxis More recently, many studies have touted the value of antibacterial prophylaxis with fluoroquinolones (eg, ciprofloxacin [Cipro], ofloxacin [Floxin], and levofloxacin [Levaquin]) in neutropenic patients. However, no single study (except for a meta-analysis of 52 trials) has demonstrated a survival advantage.

Thus, neither the NCCN nor the IDSA guidelines recommend using antibacterial prophylaxis in neutropenic patients. The NCCN guideline recommends that bacterial prophylaxis (fluoroquinolones) be considered for high-risk patients (neutropenia < 100 μL for > 7 days). Despite this lack of a strong recommendation, fluoroquinolone (mainly levofloxacin) prophylaxis is widely used at many cancer centers; the obvious downside of this trend is the emergence of resistant bacteria, which has already been observed in many institutions. Levofloxacin use has also been associated with the emergence of hypervirulent *C difficile* enterocolitis.

***Pneumocystis jirovecii* pneumonia** In patients at risk for *P jirovecii* pneumonia (patients undergoing allogeneic hematopoietic cell transplantation [HCT], those with lymphoma, or those receiving steroids), TMP-SMZ, administered for only 2 or 3 days per week, can reduce the incidence of infection.

Antifungal prophylaxis

Fluconazole, itraconazole, micafungin (Mycamine), and posaconazole (Noxafil) have all been shown to lower the incidence of invasive fungal infection when used as prophylaxis in the HCT setting. In a retrospective study, low-dose conventional amphotericin B has also been associated with a lower incidence of infection. Fluconazole, however, has no activity against molds. Itraconazole is limited by its gastrointestinal and hepatic toxicities. Posaconazole has been shown to prevent both *Candida* and *Aspergillus* infections in both neutropenic AML (acute myelogenous leukemia) and MDS (myelodysplastic syndrome) patients and the high-risk allogeneic HCT recipient with graft-vs-host disease (GVHD). Antifungal prophylaxis should be reserved for those patients at highest risk for invasive fungal infection—ie, HCT and high-risk leukemia patients undergoing high-dose chemotherapy (see also "Prevention" section under "Fungal infections").

Antiviral prophylaxis

Acyclovir Patients at risk for mucositis (ie, those undergoing induction therapy for leukemia or lymphoma or HCT) who have evidence of prior HSV infection (positive serology) can receive prophylaxis with twice-daily IV acyclovir (see Table 1 for dose).

Ganciclovir has been shown to be an effective "preemptive" antiviral in preventing CMV interstitial pneumonia in allogeneic HCT recipients who demonstrate evidence of viremia by polymerase chain reaction (PCR), antigen testing, or positive blood cultures (see section on "Viral infections").

PNEUMONIA

A significant number of infections in cancer patients are due to pneumonia. For example, 25% of documented infections in patients with nonlymphocytic leukemia are caused by pneumonia. Also, 50% of allogeneic HCT recipients will develop pneumonia.

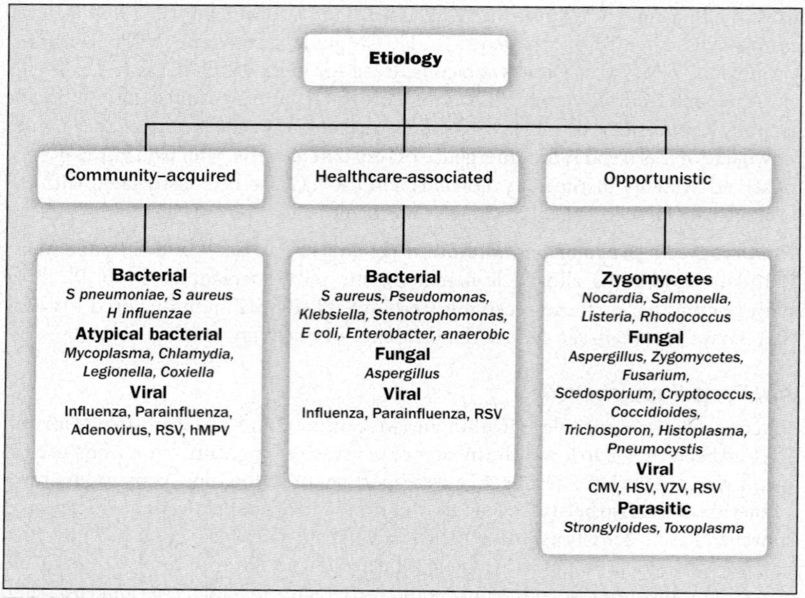

FIGURE 3: Pneumonia in a neutropenic/immunocompromised host.

RSV = respiratory syncytial virus; hMPV = human metapneumovirus; CMV = cytomegalovirus; HSV = herpes simplex virus; VZV = varicella zoster virus

ETIOLOGY AND RISK FACTORS

Some of the risk factors that predispose cancer patients to pneumonia are cellular and humoral immune deficiencies, neutropenia, impaired tracheobronchial clearance, use of antibiotics and steroids, and surgery.

Etiologic agents The etiologic agents responsible for pneumonia in the cancer patient run the gamut of most bacterial, fungal, and viral organisms (Figure 3).

Noninfectious processes mimicking pneumonia Numerous noninfectious processes can mimic pneumonia in cancer patients. They include congestive heart failure, aseptic emboli, metastatic disease, adult respiratory distress syndrome, diffuse alveolar hemorrhage, a periengraftment infiltrate, radiation injury, hypersensitivity disorders and reactions, and trauma.

Pinpointing the pathogen Certain characteristics of each cancer patient may help predict the specific etiologic agent.

Type of immunosuppression One characteristic that is particularly useful is the type of immunosuppression that the patient is experiencing. This depends on the type of neoplastic disease (eg, lymphoma, leukemia) and, more importantly, the type of therapy (eg, chemotherapy, radiation therapy, allogeneic HCT). For example, certain gram-negative and gram-positive bacteria are more prevalent during neutropenia, whereas other bacteria (*S pneumoniae*, *Haemophilus influenzae*) are more common with a humoral immune deficiency, such as occurs after splenectomy.

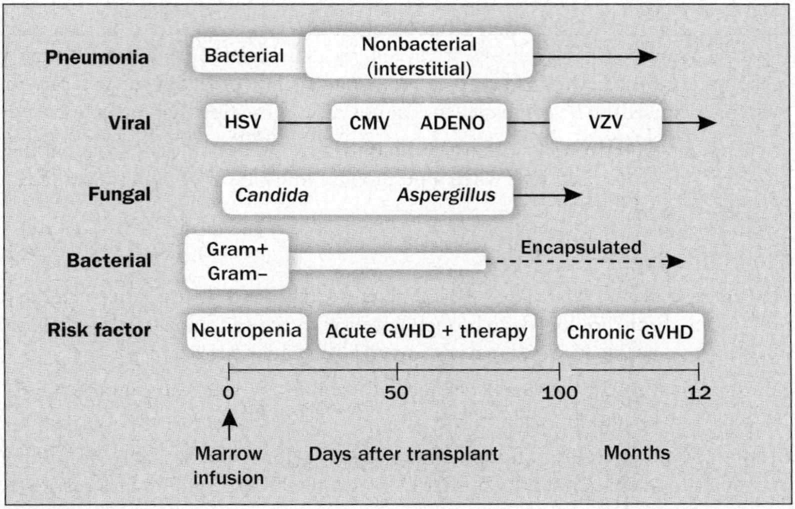

FIGURE 4: Timing of infectious syndromes after bone marrow transplantation.

ADENO = adenovirus; CMV = cytomegalovirus; GVHD = graft-vs-host disease; HSV = herpes simplex virus; VZV = varicella zoster virus

Adapted, with permission, from Meyers JD: Infections in marrow recipients, in Mandell GL, Doublas RG, Bennett JE (eds): Principles and Practice of Infectious Diseases, 2nd ed, pp 1674–1676. New York, Wiley, 1985.

Timing of pneumonia Another important characteristic is the timing of the pneumonia; in other words, the phase of the immunosuppression can help predict the etiology. For example, an interstitial pneumonia occurring during the first 30 days after allogeneic HCT would not be expected to be due to CMV (Figure 4).

Other factors Finally, other factors such as the duration of neutropenia, prior antimicrobial therapy, other agents (such as steroids and alemtuzumab [Campath]) used, and the specific local microbiota help in prediction. For example, if an allogeneic HCT patient receiving steroids for GVHD develops nodular infiltrates after weeks of broad-spectrum antibacterial antibiotics, an *Aspergillus* species would be highly suspected.

SIGNS AND SYMPTOMS

Although a productive cough is almost always present in a normal host with pneumonia, often neither a cough nor sputum is seen in an immunocompromised cancer patient with such an infection.

Fever, however, is almost invariably present in the cancer patient with pneumonia and, by itself, should prompt a workup for pneumonia.

Other possible symptoms include shortness of breath, pleuritic chest pain, and hemoptysis.

DIAGNOSIS

Because pneumonia can progress rapidly and result in high morbidity and mortality in the compromised host, and because the etiologic agent is often difficult to ascertain, the clinician needs to be aggressive in diagnosing and treating these infections.

The diagnosis of pneumonia is most commonly made by a simple chest radiograph. However, there are occasions when a pulmonary infiltrate or small nodular lesion is seen only on a CT scan.

Etiologic diagnosis

An etiologic diagnosis is made by the following procedures: sputum (expectorated or induced), bronchoscopy with bronchoalveolar lavage and transbronchial biopsy, transthoracic needle biopsy/aspiration, open lung biopsy, and serologies.

Sputum An adequate sputum specimen is difficult to obtain from cancer patients, especially during neutropenia.

Bronchoscopy with bronchoalveolar lavage is a much more sensitive technique than sputum analysis but may miss the organism when the pulmonary disease is peripheral or nodular.

Transthoracic needle biopsy/aspiration under CT guidance may be helpful if the lesion is proximal but may be contraindicated in a severely thrombocytopenic patient. This procedure is indicated when there is a focal/nodular lesion in the periphery.

Open lung biopsy is the most definitive diagnostic procedure but also the most invasive. It is still not clear whether the information obtained by open biopsy improves overall survival. The less invasive thoracoscopic open lung biopsy is becoming more popular than open lung biopsy.

Smears and cultures Both fluid and tissue specimens should be sent for bacterial smears (including acid-fast bacilli and modified acid-fast bacilli) and cultures (including those for anaerobes, acid-fast bacilli, and *Legionella* organisms), fungal smears (potassium hydroxide) and cultures, direct fluorescent antibody test for viruses, cytology (for viral inclusions and silver stains for fungi and *P jirovecii*), and histopathology.

Diagnostic approach to pneumonia is depicted in Figure 5 using risk stratification (low vs high risk). Patients with suspected pneumonia should undergo an aggressive etiologic workup along with broad-spectrum empiric antimicrobial treatment. Preemptive antifungal therapy should be based on risk. Treatment is then tailored accordingly.

TREATMENT

The therapeutic approach to pneumonia in the cancer patient should take into consideration the category of immunosuppression (neoplastic disease and immunosuppressive therapy), as well as the timing of onset and the pattern of the pneumonia.

EMPIRIC ANTIBIOTIC THERAPY

In neutropenic patients experiencing their first fever and localized pulmonary infiltrates, one can justify initiating empiric therapy similar to that used for febrile, neutropenic patients (see previous discussion), because the majority of pneumonias in this setting are caused by gram-negative bacteria. However, in other situations, such as pneumonia that has a later onset, develops after empiric antibiotics have been initiated, is more aggressive or severe, occurs in a more severely compromised host (eg, a patient who has had allogeneic HCT), or is characterized by a diffuse or interstitial infiltrate, one should proceed to immediate bronchoscopy with bronchoalveolar lavage (and possibly transbronchial biopsy).

ADDITIONS TO EMPIRIC THERAPY

If no diagnosis is forthcoming after bronchoscopy and bronchoalveolar lavage, additions to empiric therapy should be made.

Anaerobic, gram-positive, and *Legionella* coverage Certainly, anaerobic coverage should be considered, as well as gram-positive coverage. *Legionella* coverage should be added, especially if warranted by the epidemiologic setting.

Antifungal and antituberculous therapy Finally, antifungal therapy should be initiated if there is no response to antibacterial therapy and especially if there are nodular or cavitary lesions. In addition, if such lesions are present and/or the epidemiologic setting is compatible, antituberculous therapy should be added.

Further diagnostic procedures If bronchoscopy with bronchoalveolar lavage does not reveal an etiology and the pneumonia is progressing despite empiric therapy, consideration should be given to transthoracic needle biopsy/aspiration and open lung biopsy. As mentioned previously, if there is a peripheral, focal lesion, transthoracic needle biopsy/aspiration can be attempted.

The ultimate diagnostic procedure is open biopsy, but because its contribution to increased survival is unknown, the decision to proceed with this most invasive procedure must be undertaken carefully.

SPECIFIC ANTIMICROBIAL THERAPY

A specific treatment approach is suggested in Figure 6 based on whether treatment is empiric or targeted.

PREVENTION

Methods to prevent pulmonary infections fall into the following categories: colonization prevention, antimicrobial prophylaxis (and preemptive treatment), vaccination, and immunomodulation.

The simplest method of colonization prevention is hand-washing.

Other colonization prevention methods, such as protective environments, are discussed in the previous section.

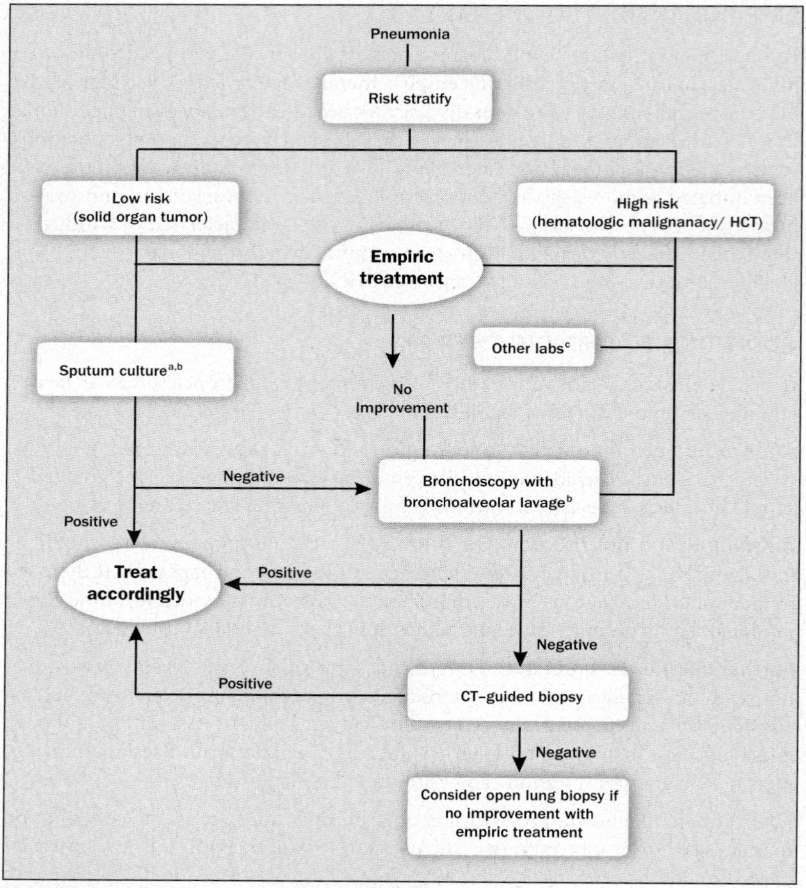

FIGURE 5: Diagnostic approach to pneumonia.

[a] Sputum cultures are usually not available or useful in most cases and should not be solely relied upon. There should be no delay in proceeding to bronchoscopy.
[b] Stains such as Gram, KOH (potassium hydroxide), and AFB (acid-fast bacilli) and cytology such as GMS (Gomori methenamine silver) and PAS (periodic acid Schiff) should be performed on respiratory samples.
[c] Consider fungal markers and serologies for various organisms based on history: *Legionella* urine antigen, *Aspergillus galactomannan*, (1-3)-beta-D-glucan assay, serologies for histoplasmosis, *Coccidioides, Cryptococcus*, Q fever.
HCT = hematopoietic cell transplant

With regard to pulmonary pathogens, HEPA-filtered rooms can eliminate *Aspergillus* spores from the immediate environment. Water supplies can be checked for *Legionella* contamination and/or adequate disinfection maintained (eg, chlorination, copper/silver ionization, temperature [60°C]).

Antimicrobial prophylaxis is discussed in the previous section.

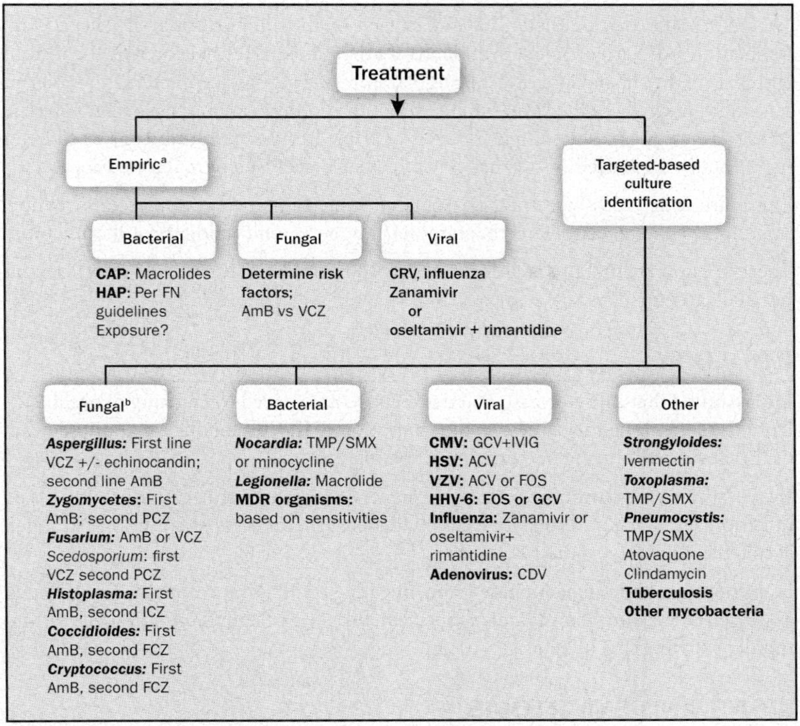

FIGURE 6: Antimicrobial treatment approach.

[a] Empiric treatment should be directed by patient risk factors.

[b] Surgical intervention with zygomycosis/aspergillosis, and removal of central venous catheter for fusariosis.

Note: ACV = acyclovir; AmB = amphotericin B products; CAP = community-acquired pneumonia; CDV = cidofovir; CMV = cytomegalovirus; CRV = community respiratory virus; FN = febrile neutropenia; FOS = foscarnet; FCZ = fluconazole; GCV = ganciclovir; HAP = healthcare-associated pneumonia; HHV-6 = human herpes virus 6; HSV = herpes simplex virus; ICZ = itraconazole; IVIG = intravenous immune globulin; MDR = multidrug resistant; PCZ = posaconazole; TMP/SMX = trimethoprim/sulfamethoxazole; VCZ = voriconazole; VZV = varicella zoster virus

The influenza and pneumococcal (killed) vaccines should be administered to cancer patients.

Immunomodulators, such as granulocyte colony-stimulating factor (G-CSF, filgrastim [Neupogen]) and granulocyte-macrophage colony-stimulating factor (GM-CSF, sargramostim [Leukine]), may help reduce infection by decreasing the duration of neutropenia.

CATHETER-ASSOCIATED INFECTIONS

Chronic indwelling right atrial catheters are commonly placed in cancer patients, as they permit frequent, long-term vascular access for drug and blood product administration, hyperalimentation, and blood drawing.

Hickman and Broviac catheters have an exit site on the skin surface, are anchored with a subcutaneous Dacron felt cuff, and have a subcutaneous tunnel entering the venous system (via the subclavian, external jugular, internal jugular, cephalic, saphenous, or femoral veins), where they lead into the superior or inferior vena cava or right atrium. These catheters can have single, double, or triple lumens. Another type of catheter has a totally implanted port (Port-A-Cath) that is accessed percutaneously.

There are four types of catheter-associated infections: exit-site infections, tunnel infections, catheter-associated bacteremia/fungemia, and septic thrombophlebitis.

There are approximately 0.4 infections per 100 catheter-days and 0.26 bacteremias per 100 catheter-days.

ETIOLOGY

It is assumed that catheter-associated infections are caused by tracking of organisms from the skin along the catheter, contamination of the lumen during manipulation, or direct seeding during bacteremia/fungemia.

By far, the most common microorganisms associated with catheter-associated infections are coagulase-negative staphylococci. The next most common pathogen is coagulase-positive *S aureus*.

Less common pathogens include gram-negative bacilli, gram-positive bacilli (such as *Corynebacterium* JK and *Bacillus* species), fungi (especially *Candida* species), and rapidly growing mycobacteria.

SIGNS AND SYMPTOMS

Exit-site infections may be manifested by local erythema, warmth, and tenderness. Purulent drainage may be present.

Tunnel infections are characterized by tenderness along the subcutaneous track.

Catheter-associated bacteremia/fungemia usually displays no local findings. A fever may be the only sign, but other signs and symptoms of sepsis or even full-blown septic shock syndrome may be present.

Likewise, septic thrombophlebitis may have no findings, except those associated with sepsis or venous thrombosis (edema).

DIAGNOSIS

In any cancer patient with a right atrial catheter who becomes febrile or is shown to be bacteremic or fungemic, a catheter-associated infection should be suspected. Without the signs or symptoms of an exit-site or tunnel infection, however, a diagnosis may be difficult.

Cultures Two blood cultures should be drawn: one from the catheter and one from a peripheral vein. There are two methods that may be helpful in making a diagnosis of right atrial catheter infection. Both depend upon drawing both (catheter and peripheral vein) blood cultures simultaneously. In the first method, quantitative colony counts are determined from both cultures. If the catheter colony counts are several-fold (3- to 10-fold) higher than the colony count from the peripheral vein, it suggests a catheter-associated infection. The second method, differential time to positivity (DTP), requires an automated continuously monitored blood culture system, which determines the time at which a blood culture turns positive. If the catheter culture turns positive at least 2 hours before the peripheral vein culture, it suggests a catheter-associated infection. A catheter infection should be assumed when the organism isolated is a coagulase-negative *Staphylococcus, Corynebacterium, Bacillus,* or *Candida* species or a mycobacterium.

If signs are consistent with an exit-site or tunnel infection, an attempt should be made to culture any exit-site drainage.

TREATMENT

Catheter removal

Although it was once believed that all catheters had to be removed to eradicate infection, it is now clear that many catheters can be salvaged. An exception to this guideline would be if the organism isolated is *Corynebacterium* JK, a *Bacillus* species, a *Candida* organism, or a rapidly growing mycobacterium. Some physicians would add to this list *S aureus*, vancomycin-resistant enterococci (VRE), *P aeruginosa*, polymicrobial bacteremia, and *Fusarium* species. The catheter also should be removed in patients with septic thrombophlebitis or evidence of septic emboli. A tunnel infection or pocket-space abscess should prompt catheter removal as well. Finally, fever or bacteremia that persists (> 72 hours) after therapy has been initiated necessitates removal of the catheter if there is no other source of infection.

Antibiotic therapy

Empiric therapy If a catheter-associated infection is suspected, vancomycin should be initiated empirically. If the patient is known to be colonized with VRE empiric therapy with quinupristin/dalfopristin (Synercid) or linezolid (Zyvox) should be considered.

Two new antimicrobial agents with activity against MRSA and VRE have been approved: daptomycin (Cubicin) and tigecycline (Tygacil). Both drugs have activity against MRSA and VRE, but they are approved only for MRSA infections. Although some of these new agents have shortcomings (eg, the activity of daptomycin is neutralized by surfactant in the lungs and emergence of resistance while on this antibiotic), they enlarge our armamentarium for fighting these resistant gram-positive infections.

Specific therapy When a microorganism has been isolated and tested for sensitivity, specific antimicrobial therapy should be added. If the catheter is left in place, a minimum of 14 days of parenteral (not oral) therapy should be administered through the catheter (rotating through each port), and follow-up cultures should be obtained.

Search for infectious metastasis

Whether or not the catheter is removed, if the patient remains febrile, a search for sources of metastatic infection (lungs, liver, spleen, brain, heart valves) should be initiated.

There are treatment concerns with alternative agents for the treatment of *C difficile* enterocolitis. They include resistance with rifaximin *(Johnson S et al: Clin Infect Dis 44:846–848, 2007)* and noninferiority of nitazoxanide (Alinia) to metronidazole *(Musher DM et al: Clin Infect Dis 43:421–427, 2006)*. The use of probiotics is cautioned due to the potential for more invasive disease in the immunocompromised patient. Studies of probiotic *Saccharomyces boulardii* have been inconclusive *(Cohen SH et al: Infect Control Hosp Epidemiol 31:431–455, 2010)*.

Fibrinolytics and anticoagulants

The use of fibrinolytics and anticoagulation is controversial. Anticoagulation is indicated in cases of septic thrombophlebitis when the deep venous system is involved.

C DIFFICILE–ASSOCIATED DIARRHEA

Although many infectious complications involve the GI tract and abdomen in cancer patients, *C difficile*-associated diarrhea and typhlitis are the most important clinically.

Diarrhea is common in the cancer patient during chemotherapy. One of the most common causes of diarrhea is antibiotic-associated colitis. By far, the predominant etiology of antibiotic-associated colitis is *C difficile*. *C difficile* may also be contracted in the community.

ETIOLOGY AND RISK FACTORS

Antibiotics The major risk factor for *C difficile*–associated diarrhea is treatment with antibiotics, especially broad-spectrum β-lactams with activity against enteric bacteria, quinolones, and clindamycin. Antibiotic therapy causes a disruption in the normal bacterial flora of the colon. Pathogenic strains then produce toxins that cause diarrhea and pseudomembranous colitis.

Other risk factors include surgery (primarily colonic, gastric, and pelvic), colon carcinoma, leukemia, and uremia. Obviously, the hospitalized cancer patient undergoing chemotherapy and/or surgery and receiving broad-spectrum antibiotics is most vulnerable to this infection.

SIGNS AND SYMPTOMS

Infection with *C difficile* can be asymptomatic. When signs and symptoms do occur, they may range from mild to moderate diarrhea with lower abdominal pain, to colitis without pseudomembranous formation, to pseudomembranous colitis, to fulminant colitis. Fulminant colitis may be associated with toxic megacolon and even perforation of the viscus and peritonitis. On occasion, a patient may present with just abdominal pain or fever and no diarrhea.

Pseudomembranes may be absent in mild disease but usually are present in severe disease and are easily recognized on sigmoidoscopic or colonoscopic examination as adherent yellow plaques that may coalesce over large areas.

DIAGNOSIS

The development of diarrhea or even abdominal pain or fever in a cancer patient should prompt a work-up for *C difficile*–associated diarrhea.

The laboratory diagnosis of *C difficile* infection depends on the demonstration of *C difficile* toxins in the stool. The gold standard is the stool cytotoxin test, a tissue-culture assay that demonstrates cell rounding by *C difficile* toxin B.

Another test that can demonstrate *C difficile* toxins (A and/or B) in the stool is an enzyme immunoassay. It is less expensive and faster than the cytotoxin test and does not need to be performed by specially trained laboratory personnel.

Although a stool culture for *C difficile* may also be obtained, it has less significance in making the diagnosis.

TREATMENT

INITIAL MANAGEMENT

The initial step in the management of *C difficile*–associated diarrhea is to discontinue antibiotic therapy. Patients may not require any other therapy. However, stopping antibiotics in a cancer patient may not be possible or the patient may be severely ill from the colitis. In these instances, specific anti–*C difficile* therapy is required.

Specific antibiotic therapy

Metronidazole and vancomycin Metronidazole (500 mg PO tid) and vancomycin (125 mg PO qid), both given for 10 to 14 days, are the drugs of choice. Metronidazole is preferred because it is less expensive. However, in the case of suspected moderate to severe enterocolitis, vancomycin is the drug of choice.

For the patient who cannot tolerate oral medications, IV metronidazole (500 mg q8h) can be given. IV vancomycin should not be used, as high intraluminal levels cannot be attained. A vancomycin retention enema may be useful for cases of ileus. For a severe complicated episode (hypotension or shock, ileus, megacolon), it is recommended to use vancomycin (500 mg orally four times per day or by nasogastric tube) plus metronidazole (500 mg every 8 hours intravenously). Vancomycin retention enemas should be added for complete ileus.

Other agents that might be used for treatment include rifamixin and nitazoxanide (Alinia). Bacitracin (25,000 U PO qid) and cholestyramine (4 g PO qid) may be used as adjuncts.

Surgical therapy Subtotal colectomy with ileostomy may be required for severe *C difficile* enterocolitis. Monitoring serum lactate and white blood cell counts (non-neutropenic) may help in making the decision to operate.

Probiotics should be avoided in neutropenic patients.

Caution Use of metronidazole beyond the first relapse is not recommended.

TREATMENT OF RELAPSE

Relapse occurs in 10% to 20% of patients. Mild cases may not need to be treated. If treatment is indicated, a repeat 7- to 14-day course of either metronidazole or vancomycin may be administered. If the infection persists after repeated therapy, longer courses (4 to 6 weeks) followed by a gradual tapering of the dose may be helpful.

PREVENTION

Patients with *C difficile*–associated diarrhea and those who are known carriers should be placed in "contact isolation"; ie, the use of gloves, gowns, and careful hand-washing should be instituted.

During outbreaks, the use of sodium hypochlorite to disinfect contaminated surfaces has been recommended.

Antibiotic prophylaxis of high-risk patients or carriers is not recommended.

TYPHLITIS

Typhlitis (necrotizing enterocolitis) occurs in patients who are severely neutropenic, usually in the setting of chemotherapy. Pathologically, the areas of involvement include the cecum and terminal ileum. Typhlitis is a broad-spectrum disease characterized by bowel wall edema, diffuse or patchy necrosis involving the mucosa alone or the full thickness of the bowel wall, mucosal ulcerations, hemorrhage, inflammatory infiltrates, and infiltration of the bowel wall by bacteria or fungi. Mild cases are self-limiting when treated with bowel rest/antibiotics. Death may occur in severe cases.

SIGNS AND SYMPTOMS

Signs and symptoms of typhlitis can be nonspecific but usually include fever, abdominal pain (typically in the right lower quadrant), and abdominal distention. The patient may have diarrhea (sometimes bloody), nausea, and vomiting or may demonstrate signs and symptoms consistent with those of acute appendicitis.

There may be abdominal guarding and rebound tenderness, diminished bowel sounds, or even a mass in the right lower quadrant of the abdomen.

DIAGNOSIS

Radiographs or CT scans of the abdomen may demonstrate a thickened cecum, mass, or even gas within the colon wall.

TREATMENT

Mortality from typhlitis is high (> 50%), and therapy is controversial. However, broad-spectrum antibiotics covering both gut aerobes and anaerobes and resection of necrotic bowel are recommended.

FUNGAL INFECTIONS

Fungal infections are a leading cause of morbidity and mortality in cancer patients. These infections pose a formidable management challenge, in that diagnosis is often difficult to make at an early stage and, therefore, appropriate treatment may be delayed.

ETIOLOGY AND RISK FACTORS

***Candida* species** The most common fungal infections in cancer patients are caused by *Candida* species. Of the candidal pathogens found in these patients, *C albicans* is the most common. However, more recently other *Candida* species, such as *C tropicalis, C glabrata, C parapsilosis, C krusei,* and *C lusitaniae,* have become more prevalent. This finding is significant, as many of these species can be resistant to fluconazole (*C krusei, C glabrata, C lusitaniae*) and echinocandins (*C parapsilosis, C guilliermondii*).

Major risk factors for candidal infections include neutropenia, a breakdown in physical defense barriers (such as mucositis induced by chemotherapy and radiation therapy), broad-spectrum antibiotics, immune dysfunction (caused by chemotherapy and steroids), surgery (especially GI surgery), long-term indwelling vascular catheters, and poor nutritional status/total parenteral nutrition.

Aspergillus species is a less common cause of infection in cancer patients than candidal organisms but is more virulent. The most common of the *Aspergillus* species is *A fumigatus*, followed by *A flavus, A niger,* and *A terreus.*

Risk factors for *Aspergillus* infections include severe immunosuppression (primarily allogeneic HCT), steroid therapy, antitumor necrosis factor therapy, GVHD, and environmental exposure.

Other fungi Other fungal pathogens in the cancer patient include *Fusarium, Trichosporon, Zygomycetes,* and *Scedosporium* species; *Cryptococcus*; and the dematiaceous/pigmented fungi (eg, *Bipolaris spicifera, Cladosporium bantianum*).

Finally, the endemic fungi, *Coccidioides immitis* and *Histoplasma capsulatum*, are often more virulent and aggressive than other fungi in the immunocompromised host.

SIGNS AND SYMPTOMS

Candidiasis

Candidiasis can present as a wide spectrum of diseases, from mucosal infection to disseminated and invasive disease.

Oropharyngeal candidiasis can present as classic thrush with beige plaques. It may be painful, as there may be a concurrent mucositis due to the ablative chemotherapy. Oropharyngeal candidiasis may extend into the esophagus as esophagitis, which may manifest as odynophagia. Epiglottitis may present as odynophagia and laryngeal stridor.

Candidemia may present simply as an asymptomatic fever or may result in a full-blown septic shock syndrome (acute disseminated candidiasis). In contrast, chronic disseminated candidiasis, which involves the chronic, indolent infection of different organs, such as the liver, spleen, and kidneys, may be manifested by fever alone.

Aspergillosis

Invasive aspergillosis most commonly involves the lungs and sinuses. However, it can also disseminate to the brain (and may be the most common cause of brain abscesses in HCT patients). Less commonly, *Aspergillus* can disseminate to other organs, including the skin.

Signs and symptoms of invasive pulmonary aspergillosis include pleuritic pain, pulmonary hemorrhage, hemoptysis, and cavitation. The chest radiograph or CT scan may demonstrate pulmonary nodular infiltration and/or cavitary lesions.

Patients with sinusitis may have few signs (swelling) or symptoms (pain), especially if they are neutropenic.

Patients with brain abscesses may have headaches and neurologic signs consistent with the specific site of the lesion.

Skin involvement may present as necrotizing skin nodules or ulcers.

Other infections

The signs and symptoms of *Fusarium* infections are similar to those of aspergillosis; pulmonary infiltrates, sinusitis, and cutaneous lesions are prominent.

Trichosporon infections are similar to *Candida* infections in that they can cause disseminated disease in multiple organs.

Zygomycetes infections cause sinopulmonary disease.

Scedosporium species are similar to *Aspergillus* species in their structure and predilection for the respiratory tract.

C immitis and *H capsulatum* also target the lungs but can disseminate to other organs.

Cryptococcus infections can cause pneumonia or cellulitis.

DIAGNOSIS

Diagnosis of fungal infection in the cancer patient requires documentation by culture or histologic examination.

Candidiasis Although the diagnosis of oropharyngeal candidiasis often is made on clinical grounds, the lesions should be scraped for microscopic examination and culture. Biopsy of esophageal lesions via endoscopy should be performed to confirm *Candida* (as opposed to HSV or CMV) as the etiology of the infection.

A positive blood culture for *Candida* (especially a species other than *C albicans*) should never be considered a "contaminant" and often implies a right atrial catheter infection. Less likely to result in positive blood cultures are chronic, deep-seated infections, such as hepatosplenic candidiasis. Such infections require biopsy for confirmation.

***Aspergillus* species,** like other species, such as *Zygomycetes* and dematiaceous fungi, are rarely found in the bloodstream and requires tissue sampling for diagnosis. Occasionally, bronchoalveolar lavage fluid or sinus drainage will yield *Aspergillus*, but often a lung biopsy is required. Recently, an *Aspergillus galactomannan* enzyme immunoassay test has become available for the diagnosis of invasive aspergillosis. Unfortunately, it is not clear that it is a sufficiently sensitive (especially in patients receiving antifungal agents) or predictive test for the disease. There are also two other diagnostic tests now available: the glucan assay (for [1,3]-β-d-glucan) and the *Aspergillus* DNA PCR. Unfortunately, there are a paucity of data and a lack of experience with these assays to determine their utility in diagnosing and predicting invasive fungal infection in patients at highest risk.

***Fusarium*, *Scedosporium*, and *Trichosporon* species,** in contrast to *Aspergillus* species, are often isolated from the bloodstream.

Skin lesions Any skin lesion should be suspected of being of fungal origin and should be biopsied, cultured, and examined histologically.

Search for sites of infection When a fungal infection is suspected or documented, a search for possible sites of infection should ensue. For a blood culture that grows a *Candida* species, the intravascular catheter should, in most cases, be removed for diagnostic as well as therapeutic reasons, and the catheter tip should be cultured. A CT scan of the abdomen should be obtained. In cases of suspected *Aspergillus* infection, in addition to a CT scan of the chest, a CT scan of the brain and sinuses should be performed.

TREATMENT

ANTIFUNGAL AGENTS

There are now three major groups of antifungal agents: 1) the polyenes (amphotericin B deoxycholate and its lipid formulations [amphotericin B lipid complex, liposomal amphotericin B, amphotericin B cholsteryl sulfate]); 2) the azoles (fluconazole, itraconzaole, voriconazole, posaconazole); and 3) the echinocandins (caspofungin, micafungin, anidulafungin [Eraxis]).

Amphotericin B deoxycholate has been the standard therapy for invasive fungal infection for 50 years. It is fungicidal and has a broad spectrum of activity against yeasts and molds, including the *Zygomycetes*. It is thought to be less active against *A terreus, Scedosporium*, C *guilliermondii*, and C *lusitaniae*. However, it is limited by its nephrotoxicity and infusional toxicity. The lipid formulations are less nephrotoxic but much more expensive than the other formulations.

The azoles are not nephrotoxic. The first-generation azoles (fluconazole and itraconazole) are considered fungistatic, whereas the extended-spectrum azoles (voriconazole and posaconazole) are considered more fungicidal. Fluconazole is well absorbed orally and can be administered orally or intravenously but is not active against molds and certain *Candida* species (*C krusei*). Itraconazole is hepatotoxic and is not well absorbed when orally administered. Voriconazole is well absorbed orally and can also be administered intravenously. It is broadly active against most *Candida* species and most molds, with the exception of the *Zygomycetes*. Posaconazole can only be orally administered and is well absorbed. It is broadly active against most *Candida* species and most molds, including the *Zygomycetes*. Drawing azole levels should be considered for itraconazole, voriconazole, and posaconazole.

The echinocandins are the least toxic of the antifungal agents. They can only be administered intravenously. They are said to be fungicidal against yeasts but fungistatic against molds.

Candidiasis

Local mucosal candidiasis In patients with local mucosal candidiasis (including esophagitis), oral fluconazole or itraconazole can be used. If the patient has difficulty in taking oral medication, IV fluconazole should be used. If the patient was receiving prophylactic fluconazole when candidiasis developed, there is a high likelihood that the causative *Candida* species may be azole-resistant, and either an echinocandin or a lipid formulation of amphotericin B should be used.

Candidemia If candidemia is documented, the intravascular catheter should be removed. This step should be followed by the administration of an antifungal for at least 2 weeks after the last positive blood culture is obtained and all signs and symptoms have resolved. Although fluconazole has been shown to be an effective and safe agent in the treatment of candidemia, there are certain circumstances in which an alternative (an echinocandin or a lipid formulation of amphotericin B) might be preferable. These situations would include hemodynamic instability, neutropenia, or high suspicion of azole resistance (eg, a patient who is colonized with a resistant *Candida* species or has been on recent fluconazole prophylaxis or treatment).

Disseminated, deep-seated candidiasis (eg, hepatosplenic infection) Although the standard of therapy for deep-seated candidiasis has been long-term therapy with amphotericin deoxycholate, it has been limited by nephrotoxicity. Thus, the lipid formulations of amphotericin B have allowed higher cumulative doses with a lower nephrotoxic potential. The azoles (fluconazole, voriconazole) have the advantage of convenient (ie, oral) administration and good absorption, with little toxicity. The echinocandins also have been shown to be effective against this infection.

Aspergillosis

Antifungal therapy Amphotericin B deoxycholate (1.0 to 1.5 mg/kg/d) had been the standard therapy for invasive aspergillosis. However, voriconazole led to better responses, improved survival, and fewer adverse events than did amphotericin B when used as initial therapy in patients with invasive aspergillosis. Thus, voriconazole is the standard therapy for invasive aspergillosis. Amphotericin B lipid complex, amphotericin B cholesteryl sulfate, liposomal amphotericin B, posaconazole, and caspofungin can be used. All of these formulations are less nephrotoxic than amphotericin B deoxycholate.

Surgical removal of infected sites In addition to antifungal therapy, it is important to attempt surgical removal of infected sites, if at all feasible. Sinus surgery should be performed. Resection of pulmonary lesions should be attempted if there are only one or two limited, discrete lesions.

Infections with other fungi

Although amphotericin B is the drug of choice for most invasive fungal infections, there are exceptions. *Scedosporium* and *Fusarium* species are often resistant to amphotericin B, and voriconazole may be the drug of choice for these infections. Voriconazole, however, is not active against *Zygomycetes* species, and if an infection with this organism is suspected or documented, amphotericin B deoxycholate, an amphotericin B lipid formulation, or posaconazole should be used. The dematiaceous/pigmented fungi also may be better treated with itraconazole. For *Trichosporon* infections, voriconazole may be more effective than amphotericin B.

> Obtaining *Aspergillus galactomannan* from bronchoalveolar lavage may be more sensitive than obtaining serum for detection of pulmonary aspergillosis. However, a higher index cutoff may be used to avoid overdiagnosis *(Hsu LY et al: BMC Infect Dis 10:44, 2010).*

PREVENTION

Because invasive fungal infection occurs with high frequency in the setting of HCT, most prophylactic studies have been performed in HCT recipients. Thus, the following recommendations apply mainly to this group, although prophylaxis can be justified when the incidence of these infections in any population is high enough.

Fluconazole Two randomized, placebo-controlled studies using prophylactic fluconazole (400 mg/d) have demonstrated a decrease in invasive and superficial *C albicans* infections. One study showed a reduction in mortality. As fluconazole is not active against *C krusei, C glabrata,* or *Aspergillus* species, there is concern that its prophylactic use will increase the incidence of these resistant fungi. Some authors have reported such an occurrence.

Micafungin has been approved for use as an antifungal (candidiasis) prophylactic agent in HCT. There was also a trend toward protection against *Aspergillus* infection with micafungin, although it was not significant.

Itraconazole has been shown to be an effective antifungal prophylactic agent in HCT, but no survival benefit has been demonstrated, possibly because of the toxic GI effects and hepatotoxicity associated with this agent.

Low-dose amphotericin B was observed, in a retrospective study, to decrease the incidence of *Candida* infection. However, this regimen only delayed the onset of *Aspergillus* infections.

Posaconazole has been shown to be effective antifungal prophylaxis in two settings: (1) neutropenic AML and MDS patients; and (2) allogeneic HCT recipients with GVHD.

Voriconazole has been shown to be as efficacious as fluconazole. However, it did not result in a significant prevention of aspergillosis or demonstrate a survival benefit.

Other prophylactic regimens have been used in small numbers of patients, with varying degrees of success. They include aerosolized amphotericin B, intranasal amphotericin B, and amphotericin B lipid complex.

The prophylactic regimen of choice in HCT might be an echinocandin (eg, micafungin) initially (while the patient is neutropenic and hospitalized) followed by an oral azole (eg, posaconazole) administered to those outpatients who remain at high risk for mold infections.

HEPA filtration Other than using prophylactic antifungals, there is little that can be done to prevent fungal infections in cancer patients. The one possible exception is the use of HEPA filtration, which can eliminate *Aspergillus* spores from the environment. However, most patients emerge from this environment still possessing the same risk factors (steroids, GVHD) for aspergillosis.

VIRAL INFECTIONS

Opportunistic viral infections are a particular problem in cancer patients who undergo HCT and those with hematologic cancers. Accurate diagnosis of viral infections is important, as treatment is available for many of them.

ETIOLOGY

As mentioned previously, viral infections in cancer patients are caused predominantly by herpesviruses (HSV, VZV, CMV, and EBV). The herpesvirus infections usually are reactivations of latent infections. Respiratory viruses that infect cancer patients include respiratory syncytial virus, influenza viruses A and B, parainfluenza virus, rhinovirus, and adenovirus.

SIGNS AND SYMPTOMS

Although all of the herpesviruses can cause fever and a septic picture, HSV usually presents as mucositis or a vesicular rash, VZV presents as a vesicular rash in a dermatomal distribution, and CMV, in the HCT setting, presents as interstitial pneumonia. When HSV or VZV disseminates, each virus can cause disseminated cutaneous lesions or visceral (liver, lung, brain) involvement. VZV infection can present with GI symptoms, such as epigastric or general abdominal pain.

DIAGNOSIS

To make a specific viral etiologic diagnosis, tissue or fluid must be obtained from the infected site and processed for histologic/cytologic examination and culture.

Vesicular skin lesions When a cancer patient presents with a vesicular rash, it is invariably due to either HSV or VZV. If the distribution of lesions is in a dermatomal pattern, a clinical diagnosis of VZV can be made. However, if there is cutaneous dissemination, the vesicular lesions should be aspirated (and sent for viral culture) or scraped down to the base, smeared on a glass slide, and sent for direct fluorescent antibody staining (for HSV and VZV).

Visceral involvement When there is visceral involvement with HSV, VZV, or CMV, biopsy material is examined for inclusions and is submitted for culture.

Respiratory infection For the respiratory viruses, diagnosis is usually made by examination of bronchoalveolar lavage fluid (obtained by bronchoscopy) or biopsy (obtained by transbronchial, percutaneous thoracic, thoracoscopic, or open lung biopsy). In the special case of CMV interstitial pneumonitis in the HCT setting, diagnosis of infection (prior to disease onset) can be made by detection of antigens or virus in the bloodstream, in addition to evidence of the virus in bronchoalveolar lavage fluid. PCR is available for various community respiratory virus (eg, adenovirus, parainfluenza, influenza, respiratory syncytial virus, and metapneumovirus).

CNS involvement can be determined by PCR performed on the cerebrospinal fluid for the following agents: HSV, VZV, human herpesvirus 6 (HHV-6), CMV, and adenovirus.

Antibody testing is of little use in the diagnosis of viral infection in the cancer patient.

Evidence of CMV viremia, which is utilized to initiate preemptive therapy, can be determined by PCR, antigen detection, or blood (shell-vial) culture.

TREATMENT

HSV infection Localized HSV infection is usually treated with acyclovir, 5 mg/kg IV q8h. If there is dissemination, a dose of 10 mg/kg q8h can be used, and if there is CNS involvement, up to 15 mg/kg IV q8h can be utilized. If acyclovir-resistant HSV is suspected, foscarnet (Foscavir) can be used (see Table 1 for doses). However, this is a nephrotoxic drug.

VZV infection is usually treated with acyclovir, administered at a dose of 10 mg/kg IV q8h.

CMV infection is treated with ganciclovir or foscarnet. Ganciclovir is the drug of choice but is toxic to bone marrow.

In the HCT setting, "preemptive" treatment (treatment to prevent disease after evidence of infection is obtained) consists of ganciclovir, 5 mg/kg IV bid for 7 days followed by 5 mg/kg/d IV for another 3 to 5 weeks. Actual treatment of CMV interstitial pneumonia consists of ganciclovir, 5 mg/kg IV q12h, along with immunoglobulin, 500 mg/kg IV every other day for 21 days

In April 2009, novel H1N1 influenza A virus emerged and led to a worldwide pandemic. During the 2009–2010 influenza season, novel H1N1 was the dominant circulating influenza virus; < 1% of characterized viruses were seasonal A (H1), A (H3), and influenza B viruses. A total of 64 oseltamivir (Tamiflu)-resistant 2009 H1N1 viruses were identified in the United States; prior treatment or chemoprophylaxis with oseltamivir was noted in 81%. All strains were sensitive to zanamivir (Relenza). Oral neuraminidase inhibitors are the treatment of choice for 2009 H1N1. In patients having issues with oral absorption, IV peramivir should be considered. IV zanamivir may be considered in patients suspected or confirmed to be infected with oseltamivir-resistant H1N1 strain (*H275Y* mutation) and can be obtained for compassionate use from the manufacturer. Inhaled zanamivir should be avoided in patients requiring mechanical ventilation *(Centers for Disease Control and Prevention. Available at http://www.cdc.gov/mmwr/preview/mmwrhtml/mm5914a3.htm. Accessed May 25, 2010)*. The interim CDC recommendations for the 2008–2009 season follow: for seasonal H1N1, use zanamivir or oseltamivir plus rimantadine. For H3N2 and influenza B, use only zanamivir or oseltamivir *(Centers for Disease Control and Prevention. Available at http://www.cdc.gov/H1N1flu/recommendations.htm#c. Accessed May 25, 2010)*.

(induction phase). Maintenance therapy (for as long as immunosuppression is present) consists of ganciclovir, 5 mg/kg/d IV for 5 days each week, and immunoglobulin, 500 mg/kg IV every week.

Foscarnet can be used instead of ganciclovir if there is marrow toxicity but poses a potential risk of nephrotoxicity.

For CMV infection resistant to both ganciclovir and foscarnet, cidofovir (Vistide) can be used.

HHV-6 infection/disease can be treated with ganciclovir, foscarnet, or cidofovir.

Respiratory viral infection Among the respiratory viruses, there is specific antiviral therapy only for respiratory syncytial virus and influenza A. Ribavirin (Virazole), 1.1 g/d by aerosol (20 mg/mL), has been used for respiratory syncytial virus (but has not been shown to be effective) and rimantadine (Flumadine) or amantadine (Symmetrel), both 100 mg PO bid, for influenza A. Zanamivir (Relenza) and oseltamivir (Tamiflu, 75 mg PO bid) can be used for both influenza A and B. Finally, cidofovir has been used (but not FDA approved) for adenovirus infection.

PREVENTION

Herpesvirus infections

Acyclovir HSV and VZV reactivate with great frequency in cancer patients undergoing chemotherapy and/or radiation therapy. This finding is especially true in the HCT population, in which 80% of HSV-seropositive patients and up to 40% of VZV-seropositive patients have a reactivation of HSV or VZV. Therefore, in HSV-seropositive HCT patients, prophylactic acyclovir is indicated. Any HSV infection that occurs during acyclovir prophylaxis should be considered resistant to acyclovir. Acyclovir has also been shown to reduce the incidence of CMV infection after HCT. It is now recommended by some to extend HSV prophylaxis for 1 year or longer for patients with allogeneic HCT or GVHD. In patients exposed to VZV, acyclovir should be given at a dose of 800 mg (adults) or 20 mg/kg (pediatrics, maximum 800 mg/dose) four times daily on days 3 to 22 after exposure.

Ganciclovir is generally considered too (marrow) toxic to be used as universal prophylaxis against CMV. Thus, the preemptive approach was developed to focus on only treating those who had evidence of CMV infection (viremia) as determined by PCR, antigen detection, or blood (shell-vial) culture. This approach allows treatment of viremia before it evolves into CMV disease (interstitial pneumonitis).

CMV-seronegative blood support In the small group of HCT recipients who are CMV-seronegative, the use of CMV-seronegative blood support has been shown to reduce CMV infection dramatically.

Varicella and VZV vaccines (Varivax) should not be given to those with hematologic malignancies, malignant neoplasms, or immunodeficiencies. The exception is with varicella vaccine in those with childhood leukemia in remission for 1 year, when selected criteria are met.

Influenza

Influenza vaccine Although the efficacy of the influenza vaccine is unknown in the HCT setting, it should be administered to all cancer patients.

Rimantadine, amantadine, zanamivir, or oseltamivir can be given prophylactically during an outbreak of influenza.

SUGGESTED READING

ON FEVER AND NEUTROPENIA

National Comprehensive Cancer Network: Prevention and Treatment of Cancer-related Infections. V.2.2009. Available at http://www.nccn.org/professionals/physician_gls/PDF/infections.pdf. Accessed May 25, 2010.

ON PNEUMONIA

American Thoracic Society; Infectious Diseases Society of America: Guidelines for the management of adults with hospital-acquired, ventilator-associated, and healthcare-associated pneumonia. Am J Respir Crit Care Med 171:388–416, 2005.

Mandell LA, Wunderink RG, Anzueto A, et al: Infectious Diseases Society of America/American Thoracic Society consensus guidelines on the management of community-acquired pneumonia in adults. Clin Infect Dis 44(suppl 2):S27–S72, 2007.

ON CATHETER-ASSOCIATED INFECTIONS

Mermel LA, Allon M, Bouza E, et al: Clinical practice guidelines for the diagnosis and management of intravascular catheter-related infection: 2009 Update by the Infectious Diseases Society of America. Clin Infect Dis 49:1–45, 2009.

ON *C DIFFICILE*–ASSOCIATED DIARRHEA

Cohen SH, Gerding DN, Johnson S, et al: Clinical practice guidelines for Clostridium difficile infection in adults: 2010 Update by the Society for Healthcare Epidemiology of America (SHEA) and the Infectious Diseases Society of America (IDSA). Infect Control Hosp Epidemiol 31:431–455, 2010.

Mermel LA, Allon M, Bouza E, et al: Clinical practice guidelines for the diagnosis and management of intravascular catheter-related infection: 2009 Update by the Infectious Diseases Society of America. Clin Infect Dis 49:1–45, 2009.

ON FUNGAL INFECTIONS

Pappas PG, Kauffman CA, Andes D, et al: Clinical practice guidelines for the management of candidiasis: 2009 update by the Infectious Diseases Society of America. Clin Infect Dis 48:503–535, 2009.

Walsh TJ, Anaissie EJ, Denning DW, et al: Treatment of aspergillosis: Clinical practice guidelines of the Infectious Diseases Society of America. Clin Infect Dis 46:327–360, 2008.

ON VIRAL INFECTIONS

Harper SA, Bradley JS, Englund JA, et al: Seasonal influenza in adults and children–Diagnosis, treatment, chemoprophylaxis, and institutional outbreak management: Clinical practice guidelines of the Infectious Diseases Society of America. Clin Infect Dis 48:1003–1032, 2009.

Abbreviations in this chapter

CDC = Centers for Disease Control and Prevention; EORTC = European Organisation for Research and Treatment of Cancer; IDSA = Infectious Diseases Society of America; NCCN = National Comprehensive Cancer Network; NCIC = National Cancer Institute of Canada

CHAPTER 40

Fluid complications

Frederic W. Grannis, Jr., MD, and Lily Lai, MD

FLUID COMPLICATIONS

MALIGNANT PLEURAL EFFUSION

Malignant pleural effusion complicates the care of approximately 150,000 people in the United States each year. The pleural effusion is usually caused by a disturbance of the normal Starling forces regulating reabsorption of fluid in the pleural space, secondary to obstruction of mediastinal lymph nodes draining the parietal pleura. Tumors that metastasize frequently to these nodes (eg, lung cancer, breast cancer, and lymphoma) cause most malignant effusions. It is, therefore, puzzling that small-cell lung cancer infrequently causes effusions. Primary effusion lymphomas caused by human herpesvirus 8 and perhaps Epstein-Barr virus (EBV) are seen in patients with AIDS.

Pleural effusion restricts ventilation and causes progressive shortness of breath by compression of lung tissue as well as paradoxical movement of the inverted diaphragm. Pleural deposits of tumor cause pleuritic pain.

Pleural effusions more commonly occur in patients with advanced-stage tumors, who frequently have metastases to the brain, bone, and other organs, physiologic deficits, malnutrition, debilitation, and other comorbidities. Because of these numerous clinical and pathologic variables, it is difficult to perform trials in patients with pleural effusions. For the same reason, it is often difficult to predict a potential treatment outcome for the specific patient with multiple interrelated clinical problems.

William generated survival curves for more than 8,000 patients with non–small-cell lung cancer (NSCLC) with pleural effusion (ie, stage IIIB) from the SEER database and showed that long-term survival is uncommon in this group. The median survival time is approximately 3 months.

DIAGNOSIS

The new onset of pleural effusion may herald the presence of a previously undiagnosed malignancy or, more typically, complicate the course of a known tumor. Malignant pleural effusions can lead to an initial diagnosis of cancer in patients. In Nantes, France, pleural effusion was the first symptom of cancer in 41% of 209 patients with malignant pleural effusion; lung cancer in men (42%) and ovarian cancer in women (27%).

Sarkar et al have introduced a simple bedside test that allows identification of exudative effusion at the time of thoracentesis. They added 10 mL of 30% hydrogen peroxide to 200 mL of pleural effusion. When catalase is present (exudates), the effusion foams. None of 32 transudates produced foam, whereas all 52 exudates produced profuse bubbles. The test is not accurate if blood contaminates the fluid ***(Sarkar S et al: Clin Chim Acta 405:83–86, 2009).***

Thoracentesis

The first step in management in almost all cases is thoracentesis. An adequate specimen should be obtained and sent for cell count; determination of glucose, protein, lactate dehydrogenase (LDH), and pH; and appropriate cultures and cytology. Chest pressure and pain during thoracentesis can occur when lung elastance is reduced and pleural pressures are markedly negative. Such pain suggests a "trapped" lung and signals an increased risk of postthoracentesis pulmonary edema.

The Light criteria (LDH > 200 U/L; pleural-serum LDH ratio > 0.6; and pleural-serum protein ratio > 0.5) help categorize pleural effusions as exudates. The majority of undiagnosed exudates are eventually diagnosed as malignant, whereas < 5% of transudates are shown to be caused by cancer. Transudates may be misclassified as exudates following dehydration or diuresis and if there are erythrocytes (LDH) in the fluid. Brain natriuretic protein levels are markedly elevated in effusions secondary to congestive heart failure.

Because it is sometimes difficult to prove the malignant nature of an effusion, many molecular tests on pleural fluid have been investigated. Multiple reports measure pleural tumor marker proteins, glycosaminoglycans, cadherins, matrix metalloproteins, cytokines, telomerase, mRNA, exosomes, and serum and pleural DNA methylation patterns, but to date, no test or panel of tests can reliably diagnose malignant effusions.

Investigators in Cambridge, England, report that thickening of the pleura > 1 cm, pleural nodularity, and diaphragmatic thickening > 7 mm on either CT or ultrasonography suggest malignant effusion.

A negative cytology result is not uncommon and does not rule out a malignant etiology. If cytology is negative in an exudative effusion, approximately 25% will have a positive cytology on a second thoracentesis; blind pleural biopsy may increase the yield to nearly 50%. This low diagnostic yield can be improved by CT or ultrasonographic guidance of needle biopsy.

PET scan may be positive with malignant pleural effusion; a high SUV (standard uptake value) is an adverse prognosticator. Kwek et al, from Massachusetts General Hospital, reported that PET scans performed on nine patients, an average of 22 months following talc pleurodesis, showed focal nodular fluorodeoxyglucose uptake in the pleura (mean standard error of mean 5.4; range: 1.2–16).

Thoracoscopy

Thoracoscopic examination performed with the patient under either general or local anesthesia and using rigid or partly flexible thoracoscopes offers a very high sensitivity, specificity, and diagnostic accuracy with a low complication rate. It allows comprehensive visualization of one pleural cavity, coupled with the opportunity to biopsy areas of disease. This method provides a definitive diagnosis and allows the pathologist to suggest possible sites of primary disease based on the histopathology. There was no incidence of later development of a malignant pleural effusion following a benign thoracoscopic study in 25 patients at the Lahey Clinic. Furthermore, this technique permits the diagnosis and staging of malignant mesothelioma if it is the cause of the effusion. Thoracoscopy also offers the opportunity for simultaneous treatment.

Gaspari et al of Milan, Italy, report an 89% success rate following video-assisted thoracic surgery (VATS) talc pleurodesis in breast cancer patients with malignant pleural effusion. Biopsies taken during VATS showed that receptor status and c-*erb*B2 status changed from negative to positive in 15% of patients.

Bronchoscopy

Bronchoscopy may be helpful when an underlying lung cancer is suspected, especially if there is associated hemoptysis, a lung mass, atelectasis, or a massive effusion. It may also be useful when there is a cytologically positive effusion with no obvious primary tumor.

PROGNOSIS

Prognosis of patients with malignant pleural effusion varies by primary tumor. For example, median survival for patients with lung cancer is 3 months, whereas it is 10 months for patients with breast cancer. Median survival is also shorter in patients with encasement atelectasis (3 months).

TREATMENT

Initial Treatment

Because the specific clinical circumstances may vary markedly in different patients, treatment must be individualized to provide the best palliation for each patient. Generally, there are many different methods available for the treatment of malignant effusions, and there is little compelling evidence to guide clinicians in the choice of the best methods. Accordingly, treatment decisions must be made with careful reference to the status of the patient and the skills and equipment available in the local community. In general, malignant pleural effusion should be treated aggressively as soon as it is diagnosed. In most cases, effusion will rapidly recur after treatment by thoracentesis or tube thoracostomy alone. If the clinician decides to administer systemic chemotherapy for the underlying primary malignancy, in tumors such as breast cancer, lymphoma, and small-cell lung cancer, it is important to monitor the patient carefully for recurrent effusion and to treat such recurrences immediately. There are few published data to document the chance of success in clearance of malignant pleural effusions with systemic chemotherapy.

If a malignant pleural effusion is left untreated, the underlying collapsed lung will become encased by tumor and fibrous tissue in as many as 10% to 30% of cases. Once this encasement atelectasis has occurred, the underlying lung is "trapped" and will no longer reexpand after thoracentesis or tube thoracostomy. Characteristically, the chest x-ray in such cases shows resolution of the pleural effusion after thoracentesis, but the underlying lung remains partially collapsed. This finding is often misinterpreted by the inexperienced clinician as evidence of a pneumothorax, and a chest tube is placed. The air space persists and the lung remains unexpanded, even with high suction and pulmonary physiotherapy. Allowing the chest tube to remain in place can worsen the situation, resulting in bronchopleural fistulization and empyema. In some cases, a trapped lung on an initial chest x-ray will have delayed reexpansion following chest tube or small pleural catheter drainage.

Intrapleural alteplase (in doses between 10 and 100 mg diluted in 50 to 150 mL of saline) has been used with success in some patients with gelatinous or loculated effusions without systemic bleeding complications.

Physical techniques

To avoid encasement atelectasis, pleural effusion should be treated definitively at the time of initial diagnosis. Multiple physical techniques of producing adhesions between the parietal and visceral pleurae, obliterating the space, and preventing recurrence have been used. They include open or thoracoscopic pleurectomy, gauze abrasion, or laser pleurodesis. Surgical methods have not been demonstrated to have any advantage over simpler chemical pleurodesis techniques in the treatment of malignant effusions. Gauze abrasion can easily be employed when unresectable lung cancer with associated effusion is found at the time of thoracotomy.

A randomized, prospective study from Ljubljanska, Slovenia, of 87 patients with malignant pleural effusion secondary to breast cancer showed that the thoracoscopic mechanical abrasion pleurodesis was equivalent to talc pleurodesis in those with normal pleural fluid pH and superior in patients with a low pH.

In Thessaloniki, Greece, 34 patients with symptomatic recurrent malignant pleural effusions had a chest tube placed followed by pleurodesis with erythromycin. Success was evaluated after 90 days. A complete response (ie, no reaccumulation of pleural fluid after 90 days) was seen in 79.4%, and a partial response (ie, reaccumulation but without symptoms and not requiring drainage) was seen in another 8.8%. Recurrence with necessity for re-intervention was seen in 11.8%. All patients experienced pleurodynia during administration. Sinus tachycardia and mild hypertension were also observed. The investigators concluded that erythromycin is effective and safe as a sclerosing agent for pleurodesis in patients with malignant pleural effusions *(Balassoulis G et al: Am J Clin Oncol 31:384–389, 2008)*.

Chemical agents

Multiple chemical agents have been used.

Tetracycline Tetracycline pleurodesis results in a lower incidence of recurrence when compared with tube thoracostomy alone but often causes severe pain. Tetracycline is no longer commercially available in the United States.

Doxycycline and minocycline are probably equivalent in efficacy to tetracycline.

Bleomycin Intrapleural bleomycin, in a dose of 60 U, has been shown to be more effective than tetracycline and is not painful, but it is costly. Absorption of the drug can result in systemic toxicity. Combined use of tetracycline and bleomycin has been demonstrated to be more efficacious than the use of either drug singly.

Talc pleurodesis was first introduced by Bethune in the 1930s. The first use of talc in malignant pleural effusion was by John Chambers in 1958. Talc powder (Sclerosol Intrapleural Aerosol) has demonstrated efficacy in numerous large studies, preventing recurrent effusion in 70% to 92% of cases. Talc is less painful than tetracycline. Cost is minimal, but special sterilization techniques must be mastered by the hospital pharmacy. Talc formulations may have significant differences in the size of particles. Smaller particles may be absorbed and disseminated systemically and may contribute to the increased incidence of adult respiratory distress syndrome (ARDS) or substantial hypoxemia. Talc has also been shown to cause decreases in forced vital capacity (FVC), forced expiratory volume in one second (FEV_1), and diffusing capacity long term.

Talc can be insufflated in a dry state at the time of thoracoscopy or instilled as a slurry through a chest tube. The dose should be restricted to no more than 5 g. A prospective phase III intergroup trial of 501 patients randomized to receive thoracoscopic talc vs talc slurry pleurodesis showed similar efficacy in each arm, with increased respiratory complications (14% vs 6%) but less fatigue and higher patient ratings in the insufflation group.

Multiloculated effusions may follow talc use. It is important to ensure that talc does not solidify and form a concretion in the chest tube, thus preventing the drainage of pleural fluid and complete reexpansion of the lung following pleurodesis. Such an event is more likely when small-bore chest tubes are used.

Pleurodesis technique With talc pleurodesis, a 24- to 32-French tube has customarily been inserted through a lower intercostal space and placed on underwater seal suction drainage until all fluid is drained and the lung has completely reexpanded. Because severe lung damage can be produced by improper chest tube placement, it is imperative to prove the presence of free fluid by a preliminary needle tap and to enter the pleural space gently with a blunt clamp technique, rather than by blind trocar insertion. If there is any question about the presence of loculated effusion or underlying adhesions, the use of CT or sonography may enhance the safety of the procedure. In the case of large effusions, especially those that have been present for some time, the fluid should be drained slowly to avoid reexpansion pulmonary edema.

Significant complications can occur with both thoracentesis and chest tube thoracostomy. These procedures should not be performed by inexperienced practitioners without training and supervision.

Premedications If doxycycline or talc is to be used, the patient should be premedicated with narcotics. Intrapleural instillation of 20 mL of 1% lidocaine before administration of the chemical agent may help reduce pain.

Following instillation of the chemical agent, the chest tube should remain clamped for at least 2 hours. If high-volume drainage persists, the treatment can be repeated. The chest tube can be removed after 2 or 3 days if drainage is < 300 mL/d.

Follow-up x-rays at monthly intervals assess the adequacy of treatment and allow early retreatment in case of recurrence.

Alternative approaches Use of fluid-sclerosing agents and outpatient pleurodesis has been advocated by some investigators and has the potential for reducing hospital stay and treatment cost. Patz performed a prospective, randomized trial of bleomycin

Schneider et al, from Heidelberg, Germany, reported on 100 patients with tunneled pleural catheters. The mean residence time of the catheter was 70 days. Spontaneous pleurodesis was achieved in 29 patients. The rate of empyema was 4%. The investigators identified three groups that seemed to benefit: (1) patients with the intraoperative finding of a trapped lung in diagnostic VATS procedures; (2) patients after repeated thoracentesis or previously failed attempts at pleurodesis; and (3) patients with a limited life span due to underlying disease *(Schneider T et al: Thorac Cardiovasc Surg 57:42–46, 2009).*

vs doxycycline (72% bleomycin vs 79% doxycycline) pleurodesis via a 14-French catheter and found no difference in efficacy. Aglayan, in Istanbul, Turkey, evaluated iodopovidone via either chest tube or a small-bore catheter in 41 patients. Complete and partial successes were observed in 60% and 27%, respectively. Results did not differ by diameter of the tube. (Because of the risk of iodine toxicity with renal failure and seizures, such use of iodopovidone should be limited to 2% solutions and should not be used in patients taking amiodarone or with prolonged use of topical iodine wound treatments.)

Other approaches that must be considered experimental at this time include quinacrine, silver nitrate, powdered collagen, and distilled water, as well as various biologic agents, including *Corynebacterium parvum,* OK-432, tumor necrosis factor, interleukin-2 (Proleukin), interferon-α (Intron A, Roferon-A), interferon-β (Betaseron), and interferon-γ (Actimmune).

Treatment of encasement atelectasis

If encasement atelectasis is found at thoracentesis or thoracoscopy, tube thoracostomy and pleurodesis are futile and contraindicated.

Management options

Surgical decortication has been advocated for this problem. This potentially dangerous procedure may result in severe complications, however, such as bronchopleural fistula and empyema.

Pleuroperitoneal shunts The Royal Brompton Hospital, London, group reported experience with pleuroperitoneal shunts in 160 patients with malignant pleural effusion and a trapped lung. Effective palliation was achieved in 95% of patients; 15% of patients required shunt revisions for complications.

Intermittent thoracentesis, as needed to relieve symptoms, may be the best option in patients with a short anticipated survival.

Catheter drainage Another new option is to insert a tunneled, small-bore, cuffed, silicone catheter (PleurX pleural catheter, Denver Biomaterials, Inc., Denver, Colorado) into the pleural cavity. The patient or family members may then drain fluid, using vacuum bottles, whenever recurrent effusion causes symptoms.

Kakuda reported on placement of 61 PleurX pleural catheters in 50 patients with malignant pleural effusions at City of Hope; 34% had lung cancer and 24% had breast cancer. There were no operative deaths. In cases where the catheter was placed under thoracoscopic control, 27 of 38 patients (68%) had encasement atelectasis visualized.

A total of 81% had a good result with control of effusion, with subsequent catheter removal (19%) or intermittent drainage for > 1 month or until death (62%). A total of 5% of patients had major complications, including empyema and tumor implant. These catheters can also be inserted using the Seldinger technique with the patient under local anesthesia. Tremblay et al placed 250 PleurX pleural catheters by percutaneous technique in patients under local anesthesia. No further pleural intervention was required during the lives of 90% of the patients. The median overall survival was 144 days, and spontaneous pleurodesis occurred in 43%. Subsequent studies showed that 70% of patients who had full lung expansion had spontaneous pleurodesis, with lifetime control of pleural effusion in 92%. They also reported good results in patients with mesothelioma effusions.

Chemotherapy options depend on the cell type of the tumor and the general condition of the patient. Although intrapleural chemotherapy offers the possibility of high-dose local therapy with minimal systemic effects, only a few, small pilot studies utilizing mitoxantrone, doxorubicin, and hyperthermic cisplatin have been published.

Ang and colleagues from Singapore reported longer mean survival (12 vs 5 months) when systemic chemotherapy was given to 71 patients who initially presented with malignant pleural/pericardial effusions. New studies in this area are much needed.

In Taiwan, Su et al treated 27 patients with NSCLC presenting with a malignant pleural effusion using a regimen of intrapleural cisplatin and gemcitabine (Gemzar), followed by radiotherapy (7,020 cGy in 39 fractions), and completed treatment with IV docetaxel (Taxotere). Only two patients experienced recurrent pleural effusion. The median disease-free and overall survival times were 8 and 16 months, respectively, and 63% of patients were alive at 1 year.

Seto et al, from the National Kyushu Cancer Center, Fukuoka, Japan, reported a single-arm series of 80 patients with previously untreated malignant pleural effusions from NSCLC. The patients had a chest tube placed and were given 25 mg of cisplatin in 500 mL of distilled water intrapleurally. Toxicity was acceptable. Median time of drainage was 4 days. A total of 34% had a complete response and 49% had a partial response, for an overall response rate of 83%. A striking finding in this study was that the median survival time of all patients was 239 days, a longer survival than seen in comparable patients treated with pleurodesis. The authors recommend a phase III study.

Radiation therapy may be indicated in some patients with lymphoma but has limited effectiveness in other tumor types, particularly if mediastinal adenopathy is absent.

Chylothorax (in the absence of trauma) is usually secondary to cancer, most frequently lymphoma. An added element of morbidity is conferred by the loss of protein, calories, and lymphocytes in the draining fluid. Chylothorax secondary to lymphoma is usually of low volume and responds to talc pleurodesis in combination with radiotherapy or chemotherapy. Gross et al, from Sao Paulo, Brazil, reported an overall survival rate of 5.6 months for patients with simultaneous ascites and malignant pleural effusions vs 7.8 months in patients without ascites. They observed that success rates for talc pleurodesis were equal and concluded that concomitant ascites did not influence the effectiveness of palliative surgical management of pleural effusion in patients with malignancies.

PERICARDIAL EFFUSION

Pericardial effusion develops in 5% to 15% of patients with cancer and is sometimes the initial manifestation of malignancy. Most pericardial effusions in cancer patients result from obstruction of the lymphatic drainage of the heart secondary to metastases. The typical presentation is that of a patient with known cancer who is found to have a large pericardial effusion without signs of inflammation. Bloody pericardial fluid is not a reliable sign of malignant effusion.

The most common malignant causes of pericardial effusions are lung and breast cancers, leukemias (specifically acute myelogenous, lymphoblastic, and chronic myelogenous leukemia [blast crisis]), and lymphomas. At Boston City Hospital, 39% of children with moderate to large pericardial effusions had malignant effusions.

Not all pericardial effusions associated with cancer are malignant, and cases with negative cytology may represent as many as half of cancer-associated pericardial effusions. Such effusions are more common in patients with mediastinal lymphoma, Hodgkin lymphoma, or breast cancer. Other nonmalignant causes include drug-induced (eg, sirolimus [Rapamune] or docetaxel) or postirradiation pericarditis, tuberculosis, collagen diseases, uremia, and congestive heart failure. Many effusions that initially have negative cytology will become positive over time.

Tamponade occurs when fluid accumulates faster than the pericardium can stretch. Compression of all four heart chambers ensues, with tachycardia and diminishing cardiac output. Fluid loading can counteract intrapericardial pressure temporarily. Reciprocal filling of right- and left-sided chambers with inspiration and expiration, secondary to paradoxical movement of the ventricular septum, is a final mechanism to maintain blood flow before death.

DIAGNOSIS

A high index of suspicion is required to make the diagnosis of pericardial effusion.

Signs and symptoms

Dyspnea is the most common symptom. Patients may also complain of chest pain or discomfort, easy fatigability, cough, and orthopnea or may be completely asymptomatic. Signs include distant heart sounds and pericardial friction rub. With cardiac tamponade, progressive heart failure occurs, with increased shortness of breath, cold sweats, confusion, pulsus paradoxus > 13 mm Hg, jugular venous distention, and hypotension.

Chest x-ray

Chest radiographic evidence of pericardial effusion includes cardiomegaly with a "water bottle" heart; an irregular, nodular contour of the cardiac shadow; and mediastinal widening.

Electrocardiogram (ECG)

ECG shows nonspecific ST- and T-wave changes, tachycardia, low QRS voltage, electrical alternans, and atrial dysrhythmia.

Pericardiocentesis and echocardiography

An echocardiogram not only can confirm a suspected pericardial effusion but also can document the size of the effusion and its effect on ventricular function. Vignon reported on the accuracy of echocardiography performed by noncardiologist residents with limited training in an ICU and concluded that brief and limited training of noncardiologist ICU residents with no prior training in ultrasound methods appears "feasible and efficient" to address simple clinical questions about using echocardiography and was specifically useful in the diagnosis of pleural and pericardial effusions. A pericardial tap with cytologic examination (positive in 50% to 85% of cases with associated malignancy) will confirm the diagnosis of malignant effusion or differentiate it from other causes of pericardial effusion. Serious complications, including cardiac perforation and death, can occur during pericardiocentesis, even when performed with echocardiographic guidance by experienced clinicians.

Tumor markers/staining and cytogenetics

Tumor markers or special staining and cytogenetic techniques may improve the diagnostic yield, but ultimately an open pericardial biopsy may be necessary. Szturmowicz, et al, from Warsaw, Poland, studied pericardial fluid carcinoembryonic antigen (CEA) and CYFRA 21-1 levels in 84 patients with pericardial effusion. There were significant differences in patients with malignant vs benign effusions with both tests. With cutoff points of > 100 ng/mL for CYFRA 21-1 and > 5 ng/mL for CEA, 14 of 15 patients with malignant pericardial effusion with negative cytologic results had a positive result on one or both tests.

CT and MRI

CT and MRI as diagnostic adjuncts may provide additional information about the presence and location of loculations or mass lesions within the pericardium and adjacent structures. Restrepo et al have published a comprehensive, well-illustrated description of CT features of pericardial tamponade.

Cardiac catheterization

This may occasionally be of value to rule out superior vena caval obstruction, diagnose microvascular tumor spread in the lungs with secondary pulmonary hypertension, and document constrictive pericarditis before surgical intervention. In experimental animals, pericardial fluid has been aspirated by femoral vein catheterization and needle puncture of the right atrial appendage from within. This technique has not been used in humans.

Pericardioscopy

This allows visualization and biopsy at the time of subxiphoid or thoracoscopic pericardiotomy and can improve the diagnostic yield.

PROGNOSIS

In general, cancer patients who develop a significant pericardial effusion have a high mortality, with a mean time to death of 2.2 to 4.7 months. However, about 25% of selected patients treated surgically for cardiac tamponade enjoy a 1-year survival.

Investigators in Barcelona, Spain, studied the effects of volume expansion in patients with large pericardial effusions and pericardial tamponade. They administered 500 mL of normal saline over 10 minutes and measured hemodynamic and echocardiographic parameters. A total of 57% had tamponade on physical exam, and 20% were hypotensive. Volume expansion resulted in increases in mean arterial, intrapericardial, right atrial, and left ventricular end-diastolic pressures. The cardiac index increased by > 10% in 47% of patients, remained unchanged in 22%, and decreased in 31%. No patient had clinical complications. Predictors of improved hemodynamics were a pressure below 100 mm Hg and a low cardiac index. The authors concluded that in approximately half of patients with cardiac tamponade, particularly those with low blood pressure, cardiac output will increase after volume overload *(Sagrista-Sauleda J et al: Circulation 117:1545–1549, 2008).*

TREATMENT

General concepts

As is the case with malignant pleural effusion, it is difficult to evaluate treatments for pericardial effusion because of the many variables. Because malignant pericardial effusion is less common than malignant pleural effusion, it is more difficult to collect data in a prospective manner. Certain generalizations can, however, be derived from available data:

- All cancer patients with pericardial effusion require a systematic evaluation and should not be dismissed summarily as having an untreatable and/or terminal problem.
- Ultimately, both the management and natural course of the effusion depend on (1) the underlying condition of the patient, (2) the extent of clinical symptoms associated with the cardiac compression, and (3) the type and extent of the underlying malignant disease.

General treatment approaches

Asymptomatic, small effusions may be managed with careful follow-up and treatment directed against the underlying malignancy. On the other hand, cardiac tamponade is a true oncologic emergency. Immediate pericardiocentesis, under echocardiographic guidance, may be performed to relieve the patient's symptoms. A high failure rate is anticipated because the effusion rapidly recurs unless steps are taken to prevent it. Therefore, a more definitive treatment plan should be made following the initial diagnostic/therapeutic tap.

In patients with symptomatic, moderate-to-large effusions who do not present as an emergency, therapy should be aimed at relieving symptoms and preventing recurrence of tamponade or constrictive pericardial disease. Patients with tumors responsive to chemotherapy or radiation therapy may attain longer remissions with appropriate therapy.

There are two theoretical mechanisms for control of pericardial effusion: (1) creation of a persistent defect in the pericardium allowing fluid to drain out and be reabsorbed by surrounding tissues or (2) sclerosis of the mesothelium, resulting in the formation of fibrous adhesions that obliterate the pericardial cavity.

Postmortem studies have demonstrated that both of these mechanisms are operative. The fact that effusions can recur implies that there is either insufficient damage to the mesothelial layer or that rapid recurrence of effusion prevents coaptation of visceral and parietal pericardium and prevents the formation of adhesions. This, in turn, would suggest that early closure of the pericardial defect can result in recurrence.

Treatment methods

Various methods can be used to treat malignant pericardial effusion.

Observation Observation alone may be reasonable in the presence of small asymptomatic effusions.

Pericardiocentesis is useful in relieving tamponade and obtaining a diagnosis. Echocardiographic guidance considerably enhances the safety of this procedure. Ninety percent of pericardial effusions will recur within 3 months after pericardiocentesis alone.

Pericardiocentesis and percutaneous tube drainage can now be performed with low risk and are recommended by some clinical groups. Marcy et al, of Nice, France, reviewed multiple, well-illustrated percutaneous methods for management of malignant pericardial effusions. Problems that may occur include occlusion or displacement of the small-bore tubes, dysrhythmia, recurrent effusion, and infections. Mayo Clinic cardiologists recommend initial percutaneous pericardiocentesis with extended catheter drainage as their technique of choice.

Intrapericardial sclerotherapy and chemotherapy following percutaneous or open drainage have been reported to be effective treatments by some groups. Problems include pain during sclerosing agent treatments and recurrence of effusions. Good results have been reported with instillation of a number of agents, including bleomycin (10 mg), cisplatin (30 mg), mitomycin (2 mg), thiotepa (1.5 mg), and mitoxantrone (10 to 20 mg). Agents are selected based on their antitumor or sclerosing effect.

Martinoni et al, from Milan, Italy, reported on the use of intrapericardial administration of thiotepa (15 mg on days 1, 3, and 5) following placement of a pericardial drainage catheter in 33 patients with malignant pericardial effusion. There were three recurrent effusions (9.1%). The medial survival was 115 days. They concluded that this protocol is safe, well tolerated, and improves the quality and duration of life.

Pericardiocentesis and balloon pericardial window After percutaneous placement of a guidewire following pericardiocentesis, a balloon-dilating catheter can be placed across the pericardium under fluoroscopic guidance and a window created by balloon inflation.

At the National Taiwan University, cardiologists performed percutaneous double-balloon pericardiotomy in 50 patients with cancer and pericardial effusion and followed their course using serial echocardiograms. Success without

Kunitoh et al, from the National Cancer Center Hospital in Tokyo, performed a randomized controlled trial in 80 patients who had undergone pericardial drainage for malignant pericardial effusion. These patients were then randomized to receive either observation alone (A) after drainage or intrapericardial bleomycin instillation (15 mg followed by 10 mg every 48 hours [B]). Drainage tubes were removed when daily drainage was 20 mL or less. Survival with control of malignant pleural effusion at 2 months was 29% in arm A and 46% in arm B (P = .08); the median survival was 79 days vs 119 days *(Kunitoh H et al: Br J Cancer 10:464–469, 2009).*

recurrence was achieved in 88%. Fifty percent of patients died within 4 months, and 25% survived to 11 months.

Subtotal pericardial resection is seldom performed today. Although it is the definitive treatment, in that there is almost no chance of recurrence or constriction, higher morbidity and longer recovery time render this operation undesirable in patients who have a short anticipated survival. Its use is restricted to cancer patients with recurrent effusions who are in good overall condition and are expected to survive for up to 1 year.

Limited pericardial resection (pericardial window) via anterior thoracotomy or a thoracoscopic approach has a lower morbidity than less invasive techniques, but recovery is delayed. There is a low risk of recurrence. Cardiac herniation is possible if the size of the opening in the pericardium is not carefully controlled.

At City of Hope, Cullinane et al reported on 62 patients with malignant disease who had a surgical pericardial window created for management of pericardial effusion. Windows were created either thoracoscopically (32) or by subxiphoid (12) or limited thoracotomy (18) approaches. Primary tumors included NSCLC, breast, hematologic, and other solid-organ malignancies. Three recurrent effusions (4.8%) required reoperations. Eight patients (13%) died during the same admission as their surgical procedure. The median survival was much shorter for patients with NSCLC (2.6 months) than for patients with breast cancer (11 months) or hematologic malignancy (10 months). The surgical pericardial window is a safe and durable operative procedure that may provide extended survival in certain subgroups of cancer patients.

Subxiphoid pericardial resection can be performed with the patient under local anesthesia and may be combined with endoscopic instrumentation, tube drainage, and/or pericardial sclerosis.

Subxiphoid pericardioperitoneal window through the fused portion of the diaphragm and pericardium has been developed to allow continued drainage of pericardial fluid into the peritoneum. Experience with this procedure is limited.

Technical factors Prior pleurodesis for malignant pleural effusion makes an ipsilateral transpleural operation difficult or impossible. In lung cancer patients, major airway obstruction may preclude single-lung anesthesia and, thus, thoracoscopic pericardiectomy. Prior median sternotomy may prohibit the use of a subxiphoid approach.

Complications A 30-day mortality rate of 10% or higher has been reported for all of these modalities but is related more to the gravity of the underlying tumor and its sequelae. A small percentage of patients will develop severe problems with pulmonary edema or cardiogenic shock following pericardial decompression. The mechanisms of these problems are poorly understood. Late neoplastic pericardial constriction can occur following initially successful partial pericardiectomy. Patients with combined malignant pericardial and pleural effusions will often have relief of recurrent pleural effusion following control of pericardial effusion, perhaps because reducing systemic venous pressure results in reduced production of pleural fluid. Simultaneous pleurodesis in the left side of the chest following pericardial window might increase the incidence of recurrent pericardial effusion and should be avoided.

Radiotherapy External-beam irradiation is utilized infrequently in this clinical setting but may be an important option in specialized circumstances, especially in patients with radiosensitive tumors who have not received prior radiation therapy. Responses ranging from 66% to 93% have been reported with this form of treatment, depending on the type of associated tumor.

Chemotherapy Systemic chemotherapy is effective in treating pericardial effusions in patients with lymphomas, hematologic malignancies, or breast cancer. Long-term survival can be attained in these patients. If the pericardial effusion is small and/or asymptomatic, invasive treatment may be omitted in some of these cases. Data regarding the effectiveness of systemic chemotherapy or chemotherapy delivered locally in prevention of recurrent pericardial and pleural effusion are limited. New studies in this area are badly needed.

Biologic therapy with various agents is in the early stages of investigation.

MALIGNANT ASCITES

Malignant ascites results when there is an imbalance in the secretion of proteins and cells into the peritoneal cavity and absorption of fluids via the lymphatic system. Greater capillary permeability as a result of the release of cytokines by malignant cells increases the protein concentration in the peritoneal fluid. Recently, several studies have demonstrated higher levels of vascular endothelial growth factor (VEGF), a cytokine known to cause capillary leak, in the sera and effusions of patients with malignancies.

SIGNS AND SYMPTOMS

Patients with malignant ascites usually present with anorexia, nausea, respiratory compromise, and immobility. Complaints of abdominal bloating, heaviness, and ill-fitting clothes are common. Weight gain despite muscle wasting is a prominent sign.

DIAGNOSIS

A malignant etiology accounts for only 10% of all cases of ascites. Nonmalignant diseases causing ascites include liver failure, congestive heart failure, and occlusion of the inferior vena cava or hepatic vein. About one-third of all patients with malignancies will develop ascites. Malignant ascites has been described with many tumor types but is most commonly seen with gynecologic neoplasms (~50%), GI malignancies (20% to 25%), and breast cancer (10% to 18%). In 15% to 30% of patients, the ascites is associated with diffuse carcinomatosis of the peritoneal cavity.

Physical examination

Physical examination does not distinguish whether ascites is due to malignant or benign conditions. Patients may have abdominal fullness with fluid wave, anterior distribution of the normal abdominal tympany, and pedal edema. Occasionally, the hepatic metastases or tumor nodules studding the peritoneal surface can be palpated through the abdominal wall, which has been altered by ascitic distention.

Radiologic studies

Radiographs

Ascites can be inferred from plain radiographs of the abdomen. Signs include a ground-glass pattern and centralization of the intestines and abdominal contents.

Ultrasonography

Abdominal ultrasonography has been shown to be the most sensitive, most specific method for detecting and quantifying ascites. It also permits delineation of areas of loculation.

Success at removing peritoneal fluid in patients was markedly better with ultrasonographic assistance, as demonstrated in a randomized trial. Ultrasonography improved the physician's ability to aspirate ascites from 67% (27 of 44 patients) to 95% (40 of 42 patients).

CT

Abdominal and pelvic CT is effective in detecting ascites. In addition, CT scans may demonstrate masses, mesenteric stranding, omental studding, and diffuse carcinomatosis. IV and oral contrasts are necessary, thus increasing the degree of invasiveness of this modality.

Paracentesis

After the diagnosis of peritoneal ascites has been made on the basis of the physical examination and imaging, paracentesis should be performed to characterize the fluid. The color and nature of the fluid often suggest the diagnosis. Malignant ascites can be bloody, opaque, chylous, or serous. Benign ascites is usually serous and clear.

Analysis of the fluid should include cell count, cytology, LDH level, proteins, and appropriate evaluation for infectious etiologies. In addition, the fluid can be sent for the determination of tumor markers, such as CEA, CA-125, *p53*, and human chorionic gonadotropin-β (hCG-β). The hCG-β level is frequently elevated in malignancy-related ascites and has been combined with cytology to yield an 89.5% efficiency in diagnosis. The use of DNA ploidy indices allowed a 98.5% sensitivity and a 100% sensitivity in the identification of malignant cells within ascitic fluid. The use of the telomerase assay, along with cytologic evaluation of the ascitic fluid contents, has a 77% sensitivity in detecting malignant ascites.

Laparoscopy

Several studies have utilized minimally invasive laparoscopy as the diagnostic tool of choice. The fluid can be drained under direct visualization, the peritoneal cavity can be evaluated carefully, and any suspicious masses can be biopsied at the time of the laparoscopy.

PROGNOSIS

The presence of ascites in a patient with malignancy often portends end-stage disease. The median survival after the diagnosis of malignant ascites ranges from 7 to 13 weeks. Patients with gynecologic and breast malignancies have a better overall prognosis than patients with GI malignancies.

TREATMENT

Medical therapy

Traditionally, the first line of treatment is medical management. Medical therapies include repeated paracentesis, fluid restriction, diuretics, chemotherapy, and intraperitoneal sclerosis.

Repeated paracentesis

Repeated paracentesis, probably the most frequently employed treatment modality, provides significant symptomatic relief in the majority of cases. The procedure is minimally invasive and can be combined with abdominal ultrasonography to better localize fluid collections. High-volume paracentesis has been performed without inducing significant hemodynamic instability and with good patient tolerance.

After paracentesis, 78% of all patients reported relief of their symptoms, especially in the areas of abdominal bloating, anorexia, dyspnea, insomnia, and fatigue. In addition, overall quality of life improved after paracentesis.

Significant morbidity occurs with repeated taps and becomes more severe with each tap necessary to alleviate symptoms. Ascitic fluid contains a high concentration of proteins. Routine removal of ascites further depletes protein stores. The removal of large volumes of fluid also can result in electrolyte abnormalities and hypovolemia. In addition, complications can result from the procedure itself. They include hemorrhage, injury to intra-abdominal structures, peritonitis, and bowel obstruction. Contraindications to repeated paracentesis are viscous loculated fluid and hemorrhagic fluid.

With the placement of an intraperitoneal port, used also for the instillation of intraperitoneal chemotherapy, removal of ascitic fluid is possible without the need for repeated paracentesis. Other possible catheters for use in repeated paracentesis include PleurX and Tenckoff catheters (used for intraperitoneal dialysis). Placement of a semipermanent catheter minimizes the risk of injury to intra-abdominal structures. However, the benefits are tempered by increased infectious risks as well as the possibility of a nonfunctioning catheter requiring removal and replacement.

Diuretics, fluid and salt restriction

Unlike ascites from benign causes such as cirrhosis and congestive heart failure, malignant ascites responds poorly to fluid restriction, decreased salt intake, and diuretic therapy. The most commonly used diuretics (in patients who may have some response to diuretic treatment) are spironolactone (Aldactone) and amiloride (Midamor). Patients with massive hepatic metastases are most likely to benefit from spironolactone.

The onset of action for spironolactone is delayed (3–4 days), whereas the effects of amiloride are seen after 24 hours. The most common complications associated with these diuretics are painful gynecomastia, renal tubular acidosis, and hyperkalemia.

Chemotherapy

Chemotherapy, both systemic and intraperitoneal, has had some success in the treatment of malignant ascites. The most commonly used agents are cisplatin and

A randomized phase II/III study evaluated the trifunctional antibody directed at adhesion molecules (catumaxomab) in 258 patients with refractory malignant ascites from epithelial cancers. The study demonstrated improvements in puncture-free survival (a measure of decreased frequency of paracentesis) as well as longer duration between paracentesis in the patients who received the antibody. Treatment was well tolerated with moderate but manageable toxicities *(Heiss MM et al: Int J Cancer 127:2209–2221, 2010).*

mitomycin. Intraperitoneal hyperthermic chemotherapy has been used with some efficacy in GI malignancies to decrease recurrence of ascites as well as to prevent the formation of ascites in patients with peritoneal carcinomatosis.

Sclerotherapy

Sclerosing agents include bleomycin (60 mg/50 mL of normal saline) and talc (5 g/50 mL of normal saline). Responses are seen in ~30% of patients treated with these agents.

Theoretically, intraperitoneal chemotherapy and sclerosis obliterate the peritoneal space and prevent future fluid accumulation. If sclerosis is unsuccessful, it may produce loculations and make subsequent paracentesis difficult.

Other therapies

Experimental models and early clinical trials have shown that an intraperitoneal bolus of tumor necrosis factor (45–350 μg/m^2) given weekly may be effective in resolving malignant ascites. Other cytokines, including interferon-α, have had varying success. A randomized, prospective trial definitively addressing the role of cytokines and other biologic treatments in the management of malignant ascites has yet to be completed. Intraperitoneal injection of antibodies directed at VEGF has shown promise in decreasing ascites in early-phase clinical trials but further studies are needed.

Surgical techniques

Limited surgical options are available to treat patients who have refractory ascites after maximal medical management, demonstrate a significant decrease in quality of life as a result of ascites, and have a life expectancy of > 3 months.

Peritoneovenous shunts

These have been used since 1974 for the relief of ascites associated with benign conditions. In the 1980s, shunting was applied to the treatment of malignant ascites.

The LeVeen shunt contains a disc valve in a firm polypropylene casing, whereas the Denver shunt has a valve that lies within a fluid-filled, compressible silicone chamber. Both valves provide a connection between the peritoneal cavity and venous system that permits the free flow of fluid from the peritoneal cavity when a 2- to 4-cm water pressure gradient exists.

Success rates vary with shunting, depending on the nature of the ascites and the pathology of the primary tumor. Patients with ovarian cancer, for example, do very well, with palliation achieved in ≥ 50% of cases. However, ascites arising from GI malignancies is associated with a poorer response rate (10%–15%).

Candidates for shunt placement should be carefully selected. Cardiac and respiratory evaluations should be performed prior to the procedure. Shunt placement is *contraindicated* in the presence of the following:

- a moribund patient whose death is anticipated within weeks
- peritonitis
- major organ failure
- adhesive loculation
- thick, tenacious fluid.

Complications of shunting

Initial concerns about the use of a shunt in the treatment of malignant ascites centered on intravascular dissemination of tumor. In practice, there has been little difference in overall mortality in patients with and without shunts.

Disseminated intravascular coagulation During the early experience with shunting, particularly in cirrhotic patients, symptomatic clinical disseminated intravascular coagulation (DIC) developed rapidly and was a major source of morbidity and mortality. However, overwhelming DIC occurs infrequently in the oncologic population.

The pathophysiology of DIC has been studied extensively and is thought to be multifactorial. The reinfusion of large volumes of ascitic fluid may cause a deficiency in endogenous circulating coagulation factors by dilution. Secondarily, a fibrinolytic state is initiated by the introduction of soluble collagen (contained within the ascitic fluid) into the bloodstream, leading to a DIC state. Infrequently, full-blown DIC results and requires ligation of the shunt or even shunt removal. Discarding 50% to 70% of the ascitic fluid before establishing the peritoneovenous connection may prevent this complication but may increase the risk of early failure due to a reduced initial flow rate.

Commonly, coagulation parameters are abnormal without signs or symptoms. In some institutions, these laboratory values are so consistently abnormal that they are used to monitor shunt patency. Abnormalities most commonly seen include decreased platelets and fibrinogen and elevated prothrombin time, partial thromboplastin time, and fibrin split products.

Other common complications include shunt occlusion (10%–20%), heart failure (6%), ascitic leak from the insertion site (4%), infection (< 5%), and perioperative death (10% to 20% when all operative candidates are included).

Shunt patency may be indirectly correlated with the presence of malignant cells. One study found that patients with positive cytology results had a 26-day shunt survival, as compared with 140 days in patients with negative cytology results. Other studies have failed to demonstrate a correlation between ascites with malignant cells and decreased survival.

Clearly, shunting is not a benign procedure, but in carefully selected patients who have not responded to other treatment modalities and who are experiencing symptoms from ascites, it may provide needed palliation. Because of the limited effectiveness of peritoneovenous shunts, patients should be carefully selected prior to shunt placement.

Radical peritonectomy

Other surgical procedures used to treat malignant ascites have been proposed. They include radical peritonectomy combined with intraperitoneal chemotherapy. This is an extensive operation with significant morbidity, although initial results appear to demonstrate that it decreases the production of ascites. To date, no randomized trial has demonstrated that radical peritonectomy increases efficacy or survival.

SUGGESTED READING

ON MALIGNANT PLEURAL EFFUSION

Dresler CM, Olak J, Herndon JE 2nd, et al: Phase III intergroup study of talc poudrage vs talc slurry sclerosis for malignant pleural effusion. Chest 127:909–915, 2005.

Du Rand I, Maskell N, eds: British Thoracic Society Pleural Disease Guideline 2010. Thorax 65(Suppl 2):ii1–ii76, 2010.

Feller-Kopman D, Parker MJ, Schwartzstein RM: Assessment of pleural pressure in the evaluation of pleural effusions. Chest 135:201–209, 2009.

Gasparri R, Leo F, Veronesi G, et al: Video-assisted management of malignant pleural effusion in breast carcinoma. Cancer 106:271–276, 2006.

Hsu LH, Soong TC, Feng AC, et al: Intrapleural urokinase for the treatment of loculated malignant pleural effusions and trapped lungs in medically inoperable cancer patients. J Thorac Oncol 1:460–467, 2006.

Paschoalini Mda S, Vargas FS, Marchi E, et al: Prospective randomized trial of silver nitrate vs talc slurry in pleurodesis for symptomatic malignant pleural effusions. Chest 128:684–689, 2005.

Steger V, Mika U, Toomes H, et al: Who gains most? A 10-year experience with 611 thoracoscopic talc pleurodeses. Ann Thorac Surg 83:1940–1945, 2007.

Tan C, Sedrakyan A, Browne J, et al: The evidence on the effectiveness of management for malignant pleural effusion: A systematic review. Eur J Cardiothorac Surg 29: 829–838, 2006.

Tremblay A, Mason C, Michaud G: Use of tunnelled pleural catheters for malignant pleural effusions in patients fit for pleurodesis. Eur Respir J 30:759–762, 2007.

Vignon P, Dugard A, Abraham J, et al: Focused training for goal-oriented hand-held echocardiography performed by noncardiologist residents in the intensive care unit. Intensive Care Med 33:1795–1799, 2007.

Warren WH, Kalimi R, Khodadadian LM, et al: Management of malignant pleural effusions using the Pleur (x) catheter. Ann Thorac Surg 85:1049–1055, 2008.

William WN Jr, Lin HY, Lee JJ, et al: Revisiting stage IIIB and IV non-small cell lung cancer: Analysis of the surveillance, epidemiology, and end results data. Chest 136:701–709, 2009.

ON PERICARDIAL EFFUSION

Maisch B, Seferovic PM, Ristic AD, et al: Guidelines on the diagnosis and management of pericardial diseases executive summary: The Task Force on the Diagnosis and Management of Pericardial Diseases of the European Society of Cardiology. Eur Heart J 25:587–610, 2004.

McDonald JM, Meyers BF, Guthrie TJ, et al: Comparison of open subxiphoid pericardial drainage with percutaneous catheter drainage for symptomatic pericardial effusion. Ann Thorac Surg 76:811–816, 2003.

Neragi-Miandoab S, Linden PA, Ducko CT, et al: VATS pericardiotomy for patients with known malignancy and pericardial effusion: Survival and prognosis of positive cytology and metastatic involvement of the pericardium: A case control study. Int J Surg 6:110–114, 2008.

Restrepo CS, Lemos DF, Lemos JA, et al: Imaging findings in cardiac tamponade with emphasis on CT. Radiographics 27:1595–1610, 2007.

Sagristà-Sauleda J, Angel J, Sambola A, et al: Hemodynamic effects of volume expansion in patients with cardiac tamponade. Circulation 117:1545–1549, 2008.

Swanson N, Mirza I, Wijesinghe N, et al: Primary percutaneous balloon pericardiotomy for malignant pericardial effusion. Catheter Cardiovasc Interv 71:508–509, 2008.

Tsang TS, Enrique-Sarano M, Freeman WK, et al: Consecutive 1,127 therapeutic echocardiographically guided pericardiocenteses: Clinical profile, practice patterns, and outcomes spanning 21 years. Mayo Clin Proc 77:429–436, 2002.

ON MALIGNANT ASCITES

Ayantunde AA, Parsons SL: Pattern and prognostic factors in patients with malignant ascites: A retrospective study. Ann Oncol 18:945–949, 2007.

Gushchin V, Demmy TL, Kane JM 3rd: Surgical management of metastatic peritoneal or pleural disease. Semin Oncol 34:215–225, 2007.

Rosenberg SM: Palliation of malignant ascites. Gastroenterol Clin North Am 35:189–199, 2006.

Seike M, Maetani I, Sakai Y: Treatment of malignant ascites in patients with advanced cancer: Peritoneal shunt versus paracentesis. J Gastroenterol Hepatol 22:2161–2166, 2007.

Abbreviations in this chapter

SEER = Surveillance, Epidemiology, and End Results

APPENDIX 1

Response evaluation criteria and performance scales

RECIST/SCALES

RECIST: DEFINITION OF RESPONSE

In clinical studies, formal response criteria have been developed and have gained wide acceptance. The National Cancer Institute (NCI) has proposed and implemented newer standard response criteria called Response Evaluation Criteria in Solid Tumors (RECIST). In contrast, the World Health Organization (WHO) has a different standard for assessing response. Major differences between these guidelines are outlined below.

Comparison of RECIST and WHO guidelines

Characteristic	RECIST	WHO
Objective response (OR) (LD is the longest diameter)	**Target lesions** change in sum of LDs, maximum 5 per organ up to 10 total (more than one organ)	**Measurable disease** change in the sum of the products of LDs and greatest perpendicular diameters, no maximum number of lesions specified
Complete response (CR)	Disappearance of all target lesions, confirmed at ≥ 4 weeks	Disappearance of all known disease, confirmed at ≥ 4 weeks
Partial response (PR)	≥ 30% decrease from baseline, confirmed at ≥ 4 weeks	≥ 50% decrease from baseline, confirmed at ≥ 4 weeks
Progressive disease (PD)	≥ 20% increase over smallest sum observed or appearance of new lesions	≥ 25% increase in one or more lesions or appearance of new lesions
Stable disease (SD)	Neither PR nor PD criteria met	Neither PR nor PD criteria met (no change)

PERFORMANCE SCALES

The Karnofsky performance index and WHO (Zubrod) scale are commonly used as proxy measures for quality of life. Because they measure only one dimension of the construct, they would not be considered quality-of-life measures by today's standards. However, given their historic relevance and current high frequency of usage as proxy measures, we have included them here.

Karnofsky performance index

Definition		
Able to carry on normal activity and to work	100	Normal; no complaints; no evidence of disease
	90	Able to carry on normal activity; minor signs or symptoms of disease
	80	Normal activity with effort; some signs or symptoms of disease
Unable to work; able to live at home, care for most personal needs; a varying amount of assistance is needed	70	Cares for self; unable to carry on normal activity or to do active work
	60	Requires occasional assistance but is able to care for most needs
	50	Requires considerable assistance and frequent medical care
Unable to care for self; requires equivalent of institutional or hospital care; disease may be progressing rapidly	40	Disabled; requires special care and assistance
	30	Severely disabled; hospitalization is indicated, although death is not imminent
	20	Very sick; hospitalization necessary; active supportive treatment necessary
	10	Moribund; fatal processes progressing rapidly
	0	Dead

From Karnofsky DA, Abelmann WH, Craver LF, et al: The use of the nitrogen mustards in the palliative treatment of carcinoma. Cancer 1:634–656, 1948.

WHO (Zubrod) scale

This scale is used to measure performance of which the patient is *capable*. For example, a patient in the hospital for metabolic studies may be fully capable of performing normal activities but will remain in bed through his or her own choice. Such a patient should be coded 0, "normal."

0	Normal activity
1	Symptoms but nearly fully ambulatory
2	Some bed time but needs to be in bed < 50% of normal daytime
3	Needs to be in bed > 50% of normal daytime
4	Unable to get out of bed

From Zubrod CG, Schneiderman M, Frei E III, et al: Appraisal of methods for the study of chemotherapy of cancer in man: Comparative therapeutic trial of nitrogen mustard and triethylene thiophosphoramide. J Chron Dis 11:7–33, 1960.

APPENDIX 2

Cancer information on the Internet

J. Sybil Biermann, MD

This chapter highlights selected websites that are developed especially for oncology professionals, researchers, and patients with cancer.

American Cancer Society (ACS)

www.cancer.org Basic resources, including the American Cancer Society's Cancer Facts & Figures 2010, are readily available from the home page.

American Psychosocial Oncology Society (APOS)

www.apos-society.org Psychological services/counseling from the American Psychosocial Oncology Society. APOS provides a helpline for patients, in addition to other tools and resources for health professionals.

American Society for Therapeutic Radiology and Oncology (ASTRO)

www.astro.org ASTRO represents the medical and scientific professionals who use radiation therapy to treat patients with cancer and other diseases.

American Society of Clinical Oncology (ASCO)

www.asco.org Healthcare professionals can access ASCO policies, clinical guidelines, publications, and a searchable database of abstracts.

www.cancer.net Patient information is available on more than 120 types of cancer and cancer-related syndromes.

American Society of Hematology (ASH)

www.hematology.org A comprehensive collection of articles and reviews on hematologic malignancies may be found at the ASH website.

Cancernetwork.com

www.cancernetwork.com An excellent source of reliable cancer information with free access to the full text of over 6,000 peer-reviewed medical journal articles from the pages of *ONCOLOGY* and news reports from *Oncology News International*; selected text of this handbook, *Cancer Management: A Multidisciplinary Approach*, is also available.

Centers for Disease Control and Prevention (CDC)

http://www.cdc.gov/ CDC maintains several websites for health professionals, researchers, and the public.

www.cdc.gov/nccdphp/ Information on CDC cancer prevention programs.

CenterWatch

www.centerwatch.com A worldwide directory of more than 41,000 active industry and government-sponsored trials with independent review board (IRB) approval.

Coalition of National Cancer Cooperative Groups

http://www.CancerTrialsHelp.org/ Use "TrialCheck" to locate ongoing clinical trials among the Coalition's cooperative groups: CALGB, ECOG, NCCTG, NSABP, POG, and RTOG.

National Cancer Institute (NCI)

http://cancer.gov The NCI's vast website provides information suitable to clinical practitioners, researchers, patients, and the general public. Among the cancer resources available from the home page are:

http://cancer.gov/cancerinfo/pdq/ Peer-reviewed, frequently updated summaries on cancer treatment, screening, prevention, genetics, and supportive care.

http://cancer.gov/researchandfunding A directory of NCI research tools and funding opportunities (human, animal, and genomic) for cancer researchers.

http://cancer.gov/statistics Statistical databases and resources, including cancer incidence by gender, race, ethnicity, and type of cancer.

http://cancer.gov/aboutnci/cis The Cancer Information Service offers reliable information for patients with cancer. CIS also offers a toll-free phone service (1-800-4-CANCER) for the public in English and Spanish.

http://clinicaltrials.gov A registry of approximately 25,000 clinical studies.

National Comprehensive Cancer Network (NCCN)

www.nccn.org The NCCN website provides access to the NCCN's current Clinical Practice Guidelines, links to ongoing clinical trials at member institutions, and a directory of physicians for referrals.

Oncology Nursing Society

www.ons.org/ ONS is a professional organization of over 37,000 registered nurses and other healthcare providers dedicated to excellence in patient care, education, research, and administration in oncology nursing.

PubMed.gov

http://www.ncbi.nlm.nih.gov/pubmed/ PubMed offers selected cancer topic searches for more than 100 different cancer topics.

SearchMedica

Searchmedica.com SearchMedica's index contains well over 1,000 websites organized into numerous therapeutic categories, including cancer. SearchMedica allows users to refine results by content category such as Research/Reviews, Practical Articles and News, Patient Education Materials, and Practice Guidelines.

Society for Integrative Oncology (SIO)

www.sio.org The Society for Integrative Oncology (SIO) is a multidisciplinary organization for health professionals committed to the study and application of complementary therapies and botanicals for cancer patients.

Surveillance, Epidemiology, and End Results Program (SEER)

http://seer.cancer.gov/ The NCI's SEER program collects and publishes cancer incidence and survival data from population-based cancer registries covering approximately 26% of the US population.

Additional Resources

www.aacr.org American Association for Cancer Research

www.acr.org The American College of Radiology

www.askcnet.org/dataq/cancer.htm State and regional cancer registries

www.leukemia-lymphoma.org The Leukemia & Lymphoma Society

www.mdlinx.com/HemeOncLinx/ MdLinx provides daily summaries of hematology/oncology articles culled from a wide variety of professional publications.

www.mskcc.org/aboutherbs An excellent resource for information on commonly used herbs and botanicals from the Memorial Sloan-Kettering Cancer Center site. General information on health-related frauds can be found at www.quackwatch.org.

www.naaccr.org North American Association of Central Cancer Registries

www.nidcr.nih.gov/oralhealth/topics/cancertreatment Resources on cancer treatment and oral health for health professionals and patients.

www.oncolink.com News articles, fact sheets, and annotated links to cancer-related information at other websites; maintained by The University of Pennsylvania.

International Resources

www.eortc.be/ European Organisation for Research and Treatment of Cancer

www.iarc.fr International Agency for Research on Cancer

www.macmillan.org.uk Macmillan Cancer Support

APPENDIX 3

Selected cancer drugs and indications

NEWLY APPROVED OR NEWLY LABELED BY THE US FOOD AND DRUG ADMINISTRATION, OCTOBER 2009 – SEPTEMBER 2010

Product (Generic) Name	Trade Name	Indication
RASBURICASE	ELITEK	Initial management of plasma uric acid levels in pediatric and adult patients with leukemia, lymphoma, and solid tumor malignancies who are receiving anticancer therapy expected to result in tumor lysis and subsequent elevation of plasma uric acid
PAZOPANIB HYDROCHLORIDE	VOTRIENT	Treatment of patients with advanced renal cell carcinoma (RCC)
OFATUMUMAB	ARZERRA	Treatment of patients with chronic lymphocytic leukemia (CLL) refractory to fludarabine (Fludara) and alemtuzumab (Campath)
ROMIDEPSIN	ISTODAX	Treatment of cutaneous T-cell lymphoma (CTCL) in patients who have received at least one prior systemic therapy
LAPATINIB DITOSYLATE	TYKERB	In combination with letrozole (Femara) for the treatment of postmenopausal women with hormone receptor–positive metastatic breast cancer that overexpresses the HER2 receptor for whom hormonal therapy is indicated. Tykerb in combination with an aromatase inhibitor has not been compared with a trastuzumab (Herceptin)-containing chemotherapy regimen for the treatment of metastatic breast cancer.

For additional information and an up-to-date listing of newly approved oncology drugs, see FDA's "What's New From the Office of Oncology Drug Products" at http://www.fda.gov/AboutFDA/CentersOffices/CDER/ucm093885.htm.

Product (Generic) Name	Trade Name	Indication
RITUXIMAB	RITUXAN	Treatment of patients previously untreated for CD20-positive chronic lymphocytic leukemia (CLL) in combination with fludarabine (Fludara) and cyclophosphamide (FC)
TRIPTORELIN PAMOATE	TRELSTAR	Palliative treatment of advanced prostate cancer
ERLOTINIB	TARCEVA	Maintenance treatment of patients with locally advanced or metastatic non–small-cell lung cancer whose disease has not progressed after 4 cycles of platinum-based first-line chemotherapy
SIPULEUCEL-T	PROVENGE	Autologous cellular immunotherapy indicated for the treatment of asymptomatic or minimally symptomatic metastatic castration-resistant (hormone-refractory) prostate cancer.
CABAZITAXEL	JEVTANA	In combination with prednisone for the treatment of patients with hormone-refractory metastatic prostate cancer previously treated with a docetaxel (Taxotere)-containing treatment regimen
NILOTINIB	TASIGNA	Treatment of patients with newly diagnosed Philadelphia chromosome–positive chronic myeloid leukemia (Ph+ CML) in chronic phase. The effectiveness of Tasigna is based on major molecular response and cytogenetic response rates. The study is ongoing and further data will be required to determine long-term outcome.

APPENDIX 4

Selected chemotherapy agents: Uses, dosages, and toxicities

Emiliano Calvo, MD, PhD, and Antonio Calles, MD

Drug and its uses	Dosages	Toxicities
Albumin-bound (nab) paclitaxel Breast cancer (relapse)	260 mg/m² IV over 30 min every 3 wk	Bone marrow depression, sensory neuropathy, arthralgia/myalgia, asthenia, abnormal ECG, alopecia
Alemtuzumab Chemotherapy-refractory B-cell CLL	Rapid daily-dose escalation, until tolerated, from 3 mg/d, and then 10 mg/d, to the recommended maintenance dose of 30 mg IV over 120 min, 3 times per wk on alternate days for up to 12 wk	Pancytopenia, infusion reaction, opportunistic infections, skin rash, nausea/vomiting
Altretamine Ovarian, lung, breast, and cervical cancers, NHL	4–12 mg/kg/d or 260 mg/m², PO divided in 3–4 doses for 14–21 d of a 28-d regimen	Nausea and vomiting, bone marrow depression, paresthesias, CNS toxicity
Asparaginase ALL, CML, AML	6,000 IU/m² IM 3 times weekly for 9 doses or 100 IU/kg/d IV for 10 continuous days, starting on Day 22 of treatment; usually given with vincristine and prednisone	Allergic reactions (fever, chills, skin rash, anaphylaxis), nausea and vomiting, anorexia, liver dysfunction, CNS depression, coagulopathy, hyperglycemia
Bendamustine CLL, B-cell NHL (relapse)	IV: 100 mg/m² on D 1 and D 2 of a 28-d cycle, up to 6 cycles	Bone marrow depression, fever, nausea, and vomiting

Drug and its uses	Dosages	Toxicities
Bevacizumab Breast cancer, colorectal cancer, NSCLC, renal cell carcinoma, glioblastoma (relapse)	5 mg/kg/wk IV over 60–90 min every 14–21 d	Asthenia, headache, epistaxis, proteinuria, GI perforations/ wound-healing complications, hypertension/hypertensive crisis; hemorrhage, thrombo-embolic events
Bleomycin Testicular cancer, HL, reticulum cell sarcoma, lymphosarcoma, squamous cell cancer of the head and neck, skin, cervix, vulva, and penis	10–20 U/m^2 given IV, IM, or SC weekly or twice weekly; maximum total dose, 400 U; a 2-U test dose should be given because of a possible anaphylactoid reaction	Pneumonitis and pulmonary fibrosis, fever and allergic reactions, anaphylaxis, hyperpigmentation, Raynaud's phenomenon, alopecia
Bortezomib Multiple myeloma	1.3 mg/m^2 on Days 1, 4, 8, and 11 every 3 wk	Diarrhea, peripheral neuropathy, asthenia, fever, anorexia, Mantle cell lymphoma, nausea and vomiting, rash, headache, thrombocytopenia
Busulfan CML, BMT for refractory leukemia, lymphomas	2–8 mg PO daily for remission induction; adjust dosage to WBC count; 1–3 mg PO daily for maintenance; withhold induction if WBC count < 15,000/μL; resume therapy when WBC count > 50,000/μL	Bone marrow depression, pulmonary fibrosis, aplastic anemia, amenorrhea, gynecomastia, skin hyperpigmentation
Cabazitaxel Hormone-refractory metastatic prostate cancer previously treated with docetaxel regimens	25 mg/m^2 IV every 3 weeks in combination with prednisone 10 mg PO daily throughout cabazitaxel treatment. Premedicate 30 minutes before each dose with antihistamine, corticosteroid, and H2 antagonist.	Febrile neutropenia (primary G-CSF prophylaxis should be considered in high-risk patients), nausea, vomiting, diarrhea, renal failure, hypersensitivity reactions
Capecitabine Breast cancer (relapsed), colorectal cancer, and other GI malignancies	1,250 mg/m^2 bid PO with food (2 wk on drug, 1 wk of rest)	Diarrhea, stomatitis, nausea and vomiting, fatigue, hand-foot syndrome, bone marrow depression (minimal)
Carboplatin[a] Ovarian cancer; endometrial, head and neck, lung, testicular, and breast cancers; relapsed acute leukemia, NHL	Single agent: 360 mg/m^2 IV every 4 wk Combination: 300 mg/m^2 IV every 4 wk Calvert formula: Total dose (mg) = Target AUC × (GFR + 25)	Bone marrow depression, nausea and vomiting, peripheral neuropathy, ototoxicity

[a]Total carboplatin dose calculation based on IDMS-measured serum creatinine using the Calvert formula may result in overestimation of the GFR in some patients with normal renal function, and therefore increased drug-related toxicity. When actual GFR measurements are made to assess renal function, carboplatin can be safely dosed as outlined in the package insert (see: *ctep.cancer.gov/content/docs/Carboplatin_Information_Letter.pdf*).

Drug and its uses	Dosages	Toxicities
Carmustine Brain tumor, multiple myeloma, HL, NHL, melanoma, BMT for refractory solid tumors and lymphomas	150–200 mg/m^2 IV every 6–8 wk	Delayed bone marrow depression, nausea and vomiting, reversible hepatotoxicity, local phlebitis, pulmonary and renal damage (high dose)
Cetuximab KRAS wild type colorectal cancer, head and neck cancer	400 mg/m^2 IV over 120 min, loading dose, and 250 mg/m^2 IV over 60 min every 7 d, as maintenance	Skin rash, infusion reaction, asthenia, diarrhea, nausea
Chlorambucil CLL, HL, NHL, ovarian cancer, choriocarcinoma, lymphosarcoma	0.1–0.2 mg/kg PO daily for 3–6 wk as required (usually 4–10 mg/d) or intermittent 0.4 mg/kg every 3–4 wk; increase by 0.1 mg/kg until control of disease or toxicity	Bone marrow depression, gonadal dysfunction, leukemia, hyperuricemia, pulmonary fibrosis
Cisplatin Testicular, ovarian, bladder, uterine, cervical, and lung cancers, squamous cell cancer of the head and neck, sarcoma, NHL	50 mg/m^2 IV or more every 3 wk; or 20 mg/m^2 IV daily for 4–5 d every 3–4 wk; give vigorous hydration before and after chemotherapy	Renal damage, nausea and vomiting, electrolyte disturbance, peripheral neuropathy, bone marrow depression, ototoxicity, radiosensitizer
Cladribine Hairy-cell leukemia, NHL, mycosis fungoides, AML, CML, CLL	0.09 mg/kg/d (4 mg/m^2/d) by continuous IV infusion for 7 consecutive days	Bone marrow depression, febrile episodes, rash, infections, septicemia
Cyclophosphamide AML, ALL, CLL, HL, and NHL, multiple myeloma, mycosis fungoides, neuroblastoma, ovarian and breast cancers, retinoblastoma, lung, testicular, and bladder cancers, sarcoma	40–50 mg/kg IV in divided doses over 2–5 d to start, followed by 10–15 mg/kg IV every 7–10 d; or 3–5 mg/kg IV twice weekly; or 1–5 mg/kg/d PO	Bone marrow depression, hemorrhagic cystitis, immunosuppression, alopecia, stomatitis, SIADH
Cytarabine (Ara-C) AML, ALL, CML, NHL, CNS leukemia (intrathecal)	AML induction: 100 mg/m^2/d by continuous IV infusion on Days 1–7; or 100 mg/m^2 IV every 12 h on Days 1–7 Relapsed ALL: 3 g/m^2 IV over 1–3 h every 12 h for 4 doses	Bone marrow depression, nausea and vomiting, diarrhea, arachnoiditis (intrathecal), stomatitis, hepatic dysfunction, fever, conjunctivitis, confusion, somnolence, cerebellar toxicity

Drug and its uses	Dosages	Toxicities
Dacarbazine Malignant melanoma, HL, soft-tissue sarcomas, neuroblastoma	Melanoma: 2.0–4.5 mg/kg/d IV for 10 d every 4 wk; or 250 mg/m^2/d IV for 5 d every 3 wk HL: 375 mg/m^2 IV on D 1, repeated every 15 d (single agent); 150 mg/m^2/d IV for 5 d every 4 wk (combination therapy)	Bone marrow depression, nausea and vomiting, flu-like syndrome, transient hepatotoxicity, local irritation, facial flushing, alopecia
Dactinomycin Testicular cancer, gestational trophoblastic tumors, Wilms' tumor, rhabdomyosarcoma, Ewing sarcoma	0.010–0.015 mg/kg IV daily for 5 d every 3 wk (usual adult dose, 0.5 mg) or 2 mg/m^2 IV as a single dose every 3–4 wk	Stomatitis, bone marrow depression, anorexia, nausea and vomiting, diarrhea, alopecia, skin changes, anaphylactoid reaction
Dasatinib CML, Ph+ ALL	140 mg/d (divided doses; 70 mg bid) or 100 mg/d PO (chronic phase CML)	Fluid-retention events (eg, pleural effusion); GI events: diarrhea, nausea, abdominal pain, vomiting; bleeding events; hematologic toxicities: neutropenia, thrombocytopenia, anemia
Daunorubicin AML, ALL	Remission induction: 30–45 mg/m^2/d IV for 3 d in combination therapy; total cumulative dose, 550 mg/m^2	Bone marrow depression, cardiotoxicity, alopecia, nausea and vomiting, diarrhea, stomatitis, fever, dermatitis at previously irradiated sites, red urine, anaphylactoid reaction
DaunoXome (liposomal daunorubicin) Kaposi sarcoma, ALL, AML	Liposomal preparation: 40 mg/m^2 IV every 2 wk	
DepoCyt (liposomal cytarabine) CNS leukemia/lymphoma	Intrathecal: DepoCyt, 50 mg over 1–5 min every 14 d, with dexamethasone, 4 mg PO bid × 5 d	
Docetaxel Breast, NSCLC, prostate, ovarian, pancreatic, head and neck, esophagus, stomach, cervical, Kaposi sarcoma, uterine, and bladder cancers	60–100 mg/m^2 IV over 1 h every 21 d or up to 42 mg/m^2 IV every wk	Bone marrow depression, fluid retention, hypersensitivity reaction, paresthesias, rash, alopecia, myalgias
Doxil (liposomal doxorubicin) Ovarian cancer (refractory to paclitaxel- and platinum-based regimens), Kaposi sarcoma, breast cancer, multiple myeloma	50 mg/m^2 IV every 4 wk 20 mg/m^2 IV every 3 wk	Bone marrow depression, hand-foot syndrome, infusional reactions

Drug and its uses	Dosages	Toxicities
Doxorubicin ALL, AML, breast, ovarian, bladder cancers, HL, NHL, SCLC, gastric cancer, sarcoma, Wilms' tumor, neuroblastoma, thyroid cancer, soft-tissue and bone sarcomas	60–90 mg/m² single IV injection every 21 d, 20–30 mg/m²/d IV for 3 d every 3–4 wk, or 20 mg/m² IV weekly; total cumulative dose of 550 mg/m²; reduce dose for liver dysfunction	Bone marrow depression, cardiotoxicity, stomatitis (continuous infusion), alopecia, nausea and vomiting, diarrhea, fever, dermatitis at previously irradiated sites, red urine, anaphylactoid reaction
Epirubicin Breast cancer	100 mg/m² IV on Day 1 or 60 mg/m² IV on Days 1 and 8 in combination therapy	Bone marrow depression, cardiotoxicity, stomatitis, alopecia
Erlotinib NSCLC, pancreas	150 mg/d PO 100 mg/d PO (pancreatic cancer)	Acne-form skin rash, diarrhea, anorexia, fatigue, dyspnea
Estramustine Prostate, renal cell carcinomas	14 mg/kg/d PO in 3–4 equally divided doses; 300 mg/d IV for 3–4 wk, followed by 300–450 mg/wk IV over 3–8 wk	Bone marrow depression, ischemic heart disease, thromboembolism, thrombophlebitis gynecomastia, nausea and vomiting, hepatotoxicity
Etoposide Testicular cancer (refractory) SCLC, HL, NHL, AML, gestational trophoblastic tumors For both indications, given with combination therapy and repeated every 3–4 wk	<u>Testicular:</u> 50–100 mg/m²/d IV for 5 d or 100 mg/m²/d IV on Days 1, 3, and 5 <u>Lung:</u> 35–50 mg/m²/d IV for 5 d or 100 mg/m²/d PO for 5 d	Bone marrow depression, nausea and vomiting, diarrhea, fever, hypotension with rapid infusion, alopecia, rash, AML (late effect)
Everolimus Renal cell carcinoma (progression to TKI)	10 mg/d PO	Stomatitis, infections, asthenia, diarrhea, pneumonitis, dyslipidemia, hyperglycemia, elevated serum creatinine
Floxuridine GI adenocarcinomas metastatic to liver, including oral, pancreatic, biliary, colon, and hepatic cancers, and metastatic breast cancer	0.1–0.6 mg/kg/d over several days via continuous arterial infusion supplying well-defined tumor; treatments given over 1–6 wk	Stomatitis and GI ulcers, bone marrow depression, abdominal pain, nausea and vomiting, diarrhea, liver dysfunction (transient)
Fludarabine CLL, AML, NHL (low-grade)	25 mg/m²/d IV over 30 min for 5 d; repeat every 28 d	Bone marrow depression, nausea and vomiting, fever, malaise, pulmonary infiltrates, tumor lysis syndrome, CNS effects (high dose)

Drug and its uses	Dosages	Toxicities
Fluorouracil Colon, rectal, stomach, pancreatic, breast, head and neck, renal cell, prostate, and ovarian cancers, squamous cell carcinomas of esophagus, basal and squamous cell carcinoma of skin (topical), hepatic cancer (intra-arterial)	<u>Loading dose:</u> 300–500 mg/m^2; or 12 mg/kg IV daily for 3–5 d, followed by weekly maintenance <u>Maintenance:</u> 10–15 mg/kg IV weekly, as toxicity permits <u>Infusion:</u> 20–25 mg/kg by continuous IV over 24 h for 4–5 d, every 4 wk	Stomatitis and GI ulcers (infusion), bone marrow depression (bolus), diarrhea, nausea and vomiting, esophagitis, angina, cerebellar ataxia, radiosensitizer
Gefitinib NSCLC	250 mg/d PO	Acne-form skin rash, diarrhea, transaminitis, asthenia, nausea/vomiting, interstitial lung disease
Gemcitabine Pancreatic, lung, breast, ovarian, and bladder cancers	1,000 mg/m^2 IV over 30 min, once weekly for up to 7 wk (or until toxicity necessitates reducing or withholding a dose), followed by 1 wk of rest <u>Subsequent cycles</u>: Infusions once weekly for 3 consecutive wk out of every 4 wk	Bone marrow depression, transient fever, flu-like syndrome, skin rash, mild nausea and vomiting
Gliadel wafers Glioblastoma multiforme	Up to 8 in brain cavity created by tumor removal	Fever, pain, and abnormal healing
Hydroxyurea CML, acute leukemia (emergent treatment), head and neck cancer, ovarian cancer, melanoma, essential thrombocytosis, polycythemia vera	<u>Intermittent:</u> 80 mg/kg PO every third day <u>Continuous:</u> 20–30 mg/kg PO daily	Bone marrow depression, mild nausea and vomiting, skin rashes, radiosensitizer
Ibritumomab CD20+ low grade follicular B-cell NHL (relapse)	<u>Dosimetric step:</u> Rituximab 250 mg/m^2 IV; 5 mCi In-111 Ibritumomab on Day 1 <u>Therapeutic step:</u> Day 7, 8, or 9 Rituximab 250 mg/m^2 IV; 0.4–0.3 mCi/kg Y-90 Ibritumomab	Myelosuppression, infection, GI symptoms, MDS/AML
Idarubicin AML, CML (blast phase), ALL	12 mg/m^2/d IV for 3 d every 3 wk in combination therapy	Bone marrow depression, nausea and vomiting, stomatitis, alopecia, cardiotoxicity
Ifosfamide Germ-cell testicular cancer, sarcoma, NHL, lung cancer	1.2 g/m^2/d via slow IV infusion for 5 consecutive days; repeat every 3 wk; give with mesna	Bone marrow depression, hemorrhagic cystitis, confusion, somnolence

Drug and its uses	Dosages	Toxicities
Imatinib CML, GIST, Ph+ ALL, dermatofibrosarcoma protuberans, mastocytosis, MDS/MPD	400 mg/d PO in chronic-phase CML and GIST and 600 mg/d PO for CML in accelerated phase or blast crisis/800 mg/d PO (DFSP)	Nausea and vomiting, edema and fluid retention, myalgias, diarrhea, myelosuppression, transaminitis
Irinotecan Colorectal cancer, lung, ovarian, and cervical cancers	125 mg/m^2 IV over 90 min once weekly for 4 wk; then 2 wk rest or 350 mg/m^2 every 21 d or 180 mg/m^2 every 2 wk	Bone marrow depression, diarrhea, nausea and vomiting, anorexia, weight loss
Lapatinib HER2-positive metastatic breast cancer	1,250 mg PO qd × 21 d in combination with capecitabine 2,000 mg/m^2/d PO (divided doses) on D 1–14 of a repeating 21-d cycle	Diarrhea, hand-foot syndrome, nausea, rash, vomiting, fatigue, LVEF decrease, pneumonitis, QT prolongation
Lenalidomide Multiple myeloma (relapse)	10 mg/d PO	Birth defects, neutropenia and thrombocytopenia, thrombosis
Lomustine Brain tumors, HL, GI carcinomas, NSCLC	130 mg/m^2 PO every 6 wk; adjust dose in combination chemotherapy	Delayed bone marrow depression, nausea and vomiting, reversible hepatotoxicity, pulmonary and renal damage, neurologic reactions, leukemia
Mechlorethamine HL, NHL, CML, CLL, mycosis fungoides, bronchogenic carcinoma, lymphosarcoma, polycythemia vera, malignant effusions (intracavitary)	0.4 mg/kg ideal body weight given as single dose or in divided doses of 0.1–0.2 mg/kg/d	Bone marrow depression, nausea and vomiting, local phlebitis, severe skin necrosis if extravasated, gonadal dysfunction
Melphalan Multiple myeloma, breast and ovarian cancers, sarcoma, testicular and lung cancers	<u>Continuous therapy:</u> 6 mg PO daily for 2–3 wk, no therapy for 2–4 wk, then maintenance with 2–4 mg PO daily <u>Pulse:</u> 10 mg/m^2 PO daily for 4 d every 4–6 wk	Bone marrow depression, anorexia, nausea and vomiting, gonadal testicular dysfunction, leukemia
Mercaptopurine ALL, CML, AML	1.5–2.5 mg/kg/d PO (100–200 mg in average adult) until response or toxic effects are seen; may increase dose to 5 mg/kg/d; adjust for maintenance dose; reduce dose by 50%–75% if given with allopurinol or if renal or hepatic insufficiency ensues	Bone marrow depression, nausea and vomiting, anorexia, diarrhea, cholestasis

Drug and its uses	Dosages	Toxicities
Methotrexate Breast, head and neck, GI, and lung cancers, ALL, CNS leukemia (intrathecal), gestational trophoblastic tumors, NHL (advanced stage), Burkitt lymphoma, osteosarcoma, mycosis fungoides	Numerous dosing schedules with combination therapy: Low dose: 2.5–5.0 mg PO daily; or 5–25 mg/m^2 PO, IM, IV twice weekly; or 50 mg/m^2 IV every 2–3 wk High dose: 1–12 g/m^2 IV with leucovorin rescue every 1–3 wk Intrathecal: 5–10 mg/m^2 (up to 15 mg) every 3–7 d	Mucositis, GI ulceration (may produce hemorrhage or perforation), bone marrow depression, pulmonary fibrosis (previously irradiated area), nerve root irritation and convulsion (intrathecal), liver cirrhosis and osteoporosis (chronic therapy), renal damage (high dose), diarrhea, skin erythema
Mitomycin Gastric, colorectal, anal cancer, pancreatic adenocarcinomas, NSCLC, breast, uterine, cervical, and head and neck cancers	20 mg/m^2 IV every 6–8 wk as a single agent or 5–10 mg/m^2 IV every 6 wk in combination therapy	Bone marrow depression (cumulative), nausea and vomiting, anorexia, alopecia, stomatitis, fever, pulmonary fibrosis
Mitoxantrone AML, prostate, ALL, CML, breast and ovarian cancers	Remission induction: 12 mg/m^2/d IV for 3 d, in combination with Ara-C	Bone marrow depression, cardiotoxicity, alopecia, stomatitis, nausea and vomiting, blue urine and sclera
Nilotinib CML	Newly diagnosed CML-chronic phase: 300 mg PO twice daily. Resistant or intolerant CML-chronic phase or accelerated phase: 400 mg PO twice daily	Myelosuppression, hyperbilirubinemia, rash, pruritus, nausea, headache, fatigue, constipation, elevated lipase, QTc prolongation
Ofatumumab CLL refractory to fludarabine and alemtuzumab	12 doses administered as follows: 300 mg initial dose, followed 1 week later by 2,000 mg weekly for 7 doses, followed 4 weeks later by 2,000 mg every 4 weeks for 4 doses. Premedicate with acetaminophen PO, antihistamine PO or IV, and corticosteroids IV.	Neutropenia, infection, infusion reaction, fatigue, rash
Oxaliplatin Colorectal, ovarian cancers	85 mg/m^2 oxaliplatin and 200 mg/m^2 leucovorin (IV) IV infusion over 120 min on D 1 followed by 400 mg/m^2 5-FU IV bolus, then 600 mg/m^2 5-FU by IV infusion over 22 h. On D 2, 200 mg/m^2 IV over 120 min IV, followed by 400 mg/m^2 5-FU IV bolus, 600 mg/m^2 5-FU IV infusion over 22 h. Repeat every 2 wk	Bone marrow depression, diarrhea, nausea and vomiting, neuropathies exacerbated by cold exposure, pharyngolaryngeal dysesthesia, pulmonary toxicity

Drug and its uses	Dosages	Toxicities
Paclitaxel Ovarian cancer (relapsed), NSCLC (in combination with cisplatin), Kaposi sarcoma, breast cancer, head and neck, gastric, colon, esophagus, uterine, prostate, bladder cancers, and melanomas	135–175 mg/m² by IV infusion (ranging from 3–96 h) every 3 wk or 80 mg/m² IV every wk	Bone marrow depression, peripheral neuropathy, alopecia, mucositis, anaphylaxis, dyspnea, myalgias
Panitumumab KRAS wild type colorectal cancer	6 mg/kg IV over 60 minutes every 14 days	Skin rash, hypomagnesemia, paronychia, fatigue, infusion reactions, nausea/vomiting, diarrhea
Pazopanib Renal cell cancer	800 mg PO once daily, without food	Diarrhea, hypertension, hair color change, nausea/vomiting, fatigue, anorexia
Pemetrexed Mesothelioma, NSCLC	500 mg/m² IV over 10 min every 21 d. Premedication needed with corticosteroid and vitamin supplementation	Bone marrow depression, stomatitis/pharyngitis, rash/skin desquamation, diarrhea
Pentostatin Hairy-cell leukemia, ALL, CLL, lymphoblastic lymphoma, mycosis fungoides	4 mg/m² IV over 30 min every other wk or for 3 consecutive wk; give vigorous hydration before and after chemotherapy	Nephrotoxicity, CNS depression, bone marrow depression, nausea and vomiting, conjunctivitis
Pralatrexate Relapsed and refractory T-cell lymphoma (PTCL)	30 mg/m² administered as an IV push over 3 to 5 min once weekly in 7-week cycles. Supplement with Vitamin B-12, 1 mg IM every 8–10 weeks and folic acid 1.0–1.25 mg PO daily	Mucositis, thrombocytopenia, nausea, fatigue, febrile neutropenia
Procarbazine HL, NHL, brain tumors, lung cancer	Single agent: 4–6 mg/kg/d PO until maximum response HL (MOPP): 100 mg/m²/d PO for 14 d	Bone marrow depression, nausea and vomiting, lethargy, depression, paresthesias, headache, flu-like symptoms
Rituximab CD20-positive B-cell NHL, CLL	375 mg/m² IV infusion (50–100 mg/h) once weekly in combination with fludarabine and cyclophosphamide. Rituxamab 375 mg/m² (first cycle) and 500 mg/m² in cycles 2–6	Infusion reactions, asthenia, headache, skin rash/pruritus, leukopenia/infection, nausea, tumor lysis syndrome, hepatitis B reactivation, PML

Drug and its uses	Dosages	Toxicities
Romidepsin Cutaneous T-cell lymphoma refractory to 1 prior systemic therapy	14 mg/m^2 IV over 4 hours on Days, 1, 8, 15 of a 28-day cycle	Myelosuppression, QT prolongation (make sure magnesium and potassium are normal prior to administration), nausea, fatigue
Sipuleucel-T Asymptomatic or minimally symptomatic metastatic castrate-resistant (hormone-refractory) prostate cancer	Administer 3 doses at approximately 2-week intervals. Premedicate patients with acetaminophen and antihistamine. Infuse sipuleucel-T IV over a period of 60 minutes. Each dose contains a minimum of 50 million autologous CD54+ cells activated with PAP-GM-CSF suspended in 250 mL of Lactated Ringer's Injection.	Chills, fever, back pain, nausea, joint ache, headache
Sorafenib Renal cell cancer, hepatocellular carcinoma	400 mg bid PO	Diarrhea, nausea, stomatitis, asthenia, cardiac ischemia, hand-foot syndrome, hypertension, bleeding, anorexia
Streptozocin Pancreatic islet-cell, carcinoid, colon, hepatoma, NSCLC, HL	<u>Daily:</u> 500 mg/m^2 IV for 5 d every 6 wk until maximum benefit or toxicity <u>Weekly:</u> 1,000 mg/m^2 IV weekly for first 2 wk, then escalate dose to response or toxicity, not to exceed a single dose of 1,500 mg/m^2	Renal damage, nausea and vomiting, diarrhea, altered glucose metabolism, liver dysfunction
Sunitinib Renal cell cancer, GIST	50 mg/d PO for 4 wk, then 2-wk rest period	Diarrhea, nausea, stomatitis, asthenia, skin discoloration, hand-foot syndrome, hypertension, bleeding, anorexia
Temozolomide Glioblastoma, anaplastic astrocytoma (relapsed), renal cell cancer, melanoma	150–200 mg/m^2/d PO for 5 d every 28 d 75 mg/m^2 PO/d concomitant with radiotherapy	Bone marrow depression, nausea and vomiting
Temsirolimus Renal cell cancer	25 mg IV weekly over 30–60 mins	Rash, asthenia, mucositis, edema, dyslipidemia, hyperglycemia, elevated serum creatinine. Rarely, interstitial lung disease

Drug and its uses	Dosages	Toxicities
Teniposide Relapsed ALL in children, SCLC	ALL: 100 mg/m^2 once or twice weekly or 20–60 mg/m^2/d for 5 d in combination with Ara-C Lung: 80–90 mg/m^2/d for 5 d as a single agent	Bone marrow depression, nausea and vomiting, alopecia, hypotension with rapid infusion, increased liver enzymes, AML (late effect)
Thalidomide Multiple myeloma	200 mg/d PO	Birth defects, thrombotic events, somnolence, peripheral neuropathy, neutropenia
Thioguanine AML, ALL, CML, advanced colorectal cancer, multiple myeloma	2 mg/kg/d PO until response or toxic effects are seen; may cautiously increase to 3 mg/kg/d	Bone marrow depression, liver damage, stomatitis
Thiotepa Ovarian, breast, and superficial bladder cancers, HL, CML, CLL, bronchogenic carcinoma, malignant effusions (intracavitary), BMT for refractory leukemia, lymphomas	IV: 0.3–0.4 mg/kg by rapid IV infusion Intravesical: 60 mg/60 mL sterile water instilled and retained in bladder for 2 h; repeat weekly for 4 wk Intracavitary: 0.6–0.8 mg/kg	Bone marrow depression, nausea and vomiting, mucositis, skin rashes
Topotecan Cervical cancer, ovarian cancer (relapsed), SCLC (relapsed), MDS, CMML	1.5 mg/m^2 IV over 30 min for 5 consecutive days at 21-d intervals or 2.3 mg/m^2/d PO for 5 consecutive days every 21 d	Bone marrow depression, fever, flu-like symptoms, nausea and vomiting
Tositumomab CD20+ low grade follicular or transformed NHL (relapse)	Dosimetric step: Day 1: Tositumomab 450 mg IV over 60 min; I-131 tositumomab (5 mCi and 35 mg tositumomab) IV over 20 min Therapeutic step: Days 7–14: Tositumomab 450 mg IV over 60 min; I-131 tositumomab calculated	Myelosuppression, hypothyroidism, second malignancies
Trastuzumab HER2-overexpressing breast cancer	4 mg/kg IV over 90 min, loading dose, and 2 mg/kg IV over 30 min every 7 d, as maintenance or 8 mg/kg loading dose and 6 mg/kg every 21 d as maintenance	Cardiac failure, infusion reaction, diarrhea
Valrubicin Bladder	800 mg intravesically once a wk for 6 wk	Local bladder symptoms

Drug and its uses	Dosages	Toxicities
Vinblastine HL, NHL, gestational trophoblastic tumors, testicular and breast cancers, mycosis fungoides, Kaposi sarcoma, histiocytosis X, bladder and renal cancers, NSCLC, CML (blast crisis)	4–12 mg/m^2 IV as a single agent every 1–2 wk; titrate dose to myelosuppression; adjust for hepatic insufficiency	Bone marrow depression, nausea and vomiting, ileus, alopecia, stomatitis, myalgias, vesication
Vincristine ALL, HL, NHL, rhabdomyosarcoma, neuroblastoma, Wilms' tumor, multiple myeloma, sarcomas, breast cancer	0.4–1.4 mg/m^2 IV weekly; maximum total dose, 2 mg/wk; reduce dose for hepatic insufficiency	Peripheral neuropathy, ileus, abdominal pain, SIADH, bone marrow depression (mild)
Vinorelbine NSCLC, breast, ovarian, head and neck cancers, HL	30 mg/m^2 IV over 10 min; repeat weekly	Peripheral neuropathy, bone marrow depression, nausea, vomiting, hepatic dysfunction

Abbreviations

ALL = acute lymphoblastic leukemia
AML = acute myelogenous leukemia
AUC = area under the curve
BMT = bone marrow transplantation
CLL = chronic lymphocytic leukemia
CML = chronic myelogenous leukemia
CMML = chronic myelomacrocytic leukemia
EGFR = epidermal growth factor receptor
5-FU = fluorouracil
GFR = glomerular filtration rate
GIST = gastrointestinal stromal tumor
GM-CSF = granulocyte-macrophage colony stimulating factor
HL = Hodgkin lymphoma
IDMS = isotope dilution mass spectrometry
MDS = myelodysplastic syndromes
MOPP = mechlorethamine, Oncovin, procarbazine, and prednisone
NHL = non-Hodgkin lymphoma
NSCLC = non–small-cell lung cancer
PAP = prostatic acid phosphatase
PTCL = peripheral T-cell lymphoma
SCLC = small-cell lung cancer
SIADH = syndrome of inappropriate antidiuretic hormone secretion
WBC = white blood cell

Index

C

D

E

M

N

O

P

Q

R

S

T